Desk Reference of Clinical Pharmacology

Second Edition

Desk Reference of Clinical Pharmacology

Second Edition

Manuchair Ebadi, Ph.D., FACCP

Chester Fritz Distinguished Professor
of Pharmacology and Clinical Neuroscience

Associate Vice President for Medical Research

University of North Dakota School of Medicine and Health Sciences
Grand Forks, North Dakota

CRC Press
Taylor & Francis Group
Boca Raton London New York

CRC Press is an imprint of the
Taylor & Francis Group, an informa business

CRC Press
Taylor & Francis Group
6000 Broken Sound Parkway NW, Suite 300
Boca Raton, FL 33487-2742

Printed in the United States of America on acid-free paper
10 9 8 7 6 5 4 3 2 1

International Standard Book Number-10: 1-4200-4743-4 (Hardcover)
International Standard Book Number-13: 978-1-4200-4743-1 (Hardcover)

Library of Congress Cataloging-in-Publication Data

Ebadi, Manuchair S.
Desk reference of clinical pharmacology / author, Manuchair Ebadi. -- 2nd ed.
p. ; cm.
Rev. ed. of: CRC desk reference of clinical pharmacology / Manuchair Ebadi. c1998.
Includes bibliographical references and index.
ISBN-13: 978-1-4200-4743-1 (hardcover : alk. paper)
ISBN-10: 1-4200-4743-4 (hardcover : alk. paper)
1. Clinical pharmacology--Handbooks, manuals, etc. I. Ebadi, Manuchair S. CRC desk reference of clinical pharmacology. II. Title.
[DNLM: 1. Pharmaceutical Preparations--administration & dosage--Handbooks. 2. Drug Therapy--Handbooks. 3. Pharmacokinetics--Handbooks. 4. Pharmacology, Clinical--Handbooks. QV 735 E15d 2007]

RM301.12.E23 2007
615'.1--dc22 2007010014

Visit the Taylor & Francis Web site at
http://www.taylorandfrancis.com

and the CRC Press Web site at
http://www.crcpress.com

Dedication

This book is humbly and reverently dedicated
to the honored memory of my beloved parents,
Ali Ebadi Shahmirzadi and Rogieh Djavadi Ebadi Shahmirzadi.

In books lie the soul of the whole past time, the articulate audible voice of the past when the body and material substances of it has altogether vanished like a dream.

Thomas Carlyle

CONTENTS

Preface to the First Edition

Hippocrates (460–377 B.C.) lamented, "Life is short, and the art long; the occasion fleeting; experience fallacious; and judgment difficult." New drugs and novel avenues of treatment are emerging rapidly, requiring constant vigilance to remain informed.

The *CRC Desk Reference of Clinical Pharmacology*, designed and prepared specifically for physicians and other members of the health-care delivery team, contains more than 2000 entries appearing under three broad categories:

I. **Short reviews** (1%) dealing with important topics of clinical pharmacology such as the pharmacokinetic basis of therapeutics, pharmacodynamic principles, and drug–drug interactions. In addition, major areas of therapeutics such as antiemetic drugs, antihistaminics, calcium channel blocking agents, and nonsteroidal antiinflammatory agents have been reviewed. The diagrams and tables not only cover major areas of therapeutics but also deal with multiple medications. For example, Table 1 summarizes the pharmacological properties of acetohexamide, chlorpropamide, glipizide, glyburide, tolazamide, and tolbutamide, the orally effective hypoglycemic agents. Table 2 summarizes the analgesic, antipyretic, antiinflammatory, and uricosuric properties of all nonsteroidal antiinflammatory agents. Figure 1 deals with pharmacokinetic principles such as absorption, distribution, tissue binding, biotransformation, and elimination of drugs. Figure 2 deals with 5-fluorouracil, dacarbazine, cytarabine, methotrexate, vincristine, vinblastine, bleomycin, actinomycin D, and doxorubicin exerting their effects at G_1 phase, S phase, G_2 phase, and miotic phase of the cell cycle, respectively.

II. **Abstract-length entries** (39%) providing a short description of every medication in use today.

III. **Short dictionary-style entries** (60%) describing in one sentence the exact therapeutic use of a medication. For example: "Halcinonide, a topical adrenocorticoid with antiinflammatory properties is indicated in inflammation of acute and chronic corticosteroid-responsive dermatoses."

Each entry gives the name of the drug, its classification, its dosage, its indications, its mechanism of action, its pharmacokinetic properties if appropriate, its side effects, and its signs and symptoms of overdosage. The section on pharmacokinetics has been designed to be meaningful in nature. For example, if a drug is mainly eliminated unchanged, it is noted that its dose should be adjusted downward in renal failure.

Another unique feature of the book is that items of information have been given in a comprehensive fashion. For example, Table 21 provides information to be used in the treatment of hypertensive emergics. This includes provision of pharmacological properties of sodium nitroprusside, diazoxide, labetalol, nitroglycerin, phentolamine, trimethaphan, hydralazine, and nicardipine. All these drugs have their own separate entries but have also been assembled in a meaningful fashion in one place.

The author expresses his heart-felt appreciation and gratitude to Professor Gerald A. Kerkut of the University of Southampton and David Grist of CRC Press LLC for the confidence rendered and for the kind invitation to prepare a volume on clinical pharmacology. Their valuable guidance, direction, and support have been immense and are gratefully acknowledged.

The author also acknowledges the contribution of the members of the international advisory board in the process of designing, writing, and completing this desk reference. They are:

Thomas E. Andreoli, M.D.
Professor and Chairman
Department of Medicine
University of Arkansas
College of Medicine
Little Rock, Arkansas

Ronald F. Pfeiffer, M.D.
Professor of Neurology
Director, Division of Neurodegenerative Disease
University of Tennessee
College of Medicine
Memphis, Tennessee

Franco Frashini, M.D.
Director
Department of Pharmacology and Chemotherapy
University Degli Studi di Milano
Milan, Italy

Alan C. Sartorelli, Ph.D.
Alfred Gilman Professor of Pharmacology and Epidemiology
Yale University School of Medicine
New Haven, Connecticut

Alfred M. Freedman, M.D.
Professor and Chairman of Psychiatry
Director of Psychiatric Service
Metropolitan and Flower and Fifth Hospitals and Chairman, Department of Psychiatry, Grasslands Hospital
Valhalla, New York

Arnold Schwartz, Ph.D.
Professor and Chairman
Department of Pharmacology and Cell Biophysics
University of Cincinnati
College of Medicine
Cincinnati, Ohio

Robert H. Handschumacher, Ph.D.
Professor Pharmacology
Yale University School of Medicine
New Haven, Connecticut

Howard M. Spiro, M.D.
Department of Internal Medicine
Yale University School of Medicine
New Haven, Connecticut

Elliot S. Vesell, M.D.
Evan Pugh Professor and Chairman
Department of Pharmacology
Pennsylvania State University
College of Medicine
Hershey, Pennsylvania

The author also expresses his everlasting admiration to Margaret McCall and to Lori Ann Clapper for their magnificent dedication, uncompromising diligence, and competent skills in typing the entire manuscript, and to John Enrique Mata for designing and drawing the art work. The exceptional and rare talent, skills, and expertise of Gail Renard, the project editor, and Kathy Johnson, the typesetter, in refining this volume, are gratefully and respectfully acknowledged. Thanks are also due to Cindy Carelli, Carolyn Lea, Julie Haydu, and Becky McEldowney—all of CRC—for their help and professionalism.

The author hopes that by providing simple and unique diagrams, comprehensive tables, and more than 2000 entries, the *CRC Desk Reference of Clinical Pharmacology* will become a valuable and essential reference book for physicians and other members of the medical profession in their quest to alleviate the mental and physical sufferings of their fellow human beings.

M. Ebadi
Omaha, Nebraska
July 1997

Preface to the Second Edition

Since publication of the first edition of *CRC Desk Reference of Clinical Pharmacology* in 1998, dramatic discoveries in **molecular medicine,** along with rapid concomitant technological advances, have revolutionized the diagnosis and treatment of a broad range of human diseases with new medications. Given the rapid pace of new discovery, **genetic-** and **cell-based therapeutics** have now become a common part of the physicians' *armamentarium*. A few examples will be given concerning two leading causes of death—cancer and cardiovascular diseases—to illustrate this.

At the midpoint of the 20th century, our knowledge of cancer was based on epidemiology and pathology, and treatment consisted of surgery and radiation therapy. More modern views on carcinogenesis favor a genetic cause for cancer. The incidence of cancer increases sharply with age, and various models have been proposed to account for this increase. The human immune system can mount a specific response to cancer. Intense research is aimed at dissecting the intricacies of the interaction between the immune system and tumor cells.

A driving force behind this research is the idea that cancer-directed immunity can be enhanced to improve the outcome for patients with the disease. The specificity of the immune response makes **cancer immunotherapy** extremely effective because it offers the promise of reducing damage to the bystander normal tissues and lessening the severe side effects associated with cancer therapies. Another modern treatment is **monoclonal antibodies**, which exhibit a favorable pharmacokinetic profile. Pharmacokinetic variability among patients is low, which helps ensure that all patients receiving a given dose achieve appropriate exposure to the drug. Unlike many therapeutics now used in cancer patients, monoclonal antibodies are not subject to metabolic drug–drug interactions and are not substrates of the multidrug-resistant efflux pumps. The third example of emerging molecular therapeutics in cancer patients is **drugs interfering with signal transduction pathways**. Signal transduction describes the processes involved in the communication between the cell and its environment, and in the regulation of cell fate. These pathways are commonly hijacked by the genomic abnormalities that drive malignant progression. Proof of principle has now been established that targeting signal transduction pathways can be clinically beneficial. Tackling multistep carcinogenesis will most likely require combinatorial therapies: probably cytotoxic plus a signal transduction inhibitor. The fourth example of the molecular therapeutics in cancer patient is **suicide gene therapy**. The possibility of rendering cancer cells more sensitive to drugs or toxins by introducing suicide genes has two alternatives: toxin gene therapy, in which the genes for toxic products are transformed into tumor cells, and enzyme-activating prodrug therapy, in which the transgene encodes an enzyme that activates specific pro-drugs to create toxic metabolites. The latter approach, as well as suicide gene therapy and **gene-directed enzyme prodrug therapy (GDEPT)**, has also been termed ***virus-directed enzyme prodrug therapy*** and ***gene prodrug activation therapy***.

The cardiovascular diseases potentially amenable to gene therapy include:

Familial hypercholesterolemia (LDL receptor defective/absent)	LDL clearance
Dyslipidemia with no specific genetic defect	LDL clearance
Hypertension	Increase in HDL
Peripheral artery disease	Angiogenesis
Occlusive arterial disease	Cytostatic, cytotoxic, inhibition of smooth muscle cell proliferation
Thrombosis	Decreased thrombus formation, increased fibrinolysis
Hypertrophic cardiomyopathy	Normalized sarcomere function
Ischemic heart disease	Angiogenesis
Heart failure	Improved calcium handling, increased contractility
Cardioprotection	Adiopectin

The second edition of the *CRC Desk Reference of Clinical Pharmacology* is designed specifically for physicians, pharmacists, nurses, and other members of the health care delivery team. It consists of three parts.

Part One: The book still has brief, concise, and informative A–Z drug facts from abciximab to zolpidem tartrate.

Part Two: The book again presents some very novel and exciting entries not seen in any existing textbooks of pharmacology. These items will include, but not be limited to, the items listed below.

DRUG METABOLISM AND TRANSPORT

Two key aspects of how the body handles drugs and other chemicals are metabolism and transport. Metabolism is critical because it enables the body to process highly lipophilic molecules for further metabolism and eventual excretion, inactivates biologically active molecules, or detoxifies potentially toxic chemicals. Transport processes are critical because they determine the ability of drugs and other chemicals to gain access to sites of metabolism or to physiological or toxicological targets within tissues. The remarkable advances in molecular and cell biology and the development of novel *in vitro* model systems to study the various processes involved in metabolism and transport have expanded our knowledge and led to numerous new therapeutic approaches to the treatment of chemically induced toxicity and disease.

PHARMACOGENOMICS

Pharmacogenomics exists at the intersection of pharmacology and genomics. It aims to study the genetic basis of interpatient variability in response to drug therapy. Pharmacogenomics holds the promise that drugs may eventually be tailor-made for individuals and adapted to each person's genetic makeup. Environment, diet, age, lifestyle, and the disease state can all influence a patient's response to medicines, but understanding an individual's genetic makeup is thought to be the key to creating personalized drugs with greater efficacy and safety. Pharmacogenomics combines traditional pharmaceutical sciences with knowledge of genes, proteins, and single nucleotide polymorphisms. Our discussion will focus on the various technologies currently available and stress that researchers must be able to choose the technology best suited to their purposes.

ANTISENSE THERAPEUTICS

The recently completed sequencing of the human genome has demonstrated the presence of a vast number of targets for antisense oligonucleotides. So we now have thousands of targets, hundreds of preclinical animal studies, and some 20 clinical trials ongoing. Any successful trial with an antisense compound will open a floodgate of new therapies for a panoply of diseases.

THE MANAGEMENT OF EATING DISORDERS AND OBESITY

There is increasing awareness about eating disorders and their predispositions. Efforts are expanding on prevention, early identification, and intervention in eating disorders. Clinicians are developing treatment strategies incorporating newer technologies including the Internet, which might eventually reduce costs while improving access to, and effectiveness of, therapy. Regarding obesity, the greater focus is on prevention, and strategies for prevention are being evaluated. Researchers are identifying the effects of maternal behaviors during pregnancy that "imprint" the fetus for increased postnatal weight gain and obesity-associated disease complications. As we learn about such effects, we may be able to recommend behaviors for pregnant women that would reduce the future risk for their infants.

PREVENTIVE NUTRITION

Preventive nutrition incorporates dietary practices and interventions directed toward the reduction of disease risk (primary prevention), improvements in disease states already manifest (secondary prevention), and improvement in health outcomes. Preventive nutrition is a critical component not only of preventive medicine, but also of therapeutic medicine and provides approaches for preventing disease and reducing its impact once it occurs.

ADOPTIVE IMMUNOTHERAPY

Over the last decade, advances in cellular and molecular immunology have been tremendous. Our continuously improving understanding of the immune system and the appreciation of the mechanisms by which tumors and viral or bacterial infections are controlled have led to promising new treatment strategies. Adoptive transfer of tailored antigen-specific immune cells and or optimally designed immunological effector molecules is an elegant and promising approach to the establishment or restoration of protective immune responses.

CANCER CHEMOPREVENTION

Despite significant advances in cancer treatment and early detection, overall cancer incidence has increased, cancer-associated morbidity is considerable, and overall cancer survival has remained relatively flat over the past several decades. However, new technology allowing exploration of signal transduction pathways, identification of cancer-associated genes, and imaging of tissue architecture and molecular and cellular function is increasing our understanding of carcinogenesis and cancer progression. This knowledge is moving the focus of cancer therapeutics, including cancer-prevention treatments, to drugs that take advantage of cellular control mechanisms to selectively suppress cancer progression.

DRUG DELIVERY SYSTEMS IN CANCER THERAPY

The use of drug delivery systems to improve the efficacy of cancer chemotherapy remains an important strategy for achieving progress against this disease. Over the past 20 years, the number of novel therapeutic approaches has expanded from traditional small chemical medicinals to a wide variety of biomolecules, including peptide/protein- and nucleic acid-based therapeutics. All of these therapies require the administration of stable dosage forms in adequate concentrations and exposure periods to realize their potential. For the treatment of many forms of cancer, the presentation and maintenance of adequate drug concentrations to the target tissues without exposure to drug-sensitive normal tissues are the major limitations for successful chemotherapy.

IMMUNOTHERAPY OF CANCER

Tumor immunology is a scientific discipline that is driven by clinical translation. For many decades, scientists both at the bench and at the bedside have struggled with determining the role immunity may play in tumor eradication, if an for many years, the major question driving the field was whether human tumors were immunogenic. Over the last decade, literally thousands of immunogenic proteins related to tumors have been identified, resulting in a host of new targets for immunomodulation.

PROTEASOME INHIBITORS IN CANCER THERAPY

Inhibition of the proteasome in cultured cells, mostly of tumor origin, produced profound stabilization of hundreds, if not thousands, of proteins, ultimately turning on the programmed cell death machinery at concentrations that directly correlated to the intrinsic inhibition constant of the proteasome. Such observations begged further investigation of proteasome inhibition in the treatment of human cancers.

RECOMBINANT ANTIBODIES FOR CANCER THERAPY

The purpose of Recombinant Antibodies for Cancer Therapy is to present a collection of detailed protocols in recombinant antibody technology. It is primarily addressed to scientists working on recombinant antibodies as well as clinicians involved with antibody-based therapies.

SUICIDE GENE THERAPY

The area of gene therapy is vast, and both malignant and nonmalignant cells can be targeted. Gene therapy that targets malignant cells in a treatment has become known as "suicide gene therapy." Basically, this approach uses the transduction of cancer cells with a gene for a foreign enzyme that, when expressed, is able to activate a nontoxic prodrug into a highly cytotoxic drug able to kill the cancer cell population

Part Three: Includes short descriptions of conditions, diseases, and disorders and their treatments. The list includes but is not limited to the following items:

- Acute respiratory distress syndrome; treatment
- Adrenergic (sympathomimetic) compounds
- Adrenergic (sympathomimetic) receptor blocking agents
- Adrenocorticoids; topical antiinflammatory agents available as cream, gel, lotion, or ointment
- Aged patients; altered pharmacokinetic profile of
- Agranulocytosis; drug-induced
- Allergic rhinitis
- Alzheimer's disease; treatment of
- Aminoglycoside antibiotics
- Analgesics; narcotics
- Analgesics; non-narcotic agents
- Androgenic steroids
- Anesthetics; inhalation
- Angiotensin-converting enzyme (ACE) inhibitors for hypertension
- Anorexia nervosa and bulimia nervosa; treatment of
- Antacids
- Antianxiety agents
- Antibacterial drugs of choice
- Antidepressants
- Antidiarrheal medication
- Antidiuretic hormone
- Antidotes
- Antiemetic preparations
- Antihistamines (H_1 receptor antagonists)
- Antihypertensive medications
- Antineoplastic agents
- Antiparasitic medications and their side effects
- Antipsychotics
- Antiviral agents
- Arrhythmias
- Arthritis and degenerative joint disease; treatment of
- Asthma; treatment of
- Autonomic receptors
- Benzodiazepines; uses of
- Beta-adrenergic-receptor-blocking agents
- Bioavailability of drugs; factors influencing
- Botulinum toxin A; uses of
- Bronchodilators; β-adrenergic agonists for the treatment of asthma
- Calcium-channel blockers for the treatment of hypertension
- Calcium products
- Cephalosporins
- Cerebroactive medications
- Chlamydial infections; treatment of
- Cholinergic drugs; uses in medicine
- Cholinergic-receptor-blocking agents; uses of
- Cirrhosis; treatment of
- Congestive heart failure; treatment of
- Constipation; drug-induced
- Corticosteroids; uses for
- Crohn's disease; treatment of
- Cytokines; their actions
- Dermatological disorders; treatment with retinoids
- Diabetes mellitus; treatment of non-insulin-dependent cases
- Diarrhea; drug-induced
- Diuretics
- Duodenal ulcers; treatment of
- Enzymes and hormones of gastrointestinal tract; actions of
- Epileptic seizures; treatment of
- Erectile dysfunction; treatment of
- Ergot alkaloids
- Estrogenic preparations
- Expectorants; drugs that increase respiratory tract fluid
- Fungal infections; treatment of
- Gastroesophageal reflux disease (GERD); treatment of
- Gaucher's disease; treatment of
- Gene therapy; e.g., for acquired immune deficiency syndrome (AIDS)
- Gilles de la Tourette's syndrome; treatment of
- Glaucoma; treatment for
- Gonorrhea; treatment of
- Gout; treatment of
- Heart failure; treatment of
- Hemostatic mechanisms and drugs influencing them
- Hiccup; treatment of
- Hirsutism; treatment of
- Human immunodeficiency virus (HIV) infection; treatment for
- Huntington's disease; the search for treatment continues

Hyperglycemia; drug-induced
Hypertension; treatment of
Hypertensive emergencies; treatment of
Hypnotics
Hypoglycemia; drug-induced
Hypothalamic hormones
Immunization; agents used in
Immunosuppressive medications
In vitro fertilization; drugs for
Insomnia; treatment with benzodiazepines
Insulin preparations
Iodine-containing products
Ischemic stroke; treatment of
Laxatives
Legionnaires' disease; treatment of
Lipid-lowering drugs
Local anesthetics
Lower respiratory tract infections; treatment of
Macrolide antibiotics
Manic symptoms; drug-induced
Migraine headaches; treatment of
Monoamine oxidase inhibitors; contemporary treatment of depression
Multiple sclerosis; treatment of
Myasthenia gravis; treatment of
Mycoses; treatment of deep-seated organisms
Myoclonus; treatment of
Narcolepsy; treatment of
Neurotransmitters and their receptor subtypes
Newborns; undeveloped pharmacokinetic profile
Nitrate products
Nondepolarizing neuromuscular blocking drugs
Nonsteroidal antiinflammatory drugs
Nursing infants; pharmacology of
Obesity; treatment of
Oculotoxicity; drug-induced
Opioid peptides
Opioids; receptor agonists and antagonists
Oral hypoglycemic agents
Orphan drugs; proposed uses of
Osteoporosis; treatment of
Otitis media; treatment of
Ototoxicity; drug-induced
Ovulation; drugs to induce
Pancreatic enzymes preparations
Panic disorder; treatment of
Parasitic infections; treatment of
Parkinson's disease; treatment of
Penicillins
Peptic ulcer; treatment of
Photosensitivity; medication-induced
Psychiatric symptoms caused by drugs
Psychotropic medications; side effects of
Pulmonary toxicity; drug-induced
Quinolone and fluoroquinolone antibiotics
Radiopaque agents
Restless legs syndrome; treatment of
Retinoids
Seizures; treatment of
Serotonin receptor subtypes
Sexual dysfunction caused by drugs
Sexually transmitted diseases; treatment of
Shingles; treatment of
Sinusitis; treatment of
Stuttering; treatment of
Suicide; prevention of
Sulfonamides
Syphilis; treatment of
Tetracyclines
Thrombolytic agents; a need for improvement
Thyroid preparations
Trace minerals essential for health
Traveler's diarrhea; prevention of
Tuberculosis; treatment of
Upper respiratory tract infection; treatment of
Urinary tract infections; treatment of
Uveitis; management of
Vaginal candidiasis; treatment of
Vasodilators; effects on cardiac output (CO)
Vitamins; their coenzymatic functions
Vomiting caused by antineoplastic agents
Wilson's disease; treatment of
Wound infection and sepsis in surgical patients; treatment of

Every attempt has been made to be comprehensive, authoritative, and accurate in the expanded and improved second edition of the *CRC Desk Reference of Clinical Pharmacology*. The first five chapters present discussions of the **Pharmacokinetic Basis of Therapeutics**, **Concepts of Pharmacodynamics**, and the **Principles of Drug–Drug Interactions and Drug–Food Interactions**. Moreover, whenever possible, the interactions among herbal alternative medicines, and modern therapeutics have been outlined.

The author expresses his heartfelt appreciation to many physicians including his son **Mark Ebadi, M.D.**, board certified in internal medicine from Northwestern University, Chicago and in allergy and immunology from National Jewish Hospital, Denver, who suggested items for inclusion, avenues for improvement, and lit the path for writing and improving this second edition to be used by those healers who extend the attributes of the Lord Almighty in alleviating the physical and mental sufferings of their fellow human beings.

M. Ebadi, Ph.D., FACCP
Grand Forks, North Dakota

Acknowledgments for the Second Edition

The author expresses his appreciation to **Dr. Judith E. Spiegel**, Senior Editor of Life Sciences for CRC Press, for the gracious invitation to prepare this second edition, and to **Gail Renard**, the production editor, for polishing and refining the book. The author remains eternally grateful and in awe of Gail's judgment and titanic contributions to restructuring and refining five books for him in an admirable fashion.

The author expresses his loving tribute to his two sons, **John Ebadi, Ph.D.** (specializing in Oriental medicine and Eastern healing art) and **Mark Ebadi, M.D.** (specializing in Western medicine and Western healing art), for their input on how to bridge past and present medical wisdom and how to respect not only the immense contributions of many ancient cultures but also the amazing advances made by physicians today to the well being of human beings in their quest to prevent disease, prolong life, and reduce morbidity.

The author remains indebted to **Victoria Swift**, the director of the art department at the University of North Dakota School of Medicine and Health Sciences, for her ingenuity in design and graphic arts in completing many of the diagrams.

The author remains beholden to **Leah Beth Gustafson**, a Presidential Scholar from the University of North Dakota, for gathering materials from world literature to prepare this new edition.

The author also remains beholden to **Angela Mae Williams**, a Presidential Scholar from the University of North Dakota, for editing the typed materials with her eagle eye and brilliant mind.

The author remains indebted to **JoAnn Johnson** for being as dependable as the rising sun and the beating heart in completing whatever tasks need completion.

The author extends his heartfelt salutation and felicitation to **Dani Stramer** for her devotion, loyalty, and perfectionism in completing all her obligations in a majestic fashion. Her dedication, skill, and determination made this edition a magnificent achievement in therapeutics.

It is with affection and gratitude that the author honors his teachers and mentors: **Carl B. Camras, M.D., Arnold L. Frizzle, Ph.D., Delta W. Gier, Ph.D., Joseph P. Gilmore, Ph.D., John M. Hamilton, Ph.D., Thomas Hernandez, M.D./Ph.D., Woodbridge O. Johnson, Jr., Ph.D., Robert B. Kugel, M.D., Ernest E. McCoy, M.D., Robert Eli Long, Ph.D., Russell J. Reiter, Ph.D.,** and **Paul M. Scott, Ph.D.,** for inspiring him to learn. And he salutes his students for encouraging him to teach.

The author extends his undying respect to the Honorable **Byron L. Dorgan**, U.S. senator from North Dakota, and to the Honorable **John Hoeven**, the governor of North Dakota, for their support and extending arms of friendship whenever needed in supporting the author's numerous research programs at the University of North Dakota.

The author salutes **Charles E. Kupchella, Ph.D.**, president of the University of North Dakota; **Peter Alfonso, Ph.D.**, vice president for research, the University of North Dakota; **H. David Wilson, M.D.**, dean and vice president for health affairs, University of North Dakota School of Medicine and Health Sciences, **Joshua Wynne, M.D., M.B.A., M.P.H.**, executive associate dean, University of North Dakota School of Medicine and Health Sciences, and **Randy Eken**, associate dean for administration and finance, University of North Dakota School of Medicine and Health Sciences, for confidence displayed in the author's talent and supporting him whenever needed.

The author remains humbled and in awe of hundreds of physicians who read and made the first edition a success but also reviewed the book, lit the path, and gave direction on how to write the revised edition.

NOTICE

The indications and dosages of all drugs in this book have been recommended in the medical literature and conform to the practices of the general medical community. The medications described do not necessarily have specific approval by the U.S. Food and Drug Administration for use in the diseases and dosages for which they are recommended. The package insert for each drug should be consulted for use and dosage as approved by the PDA. Because standards for usage change, it is advisable to keep abreast of revised recommendations, particularly concerning new drugs.

The Author

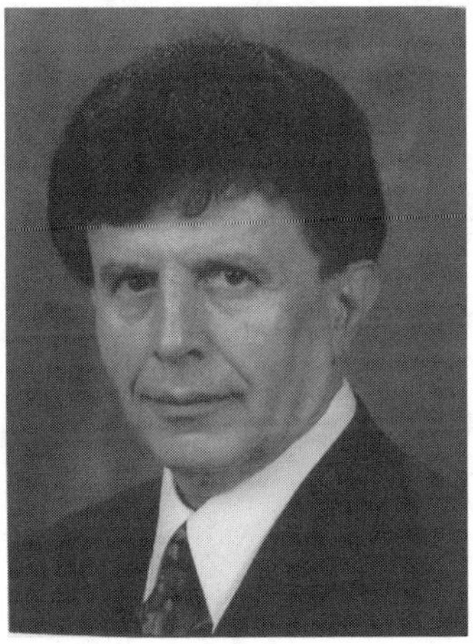

Manuchair Ebadi earned a B.S. degree in chemistry from Park University (Parkville, MO, 1960), an M.S. degree in pharmacology from the University of Missouri College of Pharmacy (Kansas City, 1962), and a Ph.D. degree in pharmacology from the University of Missouri College of Medicine (Columbia, 1967). He completed his postdoctoral training in the Laboratory of Preclinical Pharmacology at the National Institute of Mental Health (Washington, DC, 1970), under the able direction of Erminio Costa, M.D., an eminent member of the National Academy of Sciences.

Dr. Ebadi served as chairman of the Department of Pharmacology at the University of Nebraska College of Medicine from 1970 until 1988, and subsequently as professor of pharmacology, neurology, and psychiatry from 1988 through 1999. In July of 1999, he was appointed professor and chairman of the Department of Pharmacology and Toxicology at the University of North Dakota School of Medicine and Health Sciences. In September of 1999, Dr. Ebadi became professor and chairman of the newly created Department of Pharmacology, Physiology, and Therapeutics; in November 1999, he became professor of neuroscience; and in December 1999, he was appointed associate dean for research and program development. In September 2000, Dr. Ebadi was appointed director of the Center of Excellence in Neurosciences at the University of North Dakota School of Medicine and Health Sciences, and in March 2002, associate vice president for medical research at the University of North Dakota.

During his academic career, Professor Ebadi has received 36 awards, including the Burlington Northern Faculty Achievement Award (1987) and the University of Nebraska's systemwide Outstanding Teaching and Creative Activity Award (1995), and was inducted into the Golden Apple Hall of Fame (1995) for having received 11 Golden Apple awards from the national Golden Apple Foundation for excellence in teaching. He is a member of 18 research and scholarly societies including Alpha Omega Alpha Honor Medical Society.

In 1976, Dr. Ebadi became the Mid-America State Universities Association's (MASUA) honor lecturer; in 1987, he received an award for "meritorious contributions to pharmaceutical sciences" from the University of Missouri Alumni Association; in 1995, he was honored by a resolution and commendation of the board of regents of the University of Nebraska for having developed a sustained record of excellence in teaching, including creative instructional methodology; and in 1996, he received the Distinguished Alumni Award from Park University, his alma mater. In November 2002, Dr. Ebadi received a recognition award in appreciation of his outstanding contribution to the UND School of Medicine. In May 2003, Dr. Ebadi received the Outstanding Block Instructor Award for outstanding performance "in the encouragement, enrichment, and education of tomorrow's physicians." In 2003, he was elected to the prestigious Cosmos Club (Washington, DC) for individuals who have distinguished themselves in art, literature, or science.

Professor Ebadi discovered and characterized brain metallothionein isoforms in 1983 and subsequently showed that they are able to scavenge free radicals implicated in Parkinson's disease. In addition, he showed that metallothionein averts α-synuclein nitration, enhances the elaboration of coenzyme Q10, increases the activity of complex I, enhances the synthesis of ATP, and as an antioxidant is 50 times more potent than glutathione. His research programs have been supported in the past and currently by the National Institute on Aging (AG 17059-06); the National Institute of Environmental Health Sciences (NIEHS 03949); the National Institute of Child Health and Human Development (NICHD 00370); the National Institute of Neurological Disorders and Stroke (NINDS 08932, NINDS 34566, and NINDS 40160); and the Office of National Drug Control Policy, Counter Drug Technology Assessments Center (DATM 05-02-C-1252).

Professor Ebadi has written ten books. The *Pharmacology* text was translated into Japanese in 1987 (Medical Science International Ltd., Tokyo); the *Core Concepts in Pharmacology* was translated into Chinese in 2002 (Ho-Chi Book Publishing of Taiwan); and the *Pharmacodynamic Basis of Herbal Medicine* (CRC Press, 2002) became a best seller.

In 2005 Dr. Ebadi, along with Professor Ronald F. Pfeiffer, M.D., published a book entitled *Parkinson's Disease*, which received excellent reviews in *JAMA* (293, 2281, 2005), and in the *New England Journal of Medicine* (352, 1304, 2005), and won first prize in the neurology category of the 2006 British Medical Association's Book Competition.

On February 26, 2004, Dr. Ebadi received the University of North Dakota Foundation's Thomas J. Clifford Faculty Achievement Award for Excellence in Research and, on September 7, 2004, he received from President Charles E. Kupchella, the designation of Chester Fritz Distinguished Professor of Pharmacology and of Clinical Neuroscience, the highest honor bestowed by the University of North Dakota.

On July 21, 2005, Dr. Ebadi received the Pendelton Honor from Eugene DeLorme, J.D., director of Indians into Medicine Programs; from Dr. David Gipp, president of United Indian Nations; and from Dr. Frank Williams, vice president of the tribal board in appreciation of his providing research support for the Indian nations. Dr. Ebadi has served as a member of the United States Pharmacopoeia convention since 1970. On March 2, 2006, Dr. Ebadi was appointed senior advisor to the president of the University of North Dakota.

How to Use This Book

This book may be used as an encyclopedia of medications in which compounds appear under their generic names in alphabetical order from *Abacavir sulfate,* to *Zopiclone*, the first compound of the cyclopytolone class possessing anticonvulsant, anxiolytic, muscle relaxant, and sedative properties. Furthermore, in the index, all drugs, including their generic names and multiple trade names, appear in alphabetical order.

This book may also be used as a textbook with its introductory materials such as the pharmacokinetic basis of therapeutics, the pharmacodynamic basis of therapeutics, and adverse reactions and drug–drug interactions, which have been presented in a review format. In addition, many important and often-used medications (for example, androgens, antacids, antiemetic agents, antihistamines, barbiturates, benzodiazepine derivatives, calcium-channel blockers, cathartics, cephalosporins, chemoprotectants, corticosteroids, cytokines, digitalis, folic acid antagonists, general anesthetics, insulin preparations, iron preparations, laxatives, levodopa–carbidopa, nitrates–nitrites, penicillins, salicylates and allied medications, tetracyclines, thiazide diuretics, and vitamins) have been described in detail. The tables and figures summarize and illustrate in an attractive fashion information about major areas of therapeutics. In addition, medications have been covered under multiple headings to make the search for them simple and to make their descriptions informative. For example, aspirin is found in the sections on acetylsalicylic acid, nonsteroidal antiinflammatory agents, and salicylates and allied compounds.

The orientation articles, which the reader will find enclosed in boxes throughout the text, summarize the treatment of common disorders/diseases including Alzheimer's disease, arrhythmias, arthritis, asthma, congestive heart failure, constipation, Crohn's disease, duodenal ulcer, erectile dysfunction, fungal infections, Gaucher's disease, Gilles de la Tourette syndrome, glaucoma, gonorrhea, gout, heart failure, human immunodeficiency virus (HIV) infection, Huntington's disease, hypertension, insomnia, Legionnaires' disease, mania, migraine, multiple sclerosis, mycoses, narcolepsy, obesity, osteoporosis, otitis media, panic disorder, parasitic infections, Parkinson's disease, peptic ulcer, seizure disorders, sinusitis, syphilis, upper respiratory tract infections, urinary tract infections, uveitis, vaginal candidiasis, and Wilson's disease.

Orientation articles provide an encyclopedic listing of medications dealing with aminoglycoside antibiotics, analgesics, androgens, angiotensin-converting enzyme inhibitors, antianxiety agents, antibacterial drugs, antidepressants, antidiarrheal medications, antidotes, antiemetics, antipsychotics, antiviral agents, diuretics, estrogen preparations, expectorants, laxatives, lipid-lowering drugs, orphan drugs, radiopaque agents, sulfonamides, tetracyclines, thrombolytic agents, and many others.

In many cases, newly introduced medications, such as the use of melatonin for sleep disorders, have been included. Discussion of some novel medications, such as tizanmidine for the treatment of spasticity or urapidel for the treatment of hypertension, has been provided. Discussion of the rapidly growing family of peptides, such as trefoil peptides, with a possible healing factor for peptic ulcers and inflammatory bowel diseases, and many other novel avenues of therapeutics have been introduced. Whenever possible, the descriptions of medications have been given in concise form and in a nugget fashion.

LIST OF ORIENTATION ARTICLES

List of Tables

List of Figures

1

The Pharmacokinetic Basis of Therapeutics

Poisons and medicine are oftentimes the same substance given with different intents.

Peter Mere Latham

The primary objectives of therapy should be to prevent and cure disease. If these goals are not achievable, the secondary objectives should be to use drugs that mitigate the progressive, devastating, or disabling aspects of disease. The nature of the disease then determines the amount of drug or drugs to be given and the duration of therapy.

The successful prevention, cure, or treatment of a disease depends on using sufficient amounts of drugs that obtain the desirable effects, while at the same time avoiding harmful side effects.

Advances in our understanding of pharmacology and therapeutics have broadened our appreciation of (1) the mechanisms involved in the disposition of drugs by the body, (2) the inherent ability of drugs to modify the physiologic integrity of the host, and (3) the nature of drug interactions. By being aware of these pharmacologic principles, applying them fully, and remaining vigilant concerning the countless interactions between drugs and the ailing body, the side effects of numerous drugs can be substantially reduced.

Pharmacokinetic principles, which deal with the **absorption, distribution, binding, biotransformation,** and **excretion** of drugs and their metabolites in the body (Figure 1.1), are the topic of this chapter.

ADMINISTRATION OF DRUGS

Drugs are administered as a **solid** in the form of capsules, tablets, and pills (e.g., clonidine), a **volatile liquid** (e.g., halothane and enflurane), a **solution** (e.g., chlorpromazine), an **aerosol** (e.g., beclomethasone), a **gas** (e.g., oxygen and nitrous oxide), and a **crystalline suspension** (e.g., insulin). The route of administration is chosen based on the desired onset and duration of action of the drug, the nature of the drug, any special circumstances, and the bioavailability of the drug.

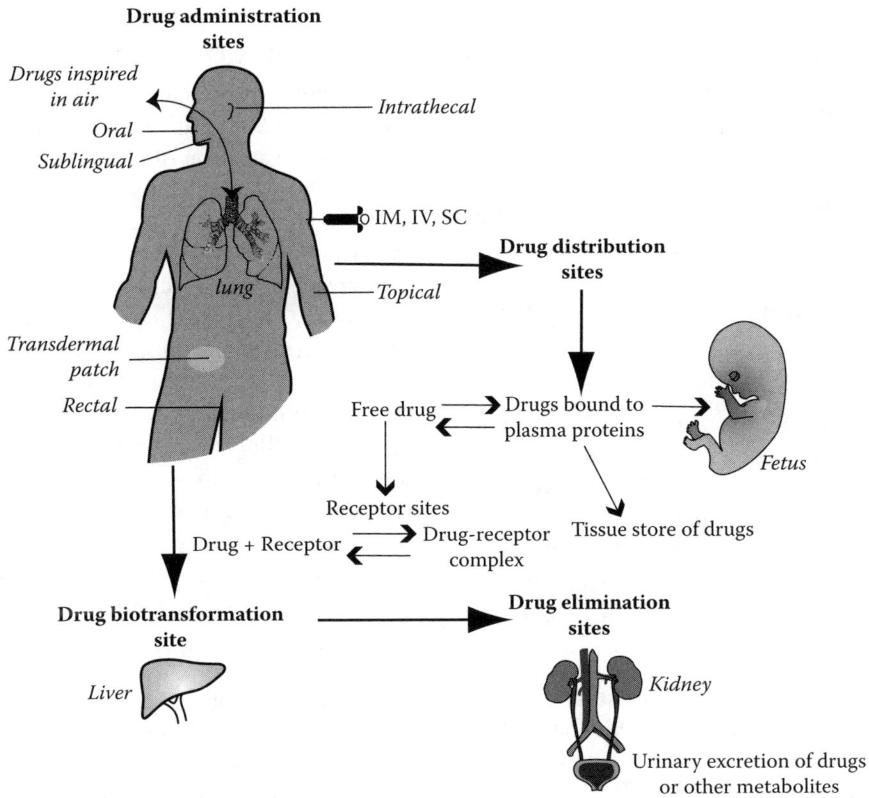

FIGURE 1.1 Pharmacokinetic basis of therapeutics; IM—intramuscular; IV—intravenous; SC—subcutaneous.

In life-threatening conditions, or in circumstances requiring an immediate onset of action, drugs must be administered directly into the general circulation. For instance, in **diabetic ketoacidosis**, large doses of insulin (2 units/kg initially, divided intravenously and subcutaneously, followed by 1 unit/kg subcutaneously every 2 hours) are given until the concentration of glucose in the blood approaches normal values. In **hypocalcemic tetany**, calcium gluconate is administered as a 10% solution delivering 0.45 mEq of Ca^{2+}/ml.

Duration of Action

If a long duration of action is desirable, one may administer a drug either continuously or in a long-acting form, or both. For example, in treating pneumococcal meningitis, 20 to 40 million units of **penicillin G** are either given daily by constant-infusion drip or divided into doses and given by intravenous bolus at 2- to 3-h intervals. **Penicillin G procaine suspension** (e.g., Crysticillin, Duracillin, Wycillin), which is soluble in water only to 0.4%, is designed for deep intramuscular injection and slow absorption from the site of injection.

Nature of the Drugs

Proteinaceous drugs, such as insulin for diabetes mellitus, growth hormone for hypopituitary dwarfism, and oxytocin in dysfunctional labor, are destroyed in the stomach, and therefore are not given orally. The first drug in milk will be obtained from a transgenic goat, owned by GTC Biotherapeutics, headquartered in Framingham, MA. The animal secretes a valuable pharmaceutical protein in its milk. Initially, GTC generated transgenic goats by microinjecting into the developing nucleus of a one-cell embryo a gene encoding the desired human protein (along with DNA that promotes activation of that gene in milk). Such embryos were transferred into female goats, which produced offspring that were then tested for the presence of the newly integrated gene. The milk of these "founder" animals contains the therapeutic protein, which must then undergo a purification process. The mature transgenic animals were bred usually with nontransgenic goats as a first step toward producing a herd.

Special Circumstances

Drugs are applied to the mucous membranes of the conjunctiva, nasopharynx, and vagina to achieve local effects. On the other hand, the antidiuretic hormone **lypressin** (Diapid) is given by nasal spray, but the intention is to produce systemic effects. For the treatment of meningeal leukemia, **cytosine arabinoside** is injected directly into the spinal subarachnoid space. In osteoarthritis, **corticosteroids** are given by intraarticular injection.

Drug Delivery by Iontophoresis or Phonophoresis

The topical application of drugs may be enhanced by decreasing the barrier function of the stratum corneum and by using either **iontophoresis** (by electrical field) or **phonophoresis** (by ultrasound). Phonophoresis has been used for the topical application of many medications, including **dexamethasone** (for inflammatory conditions), **zinc oxide** and **tannic acid** (for herpes simplex), **benzydamine** (for sports-related injuries), **benzoic acid** (for fungal infections), **hydrocortisone** (for inflamed digital/joints/subdeltoid bursitis), **phenylbutazone** (for arthrosynovitis), **thiodyne** (for vertebral osteochondrosis), and **interferon** (for herpetic keratitis).

Liposomal Drug Delivery System

Utilizing the concept that the key function of the plasmalemma is to exclude the external environment, liposomes were developed to carry **soluble** as well as **lipophilic drugs**.

Clinical studies have shown that liposomes are able to effectively encapsulate and deliver a number of drugs, including **daunorubicin** (an antineoplastic agent), **orgiprenaline** (a bronchodilator), **indium** (a gamma-imaging agent), and **amphotericin B** (for systemic mycosis). A major therapeutic advantage of liposomes is their ability to enhance the bioavailability of a drug, alter the tissue distribution of an agent, or prolong the release of a substance in the body.

Bioavailability

The physiochemical nature of certain drugs may rule out oral administration, and hence these drugs are considered to have subnormal oral bioavailability. For example, nitroglycerin is given sublingually in the treatment of angina pectoris because it is catabolized very rapidly in the liver if it is given orally (see Figure 1.2).

ABSORPTION OF DRUGS

The various lipoid barriers of the gastrointestinal tract, the kidney tubules, and the central nervous system (CNS) allow the absorption of essential nutrients, guard against the uncontrollable disposal of electrolytes and other substances, and prevent the entrance of potentially toxic materials.

To reach its site of action (the **receptor**), a drug may have to traverse a succession of membranes. For example, **phenytoin**, when administered orally, must cross the gastrointestinal epithelium, the blood–brain barrier, the plasma membrane, and finally the membranes of subcellular organelles of neurons. An understanding of how drugs traverse various cellular and subcellular membranes is of clinical significance, in terms of attaining the desired therapeutic level of an administered agent.

Multiple **physical and chemical factors** influence the rate and extent of absorption of drugs. These include:

Physiochemical factors

- Molecular weight
- The degree of ionization under physiologic conditions
- Product formulation characteristics
- Disintegration and dissolution rates for solid dosages
- Drug release characteristics for timed-release preparations

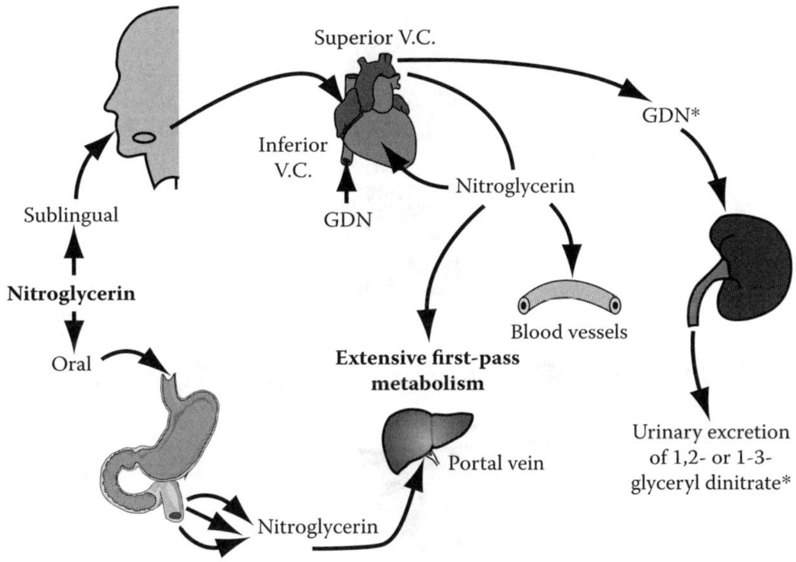

FIGURE 1.2 In order to avoid extensive hepatic first-pass metabolism, nitroglycerin is given sublingually. *GDN = 1,2- or 1-3-glyceryl dinitrate; V.C. = vena cava.

Patient factors

- The surface area available for absorption
- Gastric and duodenal pH
- The gastric emptying time
- Bile salt pool size
- Bacterial colonization of the gastrointestinal tract
- The presence and extent of underlying diseases

Lipid-soluble substances traverse the membrane by dissolving in the lipoid phase, and the lipid-insoluble substances penetrate only when they are small enough to pass through the pores. The absorption of large lipid-insoluble substances such as sugars and amino acids is accomplished by **specialized transport processes**.

DRUG PARTICLE SIZE

The rate of dissolution of a drug increases significantly as the size of the drug particle decreases. For example, the reduction in particle size of digoxin from 3 to 1 mm^3 increases the **surface area** of drug particles exposed to solution by as much as 300%. The more soluble drugs are absorbed faster and more completely than the relatively insoluble ones. The **oral bioavailability** of numerous drugs has been increased by a reduction in particle size. On the other hand, decreasing particle size is not advantageous for compounds such as **penicillin G** and **erythromycin**, which tend to decompose in the gastrointestinal tract.

BUCCAL AND SUBLINGUAL ABSORPTION

Compared with other routes of administration, different mucosa that line the oral cavity (**buccal** and **sublingual** sites of drug administration) offer advantages that include: (1) being noninvasive, (2) producing a rapid onset of action, (3) providing high blood levels, (4) avoiding first-pass effects, and (5) circumventing the exposure of drugs to the acidic and digestive fluid of the stomach. In addition, drugs may be easily applied (cheeked), sufficiently localized, and, if necessary, readily retrieved.

Drug absorption from the oral cavity occurs through the **passive diffusion** of the nonionized form from an aqueous phase to one that is lipid in nature. In addition, there is also evidence for the **carrier-mediated transport** of drugs, whereby the **levo isomers**, but not the dextro isomers, of many drugs are absorbed.

INTRANASAL DELIVERY

The intranasal route of administration is best for those drugs that either undergo **extensive degradation** or are **poorly absorbed** after oral administration.

Drugs that are routinely administered intranasally include peptides such as **vasopressin** and its analog **desmopressin**, **luteinizing hormone-releasing hormone**, **buserelin**, **leuprolide**, nafarelin, and **oxytocin**.

RECTAL ADMINISTRATION

The oral administration of drugs, which is the route of choice, is impractical or impossible to use under certain circumstances, such as in conditions causing nausea and vomiting in patients with convulsions, just before surgery, and in uncooperative patients. The rectal route is also desirable for inducing anesthesia in children. However, the relatively smaller surface area for absorption is often less than that available for orally administered drugs. To overcome this problem, absorption-promoting agents such as **surfactants, sodium salicylate**, and **enamines** are coadministered with the drugs.

If a drug undergoes an extensive **first-pass metabolism** (e.g., **morphine**, **metoclopramide**, **ergotamine**, or **lidocaine**), rectal administration may produce an even higher plasma level. The prolonged rectal administration of multiple drugs may produce local irritation or even rectal ulceration.

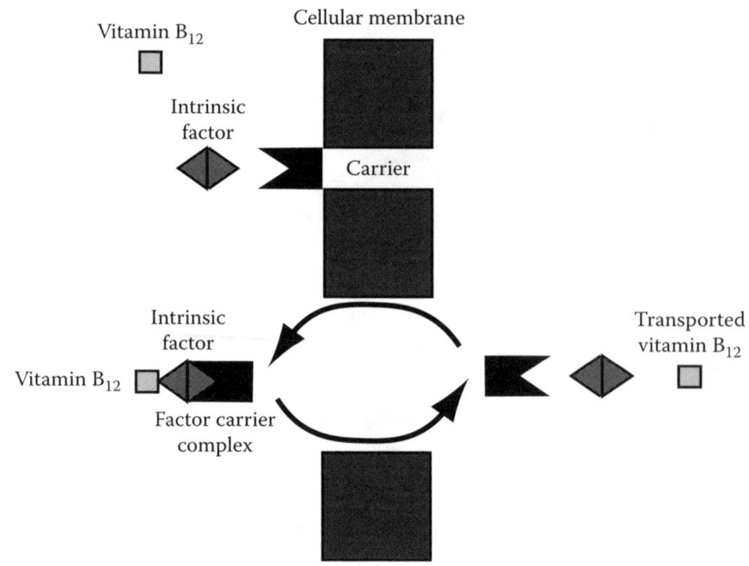

FIGURE 1.3 A carrier-mediated transport of vitamin B_{12}.

TRANSPORT MECHANISMS

Passive Diffusion

Passive diffusion takes place when a drug molecule moves from a region of relatively high concentration to low concentration without requiring energy. The diffusion and movement of drugs continue until equilibrium has been achieved on both sides of the membrane. This equilibrium is achieved faster with highly permeable and hence lipid-soluble drugs, and when the membrane has a large surface area.

Carrier-Mediated Transport

A substance to be carried forms a complex with a component of the membrane on one side; the complex is then carried through the membrane, the drug or substance is released, and the carrier returns to the original surface and state to repeat the process. The carrier shows specificity; for instance, **L-dopa** but not D-dopa is transported.

Facilitated Transport

Facilitated transport is essentially the same as carrier-mediated transport, except that, besides a carrier molecule, another transport facilitator is essential. For example, **vitamin B_{12}** attaches to the **intrinsic factor**, and the vitamin B_{12} intrinsic factor complex then attaches to the carrier molecule and is transported. This transport process does not require energy and does not proceed against a concentration gradient (Figure 1.3).

Ion Pair Transport

For ion pair transport to take place, **organic anions** combine with **organic cations** to form a neutral complex, which is then transported through the membrane by passive diffusion.

Pinocytosis

In pinocytosis, the transport of water-insoluble substances such as **vitamins A, D, E**, and **K** is accomplished in the following manner. First, they are engulfed by the membranes; they are then dissolved in the membranes and released unchanged in the inside compartment.

RECEPTOR-MEDIATED ENDOCYTOSIS

Receptor-mediated endocytosis is the process of **ligand movement** from the extracellular space to the inside of the cell by the interaction of the ligand with a specific **cell-surface receptor**. Receptors bind the ligand at the surface, internalize it by means of coated pits and vesicles, and ultimately release it into an acidic endosomal compartment (Figure 1.4).

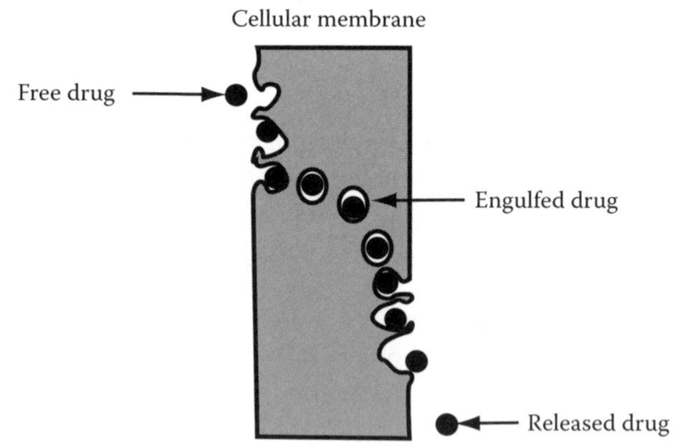

FIGURE 1.4 A mechanism for transport of water-insoluble vitamins.

OTHER FACTORS CONTROLLING THE RATE OF ABSORPTION OF DRUGS

In addition to the **lipid–water partition coefficient**, other factors that control the rate of absorption of drugs are the **degree of ionization**, the **surface area**, **blood flow** through the region, and the **gastric emptying time**.

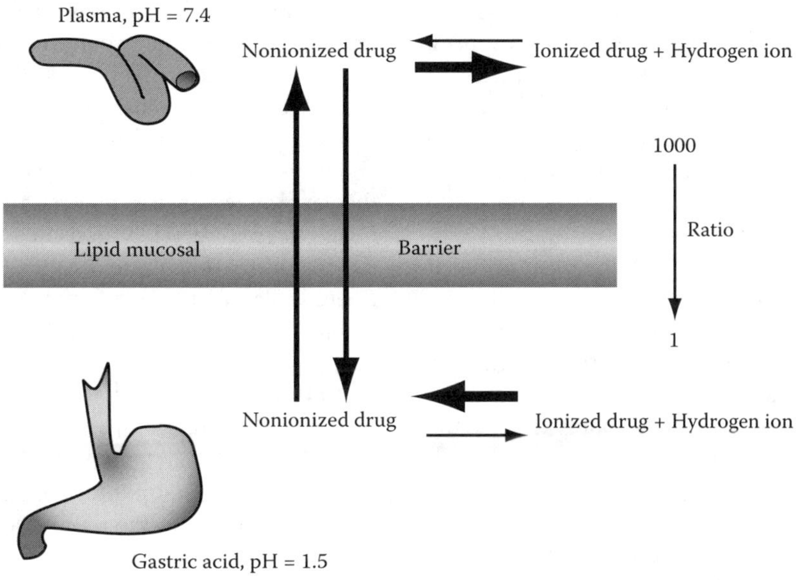

FIGURE 1.5 Drugs are absorbed in nonionized forms.

Degree of Ionization

The **degree of ionization** of drugs and the **pH of the internal medium** play important roles in the transfer of drugs across biologic membranes. Most drugs are either weak acids or bases. Therefore, in solution, they exist in nonionized and ionized forms. The nonionized forms of various compounds are more lipid soluble and can penetrate the cellular membranes (Figure 1.5). The **rate of passage** of many drugs across various membranes becomes a function of the **negative logarithm of the dissociation constant** (pK_a) of the drug and the **pH of the internal medium**. This concept is derived from the **Henderson–Hasselbalch equation**.

For example, **phenytoin** is absorbed primarily from the upper intestinal tract. Phenytoin is an acid with a pK_a of 8.3 to 9.2 and is insoluble at the pH of gastric juice (2.0). Therefore, it cannot be absorbed significantly from the stomach. On passage into the small intestine, where the pH is less acidic (7 to 7.5), phenytoin is absorbed in a nonionized form.

At the duodenal pH of 7.0, 96.9% of the phenytoin is in the nonionized form, which favors its absorption. The absorption of phenytoin is greatest in the duodenum and decreases in the lower parts of the small intestine. The absorption from the cecum and the large intestine is severalfold lower than that in the duodenum.

Again, using the Henderson–Hasselbalch equation, one finds that **acetylsalicylic acid** (pK_a 3) is 99% and 91% nonionized at the pH of 1 and 2, respectively. Therefore, according to this model, acetylsalicylic acid (aspirin)is best absorbed when the pH of the stomach is highly acidic. This high acidity, however, limits its aqueous solubility.

Surface Area

The influence of ionization on drug absorption is important only in circumstances in which biologic pHs vary dramatically, such as those in the stomach (varying from 1.4 to 7.0) and the urine (varying from 4.5 to 7.5). The changes in pH in other biologic fluids are considerably smaller. Because both ionized and nonionized drugs are absorbed from subcutaneous and intramuscular sites of injection, ionization does not appear to play as important a role in the passage of drugs across the capillary wall. Finally, although drugs such as acetylsalicylic acid are best absorbed from an acidic medium such as that in the stomach, most of the aspirin is nevertheless absorbed in the upper small intestine, which has a considerably greater absorptive surface. The **total absorptive area** of the small intestine and its microvilli has been estimated to exceed 200 m^2 for the intestine versus 1 m^2 for the stomach. Similarly, the **perfusion rate** of the intestine is considerably greater than that of the stomach. In fact, most drugs, whether nonionized or ionized, and whether acidic, basic, or neutral, are absorbed mostly from the small intestine. Consistent with this is the observation that buffered acetylsalicylic acid preparations are dissolved faster and absorbed better mostly in the intestine. Similarly, patients with **achlorhydria** or those who have undergone gastrectomy have little difficulty with the absorption of orally ingested drugs.

Blood Flow

The absorption of drugs in solution from intramuscular and subcutaneous sites of injection is limited by the **perfusion rate**. Failure to recognize this important concept has resulted in patient death. For example, **morphine sulfate** is often administered subcutaneously in a dose of 10 mg per 70 kg of body weight. This dose is sufficient to produce analgesia in 70% of patients with moderate to severe pain. However, in the setting of circulatory collapse and shock (e.g., septic shock in bacteremia due to release of endotoxin) in which the peripheral circulation may be impaired, morphine is not absorbed. Cases have been reported in which the lack of analgesia prompted the additional injection of morphine, all of which remained at the injection site and in the subcutaneous capillary bed. When the peripheral circulation improved, the massive amount of morphine that had collected became absorbed and death ensued, primarily due to respiratory depression.

Increasing the blood flow enhances the absorption of drugs, whereas decreasing the blood flow reduces absorption. Massaging the site where a drug has been administered therefore increases the rate of absorption, whereas placing an ice pack on the site retards it. One may take advantage of this concept and deliberately retard the absorption of drugs by reducing the peripheral circulation. For instance, local anesthetics are often combined with a vasoconstricting substance such as epinephrine and injected as a mixture. The epinephrine causes vasoconstriction, hence producing a bloodless field of operation. Epinephrine prevents the rapid absorption of local anesthetics and thus both enhances their duration of action and prevents systemic toxicity.

Gastric Emptying Time

Because drugs are mostly absorbed from the upper part of the small intestine, the rate of gastric emptying plays a crucial role in drug absorption. If rapid absorption is desired, drugs should be taken on an empty stomach. Meals, especially those with a high fat content, retard absorption. The desire for rapid absorption of drugs necessitates that the interactions between food and drugs be monitored carefully.

Drugs such as **clindamycin** and **lincomycin** should be taken on an empty stomach. Only 20 to 35% of clindamycin and lincomycin is absorbed from the gastrointestinal tract, and taking these agents with a meal further hinders their absorption and produces a plasma concentration of antibiotics that is ineffective.

The **tetracyclines** should be taken orally 1 hour before or 2 hours after meals. Absorption of these agents is impaired by the presence of milk and milk products and by the concomitant administration of aluminum hydroxide gels, sodium bicarbonate, calcium and magnesium salts, or iron preparations because of the chelation of divalent and trivalent cations by these agents.

Anticholinergic drugs such as **propantheline** should be taken 1 hour before meals. Anticholinergic drugs are able to inhibit the secretion of gastric juice, which is ordinarily stimulated by food.

Hepatic First-Pass Effect

By far the most important reason for an inadequate plasma concentration following the oral or parenteral administration of a drug is the **first-pass effect**, which consists of the loss of a drug as it passes through the liver for the first time. For example, **nitroglycerin**, which is used in the management of patients with angina pectoris, is given sublingually. Taken orally, nitroglycerin is rapidly inactivated in the liver, and the resulting concentration is inadequate to be of immediate value to the patient. Sublingually administered nitroglycerin bypasses the liver and enters the superior vena cava, whereupon it perfuses the coronary circulation (Figure 1.2). Besides nitroglycerin, there are other drugs that exhibit extensive first-pass hepatic elimination and hence have a very low oral bioavailability. These include **desipramine**, **morphine**, **propranolol**, **lidocaine**, and **verapamil**. The first-pass effect can at times be overcome by raising the dose, as is done with desipramine and propranolol.

DISTRIBUTION OF DRUGS

Whether given orally or parenterally, drugs are distributed nonuniformly throughout the body. Factors that regulate this distribution are the **lipophilic characteristics** of the drugs, the **blood supply** to the tissues, and the **chemical composition** of various organs and tissues. The distribution of drugs not only influences their **onset of action** but also at times determines their **duration of action**. For example, **thiopental**, an intravenous anesthetic, produces unconsciousness 10 to 20 s after its administration, and consciousness returns in 20 to 30 min. The rapid onset of action is due to the rapid transport of thiopental to the brain. The short duration of action stems from its subsequent redistribution to other tissues, such as muscle and fat.

BINDING OF VARIOUS DRUGS TO PLASMA PROTEINS

In an ideal therapeutic regimen, a sufficient amount of the drug should reach the locus of action (receptor site) in order to bring about the desired effect, but not so much as to produce toxicity. Furthermore, the drug should not disappear too rapidly from the locus of action, or the therapeutic effects will be transient and hence of limited value. The binding of drugs to plasma proteins and various subcellular components tends to accomplish these objectives. Human plasma contains over 60 different proteins, and the most abundant one is **albumin**. Other significant proteins include **prealbumin, lipoproteins**, and various **globulins**. A number of plasma proteins, especially albumin, have shown a high affinity for binding drugs, so that, at a given total plasma concentration, only a portion of the total amount of drug is free in the plasma water. The remainder is bound to plasma proteins, and in this form does not exert any pharmacologic effects.

The interaction between proteins and a drug is governed by the **law of mass action**, in that the proportion of bound drug remains constant, provided the binding sites are not saturated. With the possible exception of **valproic acid** and **disopyramide**, the saturability of binding sites does not occur within therapeutic ranges.

The interaction between drug and protein is not a chemical one but a reversible attachment that is achieved by various forces, including **electrostatic, London– van der Waals**, and **hydrogen binding**, or some combination of these. This drug–protein complex is readily reversible (the half-life being on the order of milliseconds). There is a continuous shift of bound to unbound drugs (see Figure 1.1), and, unlike receptor binding, no pharmacologic response occurs as a result of the association. The binding sites of endogenously occurring acidic substances (e.g., **bilirubin**, **vitamin C**, and **bile acids**) and acidic drugs (e.g., **phenylbutazone**, **penicillins**, **sulfonamides**, **warfarin**, and **salicylic acid**) is the N-terminal amino acid. The basic drugs (e.g., **diphenhydramine**, **streptomycin**, **chloramphenicol**, and **coumarin anticoagulants**) bind nonspecifically.

Albumin

Albumin has two binding sites: **Site I** binds structurally unrelated substances (e.g., **warfarin**, **phenytoin**, and **sulfonamides**), and **Site II,** which is more selective, binds a smaller number of drugs (i.e., **diazepam**, **phenylbutazone**, and **ibuprofen**).

Alpha$_1$-Acid Glycoprotein

Alpha$_1$-acid glycoprotein exists in concentrations that are 50 to 100 times lower than those of albumin. Basic drugs (**quinidine**, **imipramine**, **propranolo$_1$**, and **lidocaine**) bind to the single site present on alpha$_1$-acid glycoprotein.

Other Glycoproteins

Corticosteroid-binding globulin and **thyroxine-binding globulin** are both alpha globulins that possess high affinities but low capacities for their respective substrates. **Methadone** (a narcotic analgesic) binds to the gamma-, beta-, and alpha-globulins, as well as to albumin.

Lipoproteins

Lipoproteins bind a small amount of certain drugs (**imipramine**, **amitriptyline**, **nortriptyline**, **phenytoin**, and **quinidine**), which usually bind to alpha$_1$-acid glycoprotein.

The response to a drug is determined by the unbound fraction that is in the plasma water. The **concentration of unbound drug**, rather than the concentration of total drug, is often a better index of a drug's effective therapeutic level. The clinical laboratory assessment of the plasma level of a drug in most cases involves the measurement of bound-plus-unbound amounts of the agent. The greater the amount of bound drug, the less rapidly will the plasma level of unbound drug decline, as it is continuously being replenished through dissociation of the complex. The binding of drug to plasma protein is not usually a disadvantage; in fact, without such binding, the effect of most drugs would be too transient. The drugs would therefore have to be administered so frequently that the plasma concentration would oscillate between toxic and ineffective levels. Therapy is easier to control when a drug is stable in the body and the plasma concentration does not fluctuate widely.

The percentage of protein binding of drugs at therapeutic levels varies dramatically. Some drugs such as **allopurinol**, **heparin**, and **isoniazid** do not become bound. Other drugs such as **antipyrine**, **ethambutol**, and **theophylline** become bound to the extent of only 4 to 15%. Several drugs such as **ampicillin** (25%) and digoxin (23%) show low protein binding; some drugs such as **atropine** (50%) and **meperidine** (40%) show moderate protein binding, and some drugs such as **carbamazepine** (72%), **furosemide** (75%), **nitrofurantoin** (70%), and **rifampin** (85%) show high degrees of protein binding. Some drugs such as **dicumarol** (97%), **diazepam** (96%), **phenylbutazone** (98%), and **diazoxide** (96%) bind extensively to plasma proteins.

The binding sites of the protein are not unlimited and are subject to saturation. When this occurs, toxicity may develop following further drug administration because the later portion of the drug remains free. Consistent with this view is the observation that toxic manifestations of drugs are quite frequent and considerably higher in individuals suffering from hypoalbuminemia or altered plasma and tissue protein concentrations, or both.

Drugs may **alter the protein binding** of other agents. For instance, **aspirin** decreases the binding of **thyroxine**, and the binding of bilirubin is hindered by many pharmacologic agents. The more tightly bound drugs can displace the less firmly bound agents. The intensity of the effect of displaced drug on the patient will simply depend on the blood level of the free drug and its nature. At times, the effect may be highly undesirable and even fatal. Only the slight displacement of a highly bound drug such as **dicumarol** (an oral anticoagulant) by **phenylbutazone**, which has greater affinity for binding sites, can cause serious hemorrhage. Because only 3% of the anticoagulant is free, an additional displacement of 3% increases its effects by 100%.

TISSUE LOCALIZATION OF DRUGS

After a drug has been absorbed, the initial phase of its distribution into the tissues is based on **cardiac output** and **regional blood flow**. Highly perfused organs such as the brain, heart, liver, and kidney receive most of the drug. Diffusion into the interstitial compartment occurs rapidly. **Lipid-soluble** and **lipid-insoluble drugs** have different patterns of distribution; for example, **thiopental**, a highly lipid-soluble substance, distributes rapidly into the brain. Because the blood perfusion of the bone is not extensive, local blood flow may not play a role in the accumulation of **tetracycline** in bone. **Active transport** (e.g., the accumulation of **lithium** in bone) and the presence of **specific binding proteins** (e.g., thyroglobulin in the thyroid gland) are responsible for the respective accumulation of these agents at these sites.

APPARENT VOLUME OF DISTRIBUTION OF DRUGS

Volume of distribution (V_D) is defined as the amount of drug in the body in relation to the concentration of drug in the plasma:

$$V_D = \frac{\text{Amount of drug in body}}{\text{Concentration of drug in plasma}}$$

For example, if 300 mg of phenytoin is given to an epileptic patient, once equilibrium has been reached and the plasma concentration of phenytoin is 10 μg/ml, the apparent volume of distribution of phenytoin would be 30 L.

The **one-compartment model** of distribution assumes that an administered drug is homogeneously distributed throughout the tissue fluids of the body. For instance, ethyl alcohol distributes uniformly throughout the body and therefore any body fluid may be used to assess its concentration. The **two-compartment model** of distribution envisions two or multiple central or peripheral compartments. The **central compartment** includes the blood and extracellular fluid volumes of the highly perfused organs (i.e., the brain, heart, liver, and kidney, which receive three-fourths of the cardiac output); the **peripheral compartment** consists of relatively less perfused tissues such as muscle, skin, and fat depots. When distributive equilibrium has occurred completely, the concentration of drug in the body will be uniform.

The **rate of distribution** of a drug from the blood to a tissue depends on the extent of binding of that drug to plasma proteins (only free drug is able to distribute), on the ability of that drug to diffuse through tissue membrane (in general, lipophilic drugs are able to diffuse), on the degree of perfusion of that tissue (unit of blood/min/volume of tissue), and on the properties of the tissue membrane. If all other factors remain equal, the higher the tissue perfusion, the higher is the amount of drug to be diffused.

In comparing **thiopental** and **penicillin**, it is found that thiopental enters the brain more rapidly than muscle; the reverse is the case for penicillin. Thiopental is a lipophilic substance that diffuses easily into both muscle and brain. Because the perfusion of brain is higher than that of muscle, thiopental diffuses more rapidly into the brain. Penicillin is a polar substance that does not enter the brain at all. However, because the muscle capillaries are porous, they allow many drugs, including penicillin, to diffuse rapidly across the membrane.

Drugs that show **extensive tissue binding** are said to have an apparent volume of distribution many times the total body size. For example, **digoxin**, which binds to plasma protein to the extent of 23%, has an apparent volume of distribution of 8 L/kg. The volume of distribution of drugs that do not bind to plasma or tissue proteins varies between the extracellular fluid volume (16 L) and the total body water (42 L). **Insulin**, **sodium**, and **iodine** are confined to the **extracellular water**, whereas **caffeine** and **ethanol** are distributed in the **total body water**.

THE BLOOD–BRAIN BARRIER

The brain capillaries are tightly joined and covered by a footlike sheath that arises from astrocytes. Thus, a drug leaving the capillaries in the brain has to traverse not only the nonporous capillary cell wall but also the membranes of the astrocyte to reach the neurons. Such a structure, frequently referred to as the **blood–brain barrier**, tends to limit the entry of many drugs into the brain.

THE PLACENTAL BARRIER

The membrane separating fetal blood from maternal blood in the intervillous space, the **placental barrier**, resembles other membranes, in that lipid-soluble substances diffuse readily but water-soluble substances either do not or diffuse poorly. Thus, for instance, morphine-induced respiratory depression and miosis may occur in both the mother and her newborn infant. The children of narcotic-addicted mothers will be born with an addiction to narcotics.

DRUGS IN PREGNANCY AND THE NEWBORN

Pregnancy and the first weeks of life represent two physiologic situations in which there is a continual and significant change in the levels of plasma proteins, and it may therefore be necessary to adjust the doses of medications during these times.

Drug Therapy in Pregnancy

In pregnancy, the **total body fluid** increases by 8 L, of which 80% is extracellular water. The plasma volume increases by 40 to 50% (1.2–1.5 L). Consequently, in pregnancy there is an increase in plasma volume, decrease in plasma protein levels, increase in total and extracellular water compartments, and increase in total body fat. These alterations may change the volume of distribution of most drugs.

Drug Therapy in the Newborn

At birth, a full-term infant has a significantly lower plasma albumin level than do adults, and therefore the number of drug-binding sites is substantially less. This situation necessitates a reduction in the total amount of drug administered.

THE SITE OF ACTION OF DRUGS

It is generally accepted that most, but not all, drugs (e.g., antiseptics) exert their potent and specific effects by forming a bond, generally reversible, with a cellular component called a **receptor site**, which should be differentiated from **acceptor** or **silent sites** where drugs are stored. Drugs that interact with a receptor and elicit a response are called **agonists**. Drugs that interact with receptors and prevent the action of agonists are termed **antagonists**. For example, acetylcholine, which causes bradycardia, is an agonist; atropine, which blocks the action of acetylcholine and prevents bradycardia, is an antagonist. The relative effects of drugs are often judged in terms of their **potency**, which is a measure of the dosage required to bring about a response, and their **efficacy**, which is a measure of their inherent ability to exert an effect.

When the pharmacologic properties of two compounds are compared, one may prove to be more potent and efficacious than the other. For instance, as an analgesic, morphine is more potent and more efficacious than

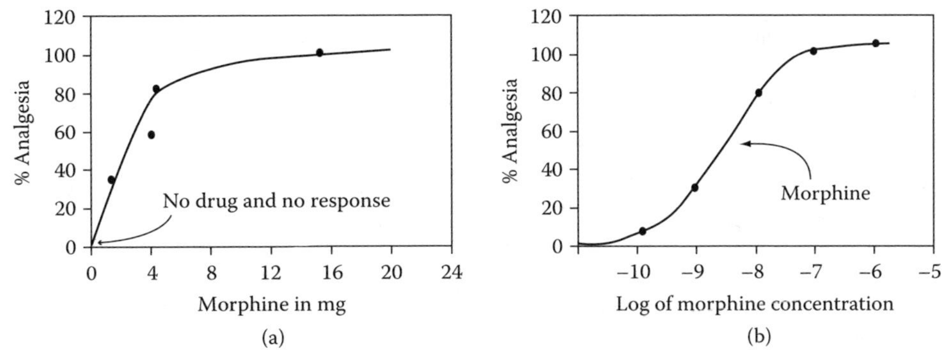

FIGURE 1.6 Examples of dose–response curves.

acetylsalicylic acid. On the other hand, two compounds may be equally efficacious but one could be more potent. Haloperidol and chlorpromazine are both efficacious neuroleptics in the management of schizophrenia, but haloperidol is more potent.

A drug's **affinity** and **intrinsic activity** also need to be differentiated. Intrinsic activity refers to a drug's ability to bind to the receptor, which results in pharmacologic actions. Affinity is a measure of the degree to which a drug binds to the receptor—whether it exerts a pharmacologic action (as an agonist) or simply blocks the receptor (as an antagonist).

NATURE AND TYPE OF PHARMACOLOGIC RECEPTOR SITES

The actions of neurotransmitters are mediated mostly through their interactions with receptors located either at **presynaptic** or **postsynaptic sites**. These receptors function in a coordinated fashion to elicit **excitation** (depolarization) or **inhibition** (hyperpolarization) within and between neuronal subsystems. A basic inadequacy in this interplay is believed to lead to pathologic states such as **Parkinson's disease** (dopamine deficiency), **Huntington's disease** (dopamine excess), **endogenous depression** (catecholamine deficiency), or **mania** (catecholamine excess).

DOSE–RESPONSE RELATIONSHIP

The relationship between the amount of drug administered (e.g., morphine), or the concentration of the administered drug in the plasma, and the magnitude of the desired response obtained (e.g., analgesia) is referred to as a **dose–response relationship**. Obviously, for example, no analgesia is obtained if no morphine exists at the receptor site (Figure 1.6a). When all the available receptor sites are occupied, hypothetically, the maximum response has been obtained **(Clark's hypothesis)**, and it may begin to produce undesirable side effects. This **linear dose–response** relationship, as depicted in Figure 1.6a, may be expressed in a logarithmic scale (Figure 1.6b). A **quantal dose–response** curve relates the frequency with which any dose of a drug evokes a fixed (all-or-none) pharmacologic response.

POTENCY AND EFFICACY

Potency refers to the lowest dose that will produce a maximum effect. **Efficacy** refers to the inherent ability to exert an effect. **Morphine** in a dose of 10 mg given subcutaneously produces analgesia, but a 2-mg dose of **dihydromorphinone** (Dilaudid) can accomplish the same degree of analgesia. Therefore, morphine and dihydromorphinone are equally efficacious, but dihydromorphinone is more potent than morphine (Figure 1.7).

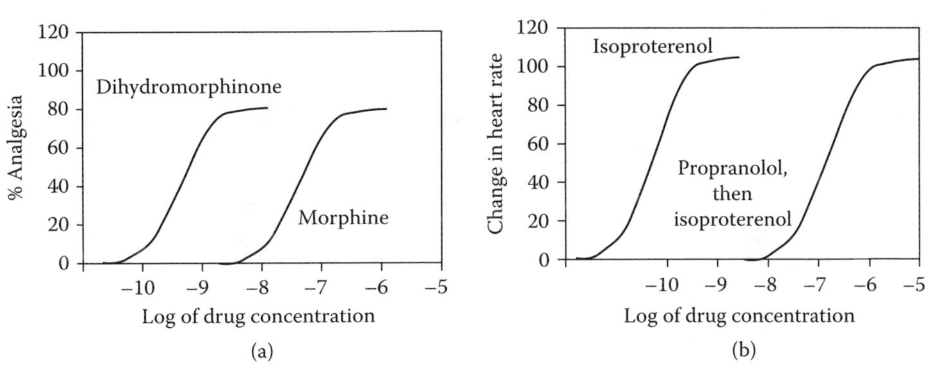

FIGURE 1.7 (a) Dihydromorphinone is more potent than morphine but is equally efficacious. (b) Propranolol is a competitive antagonist at adrenergic receptors.

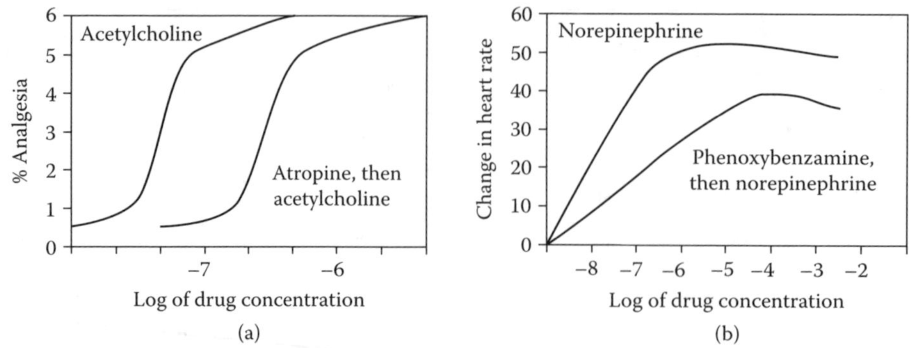

FIGURE 1.8 (a) Atropine is a competitive antagonist at cholinergic receptors. (b) Phenoxybenzamine is a noncompetitive antagonist at adrenergic receptors.

The interaction between a drug and a receptor site is similar to a reversible interaction between a substrate and an enzyme. This antagonism between agonists and antagonists is called **competitive** or **surmountable antagonism** if the inhibition is overcome by increasing the concentration of the agonist (Figure 1.8). For example, **propranolol** (a beta-adrenergic receptor antagonist) is a competitive antagonist for **isoproterenol** (a beta-adrenergic receptor agonist), and **atropine** is a competitive antagonist for **acetylcholine** at the muscarinic cholinergic receptor site. A **partial agonist** produces a lower response than a full agonist. When a maximum response is obtained by an agonist at a concentration that does not occupy all the available receptor, a **spare receptor** or high-efficacy receptor-agonist occupancy mechanism may be involved (Figure 1.9).

In examining the kinetic nature of competitive antagonists, one discovers that parallel dose–response curves possessing the same maximum effect are produced for the agonists in the presence and absence of a fixed amount of antagonists.

When an antagonist binds irreversibly to the receptor site, thus producing either permanent chemical changes or inactivation of the receptor site, or both, this is referred to as **noncompetitive antagonism** or **nonequilibrium blockade. Phenoxybenzamine**, an alpha-adrenergic receptor-blocking agent, noncompetitively and irreversibly blocks the alpha-adrenergic receptor site, preventing **norepinephrine** from exerting its full action.

PHYSIOLOGIC AND PHARMACOLOGIC ANTAGONISM

If two drugs, one an agonist and another an antagonist, bind to an identical receptor site, either producing or preventing an effect, this association is called **pharmacologic antagonism. Naloxone**, **atropine**, and **diphenhydramine** are pharmacologic and specific antagonists of **morphine**, **acetylcholine**, and **histamine** at their respective receptor sites. In **physiologic antagonism**, the drugs do not bind to the same receptor sites but produce functionally opposite

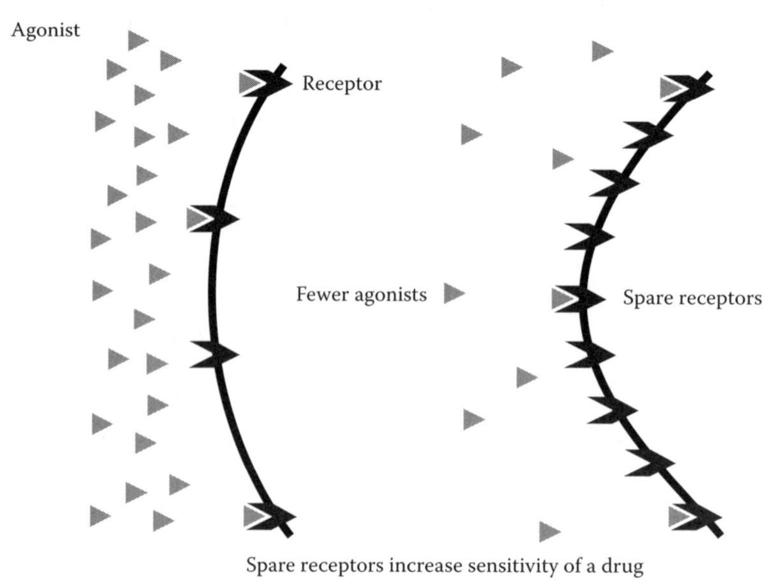

FIGURE 1.9 The concept of a spare receptor.

results. For example, histamine produces vasodilation, whereas epinephrine produces vasoconstriction; however, they interact with two separate receptor sites.

ENHANCEMENT OF DRUG ACTION

Numerous agents acting at two or more receptor sites may magnify each other's effects, producing responses that are greater than the one produced by either one of the drugs alone. For example, **angiotensin II** enhances the vasoconstricting effects of norepinephrine, and histamine augments the hypotensive effects of acetylcholine. If the quantitative summation of the effects produced by two drugs is greater than the algebraic sum of the effects produced by either drug alone, this phenomenon is called **potentiation**. For example, when taken individually, diazepam, chlorpromazine, and alcohol all cause sedation. However, when alcohol is ingested along with either diazepam or chlorpromazine, pronounced CNS depression may arise, and deaths have occurred following the injudicious combined use of these CNS depressants. In this instance, alcohol protentiates the CNS depression induced by diazepam or chlorpromazine. In depicting the potentiation of two drugs, one uses isoboles for plotting their respective effects.

THERAPEUTIC INDEX

The therapeutic index deals with the ratio of lethal doses to 50% of the population (LD_{50}) over the median minimum effective dose (ED_{50}).

$$\text{Therapeutic index} = \frac{LD_{50}}{ED_{50}}$$

The higher the therapeutic index, the safer the drug; the lower the therapeutic index, the greater the possibility of toxicity. The therapeutic index for barbiturate as a class is 10, whereas the therapeutic index for cardiac glycoside as a class is 3. Because the usual therapeutic dose of cardiac glycoside is 1 mg, death may result if only 3 mg has been administered.

BIOTRANSFORMATION

Biotransformation may be defined as the enzyme-catalyzed alteration of drugs by the living organism. Although few drugs are eliminated unchanged, urinary excretion is a negligible means of termination of the action of most drugs or poisons in the body. As a matter of fact, the urinary excretion of a highly lipid-soluble substance such as **pentobarbital** would be so slow that it would take the body a century to rid itself of the effect of a single dose of the agent. Therefore, mammalian and other terrestrial animals have developed systems that allow the conversion of most lipid-soluble substances to water-soluble ones, so that they may be easily excreted by the kidney. In general, biotransformation may be divided into two forms of metabolism: hepatic and nonhepatic (Figure 1.10).

HEPATIC DRUG METABOLISM

By far the major portion of biotransformation is carried out in the liver by **cytochrome P-450** (P-450), which is a collective term for a group of related enzymes or isoenzymes that are responsible for the oxidation of numerous drugs; **endogenous substances** such as fatty acids, prostaglandins, steroids, and ketones; and **carcinogens** such as polycyclic aromatic hydrocarbons, nitrosamines, hydrazines, and arylamines.

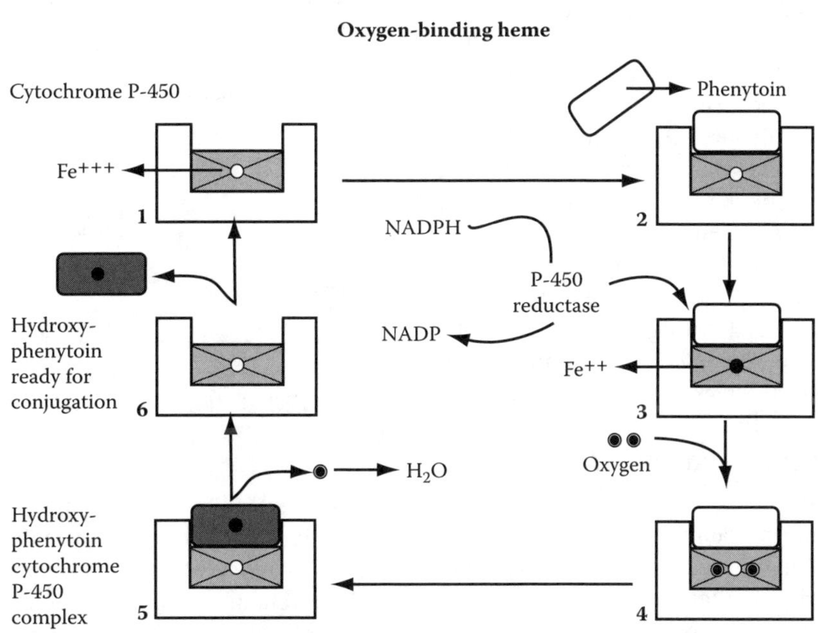

FIGURE 1.10 A simplified scheme for the mechanism of action of cytochrome P-450. NADP = nicotinamide-adenine dinucleotide phosphate; NADPH = the reduced form of NADP.

NONHEPATIC METABOLISM

Plasma

One of the drugs that is metabolized in the blood is **succinylcholine**, a muscle relaxant that is hydrolyzed by the pseudocholinesterase of liver and plasma to succinylmonocholine. The short duration of action of succinylmonocholine (5 min) is due to its rapid hydrolysis in plasma. Patients with atypical cholinesterase who cannot metabolize succinylcholine suffer pronounced apnea. **Procaine**, a local anesthetic, is also hydrolyzed by pseudocholinesterase.

Lung

The lung is involved in both the activation and inactivation of numerous physiologic and pharmacologic substances. For example, **angiotensin I** is converted to **angiotensin II** in the lung.

Intestinal Epithelium

The intestinal epithelium is capable of removing numerous agents.

MOLECULAR BIOLOGY OF MULTIPLE ISOENZYMES OF P-450

In recent years, an extensive number of complementary DNAs for the P-450 genes for humans have been isolated and sequenced. Genes that encode proteins that are less than 36% similar in their amino acid sequence belong to different families. Currently, eight different families have been identified in humans, each designated by a roman numeral. The drug-metabolizing P-450s belongs to families I, II, III, and IV. P-450s that are 70% or more similar are encoded by genes in the same subfamilies. Finally, the individual gene is designated by an arabic numeral.

During **phase I**, most drugs are inactivated pharmacologically; some remain unaltered, and some become more active and toxic. For example, phenytoin in the liver is first hydroxylated to hydroxyphenytoin (phase I) and is then conjugated with glucuronic acid (**phase II**) and excreted by the kidney as phenytoin glucuronide conjugate. During phase I, besides introducing a polar group such as an –OH group, a potential polar group may also be unmasked from the drug to be metabolized. For example, compound $R–OCH_3$ is converted to R–OH by demethylation. Codeine becomes demethylated to morphine. The free or unmasked polar group is then conjugated with glucuronate, sulfate, glycine, or acetate. With the exception of morphine 6-glucuronide, almost all conjugates lack pharmacologic activity.

SCHEME OF THE MIXED-FUNCTION OXIDATION REACTION PATHWAY

The hepatic endoplasmic reticulum possesses oxidative enzymes called **mixed-function oxidases** or **monooxygenase** with a specific requirement for both molecular oxygen and a reduced concentration of nicotinamide adenine dinucleotide phosphate (NADPH). Essential in the mixed-function oxidase system is P-450 (Figure 1.10). The primary electron donor is NADPH, whereas the electron transfer involved P-450, a flavoprotein. The presence of a **heat-stable fraction** is necessary for the operation of the system.

A drug substrate to be metabolized binds to oxidized P-450, which in turn is reduced by P-450 reductase. The drug-reduced P-450 complex then combines with molecular oxygen. A second electron and two hydrogen ions are acquired from the donor system, and the subsequent products are oxidized drug and water, with regeneration of the oxidized P-450. This process is summarized as follows:

1. NADPH + oxidized cytochrome P-450 + H^+ → reduced P-450 + $NADP^+$
2. Reduced cytochrome P-450 + O_2 → "active oxygen complex"
3. "Active oxygen complex" + drug substrate → oxidized drug + oxidized cytochrome P-450 + H_2O

NADPH + O_2 + drug substrate + H^+ → $NADP^+$ + oxidized drug + H_2O

The overall scheme for the mechanism of action of P-450 is shown in Figure 1.10.

CONSEQUENCE OF BIOTRANSFORMATION REACTIONS

The process of biotransformation usually inactivates or detoxifies, or both, the administered drugs or the ingested poisons, but other reactions may also take place.

Precursor Activation

Occasionally, an inactive precursor such as **levodopa** is converted to an active metabolite such as **dopamine**.

Metabolic Activation of Drugs

Often an active drug is converted to another pharmacologically active substance. The following table lists a few examples of this.

Drug		Active Metabolite
Mephobarbital	is demethylated to	Phenobarbital
Primidone	is oxidized to	Phenobarbital
Imipramine	is demethylated to	Desmethylimipramine
Prednisone	is reduced to	Prednisolone

CONVERSION TO METABOLITES WITH DISSIMILAR ACTIONS

In certain instances, the body converts a drug to several active metabolites possessing dissimilar pharmacologic properties. For example, phenylbutazone undergoes **aromatic hydroxylation** to produce a metabolite that has sodium-retaining and antirheumatic activities, and also undergoes **alkyl chain oxidation** to produce a metabolite with a strong uricosuric property. Thus phenylbutazone has both uricosuric and antirheumatic effects.

CONVERSION TO MORE ACTIVE PRODUCTS

The conversion of **cyclophosphamide** to **aldophosphamide** and **prednisone** to **prednisolone** are examples of active compounds that are converted to more active substances.

LETHAL SYNTHESIS

The metabolism of drugs and agents does not always lead to detoxification; occasionally, the metabolites are toxicologically more potent. Some examples of this are **sulfamethazine**, which is metabolized to N_4-acetylsulfamethazine, and **aminopyrine**, with 4-aminoantipyrine as its metabolite.

DRUG METABOLITE KINETICS

In the majority of cases, drugs are converted to metabolites, which, in the more polar and water-soluble forms, are readily excreted. Often, the concentration of a metabolite far exceeds the concentration of the drug. For example, orally administered **propranolol** is rapidly converted to 4-hydroxypropranolol, which has a concentration that is several hundred-fold higher than that of propranolol. Sometimes the metabolites are able to inhibit the further metabolism of the parent drug. For example, **phenytoin** becomes metabolized to hydroxyphenytoin. When given in higher than recommended individual doses, hydroxyphenytoin inhibits the hydroxylase system that metabolizes phenytoin, increasing its concentration in free form and its potential to produce toxicity.

The **enterohepatic circulation** may sometimes prolong the half-life of a drug. A drug that is absorbed from the gastrointestinal tract, excreted in the bile, and resorbed from the intestine is said to have undergone **enterohepatic cycling**. Drugs are delivered to the liver by both the portal vein and hepatic artery, and returned to the rest of the body by the hepatic vein. The difference between the concentration of drug transported to and removed from the liver accounts for the amount of drug metabolized or excreted, or both, in the bile. For instance, if the liver has conjugated a drug containing glucuronic acid to its metabolite, the conjugated product may appear in the bile and finally be excreted in the small intestine. However, in the intestine, the beta-glucuronidase originating from the resident flora may hydrolyze the glucuronide-drug conjugate back to the parent drug, thus allowing the parent drug to be resorbed. The continuous enterohepatic cycling will therefore increase the half-life of this agent in the body.

FACTORS THAT MODIFY THE METABOLISM OF DRUGS

Many environmental factors and pathophysiologic conditions inhibit or stimulate the activity of drug-metabolizing enzymes and hence may alter the outcome of a therapeutic regimen. Pharmacogenetics, the immaturity of drug-metabolizing enzyme systems, and drug–drug interactions are a few of the factors that have been shown to alter drug metabolism.

Pharmacogenetics

Pharmacogenetics represents the study of the hereditary variation in the handling of drugs. Pharmacogenetic abnormalities may be entirely innocuous until the affected individual is challenged with particular drugs. The **hyposensitivity** and resistance of certain individuals to coumarin anticoagulants, and the **hypersensitivity** of patients with Down's syndrome to atropine, most probably stem from abnormalities in their respective receptor sites. Acatalasia and the decrease in the activities of **pseudocholinesterase**, **acetylase**, and **glucose 6-phosphate dehydrogenase** are a few examples of enzymatic deficiencies that can lead to mild to very severe adverse reactions.

Liver Disease

The liver is the principal metabolic organ, and hepatic disease or dysfunction may impair drug elimination. Any alteration in the serum albumin or bilirubin levels and in the prothrombin time indicates impaired liver function. Similarly, skin bruising and bleeding tendency indicate decreased production of clotting factors by the liver.

The Influence of Age

Drug metabolism is qualitatively and quantitatively very deficient in **newborns**. For example, **chloramphenicol**, when used injudiciously, may cause **gray syndrome**. The mechanism of chloramphenicol toxicity is apparently the failure in the newborn to conjugate chloramphenicol with glucuronic acid due to inadequate activity of hepatic **glucuronyl transferase**. This, in combination with inadequate renal excretion of the drug in the newborn, results in a higher-than-expected plasma level of chloramphenicol. Therefore, a newborn should receive doses of chloramphenicol not greater than 25 to 50 mg per kilogram of body weight.

The **elderly** are also prone to toxicity from numerous drugs, including cardiac glycosides. A dose of digitoxin, which may be totally therapeutic and innocuous at the age of 60, may produce severe toxicity and even death at the age of 70. The abilities of the liver to metabolize drugs and of the kidney to excrete drug metabolites decline with aging.

Enzyme Induction and Inhibition

The activities of **microsomal drug-metabolizing enzymes** in humans can be enhanced by altering the levels of endogenous hormones such as androgens, estrogens, progestational steroids, glucocorticoids, anabolic steroids, norepinephrine, insulin, and thyroxine. This effect can also be elicited by the administration of exogenous substances such as drugs, food preservatives, insecticides, herbicides, and polycyclic aromatic hydrocarbons. This increase in the activities of drug-metabolizing enzymes appears to stem from an elevated rate of synthesis of the enzyme protein; hence, it is truly an enzyme-induction phenomenon.

Liver microsomal enzyme inducers that are lipid soluble at the physiologic pH can be classified into two general groups. Some, like phenobarbital, tend to stimulate all enzymes; others such as 3-methylcholanthrene, tend to be selective. The administration of phenobarbital increases the amounts of NADPH–cytochrome C reductase and P-450, and the rate of P-450 reduction. In contrast, the administration of 3-methylcholanthrene increases the amount of P-450 but neither the activity of NADPH–cytochrome C reductase nor the rate of P-450 reduction.

Clinical Implications of Enzyme Induction and Inhibition

Patients are often given several drugs at the same time. The possibility that one drug may accelerate or inhibit the metabolism of another drug should always be kept in mind. When this phenomenon occurs, the removal of an enzyme inducer could be hazardous. The following examples reveal the consequence of enzyme induction.

Phenylbutazone is an analgesic, antipyretic, uricosuric, and antiinflammatory agent. Among its side effects are activation of peptic ulcer and gastrointestinal hemorrhage. If one gives a dog large amounts of phenylbutazone, side effects such as vomiting and diarrhea with bloody stool ensue. However, if phenylbutazone treatment is continued for several days, these side effects disappear. In this case, phenylbutazone "induces" its own hydroxylation, which results in a lower plasma level of the drug and ultimately the absence of the side effects. Long-term treatment with phenylbutazone and many other drugs should be expected to result in decreased effectiveness and toxicity.

Patients who are on **anticoagulant** therapy may suffer severe hemorrhage several days after discharge from the hospital. Often, these patients are sedated with **barbiturates** during their hospitalization, which tends to stimulate the enzymes that metabolize dicumarol. The abrupt withdrawal of barbiturates after discharge tends to revert the activity of the drug-metabolizing enzymes to their prebarbiturate stage, which raises the free-circulating level of the anticoagulant and results in hemorrhage. Obviously, treatment with phenobarbital should prompt altering the maintenance dosage of anticoagulants.

RENAL EXCRETION OF DRUGS

An orally administered drug will gradually begin to be absorbed. As the amount of drug in the body increases by 50%, the amount of the drug at the absorption site should decrease by the same amount. The absorbed drug will gradually be metabolized or excreted mostly by the kidneys. Besides their renal elimination, drugs and their metabolites are eliminated in bile, breast milk, and sweat, and by the lungs.

RATE OF EXCRETION OF DRUGS BY THE KIDNEYS

The amount of a drug (and/or its metabolites) that appears in the urine depends on the amount of drug undergoing glomerular filtration, tubular secretion, and tubular resorption. **Metabolism** plays a major role in drug excretion because the metabolites are more water-soluble substances, which are excreted. Drugs are excreted when they are in their free form, but plasma protein-bound drugs and tissue-stored drugs are not excreted.

The excretion of drugs from the kidneys, like the absorption of drugs from the gastrointestinal tract, depends on lipid solubility, the degree of ionization of drugs, and the pH of the urine. Nonionized lipid-soluble drugs are resorbed and not eliminated. Generally, drugs that are bases are excreted when the urine is acidic, whereas acidic compounds are excreted in greater quantities if the urine is alkaline. For example, in **phenobarbital** (weak acid pK_a of 7.3) poisoning, alkalinization of the urine with sodium bicarbonate is helpful in eliminating the phenobarbital. In **amphetamine** toxicity, acidification of the urine with ammonium chloride is required (Figure 1.11).

Drugs that undergo both glomerular filtration and active tubular secretion have a very short half-life. **Penicillin** is

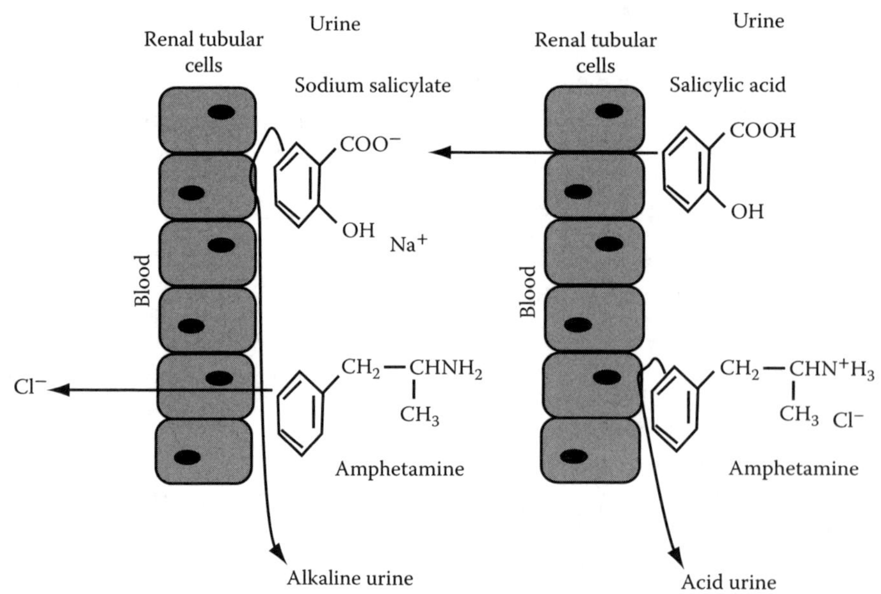

FIGURE 1.11 Elimination of drug following alkalinization or acidification of urine.

one such compound, but its half-life is prolonged by the coadministration of **probenecid**, a uricosuric drug that inhibits the tubular secretion of penicillin. Most drugs, however, have half-lives that are relatively longer than penicillin's because they undergo glomerular filtration, partial tubular resorption, and no active tubular secretion.

SIGNIFICANCE OF BLOOD FLOW ON DRUG CLEARANCE

In general, the rate of extraction of drug from blood and the rate of clearance by the kidney depend on blood flow and the ability of the kidney to extract the drug (the **extraction ratio**). If all of the drug is removed from the blood as it traverses through the kidneys, the extraction ratio is 1. The higher the blood flow, the higher is the rate of excretion of that drug, and the clearance is said to be **perfusion-rate limited**. For example, the extraction ratio of digoxin, one of the cardiac glycosides, is low, and toxicity is likely to occur in renal failure. Similarly, the hepatic extraction ratio of digitoxin is low, and toxicity is likely to occur in hepatic failure. Consequently, cardiologists have long recognized that **digitoxin** and **digoxin** should be avoided in patients suffering from liver and renal failure, respectively.

HALF-LIFE OF A DRUG

The half-life of a drug, or its elimination half-life, is the time required for its concentration in the blood to be reduced by one half. For penicillin G, the half-life is 20 min, indicating that only 50% of it remains in the blood 20 min after its intravenous administration. Both the intravenously and orally administered identical drugs have the same half-lives once they reach the general circulation. When given at regular intervals, a drug or its metabolite reaches a plateau concentration after approximately four to five half-lives. This plateau changes only if the dose or frequency of administration, or both, are altered.

2

The Pharmacodynamic Basis of Therapeutics

The desire to take medicine is perhaps the greatest feature which distinguishes men from the animals.

Sir William Osler

Pharmacodynamics may be defined as the study of the actions and effects of drugs on organ, tissue, cellular, and subcellular levels. Therefore, pharmacodynamics provides us with information about how drugs bring about their beneficial effects and how they cause their side effects.

Chapter 1 on **pharmacokinetics** discussed the processes of absorption, binding, distribution, biotransformation, and excretion of drugs. These processes are designed efficiently to ensure that a sufficient quantity of drugs reach their receptor sites to elicit the desired therapeutic effects.

Pharmacodynamics considers the sites, modes, and mechanisms of action of drugs. For example, if a patient with multiple fractures receives a subcutaneous injection of 10 to 15 mg of morphine sulfate, analgesia, sedation, respiratory depression, emesis, miosis, suppression of the gastrointestinal (GI) tract, and oliguria may ensue. These diversified effects occur at multiple peripheral and central sites and through the influence of numerous modes and mechanisms of action.

SITE OF ACTION

The receptor sites where a drug acts to initiate a group of functions is that drug's site of action. The central sites of action of morphine include the cerebral cortex, hypothalamus, and medullary center.

MODE OF ACTION

The character of an effect produced by a drug is called the **mode of action** of that drug. Morphine, by depressing the function of the cerebral cortex, hypothalamus, and medullary center, is responsible for decreasing pain perception (**analgesia**), inducing narcosis (**heavy sedation**), depressing the cough center (**antitussive effect**), initially stimulating then depressing the vomiting, and depressing respiration.

MECHANISM OF ACTION

The identification of molecular and biochemical events leading to an effect is called the mechanism of action of that drug. For instance, morphine causes respiratory depression by depressing the responsiveness of the respiratory center to carbon dioxide.

STRUCTURE–ACTIVITY RELATIONSHIP

A definite and strong relationship seems to exist between the molecular structure of most pharmacologic compounds and their inherent pharmacologic properties. For example, modifying the molecular structure of acetylcholine dramatically alters its pharmacologic properties. **Acetylcholine** mediates cholinergic function at various anatomic sites. By examining the molecular structure of acetylcholine, one notes **quaternary nitrogen** at one end of the molecule and an **ester** at the other end, separated by a two-carbon linkage. Although acetylcholine is an important physiologic agent, it is not useful as a drug, because its short-lived actions are massive and nonspecific. The various synthetic derivatives of acetylcholine differ from acetylcholine in being more resistant to hydrolysis by cholinesterase (**longer duration of action**) and possessing relatively **organ-specific action**. For example, **bethanechol chloride** is useful in treating the urinary retention, megacolon, and delayed gastric emptying that occur following vagotomy for the treatment of severe peptic ulceration.

DRUG ACTIONS UNRELATED TO STRUCTURES

In cases in which drugs exert their effects by interacting with specific receptors, structural modification dramatically alters the expected effects. However, not all drugs exert their effects by interacting with specific receptors. For example, **general anesthetics** such as **thiopental**, **halothane**, **cyclopropane**, and **nitrous oxide** have vastly dissimilar structures.

DRUG-RECEPTOR-SPECIFIC INTERACTION

Contemporary ideas of **drug action** and **specificity** are based on the assumption that the initial process in drug action is the formation of a reversible complex between the drug and a cell component generally known as the **drug receptor**. The interaction of a drug with a specific receptor site is characterized by at least three factors.

CHEMICAL AND STRUCTURAL SPECIFICITY

Any alteration in the structure of a compound alters its pharmacologic properties. For example, **nalorphine**, a narcotic antagonist, varies from **morphine**, a narcotic agonist, by the replacement of the CH_3 group on the morphine's nitrogen with the allyl radical – $CH_2CH{=}CH_2$.

STEREOISOMERIC SPECIFICITY

Only the (–) **enantiomorph** of morphine and certain other opioids can interact with (enter) the receptor site. For example, **levorphanol**, a synthetic narcotic, is 5 to 10 times more potent than morphine, but its L(+) enantiomorph **dextrorphan** is devoid of analgesic activity.

POTENCY

Drugs that interact with receptor sites may exert their effects in extremely small doses. For example, **etorphine** is 10,000 times more potent than morphine.

CELLULAR SITES OF ACTIONS OF DRUGS

Because drugs are very reactive, many elicit their effects or side effects, or both, by interacting with **coenzymes**, **enzymes**, or **nucleic acids**, as well as other macromolecules and physiologic processes such as transport mechanisms. To gain an appreciation of the complex interactions between drugs and physiologic parameters, some examples are cited.

DRUG–COENZYME INTERACTIONS

Isoniazid and Pyridoxal Phosphate

The primary drugs, first-line agents that combine the greatest level of efficacy with an acceptable degree of toxicity, in the treatment of **tuberculosis** are **isoniazid**, **ethambutol**, **pyrazinamide**, and **rifampin**. **Isoniazid** is prescribed orally in doses of 4 to 5 mg per kilogram of body weight. If pyridoxine is not given along with the isoniazid, peripheral neuritis is the most common side effect to arise. In toxic doses, optic neuritis, muscular twitching, dizziness, ataxia, paresthesias, and convulsions may occur, especially in malnourished patients. These neuropathies are thought to result from a chemical interaction between isoniazid and **pyridoxal phosphate**, and the reduced level of this important coenzyme in the body. The coadministration of **pyridoxine** with isoniazid averts these side effects.

Folic Acid and Trimethoprim-Sulfamethoxazole

In acute and chronic urinary tract infection, the combination of **trimethoprim** and **sulfamethoxazole** (Bactrim, Septra) exerts a truly synergistic effect on bacteria. The sulfonamide inhibits the utilization of ***p*-amino-benzoic acid** in the synthesis of folic acid, whereas trimethoprim, by inhibiting dihydrofolic acid reductase, blocks the conversion of dihydrofolic acid to **tetrahydrofolic acid**, which is essential to bacteria in the *de novo* synthesis of purines, pyrimidines, and certain amino acids. Because mammalian organisms do not synthesize folic acid, but require it as a vitamin in their daily diets, trimethoprim-sulfamethoxazole does not interfere with the metabolism of mammalian cells.

DRUG–ENZYME INTERACTIONS

Numerous drugs exert their effects and side effects by interacting with enzymes. Following are some examples of these interactions.

Allopurinol, Xanthine Oxidase, and Hyperuremic States

Allopurinol is used to lower uric acid levels in the treatment of primary gout, as a prophylaxis in myeloproliferative neoplastic disease, for investigational purposes in Lesch–Nyhan syndrome, and as an adjunct with thiazide diuretics or ethambutol. The mechanism of action of allopurinol is the inhibition of xanthine oxidase, which converts hypoxanthine into xanthine and in turn becomes oxidized into uric acid.

$$\text{Hypoxanthine} \xrightarrow[\text{oxidase}]{\text{Xanthine}} \text{xanthine} \xrightarrow[\text{oxidase}]{\text{Xanthine}} \text{uric acid}$$

When xanthine oxidase is inhibited by allopurinol, the plasma level of uric acid and the size of the urate pool in the body both decrease.

Drugs and Bronchial Asthma

Aminophylline (theophylline ethylenediamine), given intravenously, is used in patients with **status asthmaticus** who do not respond to epinephrine. In addition, epinephrine may be administered subcutaneously for severe acute asthma attacks. Epinephrine may also be given along with theophylline. It is thought that the bronchodilation is associated with the enhanced concentration of cyclic AMP (cAMP), which is metabolized according to the following sequence.

$$\text{ATP} \xrightarrow[\text{cyclase}]{\text{Adenylyl}} \text{cyclic AMP} \xrightarrow{\text{Phosphodiesterase}} 5'\ \text{AMP}$$

Epinephrine stimulates the beta-adrenergic receptors in the bronchioles, which in turn activates membrane-bound adenylate cyclase to synthesize more cAMP, whereas theophylline inhibits the activity of phosphodiesterase, conserving the previously synthesized cAMP.

DRUG–NUCLEIC ACID INTERACTIONS

Chemotherapeutic agents useful in the treatment of neoplastic diseases exert their therapeutic effects by modifying the synthesis or functions of nucleic acids (see chapters 51 and 58). For example, **6-mercaptopurine** inhibits purine-ring biosynthesis, **cytarabine** inhibits DNA polymerase, alkylating agents cross-link DNA, and hydroxyurea inhibits the conversion of ribonucleotides into deoxyribonucleotides. However, other pharmacologic agents such as chlorpromazine, a neuroleptic, also modify nucleic acid synthesis. One of the side effects of chlorpromazine is mild to severe agranulocytosis. **Chlorpromazine** reduces the synthesis of DNA by inhibiting the activity of thymidine kinase according to the following scheme:

$$\text{Thymidine} + \text{ATP} \xrightarrow[\text{kinase}]{\text{Thymidine}} \text{thymidine } 5'\ \text{phosphate} + \text{ADP}$$

In addition to chlorpromazine, phenylbutazone (an analgesic and antiinflammatory agent), sulfonamides (chemotherapeutic agents), chlorothiazide (a diuretic), thiouracil and methimazole (antithyroid drugs), phenytoin (an anticonvulsant), pyribenzamine (an antihistaminic), and chloramphenicol (an antimicrobial) may cause **agranulocytosis** in susceptible individuals. The incidence of this side effect is highest among those subjects with a lower than normal proliferative capacity of the bone marrow.

THE INTERACTIONS OF DRUGS WITH NEURONAL ELEMENTS

Neuropharmacology is the study of drugs that affect the nervous system and its neuronal components. The functions of the nervous system are intimately linked with the synthesis, storage, release, and uptake of many transmitters and their modulators. The beneficial effects or side effects of an extensive number of drugs are brought about through their interaction with these neurotransmitter–neuromodulator systems.

An example of this interaction is offered by **reserpine**. Reserpine may be used in conjunction with a diuretic in the treatment of mild to moderate **hypertension**. It is thought that reserpine produces this antihypertensive effect by preventing the storage of norepinephrine and hence reducing the pool of this neurotransmitter in the body. This amine-depleting action of reserpine not only brings about its beneficial effects, but also causes its side effects. For instance, reserpine may tranquilize and lead to depression (by depleting the catecholamine content in the brain) and may cause bradycardia and miosis, plus increase the motility of the GI tract (all stemming from the enhanced cholinergic activity secondary to decreased sympathetic activity). Reserpine may also increase the atrioventricular conduction time resulting from an increase in the refractory period of the atrioventricular conduction system, due to depletion of myocardial norepinephrine stores.

INTERACTION OF DRUGS WITH THE ENDOCRINE SYSTEM

Alpha-Methyldopa and Renin

Hypotension and decreased renal perfusion pressure promote the release of renin from the juxtaglomerular apparatus of the kidney. **Renin** converts angiotensin I to **antiogensin** II, a potent endogenously occurring vasoconstrictor. Catecholamine can also release renin, and this effect is blocked by **propranolol**, a beta-adrenergic-receptor-blocking agent. Drugs that alter the renin level are able to alter blood pressure. Alpha-methyldopa suppresses renin release, whereas the oral contraceptive medications have the opposite effect. In addition, other antihypertensive medications such as **captopril** specifically inhibit angiotensin-converting enzyme, hence preventing the formation of angiotensin II.

Drugs and Prolactin

The release of prolactin from the adenohypophysis is a centrally mediated event involving the **dopaminergic neurons**. Stimulation of these neurons blocks prolactin production, whereas blockade of dopaminergic function causes lactation. **Chlorpromazine**, which blocks dopamine receptors, **reserpine**, which depletes dopamine stores, and alpha-methyldopa, which forms a false transmitter such as **alpha-methyldopamine**, are all able to cause inappropriate lactation in a nonpregnant woman.

This discussion clearly emphasizes the fact that drugs do not create functions, but merely stimulate or inhibit functions already inherent in the cells. These pharmacodynamic-related interactions take place at various levels of cellular activities, including ion transport, enzymes, coenzymes, nucleic acids, and numerous other biochemical events yet to be delineated.

3

Adverse Reactions and Drug–Drug Interactions

Imperative drugging—the ordering in any and every malady—is no longer regarded as the chief function of the doctor.

Sir William Osler

On medical services, it is common for patients with **multiple medical problems** to be taking as many as 10 to 15 drugs concomitantly. It is also becoming increasingly obvious to physicians and other members of the health-care delivery team that many **drug combinations**, when used inappropriately and injudiciously, have the inherent potential to interact adversely, leading to side effects and even death.

Whether drugs are given individually or in combination, some side effects or adverse reactions are inevitable and cannot be eliminated. For example, patients undergoing treatment with antineoplastic drugs will experience expected side effects, such as hair loss. Nevertheless, many adverse effects of drugs, or **drug–drug interactions**, are either avoidable or may be substantially minimized.

The varied and complex mechanisms involved can be broadly classified as **pharmacokinetic interactions** or **pharmacodynamic interactions**. In pharmacokinetic interactions, drugs interfere with and/or alter the absorption, distribution, biotransformation, or excretion of other drugs. In pharmacodynamic interactions, which have been discussed in Chapter 2, drugs modify the intended and expected actions of other drugs. Before elaborating on the pharmacokinetic interactions, some terms will be defined.

DEFINITIONS

Iatrogenic Reactions

Iatrogenic reactions broadly refer to any adverse reactions produced unintentionally by physicians in their patients. For example, one of the side effects of many antihistaminic preparations (H_1 antagonists) such as ethanolamine derivatives (prototype: **diphenhydramine**) is heavy sedation. Although sedation may be desirable for some patients, it may interfere with daytime activities, and this needs to be considered when prescribing such medications. Other antihistaminic preparations (also H_1 antagonists) such as piperidine derivatives (prototypes: **terfenadine** or **astemizole**) have no sedative properties.

Allergic Reactions

Drug allergy refers to those drug reactions in a patient who was previously exposed to, sensitized with, and developed antibodies to that drug. The underlying immunologic mechanisms may be varied and complex, involving **anaphylactoid immediate reactions** (e.g., penicillin, due to formation of specific immunoglobulin E), **cytotoxic reactions** (e.g., drug-induced hemolytic anemias), and **delayed allergic reactions** (e.g., drug-induced contact dermatitis).

Idiosyncratic Reactions

Idiosyncrasy refers to an abnormal, unexpected, or peculiar reaction seen in only certain patients. For example, **succinylcholine** may cause prolonged apnea in patients with **pseudocholinesterase deficiency**, and **hemolytic anemia** may be seen following the administration of a number of drugs, including sulfonamides in patients with **glucose-6-phosphate dehydrogenase deficiency**. Although these reactions are inevitable when they occur unexpectedly for the first time, they may be circumvented altogether in patients who have previously shown such abnormal reactions.

Tolerance and Tachyphylaxis

Tolerance refers to decreased responses following the long-term administration of drugs. For example, after repeated **morphine** use, tolerance to all of its effects occurs, except for miosis and constipation, which continue. Morphine also no longer causes respiratory depression as readily in a tolerant patient.

Tachyphylaxis refers to a quickly developing tolerance brought about by the rapid and repeated administration of drugs. For example, indirect-acting sympathomimetic agents such as **tyramine**, which exert their effects through the release of norepinephrine, are able to cause tachyphylaxis. If norepinephrine is not present, tyramine fails to exert its effect until the supply of norepinephrine in nerve terminals has been replenished.

Although tachyphylaxis is innocuous and not regarded as a major clinical problem, not appreciating tolerance as an entity may have devastating consequences. For example, respiratory depression is not seen in a morphine-tolerant patient, and a dosage that far exceeds the normal therapeutic level is required to induce an effect. However, tolerance is lost or lessened following the discontinued administration of morphine. Therefore, in a once-tolerant patient, administering a dose of morphine that was once quite innocuous may prove fatal by causing severe respiratory depression.

Supersensitivity

Supersensitivity refers to the increased responsiveness to a drug that results either from denervation or following administration of a drug (a receptor antagonist) for a prolonged period. For example, the blocking of dopamine receptors by chlorpromazine may cause supersensitivity by upregulating dopamine receptors.

Pharmacokinetic Interactions

Drugs may affect the absorption, distribution, metabolism, or excretion of other drugs. This includes those interactions in which the gastrointestinal (GI) absorption of a drug, plasma protein binding, drug metabolism, and urinary excretion are either enhanced or inhibited.

Interaction at the Site of Absorption

The rate or extent of drug absorption from the gastrointestinal tract can be influenced in a number of ways. Following are examples of these various influences.

Alteration of Gastric pH

Iron poisoning is characterized by vomiting, abdominal pain, gastroenteritis, and shock, and, if not properly treated, severe acidosis, coma, and death eventuate. **Deferoxamine**, which binds iron, is used as the preferred chelator in treating iron poisoning. The metabolic acidosis may be appropriately treated with sodium bicarbonate. However, because deferoxamine chelates iron more effectively in an acidic medium, it should not be administered orally along with sodium bicarbonate. The ideal treatment of iron poisoning consists of gastric aspiration, followed by lavage with a phosphate solution to form insoluble iron salts. Deferoxamine should then be given intravenously or intramuscularly to chelate the iron that has been absorbed. Sodium bicarbonate may be administered intravenously. To absorb any residual iron remaining in the stomach, deferoxamine may then be instilled into the stomach.

Formation of Complex

Tetracyclines, as broad-spectrum antibiotics, are the drugs of choice in treating *Mycoplasma pneumoniae* infections. Most **tetracyclines** are absorbed to various degrees (30–100%) from the GI tract, primarily from the stomach and upper small intestine. The absorption of tetracyclines is hindered by **milk and milk products**, by numerous **antacids** such as aluminum hydroxide, sodium bicarbonate, and calcium carbonate, and by iron preparations such as ferrous sulfate. Therefore, these and similar substances should not be administered orally together with tetracycline.

Alteration in Gastric Emptying Time

Agents that reduce gastrointestinal motility and prolong gastric emptying time reduce the rate of absorption of drugs whose absorption takes place primarily in the duodenum. Furthermore, by prolonging the time poorly soluble drugs are kept in the stomach, their bioavailability may be altered. Hence, compounds with strong anticholinergic properties such as **propantheline** (for peptic diseases), **glycopyrrolate** (for asthma), **benztropine** (for parkinsonism), and **imipramine** (for depression) are potentially able to alter the absorption of other concomitantly administered drugs. The absorption of digoxin and dicumerol is altered by imipramine and other tricyclic antidepressants. On the other hand, some drugs such as antacids may speed the gastric emptying time.

Interactions at the Plasma Protein-Binding Sites

Drugs may **compete** for binding sites on the plasma or tissue protein, or may **displace** previously bound drugs. For example, **phenylbutazone** may compete with **phenytoin** for binding to albumin. Similarly, phenylbutazone (an anti-inflammatory agent) is able to displace warfarin (an anticoagulant) from its binding site and enhance the free circulating concentration of the anticoagulant. Sulfonamides (chemotherapeutic agents) are able to displace sulfonylureas (oral antidiabetic agents) and cause hypoglycemia.

Interactions at the Stage of Drug Biotransformation

Drug biotransformation usually converts the nonpolar active drugs into more water-soluble, but pharmacologically inactive, products. Drugs may stimulate or inhibit the metabolism of other drugs. These interactions may be either innocuous or detrimental to the expected therapeutic objectives.

The prolonged ingestion of alcohol or phenobarbital induces drug biotransformation. The maximum inducing effects vary from drug to drug, usually occurring and subsiding within 7 to 10 days. The sudden withdrawal of an inducing agent in some circumstances can prove fatal. For example, hypnotic sedatives accelerate the rate of metabolism of **coumarin** anticoagulants. Increased doses of coumarin may therefore have to be given in order to achieve the desired prothrombin time and therapeutic effects. The sudden withdrawal of a hypnotic–sedative agent may cause the coumarin-catabolizing enzyme to revert to the pretreatment level, and, in the presence of large concentrations of free coumarin, **hemorrhage** may ensue. Because physicians anticipate that their patients may not require hypnotic–sedatives after being discharged from the hospital, the maintenance doses of coumarin anticoagulants are gradually reduced 2 to 3 days before discharge.

On the other hand, drugs may **inhibit** the metabolism of other drugs. For example, **allopurinol** (a xanthine oxidase inhibitor that inhibits the synthesis of uric acid) increases the effectiveness of anticoagulants by inhibiting their metabolism. **Chloramphenicol** (a potent inhibitor of microsomal protein synthesis) and **cimetidine** (an H_2-receptor blocker used in acid-pepsin disease) have similar properties. In addition, drugs may **compete** with each other for metabolism. In methyl alcohol **(methanol)** poisoning, **ethyl alcohol** may be given intravenously to avert methanol-induced blindness and minimize the severe acidosis. Ethyl alcohol competes with methyl alcohol for catabolism by liver alcohol dehydrogenase. The unmetabolized and less toxic methanol is excreted unchanged in the urine.

Interactions at the Site of Excretion

Numerous drugs are able to either enhance or inhibit the excretion of other drugs. For example, **sodium bicarbonate** enhances the excretion of **phenobarbital**. Probenecid interferes with the active secretion of penicillin, and hence prolongs its half-life. Probenecid's uricosuric effects are counteracted by acetylsalicylic acid, which also possesses a uricosuric effect. When given concomitantly, both are excreted.

4

Herb–Drug Interactions

HERBS MAY MIMIC, MAGNIFY, OR OPPOSE THE EFFECTS OF MANY DRUGS

Oriental medicines, including Chinese medicine (CM), are a complex and holistic system of medical practice with its own philosophy, diagnosis, treatment systems, and pharmacology. They consider the human body in relation to its own natural, physical, and social environment. The practice of CM involves physical therapy (nonmedication) using acupuncture, moxibustion, and related disciplines such as *tuina* massage and *qi gong,* and chemical therapy using Chinese medicinal materials (CMM) of animal, mineral, and plant origin in the form of decoctions of combined CMM or related proprietary products. As most of them are from plants, medical books on CMM, throughout the ages, have conveniently referred to them as **ben cao** (herbalism).

Herbal medicines are mixtures of more than one active ingredient. The multitude of pharmacologically active compounds obviously increases the likelihood of interactions taking place. Hence, the likelihood of herb–drug interactions is theoretically higher than drug–drug interactions, if only because synthetic drugs usually contain single chemical entities. Case reports and clinical studies have highlighted the existence of a number of clinically important interactions, although cause-and-effect relationships have not always been established. Herbs and drugs may interact either pharmacokinetically or pharmacodynamically. Through induction of cytochrome P450 enzymes and/or P-glycoprotein, some herbal products (e.g., **St John's wort**) have been shown to lower the plasma concentration (and/or the pharmacological effect) of a number of conventional drugs, including **cyclosporine**, **indinavir**, **irinotecan**, **nevirapine**, **oral contraceptives**, and **digoxin**. The majority of such interactions involve medicines that require regular monitoring of blood levels. To date there is less evidence relating to the pharmacodynamic interaction. However, for many of the interactions discussed here, the understanding of the mechanisms involved is incomplete. Taking herbal agents may represent a potential risk to patients under conventional pharmacotherapy.

Herbal medicines follow modern pharmacological principles. Hence, herb–drug interactions are based on the same pharmacokinetic and pharmacodynamic mechanisms as drug–drug interactions. Pharmacokinetic interactions have been more extensively studied and *in vitro* and *in vivo* studies indicated that the altered drug concentrations by coadministered herbs may be attributable to the induction (or inhibition) of hepatic and intestinal drug-metabolizing enzymes (particularly cytochrome P450 [CYP]), and/or drug transporters such as P-glycoprotein.

Concurrent use of herbs may mimic, magnify, or oppose the effect of drugs. Plausible cases of herb–drug interactions include:

- Bleeding may occur when **warfarin** is combined with **ginkgo** (*Ginkgo biloba*), **garlic** (*Allium sativum*), **dong quai** (*Angelica sinensis*), or **danshen** (*Salvia miltiorrhiza*).
- **Mild serotonin syndrome** occurs in patients who mix **St. John's wort** (*Hypericum perforatum*) with serotonin-reuptake inhibitors.
- Decreased bioavailability of **digoxin**, **theophylline**, **cyclosporin**, and **phenprocoumon** takes place when these drugs are combined with **St. John's wort**.
- Induction of **mania** may be seen in depressed patients who mix **antidepressants** and ***Panax ginseng***.
- Exacerbation of **extrapyramidal effects** is possible with **neuroleptic drugs** and **betel nut** (*Areca catechu*).
- Increased risk of hypertension is imminent when **tricyclic antidepressants** are combined with **yohimbine** (*Pausinystalia yohimbe*).
- Potentiation of oral and topical effects of **corticosteroids** is certain by **licorice** (*Glycyrrhiza glabra*).
- Decreased blood concentration of **prednisolone** occurs when taken with the Chinese herbal product **xaio chai hu tang** (sho-saiko-to).
- Decreased concentrations of **phenytoin** is seen when its combined with the Ayurvedic syrup **shankhapushpi**.

Furthermore, anthranoid-containing plants, including **senna** (*Cassia senna*) and **cascara** (*Rhamnus purshiana*), and soluble fibers, including **guar gum** and **psyllium**, can decrease the absorption of drugs (Table 4.1).

POTENTIAL INTERACTIONS BETWEEN ALTERNATIVE THERAPIES AND WARFARIN

Alternative medicine therapies have become increasingly popular, and it has been estimated that one-third of all Americans use herbal products. In 1997, herbal medicine sales increased nearly 59%, reaching an estimated total of $3.24 billion. One particular safety concern is potential interactions of alternative medicine products with prescription medications. This issue is especially important with respect to drugs with narrow therapeutic indexes, such as **warfarin**. More food and drug interactions have been

TABLE 4.1
Herbs Interacting with Drugs

Herbs and Drugs	Results of Interaction	Comments
Betel nut (*Areca catechu*)		
Flupenthixol and procyclidine	Rigidity, bradykinesia, jaw tremor	Betel contains **arecoline**, a cholinergic alkaloid
Fluphenazine	Tremor, stiffness, akithesia	
Prednisone and salbutamol	Inadequate control of asthma	Arecoline challenge causes dose-related bronchoconstriction in patients with asthma
Chili pepper (*Capsicum* spp.)		
ACE inhibitor	Cough	Capsaicin depletes substance P
Theophylline	Increased absorption and bioavailability	
Danshen (*Salvia miltiorrhiza*)		
Warfarin	Increased INR, prolonged PT/PTT	Danshen decreases elimination of warfarin
Devil's claw (*Harpagophytum procumbens*)		
Warfarin	Purpura	—
Dong quai (*Angelica sinensis*)		
Warfarin	Increased INR and widespread bruising	Dong quai contains coumarins
Eleuthero or **Siberian ginseng** (*Eleutherococcus senticocus*)		
Digoxin	Raises digoxin concentrations	Patients exhibit unchanged ECG despite digoxin concentration of 5×2 nmol/L
Garlic (*Allium sativum*)		
Warfarin	Increased INR	Postoperative bleeding and spontaneous spinal epidural hematoma have been reported with garlic alone; garlic causes platelet dysfunction
Ginkgo (*Ginkgo biloba*)		
Aspirin	Spontaneous hyphema	Ginkgolides are potent inhibitors of PAF
Paracetamol and ergotamine/caffeine	Bilateral subdural hematoma	Subarachnoid hemorrhage and subdural hematoma have been reported with the use of ginkgo alone
Warfarin	Intracerebral hemorrhage	
Thiazide diuretic	Hypertension	This effect may be an unusual adverse reaction to the drug or herb; ginkgo alone has not been associated with hemorrhage
Ginseng (*Panax* spp.)		
Warfarin	Decreased INR	
Phenelzine	Headache and tremor, mania	
Alcohol	Increased alcohol clearance	Ginseng increases the activity of alcohol dehydrogenase and aldehyde dehydrogenase
Guar gum (*Cyamopsis tetragonolobus*)		
Metformin, phenoxymethylpenicillin, glibenclamide	Slows absorption of digoxin, paracetamol, and bumetanide; decreases absorption of metformin, phenoxymethylpenicillin, and some formulations of glibenclamide	Guar gum prolongs gastric retention
Karela or **bitter melon** (*Momordica charantia*)		
Chlorpropamide	Less glycosuria	Karela decreases glucose concentrations in blood
Licorice (*Glycyrrhiza glabra*)		
Prednisolone	Glycyrrhizin decreases plasma clearance, increases AUC, increases plasma concentrations of prednisolone	11β-dehydrogenase converts endogenous cortisol to cortisone; orally administered glycyrrhizin is metabolized mainly to glycyrrhetinic acid
Hydrocortisone	Glycyrrhetinic acid potentiates of cutaneous vasoconstrictor response	Glycyrrhetinic acid is a more potent inhibitor of 5α-, 5β-reductase and 11β-dehydrogenase than is glycyrrhizin

(*Continued*)

TABLE 4.1 (CONTINUED) Herbs Interacting with Drugs

Herbs and Drugs	Results of Interaction	Comments
Oral contraceptives	Hypertension, edema, hypokalemia	Oral contraceptive use may increase sensitivity to glycyrrhizin acid; women are reportedly more sensitive than men to adverse effects of licorice
Papaya (*Carica papaya*)		
Warfarin	Increased INR	—
Psyllium (*Plantago ovata*)		
Lithium	Decreased lithium concentrations	Hydrophilic psyllium may prevent lithium from ionizing
St. John's Wort (*Hypericum perforatu*)		
Paroxetine	Lethargy/incoherence	A similar case is described with the use of St. John's wort, alone
Trazodone	Mild serotonin syndrome	
Sertraline	Mild serotonin syndrome	
Nefazodone	Decreased theophylline concentrations	
Theophylline		
Digoxin	Decreased AUC, decreased peak and trough concentrations	Most, but not all, studies indicate that St. John's wort is a potent inhibitor of cytochrome P-450 isoenzymes
Phenprocoumon cyclosporin	Decreased AUC Decreased concentrations in serum	
Combined oral contraceptive (ethinyloestradiol and desogestrel)	Breakthrough bleeding	
Saiboku-to (Asian herbal mixture) Prednisolone	Increased prednisolone AUC	Contains all the same herbs as sho-saiko-to, and *Porio cocos*, *Magnolia officinalis*, and *Perillae* frutescens
Shankhapushipi (Ayurvedic mixed-herb syrup)		
Phenytoin	Decreased phenytoin concentrations, loss of seizure control	Multiple coadministered doses (but not single doses) decreased plasma phenytoin concentrations; single doses decreased the antiepileptic effect of phenytoin; Shankhapushpi is used to treat seizures
Sho-saiko-to or **Xiao chai hu tang** (Asian herb mixture)		
Prednisolone	Decreased AUC for prednisolone	Contains licorice (*Glycyrrhiza glabra*), *Bupleurum falcatum, Pinellia ternata, Scutellaria baicalensis, Zizyphus vulgaris, Panax ginseng,* and *Zingiber officinale*
Tamarind (*Tamarindus indica*)		
Aspirin	Increased bioavailability of aspirin	Tamarind is used as a food and a medicine
Valerian (*Valeriana officinalis*)		
Alcohol	A mixture of valepotriates reduces the adverse effect of alcohol	—
Yohimbine (*Pausinystalia yohimba*)		
Tricyclic antidepressants	Hypertension	Yohimbine alone can cause hypertension, but lower doses cause hypertension when combined with tricyclic antidepressants; effect is stronger in hypertensive than normotensive individuals

Note: ACE = angiotensin-converting enzyme; INR = international normalized ratio; PT = prothrombin time; PTT = partial thromboplastin time; ECG = electrocardiogram; PAF = platelet-activating factor; AUC = area under the concentration/time curve.

TABLE 4.2
Stages in Hemostasis

Stage	Initiator	Response or Outcome
Vascular	Tissue injury	Vasoconstriction
Platelet	Adhesion and aggregation	Plug formation
Plasma	Fibrin generation	Coagulation

Note: Hemostasis refers to a complex homeostatic mechanism within blood and on blood vessels that serves to maintain the patency of vessels after injury, while preserving the fluidity of blood.

reported for warfarin than for any other prescription medication. Multiple pathways exist for interference with warfarin, and interactions may lead to either hemorrhage or thrombotic episodes by increasing or reducing the effect of this agent. Therefore, close monitoring of therapy and knowledge of potential interactions of herbs with warfarin are extremely important.

ANTICOAGULANTS AND THROMBOLYTIC AGENTS

The clotting of blood, which protects against hemorrhage, involves the sequential initiation, interaction, and completion of several stages in hemostasis (Table 4.2).

The **adhesion** and **aggregation** of platelets are mediated via the release of **adenosine diphosphate** (ADP). An extensive number of pharmacological agents such as **acetylsalicylic acid**, **indomethacin**, **phenylbutazone**, **sulfinpyrazone**, and **dipyridamole** inhibit both **platelet aggregation** and **thrombus formation**, and thus may be of value in the treatment of **thrombotic disorders**. The **formation of fibrin** itself takes place by means of a cascading group of reactions involving numerous blood-clotting factors and is accomplished in several stages (Table 4.3).

- **Hemorrhage** may result from several causes:
- An abnormality or **deficiency of platelets** (thrombocytopenic purpuras)
- A **deficiency of clotting factors** (factors II, VII, IX, or X)
- **Vitamin K deficiency** (necessary for synthesizing clotting factors)
- **Liver diseases** that involve the synthesis of clotting factors

Increased clotting may occur in the presence of **thrombosis** (enhanced formation of fibrin), **stasis** and **phlebitis** (diminished circulation), or **embolism** (dislocation and lodging of blood clots). Although **heparin** is an extremely effective anticoagulant, it has certain limitations that are not shared by the newer thrombin inhibitors. As a result, these novel inhibitors may have advantages over heparin for use in certain clinical settings.

Thrombin activates platelets, converts fibrinogen to fibrin, activates factor XIII, which stabilizes fibrin, and activates factors V and VIII, which accelerate the generation of **prothrombinase**. Therefore, the inhibition of thrombin is essential in preventing and treating **thromboembolic disorders**.

AGGREGIN AND PLATELET AGGREGATION

Platelets circulate in blood without adhering to other platelets or to the endothelium. However, when the endothelial cells are perturbed, the platelets adhere and undergo a change in shape, and aggregate. **ADP** is known to induce

TABLE 4.3
Formation of Fibrin

Stage	Formation	Needed Factors or Precursors
One	Plasma thromboplastin	Hageman factor (XII), antihemophilic globulin (VIII), Christmas factor (IX), plasma thromboplastin antecedent (XI), calcium (IV), and platelet phospholipids
Two	Activated thromboplastin	Tissue thromboplastin (III), Stuart factor (X), proconvertin (VII), and calcium (IV)
Three	Thrombin	Prothrombin (II), proaccelerin (V), calcium (IV), and platelet
Four	Fibrin	Thrombin

Note: In fibrinolysis, **plasmin**, an endopeptidase that is converted from plasminogen by an activator, hydrolyzes; fibrin, fibrinogen, factor V, and factor VIII to their inactive products. **Hageman factor** (factor XII) converts a proactivator to the active activator. Agents such thrombin, streptokinase, and urokinase therefore enhance the formation of plasmin and, hence, have fibrin lytic properties. **Epsilon-aminocaproic acid** inhibits the activator-mediated formation of plasmin and, hence, may be used as an antidote to streptokinase-urokinase or in a defibrination syndrome when bleeding from a mucous membrane occurs.

the platelet shape change, aggregation, and exposure of fibrinogen-binding sites.

The platelet surface contains **aggregin**, a membrane protein with a molecular weight of 100 kDa, which has physical and immunochemical properties that differ from those of platelet glycoprotein IIIa.

Binding to aggregin is required in order for epinephrine-induced platelet aggregation to take place. In turn, **epinephrine** increases the affinity of ADP for its receptor. **Thrombin** stimulates platelet aggregation independent of ADP, but, by raising the level of calcium in the cytoplasm, it activates platelet **calpain**, which in turn cleaves aggregin.

VITAMIN E AND PLATELET AGGREGATION

a-Tocopherol, a **natural antioxidant**, inhibits platelet aggregation and release. The effect of vitamin E is due to a reduction in **platelet cyclooxygenase activity** and inhibition of lipid peroxide formation. It is believed that supplementing the diet with vitamin E could play a role in the treatment of thromboembolic disease, especially if it is given in conjunction with an inhibitor of platelet aggregation.

PLATELET-ACTIVATING FACTOR

A platelet-activating factor, **1-0-alkyl-2-(R)acetyl-sn- glyceryl-3-phosphocholine**, is released in the presence of shock and ischemia. The platelet-activating factor antagonist can protect the heart and brain against ischemic injury.

PLATELET-INHIBITING DRUGS

A combination of **acetylsalicylic acid** and **dipyridimole** has been found to be effective in preventing myocardial reinfarction and occlusion of aortocoronary grafts.

FIBRINOLYSIS

In fibrinolysis, **plasmin**, an endopeptidase that is converted from plasminogen by an activator, hydrolyzes fibrin, fibrinogen, factor V, and factor VIII to their inactive products. **Hageman factor** (factor XII) converts a proactivator to the active activator. Agents such as thrombin, **streptokinase**, and **urokinase** therefore enhance the formation of plasmin and hence have fibrinolytic properties. **Epsilon-aminocaproic acid** inhibits the activator-mediated formation of plasmin and so may be used as an antidote to streptokinase-urokinase, or in a defibrination syndrome when bleeding from a mucous membrane occurs.

HIRUDIN AND THROMBIN

The saliva of the **medicinal leech** contains a battery of substances that interfere with the hemostatic mechanisms of the host. One of these compounds is **hirudin**, a potent anticoagulant, which maintains the fluidity of the ingested blood and which is the most potent inhibitor of thrombin. Upon binding to thrombin, the cleavage of fibrinogen and subsequent clot formation are prevented. The potency and specificity of hirudin suggest it as a useful antithrombin III-independent alternative to heparin for the control of thrombosis.

AGENTS THAT INTERFERE WITH COAGULATION

Therapeutic agents that interfere with blood coagulation fall into four classes:

1. **Anticoagulants**, which include heparin and the **coumadin-inanedione** oral anticoagulants
2. **Thrombolytic** agents such as **streptokinase**, **urokinase**, and **recombinant tissue-type plasminogen activator**
3. **Antiplatelet** drugs, which alter the aggregating ability of platelets
4. **Defibrinogenating** agents, which remove the fibrinogen from circulating blood

ORAL ANTICOAGULANTS

The **coumarin anticoagulants** include **dicumarol**, **warfarin sodium** (coumadin sodium), **warfarin potassium** (Athrombin-K), **acenocoumarol** (Sintrom), and **phenprocoumon** (Liquamar). The **inanedione derivatives** are **phenindione** (Hedulin), **diphenadione** (Dipaxin), and **anisindione** (Miradon). The pharmacological properties of oral anticoagulants are identical qualitatively, but their pharmacokinetic parameters and their toxicities vary. **Racemic warfarin sodium** is the most widely used anticoagulant. Antithrombotic drugs are used clinically either to prevent the formation of blood clots within the circulation (anticoagulant) or to dissolve a clot that has already formed (thrombolytic).

HERBS WITH COUMARIN, SALICYLATE, OR ANTIPLATELET DRUGS

Several natural products contain substances that have coumarin, salicylate, or exhibit antiplatelet properties. Therefore, a theoretical risk for potentiation of the pharmacological activity of warfarin exists when these herbs are taken with warfarin. Herbs thought to contain coumarin or coumarin derivatives include:

- Angelica root
- Arnica flower
- Anise
- Asafoetida
- Celery
- Chamomile
- Fenugreek
- Horse chestnut
- Licorice root
- Lovage root
- Parsley
- Passionflower herb
- Quassia
- Red clover
- Rue

Meadowsweet, **poplar**, and **willow bark** contain high concentrations of salicylates, whereas **bromelain**, **clove**, **onion**, and **turmeric** have been reported to exhibit antiplatelet activity. **Borage seed oil** contains **γ-linoleic acid**, which may increase coagulation time. **Bogbean** has been noted to demonstrate hemolytic activity, and **capsicum** has been reported to cause hypocoagulability. There have been no documented case reports of an interaction of warfarin with any of these herbs. However, patients taking any products containing these herbs concurrently with medications that have anticoagulant effects, such as warfarin, should be closely monitored for signs or symptoms of bleeding.

Sweet clover also contains coumarin derivatives and therefore poses an increased risk of bleeding if given with warfarin. There have been no reports of an interaction between sweet clover and warfarin or hemorrhagic disease in humans. However, several cases of severe hemorrhage and death have been reported in cattle.

FEVERFEW

Feverfew (*Tanacetum parthenium*) is commonly used for the **treatment of migraine** headaches, arthritis, and various types of allergies. This herb is thought to exert its pharmacological activity by inhibiting serotonin release, histamine release, prostaglandin synthesis, and platelet release and aggregation. Several studies have shown feverfew to interfere with hemostasis and platelet aggregation by neutralizing platelet sulfhydryl groups, as well as preventing prostaglandin synthesis. **Parthenolide**, one of the many **sesquiterpene lactone** constituents of feverfew extract, has been shown to exert the greatest pharmacological activity.

GARLIC

Garlic (***Allium sativum***) is thought to provide several cardiovascular benefits, such as blood pressure (BP) lowering, serum lipid lowering, and antithrombotic activity. Garlic oil has been reported to interrupt **thromboxane synthesis**, thereby inhibiting platelet function.

GINGER

Ginger (***Zingiber officinale***), promoted for use in motion sickness and arthritis, has been reported to reduce platelet aggregation through the inhibition of **thromboxane synthetase**. Ginger supplements, containing amounts of ginger much greater than regularly found in food products, may lead to an increased risk of bleeding when taken with warfarin.

GINKGO

Ginkgo (***Ginkgo biloba***) is a common herbal product available in the United States and is advertised to improve **cognitive function**. Ginkgolide B, one component of ginkgo, inhibits platelet-activating factor by displacing it from its receptor-binding site, resulting in reduced platelet aggregation. Several cases of bleeding thought to be secondary to ginkgo ingestion have been reported.

COENZYME Q_{10}

Coenzyme Q_{10} (also known as **ubiquinone** or **ubidecarenone**), while not an herb, is a provitamin found in the mitochondria of plant and animal cells. It is involved in electron transport and may act as a **free-radical scavenger**, an **antioxidant**, or a **membrane stabilizer**. Coenzyme Q_{10} supplementation is primarily promoted to treat a variety of cardiovascular disorders, including:

- Heart failure
- Hypertension
- Stable angina
- Ventricular arrhythmias

Many patients with these conditions may also be prescribed warfarin. Coenzyme Q_{10} is structurally related to **menaquinone** (vitamin K) and may have procoagulant effects.

DANSHEN

Although not commonly used in the United States, danshen (the root of ***Salvia miltiorrhiza***), also known as **tan seng**, is a very popular herb recommended in the Chinese community for various cardiovascular diseases. The pharmacological effects of danshen have been described primarily *in vitro* and in animals and include:

- Hypotensive effects
- Positive inotropic effects
- Coronary artery vasodilation
- Inhibition of platelet aggregation

The available evidence contraindicates concurrent use of danshen and warfarin.

DEVIL'S CLAW

Devil's claw (***Harpagophytum procumbens***) is an expensive herbal product that has been promoted for use as an analgesic in the treatment of arthritis, gout, and myalgia. Until more is known about this possible interaction, patients taking warfarin should be advised to avoid devil's claw.

GINSENG

Three ginseng species—**American ginseng** (***Panax quinquefolius***), **Oriental ginseng** (***Panax ginseng***), and **Siberian ginseng** (***Eleutherococcus senticosus***)—have been promoted as enhancing energy, reducing the effects of stress, and improving mood. The active components of ginseng are known as **ginsenosides**, more than 20 of which have been identified. The pharmacological activity of each ginsenoside appears to vary depending on where the plant grew and the extraction techniques used. Also, data suggest that the ginsenoside composition varies widely among commercially available ginseng products. This variability makes it difficult to evaluate the safety and efficacy of ginseng products. Although the exact pharmacological actions of ginsenosides in humans are not fully understood, studies suggest that these substances may increase adrenal hormone synthesis, decrease blood glucose concentrations, and promote immunomodulation. Oriental ginseng (Ginsana) may antagonize the anticoagulant effects of warfarin.

The possible mechanism for this interaction has not been identified, and it is not known which ginsenoside or ginsenosides may be responsible.

GREEN TEA

Green tea (***Camellia sinensis***), also known as **Chinese tea**, is a popular beverage purported to prevent various cancers, treat gastrointestinal (GI) disorders, and enhance cognition. Although dried green tea leaves have been found to contain substantial amounts of **vitamin K**, brewed green tea is generally not considered a significant source of the vitamin. However, large amounts of brewed green tea may potentially antagonize the effects of warfarin.

PAPAIN

Papain is a mixture of proteolytic enzymes found in **extract of papay**a, the fruit of the **papaya tree** (***Carica papaya***). It is taken orally in the belief that it reduces edema, inflammation, herpes zoster symptoms, diarrhea, and psoriasis symptoms. The pharmacological mechanisms by which papain may affect coagulation are not known. Patients receiving warfarin should be advised to avoid papain supplementation until further information about this potential interaction becomes available (Table 4.4).

VITAMIN E

Vitamin E has received much publicity as one of several antioxidants that may be useful in treating a variety of disorders, including cardiovascular disease. Vitamin E may inhibit the oxidation of reduced vitamin K. Vitamin K oxidation is necessary for carboxylation of vitamin K-dependent clotting factors, which must occur for these clotting factors to be fully functional. Increased prothrombin times induced by combined vitamin E and warfarin therapy may be managed by discontinuing vitamin E, and, if necessary, by administering vitamin K.

Because nearly 70% of patients who use alternative therapies do not inform their health-care providers about these products, pharmacists and other health-care professionals should question all patients about their use of alternative therapies. Health-care professionals should remain vigilant for potential interactions between alternative therapies and prescription medications, especially medications with a narrow therapeutic index, and should report suspected interactions to the **FDA MedWatch program**. The FDA recently established the Special Nutritionals Adverse Event Monitoring System, a searchable database including information about suspected adverse events associated with dietary supplements or nutritional products. This database includes reports that have been submitted to MedWatch and can be accessed via the Internet (http://vm.cfsan.fda.gov/~dms/aems.html). Continued efforts by health-care professionals to recognize and report suspected interactions between prescription medications and herbal and other alternative therapies should ultimately increase knowledge and awareness of interactions and improve the quality of patient care.

TABLE 4.4
Potential and Documented Interactions of Herbs and Warfarin

Potential Increase in Risk of Bleeding	
Angelica root	Ginkgo
Arnica flower	Horse chestnut
Anise	Licorice root
Asafoetida	Lovage root
Bogbean	Meadowsweet
Borage seed oil	Onion
Bromelain	Parsley
Capsicum	Passionflower herb
Celery	Poplar
Chamomile	Quassia
Clove	Red clover
Fenugreek	Rue
Feverfew	Sweet clover
Garlic	Turmeric
Ginger	Willow bark
Documented Reports of Possible Increase in Effects of Warfarin	
Danshen	
Devil's claw	
Dong quai	
Papain	
Vitamin E	
Documented Reports of Possible Decrease in Effects of Warfarin	
Coenzyme Q_{10}	
Ginseng	
Green Tea	

Note: The coumarin anticoagulants include dicumarol, warfarin sodium (coumadin sodium), warfarin potassium (Athrombin-K), acenocoumarol (Sintrom), and phenprocoumon (Liquamar).

5

Food–Drug Interactions

INTRODUCTION

Grapefruit juice carries the American Heart Association's healthy "heart-check" food mark and contains compounds that may both reduce **atherosclerotic plaque formation** and inhibit **cancer cell proliferation**. However, unlike other citrus fruit juice, grapefruit juice interacts with a variety of prescription medications, raising the potential for concern. This is particularly worrying in that juice and medications are commonly consumed together at breakfast. This drug–food interaction seems to occur through inhibition by grapefruit juice of one of the intestinal cytochrome P-450 (CYP) enzyme systems, **cytochrome P-450 3A4** (CYP3A4). This enzyme system in the liver is well known for its involvement with drug–drug interactions. Most notably, **terfenadine**, **mibefradil**, and **cisapride** have been withdrawn from the U.S. market in recent years, in part because of deaths due to drug–drug interactions involving the hepatic CYP3A4.

BIOTRANSFORMATION

Biotransformation may be defined as the enzyme-catalyzed alteration of drugs by the living organism. Although few drugs are eliminated unchanged, urinary excretion is a negligible means of terminating the action of most drugs or poisons in the body. As a matter of fact, the urinary excretion of a highly lipid-soluble substance such as **pentobarbital** would be so slow that it would take the body a century to rid itself of the effect of a single dose of the agent. Therefore, mammalian and other terrestrial animals have developed systems that allow the conversion of most lipid-soluble substances to water-soluble ones, so that they may be easily excreted by the kidney. In general, biotransformation may be divided into two forms of metabolism: hepatic and nonhepatic.

HEPATIC DRUG METABOLISM

By far the major portion of biotransformation is carried out in the liver by **cytochrome P-450** (P-450), which is a collective term for a group of related enzymes or isoenzymes that are responsible for the oxidation of numerous drugs; endogenous substances such as fatty acids, prostaglandins, steroids, and ketones; and carcinogens such as **polycyclic aromatic hydrocarbons**, **nitrosamines**, **hydrazines**, and **arylamines**.

Nonhepatic Metabolism

Plasma

One of the drugs that is metabolized in the blood is **succinylcholine**, a muscle relaxant that is hydrolyzed by the **pseudocholinesterase** of liver and plasma to succinylmonocholine. The short duration of action of succinylcholine (5 minutes) is due to its rapid hydrolysis in plasma. Patients with atypical cholinesterase who cannot metabolize succinylcholine suffer pronounced apnea. **Procaine**, a local anesthetic, is also hydrolyzed by pseudocholinesterase.

Lung

The lung is involved in both the activation and inactivation of numerous physiological and pharmacological substances. For example, **angiotensin I** is converted to **angiotensin II** in the lung.

Intestinal Epithelium

The intestinal epithelium is capable of removing numerous agents.

MOLECULAR BIOLOGY OF MULTIPLE ISOENZYMES OF P-450

In recent years, an extensive number of complementary DNAs for the P-450 genes for humans have been isolated and sequenced. Genes that encode proteins that are less than 36% similar in their amino acid sequence belong to different families. Currently, eight different families have been identified in humans, each designated by a Roman numeral. The drug-metabolizing P-450s belongs to family I, II, III, and IV. P-450s that are 70% or more similar are encoded by genes in the same subfamily. Finally, the individual gene is designated by an Arabic numeral.

During phase I, most drugs are inactivated pharmacologically; some remain unaltered, and some become more active and toxic. For example, **phenytoin** in the liver is first hydroxylated to **hydroxyphenytoin** (phase I) and is then conjugated with glucuronic acid (phase II) and excreted by the kidney as **phenytoin glucuronide conjugate**. During phase I, besides introducing a polar group such as an –OH group, a potential polar group may also be unmasked from the drug to be metabolized. For example, compound R–OCH_3 is converted to compound R–OH by demethylation. **Codeine** becomes demethylated to **morphine**.

The free or unmasked polar group is then conjugated with glucuronate, sulfate, glycine, or acetate. With the exception of **morphine 6-glucuronide**, almost all conjugates lack pharmacological activity.

SCHEME OF THE MIXED-FUNCTION OXIDATION REACTION PATHWAY

The hepatic endoplasmic reticulum possesses oxidative enzymes called mixed-function oxidases or monooxygenase with a specific requirement for both molecular oxygen and a reduced concentration of **nicotinamide adenine dinucleotide phosphate** (NADPH). Essential in the mixed-function oxidase system is P-450. The primary electron donor is NADPH, whereas the electron transfer involves P-450, a **flavoprotein**. The presence of a heat-stable fraction is necessary for the operation of the system.

A drug substrate to be metabolized binds to **oxidized P-450**, which in turn is reduced by **P-450 reductase**. The drug-reduced P-450 complex then combines with molecular oxygen. A second electron and two hydrogen ions are acquired from the donor system, and the subsequent products are oxidized drug and water, with regeneration of the oxidized P-450. This process is summarized as follows:

1. NADPH + oxidized cytochrome P-450 + $H^+ \rightarrow$ reduced P-450 + $NADP^+$
2. Reduced cytochrome P-450 + $O_2 \rightarrow$ "active oxygen complex"
3. "Active oxygen complex" + drug substrate $\rightarrow$ oxidized drug + oxidized cytochrome P-450 + H_2O

NADPH + O_2 + drug substrate + $H^+ \rightarrow NADP^+$ + oxidized drug + H_2O.

CONSEQUENCE OF BIOTRANSFORMATION REACTIONS

The process of biotransformation usually inactivates and/or detoxifies the administered drugs or the ingested poisons, but other reactions may also take place.

Precursor Activation: Occasionally, an inactive precursor such as **levodopa** is converted to an active metabolite such as **dopamine**.

Metabolic Activation of Drugs: Often, an active drug is converted to another pharmacologically active substance. The following table lists a few examples of this.

Drug		Active Metabolite
Mephobarbital	is demethylated to	Phenobarbital
Primidone	is oxidized to	Phenobarbital
Imipramine	is demthylated to	Desmethylimipramine
Prednisone	is reduced to	Prednisolone

Conversion to Metabolites with Dissimilar Actions: In certain instances, the body converts a drug to several active metabolites possessing dissimilar pharmacological properties. For example, **phenylbutazone** undergoes aromatic hydroxylation to produce a metabolite that has sodium-retaining and antirheumatic activities, and also undergoes alkyl chain oxidation to produce a metabolite with a strong uricosuric property. Thus, phenylbutazone has both **uricosuric** and **antirheumatic effects**.

Conversion to More Active Products: The conversions of **cyclophosphamide** to **aldophosphamide** and **prednisone** to **prednisolone** are examples of active compounds that are converted to more active substances.

Lethal Synthesis: The metabolism of drugs and agents does not always lead to detoxification; occasionally, the metabolites are toxicologically more potent. Some examples of this are **sulfamethazine**, which is metabolized to **N_4-acetylsulfamethazine**, and **aminopyrine**, with **4-aminoantipyrine** as its metabolite.

DRUG METABOLITE KINETICS

In the majority of cases, drugs are converted to metabolites, which, in the more polar and water-soluble forms, are readily excreted. Often, the concentration of a metabolite far exceeds the concentration of the drug. For example, orally administered **propranolol** is rapidly converted to **4-hydroxypropranolol**, which has a concentration that is several-fold higher than that of propranolol. Sometimes the metabolites are able to inhibit the further metabolism of the parent drug. For example, **phenytoin** becomes metabolized to **hydroxyphenytoin**. When given in higher than recommended individual doses, hydroxyphenytoin inhibits the hydroxylase system that metabolizes phenytoin, increasing its concentration in free form and its potential to produce toxicity.

The **enterohepatic circulation** may sometimes prolong the half-life of a drug. A drug that is absorbed from the gastrointestinal tract, excreted in the bile, and resorbed from the intestine is said to have undergone enterohepatic cycling. Drugs are delivered to the liver by both the portal vein and hepatic artery, and returned to the rest of the body by the hepatic vein. The difference between the concentration of drug transported to and removed from the liver accounts for the amount of drug metabolized or excreted, or both, in the bile. For example, if the liver has conjugated a drug containing glucuronic acid to its metabolite, the conjugated product may appear in the bile and finally be excreted in the small intestine. However, in the intestine, the β-glucuronidase originating from the resident flora may hydrolyze the glucuronide–drug conjugate back to the parent drug, thus allowing the parent drug to be resorbed. The continuous enterohepatic cycling will therefore increase the half-life of this agent in the body.

FACTORS THAT MODIFY THE METABOLISM OF DRUGS

Many environmental factors and pathophysiological conditions inhibit or stimulate the activity of drug-metabolizing enzymes and hence may alter the outcome of a therapeutic regimen. **Pharmacogenetics**, the immaturity of drug-metabolizing enzyme systems, and drug–drug interactions are a few of the factors that have been shown to alter drug metabolism.

Pharmacogenetics

Pharmacogenetics represents the study of the **hereditary variation in the handling of drugs**. Pharmacogenetic abnormalities may be entirely innocuous until the affected individual is challenged with particular drugs. The hyposensitivity and resistance of certain individuals to **coumarin** anticoagulants and the hypersensitivity of patients with **Down's syndrome** to atropine most probably stem from abnormalities in their respective receptor sites. **Acatalasia** and the decrease in the activities of **pseudocholinesterase**, **acetylase**, and **glucose 6-phosphate dehydrogenase** are a few examples of enzymatic deficiencies that can lead to adverse reactions that are mild to very severe.

Liver Disease

The liver is the principal metabolic organ, and hepatic disease or dysfunction may impair drug elimination. Any alteration in the serum albumin or bilirubin levels and in the prothrombin time indicates impaired liver function. Similarly, skin bruising and bleeding tendency indicate decreased production of clotting factors by the liver.

The Influence of Age

Drug metabolism is qualitatively and quantitatively very deficient in newborns. For example, chloramphenicol, when used injudiciously, may cause **gray syndrome**. The mechanism of chloramphenicol toxicity is apparently the failure in the newborn to conjugate **chloramphenicol** with glucuronic acid due to inadequate activity of hepatic **glucaronyl transferase**. This, in combination with inadequate renal excretion of the drug in the newborn, results in a higher-than-expected plasma level of chloramphenicol. Therefore, a newborn should receive doses of chloramphenicol not greater than 25 to 50 mg/kg of body weight.

Elderly people are also prone to toxicity from numerous drugs, including cardiac glycosides. A dose of **digitoxin**, which may be totally therapeutic and innocuous at the age of 60, may produce severe toxicity and even death at the age of 70. The abilities of the liver to metabolize drugs and of the kidney to excrete drug metabolites decline with aging.

Enzyme Induction and Inhibition

The activities of microsomal drug-metabolizing enzymes in humans can be enhanced by altering the levels of endogenous hormones such as androgens, estrogens, progestational steroids, glucocorticoids, anabolic steroids, norepinephrine, insulin, and thyroxine. This effect can also be elicited by the administration of exogenous substances such as drugs, food preservatives, insecticides, herbicides, and polycyclic aromatic hydrocarbons. This increase in the activities of drug-metabolizing enzymes appears to stem from an elevated rate of synthesis of the enzyme protein; hence, it is truly an enzyme-induction phenomenon.

Liver microsomal enzyme inducers that are lipid soluble at the physiological pH can be classified into two general groups. Some, like phenobarbital, tend to stimulate all enzymes; others, such as **3-methylcholanthrene**, tend to be selective. The administration of phenobarbital increases the amounts of **NADPH–cytochrome C reductase** and P-450, and the rate of P-450 reduction. In contrast, the administration of 3-methylcholanthrene increases the amount of P-450 but neither the activity of NADPH–cytochrome C reductase nor the rate of P-450 reduction.

Clinical Implications of Enzyme Induction and Inhibition

Patients are often given several drugs at the same time. The possibility that one drug may accelerate or inhibit the metabolism of another drug should always be kept in mind. When this phenomenon occurs, the removal of an enzyme inducer could be hazardous. The following examples reveal the consequence of enzyme induction. Phenylbutazone is an analgesic, antipyretic, uricosuric, and antiinflammatory agent. Among its side effects are activation of peptic ulcer and gastrointestinal hemorrhage. If one gives a dog large amounts of phenylbutazone, side effects such as vomiting and diarrhea with bloody stool ensue. However, if phenylbutazone treatment is continued for several days, these side effects disappear. In this case, phenylbutazone "induces" its own hydroxylation, which results in a lower plasma level of the drug and ultimately the absence of the side effects. Long-term treatment with phenylbutazone and many other drugs should be expected to result in decreased effectiveness and toxicity.

Patients who are on anticoagulant therapy may suffer severe hemorrhage several days after discharge from the hospital. Often, these patients are sedated with barbiturates during their hospitalization, which tends to stimulate the enzymes that metabolize dicumarol. The abrupt withdrawal of barbiturates after discharge tends to revert the activity of the drug-metabolizing enzymes to their prebarbiturate stage, which raises the free-circulating level of the anticoagulant and results in hemorrhage. Obviously, treatment

TABLE 5.1
Medications with Which Grapefruit Juice Should Not Be Considered in an Unsupervised Manner

Calcium Channel Blockers	
Felodipine	
Nimodipine	
Nisoldipine	
Nitrendipine	
Pranidipine	
Immunosuppressants	
Cyclosporine	
Tacrolimus	
HMG-CoA Reductase Inhibitors[a]	
Atorvastatin	
Cerivastatin	
Lovastatin	
Simvastatin	
Antihistamines	
Ebastine	
Terfenadine	
Psychiatric Medications	
Buspirone	
Carbamazepine	
Diazepam	
Midazolam	
Triazolam	
Prokinetics	
Cisapride	
Others	
Methadone	
Sildenafil	

[a] HMG-CoA = 3-hydroxy-3-methylglutaryl coenzyme A.

with phenobarbital should prompt altering the maintenance dosage of anticoagulants.

GRAPEFRUIT JUICE ACTION ON INTESTINAL CYTOCHROME P-450 (CYP) ENZYMES

The effects of some CYP3A4 inhibitors wane with repeated administration, as they cause induction of CYP3A4 through upregulation of CYP3A messenger RNA and protein over time. However, this is not the case with grapefruit juice. Recurrent ingestion of grapefruit juice leads to a selective decrease of both CYP3A4 and CYP3A5 protein expression in enterocytes, resulting in increased drug bioavailability. Messenger RNA expression is not reduced, which suggests that this decrease in activity is not transcriptionally mediated. The mechanism of the decrease in CYP3A4 protein most likely reflects either accelerated protein degradation or reduced messenger RNA translation. It would be reasonable to suppose that one or more components of grapefruit juice cause a rapid intracellular degradation of the intestinal CYP3A4 enzyme through irreversible "suicide" inhibition. This would explain the rapid and sustained onset of inhibition by grapefruit juice. A 47% reduction in intestinal CYP3A4 concentration occurs within 4 hours of the ingestion of grapefruit juice, and grapefruit juice maintains a bioavailability-enhancing effect for up to 24 hours (see Kane and Lipsky, 2000).

Grapefruit juice also inhibits the CYP1A2 enzyme system *in vitro* but not *in vivo*. This is consistent with the understanding that its effect occurs at the level of the intestinal wall where levels of CYP2A expression are low. These CYP2A substrates studied with grapefruit juice have included **caffeine**, **theophylline**, and **coumarin** (Table 5.1).

REFERENCE

Kane, G.C. and Lipsky, J.J., Drug–Grapefruit juice interactions, *Mayo Clin. Proc.*, 75, 933–942, 2000.

A

ABACAVIR SULFATE/LAMIVUDINE

Epzicom tablets contain 600 mg abacavir (as sulfate) and 300 mg lamivudine.

ABACAVIR SULFATE/LAMIVUDINE/ZIDOVUDINE

Trizivir tablets contain 300 mg abacavir sulfate/150 mg lamivudine/300 mg zidovudine.

Abacavir is an antiretroviral/nucleoside reverse transcriptase inhibitor. It is used in the treatment of HIV-1 in combination with other antiretroviral agents. Abacavir is converted inside cells to an active metabolite, carbovir 5′-triphosphate, which is a potent inhibitor of the HIV-1 reverse transcriptase.

Abacavir is the only approved antiretroviral that is active as a guanosine analog. It is initially monophosphorylated by adenosine phosphortransferase. The monophosphate is then converted to (–)-carbovir 3′-monophosphate, which is then phosphorylated to the di- and triphosphates by cellular kinases. Carbovir 5′-triphosphate terminates the elongation of proviral DNA because it is incorporated by the reverse transcriptase into nascent DNA but lacks a 3′-hydroxyl group.

The most important adverse effect of abacavir is a unique and potentially fatal hypersensitivity syndrome. This syndrome is characterized by fever, abdominal pain, and other gastrointestinal complaints; a mild maculopapular rash; and malaise or fatigue. Respiratory complaints (cough, pharyngitis, dyspnea), musculoskeletal complaints, headache, and paresthesias are reported less commonly. Abacavir is rapidly absorbed and is metabolized to inactivate metabolites by alcohol dehydrogenase and glucuronyl transferase. Alcohol decreases the elimination of abacavir and prolongs its half-life.

ABARELIX

Plenaxis Injectable Suspension contains 113 mg of gonadotropin-releasing hormone (GnRH) antagonist. Abarelix suppresses luteinizing hormone (LH) and follicle-stimulating hormone secretion, thereby reducing the secretion of testosterone by the testes. It is injected intramuscularly, reaching a peak plasma concentration of 40.0 mg/ml three days after injection. Abarelix is used in the treatment of advanced symptomatic prostate cancer in men in whom luteinizing hormone-releasing hormone agonist therapy is not appropriate and who refuse surgical castration. Both agonists and antagonists of the GnRH receptor are used to reduce testosterone secretion. Analogs of GnRH effectively inhibit testosterone secretion by inhibiting LH secretion. GnRH "superactive" analogs, given repeatedly, downregulate the GnRH receptor and are available for treatment of prostate cancer. An extended-release form of the GnRH antagonist **abarelix** (Plenaxis) is approved for treating prostate cancer. Because abarelix does not transiently increase sex steroid production, this preparation may be especially useful in prostate cancer patients in whom any stimulus to tumor growth might have serious adverse consequences, such as patients with spinal cord metastases in whom increased tumor growth could cause paralysis. Abarelix causes prolongation of the **QT interval**. Therefore, Class IA (e.g., quinidine, procainamide), class III (e.g., amiodarone, sotalol) antiarrhythmic agents should be monitored carefully.

ABCIXIMAB
(ReoPro)

Abciximab is a glycoprotein IIb/IIIa inhibitor and binds to glycoprotein IIb/IIIA receptors on the surface of platelets, thereby preventing platelet aggregation. It is used as an adjunct to precutaneous coronary intervention (PCI) to prevent ischemic complications in patients at high risk of abrupt closure of the treated vessel. It is contraindicated in active internal bleeding.

Abciximab (ReoPro) is the Fab fragment of a humanized monoclonal antibody directed against the $\alpha_{IIb}\beta_3$ receptor. It also binds to the **vitronectin receptor** on platelets, vascular endothelial cells, and smooth-muscle cells. The antibody is used in conjunction with percutaneous angioplasty for coronary thromboses, and when used in conjunction with aspirin and heparin, has been shown to be quite effective in preventing restenosis, recurrent myocardial infarction, and death.

The major side effect of abciximab is bleeding, and the contraindications to its use are similar to those for fibrinolytic agents. The frequency of major hemorrhage in clinical trials varies from 1 to 10%, depending on the intensity of anticoagulation with heparin. Thrombocytopenia of less than 50,000 μ/L is seen in about 2% of patients and may be due to development of neoepitopes induced by bound antibody. As the duration of action is long, if major bleeding or emergent surgery occurs, platelet transfusions can reverse the aggregation defect because free antibody concentrations fall rapidly after cessation of infusion. Readministration of antibody has been performed in a small number of patients without evidence of decreased efficacy or allergic reactions.

ABORTIFACIENTS

Prostaglandins stimulate the myometrium of the gravid uterus to contract in a manner that is similar to the contractions seen in the term uterus during labor. Carboprost tromethamine, for IM use only, is administered in an initial dose of 250 mcg, with subsequent doses of 250 mcg at 2 to 4 hour intervals, and not exceeding a total dose of 12.0 mg. Dinoprostone (Prostaglandin E2) is administered by vaginal suppository (20 mg), and the subject should remain in a supine position for 10 minutes following insertion. Additional suppositories may be given every 4 hours until abortion occurs. Prostaglandins stimulate the smooth muscle of the GI tract, causing vomiting or diarrhea. **Aminopterin, mercaptopurine, azathioprine**, and **cyclophosphamide** have been known to cause miscarriage.

ACAMPROSATE CALCIUM

(Campral)

Acamprosate is a competitive inhibitor of the *N*-methyl-D-aspartate (NMDA)-type glutamate receptor that is proposed to normalize the dysregulated neurotransmission associated with chronic ethanol intake and thereby to attenuate one of the mechanisms that lead to relapse. In several European studies, acamprosate has been shown to promote abstinence either alone or in combination with naltrexone.

Acamprosate (*N*-acetylhomotaurine, calcium salt), an analog of GABA, is used widely in Europe for the treatment of alcoholism and was approved recently for use in the United States. A number of double-blind, placebo-controlled studies have demonstrated that acamprosate decreases drinking frequency and reduces relapse drinking in abstinent alcoholics. It acts in a dose-dependent manner (1.3 to 2 g/day) and appears to have efficacy similar to that of **naltrexone**. Studies in laboratory animals have shown that acamprosate decreases alcohol intake without affecting food or water consumption. Acamprosate generally is well tolerated by patients, with diarrhea being the main side effect. No abuse liability has been noted. The drug undergoes minimal metabolism in the liver, is excreted primarily by the kidneys, and has an elimination half-life of 18 hours after oral administration. Concomitant use of **disulfiram** appears to increase the effectiveness of acamprosate, without any adverse drug interactions being noted. The mechanism of action of acamprosate is obscure, although there is some evidence that it modulates the function of NMDA receptors in the brain.

Ondansetron, a 5-HT_3-receptor antagonist and antiemetic drug, reduces alcohol consumption in laboratory animals, and is currently being tested in humans. Preliminary findings suggest that ondansetron is effective in the treatment of early-onset alcoholics, who respond poorly to psychosocial treatment alone, although the drug does not appear to work well in other types of alcoholics. Ondansetron administration lowers the amount of alcohol consumed, particularly by drinkers who consume fewer than 10 drinks per day. It also decreases the subjective effects of ethanol on 6 of 10 scales measured, including the desire to drink, while at the same time not having any effect on the pharmacokinetics of ethanol.

Topiramate, a drug used for treating seizure disorders, appears useful for treating alcohol dependence. Compared with the placebo group, patients taking topiramate achieved more abstinent days and a lower craving for alcohol. The mechanism of action of topiramate is not well understood but is distinct from that of other drugs used for the treatment of dependence (e.g., opioid antagonists), suggesting that it may provide a new and unique approach to pharmacotherapy of alcoholism.

ACARBOSE

(Precose)

Alpha-glucosidase inhibitor inhibits intestinal enzymes that digest carbohydrate, thereby reducing carbohydrate digestion after meals. This lowers postprandial glucose elevation in diabetics. α-Glucosidase inhibitors reduce intestinal absorption of starch, dextrin, and disaccharides by inhibiting the action of α-glucosidase in the intestinal brush border. Inhibition of this enzyme slows the absorption of carbohydrates; the postprandial rise in plasma glucose is blunted in both normal and diabetic subjects.

α-Glucosidase inhibitors do not stimulate insulin release and therefore do not result in hypoglycemia. These agents may be considered as monotherapy in elderly patients or in patients with predominantly postprandial hyperglycemia. α-Glucosidase inhibitors typically are used in combination with other oral antidiabetic agents and/or insulin. The drugs should be administered at the start of a meal. They are poorly absorbed.

ACEBUTOLOL HYDROCHLORIDE

(Apo-Acebutolol, Gen-Acebutolol, Gen-Acebutolol Type S, Monitan, Novo-Acebutolol, Nu-Acebutolol, Rhotral)

Acebutolol is a $beta_1$ selective adrenergic receptor blocking agent that has intrinsic sympathomimetic activity with a plasma half-life of 3 to 4 hours. Propranolol has equal affinity for β_1 and β_2 adrenergic receptors; thus, it is a nonselective β adrenergic receptor antagonist. Agents such as metoprolol, atenolol, acebutolol, bisoprolol, and esmolol have somewhat greater affinity for β_1 than for β_2 receptors; these are examples of β_1-selective antagonists that, even though their selectivity is not absolute, are indicated in hypertension, to be used alone or in combination with other antihypertensive medications. Acebutolol is also indicated in the management of ventricular premature beats. The initial dose in uncomplicated mild to moderate hypertension is 400 mg. In ventricular arrhythmia, the initial dose of 200 mg twice daily may be increased gradually until optimal response is obtained (600 to 1200 mg/day), and the medication is decreased gradually in two weeks. The dose of acebutolol is lower in elderly patients (200 to 600 mg/day) and should be reduced in impairment of renal and hepatic functions.

Acebutolol is indicated in the management of hypertension and premature ventricular contractions. It is contraindicated in hypersensitivity to beta-blockers; persistently sever bradycardia; greater than first-degree heart block; congestive heart failure, unless secondary to tachyarrhythmia treatable with beta-blockers; overt cardiac failure; sinus bradycardia; cardiogenic shock. The side effects reported for acebutolol include hypotension, bradycardia, CHF, cold extremities, heart block, insomnia, fatigue, dizziness, depression, lethargy, drowsiness, forgetfulness, rash, hives, fever, alopecia, dry eyes, blurred vision, tinnitus, slurred speech, sore throat, nausea, vomiting, diarrhea, dry mouth, impotence, painful, difficult, or frequent urination, agranulocytosis, thrombocytopenia purpua, bronchospasm, dyspnea, wheezing, facial swelling, and muscle weakness.

ACENOCOUMAROL

The coumarin anticoagulants include dicumarol, warfarin sodium (coumadin sodium), warfarin potassium (Athrombin-K), acenocoumarol, and phenprocouman. Phenprocouman, acenocoumarol, and ethyl biscoumacetate are not generally available in the United States but are prescribed in Europe and elsewhere. Phenprocouman (Marcumar) has a longer plasma half-life (5 days) than warfarin, as well as a somewhat slower onset of action and a longer duration of action (7 to 14 days). It is administered in daily maintenance doses of 0.75 to 6.0 mg. By contrast, acenocoumarol (Nicoumarlone; Sinthrome) has a shorter half-life (10 to 24 hours), a more rapid effect on the prothrombin time, and a shorter duration of action (2 days). The maintenance dose is 1 to 8 mg daily. Ethyl biscoumacetate (Tromexane) has a very short half-life of 2 to 3 hours and is seldom used.

ACETAMINOPHEN AND ACETAMINOPHEN WITH CODEINE PHOSPHATE

(*N*-Acetyl-P-Aminophenol, APAP, Acephen, Anacin-3, Bromo-Seltzer, Datril, Datril 500, Tempra, Tylenol, Valadol, Valorin)

Acetaminophen is classified as a non-narcotic analgesic and antipyretic agent. Aspirin is superior to acetaminophen in treating pain of inflammatory origin. Acetaminophen is superior to aspirin in not affecting prothrombin response or producing GI ulceration. Therefore, acetaminophen is used in individuals who are allergic to aspirin; or in the presence of hemostatic disturbances, including bleeding diatheses, such as hemophilia; upper GI diseases, such as ulcer, gastritis, or hiatus hernia; or in patients who are taking anticoagulants. Acetaminophen reduces fever by acting on the hypothalamic heat-regulating centers, by blocking the actions of endogenous pyrogens, and by increasing heat dissipation through vasodilatation and sweating. It inhibits the activity of prostaglandin synthetase in the CNS, but not in the peripheral systems, which accounts for its lack of antirheumatic and antiinflammatory effects. Acetaminophen is metabolized in the liver and excreted by the kidneys mostly as glucuronate or sulfate conjugates. When given in larger-than-therapeutic doses (325 to 650 mg p.o. not exceeding 4 g daily) or in glutathione deficiency, acetaminophen may cause hepatic necrosis. Similarly, hepatotoxicity may occur in chronic alcoholics following therapeutic doses of acetaminophen. In addition, the potential hepatotoxicity of acetaminophen may increase by administration of large doses of barbiturates, hydantoins, sulfinpyrazone, carbamazepine, or rifampin when given for a prolonged period of time. Activated charcoal reduces the absorption of acetaminophen, and *N*-acetylcysteine, which provides sulfhydryl groups, is a specific antidote for acetaminophen toxicity.

ACETAZOLAMIDE

(Acetamide, Acetazolamide Sodium, AK-Zol, Albox, AK-Zol, Dehydratin, Diamox, Diamox Sequels, Diamox Sodium, Ederen, Glauconox, Glaupax, Inidrase, Ledamox, Nephramid, Ocu-zolamide, Oratrol, Storzolamide)

Acetazolamide is classified as an anticonvulsant, antiglaucomatous agent, and diuretic, and is a potent inhibitor of the enzyme carbonic anhydrase. The carbonic anhydrase inhibitors consist of acetazolamide (Diamox), ethoxzolamide (Cardrase), and dichlorphenamide (Daranide). Acetazolamide is an old agent, whereas ethoxzolamide and dichlorphenamide are newer preparations. Dichlorphenamide is the most potent carbonic anhydrase inhibitor in use today. The presence of SO_2NH_2 (sulfonamide) causes such compounds to inhibit carbonic anhydrase (CA), which catalyzes the hydration of carbon dioxide as follows:

$$CO_2 + H_2O \xrightarrow{CA} H_2CO_3 \rightleftharpoons H^+ + HCO_3^-$$

These agents inhibit carbonic anhydrase in the renal tubular cells in both the proximal and distal tubules. When the rate of hydrogen generation is reduced, HCO_3^- is lost in urine, and the patient tends to become acidotic. However, the plasma concentration of HCO_3^- is lowered and less is filtered, so the diuresis becomes less effective. In addition, the sodium output is increased because its resorption in exchange for hydrogen is limited by the decreased availability of hydrogen. With less hydrogen available, the exchange of sodium for potassium predominates, and this fosters the loss of potassium. Chloride excretion is not altered significantly. Because the aqueous humor has a high concentration of bicarbonate, carbonic anhydrase inhibitors are primarily used in the treatment of glaucoma. They are no longer used as diuretics or as antiepileptic agents.

In acute angle-closure glaucoma, dichlorphenamide (100 to 200 mg, followed by 100 mg q. 12 hours) may be used with miotics and osmotic agents to rapidly reduce intraocular tension.

ACETAZOLAMIDE

(DIAMOX)

Acetazolamide (Diamox) is the prototype of a class of agents that have limited usefulness as diuretics but have played a major role in the development of fundamental concepts of renal physiology and pharmacology. Proximal tubular epithelial cells are richly endowed with the zinc metalloenzyme carbonic anhydrase, which is found in the luminal and basolateral membranes (type IV carbonic anhydrase,

TABLE 1
Comparison of Orally Administered Sulfonylurea Hypoglycemic Agents

Characteristics	Tolbutamide	Acetohexamide	Tolazamide	Chlorpropamide	Glipizide	Glyburide
Relative potency	1	2.5	5	6	100	150
Duration of action (h)	6–10	12–18	16–24	24–72	16–24	18–24
Extent of protein binding	>98	~90	>98	~95	>98	>98
Hepatic metabolism	Yes	Yes	Yes	Yes	Yes	Yes
Urinary excretion	Yes	Yes	Yes	Yes	Yes	Yes
Fecal excretion (% of dose)	Negligible	Negligible	Negligible	Negligible	12	50
Dose (mg) range	500–3000	250–1500	100–1000	100–500	2.5–40	1.25–20
Diuretic	Yes	Yes	Yes	No	No	Yes
Antidiuretic	Yes	No	No	Yes	No	No
Disulfiram-like effects	No	No	No	Yes	No	No

an enzyme tethered to the membrane by a glycosylphosphatidylinositol linkage), as well as in the cytoplasm (type II carbonic anhydrase). Carbonic anhydrase plays a key role in $NaHCO_3$ reabsorption and acid secretion.

Carbonic anhydrase inhibitors potently inhibit (IC_{50} for acetazolamide is 10 n*M*) both the membrane-bound and cytoplasmic forms of carbonic anhydrase, resulting in nearly complete abolition of $NaHCO_3$, reabsorption in the proximal tubule. Inhibition of carbonic anhydrase is associated with a rapid rise in urinary HCO_3^- excretion to approximately 35% of filtered load. This, along with inhibition of titratable acid and NH_4^+ secretion in the collecting-duct system, results in an increase in urinary pH to approximately 8 and development of a metabolic acidosis. Although acetazolamide is used for treatment of **edema**, the efficacy of carbonic anhydrase inhibitors as single agents is low, and carbonic anhydrase inhibitors are not employed widely in this regard.

The major indication for carbonic anhydrase inhibitors is **open-angle glaucoma**. Carbonic anhydrase inhibitors also may be employed for secondary glaucoma and preoperatively in **acute angle-closure glaucoma** to lower intraocular pressure before surgery. Acetazolamide also is used for the treatment of **epilepsy**. The rapid development of tolerance, however, may limit the usefulness of carbonic anhydrase inhibitors for epilepsy.

ACETIC ACID

(Domeboro Otic, Vosol otic solution)

Acetic acid (2 drops in each ear b.i.d.) is an antibacterial and antifungal agent, which is indicated in the treatment of external ear canal infection.

ACETOHEXAMIDE

(Dimelin, Dimelor, Dymelor, Gamadiabet, Ordimel, Toyobexin)

Acetohexamide is a blood-glucose-lowering drug of the sulfonylurea class. The first-generation oral hypoglycemic agents include tolbutamide (Orinase), acetohexamide (Dymelor), tolazamide (Tolinase), and chlorpropamide (Diabinese). The second-generation oral hypoglycemic agents include glyburide (DiaBeta, Micronase), and glipizide (Glucotrol) (see Table 1 and Figure 54). These agents exert their effects initially by enhancing the secretion of insulin by b cells of the pancreas. Following several months of continuous treatment, insulin levels return to pretreatment values, whereas glucose levels remain improved. Oral hypoglycemic agents reduce the rate of hepatic glucose production, and increase the sensitivity and number of insulin receptors. Acetohexamide is an intermediate-acting sulfonylurea with a maximum hypoglycemic effect in 3 hours and a duration of action of 12 to 18 hours. It is metabolized by the liver to an active metabolite that like acetohexamide, exhibits diuretic and uricosuric effects. The recommended dose range is 250 to 1500 mg/day, and because it undergoes urinary excretion, it can accumulate in renal failure. Prolonged (4 to 10 days) hypoglycemia has been reported in neonates born to diabetic mothers who were receiving a long-acting drug at the time of delivery. Overdosage of acetohexamide causes severe hypoglycemia, which in turn may cause headache, weakness, confusion, dizziness, lethargy, convulsions, coma, or death. In elderly, debilitated, or malnourished patients, especially those with impaired renal or hepatic functions, the doses of acetohexamide should be adjusted carefully.

ACETOHYDROXAMIC ACID

(Lithostat)

Acetohydroxamic acid (250 mg p.o. t.i.d.), **an antiurolithic agent**, is indicated as an adjunctive agent in treating chronic urinary tract infections caused by urease-producing bacteria. Acetohydroxamic acid, which inhibits urease and reduces the production of ammonia, is devoid of antibacterial activity.

ACETOPHENAZINE MALEATE

(Tindal)

Acetophenazine (20 mg tablet p.o. t.i.d.; not available in injectable form) is a **neuroleptic** that exerts its antipsychotic effects by blocking the hyperactivity of dopaminergic

TABLE 2
Antipsychotic Agents

Drugs	Injectable Form	Equivalent Dose (mg)	Daily Dosage (mg)[a]	Sedation	Incidence of Movement Disorders	Anticholinergic Effects
Phenothiazines						
Aliphatic						
Chlorpromazine	Yes	50	30–800	+++	++	++
Triflupromazine	Yes	12.5	60–150	+++	++	+++
Piperidine						
Mesoridazine	Yes	25	30–400	+++	+	++
Thioridazine	No	50	150–800	+++	+	+++
Piperazine						
Acetophenazine	No	10	60–120	++	+++	++
Fluphenazine	Yes	1	1–40	+	+++	+
Perphenazine	Yes	4	12–64	+	+++	++
Prochlorperazine	Yes	8	15–150	++	+++	+
Trifluperazine	Yes	2.5	2–40	+	+++	+
Thioxanthenes						
Chlorprothixene	Yes	50	75–600	+++	++	++
Thiothixene	Yes	2	8–30	+	+++	+
Butyrophenone						
Haloperidol	Yes	1	1–15	+	+++	+
Dihydroindolone						
Molindone	No	5	15–225	+	+++	+
Dibenzoxazepine						
Loxapine	Yes	5	20–250	++	+++	+
Diphenylbutylpiperidine						
Pimozide	No	2	1–25	++	+++	++
Dibenzodiazepine						
Clozapine	No	Not available	100–90	+	—	+

Note: +++ = high; ++ = moderate; + = low; – = not present.
[a] Dosages of oral medications only.

receptors in the mesocortical and mesolimbic systems. However, by blocking dopaminergic receptors in the nigrostriatal pathway, acetophenazine causes pseudoparkinsonism, which is treated by anticholinergic drugs such as trihexyphenidyl or benztropine. Acetophenazine also possesses anticholinergic, antihistaminic, and alpha-adrenergic blocking effects. It reduces the actions of sympathomimetic amines including phenylephrine, phenylpropanolamine, and ephedrine. Acetophenazine potentiates the effects of alcohol, narcotic analgesics and barbiturates, and general, spinal, or epidural anesthetics. The combination of magnesium sulfate and acetophenazine may cause oversedation, hypotension, and respiratory depression. Acetophenazine potentiates the effects of antiarrhythmic agents (guanidine, disopyramide, or procainamide) by enhancing the incidence of cardiac arrhythmias and conduction defects; the effects of compounds possessing anticholinergic properties including amitriptyline and diphenhydramine by causing oversedation, paralytic ileus, visual disturbances, and constipation; the effects of nitrates causing hypotension; and the effects of metrizamide increasing the risk of seizures. Acetophenazine is absorbed orally, is bound to plasma protein to the extent of 90%, exerts its effects in 30 minutes, and the peak effect is seen in 2 to 4 hours. It is distributed widely in the body and its fluids, including appearing in breast milk. It is metabolized in the liver, and the metabolites are eliminated mostly in the urine and through the biliary tract in the feces. For other effects or side effects, see also the section on phenothiazine derivatives and Table 2.

ACETYLCHOLINE

Acetylcholine, an ester of choline and acetic acid, is synthesized in cholinergic neurons according to the following scheme:

$$\text{Acetyl CoA} + \text{choline} \xrightarrow[\text{acetyltransferase}]{\text{Choline}} \text{acetylcholine}$$

The acetylcholine, in turn, is hydrolyzed by both acetylcholinesterase and plasma butyrylcholinesterase. Choline is actively transported into nerve terminals (synaptosomes) by a high-affinity uptake mechanism. Furthermore, the availability of choline regulates the synthesis of acetylcholine

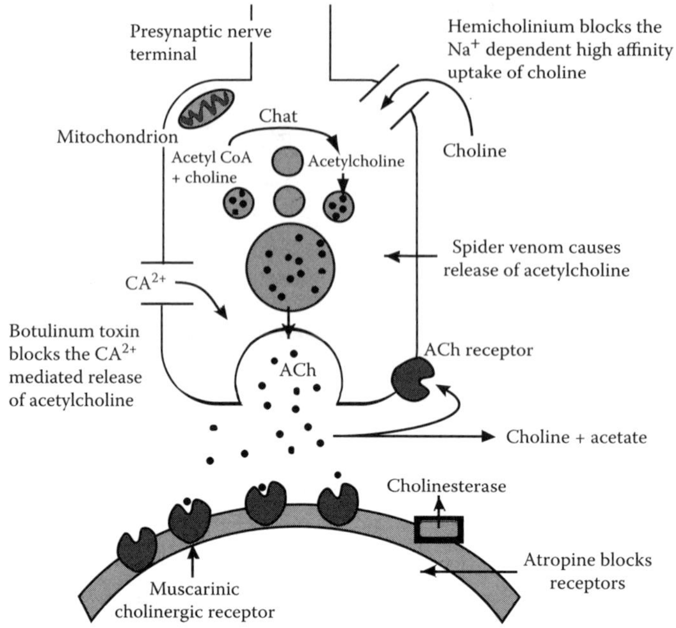

FIGURE 12 Botulinum toxin causes skeletal muscle paralysis by binding to acetylcholine receptors on the motor end plate.

(Figure 12). Hemicholinium blocks the transport of choline into synaptosomes, whereas botulinum toxin blocks the calcium-mediated release of acetylcholine. The released acetylcholine is hydrolyzed rapidly by acetylcholinesterase to choline and acetate.

Acetylcholine receptors are classified as either muscarinic or nicotinic. The alkaloid muscarine mimics the effects produced by stimulation of the parasympathetic system. These effects are postganglionic and are exerted on exocrine glands, cardiac muscle, and smooth muscle. The alkaloid nicotine mimics the actions of acetylcholine, which include stimulation of all autonomic ganglia, stimulation of the adrenal medulla, and contraction of skeletal muscle.

Dimethylphenylpiperazinium stimulates the autonomic ganglia; tetraethylammonium and hexamethonium block the autonomic ganglia; phenyltrimethylammonium stimulates skeletal motor muscle end plates; decamethonium produces neuromuscular blockade; and d-tubocurarine blocks both the autonomic ganglia and the motor fiber end plates. Among the agents cited, only d-tubocurarine is useful as a drug (skeletal muscle relaxant); the rest are useful only as research tools. Cholinesterase, found in liver and plasma, can hydrolyze other esters such as succinylcholine (a skeletal muscle relaxant). Cholinergic peripheral receptors are located on (1) postganglionic parasympathetic fibers, (2) postganglionic sympathetic fibers, (3) all autonomic ganglia, and (4) skeletal end plates.

In addition, cholinergic receptors are distributed extensively in the CNS and participate in diversified functions such as audition, vision, learning and memory, ingestive behaviors (thirst and hunger), thermoregulation, locomotor activity, diurnal rhythms, sleep, and sexual activity. Changes in cholinergic neurons have been observed in neurologic syndromes such as catalepsy, stereotypy, and tremor, and in psychiatric disorders such as depression.

Methacholine, carbachol, and bethanechol are all agents that mimic the effects of stimulation of cholinergic nerves. The two currently used derivatives of acetylcholine are bethanechol (urecholine chloride) and carbachol (Miostat). Unlike acetylcholine, both agents are resistant to hydrolysis by cholinesterase. Both are muscarinic agonists. The nicotinic action of carbachol is greater than that of acetylcholine, whereas bethanechol is devoid of nicotinic action. The cardiovascular actions of acetylcholine are vasodilation and negative chronotropic and inotropic effects. The cardiovascular effects of methacholine are more pronounced than those of acetylcholine, which in turn are greater than those of carbachol or bethanechol. The gastrointestinal effects (increase in tone, amplitude of contractions, and peristalsis) of bethanechol and carbachol are equal but greater than those of acetylcholine. The effects of carbachol and bethanechol on the urinary tract, consisting of ureteral peristalsis, contraction of the detrusor muscle of the urinary bladder, and an increase in voluntary voiding pressure, are equivalent and exceed those produced by acetylcholine.

The miotic effects of carbachol and bethanechol are greater than those of acetylcholine. Atropine is able to antagonize all cholinergic (muscarinic) effects produced by acetylcholine, methacholine, carbachol, and bethanechol. However, this antagonism is least evident with carbachol. Bethanechol is of value in the management of postoperative abdominal distention, gastric atony or stasis, and urinary retention. Carbachol (0.25 to 3.0%) may be used for the long-term therapy of noncongestive wide-angle glaucoma.

ACETYLCYSTEINE (*N*-ACETYLCYSTEINE)

Acetadote injection 20% (200mg/mL), Mucomyst solution 10% (as sodium), solution 20% (as sodium)

Acetylcysteine decreases thickness of mucous secretions in lung. As a mucolytic agent, acetylcysteine splits disulfide linkages between mucoprotein molecular complexes, decreasing their viscosity. It is used as an adjunct therapy in emphysema with bronchitis, chronic asthmatic bronchitis, tuberculosis, bronchiectasis, primary amyloidosis of the lung, pneumonia, and tracheobronchitis. In addition, it is used in pulmonary complications of cystic fibrosis and those associated with anesthetics, surgery, or care following tracheostomy.

Acetylcysteine is also used to attenuate hepatic injury from overdosing (10 to 15 g) with acetaminophen. By maintaining the hepatic level of glutathione, acetylcysteine protects the liver by acting as an alternate substrate for conjugation and hence detoxification of the reactive metabolite of acetaminophen. It is given in a dose of 140 mg/kg orally as a loading dose and then 70 mg/kg orally every four hours until acetaminophen's level becomes nontoxic.

Acetylcysteine (Fluimucil) is being tested as an immunomodulator in acquired immune deficiency syndrome (AIDS).

N-ACETYLPROCAINAMIDE

(Acecainide HCl)

N-acetylprocainamide, a metabolite of procainamide, is classified as a type III antiarrhythmic agent. It prolongs atrial and ventricular action potential durations and refractory period without depressing conduction velocity. When compared to procainamide, *N*-acetylprocainamide has distinct electrophysiologic and pharmacologic effects and does not cause lupus-like syndrome. The common side effects of *N*-acetylprocainamide are gastrointestinal disturbances, dizziness, lightheadedness, blurred vision, numbness, and tingling sensation. The majority of *N*-acetylprocainamide is excreted unchanged in the urine.

ACETYLSALICYCLIC ACID

(Aspirin)

Acetylsalicylic acid possesses analgesic, antipyretic, antiinflammatory, and uricosuric properties (see Table 3).

TABLE 3
The Pharmacologic Efficacy of Various Compounds Possessing Analgesic, Antipyretic, Uricosuric, and Antiinflammatory Actions

Specific Groups	Analgesic	Antipyretic	Antiinflammatory	Uricosuric
Salicylate derivatives				
Acetylsalicylic acid (aspirin)	*	*	*	*
Pyrazolone derivatives				
Phenylbutazone	*	*	*	*
Oxyphenbutazone	*	*	*	*
Sulfinpyrazone	0	0	0	0
Paraaminophenol derivatives				
Acetaminophen	*	*	0	0
Phenacetin	*	*	0	0
Propionic acid derivatives				
Ibuprofen	*	*	*	0
Naproxen	*	*	*	0
Fenoprofen	*	*	*	0
Flurbiprofen	*	*	*	0
Ketoprofen	*	*	*	0
Newer drugs				
Indomethacin	*	*	*	0
Sulindac	*	0	*	0
Mefenamic acid	*	0	*	0
Tolmetin	*	*	*	0
Diflunisal	*	0	*	0
Piroxicam	*	*	*	0
Diclofenac	*	*	*	0
Etodolac	*	0	*	0
Nabumetone	*	*	*	0

Note: * = possesses the property assigned; 0 = lacks the property assigned.

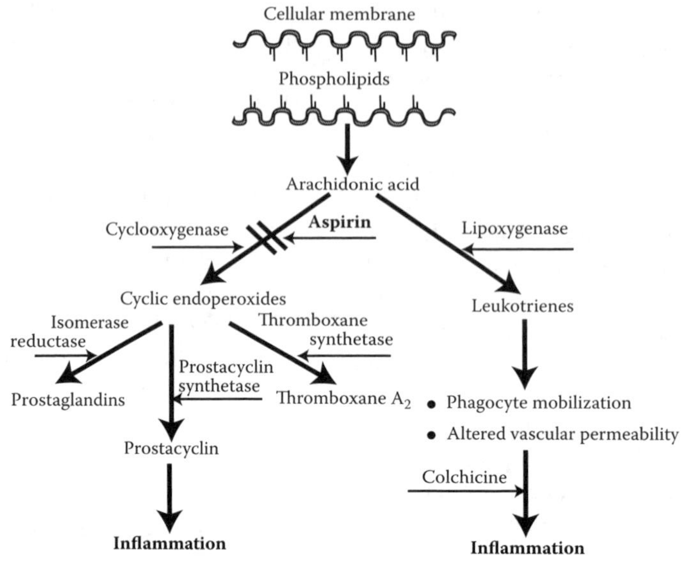

FIGURE 13 Aspirin and related compounds inhibit the enzyme **cyclooxygenase** and prevent the formation of prostaglandin endoperoxides, PGG_2 PGH^2, which are normally formed from arachidonic acid.

Unlike the narcotic analgesics such as morphine, aspirin does not depress respiration, is relatively nontoxic, and lacks addiction liability. Aspirin is a weak or mild analgesic that is effective for ameliorating short, intermittent types of pain such as neuralgia, myalgia, and toothache. It does not have the efficacy of morphine and cannot relieve the severe, prolonged, and lancinating types of pain associated with trauma such as burns or fractures. Like morphine, it produces analgesia by raising the pain threshold in the thalamus, but, unlike morphine, it does not alter the patient's reactions to pain. Because aspirin does not cause hypnosis or euphoria, its site of action has been postulated to be subcortical. In addition to raising the pain threshold, the antiinflammatory effects of aspirin may contribute to its analgesic actions. However, no direct association between the antiinflammatory and analgesic effects of these compounds should be expected. For example, aspirin has both analgesic and antiinflammatory properties, whereas acetaminophen has analgesic but not antiinflammatory properties. Furthermore, potent antiinflammatory agents such as phenylbutazone have only weak analgesic effects.

Aspirin does not alter the normal body temperature, which is maintained by a balance between heat production and dissipation. In a fever associated with infection, increased oxidative processes enhance heat production. Aspirin acts by causing cutaneous vasodilation, which prompts perspiration and enhances heat dissipation. This effect is mediated via the hypothalamic nuclei, as proved by the fact that a lesion in the preoptic area suppresses the mechanism through which aspirin exerts its antipyretic effects. The antipyretic effects of aspirin may be due to its inhibition of hypothalamic prostaglandin synthesis (Figure 13). Although aspirin-induced diaphoresis contributes to its antipyretic effects, it is not an absolutely necessary process because antipyresis takes place in the presence of atropine.

Antipyretic, Uricosuric, and Antiinflammatory Actions Small doses (600 mg) of aspirin cause hyperuricemia, but large doses (>5 gm) have a uricosuric effect. Aspirin inhibits uric acid resorption by the tubules in the kidneys. However, because of the availability of more effective uricosuric agents, aspirin is no longer used for this purpose.

Aspirin has an antiinflammatory action as well as antirheumatic and antiarthritic effects, and may therefore be used in the treatment of rheumatic fever. It is extremely effective in managing rheumatoid arthritis and allied diseases involving the joints, such as ankylosing spondylitis and osteoarthritis. It is thought that aspirin and indomethacin exert their antiinflammatory effects by inhibiting prostaglandin synthesis through the inhibition of cyclooxygenase (Figure 13). The presynthesized prostaglandins are released during a tissue injury that fosters inflammation and pain. Furthermore, aspirin reduces the formation of prostaglandin in the platelets and leukocytes, which is responsible for the reported hematologic effects associated with aspirin.

The current thinking concerning the role of aspirin in the prevention of cardiovascular disease is that it is beneficial in the event of myocardial infarction and stroke. It is effective because, in platelets, small amounts of aspirin acetylate irreversibly and bind to the active site of thromboxane A_2, a potent promoter of platelet aggregation (see Figure 14).

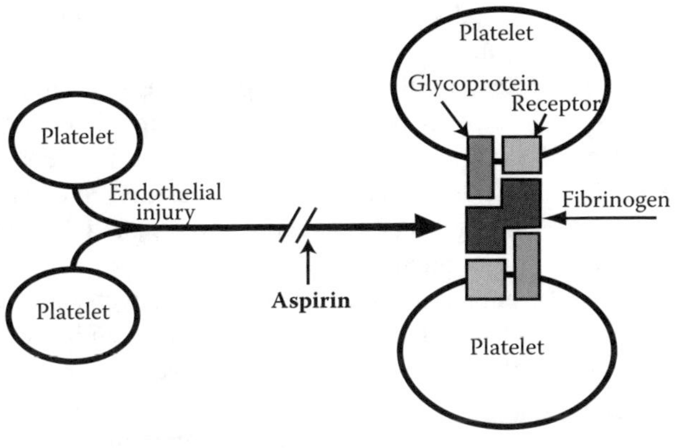

FIGURE 14 Aspirin prevents platelet aggregation and may be helpful in the treatment of thromboembolic disease.

The menstrual cycle is associated with two potentially incapacitating events: dysmenorrhea and the premenstrual syndrome. Substantial evidence indicates that the excessive production of prostaglandin F_{2a} is the major source of painful menstruation. The nonsteroidal antiinflammatory drugs approved for the treatment of dysmenorrhea are aspirin, ibuprofen, mefenamic acid, and naproxen.

Aspirin both directly and indirectly stimulates respiration. In analgesic doses, aspirin increases oxygen consumption and carbon dioxide production. However, increased alveolar ventilation balances the increased carbon dioxide production; thus, the partial pressure of CO_2 (PCO_2) in plasma does not change. In the event of salicylate intoxication (e.g., 10 to 12 g of aspirin given in 6 to 8 hours in adults, and an even smaller dosage in children whose brains are far more sensitive to salicylate intoxication), salicylate stimulates the medullary centers directly, and this causes hyperventilation characterized by an increase in the depth and rate of respiration. The PCO_2 level declines, causing hypocapnia, and the blood pH increases, causing respiratory alkalosis. The low PCO_2 then decreases the renal tubular resorption of bicarbonate and compensates for the alkalosis.

If the salicylate level continues to rise, the respiratory centers become depressed, the PCO_2 level becomes elevated, and the blood pH becomes more acidic, causing respiratory acidosis. Dehydration, reduced bicarbonate levels, and the accumulation of salicylic acid, salicyluric acid resulting from metabolism of aspirin, and lactic acid and pyruvic acid resulting from deranged carbohydrate metabolism may cause metabolic acidosis.

Although innocuous in most subjects, the therapeutic analgesic doses of aspirin may cause epigastric distress, nausea, vomiting, and bleeding. Aspirin can also exacerbate the symptoms of peptic ulcer, characterized by heartburn, dyspepsia, and erosive gastritis. An extensive number of salts have been synthesized from salicylate (e.g., calcium carbaspirin, choline salicylate, alloxipirin, and numerous buffered derivatives), and each has shown some ability to reduce the gastrointestinal toxicity of aspirin. However, other unknown factors may contribute to this undesirable gastrointestinal property of aspirin. In experimental animals, the intravenous administration of sodium salicylate or subcutaneous administration of methyl salicylate has produced petechial hemorrhage of the gastric mucosa. Furthermore, compounds possessing antiinflammatory properties (aspirin, phenylbutazone, and oxyphenbutazone) are associated with a higher incidence of gastrointestinal toxicity than those compounds devoid of antiinflammatory properties (phenacetin and acetaminophen).

Aspirin reduces the leukocytosis associated with acute rheumatic fever. When given on a long-term basis, it also reduces the hemoglobin level and the hematocrit. Aspirin use can cause reversible hypoprothrombinemia by interfering with the function of vitamin K in prothrombin synthesis. Therefore, aspirin should be used with caution in patients with vitamin K deficiency, preexisting hypoprothrombinemia, or hepatic damage; in patients taking anticoagulants; and in patients scheduled for surgery. Aspirin leads to hemolytic anemia in individuals with glucose 6-phosphate dehydrogenase deficiency. An aspirin tolerance test is used diagnostically in von Willebrand's disease because it will further prolong the bleeding time if the disease exists. Aspirin prevents platelet aggregation and may be helpful in the treatment of thromboembolic diseases. In addition to aspirin, indomethacin, phenylbutazone, sulfinpyrazone, and dipyridamole prevent platelet aggregation (see Figures 14 and 92), whereas epinephrine, serotonin, and prostaglandins promote platelet aggregation and hence are procoagulants. The erythrocyte sedimentation rate is often elevated in infections and inflammations, but aspirin therapy will yield a false negative. The supportive treatment of aspirin poisoning may include gastric lavage (to prevent the further absorption of salicylate), fluid replenishment (to offset the dehydration and oliguria), alcohol and water sponging (to combat the hyperthermia), the administration of vitamin K (to prevent possible hemorrhage), sodium bicarbonate administration (to combat acidosis), and, in extreme cases, peritoneal dialysis and exchange transfusion.

ACITRETIN

(Soriatane capsules 10 mg)

Acitretin is a second-generation retinoid. Acitretin (Soriatane) is the major metabolite of etretinate, an aromatic retinoid that formerly was approved for **psoriasis** but withdrawn from the market because of its undesirable pharmacokinetics. Acitretin has an elimination half-life of 2 to 3 days.

Retinoids include natural compounds and synthetic derivatives of retinol that exhibit vitamin A activity. Retinoids have many important functions throughout the body, including roles in vision, regulation of cell proliferation and differentiation, and bone growth, immune defense, and tumor suppression. Because **vitamin A** affects normal epithelial differentiation, it was investigated as a treatment for cutaneous disorders but was abandoned initially because of unfavorable side effects. Molecular modifications yielded compounds with vastly improved margins of safety.

First-generation retinoids include **retinol, tretinoin** (all-*trans*retinoic acid), isotretinoin (13-*cis*-retinoic acid), and **alitretinoin** (9-*cis*-retinoic acid). Second-generation retinoids, also known as **aromatic retinoids**, were created by alteration of the cyclic end group and include **acitretin**. Third-generation retinoids contain further modifications and are called **arotinoids**. Members of this generation include **tazarotene** and **bexarotene. Adapalene**, a derivative of naphthoic acid with retinoid-like properties, does not fit precisely into any of the three generations.

Retinoic acid (RA) exerts its effects on gene expression by activating two families of receptors—**retinoic acid receptors** (RARs) and the **retinoid X receptors** (RXRs)—that are members of the thyroid/steroid hormone receptor superfamily. Retinoids (ligands) bind transcription factors (nuclear receptors), and the ligand-receptor complex then binds to the promoter regions of target genes to regulate their expression. The gene products formed contribute to the desirable pharmacological effects of these drugs and their unwanted side effects. Additional complexity arises because each receptor has three isoforms (α, β, and γ) that form homo- and heterodimers. Retinoid-responsive tissues express one or more RAR and RXR subtypes in various combinations that determine activity locally. Human skin contains mainly RARα and RARβ.

ACRIVASTINE/PSEUDOEPHEDRINE HYDROCHLORIDE

(Semprex-D capsules 8 mg, Acrivastine/60 mg Pseudoephedrine)

Acrivastine is an antiviral agent and an antiherpes virus agent. Acrivastine competitively blocks histamine at H_2 receptor sites; pseudoephedrine causes vasoconstriction and subsequent shrinkage of nasal mucous membranes by alpha-adrenergic stimulation, promoting nasal drainage. Acrivastine is used in the relief of symptoms associated with seasonal allergic rhinitis. Pseudoephedrine may reduce the antihypertensive effects of agents that interfere with sympathetic activity (e.g., mecamylamine, methyldopa, reserpine, veratrum alkaloids).

Acrivastine enhances the CNS depressant effects of alcohol and other CNS depressants. Overdosage with pseudoephedrine may cause palpitations, tachycardia, pressor activity, cardiac arrhythmias, or cardiovascular collapse. These agents should not be taken with monoamine oxidase A inhibitor (MAO A inhibitor), such as **tranylcypromine.**

ACTINOMYCIN D

(Dactinomycin)

The antibiotics that bind to DNA are nonspecific to the cell-cycle phase. Actinomycin binds to double-stranded DNA and prevents RNA synthesis by inhibiting DNA-dependent RNA polymerase. It is administered intravenously in the treatment for pediatric solid tumors such as Wilms' tumor and rhabdomyosarcoma, and for gestational choriocarcinoma. Dactinomycin causes skin reactions, gastrointestinal injury, and delayed bone marrow depression (see Figure 15).

ACTIVATED CHARCOAL

(Actidose-Aqua, Arm-A-Char, Charcoaide, Charcocaps, Insta-Char, Liquid-Antidose)

Activated charcoal (1000 mg p.o. t.i.d.), is indicated for the treatment of flatulence and dyspepsia. Activated charcoal, as

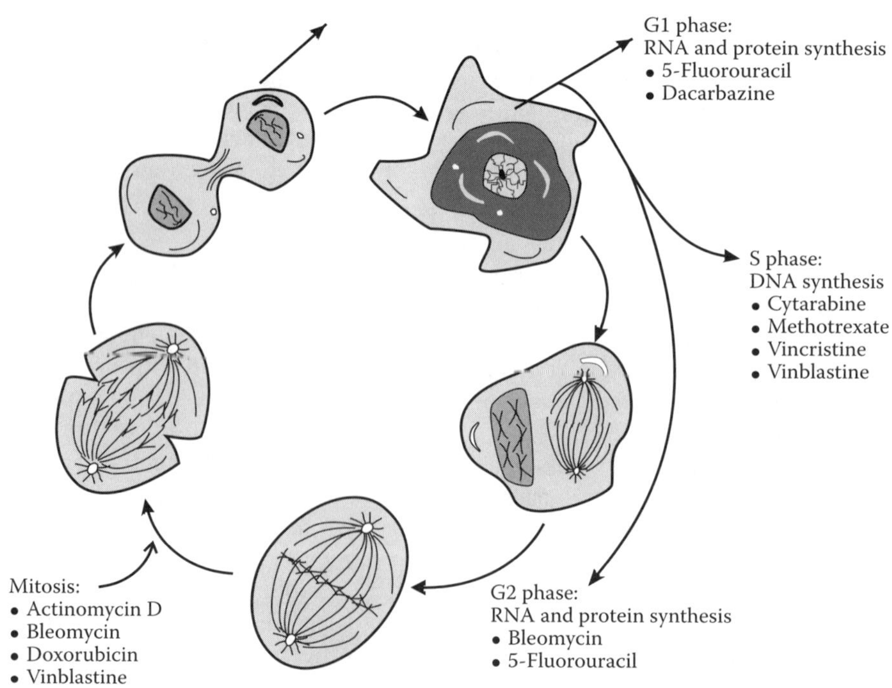

FIGURE 15 The actions of antineoplastic agents on different phases of the cell cycle.

an adsorbent (30 g in 250 ml water to make a slurry), is indicated in the treatment of overdosage from numerous medications. It absorbs intestinal gas causing discomfort, toxic and nontoxic irritants causing diarrhea, and drugs preventing their absorption, and hence toxicity.

ACUTE RESPIRATORY DISTRESS SYNDROME

Treatment of acute respiratory distress syndrome (ARDS) or acute lung injury may be defined as a condition involving impaired oxygenation. The nonpharmacologic therapies include mechanical ventilation. The pharmacologic therapies include the use of exogenous surfactant, corticosteroids, acetylcysteine (antioxidant), ketoconazole, nitric oxide, eicosanoids and their inhibitors, sodium nitroprusside (vasodilator), pentoxifylline, antiendotoxin, and anticytokine therapy and antibiotics.

ACYCLOVIR

(Acyclovir injection 50 mg/mL (as sodium))

Acyclovir is an antiviral agent and an antiherpes virus agent. The herpes virus family includes the herpes simplex virus, varicella zoster virus, cytomegalovirus, and Epstein–Barr virus. Acyclovir (Zovirax), a synthetic acyclic purine neuroside analog, has antiviral activity against the herpes viruses, especially herpes simplex type 1. It inhibits viral replication by inhibiting DNA synthesis. It interacts with the virus-induced enzyme, especially thymidine kinase and DNA polymerase (see Figure 16). Mutations that lead to

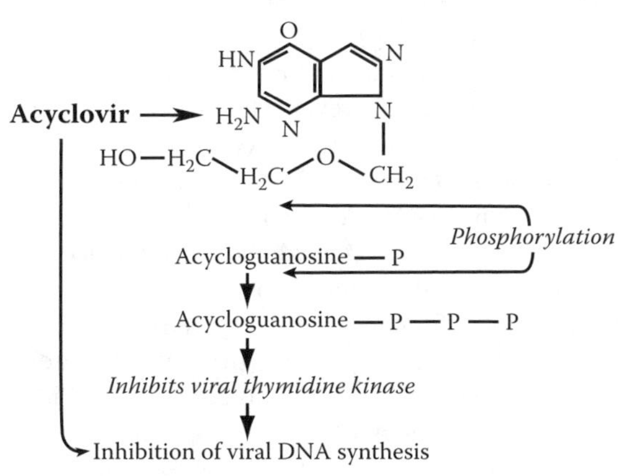

FIGURE 16 Acyclovir inhibits viral replication by inhibiting DNA synthesis.

amino acid substitutions then give rise to resistance in either enzyme. Acyclovir is effective in the treatment of herpes simplex virus type 1 and type 2 infections, including chronic and recurrent mucocutaneous herpes in the immunologically impaired host, primary and secondary genital herpes, neonatal herpes, and herpes simplex encephalitis.

In genital herpes, oral acyclovir (200 mg every 4 hours, 5 times daily for 10 days) reduces the duration of acute infection, attenuates pain and new lesion formation, and decreases but does not eliminate the recurrence of episodes. Acyclovir is effective in localized cutaneous herpes zoster infection and chicken pox infection, lessening severe itching and lesion formation.

Parenteral acyclovir (e.g., 5 mg/kg infused at a constant rate over 1 hour every 8 hours for 7 days) may be used in mucosal and cutaneous herpes simplex virus infections, and in varicella zoster infections (shingles) in immunocompromised patients and in herpes simplex encephalitis.

Acyclovir is available for topical application (Zovirax ointment 5% 50 mg/kg in a polyethylene glycol base), which may cause mucosal irritation and transient burning when applied to genital lesions.

Acyclovir is slowly absorbed from the GI tract, and peak effective plasma concentration is reached in 1.5 to 2 hours. It is widely distributed in tissues and body fluids, including brain, kidney, lung, liver, muscle, spleen, uterus, vaginal mucosa, vaginal secretions, CSF, and herpetic vesicular fluid. Acyclovir is eliminated by glomerular filtration and tubular secretion. It decreases the renal clearance of methotrexate, which is eliminated by active tubular secretion.

The side effects of oral acyclovir are nausea, diarrhea, rash, headache, and rarely nephrotoxicity or neurotoxicity. The principal dose-limiting toxicities of intravenous acyclovir are preexisting renal insufficiency, high doses (plasma level >25 μg/hour), or both. Rapid infusion, dehydration, inadequate urine flow, or nephrotoxic agents increase the risk. Probenecid decreases the renal clearance of acyclovir and prolongs its half-life, and acyclovir decreases the renal clearance of methotrexate or other agents undergoing active tubular secretion. The combined use of zidovudine and acyclovir have caused severe somnolence and lethargy.

ADALIMUMAB

(Humira injection 40 mg per 0.8 mL)

Adalimumab is another anti-TNF product of intravenous use. This recombinant human IgG1 monoclonal antibody was created by phage display technology and is approved for use in rheumatoid arthritis. Adalimumab is an immunomodulating agent. It blocks the interaction of human tumor necrosis factor (TNF)-alpha with receptors and modulates biological responses induced or regulated by TNF. Adalimumab reduces signs and symptoms and inhibits progression of structural damage in patients with moderate to severe active **rheumatoid arthritis** who have had an inadequate response to one or more disease-modifying antirheumatic drugs.

Anti-TNF Reagents

Infliximab (REMI-CADE) is a chimeric anti-TNF-α monoclonal antibody containing a human constant region and a murine variable region. It binds with high affinity to TNF-α and prevents the cytokine from binding to its receptors.

Patients with rheumatoid arthritis have elevated levels of TNF-α in their joints, whereas patients with Crohn's disease have elevated levels of TNF-α in their stools. In one trial, infliximab plus methotrexate improved the signs and symptoms of rheumatoid arthritis more than methotrexate alone. Patients with active Crohn's disease who had not responded to other immunosuppressive therapies also improved when treated with infliximab, including those with Crohn's-related fistulae. Infliximab is approved in the United States for treating the symptoms of rheumatoid arthritis, and is used in combination with methotrexate in patients who do not respond to methotrexate alone. It also is approved for treatment of symptoms of moderate to severe Crohn's disease in patients who have failed to respond to conventional therapy, and in treatment to reduce the number of draining fistulae in Crohn's disease patients. About 1 of 6 patients receiving infliximab experiences an infusion reaction characterized by fever, urticaria, hypotension, and dyspnea within 1 to 2 hours after antibody administration. Serious infections also have occurred in infliximab-treated patients, most frequently in the upper respiratory and urinary tracts. The development of antinuclear antibodies, and rarely a lupus-like syndrome, have been reported after treatment with infliximab.

Although not a monoclonal antibody, etanercept (Enbrel) is mechanistically related to infliximab because it also targets TNF-α. Etanercept contains the ligand-binding portion of a human TNF-α receptor fused to the Fc portion of human IgG_1 and binds to TNF-α and prevents it from interacting with its receptors. It is approved in the United States for treatment of the symptoms of rheumatoid arthritis in patients who have not responded to other treatments. Etanercept can be used in combination with methotrexate in patients who have not responded adequately to methotrexate alone. As with infliximab, serious infections have occurred after treatment with etanercept. Injection-site reactions (erythema, itching, pain, or swelling) have occurred in more than one-third of etanercept-treated patients.

ADAPALENE

(Differin cream 0.1%, gel 0.1%, solution 0.1%)

Adapalene, a derivative of **naphthoic acid**, is a synthetic retinoid-like compound that is available in solution, cream, and gel formulations for topical use. In addition to displaying typical retinoid effects, it also has antiinflammatory properties. Adapalene has similar efficacy to tretinoin, but unlike tretinoin, it is stable in sunlight and tends to be less irritating in nature.

Retinoids include natural compounds and synthetic derivatives of retinol that exhibit vitamin A activity. Retinoids have many important functions throughout the body, including roles in vision, regulation of cell proliferation and differentiation and bone growth, immune defense, and tumor suppression. Because vitamin A affects normal epithelial differentiation, it was investigated as a treatment for cutaneous disorders but was abandoned initially because of unfavorable side effects. Molecular modifications yielded compounds with vastly improved margins of safety. First-generation retinoids include retinol, tretinoin (all-*trans*-retinoic acid), isotretinoin (13-*cis*-retinoic acid), and alitretinoin (9-*cis*-retinoic acid). Second-generation retinoids, also known as aromatic retinoids, were created by alteration of the cyclic end group, and include acitretin. Third-generation retinoids contain further modifications and are called arotinoids. Members of this generation include **tazarotene** and **bexarotene. Adapalene**, a derivative of naphthoic acid with retinoid-like properties, does not fit precisely into any of the three generations.

Retinoic acid (RA) exerts its effects on gene expression by activating two families of receptors—retinoic acid receptors (RARs) and the retinoid X receptors (RXRs)—that are members of the thyroid/steroid hormone receptor superfamily. Retinoids (ligands) bind transcription factors (nuclear receptors), and the ligand–receptor complex then binds to the promoter regions of target genes to regulate their expression. The gene products formed contribute to the desirable pharmacological effects of these drugs and their unwanted side effects. Additional complexity arises because each receptor has three isoforms (α, β, and γ) that form homo- and heterodimers. Retinoid-responsive tissues express one or more RAR and RXR subtypes in various combinations that determine activity locally. Human skin contains mainly RARα and RARβ.

ADEFOVIR DIPIVOXIL

(Hepsera tablets 10 mg)

Adefovir is an antiviral agent that inhibits hepatitis B virus (HBV) DNA polymerase (reverse transcriptase) by competing with the natural substrate deoxyadenosine triphosphate and by causing DNA chain termination after its incorporation into viral DNA. Adefovir is indicated in the treatment of chronic hepatitis B in adults with evidence of active viral replication and evidence of persistent elevations in serum aminotransferases or histologically active disease. Adefovir dipivoxil (9-[2-[bis[(pivaloyloxy)methoxy] phosphinyl]methoxyl]ethyl]adenine, bis-POM PMEA) is a diester prodrug of adefovir, an acyclic phosphonate nucleotide analog of adenosine monophosphate.

It is inhibitory *in vitro* against a range of DNA and RNA viruses, but its clinical use is limited to HBV infections. Inhibitory concentrations for HBV range from 0.2 to 1.2 μ*M* in cell culture, and it is active against lamivudine-resistant HBV strains. Oral adefovir dipivoxil shows dose-dependent inhibition of hepad navirus replication in animal models. *In vitro* combinations of adefovir and lamivudine or other anti-HBV nucleosides show enhanced antihepadnavirus activity *in vitro*.

Adefovir dipivoxil enters cells and is deesterified to adefovir. Adefovir is converted by cellular enzymes to the diphosphate, which acts as a competitive inhibitor of viral DNA polymerases and reverse transcriptases with respect to deoxy-adenosine triphosphate and also serves as a chain terminator of viral DNA synthesis.

Adefovir dipivoxil causes dose-related nephrotoxicity and tubular dysfunction, manifested by azotemia and hypophosphatemia, acidosis, glycosuria, and proteinuria that usually are reversible months after discontinuation. The lower dose (10 mg/day) used in chronic HBV infection patients has been associated with a few adverse events (e.g., headache, abdominal discomfort, diarrhea, and asthenia) and negligible renal toxicity compared with a threefold higher dose.

ADENOSINE

(Adenocard injection 3 mg/mL, Adenoscan injection 3 mg/mL)

Adenosine slows conduction through the atrioventricular (AV) node; it can interrupt reentry pathways through AV node and restore normal sinus rhythm. Adenosine is indicated in the conversion to sinus rhythm of paroxysmal supraventricular tachycardia (PSVT), including that associated with Wolff–Parkinson–Whit syndrome. It is second- or third-degree AV black or sick sinus syndrome (except in patients with a functioning artificial pacemaker), atrial flutter, atrial fibrillation, and ventricular tachycardia.

As an **autacoid**, adenosine possesses negative chronotropic and inotropic effects, is a vasodilator in almost all vascular beds, inhibits neurotransmitter release in the CNS, causes sedation, displays anticonvulsant activity, regulates renin release, inhibits platelet aggregation, modulates lymphocyte function, induces bronchospasm, and inhibits lipolysis.

Receptors for adenosine are referred to as purinergic receptors (P1, which should be distinguished from the P2 receptors that mediate the actions of ATP in the gastrointestinal tract and vascular endothelium). Adenosine is able to modulate adenylate cyclase, similar to acetylcholine. To accomplish this, it interacts with ion channels to hyperpolarize and decrease the duration of the action potentials, and activates phospholipase C in certain tissues.

Drugs may slow automatic rhythms by altering any of the four determinants of spontaneous pacemaker discharge, increase maximum diastolic potential, decrease phase 4 slope, threshold potential, or increase action potential duration. **Adenosine** and acetylcholine may increase maximum diastolic potential, and β-adrenergic receptor antagonist (β-blockers) may decrease phase 4 slope. Block of Na^+ or Ca^{2+} channels usually results in altered threshold, and block of cardiac K^+ channels prolongs the action potential.

Adenosine (Adenocard) is a naturally occurring nucleoside that is administered as a rapid intravenous bolus for the acute termination of reentrant supraventricular arrhythmias. The effects of adenosine are mediated by its interaction with specific G-protein-coupled adenosine receptors. Adenosine activates acetylcholine-sensitive K^+ current in the atrium and sinus and AV nodes, resulting in shortening of action potential duration, hyperpolarization, and slowing of normal automaticity. Adenosine also inhibits the electrophysiological effects of increased intracellular cyclic AMP that occur with sympathetic stimulation. A major advantage of adenosine therapy is that adverse effects are short-lived because the drug is transported into cells and deaminated so rapidly. Transient asystole (lack of any cardiac rhythm whatsoever) is common but usually lasts less than 5 seconds, and is in fact the therapeutic goal. Most patients feel a sense of chest fullness and dyspnea when therapeutic doses (6 to 12 mg) of adenosine are administered.

Rarely, an adenosine bolus can precipitate bronchospasm or atrial fibrillation presumably by heterogeneously shortening atrial action potentials.

The effects of adenosine are potentiated in patients receiving **dipyridamole**, an adenosine-uptake inhibitor, and in patients with cardiac transplants owing to denervation hypersensitivity. **Methylxanthines**, such as theophylline and caffeine, block adenosine receptors; therefore, larger than usual doses are required to produce an antiarrhythmic effect in patients who have consumed these agents in beverages or as therapy.

ADOPTIVE IMMUNOTHERAPY

Over the last decade, the advances in cellular and molecular immunology have been tremendous. Our continuously improving understanding of the immune system and the appreciation of the mechanisms by which tumors and viral or bacterial infections are controlled have led to promising new treatment strategies. Adoptive transfer of tailored **antigen-specific immune cells** and/or **optimally designed immunological effector molecules** is an elegant and promising approach to the establishment or restoration of protective immune responses.

Dendritic cells (DC) are the most powerful antigen-presenting cells that induce and maintain primary immune responses *in vitro* and *in vivo*. The development of protocols for the *ex vivo* generation of DC provided a rationale to design and develop **DC-based vaccination** studies for the treatment of infectious and malignant diseases. The efficacy of antigen loading and delivery into DC is pivotal for the optimal induction of T-cell-mediated immune responses. Recently, it was shown that DC transfected with RNA coding for a **tumor-associated antigen** (TAA), or whole-tumor RNA are able to induce potent antigen- and tumor-specific T-cell responses directed against multiple epitopes. The latter technique does not require the definition of the TAA or HLA haplotype of the patients and has the potential of broad clinical application. Such a polyvalent vaccine might be able to reduce the probability of clonal tumor escape and to elicit CTL responses directed against naturally processed and presented immunodominant tumor antigens. Additional targeting of **HLA class II restricted epitopes** may further amplify and prolong the induced T-cell responses.

Dendritic cells can either be generated from progenitors such as stem cells or CD14+ monocytes, or isolated directly from the blood. Blood-derived DC are present as at least two distinct populations—myeloid and plasmacytoid DC.

Dendritic cells (DC) are important **antigen-presenting cells** (APC) that can prime naive T-cells and control **lymphocyte-mediated adaptive immune responses** with respect to magnitude, memory, and self-tolerance. Understanding the biology of these cells is central to the development of new generation immunotherapies for cancer and chronic infection.

Adoptive dendritic cell-based immunotherapy represents a promising approach to overcoming peripheral tolerance against **autologous tumor antigens** and to maintaining protective **antitumor immunity**. The translation of successful preclinical studies, however, appears to be hampered by new complexities associated with the clinical situation.

Poly(D,L-Lactide-co-glycolide) (PLGA) polymers have been used for the production of biodegradable medical sutures and for controlled drug release for decades. Useful characteristics such as *in vivo* biodegradability, an adjustable release profile, and the very high encapsulation capacity have stimulated immunologists to explore PLGA microsphere (MS) as antigen delivery systems for vaccination for more than 15 years.

Serological analysis of tumor antigens by recombinant cDNA expression cloning (Serex) allows the systematic cloning of tumor antigens recognized by the spontaneous autoantibody repertoire of cancer patients. For SEREX, cDNA expression libraries are constructed from fresh tumor specimens, packaged into λ-phage vectors and expressed recombinantly in *Escherichia coli*. Recombinant proteins expressed during the lytic infection of bacteria are transferred onto nitrocellulose membranes to be probed with diluted autologous patient serum for identification of clones reactive with high-titered IgG antibodies.

Attempts to treat patients with *tumor-reactive cytotoxic T-lymphocytes* (CTL) have been limited. This is due to the difficulty of isolating and expanding functionally active T-cells, which are present at extremely low frequencies in the peripheral blood. Recently developed multimers of the HLA-peptide complex mimic the natural ligand of the T-cell receptor and, therefore, fluorochrome-labeled multimers allow visualization and isolation of rare T-cells with defined specificity. Multimer-guided T-cell sorting permits the *in vitro* culture of antigen-specific T-cells as lines or clones. Cytolytic T-cells capable of recognizing HLA-peptide complexes endogenously processed by tumor cells are selected for further expansion because lysis of tumor cells *in vitro* is a prerequisite for effective tumor elimination *in vivo*. The expansion of tumor-reactive $CD8^+$ T-cells yields cell numbers sufficient for adoptive transfer. Tumor-reactive T-cells retain the functional activity in terms of cytolysis after expansion, encouraging their use in the immunotherapy of cancer patients. Advances in immunological monitoring provide the means to track tumor antigen-specific CTL in humans after adoptive transfer with greater specificity and sensitivity than before. Novel tools can be used not only to detect antigen-specific CTL but also to evaluate the function and phenotype of individual T-cells. Peptide major histocompatibility complexes (MHC) class I multimeric complexes are proving invaluable as fluorescent reagents for tracking of antigen-specific T-cells. The multimeric complex is constructed of four synthetic and biotinylated peptide-loaded MHC molecules, which are linked by a fluorochrome-labeled streptavidin molecule. In contrast to "indirect" assays such as limiting dilution analysis (LDA) or ^{51}Cr release assays requiring *in vitro* stimulation, this method allows direct monitoring of very low numbers of peptide-specific T-cells without the need for *in vitro* sensitization. By combining the use of multimerics with anticytokine antibodies, a more detailed picture of the tracked T-cell can be obtained.

Adoptive therapy with **allogeneic or tumor-specific T-cells** has shown substantial clinical effects for several human tumors, but the widespread application of this strategy remains a daunting task. The antigen specificity of T-lymphocytes is solely determined by the T-cell receptor (TCR) α and β chains. Consequently, genetic transfer of TCR chains may form an alternative and potentially appealing strategy to impose a desirable tumor-antigen specificity onto cytotoxic or helper T-cell populations. In this strategy, autologous or donor-derived T-cell populations are equipped with a TCR of defined reactivity in short-term *ex vivo* cultures, a reinfusion of the redirected cells is used to supply T-cell reactivity against defined tumor-specific antigens.

Reprogramming T-cell populations by **TCR gene transfer** is a new therapeutic tool for adoptive tumor immunotherapy. Gene transfer of human leukocyte antigen (HLA)-transgenic mice-derived TCR into human T-cells allows the circumvention of tolerance to tumor-associated (self) antigens (TAA). This chapter reports on the identification of the α and β chains of the heterodimeric TCR derived from a mouse T-cell clone. The related DNA fragments are inserted into a retroviral vector for heterologous expression of the TAA-specific TCR in human T-cells. Polymerase chain reaction (PCR)-based cloning protocols are provided for the tailor-made customization of murine TCR.

A major objective of immune analysis in the setting of cancer, cancer vaccination, and therapy is to accurately characterize and isolate functional T-cells elicited by a tumor. Secretion of cytokines is an important function of activated effector and memory T-cells. The **cytokine secretion assay** (CSA) directly assesses T-cells secreting cytokines after a short restimulation *in vitro*. Cells can be stained for surface markers, enabling characterization of subsets. Viable cytokine-secreting T-cells can be isolated for expansion and further functional testing or adoptive transfer. Because the method is not restricted to any antigen or MHC haplotype, it enables us to detect $CD8^+$ as well as $CD4^+$ T-cells reacting against a wide vary of tumor-associated antigens, ranging from particular known tumor antigens to whole tumor cells and crude tumor lysates. Thus, the method provides a valuable tool to analyze and isolate functional tumor-responsive T-cells according to one of their effector functions.

Monoclonal antibodies are homogeneous sets of immunoglobulins with well-defined specificity and biochemical characteristics. They were introduced into clinical practice in the early 1980s and, since then, their use has rapidly expanded. Most of the side effects observed with first-generation murine (mouse or rat) antibodies have been successfully overcome with the advent of humanized (chimeric or CDR-grafted) and, more recently, fully human antibodies.

In recent years, the development of tumor-specific recombinant antibodies fused to **immunostimulatory cytokines** such as **interleukin-2** (IL-2), interleukin-12 (IL-12), and granulocyte/macrophage colony-stimulating factor (GM-CSF) has provided a promising novel approach to cancer immunotherapy. The combined properties of specific targeting of antibodies and the immune stimulation of cytokines results in high cytokine concentration in the tumor microenvironment, and as a consequence, in an improved tumoricidal activity of the antibody and/or in a secondary effective immune response against the tumor. In the present chapter we describe strategies for the construction, expression, and *in vitro* characterization of antibody–cytokine fusion proteins with particular emphasis on antibody/IL-2 fusion proteins.

Targeted cancer therapy is a promising strategy for the treatment of this disease. In this approach, a cytotoxic agent (CA), such as a drug or a radionuclide, is attached, usually covalently, to a "**targeting**" **vehicle** (TV), which in turn is capable of recognizing specific receptor motifs on the surface of the tumor cells. Once administered systemically, the construct would localize on the tumor through the TV moiety and would release the CA cargo, resulting in the destruction of the malignant tissue. Small-molecule peptides as well as monoclonal antibodies have been used as TVs.

Graft-mediated antileukemia (GVL) activity is a major factor contributing to the success of **allogeneic hematopoietic stem transplantation** (aHCT). Recent advances have permitted the establishment of GVL activity without the need for a myeloablative conditioning regimen, thereby permitting even older and sicker patients to avail of potentially curative therapy. Use of adoptive immunotherapy by combining reduced intensity conditioning and **donor leukocyte infusion** (DLI) has resulted in strategies that can be exploited to maximize GVL effects while minimizing toxicity. These advances, combined with new molecularly targeted agents, create new possibilities to develop less toxic, curative therapy for a greater number of patients.

Bone-marrow transplantation is an approved curative treatment for many hemato- and oncologic diseases. Nevertheless, the severe acute clinical course of **graft-versus-host disease** (GVHD) after allogeneic bone-marrow transplantation is frequently fatal, and is to date not curable. Acute GVHD must, therefore, be prevented from the start of the bone-marrow transplantation by immunosuppressive medication, causing sometimes serious side effects. Therefore, new preventive strategies are tested, starting with animal experiments. Often mice are chosen for this kind of trial, and the clinical protocol of bone-marrow transplantation is transferred into the experimental settings. The first step to induce an acute GVHD is whole-body irradiation of the recipients. Several methods are available for this purpose: the most common is a ^{60}**cobalt source** (γ-irradiation); less common are a ^{137}**cesium source** (γ-irradiation) and a linear (particle) accelerator (photons). Differences between these radiation techniques can occur and can unexpectedly interfere with the results of the experiments.

GVH alloresponses mediated by **delayed donor lymphocyte infusions** (DLI) can occur in the absence of GVHD. These GVH responses are confined to the **lymphohematopoietic system** and mediate graft-versus-leukemia (GVL) reactions without causing GVHD.

ADRENOCORTICOTROPIC HORMONE (ACTH)

The adrenal steroids are divided into three major categories: glucocorticoids, mineralocorticoids, and sex hormones. The glucocorticoids mainly influence carbohydrate metabolism and, to a certain extent, protein and lipid metabolism. The main glucocorticoid is cortisol, with a daily secretion of 15 mg. The mineralocorticoids influence salt and water metabolism and, in general, conserve sodium levels. They promote the resorption of sodium and the secretion of potassium in the cortical collecting tubules, and possibly the connecting segment. They also elicit hydrogen secretion in the medullary collecting tubules. The main mineralocorticoid is aldosterone, with a daily secretion of 100 μg. Small quantities of progesterone, testosterone, and estradiol are also produced by the adrenal gland. However, they play a minor role compared to the testicular and ovarian hormones.

Adrenal glucocorticoid and androgen production are controlled predominantly by the hypothalamic–pituitary axis, whereas the production of aldosterone by the zona glomerulosa is predominantly regulated by the renin–angiotensin system and potassium concentration. The hypothalamus, pituitary, and adrenal form a neuroendocrine axis whose primary function is to regulate the production of both cortisol and some of the adrenal steroids (Figure 38).

Corticotropin-releasing factor and arginine vasopressin, which are released predominantly by the paraventricular nucleus of the hypothalamus, are important regulators of corticotropin (ACTH) release, which in turn triggers the release of cortisol and other steroids by the adrenal gland. Both the administration of certain psychoactive agents and emotional arousal originating from the limbic system are able to modify the functions of the pituitary–adrenal axis and to stimulate the synthesis of cortisol.

ACTH elicits the following effects: It enhances the synthesis of pregnenolone, activates adenylate cyclase and elevates the cyclic adenosine monophosphate level, enhances the level of adrenal steroids, especially cortisol, and reduces the level of ascorbic acid.

The level of cortisol is thought to directly control the secretion of ACTH through a negative feedback mechanism that may be directed at both the hypothalamus and the anterior pituitary gland. Conversely, a reduced concentration of cortisol or cortisol-like substances eliminates the negative effect and enhances the release of ACTH (see Figure 38).

Adrenocorticoids with topical antiinflammatory agents available as cream, gel, lotion, or ointment are

Alclometasone dipropionate	Diflucortolone valerate
Amcinonide	Flumethasone pivalate
Beclomethasone dipropionate	Fluocinolone acetonide
Betamethasone benzoate	Fluocinonide
Betamethasone dipropionate	Flurandrenolide
Betamethasone valerate	Halcinonide
Clobetasol propionate	Hydrocortisone
Clobetasone butyrate	Hydrocortisone acetate
Clocortolone pivalate	Hydrocortisone butyrate
Desonide	Hydrocortisone valerate
Desoximethasone	Methylprednisolone acetate
Dexamethasone	Mometasone furoate
Dexamethasone sodium phosphate	Triamcinolone acetonide
Diflorasone diacetate	

AGED PATIENTS: ALTERED PHARMACOKINETIC PROFILE

Pharmacokinetic Profiles	Parameters Affected
Absorption	Elevated gastric pH
	Decreased gastrointestinal blood flow
	Decreased active transport mechanisms
Distribution	Decreased total body water
	Decreased lean body mass
	Increased body fat
	Decreased serum albumin
Metabolism	Decreased liver blood flow
	Decreased liver size
	Possibly decreased enzymatic activity
Excretion	Decreased glomerular filtration rate
	Decreased renal blood flow
	Decreased tubular function
Receptors	Diminished cholinergic, alpha-1 adrenergic, and opioid receptors

Statistical analysis has firmly established four isolated but interrelated facts about the aged population.

- Longevity is increasing.
- The aged population of the world is expanding.
- The aged population may have multiple diseases and may be taking multiple medications.
- The potential of drug–drug interactions and adverse drug reactions is a conspicuous problem among the elderly.

The appreciation and application of concepts involved in geriatric pharmacology will not only reduce the incidence of potential drug-related toxicities but will also enhance the quality of life for this group of patients. As in the pediatric population, the pharmacokinetic parameters are distinct for the older age groups. Because the plasma albumin level decreases with aging, the binding of drugs to plasma protein also diminishes. Furthermore, because the total body fat increases with aging, the storage of lipid-soluble substances (silent sites) also varies. Because the total water in the body also decreases, this alters the volume of distribution of the drugs. The metabolism of some drugs is reduced, and thus their half-lives are increased. Because the glomerular filtration rate and the tubular excretion rate are diminished by the aging process, the excretion of most drugs and their metabolites is below the standard for younger patients. Consequently, the very old patient behaves pharmacokinetically very much like the very young one. However, to further complicate the situation, unlike pediatric patients, the elderly may have several diseases, including cardiovascular ones, and may be taking several agents, especially those with very narrow margins of safety (e.g., digitalis and the tricyclic antidepressants). Therefore, it is imperative that these pharmacokinetic principles be taken into consideration when prescribing medications for older patients in order to avoid undue toxicities.

AGALSIDASE BETA

(Fabrazyme)

Agalsidase is an enzyme replacement therapy that provides an exogenous source of α-galactosidase A and is used in the treatment of **Fabry's disease**.

The Lipid Storage Disorders

Fabry's disease and Gaucher's disease—for each of these disorders, affected individuals may survive into adulthood.

Fabry's disease. Fabry's disease is an inborn error of glycosphindolipid metabolism characterized by angiokeratomas (telangiectatic kin lesions), hypohidrosis, corneal and lenticular opacities, acrogaresthesia, and vascular disease of the kidney, heart, and/or brain. The disease is an X-linked recessive trait that is manifested in affected pemizygous males and has an estimated prevalence of 1 in 40,000. Atypical hemizygous males with residual α-galactosidase A activity may be asymptomatic or have late-onset, mild manifestations, usually limited to the heart. Heterozygous females are usually asymptomatic or exhibit mild manifestations.

The disease results from the deficient activity of **α-galactosidase A**, which is encoded by a gene on the long arm of the X chromosome (Xq22). The defect leads to the accumulation of neutral glycosphingolipids, primarily globotriaosylceramide, in the plasma and lysosomes of vascular endothelial and smooth-muscle cells. The progressive deposition of glycosphingolipid in vessel walls results in ischemia and infarction, the major disease manifestations. Affected males who have blood group B or AB have a more severe course due to accumulation of blood group B substance, which is normally degraded by α-galactosidase A. The cDNA and genomic sequences encoding α-galactosidase A have been characterized, and known mutations responsible for this disease include amino acid substitutions, gene rearrangements, and mRNA scheme defects.

AGGREGIN

Platelets circulate in blood without adhering to other platelets or to the endothelium. However, when the endothelial cells are perturbed, the platelets adhere and undergo a change in shape and aggregate. Adenosine diphosphate (ADP) is known to induce the platelet shape change, aggregation, and exposure of fibrinogen-binding sites (see Figure 92).

The platelet surface contains aggregin, a membrane protein with a molecular weight of 100 kDa, with physical and immunochemical properties that differ from those of platelet glycoprotein IIIa.

Binding to aggregin is required in order for epinephrine-induced platelet aggregation to take place. In turn, epinephrine increases the affinity of ADP for its receptor. Thrombin stimulates platelet aggregation independent of ADP, but by raising the level of calcium in the cytoplasm, it activates platelet calpain, which in turn cleaves aggregin.

AGMATINE

Agmatine, an endogenous vasodilating substance, has recently been identified as an endogenous clonidine-displacing substance (CDS) in mammalian brain. Agmatine, like CDS, binds to imidazoline receptors (I receptors) and alpha$_2$-adrenoceptors that stimulate the release of catecholamines from adrenal chromaffin cells in a dose-dependent manner. Although arginine decarboxylase, the enzyme which forms agmatine, has been localized in endothelial cells and endothelial cells storing agmatine, the effects of agmatine on systemic hemodynamics are unknown.

AGRANULOCYTOSIS: DRUG-INDUCED

Agranulocytosis is a symptom complex characterized by marked decrease in the number of granulocytes, and by lesions of the throat and other mucous membranes of the gastrointestinal tract, and of the skin; also called **granulocytopenia** and **Schultz's disease**.

In 1922, Werner Schultz drew attention to a syndrome of unknown cause that he had observed especially in women of middle age, and which was characterized by severe sore throat, marked prostration, extreme reduction, or even complete disappearance of the granulocytes from the blood, and, in rapid succession, sepsis and death. He considered this to be a clinical entity that he called agranulocytosis.

In agranulocytosis the most significant feature revealed by autopsy is a lack of granulocytes. Polymorphonuclear leukocytes are conspicuously absent about the necrotic lesions that may be found in the oral cavity, skin, vagina, uterus, or the gastrointestinal tract, and only plasma cells and lymphocytes are seen. The picture is that of overwhelming septicemia in a patient with no neutrophils. Drugs causing agranulocytosis include the following items.

Acetaminophen
Acetazolamide
Acetylsalicylic acid
Allopurinol
β-Lactam antibiotics
Benzodiazepines
Brompheniramine
Carbamazepine
Captopril
Ceftriaxone
Chloramphenicol
Chlorpropamide
Chlorpromazine
Cimetidine
Clindamycin
Clomipramine
Clozapine
Dapsone
Desipramine
Doxycycline
Ethacrynic acid
Ethosuximide
Fenoprofen
Flucytosine
Ganciclovir
Gentamicin
Gold salts
Griseofulvin
Hydralazine
Hydroxychloroquine
Ibuprofen
Imipramine
Indomethacin
Isoniazid
Levamisole
Lincomycin
Meprobamate
Methazolamide
Methimazole
Metronidazole
Nitrofurantoin
Oxyphenbutazone
Para-aminosalicyclic acid
Penicillamine
Pentazocine
Phenothiazines
Phenylbutazone
Phenytoin
Primidone
Procainamide
Propranolol
Propylthiouracil
Pyrimethamine
Quinine
Rifampin
Streptomycin
Sulfa antibiotics
Tocainide
Tolbutamide
Vancomycin
Zidovudine

A number of mechanisms may produce drug-induced agranulocytosis. For example, chlorpromazine and other phenothiazine derivatives (perphenazine, prochlorperazine, thioridazine, and triflupromazine) may cause agranulocytosis. The incidence of this is higher among female and elderly patients whose bone marrow has lower proliferative potential. These agents inhibit DNA polymerase, thymidylate kinase, and the incorporation of [^{3}H]thymidine into DNA. Because the phenothiazine-induced agranulocytosis is a toxic reaction, it may be prevented by carefully monitoring the status of peripheral blood.

AIDS DRUGS

See Protease Inhibitors, Stavudine, Zalcitabine, Zidovudine.

ALBUMIN

(Albuminar-5, Albutein 5%, Bumianate 5%, Plasbumin-5)

Plasma albumin (molecular weight, 66,400), the most abundant protein in the plasma, exerts 80% of the colloid osmotic pressure of blood. Albumin has two binding sites: site I binds structurally unrelated substances (e.g., warfarin, phenytoin, and sulfonamides), and site II, which is more selective, binds a smaller number of drugs (i.e., diazepam, phenylbutazone, and ibuprofen).

The percentage of protein binding of drugs at therapeutic levels varies dramatically. Some drugs such as allopurinol, heparin, and isoniazid do not become bound. Other drugs such as antipyrine, ethambutol, and theophylline become bound to the extent of only 4 to 15%. Several drugs such as ampicillin (25%) and digoxin (23%) show low protein binding; some drugs such as atropine (50%) and meperidine (40%) show moderate protein binding; and some drugs such as carbamazepine (72%), furosemide (75%), nitrofurantoin (70%), and rifampin (85%) show high degrees of protein binding. Some such as dicumarol (97%), diazepam (96%), phenylbutazone (98%), and diazoxide (96%) bind extensively to plasma proteins.

The binding sites of the protein are not unlimited and are subject to saturation. When this occurs, toxicity may develop following further drug administration, because the later portion of the drug remains free. Consistent with this view is the observation that toxic manifestations of drugs are quite frequent and considerably higher in individuals suffering from hypoalbuminemia or altered plasma and tissue protein concentrations, or both.

Drugs may alter the protein binding of other agents. For instance, aspirin decreases the binding of thyroxine, and the binding of bilirubin is hindered by many pharmacologic agents. The more tightly bound drugs can displace the less firmly bound agents. The intensity of the effect of displaced drug on the patient will simply depend on the blood level of the free drug and its nature. At times, the effect may be highly undesirable and even fatal. Only the slight displacement of a highly bound drug such as dicumarol (an oral anticoagulant) by phenylbutazone, which has greater affinity for binding sites, can cause serious hemorrhage. Because only 3% of the anticoagulant is free, an additional displacement of 3% increases its effects by 100%. The serum albumin and total protein concentrations are lower in infancy and increase to adult values by the age of 10 to 12 months.

Normal serum albumin (5% containing 130 to 160 mEq/L sodium) may be used in the treatment of a patient in shock with greatly reduced blood volume, after a burn injury, and in acute but not chronic hypoproteinemia. The use of albumin in transfusion (1 g/kg 1 to 2 hours before transfusion) is effective in hyperbilirubinemia and erythroblastosis fetalis, increasing the amount of bilirubin removed with each transfusion.

ALBUTEROL SULFATE

(Proventil, Ventolin)

Albuterol sulfate is available as a tablet (2 mg, 4 mg), solution (2 mg/5 ml), and aerosol inhaler (90 mcg/metered spray).

Albuterol selectively stimulates beta-adrenergic receptors in the lungs causing relaxation of bronchial smooth muscles, which in turn relieves bronchospasm and reduces airway resistance. The selective beta$_2$-adrenergic stimulants cause bronchodilation without cardiac acceleration. Metaproterenol and terbutaline are available in tablet form, and terbutaline is also available for subcutaneous injection. Metaproterenol and albuterol are available in metered-dose inhalers.

Inhalational selective beta$_2$-adrenergic receptor agonists (albuterol, terbutaline, fenoterol, and bitolterol) have a rapid onset of action and are effective for 3 to 6 hours. Formoterol and salmeterol are longer-acting agents (12 hours) and may prove useful in treating nocturnal symptoms.

Albuterol is used to relieve and prevent bronchospasm in patients with reversible obstructive airway disease and in individuals with exercise-induced bronchospasm. The onset of action of albuterol is 5 to 15 minutes, peak of action is 0.5 to 2 hours, and duration of action is 3 to 6 hours. Albuterol does not cross the blood–brain barrier. It must be used cautiously in patients with hyperthyroidism, diabetes mellitus, coronary insufficiency, and hypertension. The concomitant use of albuterol with monoamine oxidase inhibitors or tricyclic antidepressants should be discouraged. Glucocorticoids (beclomethasone, dexamethasone, flunisolide, or triamcinolone) may be used 15 minutes after inhalational albuterol.

ALCLOMETASONE DIPROPIONATE

(Aclovate)

Alclometasone is a topical glucocorticoid with antiinflammatory, antipruritic, and vasoconstrictive properties. It acts by inducing phospholipase A2 inhibitory proteins, thus controlling biosynthesis of potent mediators of inflammation. Alclometasone (0.05% ointment) is a topical adrenocorticoid with antiinflammatory properties that is indicated in inflammation of corticosteroid-responsive dermatoses.

ALCURONIUM

Neuromuscular blocking agents may be used to diagnose myasthenia gravis, facilitate endotracheal intubation, relieve laryngeal spasm, provide relaxation during brief diagnostic and surgical procedures, prevent bone fracture in electroconvulsive therapy, produce apnea and controlled ventilation during thoracic surgery and neurosurgery, reduce muscular spasticity in neurologic diseases (multiple sclerosis, cerebral palsy, or tetanus), and reduce the muscular spasm and pain resulting from sprains, arthritis, myositis, and fibrositis.

Skeletal muscle relaxants can be classified into four categories of depolarizing or competitive blocking agents (e.g., tubocurarine), direct-acting relaxants (e.g., dantrolene sodium), and centrally acting muscle relaxants (e.g., diazepam). Alcuronium is about twice as potent as *d*-tubocurarine, but it has a shorter duration of action. Muscular relaxation occurs 2 to 4 minutes after the injection of 0.2 mg/kg and lasts about 15 to 20 minutes. Like *d*-tubocurarine, it may lower blood pressure but does not cause histamine release. There is no evidence for any significant metabolism of alcuronium, and most of the drug is excreted unchanged in the urine, so it should be used cautiously in the presence of impaired renal function.

ALDESLEUKIN

(Proleukin)

Aldesleukin causes an enhancement of lymphocyte mitogenesis and stimulation of long-term growth of human IL-2-dependent cell lines. It produces an enhancement of lymphocyte cytotoxicity; induction of killer cell (lymphokine-activated [LAK] and natural [NAK]) activity; induction of interferon-gamma production.

Interleukin-2 (IL-2, aldesleukin, proleukin)

The isolation of a cytokine initially named T-cell growth factor, subsequently renamed IL-2, allowed the first attempts to treat cancer by producing lymphocytes specifically cytolytic for the malignant cell. IL-2 is not directly cytotoxic; rather, it induces and expands a T-cell response cytolytic for tumor cells. Clinical trials have studied the antitumor activity of IL-2 both as a single agent and with adoptive cellular therapy using IL-2-stimulated autologous lymphocytes obtained by leukopheresis, termed lymphokine-activated killer (LAK) cells. Randomized trials have not shown that the addition of LAK cells to the treatment regimen improves overall response rates. Later studies in adoptive cellular therapy have used expanded populations of lymphocytes obtained from tumor biopsies and expanded *in vitro*, so-called tumor-infiltrating lymphocytes.

Aldesleukin is indicated in the metastatic renal cell carcinoma and metastatic melanoma. Therapy with aldesleukin for injection should be restricted to patients with normal cardiac and pulmonary functions.

Aldesleukin should be administered in a hospital setting under the supervision of a qualified physician experienced in the use of anticancer agents. An intensive care facility and specialists skilled in cardiopulmonary or intensive care medicine must be available. Aldesleukin administration has been associated with hypotension and reduced organ perfusion, which may be severe and can result in death (see Figure 63).

ALDOSTERONE

The main mineralocorticoid is aldosterone, which is synthesized from 18-hydroxycorticosterone by a dehydrogenase. The consequence of 18-hydroxycorticosterone dehydrogenase deficiency is diminished secretion of aldosterone, and the clinical manifestations consist of sodium depletion, dehydration, hypotension, potassium retention, and enhanced plasma renin levels.

It is generally assumed that the intracellular content of sodium in vascular smooth muscle is increased in essential hypertension. Although the major role of aldosterone (see Figure 17) in the regulation of blood pressure is a renal one,

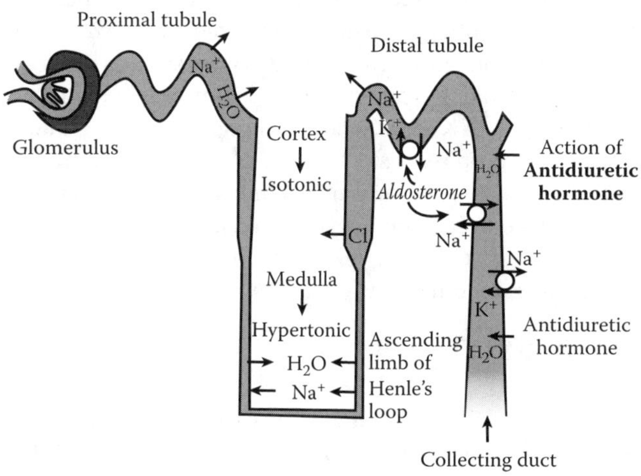

FIGURE 17 The main mineralocorticoid is **aldosterone**, which is synthesized from 18-hydroxycorticosterone by a dehydrogenase. The consequence of 18-hydroxycorticosterone dehydrogenase deficiency is diminished secretion of aldosterone, and the clinical manifestations consist of sodium depletion, dehydration, hypotension, potassium retention, and enhanced plasma renin levels.

it may also be involved in some extrarenal effects responsible for the regulation of body fluid and blood pressure. Recent studies have suggested that vascular walls specifically bind to aldosterone, and that aldosterone has a direct vasoconstrictive effect on vascular smooth muscle *in vitro*. Indeed, canrenoate potassium (Soldactone S), an aldosterone antagonist, reduces blood pressure (see Figure 24).

ALEFACEPT

(Amevive)

Alefacept interferes with lymphocyte activation and is indicated in the treatment of adult patients with moderate to severe chronic plaque psoriasis who are candidates for systemic therapy or phototherapy.

Alefacept was the first immunobiological agent approved for the treatment of moderate to severe psoriasis in patients who are candidates for systemic therapy. 3 Alefacept consists of a recombinant fully human fusion protein composed of the binding site of the leukocyte function-associated antigen 3 (LFA-3) protein and a human IgG1 Fc domain. The LFA-3 portion of the alefacept molecule binds to CD2 on the surface of T-cells, thus blocking a necessary costimulation step in T-cell activation. Importantly, because CD2 is expressed preferentially on memory-effector T-cells, naive T-cells largely are unaffected by alefacept. A second important action of alefacept is its ability to induce apoptosis of memory-effector T-cells through simultaneous binding of its IgG1 portion to immunoglobulin receptors on cytotoxic cells and its LFA-3 portion to CD2 on T-cells, thus inducing granzyme-mediated apoptosis of memory-effector T-cells.

ALEMTUZUMAB

(Campath)

Alemtuzumab is a recombinant DNA-derived humanized monoclonal antibody. Alemtuzumab binds to CD52, a non-modulating antigen that is present on the surface of essentially all B- and T-lymphocytes, a majority of monocytes, macrophages, NK cells, and a subpopulation of granulocytes. The proposed mechanism of action is antibody-dependent lysis. Alemtuzumab is indicated in the treatment of B-cell chronic lymphocytic leukemia in patients who have been treated with alkylating agents and who have failed fudarabine therapy.

ALENDRONATE SODIUM

(Fosamax)

Alendronate sodium (10 mg/day) is indicated for the treatment of **osteoporosis** in postmenopausal women and of **Paget's disease**. It acts as a specific inhibitor of osteoclast-mediated bone resorption. The osteoclasts adhere normally to the bone surface but lack the ruffled border that is indicative of active resorption. Alendronate does not interfere with osteoclast recruitment or attachment, but it does inhibit osteoclast activity. Bones examined 6 and 49 days after (^{3}H)alendronate administration showed that normal bone was formed on top of the alendronate, which was incorporated in bone matrix. Alendronate is not pharmacologically active; thus, it must be continuously administered to suppress osteoclasts on newly formed resorption surfaces. Calcium supplements, antacids, and other oral medications will interfere with absorption of Fosamax. Therefore, patients must wait at least one hour before taking Fosamax.

Several bisphosphonates are available in the United States. Etidronate sodium (Didronel) is used for treatment of Paget's disease and may be used parenterally to treat hypercalcemia. Because etidronate is the only bisphosphonate that inhibits mineralization, it has been supplanted largely by **pamidronate** and **zoledronate** for treating hypercalcemia. **Pamidronate** (Aredia) is approved for management of hypercalcemia but also is effective in other skeletal disorders. Pamidronate is available in the United States only for parenteral administration. For treatment of hypercalcemia, pamidronate may be given as an intravenous infusion of 60 to 90 mg over 4 to 24 hours.

Several newer bisphosphonates have been approved for treatment of Paget's disease. These include **tiludronate** (Skelid), **alendronate** (Fosamax), and **risedronate** (Actonel). Although the drug is approved only for treating hypercalcemia of malignancy, a single injection of zoledronate (zometa) decreased bone turnover markers for 90 days in patients with Paget's disease. Tiludronate and the potent bisphosphonate ibandronate currently are under development for treatment of women with osteoporosis, with encouraging preliminary results.

ALFENTANIL HYDROCHLORIDE

(Alfenta)

Fentanyl is a synthetic opioid related to the phenylpiperidines. The actions of fentanyl and its congeners, **sufentanil**, **remifentanil**, and alfentanil, are similar to those of other μ-receptor agonists.

Alfentanil, an opiate analgesic (8 to 50 mcg/kg IV), is indicated as an adjunct to general anesthetic in the maintenance of general anesthesia with barbiturate, nitrous oxide, and oxygen. In addition, it is used as a primary anesthetic for induction of anesthesia when endotracheal intubation and mechanical ventilation are required.

ALFUZOSIN HYDROCHLORIDE

(Uroxatral)

Alfuzosin selectively blocks alpha-adrenergic receptors in the lower urinary tract, which cause smooth muscle in the bladder neck and prostate to relax, resulting in improved urine flow and a reduction in symptoms of benign prostatic hyperplasia (BPH). It is used in the treatment of BPH. Alfuzosin is a quinazoline-based α_1 receptor antagonist with similar affinity at all of the α_1 receptor subtypes. Its bioavailability is about 64%; it has a half-life of 3 to 5 hours. The recommended dosage is one 10-mg extended-release tablet daily to be taken after the same meal each day.

Prazosin, terazosin, doxazosin, tamsulosin, and alfuzosin have been studied extensively and used widely in patients with benign prostatic hyperplasia. With the exception of tamsulosin, the comparative efficacies of each of these drugs, especially in comparison with relative adverse effects such as postural hypotension, appear similar, although direct comparisons are limited. Tamsulosin at the recommended dose of 0.4 mg daily is less likely to cause orthostatic hypotension than the other drugs. There is growing evidence that the predominant α_1-receptor subtype expressed in the human prostate is the α_1-receptor. Developments in this area will provide the basis for the selection of Ct receptor antagonists with specificity for the relevant subtype of α_1-receptor. However, the possibility remains that some of the symptoms of BPH are due to α_1-receptors in other sites, such as bladder, spinal cord, or brain.

ALGLUCERASE

(Glucocerebrosidase, Glucosylceramidase, Glucocerebrosidase-Beta-Glucosidase [Ceredase])

Alglucerase (initially 60 units/kg by infusion) is indicated for long-term endogenous enzyme (glucoslyceramidase) replacement in confirmed type I Gaucher's disease.

ALITRETINOIN

(Panretin gel 0.1%)

Alitretinoin binds to and activates all known intracellular retinoid receptor substrates. Once activated, these receptors function as transcription factors that regulate the expression of genes that control the process of cellular differentiation and proliferation of both non-rial and neoplastic cells. Alitretinoin is indicated in the topical treatment of AIDS-related **Kaposi sarcoma** (KS).

Retinoids include natural compounds and synthetic derivatives of retinol that exhibit vitamin A activity. Retinoids have many important functions throughout the body, including roles in vision, regulation of cell proliferation and differentiation and bone growth, immune defense, and tumor suppression. Because vitamin A affects normal epithelial differentiation, it was investigated as a treatment for cutaneous disorders but was abandoned initially because of unfavorable side effects. Molecular modifications yielded compounds with vastly improved margins of safety. First-generation retinoids include retinal, tretinoin (all-*trans*-ietmoic acid), isotretinoin (13-*cis*-retinoic acid), and **alitretinoin** (9-*cis*-retinoic acid). Second-generation retinoids, also known as **aromatic retinoids**, were created by alteration of the cyclic end group and include **acitretin**. Third-generation retinoids contain further modifications and are called arotinoids. Members of this generation include **tazarotene** and **bexarotene**. **Adapalene**, a derivative of naphthoic acid with retinoid-like properties, does not fit precisely into any of the three generations.

Retinoic acid (RA) exerts its effects on gene expression by activating two families of receptors—retinoic acid receptors (RARs) and the retinoid X receptors (RXRs)—that are members of the thyroid/steroid hormone receptor superfamily. Retinoids (ligands) bind transcription factors (nuclear receptors), and the ligand–receptor complex then binds to the promoter regions of target genes to regulate their expression. The gene products formed contribute to the desirable pharmacological effects of these drugs and their unwanted side effects. Additional complexity arises because each receptor has three isoforms (α, β, and γ) that form homo- and heterodimers. Retinoid-responsive tissues express one or more RAR and RXR subtypes in various combinations that determine activity locally. Human skin contains mainly RARα and RARβ.

ALLERGIC RHINITIS

Allergic rhinitis is characterized by sneezing; rhinorrhea; obstruction of the nasal passages; conjunctival, nasal, and pharyngeal itching; and lacrimation, all occurring in a temporal relationship to allergen exposure. Although commonly seasonal due to elicitation by airborne pollens, it can be perennial in an environment of chronic exposure. The incidence of allergic rhinitis in North America is about 7%, with the peak occurring in childhood and adolescence.

Drugs effective in allergic dermatitis are:

Agents	Properties
Acrivastine	Non-sedating antihistamine
Azelastine	Antihistamine
Budesonide	Topical corticosteroid
Fenoterol	β_2-Adrenergic agonist
Fluocortin butyl	Topical corticosteroid
Ketotifen	Mast cell stabilizer
Mequitazine	
Nedocromil sodium	
Oxatomide	

Avoiding the offending allergens is the best preventative treatment. The aforementioned medications are symptomatic and palliative in nature.

ALLOPURINOL SODIUM

(Zyloprim)

Allopurinol reduces the synthesis of uric acid by inhibiting the activity of xanthine oxidase (Figure 18). The reduction in the

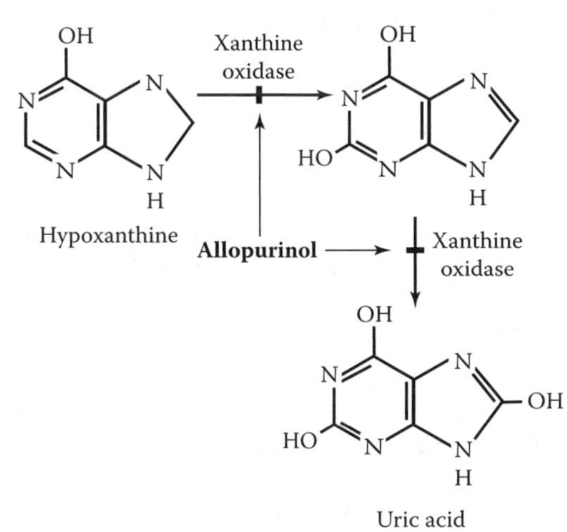

FIGURE 18 Allopurinol reduces the synthesis of uric acid by inhibiting the activity of xanthine oxidase. Not only is it used in treating the hyperuricemia associated with gout, but also in the secondary hyperuricemia associated with the use of antineoplastic agents. Allopurinol may interfere with the metabolism of antineoplastic agents. Allopurinol may interfere with the metabolism of antineoplastic agents such as **azathioprine** and **6-mercaptopurine**.

uric acid pool occurs slowly. Because xanthine and hypoxanthine are more soluble than uric acid, they are easily excreted.

Gout is a hyperuricemic state (>6 mg/dL) that is effectively diagnosed through the detection of monosodium urate crystals in the synovial fluid of the involved joint.

Conditions causing hyperuricemia include: the excessive synthesis of uric acid, the excessive synthesis of purine—precursor to uric acid—a high dietary intake of purine (shellfish, organ meat, anchovies, and wild game), diminished renal excretion of uric acid, and tissue destruction following injury or therapeutic irradiation.

Numerous agents, when used in therapeutic doses, can also cause hyperuricemia. This includes an analgesic dose of aspirin, thiazide diuretics, nicotinic acid, chronic consumption of alcohol, and antineoplastic agents.

If left untreated, the hyperuricemic state may precipitate an acute attack of gout, which first appears in metatarsal phalangeal joints. Ultimately, tophaceous deposits form in the joints and soft tissues such as the kidneys. The hyperuricemic state may be corrected either by inhibiting the synthesis of uric acid by allopurinol or by enhancing the elimination of uric acid by uricosuric agents.

Allopurinol is used not only in treating the hyperuricemia associated with gout but also in the secondary hyperuricemia associated with the use of antineoplastic agents. Therefore, allopurinol may be used in the management of patients with leukemia, lymphoma, and solid tumor malignancies who are receiving cancer therapy that causes elevations of serum and urinary uric acid levels. Allopurinol may interfere with the metabolism of antineoplastic agents such as azathioprine and 6-mercaptopurine.

Allopurinol and oxipurinol have plasma half-lives of 1 to 2 hours and 15 hours, respectively. Allopurinol is cleared by glomerular filtration, whereas oxipurinol and uric acid are reabsorbed in the kidney tubules in a similar fashion. Therefore, the addition of uricosuric drugs increases the excretion of oxipurinol and hence may reduce the effectiveness of allopurinol.

Allopurinol may cause a cutaneous reaction (3%) that is predominantly pruritic and maculopapular in nature, is accompanied by fever, malaise, or muscle ache, and the incidence increases with renal impairment. Because the onset of skin rash may be followed by severe hypersensitivity reactions, allopurinol should be discontinued by patients who develop such rashes. Patients with impaired renal function require less drug and careful observation.

ALMOTRIPTAN MALATE

(Axert)

Almotriptan is a serotonin 5-HT_1 receptor agonist that shows selectivity for vascular serotonin (5-HT) receptor subtype, causing vasoconstriction of cranial arteries. Almotriptan is indicated for an acute treatment of migraine with or without aura (see Migraine—Treatment of).

ALOSETRON

(Lotronex)

Alosetron is a 5-HT_3 receptor antagonist that inhibits serotonin receptors in the GI tract and is indicated in the treatment of irritable bowel syndrome (IBS) in women whose predominant bowel syndrome is diarrhea. The 5-HT_3 receptor participates in several important processes in the gut, including sensitization of spinal sensory neurons, vagal signaling of nausea, and peristaltic reflexes. Some of these effects in experimental models are potentially conflicting, with release of excitatory and inhibitory neurotransmitters. However, the clinical effect of 5-HT_3 antagonism is a general reduction of GI contractility with decreased colonic transit, along with an increase in fluid absorption. In general, therefore, these antagonists produce the opposite effects seen with 5-HT_4 agonists such as tegaserod. Although they also may blunt visceral sensation, a direct effect on spinal afferents has not been fully established. Alosetron was the first agent in this class specifically approved for the treatment of diarrhea-predominant IBS in women.

Alosetron is rapidly absorbed form the GI tract; its duration of action (about 10 hours) is longer than expected from its half-life of 1.5 hours. It is metabolized by hepatic enzymes. The drug should be started at 1 mg twice daily if an adequate response is not achieved.

ALPHA-METHYLDOPA

(Aldomet)

The catecholamine-synthesizing enzymes are not only able to synthesize dopamine and norepinephrine from a physiologically occurring substrate such as L-dopa but also from exogenous substrates such as alpha-methyldopa, which is converted to alpha-methyldopamine and in turn to alpha-methylnorepinephrine. Alpha-methyldopamine and alpha-methylnorepinephrine are called false transmitters and, in general (except for alpha-methylnorepinephrine), are weaker agonists (see Figure 37).

Alpha-methyldopa is used in the treatment of mild to moderate hypertension. The proposed mechanism of action is suppression of renin release, stimulation of central $alpha_2$-inhibitory adrenergic receptors ($alpha_2$-adrenergic receptor sites) such as dopamine, acetylcholine, and prostaglandins (PGE_1 and PGE_2 but not PGF_2A), and reduction of the release of norepinephrine. In addition, alpha-methyldopa reduces the peripheral vascular resistance without altering the heart rate or cardiac output. Postural hypotension is mild and infrequent. Besides reducing blood pressure, alpha-methyldopa causes sedation (interference with norepinephrine), parkinsonism (interference with dopamine), psychosis (interference with serotonin), and decreased libido and impotence (interference with norepinephrine). Alpha- methyldopa has a long onset and a short duration of action. It is especially useful in the management of hypertension complicated by renal dysfunction, because it does not alter either renal blood flow or the glomerular filtration rate. It is contraindicated in patients with liver disease and may produce hepatitis-like symptoms.

ALPHA-PROTEINASE INHIBITOR

(Human) ($Alpha_1$-PI) (Prolastin)

$Alpha_1$ proteinase inhibitor (60 mg/kg IV once weekly), is indicated for chronic replacement of $alpha_1$-antitrypsin in patients with clinically demonstrable panacinar emphysema and PIZZ, PIZ (null), or Pi (null) (null) phenotype.

ALPHA$_1$-PROTEINASE INHIBITOR (HUMAN) [α_1-PI]

(Aralast powder for injection)

Alpha$_1$-proteinase inhibitor inhibits **serine proteases** (e.g., neutrophil elastase), which are capable of degrading protein components of the alveolar walls and which are chronically present in the lung. Alpha$_1$-proteinase inhibitor is indicated in chronic augmentation therapy in patients with congenital deficiency if α_1-PI with clinically evident emphysema.

ALPRAZOLAM

(Xanax)

Alprazolam is effective in the management of anxiety disorders, panic disorder with or without agoraphobia, and anxious depression with a dosage regimen that must be individualized for each patient. Similar to benzodiazepine derivatives, alprazolam causes a dose-dependent CNS depression from mild sedation to hypnosis. Alprazolam is absorbed orally, is bound to plasma protein to the extent of 70 to 80%, possesses a half-life of 14 to 16 hours, and a volume of distribution of 1.02 to 1.20 L/kg. Both the half-life and volume of distribution are markedly increased in obese subjects. Alprazolam is metabolized to alpha-hydroxyalprazolam derivative, which is inactive (see Table 9). Alprazolam crosses the placental barrier and is found in human milk. The manifestations of overdosage include somnolence, confusion, impaired coordination, diminished reflexes, and coma. Death has been reported with large doses of alprazolam (LD50 in rats 500 to 2000 mg/kg) especially when taken with ethanol. **Flumazenil** (Mazicon), a specific benzodiazepine receptor antagonist, is effective in reversing the alprazolam-induced CNS depression, and should be complemented with other supportive therapy to aid respiration (Figure 50). The use of flumazenil is associated with the risk of precipitating seizures in susceptible individuals.

ALPRENOLOL

Alprenolol, which possesses dual beta-adrenergic receptor-blocking effects and intrinsic sympathomimetic activity, has been used widely and successfully in the treatment of hypertension, angina pectoris, and cardiac arrhythmias. The levo isomer of alprenolol has approximately one hundred times greater affinity for the beta-adrenoreceptors than the dextro isomers but has equal efficacy for their membrane-stabilizing properties. Because of this action, both isomers of alprenolol may produce a direct cardio depressant effect, including an antiarrhythmic effect unrelated to their beta-adrenergic receptor-blocking activity. Alprenolol (4 to 20 mg IV) reduces sinus tachycardia, diminishes the ventricular rate in patients with atrial fibrillation, and suppresses ventricular ectopic beats. It reduces lipolysis, and hence, free fatty acid production in hypotensive patients.

Alprenolol is completely absorbed from the gastrointestinal tract, rapidly distributed to various extravascular sites, and metabolized to 4-hydroxyalprenol, an active metabolite. Alprenolol has additive effects when used in combination with saluretic diuretics or hydralazine. It prevents sudden death in postinfarction patients, reduces persistent ventricular ectopic beats, ventricular premature beats occurring in acute myocardial infarction, and diminishes digitalis-induced ventricular arrhythmias. Therefore, alprenolol may be used with greater safety than other beta-adrenoceptor antagonists in patients with bradycardia and prolonged interval, in patients with Raynaud's phenomenon, intermittent claudication, and cold extremities. The reported side effects for alprenolol are CNS disorders such as insomnia and nightmares, gastrointestinal disorders such as esophageal stricture ulcer, and bronchospasm.

ALPROSTADIL (PROSTAGLANDIN E$_1$)

(Caverject powder for injection)

Alprostadil is used in erectile dysfunction. Alprostadil relaxes smooth muscle of ductus arteriosus. It produces vasodilation, inhibits platelet aggregation, and stimulates intestinal and uterine smooth muscle. Alprostadil induces erection by relaxation of trabecular smooth muscle and by dilation of cavernosal arteries (see Erectile Dysfunction—Treatment of).

PGE$_1$ (Alprostadil) may be used in the treatment of impotence. Intracavernous injection of PGE$_1$ causes complete or partial erection in impotent patients who do not have disorders of the vascular system or cavernous body damage. The erection lasts for 1 to 3 hours and is sufficient for sexual intercourse. PGE$_1$ is more effective than **papaverine**. The agent is available as a sterile powder that is reconstituted with water for injections (**Caverject**), although it has been superseded largely by the use of PDE$_5$ inhibitors, such as **sildenafil, tadalafil**, and **vardenafil**.

ALPROSTADIL

(Prostin VR Pediatric)

Alprostadil (0.05 to 0.1 mcg/kg/minute via infusion pump) is indicated for temporary maintenance of patency of ductus arteriosus until surgery can be performed (see Figure 61).

ALTEPLASE

(Recombinant Alteplase, Tissue Plasminogen Activator [Activase])

Alteplase (6 to 10 mg IV bolus over the first 1 to 2 minutes, then 20 mg/hour for an additional 2 hours) is indicated for lysis of thrombi obstructing coronary arteries in management of acute myocardial infarction (see Figure 44).

ALTEPLASE, RECOMBINANT

(Activase powder for injection)

Alteplase aids in dissolution of blood clots. It is indicated in the lysis of thrombi in management of acute myocardial infarction (MI) or acute massive pulmonary embolism, and management of acute ischemic stroke. Alteplase assists in restoration of function to central venous access devices as assessed by the ability to withdraw blood.

Alteplase interacts with anticoagulants (e.g., warfarin, heparin), aspirin, drugs affecting platelet function (e.g., abiciximab, dipyridamole), vitamin K antagonists: may increase the risk of bleeding; nitroglycerin: may reduce alteplase concentrations, decreasing the thrombolytic effect.

ALTRETAMINE

(Hexalen)

Altretamine is an ethyleneimine alkylating agent that is indicated as a palliative therapy of refractory ovarian cancer following treatment failure with a cisplatin- or alkylating agent-based combination. Its mechanism of action is unknown. Because the formation of the ethyleneiminium ion constitutes the initial reaction of the nitrogen mustards, it is not surprising that stable ethyleneimine derivatives have antitumor activity. Several compounds of this type, including **triethylenemelamine** (TEM) and triethylene **thiophosphoramide** (thiotepa), have been used clinically. In standard doses, thiotepa produces little toxicity other than myelosuppression; it also is used for high-dose chemotherapy regimens, in which it causes both mucosal and CNS toxicity. Altretamine (hexamethylmelamine; HMM) is mentioned here because of its chemical similarity to TEM. The methylmelamines are *N*-demethylated by hepatic microsomes with the release of formaldehyde, and there is a direct relationship between the degree of the demethylation and their activity against murine tumors.

Esters of alkanesulfonic acids alkylate DNA through the release of methyl radicals. Busulfan is of value in the treatment of chronic myelogenous leukemia and in high-dose chemotherapy. The most important pharmacologic actions of the alkylating agents are those that disturb DNA synthesis and cell division. The capacity of these drugs to interfere with DNA integrity and function and to induce cell death in rapidly proliferating tissues provides the basis for their therapeutic and toxic properties. Whereas certain alkylating agents may have damaging effects on tissues with normally low mitotic indices—for example liver, kidney, and mature lymphocytes—these tissues usually are affected in a delayed time frame. Acute effects manifest primarily against rapidly proliferating tissue. Lethality of DNA alkylation depends on the recognition of the adduct, the creation of DNA strand breaks by repair enzymes, and an intact apoptotic response. The actual mechanisms of cell death related to DNA alkylation are not yet well characterized.

In nondividing cells, DNA damage activates a checkpoint that depends on the presence of a normal p53 gene. Cells thus blocked in the G_1/S interface either repair DNA alkylation or undergo apoptosis. Malignant cells with mutant or absent p53 fail to suspend cell-cycle progress. The main toxicities of altretamine are myelosuppression and neurotoxicity. Altretamine causes both peripheral and central neurotoxicity. CNS symptoms include ataxia, depression, confusion, drowsiness, hallucinations, dizziness, and vertigo. Neurologic toxicity appears to be reversible upon discontinuation of therapy and may be prevented or decreased by concomitant administration of pyridoxine, although this remains unproven. Peripheral blood counts and a neurologic examination should be performed prior to the initiation of each course of therapy. Therapy should be interrupted for at least 14 days and subsequently restarted at a lower dose of 200 mg/m^2 daily if the white cell count falls below 2,000 cells/mm^3, or the platelet count below 75,000 cells/mm^3, or if neurotoxic or intolerable gastrointestinal symptoms occur. If neurologic symptoms fail to stabilize on the reduced dose schedule, altretamine should be discontinued. Nausea and vomiting also are common side effects and may be dose-limiting. Renal toxicity also may be dose-limiting. Other rare adverse effects include rashes, alopecia, and hepatic toxicity. Severe, life-threatening orthostatic hypotension developed in patients who received amitriptyline, imipramine, or phenelzine concurrently with altretamine.

ALUMINUM HYDROXIDE

(Alagel, AlternaGEL, Alu-cap, Aluminett, Alu-Tab, Amphojel, Dialume, Hydroxal, Nephrox, Nutrajel)

Aluminum hydroxide, an antacid with hypophosphatemic properties (500 to 1800 mg p.o.), is indicated in acid pepsin disease and in hyperphosphatemia in renal failure (see Table 4).

ALUMINUM PHOSPHATE

(Phosphaljel)

Aluminum phosphate (233 mg/5 ml to be used in 15 to 30 ml q. 2 hours between meals), by decreasing the fecal extraction of phosphate, is used as a phosphate replacement regimen.

ALZHEIMER'S DISEASE: Treatment of

Alzheimer's disease (AD), with or without comorbid conditions, is by far the leading cause of dementia. Dementia can be defined as the acquired and sustained deterioration of intellectual functions in an alert patient. It, thus, is distinguished from conditions such as mental retardation and delirium. Operationally, because of diminished cognitive ability, a demented person conducts everyday activities less well in relation to past performance. Formal criteria for dementia include the development of multiple cognitive deficits that include memory impairment and at least one of the following cognitive disturbances: aphasia, apraxia, agnosia, or a disturbance in executive functioning defined as the ability to think abstractly and to plan, initiate, sequence, monitor, and stop complex behavior. These disturbances must be sufficiently severe to cause significant impairment in social or occupational functioning, and represent a decline from a previous level of functioning. Criteria also have been proposed that do not require the presence of memory loss to accommodate disorders, such as vascular dementia, in which memory may be spared.

TABLE 4
Composition and Acid-Neutralizing Capacity of Nonprescription Antacid Preparation (Suspensions)

	Content (mg/5 ml)				
Product	**$Al(OH)_3$**	**$Mg(OH)_2$**	**$CaCO_3$**	**Simethicone**	**Acid-Neutralizing Capacity (per 5 ml)**
Maalox TC	600	300	0	0	27
Mylanta-II	400	400	0	40	25
Kudrox	500	450	0	40	25
Gelusil-II	200	200	0	25	24
Camalox	225	200	250	0	18
Di-Gel	200	200	0	20	—
Marblen	400 $MgCO_3$ + 520 $CaCO_3$		=	0	18
Alternagel	600	0	0	—	16
Silain-Gel	282	285	0	25	15
Riopan	540 magaldrate			0	15
Gelusil-M	300	200	0	25	15
Milk of Magnesia	0	390	0	0	14
Aludrox	307	103	0	—	12
Basaljel	$AL(OH)CO_3$ equivalent to 400			0	15
Gelusil	200	200	0	25	12
Wingel	180	160	0	0	10
Kolantyl gel	150	150	0	0	10
Amphojel	320	0	0	—	10
Gaviscon	31.7$Al(OH)_3$ + 137 $MgCO_3$ | Na alginate			0	15

Following the introduction of tacrine hydrochloride (Cognex®) in the United States and several other countries, researchers are pursuing two broad therapeutic strategies for AD. The first involves identifying agents or combinations of agents whose actions can compensate for the considerable cerebral damage that has typically occurred by the time the diagnosis of AD is made. Such therapeutic approaches include the development of additional cholinesterase inhibitors, agents that work on the receptors of other systems damaged by the disease process, and anti-inflammatory and immunomodulatory agents. The second and ultimately more promising strategy involves the development of approaches to retard, halt, or even prevent disease progression. Such protective approaches, which depend on the development of more effective methods for predicting and diagnosing AD, include the administration of nerve growth factor and other neurotrophins, and the use of pharmacologic or genetic interventions to limit amyloid deposition and the formation of neurofibrillary tangles.

Over 30% of patients with dementia develop a group of secondary behavioral disturbances, including depression, hallucinations and delusions, agitation, insomnia, and wandering. Because these secondary symptoms impair patients' functions, increase their need for supervision, and often influence the decision to institutionalize them, the control of these symptoms is a priority in managing AD.

Drugs used in the treatment of depression in Alzheimer's disease are:

Monoamine Oxidase Inhibitors (MAOI)
Phenelzine
Tranylcypromine

Tricyclic Antidepressants
Desipramine
Nortriptyline

Selective Serotonin Reuptake Inhibitors (SSRI)
Fluoxetine
Paroxetine
Sertraline

Drugs used in the treatment of psychosis and agitation in Alzheimer's disease are:

Classical Antipsychotics
Chlorpromazine
Haloperidol
Thioridazine

Atypical Antipsychotics
Clozapine
Risperidone

Benzodiazepines
Lorazepam
Oxazepam
Triazolam

Drugs used in the treatment of insomnia in Alzheimer's disease are:

Tricyclic Antidepressants
- Nortriptyline
- Trazodone

Benzodiazepines
- Lorazepam
- Oxazepam
- Triazolam

Antipsychotics
- Chlorpromazine
- Haloperidol
- Thioridazine

Although it is the most common form of dementia, AD-related dementia may be associated with other dementing illnesses including vascular dementia and Parkinson's disease. Other less common causes of dementia, including progressive supranuclear palsy, Huntington's disease, Pick's disease, Creutzfeldt–Jakob disease, and a variety of rare metabolic disorders, can usually be distinguished from AD by distinctive physical signs and symptoms that appear before or in tandem with the onset of cognitive impairment.

AMANTADINE

(Symmetrel)

Amantadine is 70 to 90% effective in preventing illnesses caused by circulating strains of type A influenza viruses, when administered 24 to 48 hours after onset of illness. It exerts its effects by preventing the penetration and uncoating of the virus (Figure 19). Amantadine is also useful in the treatment of mild parkinsonism, hemiparkinsonism, and drug-induced parkinsonism. Although the actions of amantadine are still not fully understood, there is some evidence that the drug inhibits the uptake of dopamine into the synaptosomes. In addition, amantadine has an indirect amphetamine-like effect, in that it releases dopamine. It augments the actions of anticholinergic medications used in patients with Parkinson's disease, and the doses of one or both should be reduced. Amantadine, which releases catecholamine, may cause insomnia, nervousness, dizziness, and ataxia when taken in toxic doses.

AMBENONIUM CHLORIDE

(Mytelase)

Ambenonium, a cholinesterase inhibitor (5 to 25 mg p.o. t.i.d.), is indicated in the symptomatic treatment of myasthenia gravis. Ambenonium results in accumulation of acetylcholine-stimulating cholinergic receptors at the myoneural junction (see Figure 12).

AMCINONIDE

(Cyclocort)

Amcinonide, a topical adrenocorticoid with antiinflammatory properties (0.1% cream, ointment, or lotion), is indicated in the treatment of inflammation of corticosteroid-responsive dermatoses.

AMIFOSTINE

(Ethyol powder for injection)

One of the goals of cancer chemotherapy is to enhance the efficacy of antineoplastic agents and at the same time protect the nonmalignant tissues using chemoprotective

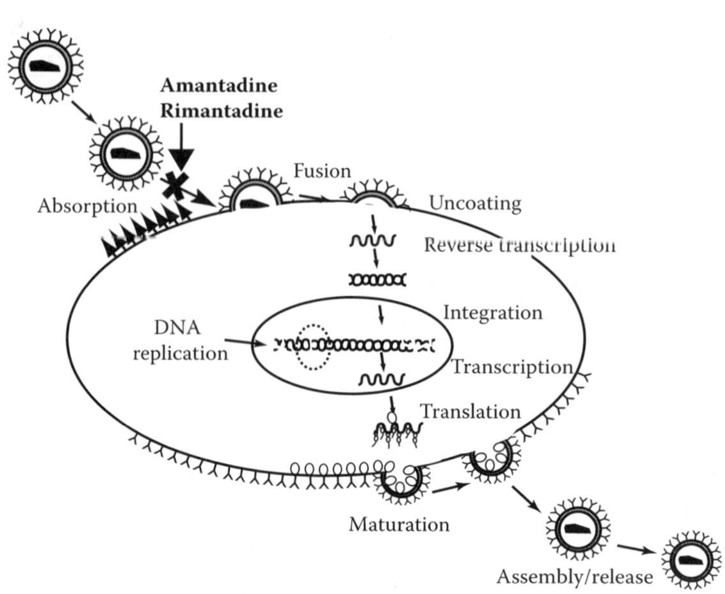

FIGURE 19 Amantadine and rimantadine, effective against RNA virus, exert their effects by preventing the penetration and uncoating of the virus.

agents. A few of the chemoenhancers and chemoprotectors are listed here:

Chemoenhancers	Chemoprotectors
Acridines	Amifostine
Amiodarone	Bismuth salts
Buthionine sulfoximine	Dexrazoxane
Calcium channel blockers	Diethyldithiocarbamate
Cyclosporine	Diuretics, phorbol esters
Ethacrynic acid	Glutathione esters
Phenothiazines	Metallothionein
Phorbol esters	Oxothiazolidine-4-carboxylate
Progesterone	Steroids
Streptozocin	Thiosulfate
Tamoxifen	
Triparanol	

Amifostine is an organic thiophosphate cytoprotective agent that can reduce the toxicity of cisplatin. It binds to and thereby detoxifies reactive metabolites of **cisplatin**. It scavenges reactive oxygen species generated by exposure to cisplatin radiation.

Amifostine prevents or reduces renal damage in patients receiving repeated cisplatin doses for advanced ovarian or non-small cell lung cancer, and reduces incidence of moderate to severe xerostomia in patients undergoing radiation of the parotid gland for head and neck. Cisplatin-induced nephrotoxicity has been largely abrogated by adequate pretreatment hydration and diuresis. Amifostine (Ethyol) is a thiophosphate cytoprotective agent that is labeled for the reduction of renal toxicity associated with repeated administration of cisplatin. It is dephosphorylated by alkaline phosphatase to a pharmacologically active free thiol metabolite. Faster dephosphorylation and preferential uptake by normal tissues results in a higher concentration of the thiol metabolite available to scavenge reactive cisplatin metabolites in normal tissues. Amifostine also is used to reduce xerostomia in patients undergoing irradiation for head and neck cancer, where the radiation port includes a substantial portion of the parotid glands. A review of the clinical status of amifostine as a cytoprotectant has been published.

Ototoxicity caused by cisplatin is unaffected by diuresis and is manifested by tinnitus and high-frequency hearing loss. The ototoxicity can be unilateral or bilateral, tends to be more frequent and severe with repeated doses, and may be more pronounced in children. Marked nausea and vomiting occur in almost all patients and usually can be controlled with 5-hydroxytryptamine (5-HT_3) antagonists, neurokinin-1 (NK1) receptor antagonists, and high-dose corticosteroids. At higher doses or after multiple cycles of treatment, cisplatin causes a progressive peripheral motor and sensory neuropathy, which may worsen after discontinuation of the drug and may be aggravated by subsequent or simultaneous treatment with taxanes or other neurotoxic drugs. Cisplatin causes mild to moderate myelosuppression, with transient leukopenia and thrombocytopenia. Anemia may become prominent after multiple cycles of treatment. Electrolyte disturbances, including hypomagnesemia, hypocalcemia, hypokalemia, and hypophosphatemia, are common. Hypocalcemia and hypomagnesemia secondary to renal electrolyte wasting may produce tetany if untreated. Routine measurement of Mg^{2+} concentrations in plasma is recommended. Hyperuricemia, hemolytic anemia, and cardiac abnormalities are rare side effects. Anaphylactic-like reactions, characterized by facial edema, bronchoconstriction, tachycardia, and hypotension, may occur within minutes after administration and should be treated by intravenous injection of epinephrine and with corticosteroids or antihistamines. Cisplatin has been associated with the development of acute myelogenous leukemia, usually 4 years or more after treatment.

AMIKACIN SULFATE

(Amikin, Elkins-Sinn, Apothecon)

Among the aminoglycosides (see Figure 88), amikacin has the broadest antimicrobial spectrum of action, and, for this reason, it is usually reserved for the treatment of serious infections due to susceptible strains of Gram-negative bacteria, including *Pseudomonas* sp., *Escherichia coli*, *Proteus* sp., *Providencia* sp., *Klebsiella* sp., *Enterobacter* sp., *Serratia* sp., and *Acinetobacter* (Mima–Herellea) sp. Amikacin is effective in bacterial septicemia including neonatal sepsis, in infections of the respiratory tract and CNS including meningitis, in intraabdominal infection including peritonitis, and in postoperative infections. Amikacin (up to 15 mg/kg/day) is given for 7 to 10 days. The patient's renal status and vestibular or auditory functions must be monitored carefully.

The aminoglycoside group includes gentamicin, tobramycin, amikacin, netilmicin, kanamycin, streptomycin, and neomycin. These drugs are used primarily to treat infections caused by aerobic Gram-negative bacteria; streptomycin is an important agent for the treatment of tuberculosis. In contrast to most inhibitors of microbial protein synthesis, which are bacteriostatic, the aminoglycosides are bactericidal inhibitors of protein synthesis. Mutations affecting proteins in the bacterial ribosome, the target for these drugs, can confer marked resistance to their action. However, most commonly, resistance is due to acquisition of plasmids or transposon-encoding genes for aminoglycoside-metabolizing enzymes or from impaired transport of drug into the cell. Thus, there can be cross-resistance between members of the class.

These agents contain amino sugars linked to an aminocyclitol ring by glycosidic bonds (Figure 88). They are polycations, and their polarity is responsible in part for pharmacokinetic properties shared by all members of the group. For example, none is absorbed adequately after oral administration, inadequate concentrations are found in cerebrospinal fluid (CSF), and all are excreted relatively rapidly by the normal kidney. Although aminoglycosides are widely used and important agents, serious toxicity limits their usefulness. All members of the group share the same spectrum of toxicity, most notably nephrotoxicity and ototoxicity, which can involve the auditory and vestibular functions of the eighth cranial nerve.

AMILORIDE HYDROCHLORIDE

(Midamor)

Amiloride interferes with sodium reabsorption at the distal tubule, resulting in increased excretion of water and sodium and decreased excretion of potassium. It is indicated in the treatment of congestive heart failure or hypertension (in combination with thiazide or loop diuretics) and diuretic-induced hypokalemia.

Triamterene (Dyrenium, Maxzide) and amiloride are potassium-sparing diuretics that inhibit renal epithelial Na^+ channels. Triamterene, amiloride, and spironolactone (Alactone), which is an aldosterone antagonist, all act in the distal tubule, where the resorption of sodium is accompanied by the transfer of potassium into the lumen contents. When sodium resorption is hindered, potassium excretion is correspondingly reduced such that more potassium is retained. The potassium-sparing diuretics are not very efficacious, as they affect only 1 to 2% of the filtered load of sodium. All are given orally and eliminated in the urine, mostly by glomerular filtration, though some active tubular secretion may occur.

Molecular cloning studies recently have revealed that the amiloride-sensitive Na+ channel consists of three subunits (alpha, beta, gamma). Although the alpha subunit is sufficient for channel activity, maximal Na^+ permeability is induced when all three subunits are coexpressed in the same cell, suggesting a minimal oligomeric structure in which one copy of each subunit is associated in a heterotrimeric protein.

Amiloride is used with thiazide or loop diuretics in hypertension, in congestive heart failure, in digitalis-induced hypokalemia, and in arrhythmias resulting from hypokalemia. Inappropriate use of amiloride may cause hyperkalemia (potassium >5.5 mEq/L), which may be fatal if not corrected, and may be more deleterious in elderly individuals and in patients with diabetes mellitus and renal impairment. The symptoms of hyperkalemia include fatigue, flaccid paralysis of the extremities, paresthesias, bradycardia, ECG abnormalities, and shock. Amiloride is not metabolized but is contraindicated in anuria, acute or chronic renal insufficiency, or in diabetic nephropathy. It should not be used with potassium preparations, and should be used cautiously with ACE inhibitors because these agents cause hyperkalemia.

The most dangerous adverse effect of Na^+-channel inhibitors is hyperkalemia, which can be life threatening. Consequently, **amiloride** and triamterene are contraindicated in patients with hyperkalemia, as well as in patients at increased risk of developing hyperkalemia (e.g., patients with renal failure, patients receiving other K^+-sparing diuretics, patients taking angiotensin-converting enzyme inhibitors, or patients taking K^+ supplements). Even aspirin can increase the likelihood of hyperkalemia patients receiving Na^+-channel inhibitors. Pentamidine and high-dose trimethoprim are used often to treat *Pneumocystis carinii* pneumonia in patients with AIDS. Because these compounds may cause hyperkalemia, this may explain the frequent occurrence of hyperkalemia in AIDS patients. Cirrhotic patients are prone to megaloblastosis because of folic acid deficiency, and triamterene, a weak folic acid antagonist, may increase the likelihood of this adverse event. Triamterene also can reduce glucose tolerance and induce photosensitization, and has been associated with interstitial nephritis and renal stones. Both drugs can cause CNS, gastrointestinal, musculoskeletal, dermatological, and hematological adverse effects. The most common adverse effects of amiloride are nausea, vomiting, diarrhea, and headache; those of triamterene are nausea, vomiting, leg cramps, and dizziness.

AMINO ACID SOLUTIONS

(Aminosyn, Aminosyn with Dextrose, Aminosyn with Electrolytes, Aminosyn-PF, Aminosyn (pH6), Aminosyn II, Aminosyn II in Dextrose, Aminosyn II with Electrolytes, Aminosyn II with Electrolytes in Dextrose, FreAmine III, FreAmine III with Electrolytes, Novamine, Novamine without Electrolytes, ProcalAmine, Travasol with Electrolytes, Travasol without Electrolytes, TrophAmine)

Amino acid solutions (1 to 1.5 g/kg IV daily) will provide nutritional support in patients with renal failure, high metabolic stress, or hepatic encephalopathy with cirrhosis or hepatitis. Amino acid injection and solution provide a substrate for protein synthesis in the protein-depleted patient or enhance conservation of body protein.

AMINOCAPROIC ACID

(Amicar)

Aminocaproic acid is a homeostatic agent that inhibits fibrinolysis to stop bleeding. Aminocaproic acid is indicated in the treatment of excessive bleeding from systemic hyperfibrinolysis and urinary fibrinolysis.

Aminocaproic acid (AMICAR) is a lysine analog that competes for lysine-binding sites on plasminogen and plasmin, thus blocking the interaction of plasmin with fibrin. It is thereby a potent inhibitor of fibrinolysis and can reverse states that are associated with excessive fibrinolysis. The main problem with its use is that thrombi that form during treatment with the drug are not lysed. For example, in patients with hematuria, ureteral obstruction by clots may lead to renal failure after treatment with aminocaproic acid. It has been used to reduce bleeding after prostatic surgery or after tooth extractions in hemophiliacs.

AMINOGLUTETHIMIDE

(Cytadren)

Aminoglutethimide (250 mg p.o. q.i.d.) is indicated in the treatment of adrenal hyperplasia from ectopic ACTH-producing tumors (see Figure 38). In addition, it has been used in medial adrenalectomy in postmenopausal metastatic breast cancer and prostate cancer, and in suppression of adrenal function in Cushing's syndrome.

Aminoglutethimide interferes with the conversion of cholesterol to delta-5-pregnenolone, effectively inhibiting the synthesis of corticosteroids, androgens, and estrogens. Therefore, by suppressing the adrenals, aminoglutethimide inhibits the growth of tumors that need estrogen to thrive.

Aminoglutethimide is an adrenal steroid inhibitor inhibiting the enzymatic conversion of cholesterol to δ^5-pregnenolone, thereby reducing the synthesis of adrenal glucocorticoids, mineralocorticoids, estrogens, and androgens. It is indicated in suppression of adrenal function in patients with **Cushing's syndrome**. **Aminoglutethimide** (AG), a first-generation type 2 aromatase inhibitor (AI), was originally developed as an anticonvulsant but was subsequently found to inhibit the synthesis of adrenocortical steroids. AG is a nonspecific, weak AI, administered as a 250-mg dose four times daily with hydrocortisone supplementation because of unwanted adrenal suppression. Because of significant toxicities related to its anticonvulsant structure and its relatively weak inhibition of aromatase, its use has declined considerably with the advent of newer AIs.

Second-generation AIs include **formestane** (4-hydroxyandrostenedione; Lentaron), a type 1 steroidal inactivator; **fadrozole**, a type 2 imidazole; and **rogletimide** (pyridoglutethimide), a type 2 inhibitor structurally similar to aminoglutethimide. Formestane was the first steroidal aromatase inactivator widely used for the treatment of breast cancer patients. Because of better aromatase inhibition *in vivo* following parenteral administration, it is administered as an intramuscular depot injection. However, formestane has also been shown to be active when given orally. It suppresses plasma sex hormone-binding globulin (SHBG), which is interpreted as an androgenic side effect. The response rates of phase II and III trials were about 25 to 40%. Due to the introduction of novel compounds, especially exemestane, formestane is not widely used today.

The third-generation inhibitors, developed in the 1990s, include the type 1 steroidal agent exemestane and the type 2 nonsteroidal imidazoles anastrozole and letrozole. Currently, third-generation AIs are most commonly used for the treatment of early-stage and advanced breast cancer.

AMINOPHYLLINE

(Theophylline Ethylenediamine)

The methylxanthines consist of aminophylline, dyphylline, enprofylline, and pentoxifylline. Aminophylline is the most widely used of the soluble theophyllines.

Epinephrine stimulates the beta-adrenergic receptors in the bronchioles, which in turn activates membrane-bound adenylate cyclase to synthesize more cyclic AMP, whereas theophylline inhibits the activity of phosphodiesterase, conserving the previously synthesized cyclic AMP (see Figure 94). In addition, recent evidence suggests that theophylline blocks the receptor for adenosine. The inhalation of adenosine can precipitate marked bronchoconstriction in asthmatic patients but shows no appreciable effects in normal subjects.

It is now recognized that adenosine receptors are linked through appropriate guanine nucleotide-binding regulatory proteins (G-proteins), not only to adenyl cyclase but also to other effector systems. Moreover, theophylline may inhibit the synthesis of prostaglandin and reduce the uptake or metabolism of catecholamines in nonneuronal tissues (see Figure 37).

Corticosteroids, which are also effective in symptomatic treatment of certain types of asthma, exert their beneficial effects in part by enhancing catecholamine effects and also by antagonizing the cholinergic actions, one of which is bronchoconstriction. Aminophylline also causes CNS stimulation, cardiac acceleration, diuresis, and gastric secretion. It is available in an oral, rectal (pediatric), or intravenous solution, which is used in the treatment of status asthmaticus. Although aminophylline is a less effective bronchodilator than beta-adrenergic agonists, it is particularly useful in preventing nocturnal asthma.

Aminophylline is a xanthine derivative that relaxes bronchial smooth muscle and pulmonary blood vessels, and stimulates central respirator drive and increases diaphragmatic contractility. It is indicated in the prevention or treatment of reversible bronchospasm associated with asthma. **Theophylline**, a methylxanthine, is among the least expensive drugs used to treat asthma and, consequently, it remains a commonly used drug for this indication in many countries. In industrialized countries, the advent of inhaled glucocorticoids, β-adrenergic receptor agonists, and leukotriene-modifying drugs has diminished theophylline use significantly, and it has been relegated to a third- or fourth-line treatment in patients whose asthma is otherwise difficult to control.

AMINOSALICYLATE SODIUM

(Para-Aminosalicylate, P.A.S.) (Nemasol Sodium, Sodium P.A.S., Tubasal)

Aminosalicylate sodium (3.3 to 4 g p.o. q. 8 hours) is indicated as an adjunctive treatment of tuberculosis. It inhibits the formation of folic acid and hence suppresses the growth and reproduction of Mycobacterium tuberculosis.

AMINOSALICYLATE SODIUM (PAS)

(Paser)

Aminosalicylate competitively antagonizes metabolism of para-aminobenzoic acid, resulting in bacteriostatic activity against Mycobacterium tuberculosis. Aminosalicylate is indicated in the treatment of tuberculosis (in combination with other antituberculous drugs) caused by susceptible strains of tubercle bacilli.

AMIODARONE

(Cordarone, Pacerone)

Amiodarone is an antiarrhythmic agent. It is indicated in the treatment of life-threatening, recurrent ventricular arrhythmias (i.e., ventricular fibrillation and hemodynamically unstable ventricular tachycardia) that do not respond to other antiarrhythmic agents. It is used only in patients with the indicated life-threatening arrhythmias because its use is accompanied by substantial toxicity. Parenteral: Initiation of treatment and prophylaxis of frequently recurring ventricular fibrillation and hemodynamically unstable ventricular tachycardia in patients refractory to other therapy; treatment of ventricular tachycardia and fibrillation when oral amiodarone is indicated but patient is unable to take oral medication.

Amiodarone exerts a multiplicity of pharmacological effects, none of which is clearly linked to its arrhythmia-suppressing properties. Amiodarone is a structural analog of thyroid hormone, and some of its antiarrhythmic actions and its toxicity may be attributable to interaction with nuclear thyroid hormone receptors. It is highly lipophilic, concentrated in many tissues, and eliminated extremely slowly; consequently, adverse effects may resolve very slowly. In the United States, the drug is indicated for oral therapy in patients with recurrent ventricular tachycardia or fibrillation resistant to other drugs. Oral amiodarone also is effective in maintaining sinus rhythm in patients with atrial fibrillation. An intravenous form is indicated for acute termination of ventricular tachycardia or fibrillation and is supplanting lidocaine as a first-line therapy for out-of-hospital cardiac arrest. Trials of oral amiodarone have shown a modest beneficial effect on mortality after acute myocardial infarction. Despite uncertainties about its mechanisms of action and the potential for serious toxicity, amiodarone now is used very widely in the treatment of common arrhythmias such as atrial fibrillation.

AMIODARONE HCL

(Cordarone)

Amiodarone is a structural analog of thyroid hormone, is highly lipophilic, concentrated in many tissues, and eliminated very slowly. Following discontinuation of chronic oral therapy, amiodarone has a biphasic elimination with an initial one-half reduction of plasma levels after 2.5 to 10 days. A much slower terminal plasma elimination phase shows a half-life of the parent compound ranging from 26 to 107 days (mean 53 days), with most patients in the 40- to 55-day range. Steady-state plasma concentrations would therefore be reached between 130 and 535 days (average 265 days).

Amiodarone (plasma concentration of 0.5 to 2.0 μg/mL) decreases conduction velocity by blocking Na^+ channels, inhibits abnormal automaticity, and prolongs the duration of action potential. Prolongation of PR, QRS, and QT intervals and sinus bradycardia are frequent during chronic therapy. Oral amiodarone is indicated in patients with recurrent ventricular tachycardia or fibrillation resistant to other drugs. In addition, it is effective in maintaining sinus rhythm in patients with atrial fibrillation. Amiodarone is metabolized to desthylamiodarone, an active antiarrhythmic agent.

Amiodarone may cause asymptomatic corneal microdeposits and inhibit the conversion of thyroxine (T4) to triiodothyronine (T3). Amiodarone has caused pulmonary toxicity (hypersensitivity pneumonitis or interstitial/alveolar pneumonitis). It is embryotoxic in that it increases fetal resorption and causes growth retardation. Amiodarone is excreted in breast milk.

AMITRIPTYLINE

(Elavil)

The dibenzapine derivatives are called tricyclic antidepressants and include imipramine (Tofranil), desipramine (Norpramin), amitriptyline (Elavil), nortriptyline (Aventyl), protriptyline (Vivactil), and doxepin (Adapin). Amitriptyline is indicated in depression; major depression with melancholia or psychotic symptoms; depressive phase of bipolar disorder; depression associated with organic disease, alcoholism, schizophrenia, or mental retardation; anorexia or bulimia associated with depression (see Figure 20).

Tricyclic antidepressants resemble the phenothiazine antipsychotics such as chlorpromazine in structure and function. Like the phenothiazine derivatives (e.g., chlorpromazine), tricyclic antidepressants (e.g., amitriptyline) may reduce the seizure threshold and precipitate seizures in epileptic patients, cause cholestatic jaundice, movement disorders, and hematologic side effects. Unlike the phenothiazine derivatives, the tricyclic antidepressants may increase motor activity, have a very slow onset and long duration of action, a relatively narrow margin of safety, and a strong anticholinergic effect. In fact, dry mouth is the most common side effect, and other anticholinergic effects such as tachycardia, loss of accommodation, constipation, urinary retention, and paralytic ileus have been reported following amitriptyline.

Imipramine is demethylated to desipramine, and amitriptyline is demethylated to nortriptyline. Both metabolites are active antidepressants. Tricyclic antidepressants bind to plasma proteins to the extent of 90%, and, because of their extensive first-pass metabolism in the liver, they have very low and variable bioavailability. In those circumstances when it is desirable to measure the plasma concentrations of these drugs, the concentrations of their active metabolites should also be measured.

Tricyclic antidepressants, like some of the phenothiazine derivatives, are sedative in nature. Those compounds containing tertiary amines (imipramine, amitriptyline, and doxepin) are the most sedative. Those compounds containing a secondary amine (nortriptyline and desipramine) are less so, and protriptyline has no sedative effect (see Table 5). Tricyclic antidepressants, like some of the phenothiazine derivatives (e.g., thioridazine), have an anticholinergic property. Amitriptyline is the strongest in this regard, and desipramine is the weakest (see Tables 5 through 7).

The tricyclic antidepressants also have cardiovascular actions. In particular, they cause orthostatic hypotension by obtunding the various reflex mechanisms involved in

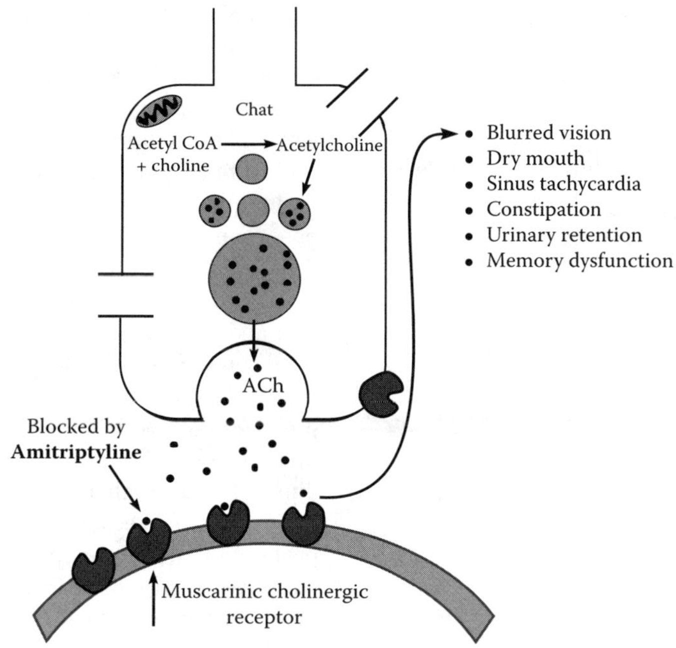

FIGURE 20 Amitriptyline, a tricyclic antidepressant, causes sedation and orthostatic hypotension. In addition, it possesses strong anticholinergic properties.

maintaining blood pressure (see Table 5). Antidepressants block the uptake of norepinephrine, serotonin, or dopamine (see Table 6) and block several receptor sites (see Table 7), causing beneficial effects as well as side effects. For example, amitriptyline blocks muscarinic cholinergic receptors causing blurred vision, dry mouth, sinus tachycardia, constipation, urinary retention, and memory dysfunction (see Figure 20). Therefore, because of its pronounced anticholinergic and potential arrhythmogenic effects, amitriptyline is contraindicated in the acute recovery phase of myocardial infarction, congestive heart failure, angina, prostatic hypertrophy, paralytic ileus, and urinary retention, and in patients undergoing surgery with general anesthetics that may cause arrhythmias (e.g., halothane) (see Table 16).

TABLE 5
Side Effects of Antidepressant Drugs

Drugs	Sedation	Insomnia	Anticholinergic Effects	Nausea	Orthostatic Hypotension
A. Tricyclic antidepressants					
Amitriptyline	+++	0	+++	0	+++
Trimipramine	+++	0	+++	0	++
Desipramine	+	+	+	0	+
Doxepin	+++	0	++	0	+++
Imipramine	++	0	++	0	++
Nortiptyline	++	0	+	0	+
Protriptyline	+	++	++	0	+
B. Second-generation antidepressants					
Amoxapine	++	0	+	0	++
Fluoxetine	0	++	0	++	0
Maprotiline	++	0	+	0	++
Trazodone	+++	0	0	+	++
Bupropion	0	++	0	+	0

Note: 0 = no side effect; + = minor side effect; ++ = moderate side effect; +++ = major side effect.

TABLE 6
The Inhibition of Monoamine Uptake by Antidepressants

Drugs	Norepinephrine	Serotonin	Dopamine
A. Tricyclic antidepressants			
Amitriptyline	±	++	0
Nortriptyline	++	±	0
Imipramine	+	+	0
Desipramine	+++	0	0
Clomipramine	+	+++	0
Trimipramine	+	0	0
Doxepine	++	+	0
B. Second-generation antidepressants			
Maprotiline	++	0	0
Amoxapine	++	0	0
Fluoxetine	0	+++	0
Bupropion	±	0	++
Mianserin	0	0	0
Trazodone	0	+	0

Note: 0 = no side effect; + = minor side effect; ++ = moderate side effect; +++ = major side effect.

AMLODIPINE

(Norvasc)

Amlodipine is a calcium-channel-blocking agent, which is indicated in the treatment of hypertension, chronic stable angina, and vasospastic (Prinzmetal or variant) angina. The ten $Ca2^{+}$ channel antagonists that are in clinical use in the United States have diverse chemical structures. Five classes of compounds have been examined: **phenylalkylamines**, **dihydropyridines**, **benzothiazepines**, **diphenylpiperazines,** and a **diarylaminopropylamine**. At present, **verapamil** (a phenylalkylamine); **diltiazem** (a benzothiazepine); **nifedipine**, **amlodipine**, **felodipine**, **isradipine**, **nicardipine**, **nisoldipine**, and **nimodipine** (dihydropyridines); and **bepridil** (a diarylaminopropylamine ether used only for refractory angina) are approved for clinical use in the United States.

Amlodipine is a dihydropyridine that has a low absorption and a prolonged effect. With a plasma half-life of 35 to 50 hours, plasma levels and effect increase over 7 to 10 days of daily administration of a constant dose. Amlodipine produces both peripheral arterial vasodilation and coronary dilation, with a hemodynamic profile similar to that of nifedipine. However, there is less reflex tachycardia with amlodipine possibly because the long half-life produces minimal peaks and troughs in plasma concentrations. Felodipine may have even greater vascular specificity than does nifedipine or **amlodipine**. At concentrations producing vasodilation, there is no negative inotropic effect. Like nifedipine, felodipine indirectly activates the sympathetic nervous system, leading to an increase in heart rate. Nicardipine has antianginal properties similar to those of nifedipine and may have selectivity for coronary vessels.

Isradipine also produces the typical peripheral vasodilation seen with other dihydropyridines, but because of its inhibitory effect on the SA node, little or no rise in heart rate is seen. This inhibitory effect does not extend to the cardiac myocytes, however, because no cardiodepressant effect is seen. Despite the negative chronotropic effect,

TABLE 7
The Affinity of Antidepressants for Various Receptors

	Receptor Affinity				
Drugs	$Alpha_1$-Adrenergic Blockade	$Alpha_2$-Adrenergic Blockade	Histaminergic (H_1) Blockade	Muscarinic Blockade	Dopaminergic (D_2) Blockade
A. Tricyclic antidepressants					
Amitriptyline	+++	±	++++	++++	0
Nortriptyline	+	0	+	++	0
Imipramine	++	0	+	++	0
Desipramine	+	0	0	+	0
Clomipramine	++	0	+	++	0
Trimipramine	++	±	+++	++	+
Doxepine	++	0	+++	++	0
B. Second-generation antidepressants					
Maprotiline	+	0	++	+	0
Amoxapine	++	±	±	0	++
Fluoxetine	0	0	0	0	0
Trazodone	++	±	±	+	0
Bupropion	0	0	0	0	0
Mianserin	++	++	+++	0	0

Note: 0 = no effect; ± = an equivocal effect; + = slight effect; ++ = moderate effect; +++ = large effect; ++++ = maximal effect.

isradipine appears to have little effect on the AV node, so it may be used in patients with AV block or combined with a β-adrenergic receptor antagonist. In general, because of their lack of myocardial depression and, to a greater or lesser extent, lack of negative chronotropic effect, dihydropyridines are less effective as monotherapy in stable angina than are verapamil, diltiazem, or a β-adrenergic receptor antagonist. Nisoldipine is more than 1000 times more potent in preventing contraction of human vascular smooth muscle than in preventing contraction of human cardiac muscle *in vitro*, suggesting a high degree of vascular selectivity. Although nisoldipine has a short elimination half-life, a sustained-release preparation has been developed that is efficacious as an antianginal agent. Nimodipine has high lipid solubility and was developed as an agent to relax the cerebral vasculature. It is effective in inhibiting cerebral vasospasm and has been used primarily to treat patients with neurological defects associated with cerebral vasospasm after subarachnoid hemorrhage.

AMLODIPINE BESYLATE/ATORVASTATIN CALCIUM

(Caduet tablets 5 mg amlodipine per 10 mg atorvastatin)

This is an antihyperlipidemic combination. Amlodipine is indicated in the treatment of hypertension, chronic stable angina, and confirmed or suspected vasospastic angina (Prinzmetal or variant angina). Statins are cholesterol-lowering agents that reversibly inhibit 3-hydroxy-3-methylglutaryl coenzyme A (HMG-CoA) reductase, which catalyzes a rate-limiting step in cholesterol biosynthesis. Statins affect serum cholesterol by inhibiting cholesterol biosynthesis in the liver, and this organ is their main target. On the other hand, exposure of extrahepatic cells in smooth muscle to these drugs may cause adverse effects. Among the statins, **pravastatin**, **fluvastatin**, **cerivastatin, atorvastatin, rosuvastatin**, and **pitavastatin** are given in a biologically active open-acid form, whereas simvastatin and lovastatin are administered as inactive prodrugs with lactone rings. The open-acid statins are relatively hydrophilic and have low membrane permeabilities. However, most of the statins in the acid form are substrates of uptake transporters, so they are taken up efficiently by the liver and undergo enterohepatic circulation.

The statins are the most effective and best-tolerated agents for treating dyslipidemia. These drugs are competitive inhibitors of HMG-CoA reductase, which catalyzes an early, rate-limiting step in cholesterol biosynthesis. Higher doses of the more potent statins (e.g., **atorvastatin** and simvastatin) also can reduce triglyceride levels caused by elevated VLDL levels. Some statins also are indicated for raising HDL-C levels, although the clinical significance of these effects on HDL-C remains to be proven.

Ammonium Chloride

Ammonium chloride, an acid-forming salt (4 to 12 g p.o. daily), is indicated in metabolic alkalosis. In addition, as an acidifying agent, it has been used as an expectorant.

AMOBARBITAL

(Amytal)

Amobarbital, a barbiturate, is used as a sedative to treat insomnia and as a preanesthetic medication. The barbiturates were used extensively in the past as hypnotic-sedatives but have been replaced by the much safer benzodiazepine derivatives (see Table 9). They do continue to be used as anesthetics (e.g., thiopental) and anticonvulsants (e.g., phenobarbital). The primary mechanism of action of barbiturates is to increase inhibition through the gamma-aminobutyric acid (GABA) system (see Figure 50). Anesthetic barbiturates also decrease excitation via a decrease in calcium conductance. The most commonly used barbiturates are thiopental (Pentothal), methohexital (Brevital), secobarbital (Seconal), pentobarbital (Nembutal), amobarbital (Amytal), and phenobarbital (Luminal).

Barbiturates are classified according to their duration of action; these are: ultra short-acting (thiopental and methohexital), short- to intermediate-acting (pentobarbital, secobarbital, and amobarbital), and long-acting (phenobarbital). The selection of a barbiturate is in part determined by the duration of action desired and by the clinical problems at hand. An ultra short-acting drug is used for inducing anesthesia. For treating epilepsy, a long-acting drug is used, whereas, in a sleep disorder, a short-acting or an intermediate-type drug is used, depending on whether patients have difficulty falling asleep or if they have difficulty staying asleep.

In general, the more lipid soluble a barbiturate derivative is, the greater is its plasma and tissue-binding capacity, the extent of its metabolism, and its storage in adipose tissues. In addition, very lipid-soluble substances have a faster onset of action and a shorter duration of action.

Barbiturates do not raise the pain threshold and have no analgesic property. In anesthetic doses, they depress all areas of the CNS, including the hypothalamic thermoregulatory system, respiratory center, and vasomotor centers, as well as the polysynaptic pathways in the spinal column. In addition, some, such as phenobarbital, but not all, are anticonvulsants. In toxic doses, barbiturates cause oliguria. They are absorbed orally and distributed widely throughout the body. Barbiturates are metabolized in the liver by aliphatic oxygenation, aromatic oxygenation, and *N*-dealkylation.

The inactive metabolites are excreted in the urine. The administration of bicarbonate enhances the urinary excretion of barbiturates that have a pKa of 7.4 (phenobarbital and thiopental). This generalization is not true of other barbiturates. The long-term administration of barbiturates activates the cytochrome P-450 drug-metabolizing system.

Acute barbiturate toxicity is characterized by automatism, or a state of drug-induced confusion, in which patients lose track of how much medication they have taken and take more. Death results from respiratory failure. The treatment of poisoning consists of support respiration, prevention of hypotension, diuresis, hemodialysis and, in the event of phenobarbital poisoning, the administration of sodium bicarbonate. Tolerance does not develop to lethal doses.

The abrupt withdrawal from barbiturates may cause tremors, restlessness, anxiety, weakness, nausea and vomiting, seizures, delirium, and cardiac arrest.

AMODIAQUINE

(Camoquin)

Amodiaquine is a congener of chlorquine that is no longer recommended for chemoprophylaxis of fulciparum malaria. It causes agranulocytosis and hepatic toxicity.

AMOXAPINE

(Asendin)

Amoxapine (50 mg p.o. t.i.d.) is a second-generation antidepressant with indications in depression associated with melancholia or psychotic symptoms, the depressive phase of bipolar disorder, depression associated with organic disease or alcoholism psychoneurotic anxiety, and mixed symptoms of anxiety or depression. It is absorbed orally, is bound to plasma proteins to the extent of 92%, distributed widely throughout the body and its fluids including milk, metabolized to 8-hydroxyamoxapine (an active metabolite), and is also excreted in the urine. Amoxapine causes mild to moderate degrees of sedation, orthostatic hypotension, and anticholinergic effects. In addition, because it blocks dopamin-ergic receptors in the striatum, it causes movement disorders (see Tables 5 through 7).

AMOXICILLIN/CLAVULANATE POTASSIUM

(Augmentin)

Augmentin is indicated in the treatment of infections of the lower respiratory tract, otitis media, sinusitis, skin and skin structure infections, UTIs, and community-acquired pneumonia caused by susceptible microorganisms.

AMOXICILLIN/LANSOPRAZOLE/ CLARITHROMYCIN

(Prevpac)

Prevpac is indicated in the eradication of *H. pylori* to reduce risk of duodenal ulcer recurrence.

AMOXICILLIN

(Amoxil)

Amoxicillin is a penicillinase-susceptible semisynthetic penicillin that resembles ampicillin (see Table 23). It is stable in acidic pH of the stomach, and is more rapidly and completely absorbed from the gastrointestinal tract than is ampicillin, which is the major difference between the two. The antimicrobial spectrum of amoxicillin is essentially identical to that of ampicillin, with the important exception that amoxicillin appears to be less effective than ampicillin for shigellosis. Clavulanic acid is a beta-lactam structurally related to the penicillins that inactivates beta-lactamase enzymes commonly found in microorganisms resistant to penicillin. The combination of amoxicillin/clavulanic acid extends the antibiotic spectrum of amoxicillin to include bacteria normally resistant to amoxicillin and other beta-lactam antibiotics. Amoxicillin is indicated in infections caused by *Philus influenzae, E. coli, P. mirabilis*, and *N. gonorrhoeae*, Gram-positive-streptococci (including *S. faecalis*), *S. pneumoniae*, and nonpenicillinase-producing staphylocci.

The broad-spectrum penicillins, such as ampicillin and amoxicillin, may cause gastrointestinal irritation. Occasionally, the overgrowth of staphylococci, *Pseudomonas*, *Proteus*, or yeasts may be responsible for causing enteritis. Because amoxicillin is more completely absorbed from the gastrointestinal tract, it causes less diarrhea than ampicillin.

AMPHETAMINE SULFATE

(Dexedrine)

Amphetamines are sympathomimetic amines with CNS stimulant activity, which are used in narcolepsy (5 to 60 mg/day in individual doses) and in attention deficit disorder in children (2.5 mg to not more than 40 mg daily). Amphetamine releases norepinephrine and, in high doses, also dopamine. It is absorbed from the gastrointestinal tract, metabolized in the liver, and is excreted unchanged in the urine. Acidification of urine shortens amphetamines' half-life, whereas alkalinization of urine prolongs it. The accumulation of hydroxy metabolite of amphetamine has been thought to cause amphetamine-induced psychosis. Therapeutic doses of amphetamine may cause insomnia, tremor, and restlessness; and toxic doses of amphetamine may cause mydriasis, hypertension, and arrhythmia. Chlorpromazine is an excellent antidote in amphetamine toxicity. The continuous use of amphetamine causes tolerance requiring higher doses, and hence there exists a high potential for its abuse.

Amphetamine should not be used with a monoamine oxidase A inhibitor such as tranylcypromine because the chance of inducing hypertension is magnified. Similar caution should be exercised with biogenic amine uptake blockers such as tricyclic antidepressants. Amphetamine is contraindicated in advanced arteriosclerosis, symptomatic cardiovascular disease, moderate to severe hypertension, hyperthyroidism, hypersensitivity or idiosyncrasy to the sympathomimetic amines, glaucoma, agitated states, history of drug abuse, and during or within 14 days following administration of MAO inhibitors (see Figure 37).

AMPHOTERICIN B

(Fungizone)

Amphotericin B (fungizone), which is ineffective in curing infections caused by bacteria, *Rickettsia*, or viruses, is either fungicidal or fungistatic, depending on the drug concentration used or the sensitivity of the particular fungus. Numerous pathogenic yeasts (*Cryptococcus neoformans*), pathogenic yeast-like organisms (*Monilia*), dimorphic fungi (*Blastomyces*), filamentous fungi (*Cladosporosium*), and other fungi are highly sensitive to amphotericin B (Figure 23).

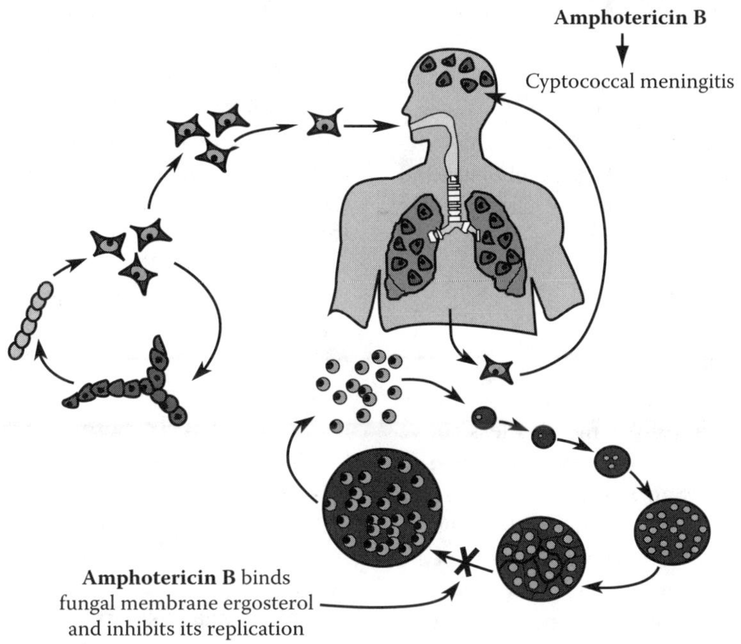

FIGURE 21 Amphotericin B, which is ineffective in ridding infections caused by bacteria, *Rickettsia*, or viruses, is either fungicidal or fungistatic, depending on the drug concentration used or the sensitivity of the particular fungus.

Furthermore, the antifungal actions of amphotericin B are enhanced by flucytosine, minocycline, or rifampin, agents otherwise devoid of antifungal activity.

Amphotericin B imposes its antifungal effects by binding to the sterol moiety of the membrane and damaging its structural and functional integrity (Figure 21). It is available in the form of a sterile lyophilized powder. Because it is insoluble in water, amphotericin B is marketed with sodium deoxycholate for dispersal in sterile water and 5% dextrose. The polyene antibiotics, amphotericin B, nystatin, and candicidin, are all poorly absorbed from the gastrointestinal tract. In the plasma, amphotericin B binds to lipoproteins including cholesterol. It is extensively metabolized, and the inactive metabolite, or metabolites, are slowly excreted in the urine.

Amphotericin B is the only polyene antibiotic given parenterally. When the intravenous route is contemplated, amphotericin B is dispersed fresh and infused slowly. It should not be administered rapidly because this causes cardiac toxicity. Heparin (1000 units) is often added to the infusion suspension to avert the risk of thrombophlebitis. Amphotericin B can also precipitate normocytic or normochromic anemia, leukopenia, and thrombocytopenia.

During the infusion of amphotericin B, the patient's temperature will rise, which may or may not be accompanied by hypotension and delirium. Often, hydrocortisone sodium succinate is added to the infusion during the initial but not the succeeding alternate-day treatment with amphotericin B.

Amphotericin B is nephrotoxic in most patients and often causes a permanent reduction in the glomerular filtration rate. Furthermore, hypokalemia may occur, requiring the oral administration of potassium chloride.

Amphotericin B has been used intrathecally in patients with coccidioidal or cryptococcal meningitis. The side effects associated with this route of administration are headache, paresthesia, nerve palsy, and visual impairment. To treat coccidioidal arthritis, amphotericin B may be injected intramuscularly, or directly into the joint (see Figure 22).

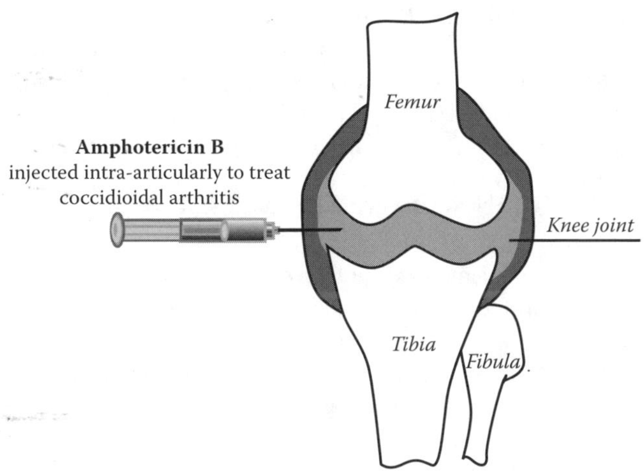

FIGURE 22 Numerous pathogenic yeasts (*Cyrptococcus neoformans*), pathogenic yeast-like organisms (*Monilia*), dimorphic fungi (*Blastomyces*), filamentous fungi (*Cladosporosium*), and other fungi are highly sensitive to amphotericin B.

AMPHOTERICIN B CHOLESTERYL SULFATE COMPLEX

(Amphotec P)

Amphotec P is indicated in the treatment of invasive **aspergillosis** when renal impairment or unacceptable toxicity precludes use of amphotericin B deoxycholate and where prior amphotericin B deoxycholate therapy has failed.

AMPICILLIN

(Amcill, Omnipen, Polycillin)

The aminopenicillins, including ampicillin, amoxicillin, and their congeners, are bactericidal for both Gram-positive and Gram-negative bacteria. They are somewhat less active than penicillin G against Gram-positive cocci sensitive to the latter agent. Ampicillin is stable in acidic pH of the stomach and is absorbed well when given orally, but its absorption is hindered by food (see Table 23). It appears in bile, undergoes enterohepatic circulation, and is excreted in the feces. Renal impairment prolongs the half-life of ampicillin, and its doses should be adjusted. Ampicillin is indicated in infections caused by susceptible strains of *Shigella, Salmonella* (including *S. typhosa*), *E. coli, Hemophilus influenzae, Proteus mirabilis, Neisseria gonorrhoeae*, and enterococci. It is also effective in the treatment of meningitis due to *N. meningitidis* and in infections caused by susceptible Gram-positive organisms, penicillin G-sensitive staphylococci, streptococci, and pneumococci. Ampicillin with probenecid is indicated in the treatment of uncomplicated urethral, endocervical, or rectal infections in adults caused by *N. gonorrhoeae*. Ampicillin sodium and sulbactam sodium are indicated in skin and skin structure infections caused by beta-lactamase-producing strains of *S. aureus, E. coli, Klebsiella* sp. (including *K. pneumoniae*), *P. mirabilis, Bacteroides fragilis, Enterobacter* sp., and *Acinetobacter caloacticus*; intra-abdominal infections caused by beta-lactamase-producing strains of *E. coli, Klebsiella* sp. (including *K. pneumoniae*), *Bacteroides* (including *B. fragilis*), and *Enterobacter* sp.; gynecological infections caused by beta-lactamase-producing strains of *E. coli* and *Bacteroides* sp. (including *B. fragilis*). High concentration of beta-lactam may cause convulsive seizures.

AMPICILLIN SODIUM/SULBACTAM SODIUM

(Unasyn)

Unasyn is indicated in the treatment of infections of skin and skin structure, intra-abdominal and gynecologic infections caused by susceptible microorganisms, and mixed infections caused by ampicillin-susceptible organisms and beta-lactamase-producing organisms.

AMPRENAVIR

(Agenerase)

Amprenavir is a protease inhibitor that is indicated in the treatment of HIV-1 infections in combination with other antiretroviral agents.

Current treatment assumes that all aspects of disease derive from the direct toxic effects of HIV on host cells, mainly CD4+T-lymphocytes. This viewpoint is based on studies demonstrating the importance of high plasma HIV RNA concentration and low CD4+ lymphocyte count as predictors of disease progression and mortality. Validation has come from evidence that treatment regimens associated with long-term suppression of HIV replication (as measured by decreased plasma HIV RNA) and repletion of peripheral CD4 cells are clinically beneficial. The goal of therapy is to suppress virus replication as much as possible for as long as possible.

HIV protease inhibitors are peptide-like chemicals that competitively inhibit the action of the virus **aspartyl protease**. This protease is a homodimer consisting of two 99-amino-acid monomers; each monomer contributes an aspartic acid residue that is essential for catalysis. The preferred cleavage site for this enzyme is the N-terminal side of proline residues especially between phenylalanine and proline. Human aspartyl proteases (i.e., renin, pepsin, gastricsin, and cathepsins D and E) contain only one polypeptide chain and are not significantly inhibited by HIV protease inhibitors. These drugs prevent proteolytic cleavage of polpolyproteins that include essential structural (pl7, p24, p9, and p7) and enzymatic (reverse transcriptase, protease, and integrase) components of the virus. This prevents the metamorphosis of HIV virus particles into their mature infectious form. Infected patients treated with HIV protease inhibitors as sole agents experienced a one hundred- to one thousand-fold mean decrease in plasma HIV RNA concentrations within 12 weeks.

The most common adverse effects associated with amprenavir are gastrointestinal, and include nausea, vomiting, diarrhea, or loose stools. Hyperglycemia, fatigue, paresthesias, and headache also have been reported. Amprenavir is the HIV protease inhibitor that is most likely to produce skin eruptions; in one study of amprenavir monotherapy, rash occurred in 5 to 35 patients over 24 weeks and began within 7 to 12 days of starting therapy. **Amprenavir** is reported to have fewer effects on plasma lipid profiles compared with ritonavir-based protease inhibitor regimens. **Fosamprenavir** has a similar toxicity profile, but gastrointestinal side effects are much less frequent than with amprenavir, and rash also may be less frequent (19% versus 27%).

AMRINONE LACTATE

(Inocor)

Agents with positive inotropic actions that may be used in the management of congestive heart failure include the cardiac glycosides (e.g., digoxin and digitoxin), dopaminergic analogs (e.g., dobutamine), phosphodiesterase inhibitors (e.g., amrinone and milrinone), angiotensin antagonists (e.g., captopril, enalapril, and lisinopril), and vasodilators (nitrates and hydralazine). Amrinone and milrinone are bipyridine derivatives and relatively selective inhibitors of the cyclic

GMP-inhibited, cyclic AMP phosphodiesterase (PDE type III) family (Figure 23). They cause vasodilation with a con-

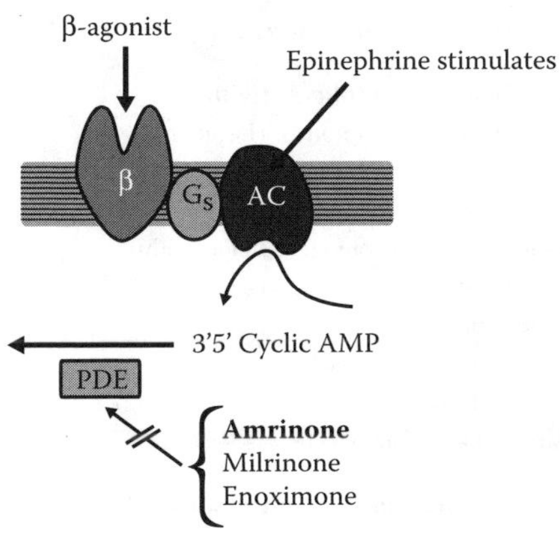

FIGURE 23 **Amrinone**, **milrinone**, and **enoximone** differ from aminophylline in that they exhibit a certain degree of selectivity for peak III phosphodiesterase, which is found predominantly in myocardial and vascular tissues. These agents exert both **positive inotropic** and **direct vasodilating actions**.

sequent fall in systemic vascular resistance, and increase both the force of contraction and velocity of relaxation of cardiac muscle. Both drugs are effective when given either as single agents or, more commonly, in combination with other oral and/or intravenous drugs for short-term treatment of patients with severe heart failure due to systolic right or left ventricular dysfunction. The elimination half-lives of amrinone (0.5 μg/kg) and milrinone (50 μg/kg) are 2 to 3 hours and 30 to 60 minutes, respectively. Thrombocytopenia occurs in 10% of patients receiving amrinone but is rare with milrinone.

AMYL NITRITE

Amyl nitrite is a highly volatile liquid that is sold in fragile glass ampules packaged in a protective cloth covering. The ampule can be crushed, which causes the rapid release of inhalable vapors. Amyl nitrite has a rapid onset of action, and its duration of action is 8 to 10 minutes. The pronounced vasodilation causes tachycardia, enhanced cardiac output, and vasoconstriction. Amyl nitrite is no longer used for the control of angina.

ANAGRELIDE
(Agrylin)

Anagrelide is an antiplatelet agent that is indicated in the treatment of thrombocythemia caused by myeloproliferative disorders; to reduce elevated platelet count and risk of thrombotic events; to relieve associated symptoms, including thrombo-hemorrhagic events.

ANAKINRA
(Kineret)

Anakinra is an immunomodular that blocks the biologic activity of interleukin-1 (IL-1) by competitively inhibiting IL-1 binding to interleukin-1 type I receptor, which is expressed in a wide variety of organs and tissues. Anakinra causes reduction in signs and symptoms, and slowing the progression of structural damage in moderately to severely active rheumatoid arthritis in patients who have failed at least one disease-modifying antirheumatic drug.

ANALGESICS: Narcotics

Methadone-Like Agonists	**Morphine-Like Agonists**
Methadone	Codeine
Propoxyphene	Hydrocodone
Meperidine-Like Agonists	Hydromorphone
Alfentanil	Levorphanol
Fentanyl	Morphine
Meperidine	Oxycodone
Sufentanil	Oxymorphone
Mixed Agonist-Antagonists	**Narcotic Antagonists**
Buprenorphine	Naloxone
Butorphanol	Naltrexone
Dezocine	
Nalbuphine	
Pentazocine	

ANALGESICS: Non-narcotic Agents

Acetaminophen	Fenoprofen
Aspirin	Magnesium salicylate
Choline salicylate	Meclofenamate
Diflunisal	Mefenamic acid
Etodolac	Naproxen
Ibuprofen	Naproxen sodium
Ketoprofen	Sodium salicylate
Ketorolac (intramuscular)	

ANASTROZOLE
(Arimidex)

Anastrozole is a selective nonsteroidal aromatase inhibitor, that lowers serum estradiol concentrations. It is indicated in advanced breast cancer in postmenopausal women with progression following tamoxifen therapy; first-line treatment of postmenopausal women with hormone receptor positive or hormone receptor unknown locally advanced or metastatic breast cancer.

Among the diverse reactions carried out by mammalian cytochrome P450S (CYPs) are *N*-dealkylation, *O*-dealkylation, aromatic hydroxylation, *N*-oxidation, *S*-oxidation, deamination, and dehalogenation. More than 50 individual CYPs have been identified in humans. As a family of enzymes, CYPs are involved in the metabolism of dietary and xenobiotic agents, as well as the synthesis of endogenous compounds such as steroids and the metabolism of bile acids, which are degradation by-products of cholesterol. In contrast to the drug-metabolizing CYPs, the

CYPs that catalyze steroid and bile acid synthesis have very specific substrate preferences. For example, the CYP that produces estrogen from testosterone, CYP19 or aromatase, can metabolize only testosterone, and does not metabolize xenobiotics. Specific inhibitors for aromatase, such as **anastrozole**, have been developed for use in the treatment of estrogen-dependent tumors. The synthesis of bile acids from cholesterol occurs in the liver where, subsequent to CYP-catalyzed oxidation, the bile acids are conjugated and transported through the bile duct and gallbladder into the small intestine. CYPs involved in bile acid production have strict substrate requirements and do not participate in xenobiotic or drug metabolism.

Anastrozole has no clinically significant effect on adrenal glucocorticoid or mineralocorticoid synthesis in postmenopausal women. It also has no effect on the adrenocorticotropic hormone-stimulated release of cortisol or aldosterone, or on plasma concentrations of luteinizing hormone or follicle-stimulating hormone. Anastrozole has been associated with a significantly lower incidence of vaginal bleeding, vaginal discharge, hot flushes, endometrial cancer, ischemic cerebrovascular events, venous thromboembolic events, and deep vein thrombosis, including pulmonary embolism. **Tamoxifen** is associated with a lower incidence of musculoskeletal disorders and fracture. In the advanced disease setting, anastrozole is as well tolerated as megestrol, although weight gain is significantly increased by megestrol compared to anastrozole. In addition, anastrozole is as well tolerated as tamoxifen, with a low rate of withdrawal due to drug-related adverse events (2%). Further, anastrozole is associated with fewer thromboembolic events and episodes of vaginal bleeding than tamoxifen.

ANDROGENS

Testosterone, the male sex hormone, is responsible for the development and maintenance of the male sex organs (the penis, prostate gland, seminal vesicle, and vas deferens) and secondary sex characteristics. In addition, testosterone has anabolic effects. Similar to progesterone, testosterone is metabolized very rapidly in the liver by the first-pass mechanism, and hence requires structural modifications in order to be effective. For example, the 17–OH group of testosterone may be modified by the addition of propionic acid, which yields testosterone propionate; cyclopentylpropionic acid, which yields testosterone cypionate; or enanthate, which yields testosterone enanthate. In addition, the 17 position may be methylated to yield methyltestosterone, or a fluorine and a methyl group may be inserted to yield fluoxymesterone. In general, these agents are more effective when given orally and have a longer duration of action than testosterone itself (Table 8).

Testosterone and its derivatives are used in the treatment of hypogonadism (eunuchoidism), hypopituitarism, accelerated growth, aging in men, osteoporosis, anemia, endometriosis, promotion of metabolism, suppression of lactation, and breast carcinoma.

TABLE 8
Examples of Anabolic and Androgenic Steroids

Steroids with Anabolic Activities
Dromostanolone propionate (Drolban)
Ethylestrenol (Maxibolin)
Methandrostenolone (Dianabol)
Nandrolone decanoate (Deca-Durabolin)
Nandrolone phenpropionate (Durabolin)
Oxandrolone (Anavar)
Oxymetholone (Adroyd)
Stanozolol (Winstrol)
Testolactone (Teslac)
Steroids with Androgenic Properties
Fluoxymesterone (Halotestin)
Methyltestosterone (Metandren)
Testosterone (Android-T)
Testosterone propionate cypionate (Depotestosterone)
Testosterone enanthate (Delatestryl)

Hormonal therapy with testosterone should be reserved primarily for patients with hypogonadal disorders. There are two important warnings about the indiscriminate use of intramuscular testosterone in patients with serum testosterone levels in the normal range. First, many impotent patients are older and may have adenocarcinoma of the prostate; thus, exogenous testosterone may accelerate the growth of the neoplasm. Second, although testosterone may induce a marked increase in libido, patients may still be unable to achieve adequate erection.

One of the side effects of testosterone compounds is masculinization in women (such as hirsutism, acne, depression of menses, and clitoral enlargement) and of their female offspring. Therefore, androgens are contraindicated in pregnant women. Prostatic hypertrophy may occur in males, which leads to urinary retention. Therefore, androgens are contraindicated in men with prostatic carcinoma.

ANGIOTENSIN

In studying the role of the renin-angiotensin system in the development of hypertension, it has become apparent that there are two systems: a tissue and a circulating renin angiotensin. The control of hypertension is focused primarily on the renin-angiotensin system in the cardiovascular system and the brain. Angiotensin-converting enzyme (ACE) is found in the lung, plasma, the brush borders of the proximal renal tubule, the endothelium of vascular beds, the brain, and the testis (see Figure 24). Its two most important actions are the inactivation of bradykinin and the conversion of angiotensin I to angiotensin II.

Receptors for angiotensin II are found in the medulla oblongata in neurons involved in the regulation of baroreceptor activity. Because studies in hypertensive patients have indicated that ACE inhibitors reduce sympathetic

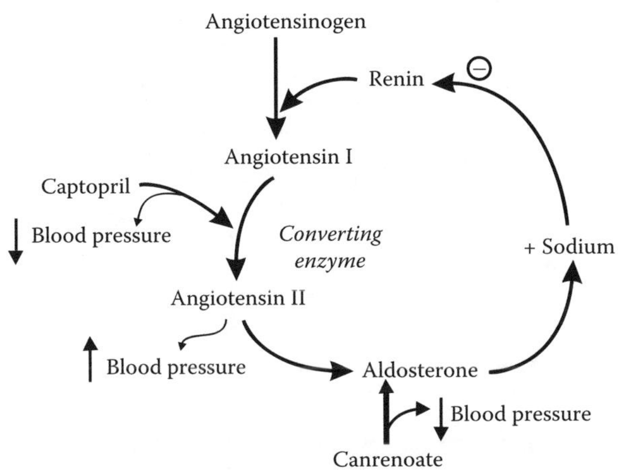

FIGURE 24 Captopril, an angiotensin-converting enzyme inhibitor, is used in hypertension and congestive heart failure.

activity and enhance baroreceptor sensitivity, it is possible that the primary hypotensive mechanism of these agents is mediated through the blockade of angiotensin II formation in the cardiovascular centers of the brain. The relationship of the renin-angiotensin-aldosterone system to bradykinin and prostaglandin production is shown in Figure 24.

ANGIOTENSIN-CONVERTING ENZYME (ACE) INHIBITORS FOR HYPERTENSION

Drugs	Initial Daily Dosages	Drugs	Initial Daily Dosages
Benazepril	10 mg	Moexipril	7.5 mg once
Captopril	25 mg bid or tid	Monopril	20 mg
Enalapril	5 mg	Perindopril	4 mg
Fornopril	10 mg	Quinapril	10 mg
Fosinopril	10 mg	Ramipril	2.5 mg
Lisinopril	10 mg	Trandolapril	1 or 2 mg once

The adverse effects of ACE inhibitors are excessive hypotension associated with volume or salt depletion. All ACE inhibitors commonly cause a dry cough and rarely may cause angioedema. Renal failure can occur in patients with bilateral renal artery stenosis. Hyperkalemia may occur in patients with renal insufficiency, diabetics with even mild renal impairment, and patients taking potassium supplements or potassium-sparing diuretics. ACE inhibitors are fetotoxic and are not recommended for use during pregnancy.

ANISINDIONE

(Miradon)

The coumarin anticoagulants include dicumarol, warfarin sodium (coumadin sodium), warfarin potassium (Athrombin-K), acenocoumarol (Sintrom), and phenprocouman (Liquamar). The inanedione derivatives are phenindione (Hedulin), diphenadione (Dipaxin), and anisindione (Miradon). Anisindione is available in a 50-mg tablet, and is used in a 300-mg dosage the first day, 200 mg the second day, 100 mg the third day, and thereafter, 25 to 250 mg daily for maintenance.

ANISTREPLASE

(Anisoylated Plasminogen-Streptokinase Activator Complex; APSAC) (Eminase)

Anistreplase, a thrombolytic enzyme (30 units by direct IV injection over 2 to 5 minutes), is indicated in the treatment of acute coronary arterial thrombosis (see Figure 94).

ANOREXIA NERVOSA AND BULIMIA NERVOSA: Treatment of

In most patients, intense dieting and compulsive exercising are the earliest signs of anorexia nervosa. In addition to amenorrhea, patients with anorexia nervosa, or bulimia nervosa, frequently complain of constipation, stomach bloating, and abdominal pain suggestive of abnormalities in gastrointestinal motility.

Although restoration of body weight and normal eating usually result in a return to normal times for gastric emptying, the short-term use of prokinetic agents such as cisapride or domperidone is indicated.

One of the most serious, and possibly irreversible, consequences of anorexia nervosa is osteoporosis, and estrogen supplementation has been advocated for its treatment.

In addition to psychotherapy, fluoxetine has offered promising results. On the other hand, serotonin uptake inhibitors, tricyclic antidepressants, and monoamine oxidase inhibitors have been shown to reduce the frequency of binge eating and vomiting, and to improve dysphoria and disturbed attitudes toward body weight and shape in patients with bulimia nervosa. Despite this, there is little knowledge regarding the mechanisms and specificity of action of these agents in bulimia nervosa.

A 24-week clinical trial of desipramine combined with individual cognitive therapy produces the best outcome.

ANTACIDS

The medical treatment of esophageal, gastric, and duodenal ulcer includes relieving the symptoms, accelerating healing, preventing complications, and preventing recurrence. Drug treatment includes the use of antacids, anticholinergic drugs, histamine H_2-receptor antagonists, and inhibitors of H^+K^+ATPase (see Figures 35 and 64).

Because acid-pepsin disease rarely occurs in the absence of gastric acid and pepsin, antacids are highly effective in its overall management. Antacids consist of a mixture of magnesium, aluminum, and calcium compounds (see Table 4). Their efficacy is based on their inherent ability to react with and neutralize gastric acid. Sodium bicarbonate, which may leave the stomach rapidly, can cause alkalosis and sodium retention. Calcium salts may produce hypercalcemia, which can be detrimental in patients with impaired renal function. Aluminum salts may decrease the absorption of tetracyclines and anticholinergic drugs.

ANTACIDS
Solid Preparations

Product	$Al(OH)_3$		$MG(OH)_2$	$CaCO_3$	Simethicone
Gelusil II	400		400	0	30
Maalox TC	600		300	0	0
Mylanta II	400		400	0	40
Riopan Plus II		Magaldrate	1080		20
Rolaids		$NaAlCO_3(OH)_2$	325		0
Tums Ex	0		0	750	0
		Liquid Preparations			
Gelusil II	400		400	0	30
Kudrox	500		450	0	40
Maalox TC	600		300	0	0
Milk of Magnesia	0		390	0	0
Mylanta II	400		400	0	40
Riopan Plus II		Magaldrate	1080		30

ANTHRACYCLINE ANTIBIOTICS
(Doxorubicin)

Anthracycline antibiotics cause unique cardiomyopathies. An acute form is characterized by abnormal electrocardiographic changes including ST-T wave alterations and arrhythmias. This is brief, and rarely a serious problem. Cineangiographic studies have shown an acute, reversible reduction in ejection fraction 24 hours after a single dose. An exaggerated manifestation of acute myocardial damage, the "pericarditis–myocarditis syndrome" may be characterized by severe disturbances in impulse conduction and frank congestive heart failure, often associated with pericardial effusion. Chronic cumulative dose-related toxicity of anthracycline antibiotics is manifested by congestive heart failure that is unresponsive to digitalis. Cardiac irradiation or administration of high doses of cyclophosphamide or another anthracycline may increase the risk of cardiotoxicity. There is evidence that cardiac damage is reduced by the concomitant administration of the iron chelator dexrazoxane (ADR-529) or by amifostine (WR-2721) or its active metabolite (WR-1065).

ANTHRA
(Anthra-Derm, Drithocreme, Drithocreme HP 1%, Dritho-Scalp, Lasan)

Anthralin, a germicide (ointment 0.1%, 0.25%, 0.4%, 0.5% 1%; cream 0.1%, 0.25%, 0.4%, 0.5%, 1%), is indicated in the treatment of quiescent or chronic psoriasis.

ANTIANXIETY AGENTS
Benzodiazepine Derivatives

Alprazolam	Clorazepate	Lorazepam
Chlordiazepoxide	Diazepam	Oxazepam
Clonazepam	Halazepam	Prazepam

Azaspirodecanedione Derivatives

Buspirone
Gepirone
Ipsapirone

The neurochemical basis for anxiety is only partially understood. Various manifestations of anxiety, such as palpitations and tremulousness, may be viewed as hyperactivity of the adrenergic system, and beta-adrenergic receptor-blocking agents are effective for the treatment of acute stress reactions, adjustment disorders, generalized anxiety, panic disorder, and agoraphobia. The discovery of the benzodiazepine-GABA receptor-chloride ionophore complex furnished additional evidence that this complex participates in the etiology and manifestation of anxiety. The fact that certain benzodiazepine receptor inverse agonists, such as beta-carboline carboxylate ethyl ester, cause anxiety substantiates the involvement of benzodiazepine-GABA receptors in the etiology and manifestations of anxiety disorders.

The introduction of novel anxiolytic agents such as buspirone, which interacts with the serotoninergic system, has suggested that serotoninergic fibers may be the final pathway through which anxiolytic effects are expressed.

Buspirone has a chemical structure that is distinct from that of the benzodiazepines. Without this structural homology, it is not surprising that buspirone does not interact with the GABA receptors. Furthermore, the clinical profile of buspirone appears to be anxioselective, with a much reduced potential for abuse.

ANTIBACTERIAL DRUGS OF CHOICE

New drugs for treatment of bacterial infections and new information about older drugs continue to become available. A few examples will be cited.

Pneumonia—Community-acquired bacterial pneumonia is frequently caused by *Streptococcus pneumoniae* (pneumococci). In the United States, more than 15% of recent isolates of *S. pneumoniae* are highly resistant to **penicillin** and increasingly resistant to **cephalosporins**, **macrolides**, and less commonly to **fluoroquinolones**. Other bacterial pathogens include *Haemophilus influenzae, Staphylococcus aureus, Klebsiella pneumoniae*, and, occasionally, other Gram-negative bacilli and anaerobic mouth organisms. "Atypical" pathogens, including *Mycoplasma pneumoniae, Chlamydia pneumoniae*, and respiratory viruses are probably the most common cause of community-acquired pneumonia.

Meningitis—The organisms most commonly responsible for community-acquired bacterial meningitis are *S. pneumoniae* and *N. meningitidis*. For treatment of meningitis in adults and in children more than two months old, pending results of cultures, high-dose **cefotaxime** or **ceftriaxone** is generally recommended, plus **vancomycin** with or without rifampin to cover resistant pneumococci.

Sepsis syndrome—For treatment of a sepsis syndrome, the choice of drugs should be based on the probable source of infection, Gram-stained smears of appropriate clinical specimens, and the immune status of the patient. The choice should also reflect local patterns of bacterial resistance. A third- or fourth-generation **cephalosporin** (**cefotaxime**, **ceftizoxime**, **ceftriaxone**, **cefepime,** or **ceftazidime**), **imipenem** or **meropenem**, or **aztreonam** can be used to treat sepsis caused by many strains of Gram-negative bacilli.

Intra-abdominal infection—For intra-abdominal or pelvic infections likely to involve anaerobes, treatment should include either **ticarcillin/clavulanic acid**, **ampicillin/sulbactam**, **piperacillin/tazobactam**, **imipenem**, **meropenem**, **cefoxitin,** or **cefotetan**, each with or without an **aminoglycoside**. When the source of bacteremia is thought to be in the biliary tract, some clinicians would use piperacillin plus metronidazole, piperacillin/tazobactam or ampicillin/sulbactam, each with or without an aminoglycoside.

Neutropenic patients—For suspected bacteremia in neutropenic patients, **ceftazidime**, **imipenem**, **meropenem,** or **cefepime**, each alone or in more seriously ill patients with an aminoglycoside (gentamicin, tobramycin or amikacin), would be a reasonable first choice.

Urinary tract infection—Acute uncomplicated cystitis in women can be effectively and inexpensively treated, before the infecting organism is known, with a three-day course of oral **trimethoprim-sulfamethoxazole**; in areas where the prevalence of *E. coli* resistant to trimethoprim-sulfamethoxazole exceeds 15 to 20%, a fluoroquinolone can be substituted.

Multiple-antibiotic-resistant enterococci—Many *Enterococcus* spp. are now resistant to penicillin and ampicillin, gentamicin or streptomycin or both, and to vancomycin. Some of these strains are susceptible *in vitro* to chloramphenicol, doxycycline or fluoroquinolones, but clinical results with these drugs have been variable.

ANTIBACTERIAL DRUGS OF CHOICE

Infecting Organism	Drug of First Choice	Alternative Drugs
	Gram-Positive Cocci	
Streptococcus, anaerobic or *Peptostreptococcus*	Penicillin G	Clindamycin; a cephalosporin; vancomycin
Streptococcus pneumoniae (pneumococcus), penicillin-susceptible (MIC <0.1 μg/mL)	Penicillin G or V; amoxicillin	A cephalosporin; erythromycin; azithromycin; clarithromycin; levofloxacin, gatifloxacin, or moxifloxacin; meropenem; imipenem; trimethoprim-sulfamethoxazole; clindamycin; a tetracycline
Penicillin-intermediate resistance (MIC <0.1 ≤2 μg/mL)	Penicillin G IV (12 million units/day for adults); ceftriaxone or cefotaxime	Levofloxacin, gatifloxacin, or moxifloxacin; vancomycin; clindamycin
Penicillin-high level resistance (MIC ≥2 μg/mL)	**Meningitis**: vancomycin + ceftriaxone or cefotaxime ± rifampin	Meropenem; imipenem
	Other infections: vancomycin + ceftriaxone or cefotaxime; or levofloxacin, gatifloxacin, or moxifloxacin	Linezolid; quinupristin/dalfopristin
	Gram-Negative Cocci	
Moraxella (Branhamella) catarrhalis	Cefuroxime; a fluoroquinolone	Trimethoprim-sulfamethoxazole; amoxicillin/clavulanic acid; erythromycin; a tetracycline; cefotaxime; ceftizoxime; ceftriaxone; cefuroxime axetil; cefixime; cefpodoxime; clarithromycin; azithromycin
Neisseria gonorrhoeae (gonococcus)	Ceftriaxone or cefixime; or ciprofloxacin, gatifloxacin, or ofloxacin	Cefotaxime; penicillin G
Neisseria meningitidis (meningococcus)	Penicillin G	Cefotaxime; ceftizoxime; ceftriaxone; chloramphenicol; a sulfonamide; a fluoroquinolone
	Gram-Positive Bacilli	
Bacillus anthracis (anthrax)	Penicillin G	Ciprofloxacin; erythromycin; a tetracycline
Bacillus cereus, subtilis	Vancomycin	Imipenem or meropenem; clindamycin
Clostridium perfringens	Penicillin G; clindamycin	Metronidazole; imipenem or meropenem; chloramphenicol
Clostridium tetani	Metronidazole	Penicillin G; a tetracycline
Clostridium difficile	Metronidazole	Vancomycin (oral)

Corynebacterium diphtheriae	Erythromycin	Penicillin G
Corynebacterium, JK group	Vancomycin	Penicillin G + gentamicin; erythromycin
Erysipelothrix rhusiopathiae	Penicillin G	Erythromycin, a cephalosporin, a fluoroquinolone
Listeria monocytogenes	Ampicillin ± gentamicin	Trimethoprim-sulfamethoxazole
	Enteric Gram-Negative Bacilli	
Bacteroides	Metronidazole or clindamycin	Imipenem or meropenem; amoxicillin/clavulanic acid; ticarcillin/clavulanic acid; piperacillin/tazobactam; ampicillin/sulbactam; cefoxitin; cefotetan; chloramphenicol; cefmetazole; penicillin G; gatifloxacin or moxifloxacin
Campylobacter fetus	Imipenem or meropenem	Gentamicin
	Enteric Gram-Negative Bacilli	
Campylobacter jejuni	Erythromycin or azithromycin	A fluoroquinolone; a tetracycline; gentamicin
Citrobacter freundi	Imipenem or meropenem	A fluoroquinolone; amikacin; a tetracycline; trimethoprim-sulfamethoxazole; cefotaxime, ceftizoxime, ceftriaxone, cefepime, or ceftazidime
Enterobacter	Imipenem or meropenem	Gentamicin, tobramycin or amikacin; trimethoprim-sulfamethoxazole; ciprofloxacin, ticarcillin, mezlocillin, or piperacillin; aztreonam; cefotaxime; ceftizoxime; ceftriaxone; cefepime or ceftazidime
Escherichia coli	Cefotaxime, ceftizoxime, ceftriaxone, cefepime, or ceftazidime	Ampicillin ± gentamicin, tobramycin, or amikacin; carbenicillin, ticarcillin, mezlocillin, or piperacillin; gentamicin, tobramycin, or amikacin; amoxicillin/clavulanic acid; ticarcillin/clavulanic acid; piperacillin/tazobactam; ampicillin/sulbactam; trimethoprim-sulfamethoxazole; imipenem or meropenem; aztreonam; a fluoroquinolone; another cephalosporin
Helicobacter pylori	Omeprazole ± amoxicillin + clarithromycin; or tetracycline HCL + metronidazole + bismuth subsalicylate	Tetracycline HCL + clarithromycin + bismuth subsalicylate; amoxicillin + metronidazole + bismuth subsalicylate; amoxicillin + clarithromycin
Klebsiella pneumoniae	Cefotaxime, ceftizoxime, ceftriaxone, cefepime, or ceftazidime	Imipenem or meropenem; gentamicin, tobramycin, or amikacin; amoxicillin/clavulanic acid; ticarcillin/clavulanic acid; piperacillin/tazobactam; ampicillin/sulbactam; trimethoprim-sulfamethoxazole; aztreonam; a fluoroquinolone; mezlocillin or piperacillin, another cephalosporin
Proteus mirabilis	Ampicillin	A cephalosporin; ticarcillin, mezlocillin or piperacillin; gentamicin, tobramycin, or amikacin; trimethoprim-sulfamethoxazole; imipenem, or meropenem; aztreonam; a fluoroquinolone; chloramphenicol
Proteus, indole-positive (including *Providencia rettgeri*, *Morganella morganii*, and *Proteus vulgaris*)	Cefotaxime, ceftizoxime, ceftriaxone, cefepime, or ceftazidime	Imipenem or meropenem; gentamicin, tobramycin, or amikacin; carbenicillin, ticarcillin, mezlocillin, or piperacillin; amoxicillin/clavulanic acid; ticarcillin/clavulanic acid; piperacillin/tazobactam; ampicillin/sulbactam; aztreonam; trimethoprim-sulfamethoxazole; a fluoroquinolone
Providencia stuartii	Cefotaxime, ceftizoxime, ceftriaxone, cefepime, or ceftazidime	Imipenem or meropenem; ticarcillin/clavulanic acid; piperacillin/tazobactam; gentamicin, tobramycin, or amikacin; carbenicillin; ticarcillin, mezlocillin, or piperacillin; aztreonam; trimethoprim-sulfamethoxazole; a fluoroquinolone
Salmonella typhi (typhoid fever)	A fluoroquinolone or ceftriaxone	Chloramphenicol; trimethoprim-sulfamethoxazole; ampicillin; amoxicillin; azithromycin
Other *Salmonella*	Cefotaxime or ceftriaxone or a fluoroquinolone	Ampicillin; amoxicillin; trimethoprim-sulfamethoxazole; chloramphenicol

Serratia	Imipenem or meropenem	Gentamicin or amikacin; cefotaxime, ceftizoxime, ceftriaxone, cefepime, or ceftazidime; aztreonam; trimethoprim-sulfamethoxazole; carbenicillin, ticarcillin, mezlocillin, or piperacillin; a fluoroquinolone
Shigella	A fluoroquinolone	Azithromycin; trimethoprim-sulfamethoxazole; ampicillin; ceftriaxone
Yersinia enterocolitica	Trimethoprim-sulfamethoxazole	A fluoroquinolone; gentamicin, tobramycin, or amikacin; cefotaxime or ceftizoxime
	Other Gram-Negative Bacilli	
Acinetobacter	Imipenem or meropenem	An aminoglycoside; ciprofloxacin; trimethoprim-sulfamethoxazole; ticarcillin, mezlocillin, or piperacillin; ceftazidime; minocycline; doxycycline; sulbactam; polymyxin
Aeromonas	Trimethoprim-sulfamethoxazole	Gentamicin or tobramycin; imipenem; a fluoroquinolone
Bartonella henselae or *Quintana* (bacillary angiomatosis)	Erythromycin	Doxycycline; azithromycin
Bartonella henselae (cat scratch bacillus)	Azithromycin	Ciprofloxacin; erythromycin; trimethoprim-sulfamethoxazole; gentamicin; rifampin
Bordetella pertussis (whooping cough)	Erythromycin	Azithromycin or clarithromycin; trimethoprim-sulfamethoxazole
Brucella	A tetracycline + rifampin	A tetracycline + streptomycin or gentamicin; chloramphenicol ± streptomycin; trimethoprim-sulfamethoxazole ± gentamicin; ciprofloxacin ± rifampin
Burkholderia cepacia	Trimethoprim-sulfamethoxazole	Ceftazidime; chloramphenicol; imipenem
Burkholderia (Pseudomonas) mallei (glanders)	Streptomycin + a tetracycline	Streptomycin + chloramphenicol; imipenem
Burkholderia (Pseudomonas) pseudomallei (melioidosis)	Imipenem; ceftazidime	Meropenem; chloramphenicol + doxycycline + trimethoprim-sulfamethoxazole; amoxicillin/clavulanic acid
Calymmatobacterium granulomatis (granuloma inguinale)	Trimethoprim-sulfamethoxazole	Doxycycline or ciprofloxacin ± gentamicin
Capnocytophaga canimorsus	Penicillin G	Cefotaxime; ceftizoxime; ceftriaxone; imipenem or meropenem; vancomycin; a fluoroquinolone; clindamycin
Eikenella corrodens	Ampicillin	An erythromycin; a tetracycline; amoxicillin/clavulanic acid; ampicillin/sulbactam; ceftriaxone
Francisella tularensis (tularemia)	Streptomycin	Gentamicin; a tetracycline; chloramphenicol; ciprofloxacin
Fusobacterium	Penicillin G	Metronidazole; clindamycin; cefoxitin; chloramphenicol
Gardnerella vaginalis (bacterial vaginosis)	Oral metronidazole	Topical clindamycin or metronidazole; oral clindamycin
Haemophilus ducreyi (chancroid)	Azithromycin or ceftriaxone	Ciprofloxacin or erythromycin
Haemophilus influenzae		
Meningitis, epiglottitis, arthritis, and other serious infections	Cefotaxime or ceftriaxone	Cefuroxime (not for meningitis); chloramphenicol; meropenem
Upper respiratory infections and bronchitis	trimethoprim-sulfamethoxazole	cefuroxime; amoxicillin/clavulanic acid; cefuroxime axetil; cefpodoxime; cefaclor; cefotaxime; ceftizoxime; ceftriaxone; cefixime; a tetracycline; clarithromycin; azithromycin; a fluoroquinolone; ampicillin or amoxicillin
Legionella species	Azithromycin or a fluoroquinolone ± rifampin	Doxycycline ± rifampin; trimethoprim-sulfamethoxazole; erythromycin
Leptotrichia buccalis	Penicillin G	A tetracycline; clindamycin; erythromycin
Pasteurella multocida	Penicillin G	A tetracycline; a cephalosporin; amoxicillin/clavulanic acid; ampicillin/sulbactam
Pseudomonas aeruginosa		
Urinary tract infection	Ciprofloxacin	Levofloxacin; carbenicillin, ticarcillin, piperacillin, or mezlocillin; ceftazidime; cefepime; imipenem or

		meropenem; aztreonam; tobramycin; gentamicin; amikacin
Other infections	Ticarcillin, mezlocillin, or piperacillin + tobramycin, gentamicin, or amikacin	Ceftazidime, imipenem, meropenem, aztreonam, cefepime + tobramycin, gentamicin, or amikacin; ciprofloxacin
Spirillum minus (rat bite fever)	Penicillin G	A tetracycline; streptomycin
Stenotrophomonas maltophilia	Trimethoprim-sulfamethoxazole	Minocycline; a fluoroquinolone
Streptobacillus moniliformis (rat bite fever; Haverhill fever)	Penicillin G	A tetracycline; streptomycin
Vibrio cholerae (cholera)	A tetracycline	A fluoroquinolone; trimethoprim-sulfamethoxazole
Vibrio vulnificus	A tetracycline	Cefotaxime
Yersinia pestis (plague)	Streptomycin ± a tetracycline	Chloramphenicol; gentamicin; trimethoprim-sulfamethoxazole
	Acid Fast Bacilli	
Mycobacterium tuberculosis	Isoniazid + rifampin + pyrazinamide ± ethambutol or streptomycin	A fluoroquinolone; cycloserine; capreomycin or kanamycin or amikacin; ethionamide; para-aminosalicyclic acid; ± clofazimine
Mycobacterium kansasii	Isoniazid + rifampin ± ethambutol or streptomycin	Clarithromycin or azithromycin; ethionamide; cycloserine
Mycobacterium avium complex	Clarithromycin or azithromycin + ethambutol ± rifabutin	Ciprofloxacin; amikacin
Prophylaxis	Clarithromycin or azithromycin ± rifabutin	
Mycobacterium fortuitum/chelonae complex	Amikacin + clarithromycin	Cefoxitin; rifampin; a sulfonamide; doxycycline; ethambutol; linezolid
Mycobacterium marinum (balnei)	Minocycline	Trimethoprim-sulfamethoxazole; rifampin; clarithromycin; doxycycline
Mycobacterium leprae (leprosy)	Dapsone + rifampin ± clofazimine	Minocycline; ofloxacin; sparfloxacin; clarithromycin
	Actinomycetes	
Actinomyces israelii (actinomycosis)	Penicillin G	A tetracycline; erythromycin; clindamycin
Nocardia	Trimethoprim-sulfamethoxazole	Sulfisoxazole; amikacin; a tetracycline; imipenem or meropenem; cycloserine; linezolid
Rhodococcus equi	Vancomycin ± a fluoroquinolone, rifampin, imipenem, or meropenem; amikacin	Erythromycin
Tropheryma whippelii (agent of Whipple's disease)	Trimethoprim-sulfamethoxazole	Penicillin G; a tetracycline
	Chlamydiae	
Chlamydia psittaci (psittacosis; ornithosis)	A tetracycline	Chloramphenicol
Chlamydia trachomatis (trachoma)	Azithromycin	A tetracycline (topical plus oral); a sulfonamide (topical plus oral)
	Erythromycin (oral or IV)	A sulfonamide
(Inclusion conjunctivitis)	Erythromycin	A sulfonamide
(Pneumonia)	Azithromycin or doxycycline	Erythromycin; ofloxacin; amoxicillin
(Urethritis, cervicitis)	A tetracycline	Erythromycin
(Lymphogranuloma venereum)		
Chlamydia pneumoniae (TWAR strain)	Erythromycin; a tetracycline; clarithromycin or azithromycin	A fluoroquinolone
	Ehrlichia	
Ehrlichia chaffeensis	Doxycycline	Chloramphenicol
Ehrlichia ewingii	Doxycycline	
Ehrlichia phagocytophila	Doxycycline	Rifampin
	Mycoplasma	
Mycoplasma pneumoniae	Erythromycin; a tetracycline; clarithromycin or azithromycin	A fluoroquinolone
Ureaplasma urealyticum	Erythromycin	A tetracycline; clarithromycin; azithromycin; ofloxacin

Rickettsia—Rocky Mountain spotted fever, endemic typhus (murine), epidemic typhus (louse-borne), scrub typhus, (Orientia tsutsugamushi), trench fever, Q fever	Doxycycline	Chloramphenicol; a fluoroquinolone; rifampin
	Spirochetes	
Borrelia burgdorferi (Lyme disease)	Doxycycline; amoxicillin; cefuroxime axetil	Ceftriaxone; cefotaxime; penicillin G; azithromycin; clarithromycin
Borrelia recurrentis (relapsing fever)	A tetracycline	Penicillin G
Leptospira	Penicillin G	A tetracycline
Treponema pallidum (syphilis)	Penicillin G	A tetracycline; ceftriaxone
Treponema pertenue (yaws)	Penicillin G	A tetracycline

Type	Drug	Common Uses	Side Effects
Aminoglycosides			
	Amikacin	Infections caused by Gram-negative bacteria, such as *E. coli* and *Klebsiella*	Hearing loss
	Gentamicin		Dizziness
	Kanamycin		Kidney damage
	Neomycin		
	Netilmicin		
	Streptomycin		
	Tobramycin		
Carbecephem			
	Loracarbef		
Carbapenems			
	Ertapenem	Gangrene, sepsis, pneumonia, abdominal and urinary infections, and (except for ertapenem) Pseudomonas infections	Seizure
	Imipenem/cilastatin		Confusion
	Meropenem		
Cephalosporins, 1st generation			
	Cefadroxil	Skin and soft tissue infections	Gastrointestinal upset and diarrhea
	Cefazolin		Nausea
	Cephalexin		Allergic reactions
Cephalosporins, 2nd generation			
	Cefaclor	Some respiratory and abdominal infections	Gastrointestinal upset and diarrhea
	Cefamandole		Nausea
	Cefotetan		Allergic reactions
	Cefoxitin		
	Cefprozil		
	Cefuroxime		
Cephalosporins, 3rd generation			
	Cefixime	Broad coverage of many bacteria for people with mild to moderate infections (oral) and serious illness (by injection)	Gastrointestinal upset and diarrhea
	Cefdinir		Nausea
	Cefditoren		Allergic reactions
	Cefoperazone		
	Cefotaxime		
	Cefpodoxime		
	Ceftazidime		
	Ceftibuten		
	Ceftizoxime		
	Ceftriaxone		

Cephalosporins, 4th generation			
	Cefepime	Serious infections, particularly in people with a weakened immune system	Gastrointestinal upset and diarrhea Nausea Allergic reactions
Macrolides			
	Azithromycin Clarithromycin Dirithromycin Erythromycin Troleandomycin	Streptococcal infections, syphilis, respiratory infections, mycoplasmal infections, Lyme disease	Nausea, vomiting, and diarrhea (especially at higher doses) Jaundice
Monobactam			
	Aztreonam	Infections caused by Gram-negative bacteria	Allergic reactions
Penicillins			
	Amoxicillin Ampicillin Carbenicillin Cloxacillin Dicloxacillin Nafcillin Oxacillin Penicillin G Penicillin V Piperacillin Ticarcillin	Wide range of infections; penicillin used for streptococcal infections, syphilis, and Lyme disease	Nausea, vomiting, and diarrhea Allergy with serious anaphylactic reactions Brain and kidney damage (rare)
Polypeptides			
	Bacitracin Colistin Polymyxin B	Ear, eye, skin, or bladder infections; usually applied directly to the skin or eye; rarely given by injection	Kidney and nerve damage (when given by injection)
Quinolones			
	Ciprofloxacin Enoxacin Gatifloxacin Levofloxacin Lomefloxacin Moxifloxacin Norfloxacin Ofloxacin Trovafloxacin	Urinary tract infections, bacterial prostatitis, bacterial diarrhea, gonorrhea	Nausea (rare) Nervousness, tremors, seizures Inflammation or rupture of tendons
Sulfonamides			
	Mafenide Sulfacetamide Sulfamethizole Sulfasalazine Sulfisoxazole Trimethoprim-sulfamethoxazole	Urinary tract infections (except sulfasalazine, sulfacetamide, and mafenide); mafenide is used topically for burns	Nausea, vomiting, and diarrhea Allergy (including skin rashes) Crystals in urine (rare) Decreases in white blood cell count Sensitivity to sunlight
Tetracyclines			
	Demeclocycline Doxycycline Minocycline Oxytetracycline Tetracycline	Syphilis, chlamydial infections, Lyme disease, mycoplasmal infections, rickettsial infections	Gastrointestinal upset Sensitivity to sunlight Staining of teeth Potential toxicity to mother and fetus during pregnancy

Miscellaneous antibiotics			
	Chloramphenicol	Typhoid and other Salmonella infections, meningitis	Severe decrease in white blood cell count (rare)
	Clindamycin	Streptococcal and staphylococcal infections, respiratory infections, lung abscess	Severe diarrhea
	Ethambutol	Tuberculosis	Vision disturbances
	Fosfomycin	Bladder infections	Diarrhea
	Isoniazid	Tuberculosis	Nausea and vomiting Jaundice
	Linezolid	Serious infections caused by Gram-positive bacteria that are resistant to other antibiotics	Nausea Headache Diarrhea Low platelet count
	Metronidazole	Vaginitis caused by Trichomonas or Gardnerella; pelvic and abdominal infections	Nausea Headache (especially if taken with alcohol) Metallic taste Dark urine
	Nitrofurantoin	Urinary tract infections	Nausea and vomiting Allergy
	Pyrazinamide	Tuberculosis	Liver dysfunction Gout (occasional)
	Quinupristin/dalfor-pristin	Serious infections caused by Gram-positive bacteria that are resistant to other antibiotics	Aching muscles and joints
	Rifampin	Tuberculosis and leprosy	Rash Liver dysfunction Red-orange saliva, sweat, tears, and urine
	Spectinomycin	Gonorrhea	Allergy Fever
	Vancomycin	Serious infections resistant to other antibiotics	Flushing, itching

ANTIEMETIC AGENTS

The physiologic purpose of nausea is to discourage food intake, and vomiting is meant to expel food or other toxic substances present in the upper part of the gastrointestinal tract. Protracted vomiting may not only cause electrolyte imbalance, dehydration, or a malnutrition syndrome but also lead to mucosal laceration and upper gastrointestinal hemorrhage (Mallory–Weiss syndrome).

Nausea and vomiting may occur when the stomach is overly irritated, stimulated, or distended (from overeating). In addition, they may occur when the chemoreceptor trigger zone for emesis or the vomiting center, or both, are directly stimulated.

Pharmacologic agents such as aspirin and levodopa may cause vomiting by directly irritating the stomach. Agents such as aminophylline, isoniazid, reserpine, anti-inflammatory steroids, and caffeine may also elicit vomiting in susceptible individuals by causing the release of hydrochloric acid. This drug-induced emesis may be avoided by having patients take the drugs with meals. Antiemetics are not effective in rectifying these conditions, and their use is not justified.

In addition to agents that stimulate or irritate the stomach, many other factors may be responsible for inducing emesis centrally. The central control of vomiting is vested in two areas:

1. The vomiting center, which is located in the lateral reticular formation in the midst of a group of cells governing activities such as salivation and respiration
2. The chemoreceptor trigger zone, which is a narrow strip along the floor of the fourth ventricle located close to the vomiting center

The functions of these two areas are distinct but interdependent. The vomiting center is activated by impulses that originate from the gastrointestinal tract and other peripheral structures. In addition, there are unidentified tracts that extend from the cerebral cortex to the vomiting center, such that emotional trauma and unpleasant olfactory and visual stimuli may cause nausea and vomiting.

Stimulation of the vestibular apparatus that responds to movements of the head, neck, and eye muscles may also cause nausea and vomiting by stimulating the vomiting center. On the other hand, circulating chemicals, toxins, viruses, and ions may provoke nausea and vomiting by first stimulating the chemoreceptor zone for emesis, which in turn stimulates the vomiting center.

The nausea and vomiting associated with circulating physical agents (radiation therapy and virus particles) and chemical agents (toxins and cancer chemotherapeutic agents) are treated with phenothiazine derivatives such as chlorpromazine, perphenazine, prochlorperazine, promethazine, triethylperazine, and triflupromazine. These agents block the dopamine receptors in the area postrema (see Figure 73).

A new class of antiemetic agents, the serotonin receptor antagonists, has been identified. These agents could be clinically useful in a wide range of areas. Selective antagonists of the serotonin (5-hydroxytryptamine) type 3 (5-HT_3) receptor such as batanopride, granisetron, ondansetron, or zacopride have proved in early clinical trials to be potent antiemetic agents in patients undergoing cytotoxic chemotherapy. Their efficacy has been shown to be comparable or superior to that of conventional phenothiazine antiemetics. The toxic effects observed so far with these agents have been modest (see Figure 73).

The specific and rational use of antiemetic agents depends on the nature of the emesis-inducing problem. Psychogenically induced vomiting is best controlled by sedatives and antianxiety agents such as

- Phenobarbital
- Buclizine (Softran) (also has antihistaminic properties)
- Hydroxyzine (Atarax) (also has antihistaminic properties)

The nausea and vomiting produced by motion sickness are best treated with antihistaminic agents that have a considerable amount of anticholinergic activity. Examples include:

- Chlorpheniramine (Chlor-Trimeton)
- Diphenhydramine (Benadryl)
- Dimehydrinate (Dramamine)
- Cyclizine (Marizine)
- Meclizine (Bonamine)
- Promethazine (Phenergan), a phenothiazine derivative that has no antipsychotic properties and has predominantly antihistaminic properties
- Diphenidol (Vontrol)
- Trimethobenzamide (Tigan)

The nausea and vomiting associated with chemicophysical agents that stimulate the chemoreceptor trigger zone for emesis are best treated with a phenothiazine derivative. With the exception of thioridazine (Mellaril), all have antiemetic effects, and the ones most often used are:

- Chlorpromazine (Thorazine)
- Fluphenazine (Prolixin, Permitil)
- Perphenazine (Trilafon)
- Promazine (Sparine)
- Promethazine (Phenergan)
- Thiethylperazine (Torecan)
- Triflupromazine (Vesprin)
- Prochlorperazine (Compazine)

Phenothiazine derivatives depress the chemoreceptor trigger zone for emesis, and large doses also inhibit the vomiting center. It has been reported that thiethylperazine depresses both the chemoreceptor trigger zone and the vomiting center (see Figure 73).

Radiation-induced emesis, or uncontrolled vomiting in patients undergoing radiation therapy, may necessitate either discontinuation of the treatment or prophylactic treatment with phenothiazine antiemetics.

Antineoplastic agents such as nitrogen-mustard or cisplatin may cause disabling nausea and severe vomiting. Triflupromazine has been shown to be more effective than chlorpromazine in controlling these symptoms. Recent studies have suggested that the naturally occurring cannabinoid (marijuana) or synthetic cannabinoids (Nabilone) are also effective in combating the vomiting associated with cancer chemotherapeutic agents. Besides their antiemetic effects, cannabinoids increase appetite, cause euphoria, and are analgesics. These properties are useful in a patient who is in the terminal stages of cancer.

Postoperative nausea and vomiting are directly related to the type and dose of the anesthetic used. It has been shown that the use of a muscle relaxant, which substantially reduces the amount of anesthetic needed, lessens the incidence and intensity of postoperative nausea and vomiting. However, most of the phenothiazines may be used to control postoperative emesis.

The nausea and vomiting associated with the first trimester of pregnancy are benign and self-limiting in nature. If at all possible, no medications should be used. If absolutely necessary, antihistaminics (meclizine and trimethobenzamide) may be effective. Pyridoxine (vitamin B_6) should not be prescribed, as it may predispose the infant to vitamin B_6-dependent syndrome.

ANTIEMETIC PREPARATIONS

Antihistaminic-Anticholinergic Agents

Benzquinamide	Dimenhydrinate	Meclizine	Scopolamine
Buclizine	Diphenhydramine	Promethazine	Trimetho-
Cyclizine	Hydroxyzine	Pyrilamine	benzamide

Benzodiazepines
Diazepam
Lorazepam

Butyrophenones
Droperidol
Haloperidol

Cannabinoids
Dronabinol
Nabilone

Corticosteroids
Dexamethasone
Methylprednisolone

Non-phenothiazine Dopamine Receptor Antagonist
Metoclopramide

Phenothiazine Dopamine Receptor Antagonists

Chlorpromazine	Promazine
Fluphenazine	Thiethylperazin
Prochlorperazine	

Serotonin Receptor Antagonists

Batanopride	Ondansetron
Granisetron	Zacopride

ANTIHEMOPHILIC FACTOR

(AHF, Hemoni M, Humáte-P, Koáte-HP, Koáte-HS, Koáte-HT, Monoclate, Profilate OSD)

Antihemophilic factor, a blood derivative, is indicated for the treatment of hemophilia A (factor VIII deficiency). Antihemophilic factor replaces deficient clotting factors that convert prothrombin to thrombin (see Tables 17 and 18).

ANTIHISTAMINIC AGENTS

The diversified actions of histamine are brought forth through their interaction with different types of receptors, which are described in the following sections.

Histamine$_1$ Receptors

Histamine$_1$ (H_1) receptors mediate such actions as bronchoconstriction and the contraction of smooth muscle in the gastrointestinal tract. These effects are blocked by classic antihistaminics such as pyrilamine. Examples of other H_1-receptor blocking agents are:

Ethanolamine derivatives
- Diphenhydramine hydrochloride (Benadryl)
- Dimenhydrinate (Dramamine)
- Carbinoxamine maleate (Clistin)

Ethylenediamine derivatives
- Pyrilamine maleate
- Tripelennamine hydrochloride
- Tripelennamine citrate

Alkylamine derivatives
- Chlorpheniramine maleate (Chlor-Trimeton)
- Brompheniramine maleate (Dimetane)

Piperazine derivatives
- Hydroxyzine hydrochloride (Atarax)
- Hydroxyzine pamoate (Vistaril)
- Cyclizine hydrochloride (Marezine)
- Meclizine hydrochloride (Antivert)

Phenothiazine derivatives
- Promethazine hydrochloride (Phenergan)

Piperidine derivatives (Second-generation antihistaminics)
- Terfenadine (Seldane)
- Astemizole (Hismanal)

The pharmacologic characteristics of H_1-receptor antagonists are qualitatively similar in that they antagonize (competitive H_1 blockers) the histamine-mediated bronchoconstriction, vasodilation, and enhanced capillary permeability. Some of these agents also have anticholinergic properties. Diphenhydramine has strong atropine-like effects, whereas pyrilamine has weak anticholinergic effects (see Figures 59 and 72).

Some antihistaminics such as benztropine (Cogentin) are used in the treatment of parkinsonism and in controlling neuroleptic-induced pseudoparkinsonism. Furthermore, diphenhydramine is most effective in reversing neuroleptic-induced dystonia. The usefulness of these agents in the management of these extrapyramidal disorders is related to their anticholinergic effects. Some antihistaminics such as cyproheptadine (Periactin) also block serotonin-receptor sites. As a result, they have been advocated for use in patients with allergic dermatitis characterized by urticaria or pruritus, or both.

Some antihistaminics, such as promethazine and diphenhydramine, have local anesthetic properties. They may be used substitutively in patients who are allergic to both amide and ester types of local anesthetics. Some phenothiazine antihistaminics, such as promethazine, have alpha-adrenergic blocking effects. Therefore, like phenothiazine neuroleptics, promethazine may cause orthostatic hypotension.

Besides the specific uses discussed, the general therapeutic uses of antihistaminics include allergic reactions such as urticaria, allergic rhinitis, motion sickness, vestibular disturbances, and the nausea and vomiting associated with pregnancy.

The most common side effect of the antihistaminics is sedation, and all of them cause it to varying degrees. For example, diphenhydramine, dimenhydrinate, and promethazine cause marked sedation, but pyrilamine produces only moderate sedation. Chlorpheniramine, meclizine, and cyclizine have mild sedative properties, while terfenadine, astemizole, loratadine, and cetirizine are nonsedating.

The acute poisoning that occurs with most antihistaminics does not cause severe CNS depression as would be expected based on their sedative properties, but is manifested by mydriasis, fever, flushing, CNS excitement, hallucinations, ataxia, athetosis, and convulsions. Some of these effects, which resemble those of atropine poisoning, may be due to their anticholinergic properties. Diazepam is an effective antidote to poisoning and should be used to reverse the CNS excitement and convulsions.

Histamine$_2$ Receptors

Stimulation of the H_2 receptors elicits a variety of responses, the most widely studied of which is gastric acid secretion from the parietal cells of the gastric glands (see Figure 23). However, many other effects mediated by H_2 receptors are manifested in peripheral tissues. These include the positive chronotropic action in the auricular muscle, the inotropic action in the ventricular muscle, and the lipolytic effect in fat cells. In addition, the extensive use of cimetidine has led to the synthesis and marketing of more specific and efficacious analogs with pharmacologic properties that are outlined in Table 8 and Figure 23. Examples of the various H_2-receptor blocking agents are:

Imidazole derivatives
- Cimetidine and etintidine

Furan derivatives
- Ranitidine and nizatidine

Guanidinothiazole derivatives
- Famotidine

Piperidinomethylphenoxy derivatives
- Roxatidine acetate and roxatidine

Histamine$_3$ Receptors

H_3 receptors suppress gastric acid secretion, and this is evoked by cholinergic stimuli. H_3 receptors exist outside the parietal cells and seem to be located on cholinergic and nonadrenergic noncholinergic neurons of the myenteric plexus, where they inhibit the release of neurotransmitters. The agonist and antagonist for H_3 receptors are alpha-methylhistamine and thioperamide, respectively.

ANTIHISTAMINES (H_1-receptor antagonists)

Alkylamine Class
Brompheniramine maleate
Chlorpheniramine maleate
Dexchlorpheniramine maleate

Ethanolamine Class
Carbinoxamine maleate
Clemastine fumarate
Diphenhydramine hydrochloride

Ethylenediamine Class
Pyrilamine maleate
Tripelennamine hydrochloride

Phenothiazine Class
Methdilazine hydrochloride
Promethazine hydrochloride
Trimeprazine

Piperidine Class
Azatadine maleate
Cyproheptadine hydrochloride
Diphenylpyraline hydrochloride
Phenindamine tartrate

Newer Products
Astemizole
Terfenadine
Loratadine

Astemizole, terfenadine, and loratadine are devoid of sedative or anticholinergic properties.

ANTIHYPERTENSIVE MEDICATIONS

An elevated arterial pressure is probably the most important public health problem in developed countries. It is common, asymptomatic, readily detectable, usually easily treatable, and often leads to lethal complications if left untreated. To make rational use of antihypertensive drugs, the sites and mechanisms of their action must be understood. In general, there are six classes of drugs: diuretics, antiadrenergic agents, vasodilators, calcium entry blockers, antitensin-converting enzyme (ACE) inhibitors, and angiotensin-receptor antagonists.

Alpha-1-Adrenergic Receptor-Blocking Agents

Doxazosin
Prazosin hydrochloride
Terazosin

Beta-1-Adrenergic Receptor-Blocking Agents

Acebutolol
Atenolol
Betaxolol
Carteolol
Metoprolol tartrate
Nadolol
Penbutolol
Pindolol
Propranolol hydrochloride
Timolol maleate

Angiotensin-Converting Enzyme Inhibitors

Benazepril
Captopril
Enalapril maleate
Fosinopril
Lisinopril
Ouinapril
Ramipril

Calcium Channel Antagonists

Diltiazem hydrochloride
Felodipine
Isradipine
Nicardipine
Nifedipine
Verapamil hydrochloride

Diuretics

Thiazides and Related Sulfonamide Diuretics

Bendroflumethiazide
Benzthiazide
Chlorothiazide sodium
Chlorthalidone
Cyclothiazide
Hydrochlorothiazide
Hydroflumethiazide
Indapamide
Methyclothiazide
Metolazone
Polythiazide
Quinethazone
Trichlormethiazide

Loop Diuretics

Bumetanide
Ethacrynic acid
Furosemide

Potassium-Sparing Agents

Amiloride hydrochloride
Spironolactone
Triamterene

Central-Acting Adrenergic Inhibitors

Clonidine hydrochloride
Guanabenz acetate
Guanfacine
Methyldopa

Peripheral-Acting Adrenergic Antagonists

Guanadrel sulfate
Guanethidine monosulfate
Reserpine

Vasodilators

Hydralazine hydrochloride
Minoxidil

ANTINEOPLASTIC AGENTS

Alkylating Agents (and Trade Names)

Busulfan (Myleran)
Carmustine (BCNU)
Chlorambucil (Leukeran)
Cyclophosphamide (Cytoxan)
Hexamethylmelamine (Hexastat)
Ifosfamide (Ifex)
Lomustine (CCNU)
Mechlorethamine (HN_2, nitrogen mustard)
Melphalan (L-phenylalanine mustard)
Semustine (MeCCNU)
Streptozocin (Streptozotocin)
Thiotepa (Triethylenethiophosphoramide)

Antimetabolites (and Trade Names)

Cladribine (2-Chloro-deoxyadenosine)
Cytarabine
Floxuridine (Ara-C)
Fludarabine phosphate (5-Fluorodeoxyuridine)
Fluorouracil (F-ara-A fludara)
(5-Fu)
Methotrexate (Amethopterin)
PALA (Sparfosate)
Pentostatin (2-Deoxy-coformycin)
Purinethol (6-MP Mercaptopurine)
Thioguanine (6-TG 6-thioguanine)

Natural Products (and Trade Names)

Asparaginase (L-Asnase)	Idarubicin (Mitomycin C)
Bleomycin (Bleo)	Mitomycin (Mithramycin)
Camptothecin	Plicamycin (Paclitaxel)
Dactinomycin (Actinomycin D)	Taxol (VM-26)
Daunorubicin (Daunomycin)	Teniposide (Vincaleukoblastine velban)
Doxorubicin (Adriamycin)	
Epirubicin	Vinblastine (Oncovin)
Etoposide (VP-16 VePesid)	Vincristine
Homoharringtonine (HHT)	Vindesine

Miscellaneous (and Trade Names)

Amsarcrine (m-AMSA)	Hydrea (Hydroxyurea)
Carboplatin (CBDCA)	Mitoxantrone (Novantrone DHAQ)
Cisplatin (Paraplatin)	
Dacarbazine (DDP) (DIC DTIC)	Procarbazine (MIH Natulan)

Hormones and Antagonists

Adrenocorticosteroids
Androgens
Antiandrogen
Antiestrogen
Estrogens
Gonadotropin-releasing hormone analog
Progestins

ANTIPARASITIC MEDICATIONS AND THEIR SIDE EFFECTS

Albendazole
Diarrhea; abdominal pain; migration of ascaris through mouth and nose; leukopenia; alopecia; increased serum transaminase activity

Benznidazole
Allergic rash; dose-dependent polyneuropathy; gastrointestinal disturbances; psychic disturbances

Bithionol
Photosensitivity reactions; vomiting; diarrhea; abdominal pain; urticaria; leukopenia; toxic hepatitis

Chloroquine HCl and Chloroquine Phosphate
Pruritus; vomiting; headache; confusion; depigmentation of hair; skin eruptions; corneal opacity; weight loss; partial alopecia; extraocular muscle palsies; exacerbation of psoriasis, eczema, and other exfoliative dermatoses; myalgias; photophobia; irreversible retinal injury (especially when total dosage exceeds 100 grams); discoloration of nails and mucus membranes; nerve-type deafness; peripheral neuropathy and myopathy; heart block; blood dyscrasias; hematemesis

Crotamiton
Rash; conjunctivitis; photosensitivity reactions; vomiting; diarrhea; abdominal pain; urticaria; leukopenia; toxic hepatitis

Dehydroemetine
Cardiac arrhythmias; precordial pain; muscle weakness; cellulitis at site of injection; diarrhea; vomiting; peripheral neuropathy; heart failure; headache; dyspnea

Diethylcarbamazine Citrate USP
Severe allergic or febrile reactions in patients with microfilaria in the blood or the skin; GI disturbances; encephalopathy

Diloxanide Furoate
Flatulence; nausea; vomiting; diarrhea; diplopia; dizziness; urticaria; pruritus

Eflornithine
Anemia; leukopenia; diarrhea; thrombocytopenia; seizures; hearing loss

Flubendazole—similar to mebendazole

Furazolidone
Nausea; vomiting; allergic reactions, including pulmonary infiltration; hypotension; urticaria; fever; vesicular rash; hypoglycemia; headache; hemolytic anemia in G-6-PD deficiency and neonates; disulfiram-like reaction with alcohol; MAO-inhibitor interactions; polyneuritis

Halofantrine
Diarrhea; abdominal pain; pruritus

Iodoquinol
Rash; acne; slight enlargement of the thyroid gland; nausea; diarrhea; cramps; anal pruritus; optic atrophy; loss of vision; peripheral neuropathy after prolonged use in high dosage (for months); iodine sensitivity

Ivermectin
Mazzotti-type reaction seen in onchocerciasis, including fever; pruritus; tender lymph nodes; headache; joint and bone pain; hypotension

Lindane
Eczematous rash; conjunctivitis; convulsions; aplastic anemia

Malathion
Local irritation

Mebendazole
Diarrhea; abdominal pain; migration of ascaris through mouth and nose; leukopenia; agranulocytosis; hypospermia

Mefloquine
Vertigo; lightheadedness; nausea; other gastrointestinal disturbances; nightmares; visual disturbances; headache; confusion; psychosis; hypotension; convulsions; coma

Meglumine Antimoniate—similar to stibogluconate sodium

Melarsoprol
Myocardial damage; albuminuria; hypertension; colic; Herxheimer-type reaction; encephalopathy; vomiting; peripheral neuropathy; shock

Metronidazole
Nausea; headache; dry mouth; metallic taste; vomiting; diarrhea; insomnia; weakness; stomatitis; vertigo; paresthesias; rash; dark urine; urethral burning; disulfiram-like reaction with alcohol; seizures; encephalopathy; pseudomembranous colitis; ataxia; leucopenia; peripheral neuropathy; pancreatitis

Niclosamide
Nausea; abdominal pain

Nifurtimox
Anorexia; vomiting; weight loss; loss of memory; sleep disorders; tremor; paresthesias; weakness; polyneuritis; convulsions; fever; pulmonary infiltrates and pleural effusion

Ornidazole
Dizziness; headache; gastrointestinal disturbances; reversible peripheral neuropathy

Oxamniquine
Headache; fever; dizziness; somnolence; nausea; diarrhea; rash; insomnia; hepatic enzyme changes; ECG changes; EEG changes; orange-red discoloration of urine; seizures; neuropsychiatric disturbances

Paromomycin
GI disturbances; eighth-nerve damage (mainly auditory); renal damage

Pentamidine Isethionate
Hypotension; hypoglycemia often followed by diabetes mellitus; vomiting; blood dyscrasias; renal damage; pain at injection site; GI disturbances; may aggravate diabetes; shock; hypocalcemia; liver damage; cardiotoxicity; delirium; rash; Herxheimer-type reaction; anaphylaxis; acute pancreatitis; hyperkalemia

Permethrin
Burning; stinging; numbness; increased pruritus; pain; edema; erythema; rash

Praziquantel
Malaise; headache; dizziness; sedation; abdominal discomfort; fever; sweating; nausea; eosinophilia; fatigue; pruritus; rash
Primaquine Phosphate USP
Hemolytic anemia in G-6-PD deficiency neutropenia; GI disturbances; methemoglobinemia in G-6-PD deficiency; CNS symptoms; hypertension; arrhythmias
Proguanil
Oral ulceration; hair loss; scaling of palms and soles; hematuria (with large doses); vomiting; abdominal pain; diarrhea (with large doses)
Pyrantel Pamoate
GI disturbances; headache; dizziness; rash; fever
Pyrethrins and Piperonyl Butoxide
Allergic reactions
Pyrimethamine
Blood dyscrasias; folic acid deficiency; rash; vomiting; convulsions; shock; possibly pulmonary eosinophilia
Quinacrine HCl
Dizziness; headache; vomiting; diarrhea; yellow staining of skin; toxic psychosis; insomnia; bizarre dreams; blood dyscrasias; urticaria; blue and black nail pigmentation; psoriasis-like rash; acute hepatic necrosis; convulsions; severe exfoliative dermatitis; ocular effects similar to those caused by chloroquine
Quinine Dihydrochloride and Sulfate
Cinchonism (tinnitus, headache, nausea, abdominal pain, visual disturbance); deafness; hemolytic anemia; other blood dyscrasias; photosensitivity reactions; hypoglycemia; arrhythmias; hypotension; drug fever; blindness; sudden death if injected too rapidly
Spiramycin
GI disturbances; allergic reactions
Stibogluconate Sodium
Muscle pain and joint stiffness; nausea; transaminase elevations; T-wave flattening or inversion; weakness; colic; liver damage; bradycardia; leukopenia; diarrhea; rash; pruritus; myocardial damage; hemolytic anemia; renal damage; shock; sudden death
Suramin Sodium
Vomiting; pruritus; urticaria; paresthesias; hyperesthesia of hands and feet; photophobia; peripheral neuropathy; kidney damage; blood dyscrasias; shock; optic atrophy
Thiabendazole
Nausea; vomiting; vertigo; leukopenia; crystalluria; rash; hallucinations; olfactory disturbance; erythema multi forme; Stevens–Johnson syndrome; shock; tinnitus; intrahepatic cholestasis; convulsions; angioneurotic edema
Tinidazole
Metallic taste; nausea; vomiting; rash
Trimetrexate (with "leucovorin rescue")
Rash; peripheral neuropathy; bone marrow depression; increased serum aminotransferase concentrations
Tryparsamide
Nausea; vomiting; impaired vision; optic atrophy; fever; exfoliative dermatitis; allergic reactions; tinnitus

ANTIPSYCHOTICS

Butyrophenone	Loxapine
Haloperidol	Dihydroindolone
Dibenzoxapine	Molindone
Clozapine	
Phenothiazines (Alipathic)	
Chlorpromazine	
Phenothiazines (Piperazine)	
Acetophenazine	Prochlorperazine
Fluphenazine	Trifluoperazine
Perphenazine	
Phenothiazines (Piperidine)	
Mesoridazine	Chlorprothixene
Thioridazine	Thiothixen
Thioxanthenes	

ANTIPYRINE/BENZOCAINE/GLYCERIN/ DEHYDRATED

(Benzocaine otic solution)

This is an otic preparation that is an analgesic and decongestant, which is indicated in the removal of cerumen, and in the treatment of acute otitis media of various etiologies.

ANTISENSE THERAPEUTICS

During the past decade, only one antisense-based therapy has received full Food and Drug Administration (FDA) approval. **Vitravene™**, developed by Isis Pharmaceuticals, was the first drug based on antisense technology to be successfully commercialized and used in treatment. The therapeutic area it is used in is a small niche related to the treatment of **preventing blindness in acquired immunodeficiency syndrome** (AIDS) patients by inhibiting **cytomegalovirus-induced retinitis**. The success of Vitravene, however, showed that antisense could be taken all the way through the FDA-approval process and provide those patients taking it with a vitally important effect.

Antisense oligonucleotides (AS-ODNs) are designed to bind and inactivate specific mRNA sequences inside cells. The potential uses for AS-ODNs are vast because RNA is so ubiquitous and abundant. With the publication of the human genome sequence, we now have such a wide open access to the sequences of genes that antisense can, in theory, be applied to almost every known gene to inhibit its mRNA. Inhibiting mRNA prevents specific proteins from being produced. Although routine human therapy may have been difficult to achieve, at a scientific level, antisense gene knockdown has become one of the fastest ways to study new therapeutic targets.

The appeal of antisense is that it potentially provides highly specific, nontoxic effects for safe and effective therapeutics of an enormous number of diseases including **AIDS**, **Crohn's disease**, **pouchitis**, **psoriasis**, **cancers**, **diabetes**, **mulitiple sclerosis**, **muscular dystrophy**, **restenosis**, **asthma**, **rheumatoid arthritis**, **hepatitis**, **skin diseases**, **polycystic kidney disease**, and **chronic cardiovascular disease**, such as **hypertension**, **restenosis**, and **heart failure**. Successes in phase I have shown that antisense therapy consistently has excellent safety results.

Over a span of more than two decades, antisense strategies for **gene therapy** have expanded from AS-ODNs solely to the addition of ribozymes and, more recently, to the inclusion of small interfering RNAs (siRNAs). Antisense therapeutics has also experienced its phases of high expectation, sudden disappointment, and meticulous rediscovery, while maintaining its status as a viable and effective gene therapy approach. With the discovery of **RNA interference** (RNAi) and development in delivery of these gene drugs, more preclinical and clinical investigations are anticipated to take place in the near future to finally fulfill the promise of antisense therapeutics in humans.

ANTITHROMBIN III

(Heparin Cofactor I) (Antativ, Thrombate III)

Antithrombin III, an anticoagulant and antithrombotic agent (50 to 100 IU/min IV), is indicated for prophylaxis and adjunct treatment of thromboembolism associated with hereditary antithrombin III deficiency (see also Tables 17 and 18).

ANTI-THYMOCYTE

(Thymoglobulin)

Anti-thymocyte globulin is an immune globulin, which is indicated in the treatment of acute allograft rejection in renal transplantation. Immunosuppressive drugs are used to dampen the immune response in organ transplantation and autoimmune disease. In transplantation, the major classes of immunosuppressive drugs used today are: (1) glucocorticoids, (2) calcineurin inhibitors, (3) antiproliferative/antimetabolic agents, and (4) biologics (antibodies). These drugs have met with a high degree of clinical success in treating conditions such as acute immune rejection of organ transplants and severe autoimmune diseases. However, such therapies require lifelong use and nonspecifically suppress the entire immune system, exposing patients to considerably higher risks of infection and cancer.

Induction therapy with polyclonal and monoclonal antibodies (mAbs) has been an important component of immunosupression when the beneficial effect of antilymphocyte globulin (ALG) in the prophylaxis of rejection in renal transplant recipients was demonstrated. Over the past 40 years, several polycolonal antilymphocyte preparations have been used in renal transplantation; however, only two preparations are currently FDA approved: **lymphocyte immune globulin** (ATGAM) and **antithymocyte globulin** (Thymoglobulin).

ANTIVIRAL AGENTS

Antiherpes Virus Agents

Acyclovir (ACV, acycloguanosine)
Famciclovir (FCV)
Foscarnet (PFA, phosphonoformate)
Ganciclovir (GCV, DHPG)
Idoxuridine (IDUR)
Sorivudine (BV-ara-U, brovavir)
Trifluridine (TFT, trifluorothymidine)
Valacyclovir
Vidarabine (ara-A, adenine arabinoside)

Antiretroviral Agents

Didanosine (ddI)
Stavudine (d4T)
Zalcitabine (ddC)
Zidovudine (AZT, ZDV, azidothymidine)

Other Antiviral Agents

Amantadine	Ribavirin
Interferon alpha (interferon alfa)	Rimantadine

APOMORPHINE HCL

Ipecac is a mixture of the alcohol-soluble alkaloid that is obtained from the South American plant *Cephaelis ipecacuanha*, and is used solely in the form of syrup of ipecac. Apomorphine hydrochloride (5 mg sc) and copper sulfate are also emetics. Syrup of ipecac and copper sulfate cause emesis by locally irritating the stomach, whereas apomorphine stimulates the chemoreceptor trigger zone for emesis located in the caudal portion of the fourth ventricle (area postrema), which in turn stimulates the vomiting center in the lateral reticular formation of the medulla (see Figure 73). Results are usually obtained within 5 to 10 minutes after parenteral administration. Apomorphine and other emetics should not be used in cases of poisoning with corrosive agents; in shock or coma; and in narcosis resulting from opiates, barbiturates, alcohol, or other CNS depressants. Overdosage with apomorphine may cause circulatory failure, which is reversed by naloxone.

APRACLONIDINE HYDROCHLORIDE

(Iopidine)

Apraclonidine, an alpha-adrenergic receptor-blocking agent that reduces intraocular pressure (one drop in the eye 1 hour before initiation of laser surgery on the anterior segment, followed by one drop immediately upon completion of surgery), is indicated for prevention or control of intraocular pressure elevations after argon laser trabeculoplasty or iridotomy.

Apraclonidine (Iopidine) is a relatively selective α_2-receptor agonist that is used topically to reduce intraocular pressure. It can reduce elevated as well as normal intraocular pressure, whether accompanied by glaucoma or not. The reduction in intraocular pressure occurs with minimal or no effects on systemic cardiovascular parameters; thus, apraclonidine is more useful than clonidine for ophthalmic therapy. Apparently, apraclonidine does not cross the blood–brain barrier. The mechanism of action of apraclonidine is related to α_2-receptor-mediated reduction in the formation of aqueous humor.

The clinical utility of apraclonidine is most apparent as a short-term adjunctive therapy in glaucoma patients whose intraocular pressure is not well controlled by other pharmacological agents such as β-receptor antagonists, parasympathomimetics, or carbonic anhydrase inhibitors. The drug also is used to control or prevent elevations in intraocular pressure that occur in patients after laser trabeculoplasty or iridotomy.

APREPITANT

(Emend)

Aprepitant is an antiemetic/antivertigo agent. Aprepitant is used in combination with other antiemetic agents for the prevention of acute and delayed nausea and vomiting associated with initial and repeat courses of highly emetogenic cancer chemotherapy, including high-dose cisplatin.

The nausea and vomiting associated with cisplatin has two components: an acute phase that universally is experienced (within 24 hours after chemotherapy), and a delayed phase that affects only some patients (on days 2 to 5). 5-HT-receptor antagonists are not very effective against delayed emesis. Antagonists of the NK_1 receptors for substance P, such as aprepitant (Emend), have antiemetic effects in delayed nausea and improve the efficacy of standard antiemetic regimens in patients receiving multiple cycles of chemotherapy. Substance P belongs to the tachykinin family of neurotransmitters and is in vagal afferent fibers innervating area postrema. The tachykinins represent a novel, promising target for new antinauseant drugs.

Aprepitant is supplied in 80- and 125-mg capsules and is administered for 3 days in conjunction with highly emetogenic chemotherapy along with a $5\text{-}HT_3$-receptor antagonist and a corticosteroid. The recommended adult dosage of aprepitant is 125 mg administered 1 hour before chemotherapy on day one, followed by 80 mg once daily in the morning on days two and three of the treatment regimen.

APROBARBITAL

(Alurate)

Aprobarbital, a barbiturate sedative-hypnotic (40 to 80 mg p.o. h.s.), is indicated in the management of mild to severe insomnia (see also Barbiturates).

APROTININ

(Trasylol)

Aprotinin, a protease inhibitor (10,000 units or 1.4 mg by IV injection), is indicated for a prophylactic reduction of preoperative blood loss and the need for blood transfusion in patients undergoing cardiopulmonary bypass during repeat coronary artery bypass graft surgery, or in selected patients undergoing initial coronary artery bypass graft surgery in whom the risk of bleeding is high because of impaired hemostasis or in whom transfusion is unavailable or unacceptable.

ARGATROBAN

Argatroban is a thrombin inhibitor. It binds reversibly to a thrombin active site, exerting its anticoagulant effects by inhibiting thrombin-catalyzed or induced reactions, including activation of coagulation factors V, VIII, and XIII, protein C, and platelet aggregation. Argatroban is indicated as an anticoagulant for prophylaxis and treatment of thrombosis in heparin-induced thrombocytopenia; and as an anticoagulant in patients with or at risk for heparin-induced thrombocytopenia undergoing percutaneous coronary intervention.

ARIPIPRAZOLE

(Abilify)

Aripiprazole, a quinolinone derivative, is a partial agonist at dopamine D2 and serotonin 5-HT1A receptors, and antagonist at serotonin 5-HT2A receptor. Aripiprazole is indicated in the treatment of schizophrenia; and treatment of acute manic and mixed episodes associated with bipolar disorder.

No one drug or combination of drugs selectively affects a particular symptom complex in groups of psychotic patients. Although individual patients may apparently respond better with one agent than another, this can be determined only by trial and error. It is sometimes claimed that certain agents (particularly newer antipsychotic drugs) are specifically effective against "negative" symptoms in psychotic disorders (e.g., abulia, social withdrawal, and lack of motivation). However, evidence supporting this proposal remains inconsistent, and such benefits usually are limited. Generally, "positive" (irrational thinking, delusions, agitated turmoil, hallucinations) and "negative" symptoms tend to respond or not respond together with overall clinical improvement. This tendency is well documented with typical neuroleptics as well as modern atypical antipsychotic agents. It is clear that **aripiprazole**, **clozapine**, **quetiapine**, and **ziprasidone** induce less bradykinesia and other parkinsonian effects than do typical neuroleptics. In addition, **aripiprazole** and **ziprasidone** are minimally sedating. Minimizing such side effects is sometimes interpreted clinically as specific improvement in impoverished affective responsiveness and energy level.

ARRHYTHMIAS

Any departure from the normal sinus rhythm imposes a hemodynamic disadvantage on cardiac function. Cardiac arrhythmias may be caused by a damaged heart, such as that produced by myocardial infarction resulting from some abnormality in the blood supply to the pacemaker cells or conducting tissues, or both. In addition, fatal arrhythmias may be caused by the injudicious use of numerous drugs, including digitalis, anesthetics, antidepressants with anticholinergic effects (e.g., amitrip-tyline), and neuroleptics with anticholinergic effects (e.g., thioridazine). Fortunately, effective antiarrhythmic agents, electrical defibrillators, and pacers can suc-cessfully reverse cardiac arrhythmias.

At the SA node, electrical impulses generate a cardiac contraction at regular intervals and with a frequency of one beat per second. This impulse then spreads rapidly through the atria and enters the AV node. The conduction through the AV node takes 0.2 seconds, which is relatively slow. The impulse then propagates over the His-Purkinje system and contracts the entire ventricular muscle in

0.1 seconds in an anatomically synchronous and hemodynamically effective fashion. Arrhythmias deviate from this pattern and result from abnormalities in either impulse generation or impulse conduction, whereby the normal impulse conduction rate is slowed somewhere in the specialized conducting system of the heart. This disturbance is frequently, but not always, found in the AV node or in the bundles of His (heart block), or both.

The major electrophysiologic manifestation of impulse generation is found in the properties of automaticity (slope of phase 4 or diastolic depolarization) and of impulse conduction in conduction velocity. Drugs that alter pacemaker automaticity have a direct effect on the heart rate.

Rapid diastolic depolarization leads to a rapid rate of firing, whereas a lowered slope of phase 4 diastolic depolarization elicits fewer action potentials in the same time interval. Similarly, drugs that increase conduction velocity in the heart can help alleviate heart block, whereas those that decrease conduction velocity may slow a rapid heart rate.

Drugs	Adverse Effects
	Quinidine, Procainamide, Disopyramide
Disopyramide	Anticholinergic effects (urinary retention, aggravation of glaucoma, constipation), hypotension, heart failure, tachyarrhythmias, torsade de pointes, heart block, nausea, vomiting, diarrhea, hypoglycemia, nervousness
Procainamide	Lupus-like syndrome, confusion, insomnia, GI symptoms, rash, hypotension, arrhythmias, torsade de pointes, blood dyscrasias, fever, hepatitis and hepatic failure, myopathy; IV: hypotension, heart block
Quinidine	Diarrhea and other GI symptoms, cinchonism, hepatic granulomas and necrosis, thrombocytopenia, rashes, hypotension, heart block, tachyarrhythmias, torsade de pointes, fever, lupus-like syndrome
	Flecainide, Propafenone, Moricizine
Flecainide	Bradycardia, heart block, new ventricular fibrillation, sustained ventricular tachycardia, heart failure, dizziness, blurred vision, nervousness, headache, GI upset, neutropenia
Moricizine	Bradycardia, heart failure, new ventricular fibrillation, sustained ventricular tachycardia, nausea, dizziness, headache
Propafenone	Bradycardia, heart block, new ventricular fibrillation, sustained ventricular tachycardia, heart failure, dizziness, lightheadedness, metallic taste, GI upset, bronchospasm, hepatic toxicity
	Adenosine
Adenosine	Facial flushing, transient dyspnea, chest discomfort, hypotension; may cause bronchoconstriction in patients with asthma
	Lidocaine and Similar Agents
Lidocaine	Drowsiness or agitation, slurred speech, tinnitus, disorientation, coma, seizures, paresthesias, cardiac depression (especially with excessive accumulation in heart failure or liver failure or infusions for more than 24 hours), bradycardia/asystole
Mexiletine	GI upset, fatigue, nervousness, dizziness, tremor, sleep upset, seizures, visual disturbances, psychosis, fever, blood dyscrasias, hepatitis
Tocainide	GI upset, paresthesias, dizziness, tremor, confusion, nightmares, psychotic reactions, coma, seizures, rash, fever, arthralgia, agranulocytosis, aplastic anemia, thrombocytopenia, hepatic granulomas, interstitial pneumonitis
	Amiodarone, Sotalol, Ibutilide
Amiodarone	Acute pulmonary toxicity, pulmonary fibrosis, bradycardia, heart block, new ventricular fibrillation, sustained ventricular tachycardia, torsade de pointes (unusual), hyper- or hypothyroidism, GI upset, alcoholic-like hepatitis, peripheral neuropathy, ataxia, tremor, dizziness, photosensitivity, blue-gray skin, corneal microdeposits
Ibutilide	Torsade de pointes, AV block
Sotalol	Heart block, hypotension, bronchospasm, bradycardia, torsade de pointes
	Other Agents
Bretylium	Initial hypertension, orthostatic hypotension, nausea and vomiting, increased sensitivity to catecholamines, initial increase in arrhythmias
Digoxin	Bradycardia, AV block arrhythmias, anorexia, nausea, vomiting, diarrhea, abdominal pain, headache, confusion, abnormal vision
Magnesium sulfate	Areflexia, apnea (very high doses)

ARSENIC TRIOXIDE

(Trisenox)

Arsenic trioxide is an antineoplastic agent that causes morphological changes and DNA fragmentation characteristic of apoptosis in NB4 human promyelocytic leukemia cells *in vitro*. Arsenic trioxide also causes damage or degradation of the fusion protein PML/RAR alpha. It is indicated in the treatment of refractory or relapsed acute promyelocytic leukemia (APL).

ARTHRITIS AND DEGENERATIVE JOINT DISEASE: Treatment of

Rheumatoid arthritis is an autoimmune disease. The antigen that stimulates the initial autoimmune response and the genetic mechanism that promotes its development are unknown. Once the disease process is under way, antigen–antibody complexes presumably activate the complement and elicit the release of various mediators, causing inflammation. The treatment of rheumatoid arthritis is aimed at reducing this inflammation, thereby decreasing the pain and attempting to slow the joint destruction.

In the management of arthritic conditions, drugs are chosen on an empirical basis, usually trying the least toxic substances first. The following schedule may be used in drug selection.

First choice—nonsteroidal antiinflammatory agents
- Aspirin
- Ibuprofen, tolmetin, naproxen, fenoprofen, or sulindac
- Indomethacin or phenylbutazone

Second choice—disease-modifying agents
- Gold salts
- P-Penicillamine
- Hydroxychloroquine

Third choice
- Steroids
- Immunosuppressive agents

Gold salt therapy is reserved for those patients with progressive disease who do not obtain satisfactory relief from therapy with aspirin-like drugs. The principle that underlies this therapy is that gold, which accumulates in lysosomes, decreases the migration and phagocytic activity of macrophages. Aurothioglucose, gold sodium thiomalate, or auranofin may cause toxic effects such as cutaneous reactions (from erythema to exfoliative dermatitis) as well as albuminuria, hematuria, and thrombocytopenia.

Besides the nonsteroidal antiinflammatory agents and gold, other drugs are also used for the treatment of rheumatoid arthritis. These include immunosuppressive agents, glucocorticoids, penicillamine, and hydroxychloroquine. With the exception of glucocorticoids, these drugs resemble gold salts in that they do not possess antiinflammatory or analgesic properties, and their therapeutic effects become evident only after several weeks or months of treatment.

Nonsalicylate Nonsteroidal Antiinflammatory Drugs for the Treatment of Rheumatoid Arthritis and Allied Degenerative Joint Diseases

Drugs	Half-life (hr)	Doses per Day
	Propionic Acids	
Fenoprofen	2 to 3	3 to 4
Ibuprofen	1.8 to 2.5	3 to 4
Ketoprofen	2 to 4	3 to 4
Naproxen	12 to 15	2
	Indoles	
Sulindac	16.4	2
Tolmetin	1.0 to 1.5	
	Oxicams	
Piroxicam	30 to 86	1 to 2

ARTIFICIAL TEARS

(Adapettes, Adsorbotear, Artificial Tears, Hypotears, Isopto Alkaline, Isopto Plain, Isopto Tears, Lacril Artificial Tears, Lacrisert, Liquifilm Forte, Liquifilm Tears, Lyteers, Moisture Drops, Murocel Solution, Muro Tears Solution, Neotears, Tearisol, Tears Naturale, Tears Plus)

Artificial tears, a derivative of polyvinyl alcohol or cellulose (1 to 2 drops in eye t.i.d.), is indicated in conditions where the production of tears is insufficient, or in moderate to severe dry eye syndromes, including keratoconjunctivitis sicca.

ASCORBIC ACID (VITAMIN C)

(Arco-cee, Ascorbicap, Cebid, Timecelles, Cecon Solution, Cemil, Cetane, Cevalin, Cevi-Bid, Ce-Vi-Sol, Cevita, C-Long, C-Span, Dull-C, Flavorcee, Vitacee)

Ascorbic acid, a water-soluble vitamin (100 to 250 mg p.o. daily), is indicated in the treatment of frank and subclinical scurvy; in extensive burns, delayed fracture or wound healing, postoperative wound healing; severe febrile or chronic disease states; and in prevention of ascorbic acid deficiency in those with poor nutritional habits or increased requirements. In addition, ascorbic acid has been used for potentiation of methenamine in urine acidification and as an adjunctive therapy in the treatment of idiopathic methemoglobinemia.

Vitamin C is an essential vitamin believed important for synthesis of cellular components, catecholamines, steroids, and carnitine. Vitamin C is indicated in the prevention and treatment of scurvy.

The recent Age-Related Eye Disease Study (AREDS) found a reduction in the risk of progression of some types of age-related **macular degeneration** for those randomized to receive high doses of **vitamins C** (500 mg), **E** (400 IU), **β-carotene** (15 mg), **cupric oxide** (2 mg), and **zinc** (80 mg). Interestingly, zinc has been found to be neuroprotective in a rat model of glaucoma. The mechanism appears to be mediated by heat shock proteins and may represent a novel treatment strategy for glaucoma.

ASPARAGINASE

(Elspar, Kidrolase)

Asparaginase, an antineoplastic agent (200 IU/kg/day IV for 28 days), is used in the treatment of acute lymphocytic leukemia. Whereas most normal tissues are able to synthesize L-asparagine in amounts sufficient for protein synthesis, some types of lymphoid malignancies derive the required amino acid from plasma. L-asp, by catalyzing the hydrolysis of circulating asparagine to aspartic acid and ammonia, deprives these malignant cells of the asparagine necessary for protein synthesis, leading to cell death. L-asp commonly is used in combination with other agents, including methotrexate, doxorubicin, vincristine, and prednisone for the treatment of ALL and for high-grade lymphomas. The sequence of drug administration in these combinations may be critical; for example, synergistic cytotoxicity results when methotrexate precedes the enzyme, but the reverse sequence leads to abrogation of methotrexate cytotoxicity. The latter outcome is a consequence of the inhibition of protein synthesis by L-asp, an effect that stops the progression of cells through the cell cycle and negates the effect of methotrexate, a drug that exerts its greatest effect during the DNA synthetic phase of the cell cycle.

Resistance arises through induction of asparagine synthetase in tumor cells. For unknown reasons, hyperdiploid ALL cells are particularly sensitive to L-asp.

L-Asparaginase (Elspar) is given parenterally. Three different preparations of L-asp are used clinically. Their pharmacokinetics and immunogenicity differ significantly after intravenous administration.

L-Asparaginase has minimal effects on bone marrow and gastrointestinal mucosa. Its most serious toxicities result from its antigenicity as a foreign protein and its inhibition of protein synthesis. Hypersensitivity reactions occur in 5 to 20% of patients and may be fatal.

ASPIRIN

(A.S.A., A.S.A. Enseals, Ascriptin, Aspergum, Bayer Timed-Release, Bufferin, Buffinol, Easpirin, Ecotrin, Empirin, Encaprin, Entrophen, Measurin, Zorprin)

Aspirin is indicated in the treatment of mild pain, fever, arthritis, thromboembolic disorders, transient ischemic attacks, to reduce the risk of heart attack in patients with previous myocardial infarction or unstable angina, and treatment of Kawasaki (mucocutaneous lymph node) syndrome (see Table 3 and the section on Acetylsalicylic Acid). Many of aspirin's pharmacological actions are thought to be mediated by inhibiting prostaglandin synthesis through the inhibition of cyclooxygenase (Figure 13).

The current thinking concerning the role of aspirin in the prevention of cardiovascular disease is that it is beneficial in the event of myocardial infarction and stroke. It is effective because, in platelets, small amounts of aspirin acetylate irreversibly and bind to the active site of thromboxane A_2, a potent promoter of platelet aggregation (see Figure 14).

ASTEMIZOLE

(Hismanal)

Astemizole, cetirizine, loratadine, and terfenadine are second-generation antihistaminic agents that are relatively nonsedating. Other H_1-receptor antagonists currently undergoing clinical trials are azelastine, ebastine, and levocabastine. Astemizole (10 to 30 mg p.o.) is a long-acting peripheral H_1-receptor antagonist, that does not pass across the blood–brain barrier and is devoid of anticholinergic properties. Astemizole is absorbed well from the gastrointestinal tract, is bound to plasma proteins to the extent of 96%, undergoes extensive first-pass metabolism, and the metabolites, including desmethylastemizole, are excreted in the feces. The metabolism of astemizole is inhibited by erythromycin, ketoconazole, or itraconazole, resulting in elevated levels of astemizole and desmethylastemizole, which may cause cardiac arrhythmias (prolongation of QT intervals) in individuals with a history of cardiovascular disorders, or in patients who are electrolyte imbalanced.

ASTHMA

Asthma is a disease of airways that is characterized by increased responsiveness of the tracheobronchial tree to a multiplicity of stimuli. It is manifested physiologically by a widespread narrowing of the air passages, which may be relieved spontaneously or as a result of therapy, and clinically by paroxysms of dyspnea, cough, and wheezing. Asthma is an episodic disease, acute exacerbations being interspersed with symptom-free periods. Typically, most attacks are short-lived, lasting minutes to hours, and clinically the patient seems to recover completely after an attack. However, there can be a phase in which the patient experiences some degree of airways obstruction daily. This phase can be mild, with or without superimposed severe episodes, or much more serious, with severe obstruction persisting for days or weeks, a condition known as **status asthmaticus**. In unusual circumstances, acute episodes can cause death.

ASTHMA: Treatment of

Drugs	Formulations
Newer Adrenergic Drugs	
Albuterol	Metered-dose inhaler (90 μg/puff)
	Powder inhaler (200 μg Rotacaps)
	Nebulized solution (5 mg/ml)
	Syrup or tablets
	Extended-release tablets
	(Repetabs) (4 mg)
	(Volmax) (4 mg and 8 mg)
Bitolterol mesylate	Metered-dose inhaler (370 μg/puff)
Metaproterenol	Metered-dose inhaler (650 μg/puff)
	Nebulized solution (5% solution)
	Syrup or tablets
Pirbuterol	Metered-dose inhaler (200 μg/puff)
Terbutaline	Subcutaneous (1 mg/ml)
(Brethaire)	Tablets
	Metered-dose inhaler (200 μg/puff)
Corticosteroids	
Beclomethasone dipropionate	Metered-dose inhaler (42 μg/puff)
Flunisolide	Metered-dose inhaler (250 μg/puff)
Prednisone or Prednisolone	Oral tablets (5, 10, 20 mg)
	Oral liquid (Liquid Pred, PediaPred, Prelone)
Triamcinolone acetonide	Metered-dose inhaler (100 μg/puff)
Cromolyn	Spinhaler, powder (20 mg/capsule)
	Metered-dose inhaler (800 μg/puff)
	Nebulized solution (10 mg/ml)
Theophylline, Oral	
Extended-release capsules or tablets	

ATAZANAVIR SULFATE

(Reyataz)

Atazanavir is a protease inhibitor, that inhibits HIV protease, the enzyme required to form functional proteins in HIV-infected cells. Atazanavir, in combination with other antiviral agents, is indicated for the treatment of

HIV-1 infection. Like **indinavir**, **atazanavir** frequently causes unconjugated hyperbilirubinemia, although this is mainly a cosmetic side effect and is not associated with other hepatotoxicity. Because **atazanavir** is metabolized by cytochrome (CYP3A4), concomitant administration of agents that induce this enzyme (e.g., **rifampin**) is contraindicated.

ATENOLOL

(Tenormin)

Atenolol is a beta-adrenergic blocking agent that slows heart rate, reduces cardiac output, and lowers BP. Chlorthalidone is a diuretic agent that reduces body water by increasing urine output. The combination issued in the treatment of hypertension.

Atenolol, introduced in 1976, is the most cardioselective beta-adrenergic blocking agent. The cardioselective beta-blockers are acebutolol, atenolol, and metoprolol; and the nonselective beta-blockers are alprenolol, nadolol, oxyprenolol, pindolol, propranolol, sotalol, and timolol (see Figure 37). Evidence suggests that atenolol is the most beta2-receptor-selective of the beta-blocking agents; therefore, as long as the daily dose is sufficiently low, side effects related to blockade of beta2-receptors—such as increased airway resistance, bronchospasm, prolongation of insulin-induced hypoglycemia, and cold extremities—are seen less frequently. Unlike pindolol, which has pronounced intrinsic sympathomimetic activity (ISA), atenolol is devoid of ISA activity. In contrast to beta-blockers without ISA, such as atenolol, beta-blockers with this property cause a reduction in peripheral vascular resistance with little change in cardiac output. This difference may be due to activation of peripheral $beta_2$-receptors by agents with ISA. This effect on peripheral vasculature offers advantages in the treatment of patients with peripheral vascular disease or obstructive airway disease.

Unlike propranolol, which has quinidine-like effects in that it impairs the capacity of excitable tissues to undergo depolarization, atenolol has no membrane-stabilizing effects. Most beta-adrenergic receptor blocking agents are lipid soluble, whereas atenolol, nadolol, and sotalol are water soluble. Therefore, atenolol has several advantages as an antihypertensive agent. Because it is water soluble, it is excreted relatively slowly by the kidney; therefore, it need be given no more than once daily in most cases. Furthermore, its hydrophilicity results in limited passage through the blood–brain barrier, thus resulting in fewer CNS-related side effects compared with lipophilic beta-blockers, such as acebutolol, alprenolol, metoprolol, oxyprenolol, pindolol, propranolol, and timolol. Atenolol reduces heart rate, cardiac index, and blood pressure. It has no effect on plasma volume, exchangeable sodium or potassium, or total body potassium. Like other beta-blocking agents, atenolol inhibits the release of renin, resulting in a decrease in angiotensin II production and aldosterone secretion. Atenolol reduces renal vascular resistance in hypertensive patients.

Atenolol is indicated in arteriosclerotic heart disease with angina pectoris, hypertension, cardiac arrhythmias and myocardial infarction; in hypertrophic obstructive cardiomyopathy, dissecting aneurysm of the aorta, pheochromocytoma, and in prevention of migraine headaches.

Atenolol is contraindicated in congestive heart failure, sinus bradycardia, and atrioventricular block greater than first degree. Atenolol has additive effects with drugs such as reserpine, causing depletion of catecholamine. It should be used cautiously with agents potentially exerting negative inotropic or chronotropic effects, such as calcium channel blockers. Because atenolol is excreted unchanged by the kidney, serum levels are increased in patients with impaired renal function.

ATHESIN

Athesin contains 9 mg of alfaxalone and 3 mg of alfadolone acetate per milliliter. Following intravenous administration, athesin produces sleep within 30 seconds and also causes respiratory depression and apnea. Athesin releases histamine and may cause hypersensitivity reactions such as bronchospasm.

ATOMOXETINE

(Strattera)

Atomoxetine is a psychotherapeutic agent that inhibits the presynaptic transport of norepinephrine. It is indicated in the treatment of attention-deficit/hyperactivity disorder (ADHD).

ATORVASTATIN CALCIUM

(Lipitor)

Atorvastatin is marketed in combination with the $Ca2^+$-channel blocker **amlodipine** (Caduet) for patients with hypertension or angina as well as hypercholesterolemia. Atorvastatin is an HMG-CoA reductase inhibitor that increases the rate at which the body removes cholesterol from blood and reduces the production of cholesterol by inhibiting enzymes that catalyze early rate-limiting steps in cholesterol synthesis; increases HDL; reduces LDL, VLDL, and triglycerides.

Atorvastatin is indicated in **elevated serum triglyceride**: as an adjunct to diet for the treatment of patients with elevated serum triglyceride levels (Fredrickson type IV); **heterozygous familial hypercholesterolemia** in pediatric patients: adjunct to diet to reduce total and LDL cholesterol and apolipoprotein B levels in boys and postmenarchal girls 10 to 17 years of age if, after an adequate trial of diet therapy, LDL remains 160 mg/dL or higher and there is a positive family history of premature cardiovascular (CV) disease or two or more other CV risk factors present; **homozygous familial hypercholesterolemia**: to reduce total cholesterol and LDL cholesterol in patients with homozygous familial hypercholesterolemia as an adjunct to other lipid-lowering treatments or if such treatments are unavailable.

ATOVAQUONE

(Mepron)

Atovaquone is an antiprotozoal agent (750 mg p.o. t.i.d for 21 days), that inhibits mitochondrial electron transport in metabolic enzymes of microorganisms. This may cause inhibition of nucleic acid and adenosine triphosphate synthesis. Atovaquone is indicated in the treatment of mild to moderate *Pneumocystis carinii* pneumonia in patients who cannot tolerate trimethoprimsulfamethoxazole, and in acute oral treatment of mild to moderate PCP in patients who are intolerant to trimethoprimsulfamethoxazole.

ATOVAQUONE/PROGUANIL HYDROCHLORIDE

(Malarone)

Atovaquone is an antimalarial preparation. It inhibits mitochondrial electron transport in parasites, causing inhibition of nucleic acid synthesis. Proguanil exerts its effect by means of the metabolite cycloguanil, which inhibits dihydrofolate reductase in the malarial parasite, disrupting deoxythymidylate synthesis. It is indicated in prophylaxis of *P. falciparum* in patients with severe renal impairment (Ccr less than 30 mL/min); hypersensitivity to any component of the product.

ATRACURIUM BESYLATE

(Tracrium)

Atracurium is a nondepolarizing skeletal muscle relaxant. It binds to cholinergic receptor sites and antagonizes the action of acetylcholine. At a dose of 0.5 mg/kg, it releases less histamine and produces less hemodynamic alterations than either d-tubocurarine or metocurine (see also Figure 80). Atracurium is used as an adjunct to general anesthesia in order to facilitate endotracheal intubation and to relax skeletal muscles during either surgery or mechanical ventilation. The duration of action of atracurium (30 minutes) is shorter than those of d-tubocurarine, metocurine, and pancuronium. Halothane, enflurane, or isoflurane prolongs the duration of neuromuscular blockade by atracurium by 20 to 30%.

Atracurium-induced bradycardia is more common than that produced by other skeletal muscle relaxants. The neuromuscular blocking effects of atracurium are prolonged in hypokalemia and following administration of thiazide diuretics. Hypokalemia enhances the neuromuscular blockade, possibly by hyperpolarizing the end plate membrane, increasing resistance to depolarization. Similarly, the duration of action of atracurium is prolonged by antibiotics such as aminoglycosides, bacitracin, capreomycin, colistimethate, polymyxin B, clindamycin, and lincomycin. Atracurium has an acid pH and should not be mixed in the same syringe with drugs (e.g., barbiturates) having alkaline pHs.

ATRIAL NATRIURETIC FACTOR

(ANF)

The atria contain secretory granules that increase in quantity with sodium restriction and decrease with sodium loading. Atrial extracts possess both vasodilatory and natriuretic activity that is mediated by atrial natriuretic factor, which is also known as cardionatrin, atriopeptin, atrin, or auriculin.

Atrial natriuretic factor brings about these changes by

- Increasing the glomerular filtration rate, plus increasing the renal excretion of water, sodium, chloride, magnesium, calcium, and phosphate ions
- Blunting renin release in response to a variety of stimuli
- Blocking the release of aldosterone
- Decreasing cardiac output
- Opposing the actions of catecholamines and angiotensin II
- Causing vasodilation (Figure 25).

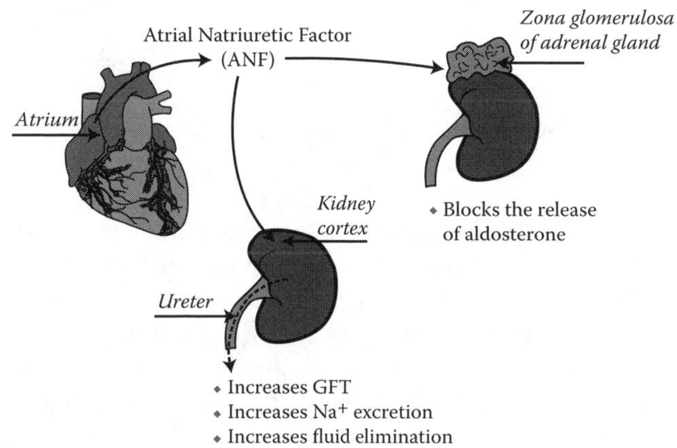

FIGURE 25 Atrial natriuretic factor (ANF) is a polypeptide hormone that is secreted mainly by the heart atria in response to increases in atrial pressure or atrial stretch.

ATROPINE SULFATE

Atropine sulfate, an anticholinergic agent with antiarrhythmic and vagolytic properties (0.5 to 1 mg by IV push), is indicated in symptomatic bradycardia and bradyarrhythmia (functional or escape rhythm). It is used preoperatively for diminishing secretions and blocking cardiac vagal reflexes and as an antidote for anticholinesterase insecticide poisoning (see Figures 18, 26, and 77).

ATROPINE SULFATE SCOPOLAMINE HYDROBOMIDE/HYOSCYAMINE SULFATE/PHENOBARBITAL

Atropine is a GI anticholinergic combination. This combination promotes peripheral anticholinergic/antispasmodic action (decreases GI motility) and provides mild sedation. It is possibly effective for treatment of irritable bowel syndrome and acute enterocolitis. It also may be useful as adjunctive therapy for duodenal ulcer.

Atropine and scopolamine are cholinergic receptor-blocking agents. They are obtained from belladonna alkaloids, as well as other synthetic anticholinergic drugs. They inhibit the actions of smooth muscle, heart, and exocrine

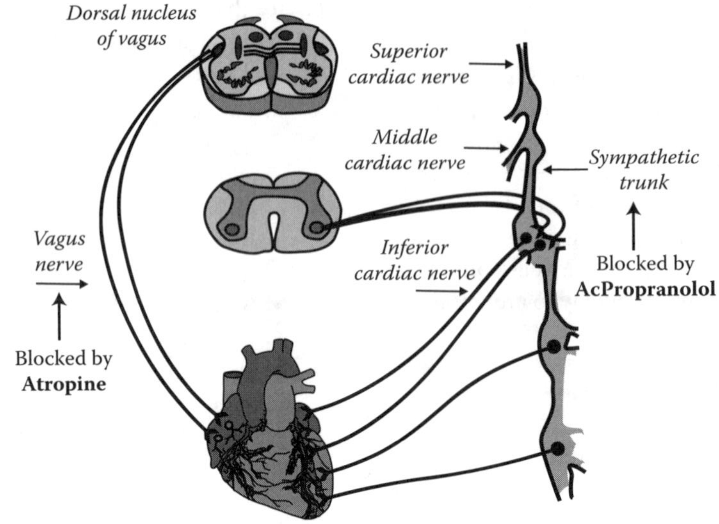

FIGURE 26 **Atropine** inhibits the actions of acetylcholine and cholinomimetic drugs at muscarinic receptors in smooth muscles, heart, and exocrine glands.

glands (see Figures 18 and 77). In addition to these peripheral effects, anticholinergic drugs, by blocking the acetylcholine receptor sites in the CNS, have pronounced CNS effects such as restlessness, irritability, excitement, and hallucinations. Scopolamine, on the other hand, depresses the CNS and, in therapeutic doses, produces fatigue, hypnosis, and amnesia. Therefore, it is used extensively in numerous medications, often in combination with antihistamines.

The pharmacologic effects of atropine in general are dose dependent. For example, in small doses, atropine depresses sweating, elevates body temperature, decreases salivary and bronchial secretions, and relaxes bronchial smooth muscles. In somewhat larger doses (1 to 3 mg), it produces mydriasis (blockade of the iris sphincter muscle), cycloplegia (blockade of the ciliary muscle), and cardiovascular effects characterized by transient bradycardia (central vagal stimulation) and tachycardia (vagal blockade at the sinoatrial node). Lacking any significant effects on circulation, atropine is often used as a preanesthetic medication to depress bronchial secretion and prevent pronounced bradycardia during abdominal surgical procedures. In still larger doses, it depresses the tone and motility of the gastrointestinal tract, the tone of the urinary bladder, and gastric secretion. Therefore, the effective doses for use in acid-pepsin diseases are preceded by numerous side effects.

Atropine is absorbed orally and crosses the placental barrier, whereupon it causes fetal tachycardia. It has been used to examine the functional integrity of the placenta. Atropine toxicity is characterized by dry mouth, burning sensation in the mouth, rapid pulse, mydriasis, blurred vision, photophobia, dry and flushed skin, restlessness, and excitement.

Physostigmine, given intravenously, counteracts both the peripheral and central side effects of atropine and other anticholinergic drugs such as thioridazine (neuroleptic), imipramine (antidepressant), and benztropine (antiparkinsonian medication). Conditions that are contraindications to the use of atropine and related drugs are glaucoma and prostatic hypertrophy, in which they cause urinary retention (see Figures 18 and 77).

AURANOFIN
(Ridauva)

Gold compounds (Figure 27) are able to prevent or suppress experimental arthritis produced by infections and chemical agents. They reduce the signs and symptoms of inflammation associated with rheumatoid arthritis. Therefore, auranofin is indicated in the management of rheumatoid arthritis in

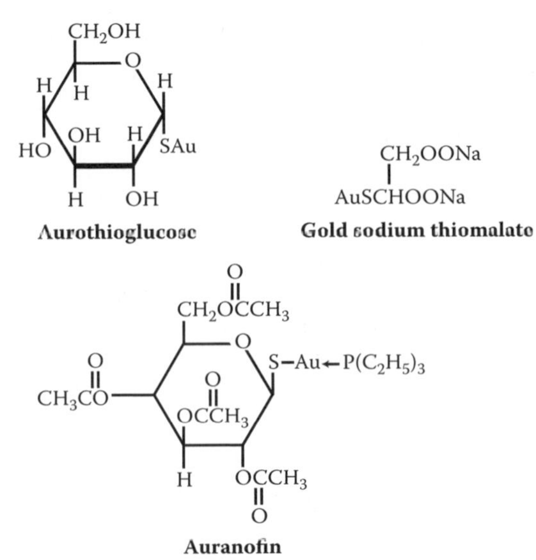

FIGURE 27 Auranofin, a gold salt with antiarthritic properties, reduces inflammation by altering the immune system.

patients who have had insufficient therapeutic response to or are intolerant of nonsteroidal antiinflammatory drugs. Gold compounds inhibit the maturation and function of mononuclear phagocytes and of T-cells, and hence suppress immune responsiveness. Decreased concentrations of rheumatoid factor and immunoglobulins are often observed in patients who are treated with gold. Unlike antiinflammatory agents, auranofin (6 mg/day) does not produce an immediate response, and beneficial effects are seen in 3 to 4 months. Steady-state concentrations of gold in plasma are proportional to the doses administered and are reached after 8 to 12 weeks of treatment. After cessation of treatment, the half-life of gold in the body is about 80 days. Auranofin is predominantly excreted in the feces. It may cause a fall in hemoglobin, leukopenia, thrombocytopenia, proteinuria, or hematuria. Therefore, it is contraindicated in patients with hematological disorders or renal impairment.

AUROTHIOGLUCOSE

(Solganal)

Chrysotherapy (gold therapy, see Figure 27) is employed in the treatment of progressive rheumatoid arthritis in patients who do not obtain satisfactory relief with nonsteroidal antiinflammatory agents. Aurothioglucose and gold sodium thiomalate are absorbed erratically when given orally and hence are administered intramuscularly.

Aurothioglucose is bound to albumin to the extent of 95% and reaches high concentration in synovial fluid of affected joints. Gold is excreted mainly by the kidneys (40 to 90%), and 10 to 40% is found in the feces. Sulfhydryl agents, such as dismercaprol, penicillamine, and *N*-acetylcysteine increase the excretion of gold. The adverse effects of aurothioglucose include hematologic abnormalities (10%), including thrombocytopenia, leukopenia, or pancytopenia. Other adverse effects include stomatitis, a metallic taste in the mouth, skin pigmentation, enterocolitis, cholestatic jaundice, peripheral neuropathy, pulmonary infiltrates, and coroneal deposition of gold (Figure 27).

AUTONOMIC RECEPTORS

	Receptor Subtype	Agonists	Antagonists
	Adrenergic Receptors		
	Alpha-1A	Epinephrine Norepinephrine Phenylephrine	Phentolamine Prazosin
	Alpha-1B	Epinephrine Norepinephrine Phenylephrine	Phentolamine Prazosin
	Alpha-2A	Epinephrine Norepinephrine Clonidine	Phentolamine Yohimbine Prazosin
	Alpha-2B	Epinephrine Norepinephrine Clonidine	Phentolamine Yohimbine
	Beta-1	Epinephrine Norepinephrine Isoproterenol	Propranolol Atenolol
	Beta-2	Epinephrine Isoproterenol Terbutaline	Propranolol
	Beta-3	Norepinephrine Epinephrine	Cyanopindolol
	Cholinergic Receptors		
Muscarinic	M_1	Acetylcholine Muscarine Carbamylcholine	Atropine Pirenzepine
	M_2	Acetylcholine Muscarine Carbamylcholine	Atropine Methoctramine
Nicotinic	Ganglionic	Acetylcholine Nicotine	Hexamethonium Mecamylamine
	Skeletal muscle	Acetylcholine Nicotine	d-Tubocurarine Succinylcholine

Note: In addition to the adrenergic and cholinergic receptor subtypes listed, other autonomic receptor subtypes have been identified, but specific agonists or antagonists to be used in medical practice are unavailable.

AZACITIDINE

(Vidaza powder for injection)

Azacitidine is a DNA demethylation agent, that causes hypomethylation of DNA and direct cytotoxicity on abnormal hematopoietic cells in bone marrow. Azacitidine is indicated in the treatment of myelodysplastic syndrome subtypes: refractory anemia or refractory anemia with ringed sideroblasts (if accompanied by neutropenia or thrombocytopenia or requiring transfusions), refractory anemia with excess blasts, refractory anemia with excess blasts in transformation, and chronic myelomonocytic leukemia.

5′-Azacitidine and the closely related investigational drug decitabine (2′-dexoy-5′-azacitidine), have antileukemic activity and induce differentiation. 5′-Azacitidine is approved for treatment of myelodysplasia, for which it induces normalization of bone marrow in 15 to 20% of patients and a reduction in transfusion requirement in one-third of patients. It becomes incorporated into RNA and DNA and inhibits methylation of DNA, inducing the expression of silenced genes. Thus, it also is used for inducing fetal hemoglobin synthesis in sickle cell anemia, although it has been largely replaced for this indication by hydroxyurea. It undergoes very rapid deamination by cytidine deaminase, the product hydrolyzing to inactive metabolites. Its major toxicities include myelosuppression and rather severe nausea and vomiting when given intravenously in large doses (150 to 200 mg/m2 per day for 5 days). In low-dose daily subcutaneous regimens for myelodysplasia, 30 mg/m2 per day, it is well tolerated.

AZATADINE MALEATE

(Optimine)

Azatadine, a histamine receptor antagonist (1 to 2 mg p.o. b.i.d.), is indicated in the treatment of rhinitis, allergy symptoms, and chronic urticaria caused by histamine (see also Figures 34 and 72).

AZATHIOPRINE

(Imuran)

Azathioprine (3 to 10 mg/kg) prevents transplant rejection. It is reserved for patients deemed unresponsive to cyclosporine and prednisone. Azathioprine is cleared to 6-mercaptopurine, which in turn can be converted to 6-mercaptopurine nucleotides leading to an inhibition of *de novo* purine synthesis or anabolism to thio-IMP, which, as a fraudulent nucleotide, can interfere with the salvage pathway of purine synthesis. Thio-IMP is subsequently converted to thio-GMP and eventually thio-GTP, leading to DNA damage upon intercalation of thio-GMP into the DNA backbone (see Figure 28). Azathioprine is a more effective immunosuppressant than is mercaptopurine (Purinethol).

Azathioprine is indicated in renal homotransplantation (five-year patient survival rate of 35%); in rheumatoid arthritis (for patients with severe, active, and erosive disease not responding to conventional therapies); and in chronic ulcerative colitis, myasthenia gravis, and Behcet's syndrome (adverse effects may offset its limited value). As with other cytotoxic drugs, azathioprine can affect rapidly growing cells, resulting in leukopenia, thrombocytopenia, and gastrointestinal toxicity. In addition, hepatotoxicity (cholestasis) has been reported. Many of the general problems of immunosuppression, such as increased risk of infections, can also occur. In addition, there is some evidence of mutagenicity and possible carcinogenicity.

AZELAIC ACID

(Azelex cream 20%)

Azelaic acid is an antibiotic agent that inhibits microbial cellular protein synthesis. It is indicated in the topical treatment of mild to moderate inflammatory acne vulgaris (cream); topical treatment of papules and pustules of mild to moderate rosacea.

AZELASTINE

Terfenadine, astemizole, loratadine, and cetirizine are second-generation antihistaminic agents that are relatively nonsedating. Other H_1-receptor antagonists currently undergoing clinical trials are azelastine, ebastine, and levocabastine.

AZELASTINE HYDROCHLORIDE

(Astelin nasal spray 137 mcg/spray)

Azelastine is an ophthalmic antihistaminic preparation. It is indicated in the treatment of symptoms of seasonal allergic rhinitis, such as rhinorrhea, sneezing, and nasal pruritus; treatment of symptoms of vasomotor rhinitis, such as rhinorrhea, nasal congestion, and postnasal drip (nasal inhalation); treatment of itching of eye associated with allergic conjunctivitis (ophthalmic).

Drug allergy may develop when H_1 antagonists are given orally but results more commonly from topical application. Allergic dermatitis is not uncommon; other hypersensitivity reactions include drug fever and photosensitization. Hematological complications such as leukopenia, agranulocytosis,

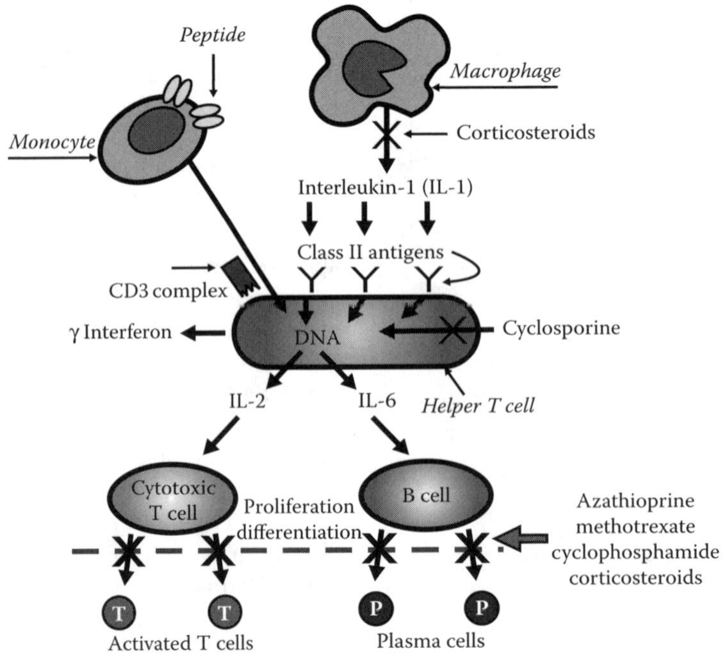

FIGURE 28 Azathioprine, a purine antagonist with immunosuppressive properties, inhibits RNA and DNA synthesis.

and hemolytic anemia are very rare. Because H_1 antihistamines cross the placenta, caution must be used when they are taken by women who are or may become pregnant. Several antihistamines (e.g., **azelastine**, **hydroxyzine**, and **fexofenadine**) showed teratogenic effects in animal studies, whereas others (e.g., **chlorpheniramine**, **diphenhydramine**, **cetirizine**, and **loratadine**) did not. Antihistamines can be excreted in small amounts in breast milk, and first-generation antihistamines taken by lactating mothers may cause symptoms in the nursing infant such as irritability, drowsiness, or respiratory depression. Because H_1 antagonists interfere with skin tests for allergy, they must be withdrawn well before such tests are performed.

AZITHROMYCIN

(Zithromax)

Azithromycin, an azalide macrolide antibiotic (500 mg p.o. as a single dose on day 1, followed by 250 mg daily on days 2 to 5; total accumulation dose is 1.5 g), is indicated in the treatment of acute bacterial exacerbations of chronic obstructive pulmonary disease caused by *Haemophilus influenzae, Moraxella (Branhamella) catarrhalis*, or *Streptococcus pneumoniae*; mild community-acquired pneumonia caused by *H. influenzae* or *S. pneumoniae*; uncomplicated skin and skin-structure infections caused by *Staphylococcus aureus, Streptococcus pyogenes*, or *S. agalactiae*; second-line therapy of pharyngitis or tonsillitis caused by *S. pyogenes*; and in nongonococcal urethritis or cervicitis caused by *Chlamydia trachomatis*.

Azithromycin is a macrolide (erythromycin, clarithromycin, and azithromycin) that interferes with microbial protein synthesis. It is indicated in the following conditions. Adults: treatment of infections of the respiratory tract, acute bacterial sinusitis, acute bacterial exacerbations of COPD, community-acquired pneumonia, *Mycobacterium avium* complex, pelvic inflammatory disease, pharyngitis/tonsillitis, skin and skin structure infections, and sexually transmitted diseases caused by susceptible organisms. Children: treatment of acute bacterial sinusitis, acute otitis media caused by susceptible organisms, community-acquired pneumonia, pharyngitis/tonsillitis caused by *S. pyogenes* in patients who cannot use first-line therapy.

AZLOCILLIN

Carbenicillin cures serious infections caused by *Pseudomonas* species and *Proteus* strains resistant to ampicillin. It is not absorbed from the gastrointestinal tract, and therefore must be administered intraperitoneally. Carbenicillin indanyl is acid stable and hence can be given orally. Ticarcillin is four times more potent than carbenicillin in treating a *Pseudomonas aeruginosa* infection, and azlocillin is ten times more potent than carbenicillin against *Pseudomonas*. Mezlocillin and piperacillin are more active against *Klebsiella* infection than is carbenicillin (see Table 23).

AZTREONAM

(Azactam)

Aztreonam, a monobactam antibiotic (500 mg to 2 g IV or IM q. 8 to 12 hours), is indicated in the treatment of urinary tract, respiratory tract, intra-abdominal, gynecological, or skin infections; or septicemia caused by Gram-negative bacteria (see Figure 74).

The antimicrobial activity of **aztreonam** differs from those of other β-lactam antibiotics and more closely resembles that of an aminoglycoside. Aztreonam has activity only against Gram-negative bacteria; it has no activity against Gram-positive bacteria and anaerobic organisms. However, activity against Enterobacteriaceae is excellent, as is that against *P. aeruginosa*. It is also highly active *in vitro* against *H. influenzae* and gonococci.

Aztreonam is administered either intramuscularly or intravenously. Peak concentrations of aztreonam in plasma average nearly 50 μg/mL after a 1-g intramuscular dose. The half-life for elimination is 1.7 hours, and most of the drug is recovered unaltered in the urine. The half-life is prolonged to about 6 hours in anephric patients.

Aztreonam generally is well tolerated. Interestingly, patients who are allergic to penicillins or cephalosporins appear not to react to aztreonam, with the exception of ceftazidime.

The usual dose of aztreonam for severe infections is 2 g every 6 to 8 hours. This should be reduced in patients with renal insufficiency. Aztreonam has been used successfully for the therapy of a variety of infections. One of its notable features is little allergic cross-reactivity with β-lactam antibiotics, with the possible exception of ceftazidime with which it has considerable structural similarity. Aztreonam is therefore quite useful for treating Gram-negative infections that normally would be treated with a β-lactam antibiotic were it not for the history of a prior allergic reaction.

B

BACAMPICILLIN HYDROCHLORIDE

(Spectrobid)

Bacampicillin, an aminopenicillin antibiotic (400 to 800 mg p.o. q. 12 hours), is indicated in the treatment of upper and lower respiratory tract, urinary tract, and skin infections caused by susceptible organisms, and in gonorrhea.

BACILLUS CALMETTE-GUÉRIN (BCG), LIVE INTRAVESICAL

(TheraCys, Tice BCG)

Bacillus Calmette-Guérin, a bacterial agent with antineoplastic properties (three reconstituted and diluted vials are injected intravesically once weekly for six weeks), is used in the treatment of *in situ* carcinoma of the urinary bladder (primary or relapsed). BCG live is a lyophilized preparation of an attenuated, live culture preparation of the Bacille Calmette-Guérin (BCG) strain of *Mycobacterium bovis* used in carcinoma *in situ* of the urinary bladder and as prophylaxis of primary or recurrent stage Ta or T1 papillary tumors following transurethral resection (TUR). Prevention of tuberculosis (TB) in the following: people not previously infected with *Mycobacterium tuberculosis*, infants and children with negative tuberculin skin tests who are at high risk of intimate and prolonged exposure to persistently untreated or ineffectively treated patients with infectious pulmonary tuberculosis, health care workers in settings where a high percentage of TB patients are infected with *M. tuberculosis* strains resistant to both isoniazid and rifampin (BCG vaccine [TICE strain, lyophilized injection]).

Bacillus Calmette-Guérin (BCG) Vaccine

This BCG vaccine (0.1 mL intradermally) is indicated in conditions where an individual has been exposed to tuberculosis, where immunity is not permanent.

BACITRACIN

(Baciquent)

Bacitracin, which inhibits cell wall synthesis, is active against Gram-positive bacteria. In combination with polymyxin and neomycin, it is often used in the treatment of topical infections as well as open infections such as infected eczema, dermal ulcers, and surgical wounds. The parenteral administration of bacitracin may cause nephrotoxicity.

BACITRACIN ZINC/NEOMYCIN/POLYMYXIN B SULFATES/HYDROCORTISONE

(Cortiporin ointment)

Used for treatment of corticosteroid-responsive dermatoses with secondary infection.

BACITRACIN ZINC/POLYMYXIN B SULFATE

(Polysporin Ophthalmic ointment)

Used for treatment of superficial ocular infections involving the conjunctiva and/or cornea, caused by susceptible organisms.

BACLOFEN

(Lioresal)

Baclofen (40 to 80 mg daily) is indicated for the alleviation of signs and symptoms of spasticity from multiple sclerosis, and for the relief of flexor spasms and concomitant pain, clonus, and muscular rigidity. Baclofen is as effective as diazepam in reducing spasticity but causes less sedation. Baclofen acts as a Gamma-aminobutyric acid (GABA) agonist at $GABA_B$ receptors (see Figure 29). Activation of receptors in the brain by baclofen results in hyperpolarization, probably increased by K+ conductance. It has been suggested that this hyperpolarization (in the cord as well as the brain) serves a presynaptic inhibitory function (Figure 29).

Baclofen is absorbed orally, reaching peak plasma concentration in 2 hours, having a half-life of 3 to 4 hours, and being excreted unchanged by the kidneys. The onset and duration of action of baclofen are 4 and 8 hours, respectively. It should be given cautiously in patients with renal impairment. The administration of baclofen via spinal catheter or lumbar puncture in a single bolus test dose of 50 to 100 mcg, or via an implantable pump for administration into the intrathecal space, has been approved for severe spasticity and pain in patients with cerebral palsy not responding to oral medications.

Several agents, many of limited efficacy, have been used to treat spasticity involving the a-motor neuron with the objective of increasing functional capacity and relieving discomfort. Agents that act in the CNS at either higher centers or the spinal cord to block spasms are **baclofen**, the **benzodiazepines**, and **tizandine**. **Botulinum toxin** and **dantrolene** act peripherally.

The most useful agent for the symptomatic treatment of spasticity in amyotrophic lateral sclerosis (ALS) is **baclofen** (lioresal), a $GABA_B$-receptor agonist. Initial doses of 5 to 10 mg/day are recommended, but the dose can be increased to as much as 200 mg/day if necessary. If weakness occurs, the dose should be lowered. In addition to oral administration, baclofen also can be delivered directly into the space around the spinal cord by use of a surgically implanted pump and an intrathecal catheter. This approach minimizes the adverse effects of the drug, especially sedation, but it carries the risk of potentially life-threatening CNS depression and should be used only by physicians trained in delivering chronic intrathecal therapy. **Tizanidine** (Zanflex) is an agonist of α_2-adrenergic receptors in the CNS. It reduces muscle spasticity and is assumed to act by increasing presynaptic

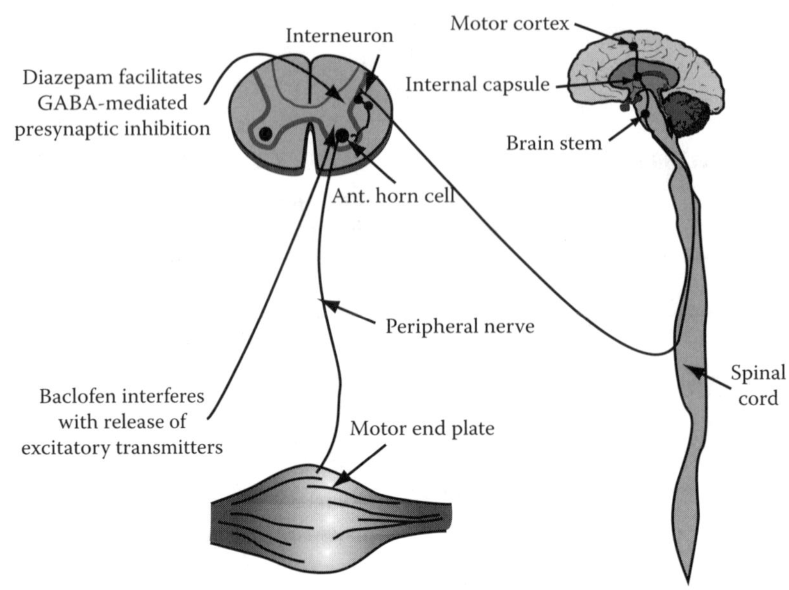

FIGURE 29 Baclofen, a skeletal muscle relaxant, acts at the spinal cord level to inhibit transmission of monosynaptic and polysynaptic reflexes.

inhibition of motor neurons. Tizanidine is used most widely in the treatment of spasticity in multiple sclerosis or after stroke, but it also may be effective in patients with ALS. Treatment should be initiated at a low dose of 2 to 4 mg at bedtime and titrated upward gradually. Drowsiness, asthenia, and dizziness may limit the dose that can be administered. **Benzodiazepines** such as clonazepam (Klonipin) are effective antispasmodics, but they may contribute to respiratory depression in patients with advanced ALS. **Dantrolene** (dantrium) also is approved in the United States for the treatment of muscle spasm. In contrast to the other agents discussed, dantrolene acts directly on skeletal muscle fibers, impairing calcium ion flux across the sarcoplasmic reticulum. Because it can exacerbate muscular weakness, it is not used in ALS but is effective in treating spasticity associated with stroke or spinal cord injury and in treating malignant hyperthermia. Dantrolene may cause hepatotoxicity, so it is important to perform liver function tests before and during therapy with the drug.

BALSALAZIDE DISODIUM

(Colazal capsule 750 mg)

Balsalazide, a GI agent, reduces inflammation of the colon by preventing local production of substances involved in the inflammatory process such as arachidonic acid.

BALSALAZINE

The idiopathic inflammatory bowel disease includes ulcerative colitis and granulomatous disease of the gastrointestinal tract (Crohn's disease). The newer derivatives of 5-aminosalicylic acid, namely balsalazine, sulfasalazine, or olsalazine, may be effective for treating ulcerative colitis but not Crohn's disease.

BANTOPRIDE

A new class of antiemetic agents, the serotonin antagonists, has been identified. These agents could be clinically useful in a wide range of areas. Selective antagonists of the serotonin (5-hydroxytryptamine) type 3 (5-HT_3) receptor such as bantopride, granisetron, ondansetron, or zacopride have proved in early clinical trials to be potent antiemetic agents in patients undergoing cytotoxic chemotherapy. Their efficacy has been shown to be comparable or superior to that of conventional phenothiazine antiemetics. The toxic effects observed so far with these agents have been modest (see Figure 73).

BARBITURATES

Barbiturates were used extensively in the past as hypnotic-sedatives, but have been replaced by the much safer benzodiazepine derivatives. They do continue to be used as anesthetics and as anticonvulsants. The primary mechanism of action of barbiturates is to increase inhibition through the GABA system. Anesthetic barbiturates also decrease excitation via a decrease in calcium conductance (see Figure 50).

The most commonly used barbiturates are thiopental (Pentothal), methohexital (Brevital), secobarbital (Seconal), pentobarbital (Nembutal), amobarbital (Amytal), and phenobarbital (Luminal).

Barbiturates are classified according to their duration of action. These are: ultra short-acting (thiopental and methohexital), short- to intermediate-acting (pentobarbital, secobarbital, and amobarbital), and long-acting (phenobarbital).

In general, the more lipid soluble a barbiturate derivative is, the greater is its plasma- and tissue-binding capacity, the extent of its metabolism, and its storage in adipose tissues.

In addition, very lipid-soluble substances have a faster onset and a shorter duration of action.

Barbiturates do not raise the pain threshold and have no analgesic property. In anesthetic doses, they depress all areas of the CNS, including the hypothalamic thermoregulatory system, respiratory center, and vasomotor centers, as well as the polysynaptic pathways in the spinal column. In addition, some, such as phenobarbital, serve as anticonvulsants, but not all are. In toxic doses, barbiturates cause oliguria.

Barbiturates are absorbed orally and distributed widely throughout the body. They are metabolized in the liver by aliphatic oxygenation, aromatic oxygenation, and N-dealkylation.

The inactive metabolites are excreted in the urine. The administration of bicarbonate enhances the urinary excretion of barbiturates that have a pK_a of 7.4 (phenobarbital and thiopental). This generalization is not true of other barbiturates. The long-term administration of barbiturates activates the cytochrome P-450 drug-metabolizing system.

Acute barbiturate toxicity is characterized by automatism, or a state of drug-induced confusion, in which patients lose track of how much medication they have taken and take more. Death results from respiratory failure. The treatment of poisoning consists of supporting respiration, prevention of hypotension, as well as diuresis, hemodialysis and, in the event of phenobarbital poisoning, the administration of sodium bicarbonate. Tolerance does not develop from lethal doses. The abrupt withdrawal from barbiturates may cause tremors, restlessness, anxiety, weakness, nausea and vomiting, seizures, delirium, and cardiac arrest.

The selection of a barbiturate is in part determined by the duration of action desired and by the clinical problems at hand. An ultra short-acting drug is used for inducing anesthesia. For treating epilepsy, a long-acting drug is used, whereas, in a sleep disorder, a short-acting or an intermediate-type drug is used, depending on whether patients have difficulty falling asleep or if they have difficulty staying asleep.

BASILIXIMAB

(Simulect powder for injection)

Basiliximab is an immunosuppressive agent that blocks the interleukin-2 receptor α-chain, which is a critical pathway in allograft rejection. Basiliximab is indicated in the prophylaxis of acute organ rejection in patients receiving renal transplantation when used as part of an immunosuppressive regimen that includes cyclosporine and corticosteroids.

BECLAMETHASONE DIPROPIONATE

(Beclovent, Vanceril)

Beclamethasone dipropionate inhaler (see Table 11) is indicated only for patients who require chronic treatment with corticosteroids for control of the symptoms of bronchial asthma. Patients require 2 inhalations, (84 mcg) 3 to 4 times/day.

Prednisone is available in oral form, and beclamethasone may be used as an aerosol, especially in children. The corticosteroids may exert their effects through multiple mechanisms, including: relaxing bronchospasm, decreasing mucous secretion, potentiating beta-adrenergic receptors, antagonizing cholinergic actions, stabilizing lysosomes, possessing antiinflammatory properties, inhibiting antibody formation, and antagonizing histamine actions.

Corticosteroids do not inhibit the release of mediators from mast cells or block the early response to allergens, but they do block the late response and the subsequent bronchial hyperresponsiveness.

Steroids such as beclamethasone dipropionate, budesonide, triamcinolone acetonide, and flunisolide are active when given topically and can control asthma without causing systemic effects or adrenal suppression. However, orally administered steroids such as prednisone, prednisolone, or methylprednisolone are still needed by some patients.

The side effects of high-dose inhalational steroids include oropharyngeal candidiasis and dysphonia. The orally administered steroids may produce osteoporosis, weight gain, hypertension, diabetes, myopathy, psychiatric disturbances, skin fragility, or cataracts.

BELLADONNA/OPIUM

(B&O supprettes No. 15A suppositories)

Contains more than a score of alkaloids, including morphine, narcotine, papaverine, and codeine, which act to relax smooth muscle, relieve pain, and cause sedation by depressant effect on cerebral cortex, hypothalamus, and medullary centers. It is indicated in the relief of moderate to severe pain associated with ureteral spasm not responsive to nonnarcotic analgesics and to space intervals between injections of opiates.

BELLADONNA (LEVOROTATORY) ALKALOIDS/ PHENOBARBITAL/ERGOTAMINE TARTRATE

(Bellamine tablets)

Belladonna agents cause inhibition of the sympathetic and parasympathetic nervous system by ergotamine and belladonna, respectively, reinforced by the synergistic activity of phenobarbital in dampening the cortical centers. These agents are indicated in the management of disorders characterized by nervous tension and exaggerated autonomic response; menopausal disorders with hot flushes, sweats, restlessness, and insomnia; cardiovascular disorders with palpitation, tachycardia, chest oppression, and vasomotor disturbances; GI disorders with hypermotility hypersecretion, "nervous stomach," diarrhea, constipation; interval treatment of recurrent, throbbing headache.

BENAZEPRIL HYDROCHLORIDE

(Lotensin tablets 5 mg)

Benazepril is an angiotensin converting enzyme (ACE) inhibitor which competitively inhibits ACE, resulting in decreased conversion of angiotensin I to angiotensin II, a potent vasoconstrictor that stimulates aldosterone secretion. It results in decreased vasopressor activity and decreased aldosterone secretion.

Benazepril, an ACE inhibitor (10 mg p.o. daily), is indicated in the treatment of hypertension (see Figure 24). Many ACE inhibitors have been synthesized. These drugs can be classified into three broad groups based on chemical structure: (1) sulfhydryl-containing ACE inhibitors structurally related to **captopril** (e.g., **fentiapril**, **pivalopril**, **zofenopril**, and **alacepril**); (2) dicarboxyl-containing ACE inhibitors structurally related to **enalapril** (e.g., **lisinopril**, **benazepril**, **quinapril**, **moexipril**, **ramipril**, **trandolapril**, **spirapril**, **perindopril**, **pentopril**, and **cilazapril**); and (3) phosphorus-containing ACE inhibitors structurally related to **fosinopril**. Many ACE inhibitors are ester-containing prodrugs that are 100 to 1000 times less potent but have a much better oral bioavailability than the active molecules.

Currently, eleven ACE inhibitors are available for clinical use in the United States. In general, they differ among themselves with regard to three properties: (1) potency, (2) whether ACE inhibition is primarily a direct effect of the drug itself or the effect of an active metabolite, and (3) pharmacokinetics (i.e., extent of absorption, effect of food on absorption, plasma half-life, tissue distribution, and mechanisms of elimination).

There is no compelling reason to favor one ACE inhibitor over another because all ACE inhibitors effectively block the conversion of angiotensin I to angiotensin II, and all have similar therapeutic indications, adverse-effect profiles, and contraindications. However, the **Quality-of-Life Hypertension Study Group** reported that although captopril and enalapril are indistinguishable with regard to antihypertensive efficacy and safety, captopril may have a more favorable effect on quality of life. Because hypertension usually requires lifelong treatment, quality-of-life issues are an important consideration in comparing antihypertensive drugs. ACE inhibitors differ markedly in tissue distribution, and it is possible that this difference could be exploited to inhibit some local renin–angiotensin systems while leaving others relatively intact. Whether site-specific inhibition actually confers therapeutic advantages remains to be established.

With the notable exceptions of fosinopril and spirapril (which display balanced elimination by the liver and kidneys), ACE inhibitors are cleared predominantly by the kidneys. Therefore, impaired renal function significantly diminishes the plasma clearance of most ACE inhibitors, and dosages of these drugs should be reduced in patients with renal impairment. Elevated plasma renin activity (PRA) renders patients hyperresponsive to ACE inhibitor–induced hypotension, and initial dosages of all ACE inhibitors should be reduced in patients with high plasma levels of renin (e.g., patients with heart failure, and salt-depleted patients).

BENDROFLUMETHIAZIDE

(Naturetin tablets 5 mg)

Bendroflumethiazide is a thiazide diuretic that enhances excretion of sodium, chloride, and water by interfering with the transport of sodium ions across the renal tubular epithelium. Bendroflumethiazide is indicated in adjunctive therapy for edema associated with congestive heart failure (CHF), hepatic cirrhosis, and corticosteroid and estrogen therapy; treatment of edema associated with various forms of renal dysfunction (e.g., nephritic syndrome, acute glomerulonephritis, chronic renal failure); management of hypertension. The thiazide diuretics are more effective antihypertensive agents than the loop diuretics, such as furosemide and bumetanide, in patients who have normal renal function. This differential effect is most likely related to the short duration of action of loop diuretics, such that a single daily dose does not cause a significant net loss of Na^+ for an entire 24-hour period. Indeed, loop diuretics are frequently and inappropriately prescribed as a once-a-day medication in the treatment not only of hypertension but also of CHF and ascites. The spectacular efficacy of the loop diuretics in producing rapid and profound natriuresis can be detrimental to the treatment of hypertension. When a loop diuretic is given twice daily, acute diuresis that occurs can be excessive and lead to more side effects than with a slower-acting, milder thiazide diuretic.

BENDROFLUMETHIAZIDE

(Naturetin)

Bendroflumethiazide, a thiazide diuretic (2.5 to 20 mg p.o. daily), is indicated in edema and hypertension (see also Table 25).

BENTIROMIDE

(Chymex)

Bentiromide, a para-aminobenzoic acid (PABA) derivative (500 mg dose p.o.), is used as a screening test for pancreatic exocrine insufficiency. Following oral administration, bentiromide is cleaved by the pancreatic enzyme chymotrypsin, causing the release of PABA.

BENZOCAINE

(Americaine, Hurricaine, Orabase with Benzocaine, Orajel, Rid-A-Pain)

Benzocaine, an ester local anesthetic (20% topical gel), is indicated as a local anesthetic for dental pain or dental procedures and as a local anesthetic for pruritic dermatoses, pruritis, or other irritations.

BENZODIAZEPINE DERIVATIVES

The anxiolytic agents consist of benzodiazepine derivatives and azaspirodecanedione derivatives. For a long period of

TABLE 9
Summary of Benzodiazepine Derivatives

Drugs	Trade Names	Dose Range (mg)	Active Metabolites	Half-Life (hrs)
Chlordiazepoxide	Librium	5–200	Desmethylchlordiazepoxide, desmoxepam, desmethyldiazepam	>100
Diazepam	Valium, Valrelease	2–40	Desmethyldiazepam	>50
Oxazepam	Serax	30–120	None	5–14
Flurazepam	Dalmane	15–30	Flurazepam aldehyde, 1-hyroxyethylflurazepam, desalkylflurazepam	>100
Chlorazepate	Tranxene	15–60	Desmethyldiazepam	>100
Prazepam	Centrax	20–60	Desmethyldiazepam	>100
Lorazepam	Ativan	2–6	None	8–25
Halazepam	Paxipam	80–160	*N*-Desmethyldiazepam	>100
Alprazolam	Xanax	0.5–4	Alpha-hydroxyalprazolam	12–15
Temazepam	Restoril	15–30	Oxazepam	8–13
Triazolam	Halcion	0.125–0.5	Insignificant	1.5–5

time, the drug treatment of anxiety disorders has been dominated by benzodiazepine derivatives (Table 9). After the advent of chlordiazepoxide in the late 1950s, many derivatives were synthesized and introduced into clinical practice. This class of antianxiety agents shares the property of binding to a benzodiazepine receptor, part of the GABA receptor–chloride channel complex whose function it modulates allosterically (see Figure 50). Not only the anxiolytic effects of the benzodiazepines but also the other activities making up their pharmacologic profile, such as the anticonvulsant, sedative, or muscle relaxant effects, seem to be mediated by the GABA-related mechanism. In addition to the direct involvement of the GABA system, in parallel or more downstream to this, several other neurotransmitters such as serotonin have been suggested as participating in different aspects of benzodiazepine action. These azaspirodecedione derivatives include buspirone, gepirone, and ipsapirone.

Benzodiazepines are of value in the treatment of anxious depressions and anxiety-tension associated with schizophrenia, as well as in patients undergoing psychotherapy. They should be used only when the symptoms are disabling, not just to alleviate stress.

Benzodiazepines are of value in alleviating the symptoms of cerebral palsy, spasticity resulting from degenerative disorders such as multiple sclerosis, tetanus, stiff-man syndrome, and backache and muscle strain. The effective doses are generally large and may be increased as the disease progresses (e.g., multiple sclerosis).

To abort an epileptic seizure, diazepam, given intravenously, is a drug of choice. Clonazepam is also effective for achieving this.

During acute withdrawal from alcohol, the intravenous administration of diazepam is recommended, usually followed by chlordiazepoxide given orally.

BENZODIAZEPINES: Uses of

Agents	Select Therapeutic Uses
Alprazolam	Anxiety disorders, agoraphobia
Brotizolam	
Chlordiazepoxide	Anxiety disorders, management of alcohol withdrawal, anesthetic premedication
Clobazam	
Clonazepam	Seizure disorders, mania, movement disorders
Clorazepate	Anxiety disorders, seizure disorders
Demoxepam	
Diazepam	Anxiety disorders, status epilepticus, muscle relaxation, anesthetic premedication
Estazolam	Insomnia
Flumazenil	Antidote to benzodiazepines
Flurazepam	Insomnia
Halazepam	Anxiety disorders
Lorazepam	Anxiety disorders, preanesthetic medication
Midazolam	Preanesthetic and intraoperative medication
Nitrazepam	
Nordazepam	
Oxazepam	Anxiety disorders
Prazepam	
Quazepam	Insomnia
Temazepam	Insomnia
Triazolam	Insomnia

Agents for which no uses have been identified have not been studied extensively.

BENZONATATE

(Tessalon capsules 100 mg)

Benzonatate is a nonnarcotic antitussive preparation that reduces cough reflex by anesthetizing stretch receptors in respiratory passages. It is indicated (100 mg p.o. t.i.d.) in symptomatic relief of cough.

BENZOYL PEROXIDE

(Benzac liquid 2.5%)

Benzoyl is an antibiotic that is indicated in the treatment of mild to moderate acne vulgaris and as an adjunct to antibiotics, retinoic acid, and sulfur or salicylic acid-containing products in treating more severe cases of acne.

Resistant strains of *P. acnes* are emerging that may respond to judicious use of retinoids in combination with antibiotics. Commonly used topical antimicrobials in acne include **erythromycin**, **clindamycin** (Cleocin-t), and **benzoyl peroxide** and antibiotic-benzoyl peroxide combinations (Benzamycin, Benzaclin, others). Other antimicrobials used in treating acne include **sulfacetamide** (Klaron), **sulfacetamide/sulfur** combinations (Sulfacet-R), **metronidawie** (Metrocream, Metro-Gel, noritate), and **azelaic acid** (Azelex). Systemic therapy is prescribed for patients with more extensive disease and acne that is resistant to topical therapy. Effective agents include **tetracycline** (sumycin, others), **minocycline** (MINOCIN, others), **erythromycin** (ERYC, others), **clindamycin** (CLEOCIN), and **trimethoprim-sulfamethoxazole** (bactrim, others). Antibiotics usually are administered twice daily, and doses are tapered after control is achieved.

Tetracycline is the most commonly employed antibiotic because it is inexpensive, safe, and effective. The initial daily dose is usually 1 g in divided doses. Although tetracycline is an antimicrobial agent, its efficacy in acne may be more dependent on its antiinflammatory activity.

Minocycline has better gastrointestinal absorption than tetracycline and may be less photosensitizing than either tetracycline or doxycycline. Side effects of minocycline include dizziness and hyperpigmentation of the skin and mucosa, serum-sickness-like reactions, and drug-induced lupus erythematosus. With all the tetracyclines, vaginal candidiasis is a common complication that is readily treated with local administration of antifungal drugs.

In healthy individuals taking oral antibiotics for acne, laboratory monitoring is not necessary. Orally administered antibiotics also may be indicated in other noninfectious conditions, including **acne rosacea**, **perioral dermatitis**, **hidradenitis suppurativa**, **autoimmune blistering diseases**, **sarcoidosis**, and **pyoderma gangrenosum**.

BENZPHETAMINE HYDROCHLORIDE

(Didrex tablets 25 mg)

Benzphetamine hydrochloride is an anorexiant that stimulates the satiety center in the brain, causing appetite suppression. It is used in 25 to 50 mg p.o. daily as a short-term (few weeks) adjunct to diet plan to reduce weight (see Amphetamine Sulfate).

BENZQUINAMIDE HYDROCHLORIDE

(Emete-Con)

Benzquinamide, a benzoquinolizine derivative (50 mg IM), is indicated in the management of nausea and vomiting associated with anesthesia and surgery.

BENZTHIAZIDE

(Aquatag, Exna, Hydrex, Marazide, Proaqua)

Benzthiazide, a thiazide diuretic (50 to 200 mg p.o. daily), is indicated in the treatment of edema and hypertension (see also Table 25).

BENZTROPINE MESYLATE

(Cogentin)

Benztropine may be used in the management of Parkinson's disease (1 to 2 mg/day), neuroleptic-induced parkinsonism (1 to 4 mg once or twice/day), and neuroleptic-induced acute dystonic syndrome (1 to 2 mg IM or IV). In parkinsonian patients, the deficiency of dopamine causes the cholinergic receptors to be hyperactive. Therefore, anticholinergic drugs may be used to mitigate some of the symptoms. These agents include: trihexyphenidyl (Artane), cycrimine (Pagitane), procyclidine (Kemadrin), biperiden (Akineton), orphenadrine (Disipal), and benztropine (Cogentin).

Neuroleptics such as chlorpromazine or haloperidol may cause parkinsonian symptoms characterized by postural instability, stooped posture, shuffling and festinating gate, or rigidity, due to enhanced muscle tone, with, at times, "cogwheel" or "ratchet" resistance to passive movements in any direction. There is also tremor at rest with regular rhythmic oscillations of the extremities, especially the hands and fingers, as well as akinesia (poverty of movement) or bradykinesia (slowness in initial volitional activities). These symptoms, which are due to blockade of dopaminergic receptor sites in the striatum, are lessened by reducing the dosage of neuroleptics and by the oral administration of anticholinergic compounds, such as trihexyphenidyl hydrochloride (Artane) or benztropine mesylate (Cogentin).

Neuroleptics such as chlorpromazine or haloperidol may cause acute dystonia, which is characterized by an exaggerated posturing of the head, neck, or jaw; by spastic contraction of the muscles of the lips, tongue, face or throat, which makes drinking, eating, swallowing, and speech difficult; by torticollis, retrocollis, opisthotonus, distress, and ultimately anoxia. Neuroleptic-induced dystonia, which may occur in children treated actively with phenothiazine derivatives for their antiemetic properties, disappears in sleep and is treated effectively with diphenhydramine hydrochloride (Benadryl), which possesses both anticholinergic and antihistaminic properties. Benztropine is also effective. Contraindications to the use of benztropine are the same as those for atropine and other anticholinergic drugs and are: glaucoma, prostatic hypertrophy, myasthenia gravis, stenosing peptic ulcer, and duodenal or pyloric obstruction. Urinary retention and tachycardia should be heeded and regarded as signs of impending toxicity.

BEPRIDIL HYDROCHLORIDE

(Vascor)

Bepridil, a calcium channel blocker (200 mg p.o. daily), is indicated in the treatment of chronic stable angina (classic effort-associated angina) in patients who are unresponsive or inadequately responsive to other antianginals (see also Table 21).

BERACTANT

(Natural Lung Surfactant) (Survanta)

Beractant, a bovine lung extract (administered by intratracheal instillation), is indicated in prevention and treatment (rescue) of respiratory distress syndrome (hyaline membrane disease) in premature infants.

BETA-ADRENERGIC-RECEPTOR-BLOCKING AGENTS

	α Blockade	β_1 Selectivity	MSA	ISA	Lipid-Solubility
Acebutolol	0	+	+	+	Low
Atenolol	0	+	0	0	Low
Betaxolol	0	+	±	0	Low
Carteolol	0	0	0	+	Low
Labetaolol	+	0	+	0	Moderate
Metoprolol	0	+	0	0	Moderate
Nadolol	0	0	0	0	Low
Penbutolol	0	0	0	+	High
Pindolol	0	0	+	+++	Moderate
Propranolol	0	0	+	0	High
Timolol	0	0	0	0	Low

MSA, membrane stabilizing activity; ISA, intrinsic sympathomimetic activity.

BETA-ARRESTIN

Two different kinases are involved in phosphorylating beta-adrenergic receptors. Protein kinase A is positively regulated by cyclic AMP and is stimulated by substances that activate adenylate cyclase. Beta-adrenergic receptor kinase (BARK) is related functionally to rhodopsin kinase and may be important for regulating neural transmission (see Figure 52). A cytosolic protein, beta-arrestin, interacts with the BARK-phosphorylated receptors and disrupts the activation of G_S by the beta receptor.

BETAMETHASONE

(Celestone)

BETAMETHASONE

(Systemic) (Celestone)

BETAMETHASONE BENZOATE

(Benisone; Uticort)

See Corticosteroids.

BETAMETHASONE BENZOATE

(Uticort)

BETAMETHASONE/CLOTRIMAZOLE

(Lotrisone cream 0.05% betamethasone (as dipropionate)/1% clotrimazole)

Betamethasone/Clotrimazole is a topical corticosteroid. Clotrimazole increases cell membrane permeability in susceptible fungi. Betamethasone has antiinflammatory, antipruritic, and vasoconstrictive actions. This combination is indicated in topical treatment of **tinea pedis**, **tinea cruris**, and **tinea corporis** caused by *Trichophyton rubrum*, *T. mentagrophytes*, *Epidermophyton floccosum*, *Microsporum canis*.

Clotrimazole is available as a 1% cream, lotion, and solution (Lotrimin, Mycelex, others), 1% or 2% vaginal cream or vaginal tablets of 100, 200, or 500 mg (Gyne-Lotrimin, Mycelex-G, others), and 10-mg troches (Mycelex, others). On the skin, applications are made twice a day. For the vagina, the standard regimens are one 100-mg tablet once a day at bedtime for 7 days, one 200-mg tablet daily for 3 days, one 500-mg tablet inserted only once, or 5 g of cream once a day for 3 days (2% cream) or 7 days (1% cream). For nonpregnant females, one 200-mg tablet may be used once a day for 3 days. Troches are to be dissolved slowly in the mouth five times a day for 14 days.

Clotrimazole has been reported to cure dennatophyte infections in 60 to 100% of cases. The cure rates in cutaneous candidiasis are 80 to 100%. In vulvovaginal candidiasis, the cure rate is usually above 80% when the 7-day regimen is used. A 3-day regimen of 200 mg once a day appears to be similarly effective, as does single-dose treatment (500 mg). Recurrences are common after all regimens. The cure rate with oral troches for oral and pharyngeal candidiasis may be as high as 100% in the immunocompetent host.

BETAMETHASONE DIPROPIONATE

(Alphatrex, Diprolene AF, Diprolene, Diprosone, Maxivate)

BETAMETHASONE DIPROPIONATE

(Diprosone)

See Corticosteroids.

BETAMETHASONE SODIUM PHOSPHATE

(BSP, Celestone Phosphate, Prelestone, Selestoject)

BETAMETHASONE SODIUM PHOSPHATE

(Celestone Phosphate)

See Corticosteroids.

BETAMETHASONE SODIUM PHOSPHATE AND ACETATE

(Celestone Soluspan)

See Corticosteroids.

BETAMETHASONE SODIUM PHOSPHATE AND BETAMETHASONE ACETATE

(Celestone Soluspan)

Betamethasone, a glucocorticoid with antiinflammatory properties, is indicated in the treatment of adrenocortical insufficiency, severe inflammation, or immunosuppression (see also Table 11 and Figure 28).

BETAMETHASONE VALERATE

(Beta-Val, Valisone)

See Corticosteroids (and Table 11).

BETAMETHASONE VALERATE

(Betatrex, Beta-Val, Valisone)

Betamethasone, a topical glucocorticoid with antiinflammatory properties (lotion, ointment 0.1%, cream 0.01%, 0.1%, aerosol solution 0.1%), is indicated in inflammation of corticosteroid-responsive dermatoses.

BETAXOLOL HYDROCHLORIDE

(Betoptic)

Betaxolol is a beta-adrenergic blocking agent that blocks beta receptors, primarily affecting the cardiovascular system (decreases heart rate, cardiac contractility, and blood pressure) and lungs (promotes bronchospasm). Ophthalmic use reduces intraocular pressure, probably by reducing aqueous production. The preparation is indicated in hypertension. Ophthalmic preparation: lowering IOP; ocular hypertension; chronic open-angle glaucoma.

Betaxolol (one drop in each eye b.i.d.), a cardioselective $beta_1$-adrenergic blocking agent, is used in chronic open-angle glaucoma and ocular hypertension. It reduces intraocular pressure by reducing the production of aqueous humor. Betaxolol is known to have caused brief discomfort, tearing, erythema, itching, photophobia, corneal sensitivity, corneal staining, keratitis, and anisocoria. Betaxolol should be used cautiously in patients with bronchial asthma, sinus bradycardia, second- or third-degree AV block, cardiac failure, and cardiogenic shock.

BETHANECHOL CHLORIDE

(Urecholine Chloride)

Bethanechol (5 mg sc) is indicated in acute postoperative and postpartum nonobstructive (functional) urinary retention and neurogenic atony of the urinary bladder with retention. The two currently used derivatives of acetylcholine are bethanechol and carbachol (Miostat). Unlike acetylcholine, both agents are resistant to hydrolysis by cholinesterase (see also Figure 12). The cardiovascular actions of acetylcholine are vasodilation and negative chronotropic and inotropic effects. The cardiovascular effects of methacholine are more pronounced than those of acetylcholine, which in turn are greater than those of carbachol or bethanechol. The gastrointestinal effects (increase in tone, amplitude of contractions, and peristalsis) of bethanechol and carbachol are equal but greater than those of acetylcholine. The effects of carbachol and bethanechol on the urinary tract, consisting of ureteral peristalsis, contraction of the detrusor muscle of the urinary bladder, and an increase in voluntary voiding pressure, are equivalent and exceed those produced by acetylcholine.

Higher than therapeutic doses of bethanechol may cause abdominal discomfort, colicky pain, belching, diarrhea, salivation, borborygmi, and a fall in blood pressure, with reflex tachycardia and bronchial constriction. Atropine (0.6 mg sc) is a specific antidote. The contraindication to larger than therapeutic doses of bethanechol are hyperthyroidism, peptic ulcer, latent or active asthma, pronounced bradycardia, atrioventricular conduction defects, vasomotor instability, coronary artery disease, epilepsy, parkinsonism, coronary occlusion, or hypotension. Bethanechol should not be used in bladder neck obstruction or mechanical obstruction of the gastrointestinal tract.

Bethanechol stimulates the parasympathetic nervous system, increasing gastric motility and tone, and may restore rhythmic peristalsis. Bethanechol is indicated in the treatment of acute postoperative and postpartum nonobstructive urinary retention and neurogenic atony of the urinary bladder with retention. Unlabeled use: diagnosis and treatment of reflux esophagitis. Bethanechol can be of value in certain cases of postoperative abdominal distention and in gastric atony or gastroparesis. The oral route is preferred; the usual dosage is 10 to 20 mg, three or four times daily. Bethanechol is given by mouth before each main meal in cases without complete retention; when gastric retention is complete and nothing passes into the duodenum, the subcutaneous route is necessary because of poor stomach absorption. Bethanechol, likewise, has been used to advantage in certain patients with congenital megacolon and with adynamic ileus secondary to toxic states. Prokinetic agents with combined cholinergic-agonist and dopamine-antagonist activity (e.g., **metoclopramide**) or serotonin-antagonist activity or serotonin-antagonist activity have largely replaced bethanechol in gastroparesis or esophageal reflux disorders.

Bethanechol may be useful in treating urinary retention and inadequate emptying of the bladder when organic obstruction is absent, as in postoperative and postpartum urinary retention, and in certain cases of chronic hypotonic, myogenic, or neurogenic bladder. α-Adrenergic receptor antagonists are useful adjuncts in reducing outlet resistance of the internal sphincter. Bethanechol may enhance contractions of the detrusor muscle after spinal injury if the vesical reflex is intact, and some benefit has been noted in partial sensory or motor paralysis of the bladder. Catheterization thus can be avoided. For acute retention, multiple subcutaneous doses of 2.5 mg of bethanechol may be administered. The stomach should be empty at the time the drug is injected. In chronic cases, 10 to 50 mg of the drug may be given orally two to four times daily with meals to avoid nausea and vomiting. When voluntary or spontaneous voiding begins, bethanechol is then slowly withdrawn.

BETHANIDINE SULFATE

Bethanidine is being investigated as an orphan drug to be used in treatment of primary ventricular fibrillation and to treat or prevent the recurrence of primary ventricular fibrillation.

BEVACIZUMAB

(Avastin injection 25 mg/mL)

Bevacizumab is a monoclonal antibody that binds to vascular endothelial growth factor, interfering with endothelial cell proliferation. It is indicated in combination with IV **5-fluorouracil** (5-FU)-based chemotherapy as first-line treatment of metastatic carcinoma of the colon or rectum. Bevacizumab (Avastin) is a humanized monoclonal antibody against vascular-endothelial growth factor (VEGF) and inhibits its interaction with the VEGFR1 and VEGFR2 receptors. Functionally, VEGF is an angiogenic growth factor that regulates vascular proliferation and permeability and inhibits apoptosis of new blood vessels. VEGF expression is increased in a variety of tumor types, including breast, ovarian, non-small cell lung, and colorectal cancer, and its expression correlates with neovascularization within tumor masses. Furthermore, in colorectal cancer, mircrovessel density is associated with progression of adenomas to carcinomas and with metastatic potential and a poor prognosis.

BEVANTOLOL

Bevantolol is a new adrenoreceptor-blocking agent with weak α_1-adrenoreceptor-blocking activity that is indicated initially in hypertension and in angina pectoris. By virtue of its apparent lack of effect on serum lipids, decrease in peripheral vascular resistance, minimal or no effect on sexual function, low incidence of CNS side effects, and absence of effects on renal function, bevantolol may offer advantages over existing treatments for patients with hypertension and angina pectoris. Bevantolol is contraindicated for patients with sinus bradycardia, greater-than-first-degree conduction block, cardiogenic shock, or overt cardiac failure.

BEXAROTENE

(Targretin gelatin capsules for oral use 75 mg)

Bexarotene is a retinoid that binds and activates retinoid X receptor subtypes (RXRα, RXRβ, RXRγ). Once activated, these receptors function as transcription factors that regulate the expression of genes that control cellular differentiation and proliferation, inhibit the growth *in vitro* of some tumor cell lines of hematopoietic and squamous cell origin, and induce tumor regression *in vivo* in some animal models. Bexarotene is indicated in refractory cutaneous T-cell lymphoma.

Retinoids include natural compounds and synthetic derivatives of retinol that exhibit vitamin A activity. Retinoids have many important functions throughout the body, including roles in vision, regulation of cell proliferation and differentiation and bone growth, immune defense, and tumor suppression. Because vitamin A affects normal epithelial differentiation, it was investigated as a treatment for cutaneous disorders but was abandoned initially because of unfavorable side effects. Molecular modifications yielded compounds with vastly improved margins of safety. First-generation retinoids include retinol, tretinoin (all-*trans*-retinoic acid), isotretinoin (13-*cis*-retinoic acid), and alitretinoin (9-*cis*-retinoic acid). Second-generation retinoids, also known as aromatic retinoids, were created by alteration of the cyclic end group, and include acitretin. Third-generation retinoids contain further modifications and are called arotinoids. Members of this generation include **tazrotene** and **bexarotene**. **Adapalene**, a derivative of naphthoic acid with retinoid-like properties, does not fit precisely into any of the three generations.

BICALUTAMIDE

(Casodex tablets for oral use 50 mg)

Bicalutamide is an antiandrogen. It inhibits the action of androgens. Bicalutamide is indicated in advanced prostate cancer in combination with a luteinizing hormone-releasing hormone (LHRH) analog. Flutamide, Bicalutamide, and Nilutamide are potent androgen receptor antagonists but have limited efficacy when used alone because the increased LH secretion stimulates higher serum testosterone concentrations. They are used primarily in conjunction with a GnRH analog in the treatment of metastatic prostate cancer. In this situation, they block the action of adrenal androgens, which are not inhibited by GnRH analogs. Survival rates in groups of patients with metastatic prostate cancer treated with a combination of a GnRH agonist and flutamide (Eulexin), bicalutamide (Casodex), or nilutamide (Nilandron) are similar to one another and to survival rates in those treated by castration. Bicalutamide is replacing flutamide for this purpose because it appears to have less hepatotoxicity and is taken once a day instead of three times a day. Nilutamide appears to have worse side effects than flutamide and bicalutamide. Flutamide also has been used to treat hirsutism in women, and it appears to be as effective as any other treatment for this purpose. However, the association with hepatotoxicity warrants cautions against its use for this cosmetic purpose.

BIMATOPROST

(Lumigan solution 0.03%)

Bimatoprost is a prostaglandin agonist. It lowers intraocular pressure by increasing outflow of aqueous humor through the trabecular meshwork and uveoscleral routes. It is indicated in the reduction of IOP in patients with open-angle glaucoma or ocular hypertension who are intolerant of other IOP-lowering agents or insufficiently responsive to other IOP-lowering medications.

BIOAVAILABILITY OF DRUGS: Factors Influencing

Physicochemical Properties of the Drugs

Solubility in aqueous and organic solvents	Crystalline and polymorphic forms
pH-solubility profile	Solvation and hydration
Lipid-water partition coefficient	Salt form
pKa	Stability in solid state and solution
Particle size and size distribution	Molecular weight

Physiologic Factors	
pH	Volume and composition of biologic fluids
Temperature	Disease state
Surface area	Sex
Surface tension	Age
Manufacturing Variables	**Environmental Factors**
Diluents	Humidity
Manufacturing factors	Temperature
Packaging	

BIPERIDEN

(Akineton tablets 2 mg [as hydrochloride], injection 5 mg/mL [as lactate])

Biperiden is a weak peripheral anticholinergic agent and possesses nicotinolytic activity. It is indicated in the control of extrapyramidal disorders secondary to neuroleptic drug therapy. Biperidine (2 mg t.i.d.) is indicated in the treatment of Parkinson's disease and drug-induced parkinsonism (2 mg t.i.d.). In parkinsonian patients, the deficiency of dopamine causes the cholinergic receptors to be hyperactive. Therefore, anticholinergic drugs may be used to mitigate some of the symptoms. These agents include: cycrimine (Pagitane), and orphenadrine (Disipal). **Trihexyphenidyl hydrochloride** (Artane), **procyclidine** (Kemadrin), **biperiden** (Akineton), and **benztropine** (Cogentin) are tertiary-amine muscarinic receptor antagonists (together with the ethanolamine antihistamine diphenhydramine [Benadryl, other]) that gain access to the CNS and can therefore be used when anticholinergics are indicated to treat parkinsonism and the extrapyramidal side effects of antipsychotic drugs.

Contraindications to the use of anticholinergic drugs in treating parkinsonism are the same as those for atropine, and are: glaucoma, prostatic hypertrophy, myasthenia gravis, stenosing peptic ulcer, and duodenal or pyloric obstruction. Urinary retention and tachycardia should be heeded and regarded as signs of impending toxicity.

BISACODYL

(Dulcolax tablets, enteric-coated 5 mg)

Bisacodyl is a laxative that is indicated in short-term treatment of constipation; evacuation of colon for rectal and bowel evaluation; preparation for delivery or surgery. **Bisacodyl** is the only diphenylmethane derivative available in the United States. It is marketed as an enteric-coated preparation (Dulcolax, Correctol, others) and as a suppository for rectal administration. The usual oral daily dose of bisacodyl is 10 to 15 mg for adults and 5 to 10 mg for children 6 to 12 years old. The drug requires hydrolysis by endogenous esterases in the bowel for activation, and so the laxative effects after an oral dose usually are not produced in less than 6 hours; taken at bedtime, it will produce its effect the next morning. Suppositories work much more rapidly, within 30 to 60 minutes. Due to the possibility of developing an atonic nonfunctioning colon, bisacodyl should not be used for more than 10 consecutive days.

Bisacodyl is mainly excreted in the stool; about 5% is absorbed and excreted in the urine as a glucuronide. Overdosage can lead to catharsis, and fluid and electrolyte deficits. The diphenylmethanes can damage the mucosa and initiate an inflammatory response in the small bowel and colon. To avoid drug activation in the stomach with consequent gastric irritation and cramping, patients should swallow tablets without chewing or crushing and avoid milk or antacid medications within 1 hour of the ingestion of bisacodyl.

BISMUTH SUBSALICYLATE

(Bismatrol tablets)

Bismuth is an antidiarrheal agent that produces antisecretory and antimicrobial effects; it may have an antiinflammatory effect. It is indicated in the treatment of indigestion without causing constipation, nausea, abdominal cramps; and for control of diarrhea, including traveler's diarrhea.

Bismuth compounds have been used to treat a variety of gastrointestinal diseases and symptoms for centuries, although their mechanism of action remains poorly understood. Pepto-Bismol (bismuth subsalicylate} is an over-the-counter preparation estimated to be used by 60% of American households. It is a crystal complex consisting of trivalent bismuth and salicylate suspended in a mixture of magnesium aluminum silicate clay. In the low pH of the stomach, the bismuth subsalicylate reacts with hydrochloric acid to form bismuth oxychloride and salicylic acid. While 99% of the bismuth passes unaltered and unabsorbed into the feces, the salicylate is absorbed in the stomach and small intestine. Thus, caution should be used in patients taking salicylates for other indications.

Bismuth is thought to have antisecretory, antiinflammatory, and antimicrobial effects. Nausea and abdominal cramps also are relieved by bismuth. The clay in Pepto-Bismol also may have some additional benefits in diarrhea, but this is not clear. Bismuth subsalicylate has been used extensively for the prevention and treatment of traveler's diarrhea, but is also effective in other forms of episodic diarrhea and in acute gastroenteritis. Today, the most common antibacterial use of this agent is in the treatment of *H. pylori*. A recommended dose of the bismuth subsalicylate (30 mL of regular strength Pepto-Bismol liquid or 2 tablets) contains approximately equal amounts of bismuth and salicylate (262 mg each). For control of indigestion, nausea, or diarrhea, the dose is repeated every 30 to 60 minutes, as needed, up to eight times a day. Bismuth products have a long track record of safety at recommended doses, although impaction may occur in infants and debilitated patients. Dark stools (sometimes mistaken for melena) and black staining of the tongue in association with bismuth compounds are caused by bismuth sulfide formed in a reaction between the drug and bacterial sulfides in the gastrointestinal tract.

BISMUTH SUBSALICYLATE/METRONIDAZOLE/ TETRACYCLINE

(Helidac)

Each of the ingredients is individually active *in vitro* against most strains of *H. pylori*.

BISOPROLOL

(Zebeta)

Bisoprolol, a beta-adrenergic receptor-blocking agent (5 mg p.o. once daily), is used in the treatment of hypertension (alone or in combination with other antihypertensives) (see also Figure 37).

BISOPROLOL FUMARATE/ HYDROCHLOROTHIAZIDE

(Ziac tablets 6.25 mg hydrochlorothiazide)

It blocks beta receptors, primarily affecting the cardiovascular system and lungs (bisoprolol); inhibits reabsorption of sodium and chloride in the ascending loop of Henle and early distal tubules (hydrochlorothiazide). The combination is indicated in the management of hypertension.

BITOLTEROL MESYLATE

(Tornalate aerosol 0.8%)

Bitolterol is a sympathomimetic agent that relaxes bronchial smooth muscle through beta$_2$-receptor stimulation. It is indicated in the prevention and treatment of reversible bronchospasm associated with asthma or other obstructive pulmonary diseases. Bitolterol is a novel β_2-agonist in which the hydroxyl groups in the catechol moiety are protected by esterification with 4-methylbenzoate. Esterases in the lung and other tissues hydrolyze this prodrug to the active form, colterol, or terbutylnorepinephrine. Animal studies suggest that these esterases are present in higher concentrations in lung than in tissues such as the heart.

Bitolterol is indicated for the prophylaxis and treatment of bronchial asthma and reversible bronchospasm. It may be used with or without concurrent theophylline or steroid therapy. The selective β_2-adrenergic stimulants cause bronchodilation without cardiac acceleration. Metaproterenol and terbutaline are available in tablet form, and terbutaline is also available for subcutaneous injection (see also Figure 94). Metaproterenol and albuterol are available in metered-dose inhalers.

Inhaled selective β_2-adrenergic receptor agonists (albuterol, terbutaline, fenoterol, and bitolterol) have a rapid onset of action and are effective for 3 to 6 hours. Formoterol and salmeterol are longer-acting agents (12 hours) and may prove useful in treating nocturnal symptoms.

The side effects of beta-adrenergic receptor agonists are tremor, tachycardia, and palpitations.

BIVALIRUDIN

(Angiomax powder for injection, lyophilized 250 mg)

Bivalirudin is a thrombin inhibitor that inhibits thrombin by reversibly binding to the catalytic site and the anion-binding exosite of circulating and clot-bound thrombin. Inhibits clot-bound and free-circulating thrombin, reducing the amount of active thrombin present for clot formation and extension. Bivalirudin is used as an anticoagulant in combination with aspirin in patients with unstable angina undergoing percutaneous transluminal coronary angioplasty (PTCA).

BLACK WIDOW SPIDER (*LATRODECTUS MACTANS*) ANTIVENIN

Black widow spider antivenin, which provides immune globulins that specifically bind black widow spider venom, is used in black widow spider bites (see also Figure 12).

BLEOMYCIN SULFATE

(Blenoxane sterile powder for injection)

Bleomycin sulfate is a mixture of cytotoxic glycopeptide antibiotics. It inhibits DNA synthesis. When administered intrapleurally, bleomycin acts as a **sclerosing agent**. It is indicated in the treatment of lymphomas (Hodgkin's and non-Hodgkin's); testicular carcinoma (e.g., embryonal cell, choriocarcinoma, teratocarcinoma); sclerosis of malignant pleural effusions (e.g., treatment, prevention); treatment of squamous cell carcinomas (e.g., head, neck). Although **bleomycin** has a number of interesting biochemical properties, its cytotoxic action results from its ability to cause oxidative damage to the deoxyribose of thymidylate and other nucleotides, leading to single- and double-stranded breaks in DNA. Studies *in vitro* indicate that bleomycin causes accumulation of cells in the G_2 phase of the cell cycle, and many of these cells display chromosomal aberrations, including chromatid breaks, gaps, and fragments, as well as translocations. Because bleomycin causes little myelosuppression, it has significant advantages in combination with other cytotoxic drugs. However, it does cause significant cutaneous toxicity, including hyperpigmentation, hyperkeratosis, erythema, and even ulceration. These changes may begin with tenderness and swelling of the distal digits and progress to erythematous, ulcerating lesions over the elbows, knuckles, and other pressure areas. Skin changes often leave a residual hyperpigmentation at these points, and may recur when patients are treated with other antineoplastic drugs.

The most serious adverse reaction to bleomycin is pulmonary toxicity, which begins with a dry cough, fine rales, and diffuse basilar infiltrates on x-ray, and may progress to life-threatening pulmonary fibrosis. Radiologic changes may be indistinguishable from interstitial infection or tumor, but may progress to dense fibrosis, cavitation, atelectasis or lobar collapse, or even apparent consolidation. Approximately 5 to 10% of patients receiving bleomycin develop clinically apparent pulmonary toxicity, and about 1% die of this complication. Most who recover experience a significant improvement in pulmonary function, but fibrosis may be irreversible.

BORIC ACID
(Borofax, Ear-Dry, Neo-Flo, Ocu-Bath, Swim Ear, Ting)

BORIC ACID AND SODIUM BORATE
(Blinx, Collyrium)

Boric acid, a topical antiinfective agent (fill ear canal with solution and plug with cotton; repeat t.i.d. or q.i.d.), is used for the treatment of external ear canal infection. In addition, 5% ointment is used for the relief of abrasions, dry skin, minor burns, insect bites, and other skin irritations.

BORTEZOMIB
(Velcade powder for injection)

It inhibits 26S proteasome, disrupting normal homeostatic mechanisms and leading to cell death. Bortezomib is indicated in the treatment of multiple myeloma in patients who received at least two prior therapies and demonstrated disease progression on the last therapy. Toxicities from the use of bortezomib have been well characterized. At the standard dose and schedule, grade 4 toxicities were rare (<4%) and grade 3 toxicities encountered in >5% of patients were as follows: thrombocytopenia (28%), fatigue (12%), peripheral neuropathy (12%), neutropenia (11%), anemia (8%), vomiting (8%), diarrhea (7%), dehydration (7%), nausea (6%), and weakness (5%). Peripheral neuropathy was encountered more frequently in patients with a prior history of neuropathy or preexisting numbness, pain, or burning. Dose reductions of bortezomib are recommended for these patients. Usually, the neuropathy improves or resolves completely after several months off treatment. Hypotension associated with the injection of **bortezomib** has been rarely encountered, and caution should be taken with patients who are volume-depleted, have a history of syncope, or who are on antihypertensive medications. Cardiac toxicity in the form of hypotension and failure has been encountered in animal studies at twice the recommended dose. Very little cardiac toxicity has been encountered in human studies.

BOSENTAN
(Tracleer tablets 62.5 mg)

Bosentan is an endothelin receptor antagonist. It antagonized endothelin (ET) receptor by binding to ET_A and ET_B receptors in the endothelium and vascular smooth muscle. Bosentan is indicated in treatment of pulmonary arterial hypertension in patients with WHO class III and IV symptoms, to improve exercise ability, and decrease the rate of clinical worsening.

BOTULINUM TOXIN TYPE A
(Botox powder for injection)

Blocks neuromuscular transmission by binding to acceptor sites on motor or sympathetic nerve terminals, entering the nerve terminals, and inhibiting the release of acetylcholine. Produces temporary chemical denervation of sweat glands and local reduction in sweating when injected intradermally. Botulinum toxin type A is indicated in the treatment of cervical dystonia; treatment of strabismus and blepharospasm associated with dystonia, including benign essential blepharospasm or VII nerve disorder in patients 12 years of age and older; treatment of severe primary axillary hyperhidrosis inadequately managed with topical agents (Botox); for temporary improvement in appearance of moderate to severe glabellar lines associated with corrugator or procerus muscle activity in patients 65 years of age or younger (Botox cosmetic).

BOTULINUM TOXIN TYPE B
(Myobloc solution, injectable 5000 units/mL)

Botulinum toxin type B interferes with neurotransmitter release by cleaving synaptic vesicle-associated membrane protein. It is indicated in reduction of severity of abnormal head position and neck pain in adult patients with cervical dystonia.

BOTULINUM TOXIN TYPE A
(Botox, Dysport)

Botulinum toxin type A is used as an orphan drug or as an investigational drug in blepharospasm and strabismus associated with dystonia in adults; cervical dystonia; dynamic muscle contracture in pediatric cerebral palsy, and essential blepharospasm; and synkinetic closure of the eyelid associated with VIII cranial nerve aberrant regeneration. Botulinum toxin produced by clostridium botulinum blocks neuromuscular conduction by binding to receptor pits on motor nerve terminals and preventing the release of acetylcholine (see Figure 12). The effect of botulinum toxin may be potentiated by aminoglycoside antibiotics or any other drug that interferes with neuromuscular transmission.

The integration of botulinum toxin into the orbicularis muscle can cause reduced blinking and lead to corneal exposure and ulceration.

BOTULINUM TOXIN A: Uses of

Dystonia: Blepharospasm	Spasticity: Multiple sclerosis
Cervical dystonia	Cerebral palsy
Spasmodic dysphonia	Head injury
Oromandibular dystonia	Paraplegia
Focal hand dystonia	Stroke
Limb dystonia	
Muscle Spasms: Hemifacial spasm	Tremor: Dystonic tremor
Facial synkinesis	Essential tremor
Masticatory spasm	Vocal tremor
	Palatal tremor (myoclonus)
Other: Bruxism	

Botulinum toxin acts selectively on cholinergic synapses to block Ca^{2+}-mediated release of acetylcholine. Unlike axotomy, botulinum toxin does not cause degeneration of the neuromuscular junction. Terminal motor axons are still capable of conducting impulses. An aqueous solution containing the botulinum toxin A, albumin, and sodium chloride is injected intramuscularly into selected muscles to produce local neuromuscular blockade.

BOTULINUM TOXIN TYPE A

(Oculinum)

Botulinum, a neurotoxin with muscle relaxant properties, is used in the treatment of strabismus (see also Figure 12).

BOTULISM ANTITOXIN, TRIVALENT (ABE) EQUINE

Botulism antitoxin, which binds and neutralizes the toxin, is used in the treatment of botulism.

BOTULISM IMMUNE GLOBULIN INTRAVENOUS (BIG-IV)

(Baby BIG powder for injection)

Botulism is an immune globulin. Botulism immune globulin contains IgG antibodies representative of the immunized donors who contribute to the plasma pool of the derived product. It is indicated in the treatment of patients younger than 1 year of age with infant botulism caused by type A or B.

BRADYKININ

As autacoids, bradykinin and kallidin increase vascular permeability, produce vasodilation, increase the synthesis of prostaglandins, and cause edema and pain. Extensive evidence exists that bradykinin and other kallidin substances contribute to the pathogenesis of the inflammatory response that occurs in acute and chronic diseases including allergic reactions, arthritis, asthma, sepsis, viral rhinitis, and inflammatory bowel diseases (see Figure 30).

BRETYLIUM TOSYLATE

(Bretylol)

Bretylium is indicated in the treatment of life-threatening ventricular arrhythmias that have failed to respond to the first-line antiarrhythmic agents such as lidocaine, and for prophylaxis and treatment of ventricular fibrillation. Bretylium initially and transiently releases norepinephrine, causing tachycardia and rise in blood pressure, but subsequently causes a chemical sympathectomy by inhibiting the release of catecholamine without reducing its concentration. Bretylium reduces heterogeneity of repolarization times, an effect that is likely to suppress reentry, blocks K^+ channels, and has no effect on automaticity. A lag time of ~2 hours has been reported between peak plasma bretylium concentrations and peak prolongation of ventricular refractoriness after an intravenous dose. This lag time suggests that bretylium will be distributed to sites in peripheral tissues prior to exerting its pharmacological effect. Bretylium is excreted unchanged by the kidneys without undergoing significant hepatic metabolism. Reduction of a maintenance infusion rate has been recommended in patients with renal failure.

BRIMONIDINE TARTRATE

(Alphagan P solution 0.15%)

Brimonidine is an alpha-adrenergic agonist that reduces aqueous humor production and increases uveoscleral outflow. It is used to lower intraocular pressure (IOP) in open-angle glaucoma or ocular hypertension. Brimonidine is another **clonidine** derivative that is administered ocularly to lower IOP in patients with ocular hypertension or open-angle glaucoma. Brimonidine is an α_2-selective agonist that reduces IOP both by

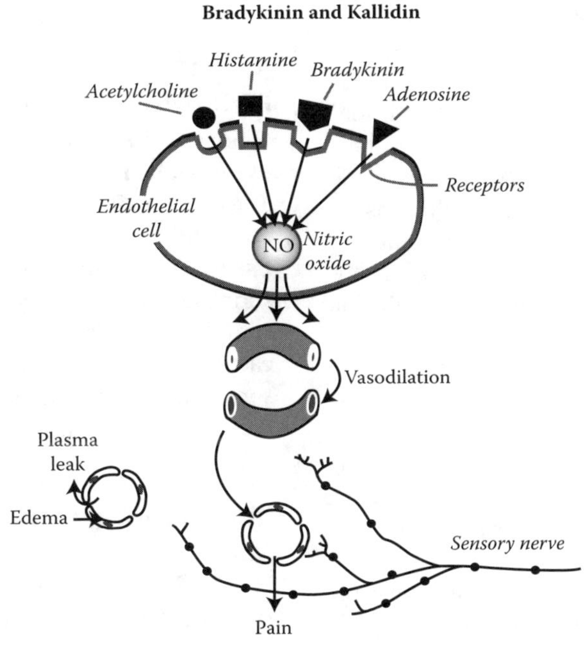

FIGURE 30 Bradykinin and kallidin increase vascular permeability, produce vasodilation, increase the synthesis of prostaglandins, and cause edema and pain.

decreasing aqueous humor production and by increasing outflow. The efficacy of brimonidine in reducing IOP is similar to that of the β-receptor antagonist **timolol**. Unlike apraclonidine, brimonidine can cross the blood–brain barrier and can produce hypotension and sedation, although these CNS effects are slight compared to those of clonidine. As with all α_2-receptor agonists, this drug should be used with caution in patients with cardiovascular disease.

BRINZOLAMIDE

(Azopt ophthalmic suspension 1%)

Brinzolamide is a carbonic anhydrase inhibitor that causes an inhibition of carbonic anhydrase in the ciliary processes of the eye decreases aqueous. It is indicated in the treatment of elevated IOP inpatients with ocular hypertension or open-angle glaucoma. The development of topical carbonic anhydrase inhibitor took many years but was an important event because of the poor side-effect profile of oral carbonic anhydrase inhibitors (CAIs). Dorzolamide (Trusopt) and **brinzolamide** both work by inhibiting carbonic anhydrase (isoenzyme II), which is found in the ciliary body epithelium. This reduces the formation of bicarbonate ions, which reduces fluid transport and thus IOP. In fact, the β-receptor antagonist timolol has been combined with the carbonic anhydrase inhibitor dorzolamide in a single medication (Cosopt).

BROMEFENAC

(Xibrom solution 0.09%)

Bromfenac decreases inflammation by blocking prostaglandin synthesis through inhibition of cyclooxygenase 1 and 2. It is indicated in the treatment of postoperative inflammation in patients who have undergone cataract surgery.

BROMOCRIPTINE MALEATE

(Parlodel)

Bromocriptine is an agonist for dopamine receptors and hence is used as an adjunct in the treatment of Parkinson's disease. As parkinsonism progresses, the activity of dopa-decarboxylase may become so reduced that it cannot adequately decarboxylate dopa to dopamine. In this case, it may be possible to stimulate the dopamine receptor sites located postsynaptically using compounds such as bromocriptine or pergolide. Bromocriptine is an ergot alkaloid that inhibits the secretion of prolactin by interfering with hypophyseal dopaminergic neurons, and has been used in the treatment of endocrine disorders such as Chiari–Frommel syndrome and Forbes–Albright syndrome. However, low-dose bromocriptine therapy is not effective in all patients. Bromocriptine has a longer duration of action than levodopa and is particularly useful in patients suffering from a high incidence of on–off phenomenon.

Bromocriptine is most effective when used with submaximal doses of levodopa. It should be regarded as an adjunct rather than as a substitute for levodopa. It is possible that more effective dopamine receptor agonists may replace bromocriptine in the future.

BROMPHENIRAMINE

(Bidhist tablets, extended-release 6 mg (as maleate))

Brompheniramine competitively antagonizes histamine at H_1-receptor sites. It is indicated in the relief of sneezing, itchy and watery eyes, itchy nose or throat, and runny nose because of hay fever (allergic rhinitis) or other respiratory allergies. VaZol is also indicated for temporary relief of runny nose and sneezing caused by the common cold; and treatment of allergic and nonallergic pruritic symptoms.

BROMPHENIRAMINE MALEATE

(Dimetane)

Brompheniramine is an alkylamine antihistaminic (H_1-receptor antagonist) agent used in allergic symptoms of rhinitis (4 to 8 mg p.o. t.i.d.). Brompheniramine is absorbed well from the gastrointestinal tract, exerts its effects in 15 to 30 minutes, and the peak of action is seen in 2 to 5 hours. It is extensively (95%) metabolized in the liver, and 5% of it is excreted unchanged by the kidneys. Clinical manifestations of overdose may include either those of CNS depression (sedation, reduced mental alertness, apnea, and cardiovascular collapse) or of CNS stimulation (insomnia, hallucinations, tremors, or convulsions). Anticholinergic symptoms, such as dry mouth, flushed skin, fixed and dilated pupils, and GI symptoms, are common, especially in children. Monoamine oxidase inhibitors inhibit the metabolism of brompheniramine, prolonging its effects. Because brompheniramine has strong anticholinergic effects, it should be used cautiously in patients with narrow-angle glaucoma, or in those with pyloroduodenal obstruction or urinary bladder obstruction from prostatic hypertrophy or narrowing of the bladder neck.

BROMPHENIRAMINE MALEATE/ PSEUDOEPHEDRINE HYDROCHLORIDE

(Lodrane liquid 4 mg brompheniramine/60 mg pseudoephedrine, Lodrane 12 D tablets 6 mg)

The combination is a respiratory agent. **Brompheniramine**: competitively antagonizes histamine at H_1-receptor sites. **Pseudoephedrine**: causes vasoconstriction and subsequent shrinkage of nasal mucous membranes by alpha-adrenergic stimulation, which promotes nasal drainage. They are indicated in temporary relief of symptoms associated with seasonal and perennial allergic rhinitis and vasomotor rhinitis, including nasal congestion.

BROMPHENIRAMINE MALEATE/PSEUDOEPHEDRINE HYDROCHLORIDE/DEXTROMETHORPHAN HBR

(Rondec-DM liquid 4 mg brompheniramine, 45 mg pseudoephedrine, 15 mg dextromethorphan)

Brompheniramine: competitively antagonizes histamine at H_1-receptor sites.

Pseudoephedrine: Causes vasoconstriction and subsequent shrinkage of nasal mucous membranes by alpha-adrenergic stimulation, which promotes nasal drainage.

Dextromethorphan: Suppresses cough by central action on the cough center in medulla.

The combination is recommended for the relief of cough and upper respiratory tract symptoms (including nasal congestion) associated with allergy or common cold.

BRONCHODILATORS: β-Adrenergic agonists for the treatment of asthma

Of the three classes of bronchodilators (β_2-adrenergic-receptor agonists, methylxanthines, and anticholinergic agents), the β_2-adrenergic-receptor agonists produce the greatest bronchodilation in patients with bronchial asthma. They are:

Intermediate-Acting (3-6 hr)			Long-Acting (>12 hr)
Albuterol	Fenoterol	Pirbuterol	Formoterol
Bitolterol	Metaproterenol	Terbutaline	Salmeterol

β_2-Adrenergic agonists are generally preferred both for the relief of acute symptoms and for the prevention of exercise-induced bronchospasm. The introduction of long-acting inhaled β_2-adrenergic agonists have overcome the principal shortcoming of the previously available drugs of this class—their limited duration of action. However, the possibility of adverse effects with regular use of β_2-adrenergic agonists has been raised.

BUCLIZINE HYDROCHLORIDE
(Bucladin S)

Buclizine (50 mg p.o. 30 minutes prior to travel) is a centrally acting antiemetic agent used for the control of the nausea, vomiting, and dizziness of motion sickness. Buclizine depresses conduction in vestibular–cerebellar pathways and hence reduces labyrinth excitability (antivertigo action), and it inhibits the chemotrigger zone for emesis (antiemetic action) (see also Figures 73 and 81).

Similar to other antihistaminic agents, buclizine possesses anticholinergic properties and hence should be used cautiously in narrow-angle glaucoma, prostatic hypertrophy, and obstruction of the gastrointestinal and urinary tracts. It has additive CNS-depressing effects with alcohol, barbiturates, anxiolytic agents, and many other medications. Buclizine should be used cautiously with ototoxic agents such as aminoglycosides because the signs of ototoxicity may become masked with buclizine.

The manifestations with buclizine overdosage may include either those of CNS depression (sedation, reduced mental alertness, apnea, and cardiovascular collapse) or of CNS stimulation (insomnia, hallucinations, tremors, or convulsions). Anticholinergic symptoms, such as dry mouth, flushed skin, fixed and dilated pupils, and GI symptoms, are common, especially in children.

Buclizine contains tartrazine, which may cause allergic reactions including asthma in susceptible individuals who also exhibit hypersensitivity to aspirin.

BUDESONIDE
(Entocort EC capsules 3 mg (micronized))

Budesonide is a corticosteroid/flucocorticoid/intranasal steroid. It exhibits a wide range of inhibitory activities against multiple cell types and mediators involved in allergic-mediated inflammation. Its indications are: Intranasal: management of seasonal and perennial allergic rhinitis symptoms in adults and children; oral inhalation: for the maintenance treatment of asthma as prophylactic therapy in adults and children and for patients requiring oral corticosteroid therapy for asthma; inhalation suspension: maintenance treatment of asthma and prophylactic therapy in children 12 months to 8 years of age; oral capsule: Crohn's disease.

BUDESONIDE
(Rhinocort)

Budesonide, an antiinflammatory corticosteroid (32 mcg/actuation and 256 mcg/daily) is indicated in the management of seasonal or perennial allergic rhinitis in adults and children.

Corticosteroids do not inhibit the release of mediators from mast cells or block the early response to allergens, but they do block the late response and the subsequent bronchial hyperresponsiveness.

Steroids such as beclomethasone dipropionate, budesonide, triamcinolone acetonide, and flunisolide are active when given topically and can control asthma without causing the systemic effects or adrenal suppression. However, orally administered steroids such as prednisone, prednisolone, or methylprednisolone are still needed by some patients.

The side effects of high-dose inhalational steroids include oropharyngeal candidiasis and dysphonia. The orally administered steroids may produce osteoporosis, weight gain, hypertension, diabetes, myopathy, psychiatric disturbances, skin fragility, or cataracts (see also Table 8).

BUMETANIDE
(Bumex tablets 0.5 mg, tablets 1 mg, tablets 2 mg, injection 0.25 mg/mL)

Bumetanide is a loop diuretic that inhibits reabsorption of sodium and chloride in proximal tubules and the loop of Henle. It is indicated in the treatment of edema associated with CHF, hepatic cirrhosis, and renal disease.

Loop Diuretics

Of the loop diuretics currently available, **furosemide** (Lasix), **bumetanide** (Bumex), and **torsemide** (Demadex) are widely used in the treatment of heart failure. Due to the increased risk of ototoxicity, ethacrynic acid (Edecrin) should be reserved for patients who are allergic to sulfonamides or who have developed interstitial nephritis on alternative drugs.

BUMETANIDE

(Bumex)

Bumetanide (0.5 to 2 mg/day p.o.), ethacrynic acid (Edecrin), furosemide (Lasix), and muzolimine are loop diuretics (see also Table 25 and Figure 17). These agents inhibit the active resorption of chloride (and sodium) in the thick, ascending medullary portion of the loop of Henle and also in the cortical portion of the loop or the distal tubule. The diuresis they produce, which is similar to that seen with the thiazides, predominantly causes a loss of chloride, sodium, and potassium, but HCO_3 excretion is not increased. Although large volumes of fluid can be excreted with the use of these agents, the ability of the kidney to produce either a dilute or concentrated urine is greatly diminished. These agents are the most efficacious of all the diuretics now in the market, usually producing about a 20% loss in the filtered load of sodium (furosemide, 15 to 30%; ethacrynic acid, 17 to 23%). Loop diuretics are ordinarily taken orally but can be given intravenously if a very rapid onset of action is sought, as when used in combination with antihypertensive medications in the management of a hypertensive crisis. Furosemide and ethacrynic acid undergo some active renal tubular secretion as well as glomerular filtration. A minor portion is excreted by the liver.

Loop diuretics are used for treating the following conditions:

- In the edema of cardiac, hepatic, or renal origin, including acute pulmonary edema and hypertensive crisis
- In acute renal failure, to maintain urine flow, though an excessive loss of extracellular fluid volume can cause a decrease in the GFR

In hypercalcemia, excessive volume depletion, hyponatremia, and hypotension are major risks associated with the use of loop diuretics, and the side effects of hypokalemia, hyperuricemia, and hyperglycemia are always present. Loop diuretics should not be used concurrently with ototoxic aminoglycoside antibiotics (i.e., streptomycin, gentamicin, kanamycin, tobramycin).

BUPIVACAINE HYDROCHLORIDE

(Marcaine)

Bupivacaine, an amide local anesthetic, is indicated in the production of local or regional anesthesia or analgesia, for oral surgery, for surgery, for diagnostic procedures, or for obstetrical anesthesia.

When a local anesthetic is injected near a nerve, it blocks the flow of electrons along the axons and eliminates the pain without loss of consciousness (see Figure 31). These effects are reversible. When administering a local anesthetic, one must remember that the larger the diameter of the nerve fiber, the more anesthetic is needed to produce anesthesia.

Epinephrine is used in combination with a local anesthetic to reduce its uptake, prolong its duration of action, produce a bloodless field of operation, and protect against systemic effects (see Figure 80). Local anesthetic solutions containing epinephrine should not be used in areas supplied by end arteries such as in the digits, ear, nose, and penis, because of the threat of ischemia and subsequent gangrene. Furthermore, under no circumstances should anesthetic solutions containing epinephrine be used intravenously in patients with cardiac arrhythmias. In general, solutions designed for multiple doses should not be used for spinal or epidural anesthesia.

Local anesthetics block the sodium channels, are cardiac depressants, and bring about a ventricular conduction defect and block that may progress to cardiac and ventilatory arrest if toxic doses are given. In addition, these agents produce

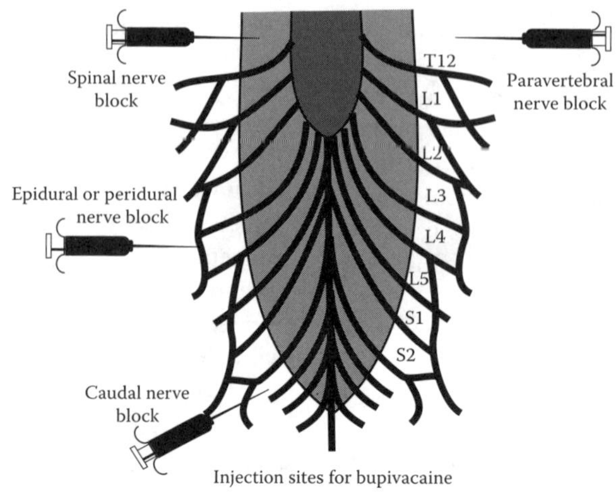

FIGURE 31 Bupivacaine, an amide local anesthetic, is sixteen times more potent than procaine and exhibits a long duration of action.

arteriolar dilation. Circulatory failure may be treated with vasopressors such as ephedrine, metaraminol (Aramine), or mephentermine (Wyamine). Artificial respiration and cardiac massage may also become necessary. Among the local anesthetics, only cocaine blocks the uptake of norepinephrine, causes vasoconstriction, and may precipitate cardiac arrhythmias.

An overdosage of local anesthetics can produce dose-dependent CNS side effects such as insomnia, visual and auditory disturbances, nystagmus, shivering, tonic–clonic convulsions, and finally fatal CNS depression. The initial CNS excitation and convulsions may be brought under control by diazepam or thiopental.

BUPRENORPHINE HYDROCHLORIDE

(Temgesic)

Buprinorphine is a semisynthetic opioid analgesic derived from thebaine. It binds readily to the opioid receptors in the CNS but dissociates from them slowly, which may be responsible for its long duration of action. Buprenorphine (0.3 mg IM) exerts its analgesic actions in 15 minutes and has a duration of action of 6 hours. It is bound to plasma proteins to the extent of 96%, is metabolized in the liver to a certain extent (*N*-dealkylmetabolite), and is excreted unchanged in the feces. Buprenorphine causes respiratory depression and elevates cerebrospinal pressure (contraindicated in head injury or conditions where intracranial pressure may be high).

Buprenorphine increases intracholedochal pressure to a similar degree as the other opiates. The adverse effects of buprenorphine are sedation, dizziness, vertigo, hypotension, hypoventilation, and miosis. Although naloxone is able to reverse several of the adverse effects of buprenorphine, it may not be as effective in reversing the respiratory depression requiring mechanical assistance of respiration.

BUPRENORPHINE

(BuprenexSubutex)

Buprenorphine is an opioid agonist–antagonist analgesic. Its analgesic effect is caused by binding to opiate receptors in the CNS. Antagonist effects decrease its abuse potential. It is indicated in tablet: treatment of opioid dependence; injection: relief of moderate to severe pain.

BUPRENORPHINE HYDROCHLORIDE/ NALOXONE HYDROCHLORIDE

(Suboxone tablets, sublingual 2 mg buprenorphine base per 0.5 mg naloxone tablets, sublingual 8 mg buprenorphine base per 2 mg naloxone)

Buprenorphine is a narcotic agonist–antagonist analgesic. **Buprenorphine**: analgesic effect caused by binding to opiate receptors in the CNS, whereas antagonist effects decrease abuse potential. **Naloxone**: possibly antagonizes opioid effects by competing for the same receptor sites. It is indicated in the treatment of opioid dependence. **Buprenorphine** is approved by the Food and Drug Administration (FDA) for the treatment of opioid addiction. Treatment is initiated with buprenorphine alone administered sublingually, followed by maintenance therapy with a combination of buprenorphine and naloxone (Suboxone) to minimize abuse potential. The partial agonist properties of buprenorphine limit its usefulness for the treatment of addicts who require high maintenance doses of opioids. However, conversion to maintenance treatment with higher doses of methadone, a full agonist, is possible.

BUPROPION HYDROCHLORIDE

(Wellbutrin)

Bupropion (100 mg p.o. b.i.d.) is indicated in the treatment of depression. It is reserved for patients who cannot tolerate or have not responded to other medications. Bupropion does not alter the uptake of serotonin, has an equivocal effect on the uptake of norepinephrine, but blocks the uptake of dopamine. Bupropion has no affinity for alpha-1 and alpha-2-adrenergic receptors, H_1-histamine receptors, muscarinic cholinergic receptors, or D_2-dopaminergic receptors. It does not cause sedation or orthostatic hypotension. However, because it is structurally related to amphetamine, it may cause insomnia, agitation, and anxiety shortly after initiation of therapy. Bupropion lowers the seizure threshold and hence is contraindicated in patients with a history of seizure disorder (see also Tables 5 through 7).

BURIMAMIDE

Histamine, as a normal constituent of the gastric mucosa, controls both microcirculation and gastric secretion. The gastric secretagogs are acetylcholine, histamine, and gastrin. The action of acetylcholine is blocked by atropine, and the action of histamine is blocked by cimetidine, burimamide, and metiamide. No specific antagonist is available for gastrin.

BUSPIRONE HYDROCHLORIDE

(BuSpar)

Buspirone (25 mg/day) is indicated in the management of anxiety disorders. The anxiolytic agents consist of benzodiazepine derivatives (see Table 9) and azaspirodecanedione derivatives, which include buspirone, gepirone, and ipsapirone. The introduction of novel anxiolytic agents such as buspirone, which interacts with the serotoninergic system, has suggested that serotoninergic fibers may be the final pathway through which anxiolytic effects are expressed.

Buspirone has a chemical structure that is distinct from that of the benzodiazepines. Without this structural homology, it is not surprising that buspirone does not interact with GABA receptors. Furthermore, the clinical profile of buspirone appears to be anxioselective, with a much reduced potential for abuse.

Several types of serotonin (5-HT) receptors exist in the mammalian brain, two of which are well characterized: 5-HT_3 and 5-HT_2 sites. The 5-HT_3 sites can be further subdivided into at least three distinct subsets, which differ in their regional distribution and functions and are currently termed 5-HT_{1A}, 5-HT_{1B}, and 5-HT_{1C} sites.

The 5-HT receptors in the hippocampus and other parts of the limbic system are primarily of the $5\text{-}HT_{1A}$ type. It is therefore tempting to speculate that drugs that display a high degree of selectivity for these receptor sites can selectively affect anxiety states. A breakthrough in that direction came with the discovery of buspirone, a drug with anxiolytic activity in humans that can help elucidate the role of 5-HT in anxiety. Buspirone, gepirone, and ipsapirone may therefore offer new therapeutic directions in the treatment of anxiety.

Buspirone is an anxiety agent but has no sedative, anticonvulsant, or muscle-relaxant properties. It binds selectively to the $5\text{-}HT_{1A}$ receptors, which are abundant in the hippocampus, a portion of the frontal cortex, and the dorsal raphe nucleus. The universal mechanism underlying its anxiolytic effects may be the inhibition of raphe-cell firing. The most common side effects of buspirone are dizziness, headache, and nervousness.

The drug is rapidly absorbed after oral administration, and peak plasma concentrations occur about 1 hour later. Buspirone is extensively metabolized, with less than 1% of an administered dose excreted unchanged. Important routes of biotransformation are hydroxylation and oxidative dealkylation, the latter yielding 1-(2-pyrimidinyl) piperazines. This metabolite has been shown to concentrate in the brain and to have pharmacologic activity, though its capacity to interact with different brain receptors appears to differ from that of buspirone.

BUSULFAN

(Myleran)

Busulfan, an alkylsulfonate, is indicated in the palliative treatment of chronic myelogenous leukemia including myeloid, myelocytic, or granulocytic leukemia. Busulfan is of no value in chronic lymphocytic leukemia, acute leukemia, or in the "blastic crisis" of chronic myelogenous leukemia. Busulfan (4 to 8 mg/day) is a cell-cycle phase, nonspecific, polyfunctional alkylating agent that interacts with cellular thiol groups without cross-linking of nucleoproteins. In treating chronic granulocytic leukemia, the initial oral dose of busulfan varies with the total leukocyte count and the severity of the disease; daily doses from 2 to 8 mg are recommended to initiate therapy and are adjusted appropriately to subsequent hematological and clinical responses. Busulfan is well absorbed after oral administration, and it disappears from the blood with a half-life of 2 to 3 hours. Almost all of the drug is excreted in the urine as methanesulfonic acid (see also Figure 15).

The most frequent and serious side effect of busulfan is bone marrow failure. Therefore, the hemoglobin, hematocrit, white blood cells, platelets, and differential counts should be monitored weekly. A rare complication of busulfan therapy is the development of bronchopulmonary dysplasia with pulmonary fibrosis. Busulfan is known to have caused cataract, hyperpigmentation of skin, adrenal insufficiency, gynecomastia, cholestatic jaundice, and myasthenia gravis.

BUTABARBITAL

(Barbased, Butalan, Buticaps, Butisol, Butartran, Sarisol No. 2)

Butabarbital, a barbiturate hypnotic sedative (15 to 30 mg p.o. t.i.d.), is indicated for causing sedation, and preoperative sedation and treating insomnia.

BUTALBITAL/ACETAMINOPHEN/CAFFEINE

(Esgic capsules 325 mg acetaminophen/40 mg caffeine/50 mg butalbital)

Butalbital has generalized depressant effect on CNS and, in very high doses, has peripheral effects. Acetaminophen has analgesic and antipyretic effects; its analgesic effects may be mediated through inhibition of prostaglandin synthetase enzyme complex. Caffeine is thought to produce constriction of cerebral blood vessels.

The combination is indicated in relief of symptom complex of tension (or muscle contraction) headache.

BUTALBITAL/ACETAMINOPHEN/ CAFFEINE/CODEINE PHOSPHATE

(Fioricet with Codeine Capsules 30 mg codeine phosphate/325 mg acetaminophen/40 mg caffeine/50 mg butalbital)

Butalbital has generalized depressant effect on CNS and, in very high doses, has peripheral effects. Acetaminophen has analgesic and antipyretic effects; its analgesic effects may be mediated through inhibition of prostaglandin synthetase enzyme complex. Caffeine is thought to produce constriction of cerebral blood vessels. Codeine binds to opiate receptors in the CNS, causing inhibition of ascending pain pathways and altering perception of and response to pain. The combination is indicated in relief of symptom complex of tension (or muscle contraction) headache.

BUTALBITAL/ACETAMINOPHEN/CAFFEINE/ CODEINE PHOSPHATE

Butalbital has generalized depressant effect on CNS and, in very high doses, has peripheral effects. Aspirin has analgesic, antipyretic, antiinflammatory, and antirheumatic effects; its analgesic and antiinflammatory effects may be mediated through inhibition of prostaglandin synthetase enzyme complex. Aspirin also irreversibly inhibits platelet aggregation. Caffeine is thought to produce constriction of cerebral blood vessels. The combination is indicated in the relief of symptom complex of tension (or muscle contraction) headache.

BUTENAFINE HYDROCHLORIDE

(Lotrimin Ultra Cream 1%, Mentax Cream 1%)

Butenafine is an antifungal agent that inhibits the biosynthesis of the ergosterol component of fungal cell membranes. It is indicated in the treatment of interdigital tinea pedis (athlete's foot); tinea corporis (ringworm); tinea cruris (jock itch); tinea (pityriasis) versicolor caused by susceptible organisms.

BUTHIONINE SULFOXIMINE

One of the goals of cancer chemotherapy is to enhance the efficacy of antineoplastic agents and, at the same time, protect the nonmalignant tissues using chemoprotective agents. Buthionine sulfoximine is a chemo-enhancing agent.

BUTOCONAZOLE NITRATE

(Femstat)

Butoconazole, a synthetic imidazole derivative with antifungal properties (2% vaginal cream with applicators to be used intravaginally at bedtime for 3 days), is indicated in the treatment of vulvovaginal candidiasis (moniliasis).

BUTOCONAZOLE NITRATE

(Femstat 3 vaginal cream 2%)

Butoconazole is a vaginal antifungal agent that increases cell membrane permeability in susceptible fungi. It is indicated for local treatment of vulvovaginal candidiasis (moniliasis).

BUTORPHANOL TARTRATE

(Stadol)

Butorphanol is a narcotic agonist with analgesic action five times more potent than morphine, and a narcotic antagonist with antagonist action 1/40 that of naloxone. Butorphanol (2 to 3 mg IM) exerts its analgesic action in 10 to 15 minutes, with a peak of action in 30 to 60 minutes, and a duration of action of 3 to 4 hours. Butorphanol is metabolized in the liver to hydroxybutorphanol, which is excreted mainly by the kidneys. Like pentazocine, butorphanol depresses respiration and increases pulmonary artery pressure, pulmonary wedge pressure, left ventricular end diastolic pressure, and systemic arterial pressure. Because it increases cardiac workload, it should be used cautiously in acute myocardial infarction, in ventricular dysfunction, or coronary insufficiency. Like morphine, butorphanol increases the cerebrospinal fluid pressure, and hence should be used cautiously in recent head injury. Naloxone is able to overcome the toxicity of butorphanol.

BUTORPHANOL TARTRATE

(Stadol injection 1 mg/mL [1 mg of tartrate salt is equal to 0.68 mg base], injection 2 mg/mL [1 mg of tartrate salt is equal to 0.68 mg base], nasal spray 10 mg/mL)

Butorphanol is an opioid agonist–antagonist analgesic potent analgesic that stimulates and inhibits opiate receptors in CNS. Antagonist effects decrease (but do not eliminate) abuse potential, and may cause withdrawal symptoms in patients with opiate dependence. It is indicated in the management of pain when use of an opioid analgesic is appropriate (parenteral/nasal); preoperative or preanesthetic medication, as a supplement to balanced anesthesia; and for relief of pain during labor (parenteral).

C

CAFFEINE

(Caffedrine tablets 200 mg)

Caffeine is an analeptic that increases calcium permeability in sarcoplasmic reticulum, inhibiting phosphodiesterase-promoting accumulation of cyclic AMP. It is indicated in fatigue and drowsiness; analgesia; apnea of premature respiratory depression.

Oral caffeine (40 to 150 mg/5 oz. brewed coffee; 100 mg in No-Doz; 150 mg in Quick Pep; and 200 mg in Caffedrine) is used to remain mentally alert, and parenteral caffeine has been used as an analeptic to treat respiratory depression. Caffeine has been used as an orphan drug in neonatal apnea. Caffeine stimulates the central nervous system (CNS) and produces cardiac stimulation, dilation of coronary and peripheral blood vessels, and constriction of cerebral blood vessels. It stimulates the skeletal muscles, enhances the secretion of gastric acid, and has diuretic properties. Caffeine exerts its various pharmacological effects by increasing calcium permeability in sarcoplasmic reticulum, by inhibiting phosphodiesterase, by raising the concentration of cyclic AMP, and by blocking adenosine receptors. Caffeine in adults is metabolized in the liver, but in neonates is excreted unchanged by the kidneys. The half-lives of caffeine in the newborn, 3-month-old infant, and 6-month-old infant are 70 hours, 15 hours, and 3 hours, respectively (see also Figure 23).

Overdosage of caffeine in a nontolerant individual causes insomnia, anxiety, diuresis, restlessness, excitement, nervousness, tinnitus, muscular tremor, headache, and scintillating scotoma.

CALCIFEDIOL

(Calderol)

Calcifediol, a vitamin D analog (300 to 350 mg p.o. weekly), is indicated in the treatment and management of metabolic bone disease associated with chronic renal failure (see also Figure 105).

CALCIPOTRIENE

(Dovonex ointment 0.005%, cream 0.005%, scalp solution 0.005%)

Calcipotriene is an antipsoriatic agent. It is a synthetic vitamin D_3 analog. In a manner similar to vitamin D, calcipotriene regulates skin cell production and development, thereby modifying the abnormal growth and production of keratinocytes, responsible for the scaly red patches characteristic of psoriasis (see Figure 105). **Calcipotriene** is indicated in the treatment of plaque psoriasis. Scalp solution: topical treatment of chronic, moderately severe psoriasis of the scalp.

Calcipotriol (calcipotriene) is a synthetic derivative of calcitriol with a modified side chain that contains a 22 to 23 double bond, a 24(*S*)-hydroxy functional group, and carbons 25 to 27 incorporated into a cyclopropane ring. Calcipotriol has comparable affinity with calcitriol for the vitamin D receptor, but it is less than 1% as active as calcitriol in regulating calcium metabolism. This reduced calcemic activity largely reflects the pharmacokinetics of calcipotriol. Calcipotriol has been studied extensively as a treatment for psoriasis, although its mode of action is not known; a topical preparation (Dovonex) is available for that purpose. In clinical trials, topical calcipotriol has been found to be slightly more effective than glucocorticoids with a good safety profile.

Calcipotriene is applied twice daily to plaque psoriasis on the body. Improvement is detectable within 1 to 2 weeks, and maximum clinical response occurs within 6 to 8 weeks. Most patients show some improvement, but complete resolution occurs in no more than 15%. Maintenance therapy usually is necessary, and tachyphylaxis does not occur. Reports of hypercalcemia with calcipotriene are rare.

CALCITONIN-HUMAN

(Cibacalcin — 0.5 mg SC; Calcitonin-Salmon, Calcimar, Miacalcin, 100 to 200 IUSC)

The thyroid gland synthesizes thyroxine (T_4) and triiodothyronine (T_3), and these hormones are involved in the regulation of growth and development, thermoregulation and calorigenesis, metabolism of carbohydrates, proteins, and lipids, and hypophyseal thyrotropin secretion (see Figure 75).

The thyroid gland also synthesizes calcitonin, which produces hypocalcemia by inhibiting bone resorption and by enhancing the urinary excretion of calcium and phosphate.

Calcitonin, a polypeptide consisting of 32 amino acids, is produced by parafollicular cells (C cells) of the thyroid gland. The secretion of calcitonin is stimulated by calcium, catecholamine, and theophylline (increased cyclic adenosine monophosphate levels), glucagon, cholecystokinin, gastrin, and cerulean.

Calcitonin is indicated for patients with moderate to severe Paget's disease, characterized by abnormal and accelerated bone formation, and for patients with hypercalcemia associated with carcinoma multiple myeloma.

CALCITRIOL

(Rocaltrol)

Calcitriol, a vitamin D analog (0.25 mcg p.o. daily), is indicated in the management of hypocalcemia in patients undergoing chronic dialysis. In addition, calcitriol (0.5 mcg IV 3 times weekly), is used in the management of hypoparathyroidism and pseudohypoparathyroidism (see Figure 105).

CALCIUM-CHANNEL BLOCKERS

Many hormones, neurotransmitters, and autacoids exert their actions by altering phosphoinositide metabolism, increasing the concentration of ionized calcium in the cytosol of their target cells, and stimulating the turnover rate of phosphatidylinositol 4,5-biphosphate (PIP_2).

Under normal conditions, the extracellular concentration of calcium is in the millimolar range (10^{-3} M), whereas its intracellular concentration is less than 10^{-7} M. The cytoplasmic concentration of calcium is increased through the actions of receptor-operated channels, voltage-activated channels, or ionic pumps. In addition, calcium can be released from internal stores (see also Figure 103).

There are two types of voltage-activated channels:

1. Low-voltage-activated channels or low-threshold channels, which are also termed T-type channels.
2. High-voltage-activated channels, which are further subdivided into L-type, N-type, and P-type channels.

T-Type Channels

T-type calcium channels (with the T standing for "transient") require only a weak depolarization for activation and carry a transient current at negative membrane potentials that inactivates rapidly during a prolonged pulse. In neurons, the T-type channel is responsible for neuronal oscillatory activity and is thought to play a role in the regulation of wakefulness and motor coordination. The pyrazine diuretic, amiloride, inhibits the T-type calcium channel.

L-Type Channels

L-type calcium channels (with the L standing for "long lasting") exist in high numbers in the skeletal muscle and require a large depolarization for activation to take place. The channels are phosphorylated prior to opening. Each channel is composed of five subunits: $alpha_1$ (molecular weight [MW] = 175 kDa), $alpha_2$ (MW = 143 kDa), beta (MW = 54 kDa), gamma (MW = 30 kDa), and delta (MW = 27 kDa). The $alpha_1$ and beta subunits contain phosphorylation sites for cyclic adenosine monophosphate (AMP)-dependent protein kinase. The $alpha_1$ subunit contains the dihydropyridine-binding sites. The L-type calcium channel is involved in the generation of action potentials and in signal transduction at the cell membrane.

N-Type Channels

The N-type channel (with the N standing for "neither T nor L or neuronal") appears to convey most of the whole-cell calcium current; it is insensitive to dihydropyridine and is blocked by omega-conotoxin. The N-type channel is involved in the release of transmitter in some, but not all, tissues, with the CNS neurons being the exception.

P-Type Channels

The P-type channels were first observed in the Purkinje cells and are inhibited by a toxin derived from a funnel-web spider poison, but not by other calcium channel-blocking agents. P-type channels are widely distributed throughout the CNS and are thought to participate in the generation of intrinsic activity as well as serving as modulators of neuronal integration and transmitter release.

Calcium-activated potassium channels increase their permeability to potassium ions in response to increases in the intracellular calcium concentration. These potassium channels couple the membrane potential to the intracellular concentration of calcium, in that a rise in the intracellular calcium level leads to an efflux of potassium ions and hence hyperpolarization of the membrane.

The secretion of neurotransmitters and neurohormones is usually triggered by a rise in the intracellular calcium concentration. However, the release of acetylcholine from the Schwann cells and renin from the juxtaglomerular apparatus is triggered by a fall in the intracellular calcium level.

Unlike skeletal muscles, which contain endogenous stores of calcium ions, both cardiac muscle and vascular smooth muscle require extracellular calcium for contractile function. Therefore, cardiac muscle and vascular smooth muscle are subject to regulation by calcium antagonists or calcium entry blockers (Figure 103 and Table 21), which are used in the treatment of hypertension, Raynaud's disease, Prinzmetal's angina, and migraine syndromes.

Calcium enters the cell through voltage-dependent channels mainly during depolarization, and this process is regulated by the cyclic AMP level. Because the cellular content of cyclic AMP depends on a series of enzymatic steps initiated by receptor stimulation and ending with cyclic AMP degradation, an increase in cellular calcium uptake can be achieved by interventions that act at any of these stages. A major mechanism for calcium transport through the sarcolemma in both directions consists of electrogenic sodium–calcium exchange, which depends on the electrochemical gradient for sodium. A reduction in this gradient leads to increased calcium uptake by the exchanger. Therefore, a great variety of agents that promote an increase in the intracellular sodium level produce positive inotropic effects.

CALCIUM-CHANNEL BLOCKERS FOR THE TREATMENT OF HYPERTENSION

Drugs

Amlodipine	Isradipine	Nifedipine
Diltiazem	Lacidipine	Nitrendipine
Felodipine	Nicardipine	Verapamil

All calcium-channel blockers cause vasodilatation, but the cardiac response to the decrease in peripheral resistance is variable. An initial reflex increase in heart rate usually occurs with the dihydropyridines (nifedipine, nicardipine, isradipine, and felodipine); verapamil and diltiazem cause little or no change in heart rate. Verapamil and diltiazem can, however, slow atrioventricular (AV) conduction and should be used with caution in patients also taking a beta-blocker; dihydropyridines generally do not affect AV conduction and can be used with a beta-blocker, which decreases reflex tachycardia. All calcium-channel blockers should be used with caution in patients with heart failure.

CALCIUM-ENTRY BLOCKERS

Calcium-entry blockers include those agents that are selective for slow calcium channels in the myocardium (slow-channel blockers), and consist of the following categories of substances:

Phenylalkylamines—verapamil, gallopamil, anipamil, desmethoxyverapamil, emopamil, falipamil, and ronipamil

Dihydropyridines—nifedipine, nicardipine, niludipine, nimodipine, nisoldipine, nitrendipine, ryosidine, amlodipine, azodipine, dazodipine, felodipine, floridipine, iodipine, isradipine, mesudipine, oxodipine, and riodipine

Benzothiazepines—diltiazem

Agents that have no perceived action on the slow calcium inward current in the myocardium (voltage clamp) consist of the diphenylpiperazines, and include cinnarizine and flunarizine.

There are also nonselective calcium-entry blockers that act at similar concentrations on both calcium channels and fast sodium channels. These agents consist of bencyclane, bepridil, caroverine, etafenone, fendiline, lidoflazine, perhexiline, prenylamine, proadifen, terodiline, and tiapamil.

Those agents that interact with calcium channels but have another primary site of action include: agents acting on sodium channels (local anesthetics and phenytoin), catecholamine receptors (benextramine, nicergoline, phenoxybenzamine, phenothiazines, pimozide, propranolol, and yohimbine derivatives), benzodiazepine receptors (diazepam and flurazepam), opiate receptors (loperamide and fluperamide), and cyclic nucleotide phosphodiesterases (amrinone, cromoglycate, and papaverine), as well as barbiturates, cyproheptadine, indomethacin, and reserpine.

Sodium–calcium exchange inhibitors include amiloride and its derivatives, specifically dantrolene, which acts on the sarcoplasmic reticulum, and ruthenium red, which acts on the mitochondria.

Calmodulin antagonists consist of the phenothiazines (trifluoperazine and chlorpromazine), local anesthetics (dibucaine), and dopamine antagonists (pimozide and haloperidol).

Calcium Entry Blockers and Their Use in Various Disorders

Hypertension

Verapamil, nifedipine, and diltiazem lower blood pressure with an efficacy comparable to that achieved by other commonly used agents. Their specific effects on the cardiovascular system are as follows:

Drugs	Heart Rate	Atrioventricular Nodal Conduction	Myocardial Contractility	Arteriolar Vasodilation
Verapamil	No change	Greatly decreased	Moderately decreased	Moderately increased
Nifedipine	Increased	—	No change	Greatly increased
Diltiazem	Decreased	Moderately decreased	Decreased	Increased

The intravenous administration of diltiazem or verapamil, or the oral or sublingual administration of nifedipine, is effective in managing hypertensive emergencies.

Myocardial Infarction

Heart failure is associated with changes in the intracellular calcium levels. The rationale for using calcium-entry blockers in preventing the secondary complications of myocardial infarction stems from the fact that these agents reduce systemic vascular resistance, afterload, myocardial contractility, blood pressure, and oxygen consumption. However, despite these effects, the efficacy of calcium-entry blockers in preventing the secondary complications of myocardial infarction or their usefulness in the context of cerebrovascular diseases such as aneurysmal subarachnoid hemorrhage needs to be established.

Angina

Beta-adrenergic blocking agents are effective for the prophylactic therapy of exertional angina pectoris by reducing heart rate and the force of myocardial contraction. However, verapamil, nifedipine, and diltiazem are also effective for the prophylactic treatment of stable exertional angina. The combination therapy with beta-blockers and calcium-entry blockers is well tolerated, effective, and safe.

Psychiatric Disorders

Verapamil has also been used in the treatment of mania, depression, maintenance control of manic depression, and schizophrenia. In addition, it has been used in the management of premenstrual syndrome, stuttering, and intoxication with phencyclidine.

Cerebrovascular Disorders

Among the various types of calcium-entry blockers, flunarizine has proved to be the most effective in the prophylaxis of migraine. It has also been shown to be beneficial in protecting brain cells against hypoxia and in preventing the constriction of cerebrovascular smooth-muscle cells. Moreover, it has been shown to be effective in the treatment of epilepsy and hemiplegia.

Parkinson's Disease

Calcium-entry blockers may induce extrapyramidal symptoms and aggravate parkinsonism.

Drug Interactions and Calcium-Entry Blockers

The following are some of the drug interactions seen with either specific calcium-entry blockers or these agents in general:

- Verapamil inhibits several oxidative routes of hepatic metabolism.
- Verapamil and diltiazem decrease the clearance of theophylline and increase its half-life.

- Calcium-channel blockers increase the toxicity of lithium, which has calcium antagonist effects itself.
- Calcium-channel blockers potentiate the negative inotropic effects of type Ia antiarrhythmic agents.
- Verapamil increases the plasma concentration of digitoxin.
- Calcium-entry blockers potentiate the hypotensive effects of prazocin.
- Calcium-entry blockers increase the plasma concentration of carbamazepine.
- Calcium-entry blockers decrease the clearance of cyclosporine.
- Calcium-entry blockers cause impaired myocardial conduction when given with enflurane and precipitate pronounced hypotension when given with halothane.

CALCIUM GLUCONATE

Calcium gluconate is indicated in hypocalcemia associated with neonatal tetany and tetany due to parathyroid difficulty, vitamin D deficiency, or alkalosis; in prevention of tetany during exchange transfusions; and in conditions related to malabsorption.

The concentration of calcium in extracellular fluids is 10^{-3} M, and the concentration of cytoplasmic calcium is 10^{-6} M. The mitochondria and microsomes contain 90 to 99% of the intracellular calcium, which is bound largely to organic and inorganic phosphates. The low cytoplasmic concentration of calcium is maintained by three calcium pump-leak-transport systems. Each pump is oriented in a direction of calcium egress from the cytosol (see also Figure 84).

Calcium functions at both extracellular and cellular sites. Its extracellular functions consist of the maintenance of normal ion products for mineralization; cofactor for prothrombin factors VII, IX, and X; and maintenance of plasma membrane stability and permeability.

Its cellular functions comprise skeletal and cardiac muscle contraction; cellular secretion; exocrine, endocrine, and neurotransmitters, neural excitation and regulation of membrane ion transport; enzyme regulation (gluconeogenesis and glycogenolysis); and cell growth and division.

The symptoms of hypocalcemia are: tetany, paresthesias, laryngospasm, muscle spasms, seizures (usually grand mal), irritability, depression, psychosis, prolonged QT interval, intestinal cramps, and respiratory arrest.

Calcium salts are contraindicated in hypercalcemia, ventricular fibrillation, and in digitalized patients, who may be predisposed to arrhythmias. Inadvertent calcium overloading may be treated by IV infusion of sodium chloride, which competes with calcium for reabsorption in the distal renal tubercle, and by furosemide (see also Figure 17).

CALCIUM POLYCARBOPHIL

(Equalactin, Fiberall, FiberCon, Mitrolan)

Calcium polycarbophil, a hydrophilic agent that absorbs water (1 g p.o. q.i.d.), is used in the treatment of constipation.

CALCIUM PRODUCTS

Preparation	mg Elemental Calcium/Tablet
Calcium Carbonate	
(40% elemental calcium)	
Cal-Sup	300
Caltrate	600
Os-Cal	500
Tums	200
Titralac	168
Generic Calcium Gluconate	58.5
(9% elemental calcium)	
Generic Calcium Lactate	84.5
(13% elemental calcium)	
Generic Dibasic Calcium Phosphate	115
(23% elemental calcium)	

CALCIUM SALTS

CALCIUM ACETATE

(Calcium Acetate Injection, Phos-Ex, Phoslo)

CALCIUM CARBONATE

(Alka-Mints, Amitone, Bio-Cal, Calcilac, Calglycine, Caltrate, Cal-Sup, Chooz, Dicarbosil, Equilet, Gustalac, Os-Cal 500, PAMA No. 1, Suplical, Titracid, Titralac, Tums, Tums E-X)

CALCIUM CHLORIDE

CALCIUM CITRATE

(Citracel)

CALCIUM GLUBIONATE

(Neo-Calglucon)

CALCIUM GLUCEPTATE

CALCIUM GLUCONATE

(Kalcinate)

CALCIUM GLYCEROPHOSPHATE

CALCIUM LACTATE

CALCIUM PHOSPHATE, DIBASIC

CALCIUM PHOSPHATE, TRIBASIC

(Posture)

The calcium salts are used in the emergency treatment of hypocalcemia, in hyperkalemia, in hypermagnesemia, and in hyperphosphatemia in end-stage renal failure. In addition, they are used in prevention of osteoporosis (see also Figure 105).

CALFACTANT

(Infasurf suspension, intratracheal 35 mg phospholipids/mL suspended in 0.9% sodium chloride solution and 0.65 mg proteins; with 26 mg phosphatidylcholine, of which 16 mg is disaturated phosphatidylcholine)

Calfactant is a lung surfactant. It is an extract of natural surfactant from calf lungs that restores lung surfactant in premature infants with lung surfactant deficiency causing respiratory distress syndrome (RDS). Calfactant is indicated in RDS in premature infants under 29 weeks of gestational age at high risk for RDS and for the treatment rescue of premature infants under 72 hours of age who develop RDS and require endotracheal intubation.

CANCER DRUG DISCOVERY AND DEVELOPMENT

The use of drug delivery systems to improve the efficacy of cancer chemotherapy remains an important strategy for achieving progress against this disease. Over the past 20 years, the number of novel therapeutic approaches has expanded from traditional small chemical medicinals to a wide variety of biomolecules, including peptide/protein- and nucleic acid-based therapeutics. All of these therapies require the administration of stable dosage forms in adequate concentrations and exposure periods to realize their potential. For the treatment of many forms of cancer, the presentation and maintenance of adequate drug concentrations to the target disease tissues without overexposure to drug-sensitive normal tissues is the major limitation for successful chemotherapy.

Systemically Administered Drugs

Although the use of drugs in the management of cancer has made a significant impact on the outcome of most types of malignancies, one of the lingering challenges in cancer therapeutics is how to influence the outcome of cancer treatment by optimal and careful application of anticancer drugs. Addressing this challenge requires the adoption of treatment strategies that employ sound pharmacologic principles in the use of anticancer agents.

The majority of drugs used in cancer treatment are administered systemically, orally, or loco-regionally. Of these, only loco-regional delivery presumes restriction of an administered drug to the site or location of the tumor. Thus, because the concentration of the antineoplastic agent at the tumor site is enhanced, systemic exposure is avoided or significantly minimized. Consequently, it is assumed that the therapeutic benefits as well as therapeutic window of the drug are improved upon. However, these assumptions are not always true because the loco-regional delivery of drugs could present unique and/or similar adverse events in comparison to systemically administered antineoplastics. Systemic delivery of cytotoxic anticancer drugs has and will continue to play a crucial role in cancer therapeutics; however, one of the major problems with this form of drug delivery is the exposure of normal tissues/organs to the administered drug. Clearly, any new strategy to enhance systemic delivery of anticancer drugs should be intended to ameliorate this problem.

Regional Administration of Antineoplastic Drugs

Regional antineoplastic drug delivery is not a new concept. Following the initial recognition that cytotoxic alkylating agents could cause shrinkage of tumor masses and a reduction in the quantity of malignant ascites in patients with advanced ovarian cancer, investigators in the 1950s instilled the drugs directly into the peritoneal cavity in an effort to treat the malignancy.

Similarly, intrathecal administration of **methotrexate** in the treatment and prevention of **meningeal leukemia**, intravesical treatment of superficial bladder cancer, and direct administration of drugs into blood vessels feeding a localized cancer, have been evaluated for more than a decade as therapeutic strategies in the management of malignant disease.

Theoretical Analyses and Simulations of Anticancer Drug Delivery

Large amounts of data on tumor cell survival as a function of exposure to anticancer drugs, drug pharmacokinetics, drug distribution in the body, and other aspects of drug delivery and effectiveness are continually being generated. Cancer therapies are becoming increasingly complex, and it is now possible to choose the time schedule of drug delivery, the site of delivery, the size, lipophilicity, release kinetics and other properties of a carrier, and numerous other options. However, it is clearly impossible to perform sufficient animal experiments or clinical trials to determine the optimal choices of all these variables. Even for drugs that have been used for decades, doses and schedules are often based on past experience and medical tradition rather than on rational analysis. These circumstances suggest an increasing need for theoretical models of anticancer drug delivery. Such models can provide a framework for synthesizing and interpreting available experimental data, and a rational basis for optimizing therapies using existing drugs and for guiding development of new drugs.

A synthesis is needed of two main bodies of anticancer drug research: studies on cellular responses to drugs, and studies on how the method of drug administration affects an animal or patient. Improved understanding is needed of the relation between the mode and schedule of therapy and the resulting drug exposure of cancer cells and normal cells that are responsible for limiting toxicities.

Biopolymers for Parenteral Drug Delivery in Cancer Treatment

Traditional chemotherapy treats tumors by systemic treatment via parenteral or oral application, by intratumoral injection, or by interstitial placement of drugs. New drug delivery systems can be used for local delivery to reduce side effects, to improve the bioavailability, or to target specific sites. Most of these specifically designed dosage forms in cancer treatment are based on polymeric materials to control the release of the active agent via dissolution, matrix erosion and degradation, diffusion, or cleavage of prodrugs. Enhanced local drug retention at the tumor site can be achieved by administration of drug-loaded monolithic polymer implants of different shapes, microparticles, or a polymeric gel vehicle. In addition, chemoembolization provides higher local therapeutic concentrations. The expression *chemoembolization* connotes a bipartite anticancer effect through occlusion of the tumor vascular bed via metal coils, ethanol, glues, or paniculate systems coupled with cytotoxic drug administration either via embolization followed by chemotherapy or embolization with microparticulate drug delivery systems.

Hydrogels in Cancer Drug Delivery Systems

Hydrogels have played a vital role in the development of controlled-release drug delivery systems. A hydrogel (also called an aquagel) is a three-dimensional (3-D) network of hydrophilic polymers swollen in water. The 3-D polymer network of a hydrogel is maintained in the form of an elastic solid in the sense that there exists a remembered reference configuration to which the system returns even after being deformed for a very long time. By definition, hydrogels usually contain water of at least 10% of the total weight. The term *hydrogel* implies that the material is already swollen in water. Dried hydrogels (or xerogels) absorb water to swell, and the size of the swollen gel depends on how much water is absorbed. A hydrogel swells for the same reason that an analogous linear polymer dissolves in water to form an ordinary polymer solution. The extent of swelling is usually measured by the swelling ratio, which is the volume (or weight) of the swollen gel divided by the volume (or weight) of the xerogel. If the weight of absorbed water exceeds 95% of the total weight, a hydrogel is often called a superabsorbent. Thus, 20 g of fully swollen superabsorbent will have 1 g or less of polymer network and 19 g or more of water (i.e., the swelling ratio is more than 20). The swelling ratio of many hydrogels can easily reach greater than 100. Despite such a large quantity of water, highly swollen hydrogels still maintain solid forms.

Microparticle Drug Delivery Systems

Tremendous opportunities exist for utilizing advanced drug delivery systems for cancer treatments. One such formulation type that has already begun to fulfill its promise is injectable microenpsulated delivery systems. Biodegradable microspheres containing leutinizing hormone-releasing hormone (LHRH) are already used for treatment of hormone-dependent cancers and precocious puberty. This product is Lupron Depot.

Polyethylene Glycol Conjugation of Protein and Small Molecule Drugs

Prior to the advent of biotechnology, use of protein drugs was largely limited to products isolated from human donor plasma such as serum albumin, immunoglobulin, and clotting factors. Use of these agents requires stringent protocols for collection, purification, and removal of infectious agents such as bacteria, virus, and, more recently, prions. Although for diabetics who require insulin, porcine sources were useful, use of animal or bacterial or other nonhuman-derived proteins was, and continues to be, complicated by the potential formation of antibodies that may rapidly clear the drug from the body or lead to anaphylactoid reactions and "allergic responses."

The ability to clone and express commercially useful quantities of recombinant human proteins in bacterial, insect cell, yeast fermentation systems, or transgenic animals has enabled the development and introduction into the marketplace of otherwise unavailable lifesaving protein drugs. Numerous recombinant human protein and biotechnology products are in clinical trials or pending regulatory agency approval.

In addition to the cloning and expression of "normal or wild-type" human proteins in the aforementioned manner, the design and production of mutant forms of human and other proteins is possible. Such "muteins" include chimeric or "humanized" mouse antibodies and a variety of fragments such as single chains, Fab and Fab_2, fusion proteins, toxins, and enzymes. Human serum albumin fusion proteins are designed to have a more prolonged circulating life than the native protein product. Human growth hormone and α-interferon human serum albumin fusions are being developed by Principia Pharmaceuticals, Inc. (Philadelphia, PA), recently acquired by Human Genome Sciences. Like nonhuman proteins, muteins may elicit an antibody or immune reaction that may or may not be clinically relevant.

With the sequencing of the human genome completed, the accelerated discovery of genes and gene products regulat-ing growth and development, as well as disease, is likely to fuel the identification of novel protein therapeutics and drug targets. For each of the protein drugs seeking development, issues related to optimum circulating life, polyethylene glycol (PEG)ylation might address dosing levels and frequency of administration, as well as safety. However, not all that could are being pursued in this fashion; when and how to apply PEG technology is itself an emerging science.

To understand PEGylation, it is essential to understand what PEG does and does not do vis-à-vis drug performance, as well as its proposed mechanisms of action.

Emulsions as Anticancer Delivery Systems

Anticancer agents are typically hydrophobic and unstable in water, making formulation development a major undertaking. For this reason, emulsion, the semihomogeneous mixture of two immiscible liquids, is an attractive dosage form for anticancer drugs. However, because of processing difficulties, lack of physiologically safe ingredients, and thermodynamic instability of the emulsion system, development of injectable emulsion formulations, particularly those containing anticancer drugs, has not been very successful. However, an intravenous (IV) emulsion containing a water-insoluble and heat-labile anticancer agent, penclomedine, was successfully developed and tested in clinical trials.

Liposomal Drug Delivery Systems for Cancer Therapy

Liposomes are currently one of the most well-studied drug delivery systems used in the treatment of cancer. They are being employed in the treatment of a wide variety of human malignancies. Their large size relative to the gaps in the vasculature of healthy tissues inhibits their uptake by these tissues, thus avoiding certain nonspecific toxicities. However, the "leaky" microvasculature supporting solid tumors allows for the uptake of these large (~ 100 nm) drug carriers and their subsequent interaction with cancer cells, or release of the encapsulated drug specifically near the tumor, where it can diffuse into the tumor in its free form. Liposomes have many other potential advantages over the corresponding free drugs, including favorable pharmacokinetic properties, where encapsulation of a usually rapidly cleared drug results in a considerable increase in the circulation lifetime for the drug. In addition, encapsulation or complexation of a normally labile therapeutic agent, such as DNA, antisense oligonucleotides, or the lactone ring of camptothecins, can protect the agent from premature degradation by enzymes in the plasma or from simple hydrolysis. The result of liposome formulation can thus be a substantial increase in antitumor efficacy when compared to the free drug or standard chemotherapy regimens.

Gliadel®: A New Method for the Treatment of Malignant Brain Tumors

Designing effective therapies for patients with malignant brain tumors represents a major challenge. Despite significant advances in neuroimaging, microsurgery, and radiation therapy, the prognosis of patients harboring malignant gliomas still remains poor. The addition of systemic chemotherapy does not provide significant impact on survival of patients. One of the reasons for such failure is that systemic chemotherapy has several limitations that reduce its effectiveness in fighting the progressive nature of CNS malignancies. First, the blood–brain barrier keeps a large number of chemotherapeutic agents from reaching the brain parenchyma. Second, the amount of drug administered is limited by variable systemic toxicities. Because the goals of chemotherapy for brain tumors should be achieving and sustaining cytotoxic concentrations of drug in the brain with minimal systemic concentrations, local delivery of these agents could result in a more effective treatment. Moreover, the notions that 80% of malignant gliomas recur within 2 cm of the original tumor site, and that extra CNS metastases are exceedingly rare, strengthen the rationale for strategies aimed at controlling local disease.

One approach for intratumoral delivery of chemotherapy is the development of polymer systems capable of sustained release of drugs to be surgically placed at the tumor site. Direct implant of drug-embedded polymers makes it possible to overcome the limitations imposed by the blood–brain barrier and to achieve high local concentrations of anticancer agents while greatly decreasing systemic toxicity. Additionally, polymer-mediated delivery of drugs provides continuous release of active drugs that, systemically, would often have a short half-life. Finally, this technology has opened the door to the testing of new therapeutic agents that, in the past, could not be used because of their systemic toxicity for the treatment of brain tumors.

Intralesional Chemotherapy with Injectable Collagen Gel Formulations

Management of solid tumors continues to be a major challenge in cancer therapy. Two traditional approaches for local disease are surgical excision and radiation therapy, although treatment of metastatic disease requires systemic chemotherapy. Researchers have explored the concept of intratumoral chemotherapy via simple injection of drugs directly into tumors as an additional option along with surgery or radiation to manage locally confined malignant tumors. However, intratumoral injection of aqueous solutions of cytotoxic agents has had only marginal success. The heterogenous blood supply and interstitial pressure in solid tumors can limit drug penetration and dispersion throughout the tumor. Moreover, aqueous drugs are rapidly cleared from the tumor mass. Thus, inclusion of drugs into slow-release systems provides an attractive alternative.

Novel drug systems developed by Matrix Pharmaceutical, Inc. have been specially designed to treat local tumors with the goal of achieving high, sustained, and homogenous intratumoral drug concentrations without the toxicities typically observed with systemically administered agents. The injectable drug systems use a carrier matrix that can be formulated with a variety of hydrophilic drugs. Two examples of this approach for therapy of solid tumors and cutaneous epitheliomas are the cisplatin/epinephrine gel (CDDP/epi) gel and the fluorouracil/epinephrine (5-FU/ epi) gel that have been extensively evaluated experimentally in clinical trials with veterinary and human patients.

Sustained-Release Drug Delivery with DepoFoam

Sustained-release drug delivery systems, which meter out the encapsulated drug aver a long period of time, augment the effectiveness of therapy in several ways. An ideal sustained-release drug delivery system prolongs the half-life of the drug while maintaining the concentration of the released drug in the therapeutic range during the entire duration of drug release. For cell-cycle phase-specific drugs in particular, prolonging the half-life of the administered drug has a profound effect on its efficacy by increasing the area under the "exposure versus time" curve for a given amount of drug at the same time, decreasing toxicity by reducing the high concentration peak of drug that otherwise occurs immediately after injection. Tissue distribution of the drug is often altered, resulting in higher concentrations and greater efficacy at the desired site, and lower exposure and toxicity elsewhere. Sustained-release formulations are an effective tool in cases where patient compliance is a problem. The feasibility of delivering treatment with fewer injections may enable outpatient treatment that can markedly improve the patient's quality of life. There are, of course, economic incentives. For parenteral products that require administration and monitoring by medical personnel, decreasing the number of injections may reduce overall treatment cost. Proprietary sustained-release formulations can extend the economic viability of a compound beyond the termination of its patent life.

Cancer Vaccines

The concept of vaccination is based on the idea that the patient's immune system is able to recognize antigens expressed by the tumor and that activation of the immune system may result in antitumor immunity. Tumor-associated antigens have been identified for a number of tumors such as melanoma and virus-associated tumors. These antigens have renewed the interest and enthusiasm for the development of cancer vaccines, and they provide the basis for antigen-specific vaccines in the form of peptide, protein, or recombinant DNA encoding for such an antigen. At present, the number of relevant tumor-associated antigens against which the patient can be vaccinated is growing, although for the majority of tumors, such tumor-associated antigens are still not identified. Cancer vaccines for these tumors may rely on the use of tumor cells themselves as the source of antigens.

Gene Therapy of Cancer

Our knowledge of the human genome and the technological development of molecular biology have enabled the development of gene therapy. Gene therapy can be defined as the introduction of genetic material into "defective" somatic cells to restore normal function and produce a therapeutic effect. Gene therapy may replace a missing gene, restore a gene function that is altered by mutation, increase the expression of a gene, introduce a new gene, or abrogate the expression of a gene. Somatic gene therapy involves the transfer of genetic material into non-germ-line cells.

Historically, somatic cell gene therapy has been thought of as a treatment and potential cure for classical inherited diseases based on single gene defects. This is in contrast to the multifactorial inherited disorders that involve multiple genes and environmental factors. In patients with single gene disorders such as hemophilia, severe combined immunodeficiency (SCID), cystic fibrosis, and Duchenne's muscular dystrophy, gene replacement therapy involving transfer of the normal gene and continued expression of the normal protein is desired. In dominantly inherited disorders where the presence of an abnormal protein interferes with the function and development of organ or tissue, selective mutation of the mutant gene could result in a therapeutic effect.

Critical requirements in gene therapy are efficient gene transfer techniques and gene expression at appropriate levels for therapy. Gene transfer can be achieved by two methods: direct transfer *in vivo* or *ex vivo*. The *in vitro* gene transfer techniques are currently most widely used for clinical trials because these techniques are generally more efficient. Various gene transfer methods, including the use of defective viruses, are currently under development. Each of these defective viruses has specific advantages and disadvantages.

Diagnosis and Treatment of Human Disease Using Telomerase as a Novel Target

Telomerase has been associated with almost 90% of all malignant human cancers, making it the most prominent molecular marker known to date. Because of its association with malignancy, telomerase is also regarded as a novel diagnostic marker and a specific target for gene therapy or chemotherapy.

Normal human somatic cells have a limited replicative life span in culture, followed by a process known as **cellular senescence** or the **Hayflick limit**. Unique structures at the end of the chromosomes (telomeres) are necessary for chromosomal integrity and overall genomic stability. Vertebrate telomeres are composed of a hexameric sequence (TTAGGG) repeated for many kilobases. Telomeres continuously shorten with successive cell divisions owing to the inability of normal DNA polymerases to replicate the ends of linear molecules. This "end replication problem" occurs on the lagging strand during DNA synthesis, leaving a gap between the final priming event and the end of the chromosome. Without appropriate mechanisms to offset telomere shortening, normal human cells proliferate for a certain number of divisions, or population doublings (PDs), followed by growth arrest or cellular senescence.

The decline in proliferative capacity correlates with progressive telomere shortening in aging cells. This shortening is counterbalanced in specific germ-line cells, stem cells, and most immortal cells through the telomere lengthening activity of telomerase. The ribonucleoprotein, telomerase, provides the necessary enzymatic activity to restore telomere length. Telomerase utilizes its associated RNA component as a template for catalyzing DNA addition at the telomere. It is a reverse transcriptase that restores telomeres by adding G-rich repeats (TTAGGG for vertebrates) to the 3′ single-stranded overhang at the end of the chromosomes. In humans, at least two components of telomerase are required for the synthesis of telomeric DNA: a protein catalytic subunit (hTERT) and an integral RNA template (hTR). hTERT is the limiting component for reconstituting telomerase activity in normal cells. This protein contains multiple reverse transcriptase motifs essential for enzymatic activity that are conserved among similar genes in diverse organisms such as *Saccharomyces cerevisiae* Est2 and *Euplotes aediculatus* pl23. Because most normal cells that undergo senescence experience telomere shortening, telomere attrition has been proposed as a primary cause of cellular aging or senescence.

With the recent FDA approval of **Vitravene**™, the first drug based on antisense technology to be commercialized, the new technology has achieved an important milestone. Although the basic questions have been addressed, there are still many unanswered questions.

Cancer Prevention

Despite significant advances in cancer treatment and early detection, overall cancer incidence has increased, cancer-associated morbidity is considerable, and overall cancer survival has remained relatively flat over the past several decades. However, new technology allowing exploration of **signal transduction pathways**, **identification of cancer-associated genes**, and **imaging of tissue architecture and molecular and cellular function** is increasing our understanding of carcinogenesis and cancer progression. This knowledge is moving the focus of cancer therapeutics, including cancer-prevention treatments, to drugs that take advantage of cellular control mechanisms to selectively suppress cancer progression.

Carcinogenesis is now visualized as a multifocal, multipath process of genetic progression occurring over a long time period and resulting in increasing loss of cellular controls. This process provides promising opportunities for **chemoprevention**, which involves using drugs, biologies, or nutrients to inhibit, delay, or reverse neoplastic progression at any time before the onset of invasive disease. Remarkable progress has been made in developing chemoprevention strategies, started by research on mechanisms of chemopreventive drugs and assays for evaluating these drugs in animal models, and led in the clinic by early studies on prevention of head and neck carcinogenesis.

Progressive disorganization provides a strong rationale for early intervention in carcinogenesis when mutations are fewer, even before tissue-level phenotypic changes are evident. However, the long latency also presents a significant challenge for prevention and treatment of early cancer. That is, cancer incidence reduction studies in subjects at relatively low risk may require thousands of subjects and many years to obtain significant and definitive results. The successful trial of **tamoxifen** as a **chemopreventive for breast cancer** illustrates the vast resources required for a primary prevention study, even when the cohort is well defined and the drug effect is already well characterized. This trial was carried out in women who at a minimum had a relative risk for breast cancer equivalent to a 60-year-old. Six thousand six hundred (6600) treated women and an equivalent number of control subjects were required to achieve a significant treatment effect.

This inherent inefficiency in validating that chemopreventive treatment results in net clinical benefit for the patient has led to intensive research efforts to develop useful biomarkers. These biomarkers include measures of neoplastic progression, drug effect (of pharmacodynamic markers), and markers that measure prognosis as well as predict responses to specific therapy. All these biomarkers have the potential to greatly augment the development of successful chemoprevention therapies, but two specific types of biomarkers will have the most immediate impact on successful chemopreventive drug development—those that measure the risk of developing invasive life-threatening disease, and those whose modulation can "reasonably predict" clinical benefit and, therefore, serve as surrogate end points for later-occurring clinical disease. Thus far, the biomarker that best measures these two phenomena is **intraepithelial neoplasia** (IEN) because it is a near obligate precursor to cancer. As precancer, it is a very good risk marker for cancer development; and as a recognized disease that is being treated, it has been validated as a surrogate end point biomarker.

IEN is a near obligate precursor to cancer. IEN occurs in most epithelial tissue as moderate to severe dysplasia, is on the causal pathway leading from normal tissue to cancer, and is close in progression to cancer (**invasive neoplasia**). Genetic progression with loss of cellular control functions is observed as the phenotype gradually changes from normal histology to early dysplasia, then to increasingly severe IEN, superficial cancers, and finally invasive disease. For example, in the breast, it is estimated that progression from atypical hyperplasia through **ductal carcinoma** *in situ* (DCIS) to adenocarcinoma requires 10 to 20 years or more. **Colorectal adenomas** may form over a period as long as 5 to 20 years, and progression from adenoma to colorectal carcinoma usually requires another 5 to 15 years. **Prostatic intraepithelial neoplasia** (PIN) may develop over approximately 20 years. From PIN to early latent cancer may take 10 or more years, and clinically significant carcinoma may not occur until 3 to 15 years later. Progression is marked in target tissues by the appearance of specific molecular and more general genotypic damage associated with increasingly severe dysplastic histology. In many cases, critical early steps include inactivation of tumor suppressors such as adenomatous polyposis coli (APC) in colon or BRCA in breast cancers, and activation of oncogenes such as *ras* in colon, lung, and pancreatic cancers. The tests for BRCA-1 and BRCA-2 can tell you if you have mutations in either of these two genes that have been connected to the development of breast and ovarian cancer. Most people do not have a BRCA gene mutation.

Progression is also influenced by factors specific to the host tissue's environment, such as the action of hormones and cytokines produced in stroma around the developing epithelial tumor, and changes in tissue structure. IEN shows these changes and provides a suitable target for treatment intervention because of its phenotypic and genotypic similarities and evolutionary proximity to invasive cancer.

The multipath, multifactorial nature of carcinogenesis is predicted by the heterogeneity that can result from processing the human genome. The 30,000 or so human genes contain as many as several hundred thousand allelic variants from single nucleotide gene polymorphisms including splicing variants. These variations are compounded another three- to fivefold by posttranslational protein modifications leading to a multitude ($>10^6$) of protein–protein interactions. Even if only a small fraction of the genome is critical to cancer, the number of possible molecules and interactions involved is enormous. This level of complexity highlights the uncertainties of using isolated molecular and cellular biomarkers to measure carcinogenesis. Moreover, this complexity is heightened by expected intra–intersubject and tissue variations.

Prospects are bright that surrogate end point biomarkers will make cancer chemoprevention studies more efficient and informative; however, hard work and exceptional dedication to sound, standardized methods will be required to assure that the application of these efforts in developing chemopreventive drugs is fruitful. The eventual acceptance of surrogate end point biomarkers may entail more than scientific rationale. Scientific and regulatory policy changes may also be required. It is often observed that candidate surrogate end point biomarkers are expressed at higher incidences than the symptomatic clinical disease that they approximate. Such will always be the case when completely unrelated end points (other causes of death) do not allow carcinogenesis to go to completion. Based on existing disease models, it is likely that all high-grade IEN-carrying confirmed genetic lesions would end in cancer if the host lived long enough. Validation like causality, is a relative term that only becomes absolute when all variables and elements of a process are known and can be studied quantitatively. It is undesirable and short sighted to require any data more rigorous than validation based on probabilistic estimates that are consistent with current medical and regulatory practice. Based on existing knowledge, we can assume that IEN and the earlier biomarkers within IEN are on one or more of the possible causal pathways to carcinogenesis. Because they sometimes precede the cancer end point by several years, there is potential for interference, diversion, a role in other biological processes, etc., that would keep these events from being ideal surrogate end point biomarkers. However, intervention to treat or prevent could be shown to provide clinical benefit, much like lipid-lowering in cardiovascular disease and viral load reduction in AIDS. If interventions show compelling efficacy against surrogate end point biomarkers and can be administered safely to populations at risk, it would seem prudent to formulate scientific and regulatory policy changes allowing the use of these biomarkers in evaluating interventions that would lead to more efficient drug approvals to prevent this dreaded disease.

CANDESARTAN CILEXETIL

(Atacand tablets 4 mg)

Candesartan is an angiotensin II receptor antagonist that antagonizes the angiotensin II effect (vasoconstriction and aldosterone secretion) by blocking the angiotensin II receptor (AT_1 receptor) in vascular smooth muscle and the adrenal gland, producing decreased blood pressure. Candesartan is indicated in the treatment of hypertension.

CANDESARTAN CILEXETIL/ HYDROCHLOROTHIAZIDE

(Atacand HCT tablets 16 mg candesartan, 12.5 mg hydrochlorothiazide, tablets 32 mg candesartan, 12.5 mg hydrochlorothiazide)

Candesartan is an antihypertensive combination. Candesartan: antagonizes the effect of angiotensin II (vasoconstriction and aldosterone secretion) by blocking the angiotensin II receptor (AT receptor) in vascular smooth muscle and the adrenal gland, producing decreased BE. Hydrochlorothiazide (HCTZ): increases chloride, sodium, and water excretion by interfering with transport of sodium ions across renal tubular epithelium.

The importance of angiotensin II in regulating cardiovascular function has led to the development of nonpeptide antagonists of the AT (angiotensin II) receptor for clinical use. **Losartan** (Cozaar), **candesartan** (Atacand), **irbesartan** (Avapro), **valsartan** (Diovan), **telmisartan** (Micardis), and **eprosartan** (Teveten) have been approved for the treatment of hypertension.

Candesartan cilexetil (Atacand): This cilexetil is an inactive ester prodrug that is completely hydrolyzed to the active form, candesartan, during absorption from the gastrointestinal tract. Peak plasma levels are obtained 3 to 4 hours after oral administration, and plasma half-life is about 9 hours. Plasma clearance of candesartan is due to renal elimination (33%) and biliary excretion (67%). Candesartan cilexetil should by administered orally once or twice daily for a total daily dosage of 4 to 32 mg.

CANNABINOID

Delta^9-Tetrahydrocannabinol (delta^9-THC) is considered to be the predominant compound in preparations of *Cannabis sativa* (marijuana, hashish, bhang) responsible for CNS effects in humans. The recognized CNS responses to these preparations include alterations in cognition and memory, euphoria, and sedation. Potential therapeutic applications of cannabis preparations include analgesia, attenuation of the nausea and vomiting of cancer chemotherapy, appetite stimulation, decreased intestinal motility of diarrhea, decreased bronchial constriction of asthma, decreased IOP of glaucoma, antirheumatic and antipyretic actions, and treatment of convulsant disorders.

CANNABINOID

(Nabilone)

Nausea and vomiting are frequent side effects of radiotherapy and cancer chemotherapy. The incidence of this is relatively low for bleomycin, vincristine, and chlorambucil, but is high for the remaining agents. In addition to prochlorperazine and metoclopramide (dopamine-receptor-blocking agents), nabilone (a cannabinoid), batanopride, granisetron, and ondansetron (all serotonin-receptor-blocking agents) have been shown to be effective in ameliorating these symptoms (see also Figure 73).

CANRENOATE POTASSIUM

(Soldactone S)

It is generally assumed that the intracellular content of sodium in vascular smooth muscle is increased in essential hypertension. Although the major role of aldosterone in the regulation of blood pressure is a renal one, it may also be involved in some extrarenal effects responsible for the regulation of body fluid and blood pressure. Recent studies have suggested that vascular walls specifically bind to aldosterone and that aldosterone has a direct vasoconstrictive effect on vascular smooth muscle *in vitro*. Indeed, canrenoate potassium (Soldactone S), an aldosterone antagonist, reduces blood pressure (Figure 24).

CANTHARIDIN

(Cantharone, Verr-Canth)

Cantharidin, a cantharide derivative with keratolytic properties (0.7% solution), is used for removal of ordinary and periungual warts.

CAPECITABINE

(Xeloda tablets 150 mg)

Capecitabine is a pyrimidine analog. It is an oral systemic prodrug that is enzymatically converted to **5-fluorouracil** (5-FU). Healthy and tumor cells metabolize 5-FU to 5-fluoro-2-deoxyuridine monophosphate (FdUMP) and 5-fluorouridine triphosphate (FUTP). These metabolites cause cell injury by two different mechanisms. First, they inhibit the formation of thymidine triphosphate, which is essential for the synthesis of DNA. Second, nuclear transcriptional enzymes can mistakenly incorporate FUTP during the synthesis of RNA. This metabolic error can interfere with RNA processing and protein synthesis. Capecitabine is indicated in the treatment of resistant metastatic breast cancer alone or in combination with **docetaxel**, and colorectal cancer.

A number of 5-PU analogs have reached the clinic. The most important of these is **capecitabine** (N4-pentoxycarbonyl-5'-deoxy-5-fluorocytidine), a drug active against colon and breast cancers. This orally administered agent is converted to 5'-deoxy-5-rruorocytidine by carboxylesterase activity in liver and other normal and malignant tissues. From that point, it is converted to 5'-deoxy-fluorodeoxyuridine by the ubiquitous cytidine deaminase. The final step in its activation occurs when thymidine phosphorylase cleaves off the 5'-deoxy sugar, leaving intracellular 5-PU. Tumors with elevated thymidine phosphorylase activity seem particularly susceptible to this drug.

Capecitabine is approved by the FDA for the treatment of (1) metastatic breast cancer in patients who have not responded to a regimen of **paclitaxel** and an anthracycline antibiotic; (2) metastatic breast cancer when used in combination with **docetaxel** in patients who have had a prior anthracycline-containing regimen; and (3) metastatic colorectal cancer for patients in whom fluoropyrimidine monotherapy is preferred. The recommended dose is 2500 mg/m^2 daily, given orally in two divided doses with food, for 2 weeks followed by a rest period of 1 week. This cycle is then repeated two more times.

Capecitabine causes much the same spectrum of toxicities as 5-FU (diarrhea, myelosuppression), but the hand–foot syndrome occurs more frequently and may require dose reduction or cessation of therapy.

CAPREOMYCIN

(Capastat sulfate powder for injection 1 g)

Capreomycin is an antituberculosis agent that interferes with protein synthesis and is indicated in the treatment of tuberculosis concomitantly with other antituberculous agents. The essential elements of the treatment of mycobacterial disease are to always treat with at least two different drugs to which the organism is susceptible and to treat for sufficient duration to prevent relapse. Drugs used in the treatment of tuberculosis can be divided into two major categories. "First-line" agents combine the greatest level of efficacy with an acceptable degree of toxicity; these include **isoniazid**, **rifampin**, **ethambutol**, **streptomycin**, and **pyrazinamide**. The large majority of patients with tuberculosis can be treated successfully with these drugs. Excellent results for patients with non-drug-resistant tuberculosis can be obtained with a 6-month course of treatment; for the first 2 months, isoniazid, rifampin, ethambutol, and pyrazinamide are given, followed by isoniazid and rifampin for the remaining 4 months. Administration of rifampin in combination with isoniazid for 9 months also is effective therapy for all forms of disease caused by strains of *Mycobacterium tuberculosis* susceptible to both agents. Occasionally, because of microbial resistance, it may be necessary to resort to "second-line" drugs in addition; thus, treatment may be initiated with 5 to 6 drugs. This category of agents includes **moxifloxacin** or **gatifloxacin**, **ethionamide**, **aminosalicylic acid**, **cycloserine**, **amikacin**, **kanamycin**, **capreomycin**, and **linezolid**. In HIV-infected patients receiving protease inhibitors and/or nonnucleoside reverse-transcriptase inhibitors, drug interactions with the rifamycins (rifampin, rifapentine, rifabutin) are an important concern. Directly observed therapy, in which a health care worker actually witnesses the ingestion of medications, improves the outcome of tuberculosis treatment regimens.

CAPSAICIN

(Capsin lotion 0.025%)

Capsaicin is a counterirritant that depletes and prevents reaccumulation of substance P, principal transmitter of pain impulses, from periphery to the CNS. Capsaicin is indicated in temporary relief of pain from rheumatoid arthritis and osteoarthritis; relief of neuralgias (e.g., pain after shingles, diabetic neuropathy). **Capsaicin** is a naturally occurring substance derived from hot chili peppers of the genus *Capsicum*.

Capsaicin interacts with the canilloid receptor (VR1) on sensory afferents. VR1 is a gated cation channel of the TRP family, modulated by a variety of noxious stimuli. Chronic exposure to capsaicin stimulates and desensitizes this channel. Capsaicin also causes local depletion of substance P, an endogenous neuropeptide involved in sensory perception and pain transmission. Capsaicin is available as a 0.025% cream (Zostrix, others) and 0.075% cream (Zostrix HP, others) to be applied three to four times daily. Capsaicin is FDA approved for the treatment of postherpetic neuralgia and painful diabetic neuropathy, although its efficacy in relieving pain is debatable.

CAPTOPRIL

(Monopril)

Captopril, an angiotensin-converting enzyme inhibitor (ACE), is indicated in the management of hypertension by itself or in combination with other antihypertensive medications, in heart failure when the patients have not responded adequately to digitalis, after myocardial infarction associated with left ventricular dysfunction, and in diabetic nephropathy (Figure 25).

In studying the role of the renin-angiotensin system in the development of hypertension, it has become apparent that there are two systems: a tissue and a circulating renin angiotensin. The control of hypertension is focused primarily on the renin-angiotensin system in the cardiovascular center of the brain. ACE is found in the lung, plasma, the brush borders of the proximal renal tubule, the endothelium of vascular beds, the brain, and the testes. Its two most important actions are the inactivation of bradykinin and the conversion of angiotensin I to angiotensin II.

Receptors for angiotensin II are found in the medulla oblongata in neurons involved in the regulation of baroreceptor activity. Because studies in hypertensive patients have indicated that ACE inhibitors reduce sympathetic activity and enhance baroreceptor sensitivity, it is possible that the primary hypotensive mechanism of these agents is mediated through the blockade of angiotensin II formation in the cardiovascular centers of the brain.

The relationship of the renin-angiotensin-aldosterone system to bradykinin and prostaglandin production is shown in Figure 30.

Captopril and other drugs in this class inhibit the converting enzyme peptidyl dipeptidase that hydrolyzes angiotensin I to angiotensin II and inactivates bradykinin, a potent vasodilator (see also Figure 24). Unlike saralasin, captopril has no pressor activity. Thus, the hypotensive activity of captopril probably results from an inhibitory action on the renin-angiotensin system and stimulating action on the kallikrein-kinin system.

Captopril is absorbed rapidly, partly metabolized to disulfide conjugate, and excreted unchanged in the urine. With the exception of fosinopril, all ACE inhibitors are eliminated by the kidneys, and their doses should be reduced in renal insufficiency. Captopril, in high doses and in renal impairment, has caused neutropenia or proteinuria.

Alteration in taste occurs with captopril, but the incidence is less with enalapril and lisinopril.

Nonsteroidal antiinflammatory agents may impair the hypotensive effects of captopril by blocking bradykinin- and prostaglandin-mediated vasodilatation. Triamterene-induced hyperkalemia is enhanced by captopril.

CAPTOPRIL/HYDROCHLOROTHIAZIDE

(Capozide 50/25 tablets 50 mg captopril and 25 mg hydrochlorothiazide)

Captopril: competitively inhibits angiotensin I-converting enzyme, resulting in the prevention of angiotensin I conversion to angiotensin II, a potent vasoconstrictor that also stimulates aldosterone secretion. This action results in a decrease in sodium and fluid retention, increase in diuresis, and a decrease in BP.

Hydrochlorothiazide (HCTZ): increases chloride, sodium, and water excretion by interfering with transport of sodium ions across renal tubular epithelium. The combination is used in the treatment of hypertension.

CARBACHOL

(Miostat)

Carbachol (1 to 2 drops into each eye t.i.d.) is indicated for lowering IOP in the treatment of glaucoma; and for causing miosis during surgery (0.5 mL of 0.01% into the anterior chamber causing miosis in 2 to 5 minutes).

Methacholine, carbachol, and bethanechol are all agents that mimic the effects of stimulation of cholinergic nerves (see also Figure 78).

The two currently used derivatives of acetylcholine are bethanechol (Urecholine chloride) and carbachol (Miostat). Unlike acetylcholine, both agents are resistant to hydrolysis by cholinesterase. Both agents are muscarinic agonists. The nicotinic action of carbachol is greater than that of acetylcholine, whereas bethanechol is devoid of nicotinic action. The cardiovascular actions of acetylcholine are vasodilation and negative chronotropic and inotropic effects. The cardiovascular effects of methacholine are more pronounced than those of acetylcholine, which in turn are greater than those of carbachol or bethanechol. The gastrointestinal effects (increase in tone, amplitude of contractions, and peristalsis) of bethanechol and carbachol are equal but greater than those of acetylcholine. The effects of carbachol and bethanechol on the urinary tract, consisting of ureteral peristalsis, contraction of the detrusor muscle of the urinary bladder, and an increase in voluntary voiding pressure, are equivalent and exceed those produced by acetylcholine.

The miotic effects of carbachol and bethanechol are greater than those of acetylcholine.

Atropine is able to antagonize all cholinergic (muscarinic) effects produced by acetylcholine, methacholine, carbachol, and bethanechol. However, this antagonist is least evident with carbachol (see also Figure 12).

Carbamates

The cholinesterase inhibitors are divided into two categories: organophosphorous compounds (such as parathion, malathion, and tetraethyl pyrophosphate [TEPP]) and the carbamates (such as naphthyl-*N*-methyl carbamate [carbaryl and Sevin]).

The clinical manifestations of acute and severe poisoning from the organophosphorous insecticides include cholinergic crisis (see also Figure 79), resulting from the stimulation of muscarinic cholinergic receptors (bronchoconstriction, salivation, sweating, lacrimation, bradycardia, hypotension, and urinary and fecal incontinence); the stimulation of nicotinic cholinergic receptors (muscular fasciculation); and the CNS effects (with initial restlessness, tremors, ataxia, and convulsions, followed by CNS depression and respiratory and circulatory depression). The treatment of a cholinergic crisis caused by organophosphorous compounds includes the administration of a cholinesterase reactivator such as a pralidoxime (2-PAM) together with atropine (see Figure 72). The poisoning stemming from antidoting with 2-PAM can be avoided in the event of carbaryl toxicity because this agent is a reversible cholinesterase inhibitor.

CARBAMAZEPINE

(Tegretol)

Carbamazepine is as effective as phenobarbital, phenytoin, and primidone in the prevention of generalized tonic–clonic seizures, but is significantly more effective than the others in the treatment of complex partial seizures. Carbamazepine is also used for the management of trigeminal neuralgia and complex partial seizures with temporal lobe symptomatology. Besides its antiepileptic effect, carbamazepine possesses sedative, anticholinergic, antidepressant, muscle relaxant, antiarrhythmic, antidiuretic, and neuromuscular transmission inhibitory actions. Therefore, it has been used in the treatment of the childhood episodic behavior disorder, multiple sclerosis, central diabetes insipidus, and dystonia. Additional clinical trials should clarify the usefulness of carbamazepine in these conditions (see Figure 32).

Carbamazepine is structurally related to phenytoin and to the tricyclic antidepressant, imipramine. The oral bioavailability of carbamazepine, which may depend on a particular pharmaceutical preparation, is 75 to 85%. After absorption, it is bound to plasma proteins to the extent of 60 to 70%. Carbamazepine is metabolized to its 10,11-epoxide and 10,11-dihydroxide derivatives, some of which are

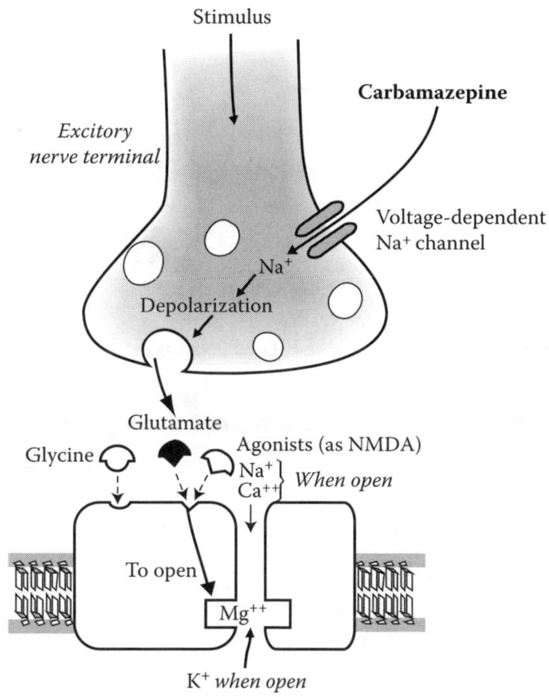

FIGURE 32 Carbamazepine inhibits seizure propagation by reduction of post-tetanic potentiation of synaptic transmission.

excreted unchanged; the other portion is conjugated with glucuronic acid. The 10,11-epoxide derivatives are active anticonvulsants.

Phenobarbital has been shown to decrease serum carbamazepine half-life and plasma concentration levels when given in combination. Significant changes in carbamazepine serum concentrations were seen within 5 days after the addition of phenobarbital to the therapeutic regimen. Conversely, carbamazepine appears to have no effect on serum phenobarbital levels. It has been reported to lower serum concentrations of primidone, but the decrease does not appear to be clinically significant. Other barbiturates (e.g., amobarbital, butabarbital, secobarbital) may interact in a manner similar to phenobarbital because of pharmacologic similarity.

Phenobarbital is thought to induce the metabolism of carbamazepine to its epoxide metabolite. Accordingly, after phenobarbital administration, decreased serum carbamazepine concentrations were accompanied by increased epoxide levels.

The mode and mechanism of carbamazepine action are similar but not identical to those of phenytoin. In high but therapeutic doses, carbamazepine decreases sodium and potassium conductances and depresses post-tetanic potentiation. Furthermore, it increases the taurine level, decreases the glutamic acid concentration, and enhances GABA ergic transmission (see Figure 32).

The most frequent CNS adverse reactions of carbamazepine are dizziness, drowsiness, and unsteadiness. In addition, it is known to have caused confusion, headache,

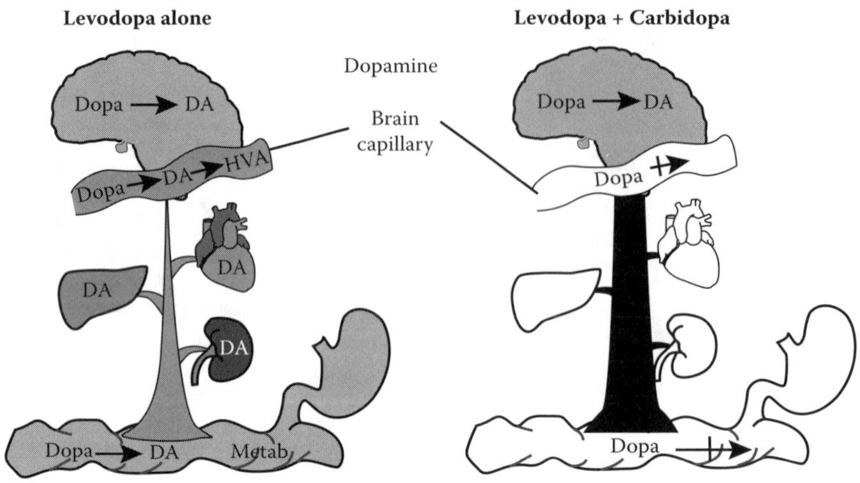

FIGURE 33 Carbidopa substantially decreases the formation of dopamine in the periphery and thus increases its formation in the brain.

fatigue, blurred vision, hallucinations, speech disturbances, abnormal involuntary movements, peripheral neuritis and paresthesias, depression with agitation, talkativeness, tinnitus, and hyperacusis (an abnormally acute sense of hearing or a painful sensitivity to sounds).

CARBENICILLIN INDANYL SODIUM
(Geocillin tablets 382 mg carbenicillin (118 mg indanyl sodium ester))

Carbenicillin is an extended-spectrum penicillin, that inhibits mucopeptide synthesis in bacterial cell wall. It is indicated in the treatment of acute and chronic infections of the upper and lower urinary tract, prostatitis, and asymptomatic bacteriuria caused by susceptible microorganisms.

Carbenicillin is indicated in the treatment of acute and chronic infections of the upper and lower urinary tract and in asymptomatic bacteriuria due to susceptible strains of *Escherichia coli, Proteus mirabilis, Morganella morganii, Providencia rettgeri, P. vulgaris, Pseudomonas, Enterobacter*, and enterococci. It is also indicated in the treatment of prostatitis due to susceptible strains of *E. coli*, enterococcus (*S. faecalis*), *P. mirabilis*, and *Enterobacter* species.

Carbenicillin cures serious infections caused by *Pseudomonas* species and *Proteus* strains resistant to ampicillin. It is not absorbed from the gastrointestinal tract, and therefore must be administered intraperitoneally. Carbenicillin indanyl is acid stable and hence can be given orally. Ticarcillin is four times more potent than carbenicillin in treating a *Pseudomonas aeruginosa* infection, and aziocillin is ten times more potent than carbenicillin against *Pseudomonas*. Mezlocillin and piperacillin are more active against *Klebsiella* infection than carbenicillin.

CARBIDOPA
(with Levodopa as Sinemet)

Carbidopa has no effect when given alone. It is used along with levodopa in the management of Parkinson's disease. When administered orally, levodopa is metabolized substantially in the gut and tissues, and very little penetrates into the brain to be converted to dopamine. The combined administration of levodopa with a peripheral dopa-decarboxylase inhibitor (carbidopa) substantially decreases the formation of dopamine in the periphery and thus increases its formation in the brain where it can work on the corpus striatum (Figure 33).

The pharmacology and advantages of the combined administration of a peripheral dopa-decarboxylase along with levodopa (e.g., Sinemet 10) are as follows: The peripheral dopa-decarboxylase inhibitors such as carbidopa do not penetrate the blood–brain barrier; hence they do not affect the formation of dopamine in the brain. Because the metabolism of levodopa in the periphery is reduced, it can therefore be given in smaller doses, and this lessens its peripheral side effects (hypotension and tachycardia). Once converted to dopamine, levodopa stimulates the chemoreceptor trigger zone for emesis located in the area postrema and causes nausea and vomiting. This side effect is reduced when levodopa is given with carbidopa. Peripheral dopa-decarboxylase inhibitors dramatically reduce the incidence of levodopa-induced tachycardia. In the presence of carbidopa, vitamin B_6 is not contraindicated. Adding vitamin B_6 may even enhance the formation of dopamine in the brain. Peripheral dopa-decarboxylase reduces the onset of the on–off phenomenon.

The appropriate starting dose for dopa-decarboxylase (Sinemet) varies among individuals. Many tolerate very well an initial dose of Sinemet 25/100, one tablet three times daily. However, older individuals, or those taking multiple medications, may tolerate only smaller initial doses, sometimes as low as one-half tablet daily. Because Sinemet 25/100 provides a higher ratio of carbidopa to levodopa and allows quicker attainment of the 75 to 100 mg of carbidopa necessary to sufficiently block the peripheral decarboxylation of levodopa to dopamine, it should be used instead of Sinemet 10/100 when initiating therapy. One can, however, later switch a patient to Sinemet 10/100 to take advantage of its lower cost. Sinemet 25/250 should not be used during the initiation of Sinemet therapy. Sinemet CR 50/200, the controlled-release form, can also be used in the initiation of therapy at an initial dose of one-half or one tablet twice daily.

CARBIDOPA/LEVODOPA/ENTACAPONE

(Stalevo 50 tablets 12.5 mg carbidopa, 50 mg levodopa, 200 mg entacapone)

Carbidopa: inhibits peripheral decarboxylation of levodopa, making more levodopa available for transport to the brain. Levodopa is a precursor of dopamine, which is deficient in parkinsonism patients. Entacapone: inhibits the enzyme that metabolizes levodopa (catechol-*O*-methyltransferase [COMT]), which increases and prolongs levodopa plasma levels. The combination is indicated in the treatment of idiopathic Parkinson disease: (1) to substitute (with equivalent strength of each of the 3 immediate-release components) for the previously administered individual products, (2) to replace immediate-release carbidopa/levodopa therapy (without entacapone) when patients experience signs and symptoms of end-of-dose "wearing-off" (only for patients taking a total daily dose of levodopa of 600 mg or less and not experiencing dyskinesias).

CARBIMAZOLE

Propylthioural, methimazole, and carbimazole exert their effects by inhibiting iodide organification and by inhibiting the formation of DIT (see also Figure 66).

These agents all possess a thiocarbamide moiety:

$$\begin{array}{c} S \\ || \\ (-N-C-R) \end{array}$$

which is essential for their antithyroid actions. The onset of their beneficial effects is slow and takes 3 to 4 weeks.

CARBINOXAMINE MALEATE

(Clistin)

Carbinoxamine compound syrup (Pennex) containing 60 mg pseudoephedrine HCl, 4 mg carbinoxamine maleate, and 15 mg dextromethorphan HBr in 0.2% alcohol is indicated for relief of cough and upper respiratory systems including nasal congestion associated usually with allergy or common cold. Carbinoxamine possesses H_1 antihistaminic activity with mild anticholinergic-sedative properties. Carbinoxamine, which is metabolized completely, has a serum half-life of 10 to 12 hours.

CARBINOXAMINE MALEATE

(Histex CT tablets, timed-release 8 mg)

Carbinoxamine competitively antagonizes histamine at H_1 receptor sites. It is indicated in the symptomatic treatment of nasal and nonnasal seasonal and perennial allergic rhinitis. Palgic tablets also are indicated for vasomotor rhinitis; allergic conjunctivitis caused by inhalant allergens and foods; mild, uncomplicated allergic skin manifestations of urticaria and angioedema; dermatographism; as therapy for anaphylactic reactions adjunctive to epinephrine and other standard measures after the acute manifestations have been controlled.

CARBINOXAMINE MALEATE/ PSEUDOEPHEDRINE HYDROCHLORIDE/ DEXTROMETHORPHAN HBR

(Histex I/E capsule)

Carbinoxamine is an antihistamine/decongestant/antitussive preparation. Carbinoxamine: competitively antagonizes histamine at H_1-receptor sites; pseudoephedrine: causes vasoconstriction and subsequent shrinkage of nasal mucous membranes by alpha-adrenergic stimulation, which promotes nasal drainage; dextromethorphan: suppresses cough by central action on the cough center in the medulla. The combination is indicated in the relief of coughs and upper respiratory tract symptoms, including nasal congestion, associated with allergy or the common cold.

CARBONIC ANHYDRASE INHIBITORS

The carbonic anhydrase inhibitors consist of acetazolamide (Diamox), ethoxzolamide (Cardrase), and dichlorphenamide (Daranide). Acetazolamide is an old agent, whereas ethoxzolamide and dichlorphenamide are newer preparations. Dichlorphenamide is the most potent carbonic anhydrase inhibitor in use today. The presence of SO_2NH_2 (sulfonamide) causes such compounds to inhibit carbonic anhydrase (CA), which catalyzes the hydration of carbon dioxide as follows:

$$CO_2 + H_2O \xrightarrow{CA} H_2CO_3 \rightleftharpoons H^+ + HCO^-_3$$

These agents inhibit carbonic anhydrase in the renal tubular cells in both the proximal and distal tubules. When the rate of hydrogen generation is reduced, HCO_3 is lost in urine and the patient tends to become acidotic. However, the plasma concentration of HCO_3 is lowered and less is filtered, so the diuresis becomes less effective. In addition, the sodium output is increased because its resorption in exchange for hydrogen is limited by the decreased availability of hydrogen. With less hydrogen available, the exchange of sodium for potassium predominates, and this fosters the loss of potassium. Chloride excretion is not altered significantly. Because the aqueous humor has a high concentration of bicarbonate, carbonic anhydrase inhibitors are primarily used in the treatment of glaucoma. They are no longer used as diuretics or as antiepileptic agents (see also Figure 17).

CARBOPLATIN

(Paraplatin lyophilized powder for injection)

Carboplatin is a platinum coordination complex that produces predominantly interstrand DNA cross-links causing equivalent lesions and biological effects. It is indicated as an initial treatment for advanced ovarian carcinoma in combination with other chemotherapy agents; and secondary treatment in palliative treatment of patients with ovarian carcinoma recurrent after prior chemotherapy.

Mechanism of action: Cisplatin, **carboplatin**, and **oxaliplatin** enter cells by diffusion, and by an active Cu^{2+} transporter. Inside the cell, the chloride atoms of cisplatin may be displaced, and the compound may be inactivated directly by reaction with nucleophiles such as thiols. Chloride is replaced by water, yielding a positively charged molecule. In the primary cytotoxic reaction, the aquated species of the drug then reacts with nucleophilic sites on DNA and proteins. Aquation is favored at the low concentrations of chloride inside the cell and in the urine. High concentrations of chloride stabilize the drug, explaining the effectiveness of chloride diuresis in preventing nephrotoxicity (see the following text). Hydrolysis of carboplatin removes the bidentate cyclobutanedicarboxylato group; this activation reaction occurs slowly.

The platinum complexes can react with DNA, forming both intrastrand and interstrand cross-links. The N7 of guanine is a particularly reactive site, leading to platinum cross-links between adjacent guanines on the same DNA strand; guanine-adenine cross-links also readily form, and may be critical to cytotoxicity. The formation of interstrand cross-links is less favored. DNA adducts formed by cisplatin inhibit DNA replication and transcription and lead to breaks and miscoding, and if recognized by p53 and other checkpoint proteins, induction of apoptosis. Although no conclusive association between platinum DNA adduct formation and efficacy has been documented, the ability of patients to form and sustain platinum adducts appears to be an important predictor of clinical response. Preclinical data suggest that the formation of the platinum-adenosine-to-guanosine adduct may be the most critical adduct in terms of cytotoxicity.

The specificity of cisplatin with regard to phases of the cell cycle appears to differ among cell types, although the effects of cross-linking are most pronounced during the S phase. Cisplatin is mutagenic, teratogenic, and carcinogenic. The use of cisplatin- or carboplatin-based chemotherapy for women with ovarian cancer is associated with a fourfold increased risk of developing secondary leukemia.

Because carboplatin is much less reactive than cisplatin, the majority of drug in plasma remains in its parent form, unbound to the proteins. Most drug is eliminated via renal excretion, with a half-life in plasma of about 2 hours. A small fraction of platinum does become irreversibly bound to plasma proteins and disappears slowly, with a half-life of 5 days or more.

Carboplatin is relatively well tolerated clinically, with less nausea, neurotoxicity, ototoxicity, and nephrotoxicity than associated with cisplatin. Instead, the dose-limiting toxicity is myeloppression, primarily evident as thrombocytopenia.

Carboplatin and cisplatin appear to be equally effective in the treatment of suboptimally debulked ovarian cancer, non-small-cell lung cancer, and extensive stage small-cell lung cancer; however, carboplatin may be less effective than cisplatin in germ cell, head and neck, and esophageal cancers. Carboplatin is an effective alternative for responsive tumors in patients unable to tolerate cisplatin because of impaired renal function, refractory nausea, significant hearing impairment, or neuropathy, but doses must be adjusted for renal function. In addition, it may be used in high-dose therapy with bone marrow or peripheral stem-cell rescue. The dose of carboplatin should be adjusted in proportion to the reduction in creatinine clearance for patients with a creatinine clearance below 60 mL/min.

CARBOPLATIN

(Paraplatin)

Carboplatin and cyclophosphamide are indicated in the treatment of advanced ovarian carcinoma. Cisplatin and carboplatin produce predominantly interstrand DNA cross-links rather than DNA-protein cross-links, and the effect is cell-cycle nonspecific. Carboplatin is not bound to plasma proteins, whereas platinum from carboplatin becomes bound to plasma protein and is eliminated slowly with a half-life of 5 days. The major route of elimination of carboplatin is the kidneys, and its doses should be reduced in renal impairment. Furthermore, the coadministration of aminoglycosides increases the chance of nephrotoxicity. Carboplatin causes anemia, neutropenia, leukopenia, and thrombocytopenia requiring transfusions. Cisplatin and, to a lesser extent, carboplatin cause emesis, which requires treatment with antiemetic agents. Alopecia, pain, and asthenia do occur (see also Figure 15).

CARBOPROST TROMETHAMINE

(Hemabate)

Carboprost is used for abortion and in refractory postpartum uterine bleeding. Prostaglandins are mostly used as abortifacients. They may be administered by vaginal suppository (Dinoprostone), which contains prostaglandin E_2; by intramuscular injection (carboprost and tromethamine), which contains 15-methyl prostaglandin F_{2a}; or by intra-amnionic administration (dinoprost and tromethamine), which contains prostaglandin F_{2a}. Other possible uses of prostaglandins may include the treatment of ductus arteriosus (prostaglandin E_1) to maintain patency (see Figure 61), and as a vasodilator. High levels of prostaglandin F_{2a} may cause dysmenorrhea, and substances such as indomethacin and ibuprofen are effective in relieving these symptoms.

CARISOPRODOL

(Soma tablets 350 mg)

Carisoprodol is a centrally acting skeletal muscle relaxant. It is indicated as an adjunctive treatment for acute, painful musculoskeletal conditions (e.g., muscle strain). Carisoprodol (350 mg p.o. t.i.d.) is indicated as an adjunct to physical therapy in acute painful musculoskeletal conditions. It causes muscular relaxation by blocking interneuronal activity in the descending reticular formation and spinal cord. Drowsiness, dizziness, vertigo, and tremor may be managed by dose reduction.

CARISOPRODOL/ASPIRIN/ CODEINE PHOSPHATE

(Soma compound with codeine tablets 200 mg Carisoprodol, 325 mg aspirin, 16 mg codeine)

Carisoprodol is a skeletal muscle relaxant/analgesic/ narcotic analgesic.

Carisoprodol: produces skeletal muscle relaxation, probably as a result of its sedative properties. Aspirin: inhibits prostaglandin synthesis, resulting in analgesia, antiinflammatory activity, and inhibition of platelet aggregation. Codeine: stimulates opiate receptors in the CNS.

This combination is used in addition to rest, physical therapy, and other measures for the relief of pain, muscle spasm, and limited mobility associated with acute, painful musculoskeletal conditions.

The abuse of meprobamate has continued despite a substantial decrease in the clinical use of the drug. **Carisoprodol** (soma), a skeletal muscle relaxant whose active metabolite is meprobamate, also has abuse potential and has become a popular "street drug." Meprobamate is preferred to the benzodiazepines by subjects with a history of drug abuse. After long-term medication, abrupt discontinuation evokes a withdrawal syndrome usually characterized by anxiety, insomnia, tremors, and, frequently, hallucinations; generalized seizures occur in about 10% of cases. The intensity of symptoms depends on the dosage ingested.

CARMUSTINE

(BICNU powder for injection 100 mg)

Carmustine is a nitrosourea that alkylates DNA and also inhibits several enzymes by carbamoylation of amino acids in proteins. Antineoplastic and toxic activities may be caused by its metabolites. Carmustine is indicated in the treatment of brain tumors, multiple myeloma, Hodgkin's and non-Hodgkin's lymphomas; adjunct to surgery and radiation in newly diagnosed high-grade malignant glioma patients; and as an adjunct in recurrent glioblastoma multiforme patients.

The nitrosoureas, which include compounds, such as 1, 3-*bis*-(2-chloroethyl)-l-nitrosourea (**carmustine**; BCNU), l-(2-chloroethyl)-3-cyclohexyl-1-nitrosourea (lomustine; CCNU), and its methyl derivative (**semustine**; methyl-CCNU), as well as the antibiotic **streptozocin** (streptozotocin), exert their cytotoxicity through the spontaneous breakdown to an alkylating intermediate, the 2-chloroethyl diazonium ion (see Figure 15).

Cytotoxic actions: The most important pharmacological actions of the alkylating agents are those that disturb DNA synthesis and cell division. The capacity of these drugs to interfere with DNA integrity and function and to induce cell death in rapidly proliferating tissues provides the basis for their therapeutic and toxic properties. Whereas certain alkylating agents may have damaging effects on tissues with normally low mitotic indices—for example, liver, kidney, and mature lymphocytes—these tissues usually are affected in a delayed time frame. Acute effects are manifest primarily against rapidly proliferating tissues. The lethality of DNA alkylation depends on the recognition of the adduct, the creation of DNA strand breaks by repair enzymes, and an intact apoptotic response. The actual mechanisms of cell death related to DNA alkylation are not yet well characterized.

In nondividing cells, DNA damage activates a checkpoint that depends on the presence of a normal p53 gene. Cells thus blocked in the G_1/S interface either repair DNA alkylation or undergo apoptosis. Malignant cells with mutant or absent p53 fail to suspend cell-cycle progression, do not undergo apoptosis, and exhibit resistance to these drugs.

While DNA is the ultimate target of all alkylating agents, a crucial distinction must be made between the bifunctional agents, in which cytotoxic effects predominate, and the monofunctional methylating agents (procarbazine, temozolomide), which have greater capacity for cross-linking of DNA strands. The latter represent a much greater threat to cellular survival than do other effects such as single-base alkylation and the resulting depurination and chain scission. On the other hand, the more frequent methylation may be bypassed by DNA polymerases, leading to mispairing reactions that permanently modify DNA sequence. These new sequence are transmitted to subsequent generations and may result in mutagenesis or carcinogenesis. Some methyl agents, such as procarbazine, are highly carcinogenic. **Carmustine** and other chloroethylnitrosoureas cause delayed and prolonged suppression of both platelets and granulocytes, reaching a nadir 4 to 6 weeks after drug administration and reversing slowly thereafter.

Both cellular and humoral immunity are suppressed by alkylating agents, which have been used to treat various autoimmune diseases. Immunosuppression is reversible at doses used in most anticancer protocols.

Carmustine is indicated in brain tumors such as glioblastoma, brain stem glioma, medulloblastoma, astrocytoma, ependymoma and metastatic brain tumors; in combination with prednisone in multiple myeloma; and as a secondary therapy in Hodgkin's disease and non-Hodgkin's lymphomas in patients who fail to respond to primary therapy. Carmustine, which does not exhibit cross resistance with other alkylating agents, exerts its antineoplastic effects by alkylating DNA and RNA and by carbamoylating amino acids and inhibiting enzymes. Carmustine crosses the blood–brain barrier readily and is excreted in the urine and in respiratory CO_2. High-dose carmustine causes myelosuppression, progressive azotema and renal failure, pulmonary infiltrates or fibrosis, and retinal hemorrhages. Cimetidine may enhance the carmustine-induced myelosuppression (see also Figure 15).

CAROTENOIDS

Carotenoids are a group of pigments that can be divided into two main classes: carotenes and xanthophylls. Carotenoids are introduced into the human body through dietary intake (mainly from fruits and vegetables and as food additives). Some are nutritionally active as precursors of vitamin A, but only approximately 10% of those identified in nature possess this property.

Aside from the nutritional context, the carotenoids have other important, well-defined functions, such as those related to their antioxidant properties (singlet oxygen quenching and scavenging oxyradicals) and their photoprotective activities, aspects that are now being considered to be of some significance in disease prevention.

CARTEOLOL HYDROCHLORIDE

(Cartrol tablets)

Carteolol is a beta-adrenergic-blocking agent that blocks beta-receptors, primarily affecting the cardiovascular system (e.g., decreases heart rate, cardiac contractility, blood pressure) and lungs (promotes bronchospasm). Ophthalmic use reduces intraocular pressure, probably by decreasing aqueous production. Carteolol is indicated in the management of hypertension; ophthalmic preparation for control of intraocular hypertension and lowering of IOP in chronic open-angle glaucoma. β-Receptor antagonists are very useful in the treatment of chronic open-angle glaucoma. Six drugs currently are available: **carteolol** (Ocupress, others), **betaxolol** (Betaoptic, others), **levobunolol** (Betagan, others), **metipranolol** (Optipranolol, others), **timolol** (Timop-TIC, others), and **levobetaxolol** (Betaxon). Timolol, levobunolol, carteolol, and metipranolol are nonselective, whereas betaxolol and levobetaxolol are selective. None of the agents has significant membrane-stabilizing or intrinsic sympathomimetic activities. Topically administered β-blockers have little or no effect on pupil size or accommodation, and are devoid of blurred vision and night blindness often seen with miotics. These agents decrease the production of aqueous humor, which appears to be the mechanism for their clinical effectiveness.

The drugs generally are administered as eye drops and have an onset in approximately 30 minutes with a duration of 12 to 24 hours. While topically administered β-blockers usually are well tolerated, systemic absorption can lead to adverse cardiovascular and pulmonary effects in susceptible patients. They, therefore, should be used with great caution in glaucoma patients at risk for adverse systemic effects of β-receptor antagonists (e.g., patients with bronchial asthma, or those with bradyarrhythmias).

CARVEDILOL

(Coreg tablets 3.125 mg)

Carvedilol is an alpha-adrenergic-blocking agent/Beta-adrenergic-blocking agent that is indicated in the management of essential hypertension; treatment of mild to severe heart failure of ischemic or cardiomyopathic origin. It reduces cardiovascular mortality in clinically stable patients who have survived the acute phase of MI and have a left ventricular ejection fraction of 40% or less.

Carvedilol (25 to 50 mg b.i.d.) is indicated in the treatment of hypertension. It is a nonselective competitive beta- and beta$_2$-adrenergic-blocking agent, with no intrinsic sympathomimetic activity but with a membrane-stabilizing action. Carvedilol lowers blood pressure by diversified mechanisms that include beta-blockade, alpha$_1$-blockade, calcium-channel blockade, and direct vasodilating effects resembling those produced by nitrates or prostaglandins. It is a lipid-soluble substance, crosses the blood–brain barrier, and produces some of the side effects seen with other beta-adrenergic-receptor-blocking agents.

Carvedilol is a third-generation FT receptor antagonist that has a unique pharmacological profile. It blocks β_1, β_2, and α_1 receptors similarly to labetalol, but also has antioxidant and antiproliferative effects. It is thought that the additional properties (e.g., antioxidant and antiproliferative effects) contribute to the beneficial effects seen in treating congestive heart failure. Carvedilol does not increase β-receptor density and is not associated with high levels of inverse agonist activity.

CASCARA SAGRADA

(Aromatic fluid extract, Cascara Sagrada fluid extract)

Cascara sagrada, an anthraquinone glycoside mixture (325 mg p.o. h.s., 1 mL fluid extract daily; or 5 mL aromatic fluid extract daily), is used in acute constipation and preparation for bowel or rectal examination.

CASPOFUNGIN ACETATE

(Cancidas powder for injection)

Caspofungin is an echinocandins/antifungal agent that inhibits synthesis of β-(1,3)-D-glucan, an integral component of fungal cell wall.

Caspofungin is indicated in the treatment of invasive aspergillosis in patients refractory to, or intolerant of, other antifungal therapies; empirical treatment for presumed fungal infections in febrile, neutropenic patients; treatment of esophageal candidiasis; treatment of candidemia and the following *Candida* infections: intra-abdominal abscesses, peritonitis, and pleural space infections.

Caspofungin has been remarkably well tolerated, with the exception of phlebitis at the infusion site. Histamine-like effects have been reported with rapid infusions. Other symptoms have been equivalent to those observed in patients receiving fluconazole in the comparator arm.

CASTOR OIL

(Alphamul, Emulsoil, Neoloid, Purge)

Castor oil, a glyceride *Ricinus communis* derivative with stimulant laxative properties (15 to 60 mL p.o.), is used for preparation for rectal or bowel examination or surgery.

Castor Oil (Apothecon, Purepac)

Irritant agents used in the treatment of constipation include cascara sagrada, castor oil, senna, rhubarb, phenolphthalein, and acetphenolisatin. Phenolphthalein is a constituent of many over-the-counter preparations, including Ex-Lax and Feen-A-Mint. Most of these agents, with the exception of castor oil, are slow in their onset of action (24 hours).

Phenolphthalein is thought to exert its effect by inhibiting the movement of water from the colon into the blood and by stimulating mucous secretion. If misused on a prolonged basis, a consequential loss of mucus may lower the plasma protein level. Castor oil is hydrolyzed to ricinoleic acid, the active cathartic. It has an onset of action of 2 to 6 hours.

The misuse of any of these agents has been shown to cause hypokalemia, dehydration, and a cathartic colon (resembling ulcerative colitis). Phenolphthalein-containing products may color alkaline urine red.

CATECHOLAMINE

Dopamine, norepinephrine, and epinephrine are classified as catecholamines and are synthesized according to the scheme depicted in Figure 37.

Tyrosine is converted to dopa by the rate-limiting enzyme, tyrosine hydroxylase, which requires tetrahydrobiopterin and is inhibited by alpha-methyltyrosine. Dopa is decarboxylated to dopamine by L-aromatic amino acid decarboxylase, which requires pyridoxal phosphate (vitamin B_6) as a coenzyme. Carbidopa, which is used with L-dopa in the treatment of parkinsonism, inhibits this enzyme (see Figure 37). Dopamine is converted to norepinephrine by dopamine beta-hydroxylase, which requires ascorbic acid (vitamin C), and is inhibited by diethyldithiocarbamate. Norepinephrine is converted to epinephrine by phenylethanolamine *N*-methyltransferase (PNMT), requiring *S*-adenosylmethionine. The activity of PNMT is stimulated by corticosteroids.

The catecholamine-synthesizing enzymes are not only able to synthesize dopamine and norepinephrine from a physiologically occurring substrate such as L-dopa, but also from exogenous substrates such as alpha-methyldopa, which is converted to alpha-methyldopamine and in turn to alpha-methylnorepinephrine. Alpha-methyldopamine and alpha-methyl-norepinephrine are called false transmitters and, in general (except for alpha-methylnorepinephrine), are weaker agonists. Alpha-methyldopa is used in the management of hypertension.

In addition to being synthesized in the peripheral nervous system, dopamine is also synthesized in the corpus striatum and in the mesocortical, mesolimbic, and tuberoinfundibular systems. Norepinephrine is synthesized and stored primarily in sympathetic noradrenergic nerve terminals, as well as in the brain and the adrenal medulla. Epinephrine is synthesized and stored primarily in the adrenal medulla, and, to a certain extent, in the hypothalamic nuclei.

In sympathetic nerve terminals, as well as the brain, the adrenal medulla, and sympathetic postganglionic terminals, there are osmophilic granules (synaptic vesicles) that are capable of storing high concentrations of catecholamine (a complex with adenosine triphosphate [ATP] and protein). The stored amines are not metabolized by the intersynaptosomal mitochondrial enzyme (monoamine oxidase).

Besides releasing norepinephrine (through exocytosis), the stimulation of sympathetic neurons also releases ATP, storage protein, and dopamine beta-hydroxylase. The released norepinephrine interacts with receptor sites located postsynaptically (alpha$_1$) to produce the desired effects.

The action of norepinephrine is terminated by reuptake mechanisms, two of which have been identified: Uptake 1 is located in the presynaptic membrane, requires energy for the transport, is sodium and temperature dependent, and is inhibited by ouabain (a cardiac glycoside), cocaine (a local anesthetic), and imipramine (an antidepressant). Uptake 2 is located extraneuronally in various smooth muscles and glands, requires energy, and is temperature dependent. Approximately 20% of the amine is either taken up by the Uptake 2 mechanism or is metabolized. There are two enzymes capable of metabolizing catecholamines. The first is monoamine oxidase (MAO), a mitochondrial enzyme that oxidatively deaminates catecholamines, tyramine, serotonin, and histamine. MAO is further subclassified as either monoamine oxidase A, which metabolizes norepinephrine and is inhibited by tranylcypromine, and monoamine oxidase B, which metabolizes dopamine and is inhibited by L-deprenyl (selegiline, see Figure 88). Catechol-*O*-methyltransferase (COMT), a soluble enzyme present mainly in the liver and kidney, is also found in postsynaptic neuronal elements. About 15% of norepinephrine is metabolized postsynaptically by COMT (see also Figure 37).

CATHARTICS

Constipation may be defined as the passage of excessively dry stools, infrequent stools, or stools of insufficient size. Constipation is a symptom and not a disease. It may be of brief duration (e.g., when one's living habits or diet changes abruptly) or it may be a lifelong problem, as occurs in congenital aganglionosis of the colon (Hirschsprung's disease). The causes of constipation are multiple and include the following:

- Functional causes
  - Fiber-deficient diets
  - Variants of irritable bowel syndrome
  - Debilitation and extreme old age
- Colonic diseases
  - Chronic obstructive lesions (e.g., tumors or strictures)
  - Ulcerative colitis
  - Collagen vascular diseases
- Rectal diseases
  - Stricture (e.g., ulcerative colitis)
  - Painful conditions (fissure or abcess)

- Neurologic diseases
  - Hirschsprung's disease
  - Spinal cord injuries and disease
  - Parkinson's disease
  - Cerebral tumors and cerebrovascular disease
- Metabolic diseases
  - Porphyria
  - Hypothyroidism
  - Hypercalcemia
  - Pheochromocytoma
  - Uremia
- Use of the following drugs may also lead to constipation:
  - Anticholinergic drugs contained in many over-the-counter medications
  - Antiparkinsonian drugs possessing anticholinergic properties (e.g., trihexyphenidyl and ethopropazine)
  - Antihistaminic drugs with anticholinergic properties (e.g., diphenhydramine)
  - Neuroleptics with anticholinergic properties (e.g., thioridazine)
  - Antidepressants with anticholinergic properties (e.g., amitriptyline)
  - Anticonvulsants with anticholinergic properties (e.g., carbamazepine)
  - Analgesics (e.g., morphine, codeine, and diphenoxylate)
  - Ganglionic blocking agents (e.g., mecamylamine hydrochloride and pempidine)
  - Antacids (calcium- or aluminum-containing compounds)

Laxatives and Cathartics

Although used interchangeably, the terms laxative and cathartic do have slightly different meanings. A laxative effect refers to the excretion of a soft, formed stool; catharsis implies a more fluid and complete evacuation.

Irritants

Irritant agents used in the treatment of constipation include cascara sagrada, castor oil, senna, rhubarb, phenolphthalein, and acetphenolisatin. Phenolphthalein is a constituent of many over-the-counter preparations, including Ex-Lax and Feen-A-Mint. Most of these agents, with the exception of castor oil, are slow in their onset of action (24 hours).

Phenolphthalein is thought to exert its effect by inhibiting the movement of water and sodium from the colon into the blood and by stimulating mucus secretion. If misused on a prolonged basis, a consequential loss of mucus may lower the plasma protein level. Castor oil is hydrolyzed to ricinoleic acid, the active cathartic. It has an onset of action of 2 to 6 hours.

The misuse of any of these agents has been shown to cause hypokalemia, dehydration, and a cathartic colon (resembling ulcerative colitis). Phenolphthalein-containing products may color alkaline urine red.

Bulk Saline Laxatives

Bulk saline laxatives fall into two categories: inorganic salts (magnesium sulfate, magnesium citrate, milk of magnesia, sodium sulfate, and sodium phosphate), and organic hydrophilic colloids (methylcellulose, carboxymethylcellulose [Metamucil], plantago seed, agar, psyllium, bran, and fruits). They exert their effects by absorbing and retaining water, increasing bulk, stimulating colonic peristaltic movements, and lubricating and hydrating the desiccated fecal materials.

Saline laxatives are more effective when administered with water. The onset of action of organic salts is relatively fast (2 to 6 hours), and that of colloids is relatively slow (1 to 3 days). These agents, which are very effective and safe, should not be used when the intestinal lumen has been narrowed. The prolonged use of saline cathartics may create problems for certain individuals. For example, magnesium salts have been known to cause hypermagnesemia, coma, and death in patients with renal insufficiency. Sodium salts may also be responsible for causing congestive heart failure.

Lubricants

Lubricants consist of mineral oil and dioctyl sodium sulfonsuccinate (Colace). Colace is used in the pharmaceutical industry as an emulsifying and dispersing substance. Both agents are taken orally. These agents, which do not influence peristalsis, soften desiccated stools or delay the desiccation of fecal materials. They are especially useful in patients with painful bowel movements resulting from inspissated stools or inflammation of the anal sphincter such as occurs with hemorrhoids or anal fissures. Colace is also useful for patients in whom the consequences of "straining at stool" may be harmful.

When used for a long time, mineral oil may come to interfere with the absorption of fat-soluble vitamins and other essential nutrients. Lipid pneumonitis may evolve if mineral oil is used as a vehicle for drugs that are taken nasally.

Other Uses of Laxatives

In Poisoning

Laxatives are used to hasten the elimination and reduce the absorption of a poison that has been taken.

Antihelmintics

Laxatives are used before and after treatment with antihelmintic drugs.

Radiology

Laxatives are used to clean the gastrointestinal tract before radiographic techniques are performed.

CEFACLOR

(Ceclor powder for oral suspension)

Cefaclor is a cephalosporin/antibiotic which inhibits mucopeptide synthesis in bacterial cell wall. It is indicated in the treatment of infections of respiratory tract, urinary tract, skin and skin structures; treatment of otitis media caused by susceptible strains of specific microorganisms. Second-generation cephalosporins have a broader spectrum than do the first-generation agents, and are active against *Enterobacter* spp., indole-positive *Proteus* spp., and *Klebsiella* spp.

Cefoxitin is a cephamycin produced by *Streptomyces lactamdurans*. It is resistant to some β-lactamases produced by Gram-negative rods. This antibiotic is less active than the first-generation cephalosporins against Gram-positive bacteria. Cefoxitin is more active than other first- or second-generation agents (except cefotetan) against anaerobes, especially *B. fragilis*. After an intramuscular dose of 1 g, concentrations in plasma are about 22 /μg/mL. The half-life is approximately 40 minutes. Cefoxitin's special role seems to be for treatment of certain anaerobic and mixed aerobic–anaerobic infections, such as pelvic inflammatory disease and lung abscess.

Cefaclor is used orally. The concentration in plasma after oral administration is about 50% of that achieved after an equivalent oral dose of cephalexin. However, cefaclor is more active against *H. influenzae* and *Moraxella catarrhalis*, although some β-lactamase-producing strains of these organisms may be resistant.

CEFADROXIL MONOHYDRATE

(Duricef, Ultracef)

Cefadroxil, a first-generation cephalosporin antibiotic (500 to 2 g p.o. daily), is indicated in urinary tract, skin, and soft-tissue infections caused by susceptible organisms.

CEFAMANDOLE NAFATE

(Mandol)

Cefamandole, a second-generation cephalosporin antibiotic (500 mg to 1 g q. 4 to 8 hours), is indicated in the treatment of serious respiratory, genitourinary, skin and soft-tissue, and bone and joint infections; in septicemia; and in peritonitis from susceptible organisms.

CEFAZOLIN SODIUM

(Ancef, Ketzol, Zolicef)

Cefazolin, a first-generation cephalosporin antibiotic (250 mg IM or IV q. 8 hours), is indicated in the treatment of serious respiratory, genitourinary, skin and soft-tissue, and bone and joint infections; and septicemia and endocarditis from susceptible organisms.

CEFDITOREN

Cefditoren is a new cephalosporin available for oral administration as the pivaloyloxy methyl ester, which is known to possess a broad spectrum of antibacterial activity.

CEFEPINE

Cefepine, the last generation of the first enhanced-potency broad-spectrum cephalosporins, possesses enhanced activity compared with other cephalosporins, and this may result from its improved penetration into the Gram-negative cell and the lower affinity of beta-lactamase for the drug.

CEFIXIME

(Suprax)

Cefixime, a third-generation cephalosporin antibiotic (400 mg p.o. daily in 1 to 2 doses), is indicated in the treatment of otitis media, acute bronchitis, acute exacerbations of chronic bronchitis, pharyngitis, and tonsillitis.

CEFMETAZOLE SODIUM

(Zefazone)

Cefmetazole, a second-generation cephalosporin antibiotic (1 to 8 g IV total dose divided q. 6 to 12 hours), is indicated in the treatment of serious respiratory, urinary, skin and soft-tissue, abdominal, and pelvic infections caused by susceptible organisms. It is also used as surgical prophylaxis.

CEFONICID SODIUM

(Monocid)

Cefonicid, a second-generation cephalosporin antibiotic (1 gm IV or IM q. 24 hours), is indicated in the treatment of serious lower respiratory, urinary tract, skin, and skin-structure infections; in septicemia; and in bone and joint infections from susceptible organisms.

CEFOPERAZONE SODIUM

(Cefobid)

Cefoperazone, a third-generation cephalosporin antibiotic (1 to 2 g q. 12 hours IM or IV), is indicated in the treatment of serious respiratory tract, intra-abdominal, gynecologic, and skin infections; in bacteremia; and in septicemia caused by susceptible organisms.

CEFOTAXIME SODIUM

(Claforan)

Cefotaxime, a third-generation cephalosporin antibiotic (1 g IV or IM q. 6 to 8 hours), is indicated in the treatment of serious lower respiratory, urinary, CNS, gynecologic, and skin infections; in bacteremia; and in septicemia caused by susceptible organisms.

CEFOTETAN DISODIUM

(Cefotan)

Cefotetan, a second-generation cephalosporin antibiotic (1 to 2 g IV or IM q. 12 hours), is indicated in the treatment of serious urinary, lower respiratory, gynecologic, skin, intra-abdominal, and bone and joint infections caused by susceptible organisms.

CEFOXITIN SODIUM

(Mefoxin)

Cefoxitin, a second-generation cephalosporin antibiotic (1 to 2 g q. 6 to 8 hours), is indicated in the treatment of serious respiratory, genitourinary, skin, soft-tissue, bone and joint, blood, and intra-abdominal infections caused by susceptible organisms.

CEFPODOXIME PROXETIL

(Vantin)

Cefpodoxime, a second-generation cephalosporin antibiotic (100 to 400 mg p.o. q. 12 hours for 7 to 14 days depending on infections), is used in the treatment of acute, community-acquired pneumonia caused by non-beta-lactamase-producing strains of *Haemophilus influenzae* or *Streptococcus pneumoniae*; in acute bacterial exacerbations of chronic bronchitis caused by non-beta-lactamase-producing strains of *H. influenzae, S. pneumoniae*, or *Moraxella catarrhalis*; in uncomplicated gonorrhea in men and women; rectal gonococcal infections in women; uncomplicated skin and skin-structure infections caused by *Staphylococcus aureus* or *Streptococcus pyogenes*; in acute otitis media caused by *S. pneumoniae*, *H. influenzae*, or *M. catarrhalis*; pharyngitis or tonsillitis caused by *Streptococcus pyogenes*; and in uncomplicated urinary tract infections caused by *Escherichia coli, Klebsiella pneumoniae, Proteus mirabilis*, or *Staphylococcus saprophyticus*.

CEFPROZIL

(Cefzil)

Cefprozil, a second-generation cephalosporin antibiotic, is indicated in the treatment of pharyngitis or tonsillitis caused by *S. pyogenes*; otitis media caused by *S. pneumoniae, H. influenzae*, and *M.(Branhamella) catarrhalis*; in secondary bacterial infections of acute bronchitis and acute bacterial exacerbation of chronic bronchitis caused by *S. pneumoniae, H. influenzae*, and *M. (B.) catarrhalis*; and in uncomplicated skin and skin-structure infections caused by *Staphylococcus aureus* and *S. pyogenes*.

CEFTAZIDIME

(Fortaz, Tazicef, Tazidime)

Ceftazidime, a third-generation cephalosporin antibiotic (1 g IV or IM q. 8 to 12 hours), is indicated in the treatment of bacteremia, septicemia, and serious respiratory, urinary, gynecologic, intra-abdominal, CNS, and skin infections from susceptible organisms.

CEFTIZOXIME SODIUM

(Cetizox)

Ceftizoxime, a third-generation cephalosporin antibiotic (1 to 2 g IV or IM q. 8 to 12 hours), is indicated in the treatment of bacteremia, septicemia, meningitis, and serious respiratory, urinary, gynecologic, intra-abdominal, bone and joint, and skin infections from susceptible organisms.

CEFTRIAXONE SODIUM

(Rocephin)

Ceftriaxone, a third-generation cephalosporin antibiotic (1 to 2 g IM or IV once daily), is indicated in the treatment of bacteremia, septicemia, and serious respiratory, urinary, gynecologic, intra-abdominal, and skin infections from susceptible organisms.

CEFUROXIME AXETIL

(Ceftin)

CEFUROXIME SODIUM

(Kefurox, Zinacef)

Cefuroxime, a second-generation cephalosporin antibiotic (750 mg to 1.5 g IM or IV q. 8 hours), is indicated in the treatment of serious lower respiratory, urinary tract, skin and skin-structure infections; in septicemia; and in meningitis caused by susceptible organisms.

CELECOXIB

(Celebrex capsules 100 mg)

Celecoxib is a selective COX-2 inhibitor/GI agent that reduces inflammation (e.g., pain, redness, swelling, heat), fever, and pain by inhibiting chemicals in the body that cause inflammation, fever, and pain. This is probably caused by the inhibition of prostaglandin synthesis, primarily via inhibition of cyclooxygenase-2 (COX-2) isoenzyme. Celecoxib is indicated in relief of symptoms of osteoarthritis; relief of symptoms of rheumatoid arthritis in adults; management of acute pain in adults; treatment of primary dysmenorrhea; and reduction of the number of adenomatous colorectal polyps in familial adenomatous polyposis (FAP), as an adjunct to usual care (e.g., endoscopic surveillance, surgery).

Three members of the initial class of COX-2 inhibitors, coxibs, were approved for use in the United States and Europe. Both **rofecoxib** and **valdecoxib** have now been withdrawn from the market in view of their adverse event profiles. Two others, **parecoxib** and **etoricoxib**, are approved in Europe but still under consideration in the United States. The newest drug in the class, **lumiracoxib**, is under consideration for approval in Europe and the United States. The relative degree of selectivity for COX-2 inhibition is lumiracoxib = etoricoxib > valdecoxib = rofecoxib » celecoxib. However, there is considerable difference in response to the coxibs among individuals, and it is not known how the degree of selectivity may relate to either efficacy or adverse effect profile, although it seems likely to be related to both. No controlled clinical trials comparing outcomes among the coxibs have been performed.

The bioavailability of oral celecoxib is not known, but peak plasma levels occur at 2 to 4 hours postdose. Celecoxib is bound extensively to plasma proteins. Little drug is excreted unchanged; most is excreted as carboxylic acid and glucuronide metabolites in the urine and feces. The elimination half-life is approximately 11 hours. The drug commonly is given once or twice per day during chronic treatment. Renal insufficiency is associated with a modest, clinically insignificant decrease in plasma concentration. Celecoxib has not been studied in patients with severe renal insufficiency. Plasma concentrations are increased by approximately 40% and 180% in patients with mild and moderate hepatic impairment, respectively, and dosages should be reduced by at least 50% in patients with moderate hepatic impairment. Significant interactions occur with fluconazole and lithium, but not with ketoconazole or methotrexate. Celecoxib is metabolized predominantly by cytochrome P450 P2C9 (CYP2C9). Although not a substrate, celecoxib also is an inhibitor of CYP2D6. Clinical vigilance is necessary during coadministration of drugs that are known to inhibit CYP2C9 and drugs that are metabolized by CYP2D6.

CELIPROLOL

Celiprolol is a potent beta$_1$-adrenergic receptor antagonist. It has intrinsic sympathomimetic action, possesses some alpha$_2$-adrenoreceptor antagonistic properties, is a direct vasodilator, and a direct bronchodilator. Celiprolol is incompletely and variably absorbed, eliminated both in bile and urine, and has a half-life of 4 to 5 hours. Celiprolol (200 to 400 mg/day) has efficacy similar to atenolol or propranolol in reducing blood pressure and is useful in hypertensive patients with asthma or bronchitis. Furthermore, celiprolol is as effective as atenolol in treating patients with stable angina.

CELL THERAPY, STEM CELLS, AND BRAIN REPAIR

As our world continues to evolve, the field of regenerative medicine follows suit. Although many modern-day therapies focus on synthetic and natural medicinal treatments for brain repair, many of these treatments and prescriptions lack adequate results or only have the ability to slow the progression of neurological disease or injury.

Cell therapy, however, remains the most compelling treatment for neurodegenerative diseases, disorders, and injuries, including **Parkinson's disease**, **Huntington's disease**, **traumatic brain injury**, and **stroke**.

Cell therapy is also unique in that it is the only therapeutic strategy that strives to replace lost, damaged, or dysfunctional cells with healthy ones. This repair and replacement may be due to an administration of exogenous cells themselves or the activation of the body's own endogenous reparative cells by a trophic, immune, or inflammatory response to cell transplantation. However, the precise mechanism of how cell therapy works remains elusive and is continuing to be investigated in terms of molecular and cellular responses, in particular. During the past 20 years, most investigations have utilized cells derived from fetal tissue as a source of transplantable cells for cell therapy, which have demonstrated an underlying proof of principle for current cell transplants for a treatment of a variety of neurological diseases and injuries, including **Huntington's disease**.

Stem cells have emerged as the leading topic regarding cell therapy. According to the National Institutes of Health, "a stem cell is a cell that has the ability to divide (self replicate) for indefinite periods–often throughout the life of the organism. Under the right conditions, or given the right signals, stem cells can give rise (differentiate) to the many different cell types that make up the organism. That is, stem cells have the potential to develop into mature cells that have characteristic shapes and specialized functions, such as heart cells, skin cells, or nerve cells."

Previous studies in fetal tissue also contributed a great deal to the discovery of **neural stem cells**. Neural stem cells are derived from fetal and adult brain, and have the ability to divide and give rise to more stem cells or to several types of precursor cells, which can then become neurons and glia. Neural stem cells in the mammalian fetal brain have been located in the subventricular zone, ventricular zone, hippocampus, olfactory bulb, cerebellum, and cerebral cortex.

A new era in stem cell research began in 1998 with the derivation of embryonic stem cells. Techniques involving embryonic stem cells have developed greatly since 1998, when scientists reported methods for deriving and maintaining these cells. Stem cells derived from embryos have also been extensively studied and have demonstrated the remarkable ability to differentiate into neurons, glia, and numerous cell types in animals. Owing to the heightened ethical concerns and governmental issues regarding embryonic and fetal tissue research, cellular research has continued to expand its search for alternative sources of stem cells. More recently, adult stem cells, which are cells obtained post-birth, have made a breakthrough in the field of stem cell research. **Adult stem cells** make identical copies of themselves for long periods of time (self-renewal), and can produce mature cell types that have specific morphologies and functions. Their primary functions are to maintain the steady state of a cell and to replace cells that die due to injury or disease. Adult stem cells usually generate an intermediate cell type or types before they become fully differentiated. The intermediate cell type is commonly called a **precursor or progenitor cell**. This progenitor cell has the capacity to produce cells of the original tissue or organ (**multipotent**). For instance, stem cells isolated from the brain will give rise to neural cells, stem cells from the heart will give rise to cardiac cells, or stem cells from the bone marrow will give rise to blood cells. In addition, the adult stem cells also have the capacity to produce cells giving rise to many different cell types, tissues, and organs regardless of the origin of the stem cell (pluripotent). For example, **stem cells from umbilical cord blood** may give rise to neural cells, cardiac muscles, or other blood cells depending upon the condition or environment of the stem cells themselves. The ability of the adult stem cells to display pluripotency is quite similar to embryonic stem cells, thus expanding our resources for stem cells for cell therapy. Adult stem cells may be obtained from many different types of tissues; however, they retain the ability to produce many tissue types as well. These cells can be harvested from donors and isolated within the laboratory, where scientists culture and grow these cells for transplantation.

Bone marrow has also been found to be rich in adult stem cells. This idea, however, is not novel; **hematopoietic stem cells** were recognized as stem cells more than

40 years ago. However, more recent research has shown that these stem cells have exercised enormous potential for cellular therapy by demonstrating the capability of neuronal and astrocytic differentiation following transplantation. Thus, studies in bone marrow have advanced cell therapy to now include brain repair as well. Bone marrow actually contains three specific stem cell populations– **hematopoietic stem cells**, **stromal cells**, and **endothelial progenitor cells**.

Another hematopoietic source that is rich in adult stem cells includes umbilical cord blood. The umbilical cord, which supports the fetus during pregnancy, is delivered with the baby, and is typically discarded. Since the first successful umbilical cord blood transplants in children with **Fanconi anemia**, the collection of cord blood and cellular therapeutic use has grown rapidly. Moreover, there are none of the ethical issues regarding the use of cord blood stem cells compared to embryonic stem cells, and the method of harvesting the stem cells from the umbilical vein poses no risk to the mother or baby, because the cord is removed and set aside prior to blood collection. From a cellular therapeutic perspective, umbilical cord blood offers many advantages. Like bone marrow, it is rich in stem cells, but is much easier to obtain than bone marrow. Fortunately, both bone marrow and umbilical cord blood stem cells have been shown to migrate and engraft to neurological sites of injury following noninvasive intravenous injection, and amazingly produce recovery of function resulting from stroke and other forms of neurological injury, which offers an extreme advantage for cell therapy with these cells.

Although the field of stem cell research has evolved into a promising therapy for brain repair, many challenges still exist. The process of identifying the desired type of stem cell in culture will involve tedious research, while developing the right biochemical environment or media is essential to ensure that the stem cell differentiates into the desired cell type. Also, once the stem cells have been transplanted, the cells must be integrated within the body's own tissue and organs and must function correctly. Yet another challenge is tissue rejection. The body's immune system must not recognize the transplanted cells as foreign. Fortunately, cord-blood-derived stem cells are considered to be more immune immature cells, thus making the incidence of tissue rejection much less than other types of transplantable cells.

However, with these challenges in mind, stem cell therapy remains one of the best "natural" candidates to help heal the human body. Despite the many challenges, many scientists believe that cell therapy will revolutionize medicine. These cell therapies may one day offer cures for cancer, Parkinson's disease, diabetes, kidney disease, multiple sclerosis, cardiovascular disease, and symptoms of stroke. Cell therapy may also fill a tremendous need for chronic pain management and **traumatic brain injury** (TBI).

Scientists have begun to recognize the amazing versatility of these primitive cells that exist for only a short period of time prior to differentiating into other cell types and tissues within the body. Because cells are the basic building blocks of the human body, it would only stand to reason that we should harness the power of these stem cells to sustain and repair the body's tissues and organs with the appropriate research.

CEPHALEXIN HYDROCHLORIDE

(Keftab)

CEPHALEXIN MONOHYDRATE

(Keflet, Keflex)

Cephalexin, a first-generation cephalosporin antibiotic (250 mg to 1 g p.o. q. 6 hours), is indicated in the treatment of respiratory, genitourinary, skin and soft-tissue, or bone and joint infections, and in otitis media caused by susceptible organisms.

CEPHALOSPORINS

Cephalosporins are structurally related to the penicillins. The nucleus of the cephalosporin, 7-aminocephalosporanic acid, resembles the nucleus of penicillin, 6-aminopenicillanic acid. Cephalosporins have a broad spectrum of antimicrobial activity and are effective against a variety of Gram-positive and some strains of Gram-negative bacteria, such as *E. coli* and *Klebsiella* and *Proteus* species. In addition, cephalosporins are effective against some strains of *Enterobacter*, *Serratia*, and *Pseudomonas*. Among the Gram-positive bacteria, the enterococci, penicillin-resistant pneumococci, and methicillin-resistant staphylococci are also resistant to cephalosporins. However, the second-generation and newer cephalosporins, such as cefamandole, cefoxitin, cefuroxime, and moxalactam, offer an even greater spectrum of activity and are more active than the first-generation cephalosporins, such as cephalothin, against Gram-negative microorganisms.

Like the penicillins, cephalosporins exert their effects by inhibiting the formation of cell walls in the bacteria (see Figure 74). Clinical resistance to some of the second- and third-generation cephalosporins has been reported. These agents are resistant to penicillinase-producing organisms (see also Table 23).

Cephalexin, cefaclor, cefadroxil, and cephradine are absorbed well from the gastrointestinal tract and thus are given orally. Cephaloridine, cephalothin, cephapirin, cefoxitin, cefotaxime, cefamandole, and cefazolin are poorly absorbed from the gastrointestinal tract and must be given parenterally. Because the cephalosporins have short half-lives, they must be administered frequently. First- and second-generation (but not third-generation) cephalosporins do not readily penetrate the CNS and, therefore, are not effective for the treatment of meningitis. The cephalosporins are eliminated by glomerular filtration and active tubular secretion, which are blocked by probenecid. The acetylated derivatives of cephalosporins, such as cephalothin and cephapirin, are metabolized in the liver to inactive metabolites.

First-generation cephalosporins consist of:

- Cephalothin (Keflin); cephalothin not absorbed orally
- Cephapirin (Cefadyl)
- Cefazolin (Ancef, Kefzol, and others)
- Cephalexin (Keflet and Keflex)
- Cefadroxil (Duricef and Ultracef)
- Cephradine (Anspor and Velocef)

Second-generation cephalosporins are:

- Cefamandole (Mandol)
- Cefoxitin (Mefoxin)
- Cefaclor (Ceclor)
- Cefuroxime (Kefurox and Zinacef)
- Cefuroxime axetil (Ceftin)
- Cefonicid (Monocid)
- Cefotetan (Cefotan)
- Ceforanide (Precef)

These are more active than first-generation cephalosporins against certain Gram-negative organisms, including *Haemophilus influenzae, Enterobacter* species, indole-positive *Proteus* species, *E. coli*, and *Klebsiella* species.

Third-generation cephalosporins are:

- Cefotaxime (Claforan)
- Ceftizoxime (Cefizox)
- Ceftriaxone (Rocephin)
- Cefoperazone (Cefobid)
- Ceftazidime (Fortaz and others)

The pharmacologic features of third-generation cephalosporins vary widely for each drug. They are effective in treating infections caused by aerobic Gram-negative organisms.

Decreased renal function affects the elimination of most third-generation cephalosporins, whereas the presence of hepatic disease does not require dose adjustment.

The cephalosporins, often in combination with aminoglycoside antibiotics, are used in suspected cases of bacteremia due to *Staphylococcus, Klebsiella,* coliform bacteria, *Proteus*, or *Pseudomonas* infection.

Cephalosporins may be used as alternative agents to penicillin G for the treatment of streptococcal and pneumococcal infections. Third-generation cephalosporins are the drugs of choice in Gram-negative bacillary meningitis. Cephalosporins are used on a very limited basis as prophylaxis prior to and following some surgical procedures that carry high risks for infections.

The adverse reactions caused by cephalosporins resemble those to be named for penicillin, and include injection-site complications, phlebitis following intravenous administration, hypersensitivity reactions, and rare anaphylactoid shock. Infrequently, nephrotoxicity does occur with some cephalosporins.

CEPHALOSPORINS

Type	Drug	Common Uses	Side Effects
Cephalosporins: 1st Generation			
	Cefadroxil	Skin and soft tissue infections	Gastrointestinal upset and diarrhea
	Cefazolin		Nausea
	Cephalexin		Allergic reactions
Cephalosporins: 2nd Generation			
	Cefaclor	Some respiratory and abdominal infections	Gastrointestinal upset and diarrhea
	Cefamandole		
	Cefotetan		Nausea
	Cefoxitin		Allergic reactions
	Cefprozil		
	Cefuroxime		
Cephalosporins: 3rd Generation			
	Cefixime	Broad coverage of many bacteria for people with mild-to-moderate infections (oral) and serious illness (by injection)	Gastrointestinal upset and diarrhea
	Cefdinir		
	Cefditoren		Nausea
	Cefoperazone		Allergic reactions
	Cefotaxime		
	Cefpodoxime		
	Ceftazidime		
	Ceftibuten		
	Ceftizoxime		
	Ceftriaxone		
Cephalosporins: 4th Generation			
	Cefepime	Serious infections, particularly in people with a weakened immune system	Gastrointestinal upset and diarrhea; Nausea; Allergic reactions

CEPHALOTHIN SODIUM
(Keflin, Seffin)

Cephalothin, a first-generation cephalosporin antibiotic (500 mg to 1 g IM or IV q. 4 to 6 hours), is indicated in the treatment of serious respiratory, genitourinary, GI, skin and soft-tissue, bone and joint infections; in septicemia; and in endocarditis and meningitis.

CEPHAPIRIN SODIUM
(Cefadyl)

Cephapirin, a first-generation cephalosporin antibiotic (500 mg to 1 g IV or IM q. 4 to 6 hours), is indicated in the treatment of serious respiratory, genitourinary, GI, skin and soft-tissue, bone and joint infections (including osteomyelitis); in septicemia; and in endocarditis.

CEPHRADINE
(Anspor, Velosef)

Cephradine, a first-generation cephalosporin antibiotic (500 mg to 1 g IM or IV b.i.d.), is indicated in the treatment of serious respiratory, genitourinary, GI, skin and soft-tissue, bone and joint infections; and in septicemia, endocarditis, and otitis media.

CEREBROACTIVE MEDICATIONS

Bamethan	Naftidrofuryl
Bencyclane	Nicergoline
Bethahistine	Nicotinic acid derivatives
Cinnarizine	Nylidrin
Citicoline	Pentoxifylline
Cyclandelate	Papaverine
Dihydroergocristine	Pinacidil
Dihydroergotoxine	Piracetam
Ebunamonine	Piribedil
Flunarizine	Raubasine
Ginkgo-biloba extracts	Suloctidil
Isoxsuprine	Vincamine

These allegedly cerebroactive and vasodilating medications have been tried in vascular disorders. Their pharmacological properties are complex, and their values remain to be established. For example, as a vasodilator, pinacidil is three- and tenfold more potent than hydralazine and minoxidil, respectively. It does not interact with alpha, beta, cholinergic, or histaminergic receptors, and also does not produce vasodilation via an indirect effect that is mediated by adenosine, prostaglandin, or endothelial-derived relaxant factor. Its vasodilating activity does not resemble that brought about by the conventional calcium-channel antagonists. Thus, pinacidil-induced vascular relaxation is a direct effect mediated by a novel mechanism.

CETIRIZINE

(Zyrtec tablets 5 mg)

Cetirizine competitively antagonizes histamine at the H_1-receptor site and is indicated in the symptomatic relief of symptoms (e.g., nasal, nonnasal) associated with seasonal and perennial allergic rhinitis; treatment of uncomplicated skin manifestations of chronic idiopathic urticaria. **Histamine** is a potent vasodilator, bronchial smooth-muscle constrictor, and stimulant of nociceptive itch nerves. In addition to histamine, multiple chemical itch mediators can act as pruritogens on C-fibers, including neuropeptides, prostaglandins, serotonin, acetylcholine, and bradykinin. Furthermore, new receptor systems such as vanilloid, opioid, and cannabinoid receptors on cutaneous sensory nerve fibers that may modulate itch offer novel targets for antipruritic therapy.

Histamine is in mast cells, basophils, and platelets. Human skin mast cells express H_1, H_2, and H_4 receptors, but not H_3 receptors. H_1 and H_2 receptors are involved in wheal formation and erythema, whereas only H_1-receptor agonists cause pruritus. Complete blockade of H_1-receptors does not totally relieve itching, and combinations of H_1 and H_2 blockers may be superior to H_1 blockers alone.

Oral antihistamines, particularly H_1-receptor antagonists, have some anticholinergic activity and are sedating, making them useful for the control of pruritus. First-generation sedating H_1-receptor antagonists include **hydroxyzine hydrochloride** (Atarax), which is given in a dose of 0.5 mg/kg every 6 hours; **diphenhydramine** (Benadryl; others); **promethazine** (Phenergan); and **cyproheptadine** (Periactin). **Doxepin** (Adapin, Sine-quan), which has tricyclic antidepressant and sedative antihistamine effects, is a good alternative for severe pruritus. A topical formulation of doxepin also is available as a 5% cream (Zonalon), which can be used in conjunction with low- to moderate-potency topical glucocorticoids. The systemic effect from topical doxepin is comparable with that of low-dose oral therapy.

Second-generation H_1-receptor antagonists lack anticholinergic side effects and are described as nonsedating largely because they do not cross the blood–brain barrier. They include **cetirizine** (Zyrtec), loratadine (Claratin), desloratidine (Clarinex), and fexofenadine hydrochloride (Allegra). Although second-generation nonsedating H_1-receptor blockers are as effective as the first-generation H_1 blockers, they are metabolized by CYP3A4 and, to a lesser extent, by CYP2D6, and should not be coadministered with medications that inhibit these enzymes (e.g., imidazole antifungals and macrolide antibiotics).

H_2-receptor blockers include cimetidine (Tagamet), ranitidine (Zantac), famotidine (Pepcid), and nizatidine (Axid). Besides their use in combination with H_1-receptor blockers for pruritus, the H_2-receptor blockers have immunomodulating effects, and this property has been exploited in children to treat warts. Drug allergy may develop when H_1 antagonists are given orally but results more commonly from topical application. Allergic dermatitis is not uncommon; other hypersensitivity reactions include drug fever and photosensitization. Hematological complications such as leukopenia, agranulocytosis, and hemolytic anemia are very rare. Because H_1 antihistamines cross the placenta, caution must be used when they are taken by women who are or may become pregnant. Several antihistamines (e.g., azelastine, hydroxyzine, and fexofenadine) showed teratogenic effects in animal studies, whereas others (e.g., chlorpheniramine, diphenhydramine, cetirizine, and loratadine) did not. Antihistamines can be excreted in small amounts in breast milk, and first-generation antihistamines taken by lactating mothers may cause symptoms in the nursing infant such as irritability, drowsiness, or respiratory depression. Because H_1 antagonists interfere with skin tests for allergy, they must be withdrawn well before such tests are performed.

Cetirizine is indicated in the treatment of pollen-associated asthma in individuals with angioedema, atopic dermatitis, and certain types of physical urticaria such as delayed pressure urticaria, dermatographia, and cold urticaria. Terfenadine, astemizole, loratadine, and cetirizine are second-generation antihistaminic agents that are relatively nonsedating. Cetirizine is a carboxylated metabolite of hydroxyzine (Vistaril), a piperazine derivative H_1-receptor antagonist. Cetirizine inhibits both histamine release and eosinophil chemotaxis during the secondary phase of the allergic response. It reduces inflammatory cell infiltration (i.e., eosinophils, neutrophils, basophils) by 75% during the late-phase response.

Cetirizine 10 mg is more potent than terfenadine 60 mg, loratadine (Claritin) 10 mg, and chlorpheniramine (e.g., Chlor-Trimeton) 6 mg, and equal in potency to diphenhydramine (e.g., Benadryl) 50 mg, hydroxyzine 25 mg, and terfenadine 180 mg. Cetirizine is absorbed well when given orally, is bound to plasma protein to the extent of 93%, does not cross the blood–brain barrier, has an elimination half-life of 7 to 10 hours, and is excreted mostly unchanged in the urine. The half-life of cetirizine is increased in renal impairment, requiring smaller dosage.

CETUXIMAB

(Erbitux injection 100 mg)

Cetuximab is an antineoplastic/monoclonal antibody that competitively inhibits binding of epidermal growth factor (EGF) to receptors, which blocks phosphorylation and activation of receptor-associated kinases, resulting in inhibition of cell growth. Cetuximab is used alone and in combination with **irinotecan** for treatment of EGF-receptor-expressing metastatic colorectal carcinoma in patients intolerant or refractory in irinotecan.

Cetuximab is a chimeric monoclonal antibody that recognizes the EGF receptor (EGFR; also ERBB1 or HER1). Activation of EGF receptor signaling through its intercellular tyrosine kinase domain produces multiple cellular events associated with proliferation, survival, and angiogenesis. EGFR expression is found in 60 to 75% of colorectal cancers, where it has been linked to tumor progression and a poor prognosis. Multiple epithelial cancers, such as breast, lung, kidney, prostate, brain, pancreas, bladder, and head and neck malignancies, also express EGFR and are potential therapeutic targets of cetuximab. Although the mechanism of tumor cell kill for cetuximab is uncertain, it is likely to involve inhibition of EGF binding and signaling, which may lead to inhibition of pro-angiogenic factors and apoptosis.

CEVIMELINE HYDROCHLORIDE

(Evoxac gelatin capsules 30 mg)

Cevimeline is a cholinergic agonist that binds to muscarinic receptors. Muscarinic agonists in sufficient dosage can increase secretion of exocrine glands, such as salivary and sweat glands, and increase tone of the smooth muscle in the GI and urinary tracts. Cevimeline relieves dry mouth in patients with **Sjogren syndrome**.

CHARCOAL, ACTIVATED

(Actidose-aqua liquid 208 mg/mL)

Charcoal inhibits GI absorption of toxic substances and is indicated in the emergency treatment of poisoning by most drugs and chemicals. Activated charcoal must be distinguished from the so-called **universal antidote**, which consists of two parts burned toast (not activated charcoal), one part tannic acid (strong tea), and one part magnesium oxide. **Activated charcoal** avidly adsorbs drugs and chemicals on the surfaces of the charcoal particles, thereby preventing absorption and toxicity. Many, but not all, chemicals are adsorbed by charcoal. For example, alcohols, hydrocarbons, metals, and corrosive are not well adsorbed by activated charcoal, and therefore, it is of little value in treating these poisonings. The effectiveness of charcoal also depends on the time since the ingestion and on the dose of charcoal; one should attempt to achieve a charcoal–drug ratio of at least 10:1. Activated charcoal also can interrupt the enterohepatic circulation of drugs and enhance the net rate of diffusion of the chemical from the body into the gastrointestinal tract. For example, serial doses of activated charcoal have been shown to enhance the elimination of theophylline and phenobarbital.

CHEMOPROTECTANTS

(e.g., Amifostine, Dexrazoxane)

One of the goals of cancer chemotherapy is to enhance the efficacy of antineoplastic agents and, at the same time, protect the nonmalignant tissues using chemoprotective agents. A few of the chemoenhancers and chemoprotectors are listed below:

Chemoenhancers	Chemoprotectors
Calcium-channel blockers	Amifostine
Phenothiazines	Thiosulfate
Cyclosporine	Diethyldithiocarbamate
Buthionine suloximime	Diuretics, phorbol esters
Tamoxifen	Bismuth salts
Triparanol	Oxothiazolidine-4-carboxylate
Acridines	Glutathione esters
Amiodarone	Steroids
Phorbol esters	Metallothionein
Streptozocin	Dexrazoxane
Progesterone	
Ethacrynic acid	

Anthyracycline antibiotics (e.g., doxorubicin) causes unique cardiomyopathies. An acute form is characterized by abnormal electrocardiographic changes, including ST-T wave alterations and arrhthymias. This is brief and rarely a serious problem. Cineangiographic studies have shown an acute, reversible reduction in ejection fraction 24 hours after a single dose. An exaggerated manifestation of acute myocardial damage, the "pericarditis–myocarditis syndrome," may be characterized by severe disturbances in impulse conduction and frank congestive heart failure, often associated with pericardial effusion. Chronic, cumulative dose-related toxicity is manifested by congestive heart failure that is unresponsive to digitalis.

Cardiac irradiation or administration of high doses of cyclophosphamide or another anthracycline may increase the risk of cardiotoxicity. There is evidence that cardiac damage is reduced by the concomitant administration of the iron chelator dexrazoxane (ADR-529) or by amifostine (WR-2721) or its active metabolite (WR-1065).

CHENODIOL

(Chenix)

Chenodiol, a bile acid with cholelitholytic properties (250 mg b.i.d. for 2 weeks), is indicated in dissolution of radiolucent cholesterol stones (gallstones) when systemic disease or age precludes surgery; and to increase bile flow in patients with bile duct prostheses or stents.

CHLAMYDIAL INFECTIONS: Treatment of

Infections	Medications
Uncomplicated urethral, endocervical, or rectal infection in adults	Doxycycline 100 mg p.o. two times daily for 7 days, or tetracycline 500 mg p.o. four times daily for 7 days
Urogenital infections during pregnancy	Erythromycin base 500 mg p.o. four times daily for 7 days, or Erythromycin ethyl succinate 800 mg p.o. four times daily for 7 days (or 400 mg p.o. four times daily for 14 days)
Conjunctivitis of the newborn	Erythromycin suspension 50 mg/kg/d p.o. in four divided doses for 14 days)
Pneumonia in infants	Erythromycin suspension 50 mg/kg/d p.o. in four divided doses for 14 days
Acute epididymo-orchitis	Amoxicillin 3.0 g p.o., or ampicillin 3.5 g p.o., or aqueous procaine penicillin G 4.8 million units IM at two sites (each along with probenecid 1.0 g p.o.), or spectinomycin 2.0 g IM or ceftriaxone 250 mg IM followed by tetracycline 500 p.o. four times daily for 10 days or Doxycycline 100 mg p.o. two times daily for 10 days

CHLORAL HYDRATE
(Noctec, Somnos)

Chloral hydrate (500 to 1000 mg taken 15 to 30 minutes before bedtime) is indicated for nocturnal sedation in patients intolerant to barbiturates or benzodiazepine derivatives. It may be used in candidates for surgery to alleviate anxiety and induce sleep without depressing respiration or cough reflex. Chloral hydrate rectal suppositories are available. The CNS depressant effects of chloral hydrate are believed to be due to trichlorethanol, its metabolite. Chloral hydrate has additive CNS-depressing effects when taken with alcohol. Chloral hydrate, when used on a chronic basis, is known to be habit forming. The toxic dose of chloral hydrate is 10 g, producing hypothermia, hypotension, slow or rapid shallow breathing, pinpoint pupils, and comatose state. In surviving individuals, hepatic and renal impairments may result.

CHLORAMBUCIL
(Leukeran)

Chlorambucil (0.1 to 0.2 mg/kg/d for 3 to 6 weeks) will provide palliation in chronic lymphocytic leukemia, malignant lymphomas including lymphosarcoma, giant follicular lymphoma, and Hodgkin's disease. In addition, it has been used in the treatment of uveitis and meningoencephalitis associated with Behcet's disease. Chlorambucil is absorbed orally, metabolized extensively, and the metabolite is excreted in the urine. It causes reversible bone-marrow suppression, hepatotoxicity with jaundice, infertility, sterility, bronchopulmonary dysplasia, seizures in susceptible individuals, and gastrointestinal problems such as oral ulceration, nausea, vomiting, or diarrhea. Chlorambucil, which is carcinogenic, mutagenic, and teratogenic, should be used cautiously in all subjects including patients with leukemia and malignant lymphomas. Radiation therapy will enhance chlorambucil-induced bone–marrow depression.

CHLORAMPHENICOL
(Chloromycetin)

Chloramphenicol is indicated for infection caused by susceptible strains of *Salmonella* species; and by *H. influenzae*, specifically, meningeal infections and rickettsiae; for the lymphogranuloma-psittacosis group and various Gram-negative bacteria causing bacteremia, meningitis, or other serious Gram-negative infections; for infections involving anaerobic organisms when *Bacteroides fragilis* is suspected; and for other susceptible organisms that have been demonstrated to be resistant to all other appropriate antimicrobial agents.

Chloramphenicol has a broad spectrum of bacteriostatic activity for many bacteria, including *Rickettsia*. It is the preferred drug in the treatment of *Salmonella* infection (e.g., typhoid fever); *H. influenzae*, meningitis, laryngotracheitis, or pneumonia not responding to ampicillin; in *Bacteroides* infections and meningococcal infections in patients allergic to penicillin; and in *Rickettsia* infections (see also Figure 88).

Chloramphenicol exerts its effects by binding to 50S ribosomal subunits and thus inhibiting bacterial protein synthesis by preventing peptide-bond formation, and by inhibiting the synthesis of mitochondrial proteins in the host. The resistance of chloramphenicol stems from the production of chloramphenicol acetyltransferase by microorganisms that metabolize the drug.

Chloramphenicol is completely absorbed from the gastrointestinal tract and is distributed widely throughout the body, including the cerebrospinal fluid. It is metabolized in the liver by glucuronyl transferase, and the metabolites are excreted by the kidneys. Newborn infants cannot metabolize chloramphenicol readily.

Chloramphenicol causes both dose-dependent and dose-independent hematologic reactions. Fatal aplastic anemia occurs in genetically susceptible patients taking chloramphenicol on a long-term basis. Reversible and dose-dependent disturbances of hemopoiesis can also arise, and are characterized by the altered maturation of red blood cells, vacuolated nucleated red blood cells in the marrow, and reticulocytopenia.

Newborn infants are deficient in glucuronyl transferase. Thus, when treating newborns, doses of chloramphenicol should not exceed 50 mg/kg per day. Large doses will precipitate gray baby syndrome, characterized by vomiting, hypothermia, gray skin tone, and shock.

CHLORAZEPATE DIPOTASSIUM

(Tranxene)

Chlorazepate, which enhances GABAergic transmission (see Figure 50), is indicated in acute alcohol withdrawal, in anxiety disorders, and as an adjunct in seizure management. Chlorazepate is hydrolyzed in the stomach to desmethyldiazepam, which is then absorbed completely and bound to plasma proteins to the extent of 80 to 95%. Desmethyldiazepam is then metabolized to oxazepam, whose inactive metabolite conjugated to glucuronic acid is excreted in the urine.

Chlorazepate potentiates the CNS-depressant effects of phenothiazines, narcotics, barbiturates, alcohol, antihistamines, monoamine oxidase inhibitors, general anesthetics, and antidepressants. Concomitant use with cimetidine and possibly disulfiram causes diminished hepatic metabolism of chlorazepate, which increases its plasma concentration.

Clinical manifestations of overdose with chlorazepate include somnolence, confusion, coma, hypoactive reflexes, dyspnea, labored breathing, hypotension, bradycardia, slurred speech, and unsteady gait or impaired coordination.

CHLORCYCLIZINE

(Mantadil)

Noscapine (Nectadon) is a naturally occurring opium alkaloid with a structure and function similar to papaverine. It is antitussive and has no analgesic or additive properties.

Diphenhydramine and chlorcyclizine are antihistaminic agents that also have antitussive properties. Dimethoxanate (Cothera) and pipazethate (Theratuss) are phenothiazine derivatives without analgesic but with weak antitussive and local anesthetic properties.

CHLORDIAZEPOXIDE

(Librium)

Chlordiazepoxide is indicated in the management of anxiety disorders for the short-term relief of symptoms of anxiety; for symptoms of acute alcohol withdrawal; and for preoperative apprehension and anxiety.

Chlordiazepoxide, a weakly basic substance, is unstable both in solution and when exposed to ultraviolet light. Thus, oral preparations are protected with opaque capsules, and solutions for parenteral injection must be prepared fresh and used immediately. The absorption of chlordiazepoxide from intramuscular sites is erratic and unpredictable. Thus, the oral and intravenous routes are used when reliable or rapid effects are desired. Chlordiazepoxide disappears from the plasma rapidly, but its metabolites, desmethylchlordiazepoxide, demoxepam, and desmethyldiazepam, are eliminated more slowly.

Chlordiazepoxide is about 94 to 97% bound to plasma proteins, and has a distribution volume of 0.3 to 0.4 L/kg in males and a somewhat larger volume in females.

The rate of elimination of chlordiazepoxide is prolonged in the elderly, the clearance in those over 60 years of age being about half that of young adults. The elderly are also more "sensitive" to the CNS effects of chlordiazepoxide; thus, they should be given smaller doses. Clearance of chlordiazepoxide is also reduced in patients with cirrhosis, as are the rate and extent of formation of desmethylchlordiazepoxide. Disulfiram inhibits the metabolism of chlordiazepoxide (see also Figure 50 and Table 9).

CHLORDIAZEPOXIDE/AMITRIPTYLINE

(Limbitrol DS 10-25 tablets 10 mg chlordiazepoxide and 25 mg amitriptyline)

Amitriptyline blocks reuptake of serotonin and norepinephrine in CNS. **Chlordiazepoxide** potentiates effects of GABA in CNS. The combination is indicated in the treatment of moderate to severe depression associated with moderate to severe anxiety.

CHLORGYLINE

Monoamine oxidase inhibitors are classified into A and B types. Monoamine oxidase A preferentially uses serotonin and norepinephrine as substrates and is inhibited by chlorgyline and harmaline. Monoamine oxidase B preferentially uses dopamine and is inhibited by selegiline (see also Figures 37 and 87).

CHLORHEXIDINE GLUCONATE

(Bactoshield solution 4% with 4% isopropyl alcohol)

Chlorhexidine is an antiseptic/germicide/mouth and throat product that provides antimicrobial effect against a wide range of microorganisms. Chlorhexidine is indicated in surgical scrub; skin cleanser; preoperative skin preparation; skin wound cleanser; hand rinse; oral rinse for gingivitis; and as an adjunct to scaling and root planning procedures for reduction of pocket depth in adults with periodontitis.

CHLOROPROCAINE

(Nesacaine)

Chloroprocaine (1 to 2% injection with methylparaben as a preservative) is indicated in the production of local anesthesia by infiltration and peripheral nerve block. Chloroprocaine without methylparaben is indicated in peripheral and central nerve block, including lumbar and caudal epidural blocks. Chloroprocaine has an onset of action of 6 to 12 minutes.

Chloroprocaine, like other local anesthetics, blocks the generation and the conduction of nerve impulses, presumably by increasing the threshold for electrical excitation in the nerve by slowing the propagation of the nerve impulse and by reducing the rate of the rise of action potential. In general, the progression of anesthesia is related to the diameter, myelination, and conduction velocity of affected nerve fibers. Clinically, the order of loss of nerve function is as follows: pain, temperature, touch, proprioception, and skeletal muscle tone.

The adverse reactions of chloroprocaine, which are dose-dependent and may result from rapid absorption from the injection site or unintentional intravascular injection, are CNS reactions (restlessness, anxiety, dizziness, tinnitus, blurred vision, tremor, and even convulsions) and cardiovascular reactions (depression of myocardium, bradycardia, hypotension, arrhythmias, and even cardiac arrest) (see also Figure 31).

CHLOROQUINE PHOSPHATE

(Aralen)

Chloroquine is indicated for prophylaxis and treatment of acute attacks of malaria due to *P. vivax*, *P. malariae*, *P. ovale*, and susceptible strains of *P. falcinarum*. It is also used for treatment of extraintestinal amebiasis. Chloroquine destroys schizonts in erythrocytes by interfering with DNA synthesis. The phosphate salts are active orally, whereas the hydrochloride salt is used for intravenous purposes. It accumulates in normal and parasitized erythrocytes. Overdosage has caused reversible corneal damage and permanent retinal damage. In toxic doses, chloroquine causes visual disturbances, hyperexcitability, convulsions, and heart block. It is an antimalarial of choice in all cases except chloroquine-resistant *Plasmodium falciparum*. In addition, it has a certain degree of effectiveness in amebiasis and in the late stages of rheumatoid arthritis. Amodiaquine (Camoquin) may be used as an alternate drug.

CHLOROTHIAZIDE

(Diuril)

Thiazides and related diuretics (see Table 25) are used in edema associated with congestive heart failure, hepatic cirrhosis, nephrotic syndrome, acute glomerulonephritis, or chronic renal failure. Thiazides are used as sole therapeutic agents, or in combination with other drugs in the management of hypertension. Thiazides in combination with amiloride or allopurinol have been used to prevent formation and recurrence of calcium nephrolithiasis in hypercalciuric and normal calciuric patients. Thiazide in combination with calcium and estrogen may be helpful in postmenopausal osteoporosis. Thiazide is useful in treating nephrogenic diabetes insipidus (see also Figure 17 and Table 25).

Thiazide diuretics, also called sulfonamide or benzothiazide diuretics, vary in their actions. For instance, the potency of hydrochlorothiazide (Hydro-Diuril and Esidrix) is ten times greater than that of chlorothiazide (Diuril), but the two drugs have equal efficacy. The duration of action of hydrochlorothiazide, which is 6 to 12 hours, is equal to that of chlorothiazide. On the other hand, chlorthalidone (Hygroton) has a duration of action lasting 48 hours. Some thiazide derivatives inhibit carbonic anhydrase, which is unrelated to their diuretic activity. Those that are active in this respect may, at sufficient doses, have the same effect on bicarbonate excretion as does acetazolamide. They cause a moderate loss of sodium (5 to 10% of the filtered load), chloride, and water, and the clearance of free water is impaired. They may cause metabolic alkalosis (resorption of bicarbonate and loss of hydrogen ions), hyperuricemia (enhanced resorption of uric acid), or hyperglycemia (inhibiting insulin release directly and due to hypokalemia).

Thiazide diuretics are used in the treatment of edema of cardiac and gastrointestinal origin and bring about a state of intravascular volume depletion. Because this depleted intravascular volume is replenished from the interstitial (edematous) sites, thiazide diuretics should not be administered too frequently. For example, hydrochlorothiazide is given every other day, and chlorthalidone is given once every 2 to 3 days. In small doses, thiazide diuretics are extremely effective in controlling essential hypertension. They exert their effects initially by bringing about volume depletion, then reduce the peripheral resistance and sensitivity of vascular receptor sites to catecholamine. Thiazide diuretics are also used in conjunction with antihypertensive medications.

Thiazides decrease the urinary calcium concentration by diminishing glomerular filtration and also enhance the urinary magnesium level. They can reduce free water formation in patients with diabetes insipidus, in whom large amounts of free water are eliminated. The loss of potassium can produce hypokalemia, which is particularly dangerous in patients receiving digitalis because it increases the risk of arrhythmias. Hypokalemia can be offset either by giving a potassium supplement (potassium chloride), or by the concurrent use of a potassium-sparing diuretic. However, only one of these measures should be adopted because hyperkalemia will result. Hyperglycemia is a potential hazard for patients with diabetes mellitus. Hyperuricemia can precipitate an acute attack of gout, but usually only in those patients who either have already had gout or have a propensity toward it. Because thiazides can cause a decrease in the GFR, they should not be used in patients whose renal function is less than one third of normal. The risk of thiazide-induced hypercalcemia should be kept in mind in patients with conditions such as malignancies or hyperparathyroidism that are associated with hypercalcemia.

CHLOROTRIANISENE

(Tace)

Chlorotrianisene is a nonsteroidal synthetic estrogen that is used in postpartum breast engorgement (12 mg 4 times/day for 7 days), vasomotor symptoms associated with menopause (12 mg/day cyclically for 30 days), atrophic vaginitis and Kraurosis vulvae (12 mg/day cyclically for 60 days), female hypogonadism (12 mg/day cyclically for 21 days), and inoperable prostate carcinoma (12 mg/day given chronically) (see also Figure 28).

CHLORPHENESINE CARBAMATE

(Maolate)

Chlorphenesine (400 to 800 mg t.i.d.) is indicated as an adjunct to rest and physical therapy for the relief of discomfort associated with acute and painful musculoskeletal conditions. Chlorphenesine-induced muscular relaxation may be related to its sedative properties because it does not exert its effects either directly on skeletal muscles or myoneural junctions.

CHLORPHENIRAMINE MALEATE

(Chlor-Trimeton)

Chlorpheniramine (4 mg q. 4 to 6 hours) is an alkylamine derivative H_1 antihistaminic agent that is indicated in perennial and seasonal allergic rhinitis; vasomotor rhinitis; allergic conjunctivitis due to inhalant allergens and foods; mild, uncomplicated allergic skin manifestations of urticaria and angioedema; amelioration of allergic reactions to blood or plasma; demographism; or as therapy for anaphylactic reactions adjunctive to epinephrine and other standard measures after the acute manifestations have been controlled.

Chlorpheniramine has anticholinergic properties and hence is contraindicated in narrow-angle glaucoma, prostatic hypertrophy, stenosing peptic ulcer, pyloroduodenal obstruction, and bladder neck obstruction. In addition, it has sedative properties, and the drug may impair alertness needed to complete hazardous tasks. Chlorpheniramine maleate (2 mg)/ codeine phosphate (10 mg)/ guaifenesin (100 mg) is indicated for its antiallergic, antitussive, expectorant, and mucolytic properties and is marketed as Tussar. Chlorpheniramine maleate/codeine phosphate/phenylephrine hydrochloride/ potassium iodide (Demi-Cof) is marketed for its antiallergic, antitussive, expectorant, and mucolytic properties to be used for the common cold associated with bronchitis. Many other preparations containing chlorpheniramine sold as Novahistine-Dh, Chem-Tuss, Anaplex-Hd, D-Allergy, Ru-Tuss, and Lantuss-forte are indicated for their antitussive properties associated with allergies and the common cold.

CHLORPHENIRAMINE MALEATE/ PHENYLEPHRINE HYDROCHLORIDE/ METHSCOPOLAMINE NITRATE

(AH-chew tablets 10 mg phenylephrine, 2 mg chlorpheniramine, 1.25 mg methscopolamine; D.A. chewable tablets 10 mg phenylephrine, 2 mg chorpheniramine, 1.25 mg methscopolamine)

The combination possesses antihistamine/decongestant/anticholinergic properties. **Chorpheniramine**: competitively antagonizes histamine at H_1-receptor sites; **phenylephrine**: stimulates postsynaptic alpha-receptors, resulting in vasoconstriction, which reduces congestion; **methscopolamine**: competitively inhibits action of acetylcholine at muscarinic receptors. The combination is indicated for temporary relief of symptoms of allergic rhinitis, casomotor rhinitis, sinusitis, and the common cold.

CHLORPHENIRAMINE MALEATE/ PSEUDOEPHEDRINE HYDROCHLORIDE/ CODEINE PHOSPHATE

(Decohistine DH liquid 10 mg codeine phosphate, 2 mg chlorpheniramine maleate, 30 mg Pseudoephedrine hydrochloride)

Chlorpheniramine is an antitussive combination. **Chlorpheniramine**: competitively antagonizes histamine at H_1-receptor sites; **pseudoephedrine**: causes vasoconstriction and subsequent shrinkage of nasal mucous membranes by alpha-adrenergic stimulation, which promotes nasal drainage; **codeine**: suppresses cough reflex. This combination is indicated in temporary relief of runny nose, sneezing, and itchy and watery eyes due to hay fever (allergic rhinitis); temporary relief of cough due to minor bronchial irritation and nasal congestion caused by common cold; and temporary relief of sinus congestion and pressure.

CHLORPROMAZINE

(Thorazine)

Chlorpromazine is indicated for the management of manifestations of psychotic disorders, to control nausea and vomiting (see Figure 73), for relief of restlessness and apprehension before surgery, for acute intermittent porphyria, as an adjunct in the treatment of tetanus, to control the manifestations of the manic type of manic–depressive illness, for relief of intractable hiccups, for the treatment of severe behavioral problems in children marked by combativeness and/or explosive hyperexcitable behavior, and in the short-term treatment of hyperactive children who show excessive motor activity with accompanying conduct disorders consisting of some or all of the following symptoms: impulsivity, difficulty sustaining attention, aggressiveness, mood lability, and poor frustration tolerance.

Chlorpromazine is well absorbed mainly from the jejunum. It is extensively metabolized in the liver, which produces several active metabolites. When given intramuscularly, the phenothiazine neuroleptics avoid metabolic degradation (first-pass metabolism), making them more beneficial as long-acting depot antipsychotics (see Table 2).

Chlorpromazine produces a tranquility characterized by a detached serenity without depression of mental faculties or clouding of consciousness. It depresses the CNS selectively by reducing input directed to the reticular formation through collaterals arriving from the sensory pathways. Chlorpromazine-induced sedation differs from that caused by barbiturates in that the patient can be easily aroused. In practice, the more sedative neuroleptics are often prescribed for agitated, overactive patients, and the less sedative agents are used for apathetic, withdrawn patients. However, sedation is not necessary for its antipsychotic property for two reasons: (1) tolerance develops to the sedative effects, and (2) fluphenazine, prochlorperazine, and trifluoperazine are excellent neuroleptics that lack pronounced sedative effects.

In general, chlorpromazine and other neuroleptics reduce spontaneous motor activity in proportion to their dosages.

The nausea and vomiting associated with circulating physical agents (radiation therapy and virus particles) or chemical agents (toxins and cancer chemotherapeutic agents) that stimulate the chemoreceptor trigger zone for emesis are treated with phenothiazine derivatives such as chlorpromazine, perphenazine, promethazine, triethylperazine, and triflupromazine. With the exception of thioridazine (Mellaril), all have antiemetic effects because they depress the chemoreceptor zone for emesis. Larger-than-therapeutic doses inhibit the vomiting center (see Figure 73).

The phenothiazine derivatives are hypothermic, and the extent of hypothermia depends on the dosage and the environmental temperature. Substances that reduce the concentrations of norepinephrine (reserpine) or block its receptor site (chlorpromazine) are hypothermic, whereas substances that increase the release of norepinephrine (amphetamine) are hyperthermic.

Phenothiazine derivatives cause postural or orthostatic hypotension. This may be more pronounced in patients with reduced vascular volume resulting from acute hemorrhage or dehydration, and when used with diuretic agents. Hypotension is more frequent with phenothiazine derivatives having either an aliphatic substitution on N10 (e.g., chlorpromazine) or a piperidine substitution on N10 (e.g., mesoridazine or thioridazine). It occurs less frequently with compounds containing a piperazine substitution (e.g., trifluoperazine). The hypotension is due to direct vasodilation and an alpha-adrenergic-receptor-blocking effect. The pressor effects of epinephrine can be reduced, blocked, or reversed by appropriate doses of chlorpromazine.

Surgical patients who are premedicated with chlorpromazine respond poorly to pressor drugs, requiring larger-than-anticipated doses. The inotropic effects of epinephrine (increase in the strength of muscular contraction) are reduced by chlorpromazine. The chronotropic effects of epinephrine (increase in the rate of contraction) are increased as the result of chlorpromazine's anticholinergic properties. The local vasoconstrictor action of epinephrine (as used with a local anesthetic) is blocked by chlorpromazine, but its hyperglycemic effect is not. The lethal effect of toxic doses of epinephrine or norepinephrine can be reversed by chlorpromazine.

Most phenothiazine neuroleptics (see Table 2) have weak anticholinergic properties. However, the anticholinergic effects of thioridazine or ethapropazine are pronounced, and all the cautions cited for atropine apply to these agents as well. Indeed, fatal tachyarrhythmias and other electrocardiographic changes such as blunting and notching of T waves, prolongation of the QT interval, increased convexity of the ST segment, and appearance of V waves have been caused through the injudicious use of thioridazine (1500 to 3600 mg/day), especially in elderly patients.

Nausea, which may be patient related, occurs frequently with psychotropic drugs, but the incidence is also high in schizophrenic patients who are receiving placebo. Furthermore, the incidence of vomiting with thioridazine, which has no antiemetic effect, is high. Dry mouth, constipation, paralytic ileus, and decreased gastric secretion, which are all due to its anticholinergic effects, may occur.

Phenothiazine derivatives have been observed to cause jaundice in 5% of the patients. The jaundice is accompanied by intense pruritus, fever, chills, nausea, epigastric or right upper quadrant abdominal pain, and malaise. The jaundice is not dose dependent, and develops after a typical delay of 2 to 3 weeks. With discontinuation of medication, the prognosis has been excellent.

Phenothiazine derivatives (thioridazine, trifluoperazine, prochlorperazine, and fluphenazine) have been known to cause reversible galactorrhea. This commonly occurs with large doses and long-term treatment. It arises because dopamine normally inhibits the release of prolactin but, by blocking dopamine receptor sites, neuroleptics nullify this action. Thioridazine causes a reversible ejaculation disorder, in that erection and orgasm occurs without ejaculation. Bromocriptine mesylate (Parlodel), a dopaminergic agonist used in the treatment of parkinsonism, has been shown to be effective in preventing postpartum lactation. Chlorpromazine, by preventing the release of insulin, may cause diabetes mellitus in a borderline individual or unstabilize a diabetic patient.

Chlorpromazine and other phenothiazine derivatives (perphenazine, prochlorperazine, thioridazine, and triflupromazine) may cause agranulocytosis. The incidence of these side effects is higher among female and elderly patients whose bone marrow has lower proliferative potential. These agents inhibit DNA polymerase, thymidylate kinase, and the incorporation of 3H-thymidine into DNA. Because the phenothiazine-induced agranulocytosis is a toxic reaction, it may be prevented by carefully monitoring the status of peripheral blood.

Dermatologic reactions following the use of phenothiazine derivatives can be divided into three categories: solar sensitivity, allergic dermatitis, and pigment retinopathy.

Solar sensitivity, which occurs only in sun-exposed areas of the body such as the hands and face, can be prevented by having patients avoid exposure to the sun.

Allergic dermatitis, which may be maculopapular, urticarial, or pruritic, should be regarded as a hypersensitivity reaction. Medication should be discontinued and other supportive therapy initiated.

Pigment retinopathy is manifested by the deposition of dot-like particles in the anterior capsular and subcapsular portion of the lens, pupillary area, cornea, conjunctiva, and retina. It is thought that, in the presence of ultraviolet light, the highly reactive metabolites of phenothiazine form free radicals that undergo covalent linkage with melanin. The synthesis of melanocyte-stimulating hormone, like that of prolactin, is stimulated following treatment with phenothiazine derivatives. These side effects may be prevented by using the lowest possible maintenance doses of neuroleptics and by observing "drug-free holidays" to reduce the endogenous concentrations of neuroleptics that have long and protracted half-lives.

A variety of neurologic syndromes, involving particularly the extrapyramidal system, occur following short- or long-term use of neuroleptic (antipsychotic) drugs. These include akathisia, dystonia, neuroleptic malignant syndrome, parkinsonism, and tardive dyskinesia.

Akathisia is characterized by an inability to sit still, by shifting of the legs and tapping of feet while sitting, and by rocking and shifting of the weight while standing. This "motoric restlessness" is not caused by agitation or anxiety, occurs more frequently among female and elderly patients, is stopped volitionally, returns spontaneously when it is not controlled consciously, and is aggravated by physical inactivity. Reducing the total dosage of neuroleptic medications and the addition of either an anticholinergic drug, one of the benzodiazepine derivatives, or propranolol have been shown to reduce the severity of akathisia. Restless legs syndrome is characterized by a creeping or crawling sensation that most frequently affects movements in sleep; it is also called nocturnal myoclonus and causes intense and repetitive muscle jerking during sleep. Treatment with 100 to 200 mg of levodopa, levodopa plus benserazide, bromocriptine, or piribedil has been reported to be beneficial in managing both movement disorders.

Dystonia is characterized by an exaggerated posturing of the head, neck, or jaw; by spastic contraction of the muscles of the lips, tongue, face, or throat, which makes drinking, eating, swallowing, and speech difficult; by torticollis, retrocollis, opisthotonus, distress, and ultimately anoxia. Neuroleptic-induced dystonia, which may occur in children treated actively with phenothiazine derivatives for their antiemetic properties, disappears in sleep and is treated effectively with diphenhydramine hydrochloride (Benadryl), which possesses both anticholinergic and antihistaminic properties.

Parkinsonian symptoms may be characterized by postural instability, stooped posture, shuffling and festinating gate, or rigidity, due to enhanced muscle tone with, at times, "cogwheel" or "ratchet" resistance to passive movements in any direction. There is also tremor at rest with regular rhythmic oscillations of the extremities, especially in the hands and fingers as well as akinesia (poverty of movement) or bradykinesia (slowness in initiating volitional activities). These symptoms, which are due to blockade of dopaminergic receptor sites in the striatum, are lessened by reducing the dosage of neuroleptics and by the oral administration of anticholinergic compounds such as trihexyphenidyl hydrochloride (Artane) or benztropine mesylate (Cogentin).

Tardive dyskinesia, which was initially called persistent dyskinesia or reversible drug-related dyskinesia, is characterized by abnormal involuntary movements frequently involving the facial, buccal, and masticatory muscles, and often extending to the upper and lower extremities, including the neck, trunk, fingers, and toes. For example, the typical abnormal facial movements include opening, protrusion, and retrieval of the tongue then closing of the mouth, chewing, licking, sucking, puckering, smacking, panting, and grimacing. Abnormal movements associated with the disorder, which may involve any part of the body, may be ballistic, athetotic, myoclonic, dyskinetic, or choreiform. The neuroleptic-induced dyskinesias, which have been reported and studied extensively in adult patients, also occur in children. It is generally believed that the pathogenesis of tardive dyskinesia relates closely to the ongoing blockade of dopamine receptor sites, which is the opposite of receptor desensitization. With continuous blockade, the dopaminergic receptors in the striatum upregulate. Following the discontinued use of neuroleptics or a reduction in dosage, the dyskinesia becomes apparent. In the therapeutic management of neuroleptic-induced tardive dyskinesia, reserpine, lithium, diazepam, baclofen (see Figure 29), and gamma-vinyl-gamma-aminobutyric acid (vigabatrin) (see Figure 104) have all been used with unsatisfactory results. Therefore, in the absence of an effective treatment, the best prevention of tardive dyskinesia is to prescribe the neuroleptics at their lowest possible doses, have patients observe drug-free holidays, and avoid prescribing anticholinergic agents solely to prevent parkinsonism.

Neuroleptic Malignant Syndrome

Among the complications of neuroleptic chemotherapy, the most serious and potentially fatal complication is malignant syndrome, which is characterized by extreme hyperthermia; "lead pipe" skeletal muscle rigidity that causes dyspnea, dysphagia, and rhabdomyolysis; autonomic instability; fluctuating consciousness; leukeocytosis; and elevated creatine phosphokinase levels.

The treatment of neuroleptic malignant syndrome consists of immediately discontinuing the neuroleptic agent and administering dantrolene sodium and dopamine-function-enhancing substances such as levodopa-carbidopa, bromocriptine, or amantadine.

Phenothiazine derivatives potentiate the CNS-depressing effects of alcohol and barbiturates and shorten the onset of action of anesthetics.

CHLORPROPAMIDE

(Diabinese)

Chlorpropamide (250 mg/day), an oral hypoglycemic agent, is indicated in the treatment of diabetic patients (see Table 1 and Figure 54). Oral hypoglycemic agents have advantages over insulin because, by releasing insulin and by decreasing the release of glucagon, they mimic physiologic processes and cause fewer allergic reactions. Furthermore, they are effective in an oral form, thus eliminating the need for daily injections. The properties of chlorpropamide are compared in Table 1 with other orally administered hypoglycemic agents. The mechanisms that underlie the hypoglycemic actions of sulfonylureas are:

- Pancreatic
    - Improved insulin secretion
    - Reduced glucagon secretion
- Extrapancreatic
    - Improved tissue sensitivity to insulin
- Direct
    - Increased receptor binding
    - Improved post-binding action
- Indirect
    - Reduced hyperglycemia
    - Decreased plasma free fatty-acid concentrations
    - Reduced hepatic insulin extraction

Sulfonylurea oral hypoglycemic agents bind to sulfonylurea receptors located on the surface of beta cells and trigger insulin releases at nanomolar concentrations (Figure 54). Sulfonylureas bind to ATP-sensitive potassium channels and inhibit potassium efflux through these channels. The inhibition of ATP-sensitive potassium channels then leads to depolarization of the beta cell; this opens voltage-dependent calcium channels and allows the entry of extracellular calcium. The rising level of cytosolic free calcium next triggers the release of insulin. An increase in the cyclic adenosine monophosphate levels in the cells can also open the voltage-dependent calcium channels, thus increasing calcium influx into the cells.

CHLORPROTHIXENE

(Taractan)

Chlorprothixene (25 to 50 mg p.o. t.i.d.) is indicated in the management of manifestations of psychotic disorders. Chlorprothixene is absorbed rapidly, distributed throughout the body, is bound to plasma protein to the extent of 90 to 95%, and is excreted mostly unchanged via the biliary tract in feces. It exerts its antipsychotic effects in part by blocking dopamine receptors in the mesolimbic and mesocortical systems; and like chlorpromazine, it produces movement disorders such as parkinsonism (see also Table 2).

CHLORTETRACYCLINE HYDROCHLORIDE

(Aureomycin)

Chlortetracycline (see Tetracycline) is an antibiotic available for eye, ear, nose, and throat preparation. For example, it is available as 1% ointment to treat conjunctivitis and blepharitis. Chlortetracycline, like other tetracyclines, possesses a wide range of antimicrobial activity against aerobic and anaerobic Gram-positive and Gram-negative bacteria, which overlaps that of many other antimicrobial drugs. They also are effective against some microorganisms that are resistant to cell-wall-active antimicrobial agents, such as *Rickettsia, Coxiella burnetii, Mycoplasma pneumoniae, Chlamydia* spp., *Legionella* spp., *Ureaplasma*, some atypical mycobacteria, and *Plasmodium* spp.

Tetracyclines are thought to inhibit bacterial protein synthesis by binding to the 30S bacterial ribosome and preventing access of aminoacryl tRNA to the acceptor site on the mRNA-ribosome complex (see also Figure 96).

CHLORTHALIDONE

(Hygroton)

Chlorthalidone in a dose of 50 to 100 mg daily is indicated in edema, and a dose of 25 mg/day is used in hypertension. The thiazide diuretics, also called sulfonamide or benzothiadiazide diuretics, vary in their actions. For instance, the potency of hydrochlorothiazide (Hydro-Diuril and Esidrix) is ten times greater than that of chlorothiazide (Diuril), but the two drugs have equal efficacy. The duration of action of hydrochlorothiazide, which is 6 to 12 hours, is equal to that of chlorothiazide. On the other hand, chlorthalidone has a duration of action lasting 48 hours. Some thiazide derivatives inhibit carbonic anhydrase, which is unrelated to their diuretic activity. Those that are active in this respect may, at sufficient doses, have the same effect on bicarbonate excretion as does acetazolamide. They cause a moderate loss of sodium (5 to 10% of the filtered load), chloride, and water, and the clearance of free water is impaired. The loss of potassium can produce hypokalemia, which is particularly dangerous in patients receiving digitalis because it increases the risk of arrhythmias. Hypokalemia can be offset either by giving a potassium supplement (potassium chloride), or by the concurrent use of a potassium-sparing diuretic. However, both measures should not be adopted together because hyperkalemia will result. Hyperglycemia is a potential hazard for patients with diabetes mellitus. Hyperuricemia can precipitate an acute attack of gout, but usually only in those patients who either have already had gout or have a propensity toward it. Because thiazides can cause a decrease in the GFR, they should not be used in patients whose renal function is less than one third of normal. The risk of thiazide-induced hypercalcemia should be kept in mind in patients with conditions such as malignancies or hyperparathyroidism that are associated with hypercalcemia (see also Table 24).

CHLORZOXAZONE

(Paraflex, Parafon Forte DSC)

Chlorzoxazone, a benzoxazole derivative with skeletal muscle relaxant properties (250 to 750 mg p.o. t.i.d.), is used as an adjunct medication in the treatment of acute and painful musculoskeletal conditions.

CHOLERA VACCINE

Cholera vaccine is a suspension of killed *Vibrio cholerae* (each millimeter contains 8 units of Inaba and Ogawa serotypes) that is used for primary immunization.

CHOLESTYRAMINE

(Questran)

Cholestyramine is indicated as adjunctive therapy to diet for the reduction of elevated serum cholesterol in patients with primary hypercholesterolemia (elevated low-density lipoprotein [LDL] cholesterol) who do not respond adequately to diet. Similarly, it is indicated for the relief of pruritus associated with partial biliary obstruction. Cholestyramine is not absorbed but binds to bile acids in the intestine, whereupon it is eliminated. To replenish the lost bile acid, cholesterol is then converted to bile acid, and this lowers the level of cholesterol (see Figure 34). Cholestyramine has also been used in the treatment of cholestasis to control the intense pruritis. It reduces the LDL level in 4 to 7 days, and the maximum effect is seen in 14 days.

Besides binding to bile acid, cholestyramine binds to numerous other drugs used in the management of cardiovascular diseases, which may be taken along with it. These include chlorothiazide, phenylbutazone, phenobarbital, anticoagulants, digitalis, and fat-soluble vitamins (A, D, E,

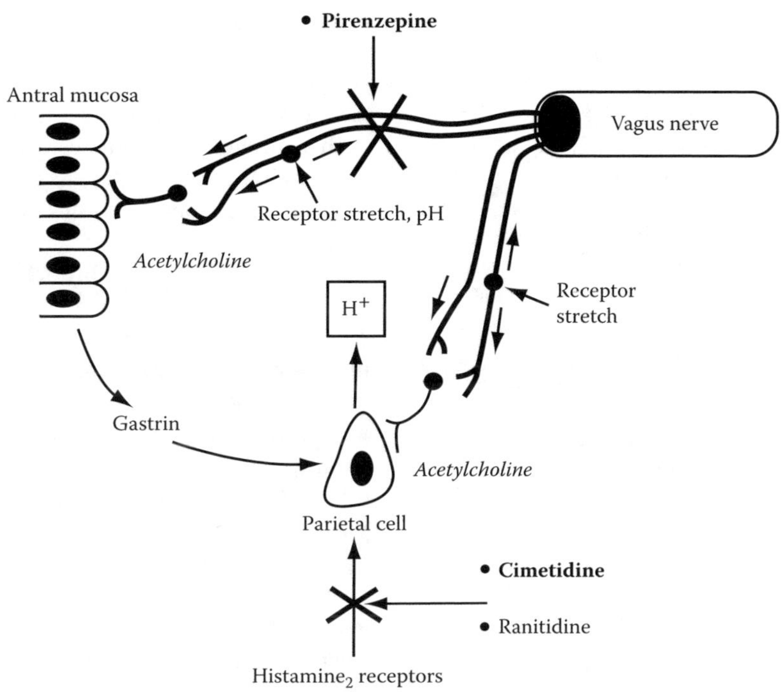

FIGURE 34 Clofibrate lowers serum triglyceride levels by accelerating catabolism of very-low-density lipoproteins.

and K). Consequently, these and similar agents should be taken 1 hour before or 4 hours after the administration of cholestyramine. Cholestyramine, which is given in large doses of 16 to 30 g per day, causes severe constipation.

CHOLINE MAGNESIUM TRISALICYLATE (Tricosal, Trilsate)

CHOLINE SALICYLATE (Arthropan)

Choline salicylate, a nonnarcotic analgesic, antipyretic, and antiinflammatory agent, is indicated in mild to moderate pain and fever, in arthritis, and in rheumatoid arthritis and osteoarthritis (see also Table 3).

CHOLINERGIC DRUGS: Uses in Medicine

Cholinomimetics

Glaucoma	**Urinary retention**
Carbachol	Bethanechol
Pilocarpine	

Muscarinic Cholinergic Receptor-Blocking Agents

Antispasmodics	**Cardiac/Pulmonary Disorders**
Atropine sulfate	Atropine sulfate
Clidinium bromide	Ipratropium bromide
Glycopyrrolate	**Mydriatic and Cycloplegic**
Isopropamide iodide	Atropine sulfate
l-hyoscyamine sulfate	Cyclopentolate hydrochloride
Methantheline bromide	Eucatropine hydrochloride
Methscopolamine bromide	Homatropine hydrobromide
Propantheline bromide	Scopolamine hydrobromide
Scopolamine hydrobromide	Tropicamide

Motion Sickness
Scopolamine hydrobromide
Anesthetic Premedication
Atropine sulfate
Glycopyrrolate
Scopolamine hydrobromide

Parkinson's Disease and Drug-induced Parkinsonism

Benztropine mesylate
Biperiden lactate
Procyclodine hydrochloride
Trihexyphenidyl hydrochloride

Cholinesterase Inhibitors

Myasthenia gravis	**Glaucoma**
Edrophonium chloride	Demecarium bromide
Neostigmine bromide	Echothiophate iodide
Pyridostigmine bromide	Isofluorophate
	Physostigmine sulfate

Autonomic drugs have extensive clinical applications. They are used in the treatment of wide-angle glaucoma, in the diagnosis of myasthenia gravis, as gastrointestinal and urinary tract stimulants in postoperative abdominal distention and urinary retention, as antidotes to poisoning from curare and the tricyclic antidepressants, as preanesthetic medications, as mydriatics, as cycloplegics, in peptic acid oversecretion to diminish the vagally mediated secretion of gastric juices, in slowing of gastric emptying, in vestibular disorders, in parkinsonism, in conjugation with local anesthetics, in hypotension and shock, in heart block to improve atrioventricular conduction and stimulate ventricular automaticity, in bronchial asthma, as a nasal decongestant, in narcolepsy, in attention deficit hyperactivity disorders, in the diagnosis and treatment of pheochromocytoma, in cardiac arrhythmias, in angina pectoris, in hypertension, in thyrotoxicosis, and in tremor. In addition, numerous drugs such as neuroleptics and antidepressants produce side effects by modifying the function of the autonomic nervous system.

CHOLINERGIC-RECEPTOR-BLOCKING AGENTS: Uses of

Tertiary Amines	
Adiphenine hydrobromide	Pyloric and biliary spasm, dysmenorrhea
Atropine sulfate	Preoperative medication; treatment of anticholinesterase poisoning
Benztropine methanesulfonate	Antagonizes extrapyramidal symptoms of the antipsychotics
Cyclopentolate	Mydriatic, cycloplegic
Dicyclomine	Alleviates gastrointestinal spasm, dysmenorrhea: pylorospasm, and biliary distention
Homatropine hydrobromide	Mydriatic and cycloplegic; anterior uveitis
Oxyphencyclimine	Antisecretory compound in peptic ulcer
Scopolamine hydrobromide	Preoperative medication
Trihexyphenidyl	Similar uses as benztropine methanesulfonate
Tropicamide	Mydriatic, cycloplegic
Quaternary Amines	
Atropine methylbromide (and methylnitrate)	Mydriatic, cycloplegic, antispasmodic in pyloric stenosis
Clidinium bromide	Spasmolytic in ulcer
Glycopyrrolate	Spasmolytic for ulcer therapy; preoperative medication
Homatropine methylbromide	In gastric acidity and spasm
Ipratropium	Chronic emphysema
Isopropamide iodine	In Zollinger–Ellison syndrome
Methantheline bromide	Spasmolytic to treat peptic ulcer
Methscopolamine bromide	Decreases gastric hyperacidity and hypermotility
Propantheline bromide	Spasmolytic in peptic ulcer
Tridihexethyl chloride	Antispasmodic, preoperative medication

CHOLINESTERASE INHIBITORS

Acetylcholine, an ester of choline and acetic acid, is synthesized in cholinergic neurons according to the following scheme:

$$\text{Acetyl CoA} + \text{choline} \xrightarrow{\text{Choline acetyltransferase}} \text{acetylcholine}$$

The acetylcholine, in turn, is hydrolyzed by both acetylcholinesterase and plasma butyrylcholinesterase. Choline is actively transported into nerve terminals (synaptosomes) by a high-affinity uptake mechanism. Furthermore, the availability of choline regulates the synthesis of acetylcholine (see Figure 12).

Hemicholinium blocks the transport of choline into synaptosome, whereas botulinum toxin blocks the calcium-mediated release of acetylcholine. The released acetylcholine is hydrolyzed rapidly by acetylcholinesterase to choline and acetate. The cholinesterase inhibitors are divided into two categories: organophosphorous compounds, such as parathion, malathion, and tetraethyl pyrophosphate (TEPP); and the carbamates, such as naphthyl-*N*-methyl carbamate (carbaryl and Sevin).

The clinical manifestations of acute and severe poisoning from the organophosphorous insecticides include cholinergic crisis, resulting from the stimulation of muscarinic cholinergic receptors (bronchoconstriction, salivation, sweating, lacrimation, bradycardia, hypotension, and urinary and fecal incontinence); the stimulation of nicotinic cholinergic receptors (bronchoconstriction, salivation, sweating, lacrimation, bradycardia, hypotension, and urinary and fecal incontinence); the stimulation of nicotinic cholinergic receptors (muscular fasciculation); and the CNS effects (with initial restlessness, tremors, ataxia, and convulsions, followed by CNS depression and respiratory and circulatory depression). The treatment of a cholinergic crisis caused by organophosphorous compounds includes the administration of a cholinesterase reactivator such as pralidoxime (2-PAM) together with atropine. The poisoning stemming from antidoting with 2-PAM can be avoided in the event of carbaryl toxicity because this agent is a reversible cholinesterase inhibitor (see Figure 79).

CHORIONIC GONADOTROPIN

(Chorex-10 powder for injection)

Chorionic is an ovulation stimulant, which stimulates production of gonadal steroid hormones by stimulating interstitial cells (Leydig cells) of the testis to produce androgens, and corpus luteum of the ovary to produce progesterone. Chorionic gonadotropin is indicated in prepubertal cryptorchidism not caused by anatomical obstruction; selected cases of hypogonadotropic hypogonadism (e.g., hypogonadism secondary to pituitary deficiency) in men; induction of ovulation in anovulatory, infertile women in whom the cause of anovulation is secondary and not caused by primary ovarian failure, and who have been appropriately pretreated with human menotropins.

Gonadotropins are purified from human urine or prepared using recombinant DNA technology. Several preparations of urinary gonadotropins have been developed. **Chorionic gonadotropin** (Pregnyl, Novarel, Profasi, others), which mimics the action of LH, is obtained from the urine of pregnant women. Urine from postmenopausal women is the source of menotropins (Pergonal, Repronex), which contain roughly equal amounts of FSH and LH, as well as a number of other urinary proteins. Because of their relatively low purity, menotropins are administered intramuscularly to decrease the incidence of hypersensitivity reactions. Urofollitropin (uFSH; Bravelle) is a highly purified FSH prepared by immunoconcentration with monoclonal antibodies and pure enough to be administered subcutaneously.

Recombinant preparations of gonadotropins are assuming an increasing role in clinical practice. Recombinant

FSH (rFSH) is prepared by expressing cDNAs encoding the α and β subunits of FSH in a mammalian cell line, yielding products whose glycosylation pattern mimics that of FSH produced by gonadotropes. The two rFSH preparations that are available (follitropin α [GONAL-F] and follitropin β [Puregon, Follistim]) differ slightly in their carbohydrate structures; both exhibit less inter-batch variability than do preparations purified from urine and can be administered subcutaneously because they are considerably purer. The recombinant preparations are more expensive than the naturally derived hormones, and their relative advantages (i.e., efficacy, lower frequency of side effects such as ovarian hyperstimulation) have not been definitively established despite much debate in the published literature.

Recombinant forms of hCG (**choriogonadotropin** alfa; Ovidrel) and LH (Luveris, Lhadi) also have been developed and are being investigated for the treatment of infertility. Providing that their cost–benefit ratios are favorable, it is likely that these recombinant gonadotropin preparations will have an increasing role in the future, possibly replacing the urinary preparations entirely. In addition, recombinant technology is likely to lead to improved forms of gonadotropins with increased half-lives or higher clinical efficacy.

CHORIONIC GONADOTROPIN, HUMAN (HCG)

(A.P.L., Chorex 5, Chorex 10, Chorigon, Choron 10, Corgonject 5, Follutein Gonic, Pregnyl, Profasi HP)

Chorionic gonadotropin, a gonadotropin with ovulation and spermatogenesis-stimulating properties (5,000 to 10,000 USP units IM), is indicated in the treatment of hypogonadotropic hypogonadism.

CHROMIC PHOSPHATE P 32

(Phosphocol P 32 suspension 15 mCi with a concentration of up to 5 mCi/mL)

Chromic is a radiopharmaceutical. It causes local irradiation by beta emission. Chromic phosphate P32 decays by beta emission with a physical half-life of 14.3 days. It is used in the treatment of peritoneal or pleural effusion caused by metastatic disease.

CHROMIUM

(Chromic Chloride injection 4 mcg/ml)

Chromium is a trace metal that helps maintain normal glucose metabolism and peripheral nerve function. It is used as a supplement to IV solutions given for total parenteral nutrition (TPN) to prevent depletion of endogenous stores and subsequent deficiency symptoms.

Nephrotoxicity is the principal dose-limiting side effect of intravenous **cidofovir**. Proximal tubular dysfunction includes proteinuria, azotemia, glycosuria, metabolic acidosis and, uncommonly, Fanconi's syndrome. Concomitant oral probenecid and saline prehydration reduce the risk of renal toxicity.

CHYMOPAPAIN

(Chymodiactin)

Chymopapain is a proteolytic enzyme with chemonucleolytic properties (2000 to 4000 pKat units per disk injected intradiskally). The maximum dose in a patient with multiple disk herniation is 8000 pKat units. The drug is indicated in the treatment of herniated lumbar intervertebral disk.

CICLOPIROX OLAMINE

(Loprox)

Ciclopirox olamine is indicated for the treatment of tinea pedis (athlete's foot), tinea cruris (jock itch), and tinea corporis (ringworm) due to *T. rubrum*, *T. mentagrophytes*, *E. floccosum*, and *M. canis*; for candidiasis (moniliasis) due to *C. albicans*; and for tinea (pityriasis) versicolor due to *M. fufur*. Loprox is available as 1% cream (water-miscible base, 1% benzyl alcohol mineral oil in 15, 30, and 90 g, and 1% lotion (water-miscible base, 1% benzyl alcohol, mineral oil, in 30 mL).

CIDOFOVIR

(Vistide injection 75 mg/mL)

Cidofovir is an antiviral agent that inhibits viral DNA synthesis by interfering with viral DNA polymerase. It is indicated in the treatment of Cytomegalovirus retinitis in patients with AIDS. Cidofovir (l-[(*S*)-3-hydroxy-2-(phosphonomethoxy)-propyl]cytosine dihydrate) is a cytidine nucleotide analog with inhibitory activity against human herpes, papilloma, polyoma, pox, and adenoviruses.

Viral infections of the skin are very common, and include verrucae [human papillomavirus (HPV)], herpes simplex (HSV), condyloma acuminatum (HPV), molluscum contagiosum (poxvirus), and chicken pox [varicella-zoster virus (VZV)]. Acyclovir (Zovirax), famciclovir (Famvir), and valacyclovir (Valtrex) frequently are used systemically to treat herpes simplex and varicella infections. Cidofovir (Vistide) may be useful in treating acyclovir-resistant HSV or VZV and other cutaneous viral infections. Topically, acyclovir, docosanol (Abreva), and penciclovir (Denavir) are available for treating mucocutaneous HSV. Podophyllin (25% solution) and podofilox (condylox; 0.5% solution) are used to treat condylomata.

CILOSTAZOL

(Pletal tablets 50 mg)

Cilostazol is an aggregations inhibitor that inhibits cellular phosphodiesterase and exhibits a higher specificity for phosphodiesterase III (PDE3). It is indicated in reduction of symptoms of intermittent claudication as indicated by an increased waling distance.

Most patients with peripheral vascular disease also have coronary artery disease, and the therapeutic approaches for peripheral and coronary arterial diseases overlap. Mortality in patients with peripheral vascular disease is most commonly due to cardiovascular disease, and treatment of coronary disease remains the central focus of therapy.

Many patients with advanced peripheral arterial disease are more limited by the consequences of peripheral ischemia than by myocardial ischemia. In the cerebral circulation, arterial disease may be manifest as stroke or transient ischemic attacks. The painful symptoms of peripheral arterial disease in the lower extremities (**claudication**) typically are provoked by exertion, with increases in skeletal muscle O_2 demand exceeding blood flow impaired by proximal stenoses. When flow to the extremities becomes critically limiting, peripheral ulcers and rest pain from tissue ischemia can become debilitating.

Most of the therapies shown to be efficacious for treatment of coronary artery disease also have a salutary effect on progression of peripheral artery disease. Reductions in cardiovascular morbidity and mortality in patients with peripheral arterial disease have been documented with antiplatelet therapy using aspirin or with ADP antagonists such as clopidogrel or ticlopidine, administration of ACE inhibitors, and treatment of hyperlipidemia. Interestingly, neither intensive treatment of diabetes mellitus nor antihypertensive therapy appears to alter the progression of symptoms of claudication. Other risk factor and lifestyle modifications remain cornerstones of therapy for patients with claudication: physical exercise, rehabilitation, and smoking cessation have proven efficacy. Drugs used specifically in the treatment of lower extremity claudication include **pentoxyfylline** and **cilostazol**. Pentoxyfylline is a methylxanthine derivative that has been termed a rheologic modifier for its effects on increasing the deformability of red blood cells. However, the effects of pentoxifylline on lower extremity claudication appear to be modest. Cilostazol is an inhibitor of PDE3 and promotes accumulation of intracellular cyclic AMP in many cells, including blood platelets. Cilostazol-mediated increases in cyclic AMP inhibit platelet aggregation and promote vasodilation.

Cilostazol treatment improves symptoms of claudication but has no effect on cardiovascular mortality. As a PDE3 inhibitor, cilostazol is placed in the same drug class as milrinone, which had been used as an inotropic agent for patients with heart failure. Milrinone therapy was associated with an increase in sudden cardiac death, and the drug was withdrawn from the market. Cilostazol, therefore, is contraindicated in patients with heart failure, although it is not clear that cilostazol itself leads to increased mortality in such patients. Cilostazol has been reported to increase nonsustained ventricular tachycardia; headache is the most common side effect. Other treatments for claudication, including **naftidrofuryl**, **proprionyl levocarnitine**, and prostaglandins, have been explored in clinical trials, and there is some evidence that some of these therapies may be efficacious.

CIMETIDINE

(Tagamet)

Cimetidine is indicated in treating duodenal ulcer, benign gastric ulcer, gastrointestinal reflux disease, pathological hypersecretory conditions, and in preventing upper GI bleeding in critically ill patients (Figure 35 and Table 10). There are two types of histamine receptors: H_1 receptors, which are blocked by agents such as diphenhydramine and other antiallergic compounds, and H_2 receptors, which are blocked by cimetidine, ranitidine (Zantac), famotidine (Pepcid), and nizatidine (Axid). Cimetidine has no effect on most H_1-receptor-mediated symptoms, such as bronchoconstriction.

The clinical use of H_2-receptor antagonists stems from their capacity to inhibit gastric acid secretion, especially in patients with peptic ulceration. Cimetidine, which is far more efficacious than anticholinergic drugs, is used in the treatment of duodenal ulcers and gastrinoma, and in patients

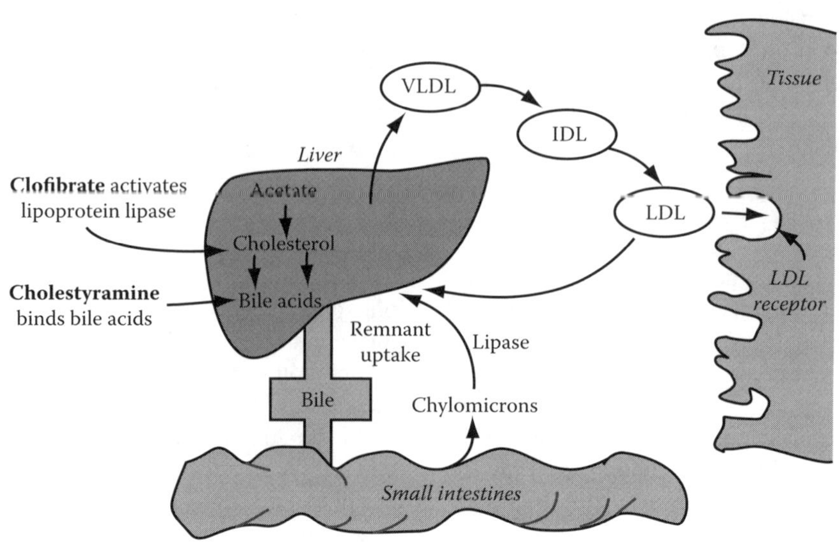

FIGURE 35 Cimetidine, a histamine$_2$-receptor antagonist, inhibits basal and nocturnal gastric acid secretion.

TABLE 10
Comparison of H_2-Receptor Antagonists

Actions	Cimetidine	Ranitidine	Famotidine
Ability to inhibit acid production	+++	+++	+++
Ability to inhibit pepsin	+++	+++	+++
Relative potency (in comparison to cimetidine)	1	5	32
Neuropsychiatric side effects	+	—	—
Pituitary stimulation	+	—	—
Antiandrogen effect	+	—	—
Inhibition of drug metabolism	++	+	—
Inhibition of cation transport	+	—	—
Frequency recommended for drug administration (doses per day)	4	2	1

suffering from gastroesophageal reflux disorders. It is absorbed orally, has a plasma half-life of 2 hours, and is excreted mainly unchanged by the kidney. Doses of cimetidine must be reduced in the presence of impaired renal function. The few and infrequent adverse effects of cimetidine use include gynecomastia (may bind to androgen receptor sites), galactorrhea (especially in patients with gastrinoma), granulocytopenia, agranulocytosis (very rare), mental confusion (especially in the elderly), restlessness, seizures, and reduced sperm count. Ranitidine is more effective than cimetidine and allegedly has fewer side effects.

CINACALCET HYDROCHLORIDE

(Sensipar tablets 30 mg)

Cinacalcet is a calcimimetic agent that lowers parathyroid hormone (PTH) levels by increasing sensing receptor to extracellular calcium. This drug is indicated in the treatment of secondary hyperparathyroidism in patients with chronic kidney disease on dialysis; and hypercalcemia in patients with parathyroid carcinoma.

Calcimimetics are drugs that mimic the stimulatory effect of calcium to inhibit PTH secretion by the parathyroid glands. By enhancing the sensitivity of the CaSR to extracellular Ca^{2+}, calcimimetics lower the concentration of Ca^{2+} at which PTH secretion is suppressed. The type II calcimimetics are phenylalkylamine derivatives that allosterically modulate the CaSR. **Cinacalcet** (Sensipar) is FDA approved for the treatment of secondary hyperparathyroidism owing to chronic renal disease and for patients with hypercalcemia associated with parathyroid carcinoma. **Cinacalcet** lowers serum PTH levels in patients with normal or reduced renal function. In clinical trials, cinacalcet at 20- to 100-mg doses lowered PTH levels in a concentration-dependent manner by 15 to 50%, and serum calcium × phosphate product by 7% compared with placebo. Cinacalcet also effectively reduced PTH in patients with primary hyperparathyroidism and provided sustained normalization of serum calcium without altering bone mineral density. Long-term control of PTH levels was achieved during a 2-year study of cinacalcet, suggesting that resistance does not develop.

Cinacalcet is available in 30-, 60-, and 90-mg tablets. Optimal doses have not been defined. The recommended starting dose for treatment of secondary hyperparathyroidism in patients with chronic kidney disease on dialysis is 30 mg once daily, with a maximum of 180 mg/day. For treatment of parathyroid carcinoma, a starting dose of 30 mg twice daily is recommended, with a maximum of 90 mg four times daily. The starting dose is titrated upward every 2 to 4 weeks to maintain the PTH level between 150 and 300 pg/mL (secondary hyperparathyroidism) or to normalize serum calcium (parathyroid carcinoma). The principal adverse event with cinacalcet is hypocalcemia. Thus, the drug should not be used if the initial serum calcium concentration is less than 8.4 mg/dL; serum calcium and phosphorus concentrations should be measured within 1 week, and PTH should be measured within 4 weeks after initiating therapy or after changing dosage.

Hypocalcemia can be diminished by initiating therapy with a low dose and gradually titrating it as necessary or adjusting the dose when vitamin D and/or phosphate binders are administered concomitantly. Patients on hemodialysis with low-calcium dialysate need to be monitored closely for hypocalcemia. Seizure threshold is lowered by significant reductions in serum Ca^{2+}, so patients with a history of seizure disorders should be monitored especially closely. Finally, adynamic bone disease may develop if the PTH level is less than 100 pg/mL, and the drug should be discontinued or the dose decreased if the PTH level falls below 150 pg/mL.

CINOXACIN

(Cinobac)

Cinoxacin, a quinolone antibiotic (1 g daily in 2 to 4 divided doses for 7 to 14 days), is indicated in initial and recurrent urinary tract infections caused by susceptible organisms (see also Figure 85).

The quinolones include: nalidixic acid (NegGram), cinoxacin, norfloxacin (Noroxin), and ciprofloxacin (Cipro). Other members of the quinolone family are pefloxacin, ofloxacin, enoxacin, and fleroxacin. The bacterial DNA gyrase is responsible for the continuous introduction of negative supercoils into DNA, and the quinolones inhibit this gyrase-mediated DNA supercoiling (see Figure 85).

Nalidixic acid and cinoxacin are bactericidal Gram-negative organisms that cause urinary tract infections. The fluoroquinolones are bactericidal and considerably more potent against *E. coli* and various species of *Salmonella*, *Shigella*, *Enterobacter*, *Campylobacter*, and *Neisseria*. Ciprofloxacin also has good activity against staphylococci, including methicillin-resistant strains. The quinolones and fluoroquinolones may produce arthropathy, and hence should not be used in prepubertal children or pregnant women.

Nalidixic acid and cinoxacin are useful only for treating urinary tract infections. Ciprofloxacin is useful for both urinary tract infections and prostatitis.

CIPROFLOXACIN

Lower respiratory tract infections account for a large proportion of prescribed antibiotics and, with emerging resistance to standard agents, the introduction of the fluoroquinolones, in particular ciprofloxacin, has provided a further component in the armamentarium. Ciprofloxacin is able to eradicate *S. pneumoniae, H. influenzae*, and *M. catarrhalis* readily. These findings suggest that the high respiratory tissue penetration of ciprofloxacin and the achievable minimum inhibitory concentrations lead to acceptable clinical outcomes in lower respiratory tract infections.

CIPROFLOXACIN

(Cipro tablets 100 mg)

Ciprofloxacin is a fluoroquinolone antibiotic that interferes with microbial DNA synthesis. It is indicated in the treatment of infections of the lower respiratory tract, skin and skin structure, bones and joints, urinary tract; gonorrhea, chancroid, and infectious diarrhea caused by susceptible strains of specific organisms; typhoid fever; uncomplicated cervical and urethral gonorrhea; women with acute uncomplicated cystitis; acute sinusitis; nosocomial pneumonia; chronic bacterial prostatitis; complicated intra-abdominal infections; reduction of incidence or progression of inhalational anthrax following exposure to aerosolized *Bacillus anthracis*. Cipro IV: Used for empirical therapy for febrile neutropenic patients.

The first quinolone, **nalidixic acid**, was isolated as a by-product of the synthesis of chloroquine. It has been available for the treatment of urinary tract infections for many years. The introduction of fluorinated 4-quinolones, such as **ciprofloxacin** (Cipro), moxifloxacin (Avelox), and gatifloxacin (Tequin) represents a particularly important therapeutic advance because these agents have broad antimicrobial activity and are effective after oral administration for the treatment of a wide variety of infectious diseases. Relatively few side effects appear to accompany the use of these fluoroquinolones, and microbial resistance to their action does not develop rapidly. Rare and potentially fatal side effects, however, have resulted in the withdrawal from the market of temafloxacin (immune hemolytic anemia), trovafloxacin (hepatotoxicity), grepafloxacin (cardiotoxicity), and clinafloxacin (phototoxicity). In all these cases, the side effects were so infrequent as to be missed by prerelease clinical trials and detected only by postmarketing surveillance.

Amoxicillin plus clavulanate is effective *in vitro* and *in vivo* for β-lactamase-producing strains of staphylococci, *H. influenzae*, gonococci, and *E. coli*. **Amoxicillin-clavulanate** plus **ciprofloxacin** has been shown to be an effective oral treatment for low-risk, febrile patients with neutropenia from cancer chemotherapy. It also is effective in the treatment of acute otitis media in children, sinusitis, animal or human bite wounds, cellulitis, and diabetic foot infections. The addition of clavulanate to ticarcillin (timentin) extends its spectrum such that it resembles imipenem to include aerobic Gram-negative bacilli, *S. aureus*, and *Bacteroides* spp. There is no increased activity against *Pseudomonas* spp. The dosage should be adjusted for patients with renal insufficiency. The combination is especially useful for mixed nosocomial infections and is used often with an aminoglycoside.

The quinolones include: nalidixic acid (NegGram), cinoxacin, norfloxacin (Noroxin), and ciprofloxacin (Cipro). Other members of the quinolone family are pefloxacin, ofloxacin, enoxacin, and fleroxacin. The bacterial DNA gyrase is responsible for the continuous introduction of negative supercoils into DNA, and the quinolones inhibit this gyrase-mediated DNA supercoiling (see Figure 85).

Nalidixic acid and cinoxacin are bactericidal Gram-negative organisms that cause urinary tract infections. The fluoroquinolones are bactericidal, and considerably more potent against *E. coli* and various species of *Salmonella, Shigella, Enterobacter, Campylobacter,* and *Neisseria*. Ciprofloxacin also has good activity against staphylococci, including methicillin-resistant strains. The quinolones and fluoroquinolones may produce arthropathy, and hence should not be used in prepubertal children or pregnant women.

Nalidixic acid and cinoxacin are useful only for treating urinary tract infections. Ciprofloxacin is useful for both urinary tract infections and prostatitis.

CIPROFLOXACIN HYDROCHLORIDE

(Ophthalmic) (Ciloxan)

Ciprofloxacin, a fluoroquinolone antibacterial agent (2 drops in the affected eye q. 15 minutes for the first six hours, then 2 drops q. 30 minutes for the remainder of the first day), is indicated for corneal ulcers caused by *P. aeruginosa, S. aureus, S. epidermidis, S. pneumoniae,* and possibly *Serratia marcescens* and *Streptococcus viridans*; and for bacterial conjunctivitis caused by *S. aureus* and *S. epidermidis*, and possibly *S. pneumoniae*.

CIPROFLOXACIN HYDROCHLORIDE/HYDROCORTISONE

(Cipro HC otic suspension 2mg ciprofloxacin, 10 mg hydrocortisone/mL)

Ciprofloxacin: interferes with microbial DNA synthesis. **Hydrocortisone:** depresses formation, release, and activity of endogenous mediators of inflammation as well as modifying the body's immune response. The combination is indicated in the treatment of acute otitis externa in adults and pediatric patients caused by susceptible strains of *P. aeruginosa*, *S. aureus*, and *Proteus mirabilis*.

CIRRHOSIS: Treatment of

Hepatic cirrhosis may be associated with portal hypertension, ascites, encephalopathy, spontaneous bacterial peritonitis, and hepatocellular carcinoma. Portal hypertension is directly responsible for the formation of esophageal varices, which may give rise to massive upper gastrointestinal bleeding. Therapy is aimed at correcting hypovolemic shock and at achieving hemostasis at the bleeding site.

Drug therapy is based on the use of agents that may decrease pressure and blood flow at the esophageal varices. This can be achieved either by the use of splanchnic vasoconstrictors (vasopressin, glypressin, or somatostatin), which decrease portal-collateral blood flow, or by drugs that decrease the vascular resistance at the intrahepatic and portal-collateral circulation (nitroglycerine), or by combination therapy. Terlipressin or glypressin is a synthetic vasopressin derivative with prolonged biological activity, which allows its administration as IV injections of 2 mg/4 hr until achieving a bleeding-free period of 24 to 48 hours.

Treatment of ascites is directed toward eliminating the intra-abdominal fluid by increasing urinary excretion of water and sodium with diuretics and through paracentesis and/or peritonea-venous shunt. The therapeutic approach to chronic hepatic encephalopathy is based on dietary protein restriction and the use of nonabsorbable disaccharides. Because spontaneous bacterial peritonitis may precipitate numerous potentially lethal complications (septic shock, progressive circulatory and renal impairment, liver failure), antibiotic administration must be started as soon as the diagnosis is established. The combination of an aminoglycoside, gentamicin or tobramycin, plus a β-lactam antibiotic, ampicillin or cefalotin, has been the most frequently used empiric antibiotic regimen in cirrhotic patients.

Hepatocellular carcinoma constitutes a frequent clinical program during the follow-up of cirrhotic patients requiring surgical treatment by liver transplantation, radiotherapy, or immunotherapy.

CISAPRIDE

(Propulsid)

Cisapride, a serotonin$_4$ receptor agonist (10 mg p.o. q.i.d.) with gastrointestinal prokinetic properties, is indicated in the symptomatic treatment of nocturnal heartburn due to gastroesophageal reflux disease.

CISATRACURIUM BESYLATE

(Nimbex injection 2 mg/mL)

Cisatracurium is a nondepolarizing neuromuscular blocking agent that binds competitively to cholinergic receptors on the motor end-plate to antagonize action of acetylcholine, resulting in block of neuromuscular transmission. Cisatracurium is indicated in intermediate-onset/intermediate-duration neuromuscular blockade for inpatients and outpatients as an adjunct to general anesthesia, to facilitate tracheal intubation, and to provide skeletal muscle relaxation during surgery or mechanical ventilation.

CISPLATIN

(Cis-Platinum) (Platinol, Platinol AQ)

Cisplatin, an alkylating agent, is indicated as an adjunctive therapy in metastatic testicular cancer; adjunctive therapy in metastatic ovarian cancer, head and neck cancers, lung cancer, and esophageal cancer, and in the treatment of advanced bladder cancer (see also Figure 15).

CITALOPRAM

Citalopram, a new serotonin uptake inhibitor (20 to 60 mg) is an effective antidepressant. Together with fluoxetine, fluvoxamine, paroxetine, and sertraline, it belongs to the group of selective serotonin reuptake inhibiting (SSRI) antidepressants (see also Tables 5 through 7 and Figure 51).

CITALOPRAM

(Celexa tablets 20 mg)

Citalopram is a selective serotonin reuptake inhibitor, that inhibits the CNS neuronal uptake of serotonin, potentiating serotonergic activity. It is used in depression.

The metabolism of most antidepressants is greatly dependent on hepatic activity. Most tricyclic antidepressants are extensively oxidized by CYP1A2. **Citalopram**, imipramine, and the meta-chlorophenylpiperidine metabolite of trazodone and nefazodone are substrates for CYP2C19, whereas duloxetine, mirtazapine, paroxetine, trazodone, and some tricyclics are substrates for CYP2D6. Nefazodone and some tricyclic and SSRI antidepressants are oxidized by CYP3A3/4. In general, CYP1A2 and CYP2D6 mediate aromatic hydroxylation, and CYP3A3/4 mediate *N*-dealkylation and *N*-oxidation reactions in the metabolism of antidepressants.

Some antidepressants not only are substrates for metabolism by CYPs but also can inhibit the metabolic clearance of other drugs, sometimes producing clinically significant drug–drug interactions. Notable inhibitory interactions include fluvoxamine with CYP1A2; fluoxetine and fluvoxamine with CYP2C9, and fluvoxamine with CYP1A2 and CYP2C19; paroxetine, fluoxetine and, less actively, sertraline with CYP2D6; norfluoxetine with CYP3A4; and fluvoxamine and nefazodone with CYP3A3/4. **Citalopram** or *S*-citalopram and venlafaxine interact much less with CYPs. Atomoxetine has weak effects on the metabolism of most other agents, but its clearance is inhibited by some SSRIs including paroxetine. Duloxetine can inhibit the metabolism of agents such as desipramine that are metabolized extensively through CYP2D6, and its own metabolism is inhibited by some SSRIs including paroxetine.

Potentially clinically significant interactions include the tendency for fluvoxamine to increase circulating concentrations of oxidatively metabolized benzodiazepines, clozapine, theophylline, and warfarin. Sertraline and fluoxetine can increase levels of benzodiazepines, clozapine, and warfarin. Paroxetine increases levels of clozapine, theophylline, and warfarin. Fluoxetine also potentiates tricyclic antidepressants and some class IC antiarrhythmics with a narrow therapeutic index (including encainide, flecainide, and propafenone). Nefazodone potentiates benzodiazepines other than lorazepam and oxazepam.

CLADRIBINE

(Leustatin Solution for Injection 1 mg/mL)

Cladribine is a purine analog. The selective toxicity of cladribine toward certain normal and malignant lymphocyte and monocyte populations is based on the relative activities of deoxycytidine kinase, deoxynucleoridase, and adenosine deaminase. In cells with a high ratio of deoxycytidine kinase to deoxynucleotidase, cladribine passively crosses the cell membrane. Cladribine is cytotoxic to actively dividing and quiescent lymphocytes and monocytes, inhibiting DNA synthesis and repair. Cladribine is used in hairy cell leukemia. Purine analogs, naturally occurring purine base, have antileukemic and immunosuppressant properties. In addition, studies on purine analogs have led to discovery of drug immunosuppresion (**azathioprine**) and antiviral chemotherapy (**acyclovir, ganciclovir, vidarabine, and zidovudine**). The hypoxanthine analog allopurinol, a potent inhibitor of xanthine oxidase, used in gout, is an important by-product of this effort. Other purine analogs have found important use in cancer therapy. These include **pentostatin** (2′-deoxycoformcycin), the first effective agent against hairy cell leukemia. Pentostatin has largely been replaced by another adenosine analog, **cladribine**, whereas the closely related fludarabine phosphate has become a standard treatment for chronic lymphocytic leukemia (CLL) and follicular lymphomas.

Cladribine (Leustatin) is administered as a single course of 0.09 mg/kg per day for 7 days by continuous intravenous infusion. Cladribine is considered the drug of choice in hairy cell leukemia. Eighty percent (80%) of patients achieve a complete response after a single course of therapy. The drug also is active in CLL, and is a secondary agent in other leukemias and low-grade lymphomas, Langerhans cell histiocytosis, cutaneous T-cell lymphomas including mycosis fungoides and the Sézary syndrome, and Waldenström's macroglobulinemia.

The major dose-limiting toxicity of cladribine is myelosuppression. Cumulative thrombocytopenia may occur with repeated courses. Opportunistic infections are common and are correlated with decreased $CD4^+$ cell counts. Other toxic effects include nausea, infections, high fever, headache, fatigue, skin rashes, and tumor lysis syndrome. Neurological and immunosuppressive adverse effects are less evident than with **pentostatin** at clinically active doses. Pentostatin, a transition-state analog of the intermediate in the adenosine deaminase (ADA) reaction, is a potent inhibitor of ADA. Its effects mimic the phenotype of genetic ADA deficiency, which is associated with severe immunodeficiency affecting both T- and B-cell functions. It was isolated from fermentation cultures of *Streptomyces antibioticus*. Inhibition of ADA by pentostatin leads to accumulation of intracellular adenosine and deoxyadenosine nucleotides, which can block DNA synthesis by inhibiting ribonucleotide reductase. Deoxyadenosine also inactivates *S*-adenosyl homocysteine hydrolase. The resulting accumulation of *S*-adenosyl homocysteine is particularly toxic to lymphocytes. Pentostatin also can inhibit RNA synthesis, and its triphosphate derivative is incorporated into DNA, resulting in strand breakage. In combination with 2′-deoxyadenosine, it is capable of inducing apoptosis in human monocytoic leukemia cells. Although the precise mechanism of cytotoxicity is not known, it is probable that the imbalance in purine nucleotide pools account for its antineoplastic effect in hairy cell leukemia and T-cell lymphomas.

Cladribine, a purine nucleoside analog, with antineoplastic properties (0.09 mg/kg daily by continuous IV infusion for 7 days), is indicated in the treatment of active hairy cell leukemia. In addition, it has been used in advanced cutaneous T-cell lymphomas, chronic lymphocytic leukemia, non-Hodgkin's lymphomas, acute myeloid leukemias, autoimmune hemolytic anemia, mycosis fungoides, or Sezary syndrome (see also Figure 15).

Cladribine has been designed to stimulate the immunodeficiency state of hereditary adenosine deaminase by causing the accumulation of deoxynucleotides in lymphocytes. Cladribine, an immunosuppressive drug, stabilizes the condition of patients with chronic progressive multiple sclerosis.

CLARITHROMYCIN

(Biaxin tablets 250 mg)

Clarithromycin is an *H. pylori* agent/macrolide, which inhibits microbial protein synthesis. Clarithromycin is indicated in the treatment of infections of the respiratory tract, skin and skin structure; treatment of disseminated atypical mycobacterial infections caused by susceptible strains of specific microorganisms; and prevention of disseminated *Mycobacterium avium* complex disease in patients with advanced HIV infection. Clarithromycin in combination with omeprazole is indicated in the treatment of patients with an active duodenal ulcer associated with *H. pylori* infection. In children it is used in acute otitis media. Macrolides are erythromycin, **clarithromycin**, and azithromycin.

Macrolide antibiotics contain a many-membered lactone ring (14-membered rings for erythromycin and clarithromycin, and a 15-membered ring for azithromycin) to which are attached one or more deoxy sugars. **Clarithromycin** differs from erythromycin only by methylation of the hydroxyl group at the 6 position, and **azithromycin** differs by the addition of a methyl-substituted nitrogen atom into the lactone ring. These structural modifications improve acid stability and tissue penetration and broaden the spectrum of activity.

Erythromycin usually is bacteriostatic, but may be bactericidal in high concentrations against very susceptible organisms. The antibiotic is most active *in vitro* against aerobic Gram-positive cocci and bacilli. Susceptible strains of *S. pyogenes, S. pneumoniae*, and viridans streptococci have MICs that range from 0.015 to 1 μg/mL. Macrolide resistance is common among streptococci. Because the mechanisms producing resistance to erythromycin affect all macrolides, cross-resistance among them is complete. The prevalence of macrolide resistance among group A streptococcal isolates, which can be as high as 40%, is related to consumption of macrolide antibiotics within the population. Macrolide resistance among *S. pneumoniae* often coexists with penicillin resistance. Only 5% of penicillin-susceptible strains are macrolide-resistant, whereas 50% or more of penicillin-resistant strains may be macrolide-resistant. Staphylococci are not reliably sensitive to erythromycin. Macrolide-resistant strains of *S. aureus* are potentially cross-resistant to clindamycin and streptogramin B (quinupris tin). Gram-positive bacilli also are sensitive to erythromycin; typical MICs are 1 μg/mL for *Clostridium perfringens*, from 0.2 to 3 μg/mL for *Corynebacterium diphtheriae*, and from 0.25 to 4 μg/mL for *Listeria monocytogenes*.

Clarithromycin is slightly more potent than erythromycin against sensitive strains of streptococci and staphylococci, and has modest activity against *H. influenzae* and *N. gonorrhoeae*. **Clarithromycin** has good activity against *M. catarrhalis, Chlamydia* spp., *L. pneumophila, B. burgdorferi, Mycoplasma pneumoniae,* and *H. pylori*.

Azithromycin generally is less active than erythromycin against Gram-positive organisms and slightly more active than either erythromycin or clarithromycin against *H. influenzae* and *Campylobacter* spp. Azithromycin is very active against *M catarrhalis, P. multocida, Chlamydia* spp., *M. pneumoniae, L. pneumophila, B. burgdorferi, Fusobacterium* spp., and *N. gonorrhoeae*. Erythromycin and **clarithromycin** inhibit CYP3A4 and are associated with clinically significant drug interactions. Erythromycin potentiates the effects of carbamazepine, corticosteroids, cyclosporine, digoxin, ergot alkaloids, theophylline, triazolam, valproate, and warfarin, probably by interfering with CYP-mediated metabolism of these drugs. Clarithromycin, which is structurally related to erythromycin, has a similar drug interaction profile. Azithromycin, which differs from erythromycin and clarithromycin because of its 15-membered lactone ring structure, and dirithromycin, which is a longer-acting 14-membered lactone ring analog of erythromycin analog, appear to be free of these drug interactions. Caution is advised, nevertheless, when using azithromycin in conjunction with drugs known to interact with erythromycin.

CLARITHROMYCIN

(Biaxin Filmtabs)

Clarithromycin, a macrolide antibiotic, is indicated in the treatment of pharyngitis or tonsillitis caused by *S. pyogenes*, acute maxillary sinusitis caused by *S. pneumoniae*, acute exacerbations of chronic bronchitis caused by *M. (Branhamella) catarrhalis* or *S. pneumoniae*, pneumonia caused by *S. pneumoniae* or *Mycoplasma pneumoniae*, acute exacerbations of chronic bronchitis caused by *H. influenzae*, and uncomplicated skin and skin-structure infections caused by *Staphylococcus aureus, Streptococcus aureus*, or *S. pyogenes*.

CLEMASTINE FUMARATE

(Dayhist-1 tablets 1.34 mg as fumarate)
(Tavist, Tavist-1)

Clemastine competitively antagonizes histamine at H_1-receptor sites and is indicated in the relief of symptoms associated with allergic rhinitis or other upper respiratory allergies, such as sneezing, rhinorrhea, pruritus, and lacrimation; and relief of mild, uncomplicated allergic skin manifestation of urticaria and angioedema.

CLIDINIUM BROMIDE

(Quarzan)

Clidinium, an anticholinergic agent with gastrointestinal, antispasmodic properties (2.5 to 5.0 mg p.o. t.i.d.), is indicated as an adjunctive therapy for peptic ulcers (see also Figure 12).

CLINDAMYCIN

(Cleocin vaginal ovules 100 mg, vaginal cream 2%)

Clindamycin is an antibiotic/antiinfective/lincosamide, which suppresses bacterial protein synthesis. It is indicated in the treatment of serious infections caused by susceptible strains of anaerobes, streptococci, staphylococci, and pneumococci; treatment of acne vulgaris (topical use); treatment of bacterial vaginosis (vaginal use) in nonpregnant women and second- or third-trimester pregnant women (Cleocin and ClindaMax only).

Clindamycin binds exclusively to the 50S subunit of bacterial ribosomes and suppresses protein synthesis. Although clindamycin, erythromycin, and chloramphenicol are not structurally related, they act at sites in close proximity, and binding by one of these antibiotics to the ribosome may inhibit the interaction of the others. There are no clinical indications for the concurrent use of these antibiotics. Macrolide resistance due to ribosomal methylation by encoded enzymes also may produce resistance to clindamycin. However, because clindamycin does not induce the methylase, there is cross-resistance only if the enzyme is produced constitutively. Clindamycin is not a substrate for macrolide efflux pumps; thus, strains that are resistant to macrolides by this mechanism are susceptible to clindamycin. Altered metabolism occasionally causes clindamycin resistance.

The reported incidence of diarrhea associated with the administration of **clindamycin** ranges from 2 to 20%. A number of patients (variously reported as 0.01 to 10%) have developed pseudomembranous colitis caused by the toxin from the organism *C. difficile*. This colitis is characterized by abdominal pain, diarrhea, fever, and mucus and blood in the stools. Proctoscopic examination reveals white-to-yellow plaques on the mucosa of the colon. This syndrome may be lethal. Discontinuation of the drug, combined with administration of metronidazole orally or intravenously, usually is curative, but relapses can occur. Agents that inhibit peristalsis, such as opioids, may prolong and worsen the condition.

Skin rashes occur in approximately 10% of patients treated with clindamycin, and may be more common in patients with HIV infection. Other reactions, which are uncommon, include exudative erythema multiforme (Stevens–Johnson syndrome), reversible elevation of aspartate aminotransferase and alanine aminotransferase, granulocytopenia, thrombocytopenia, and anaphylactic reactions. Local thrombophlebitis may follow intravenous administration of the drug. Clindamycin can inhibit neuromuscular transmission and may potentiate the effect of a neuromuscular blocking agent administered concurrently.

CLINDAMYCIN HYDROCHLORIDE
(Cleocin HCL)

CLINDAMYCIN PALMITATE HYDRCHLORIDE
(Cleocin Pediatric)

CLINDAMYCIN PHOSPHATE
(Cleocin)

Clindamycin, an aminoglycoside, is indicated in serious respiratory tract infections such as emphysema, anaerobic pneumonitis, and lung abscess; serious skin and soft-tissue infections; septicemia; intra-abdominal infections such as peritonitis and intra-abdominal abscess; infections of the female pelvis and genital tract such as endometriosis, nongonococcal tubo-ovarian abscess, pelvic cellulitis, and postsurgical vaginal cuff infection.

Aminoglycosides are bactericidal, and inhibit protein synthesis in susceptible microorganisms (see Figure 88). They exert this effect by (1) interfering with the initiation complex of peptide formation, (2) inducing the misreading of the code on the messenger RNA template, which causes the incorporation of inappropriate amino acids into peptides, and (3) rupturing the polysomes into monosomes, which become nonfunctional (see Figure 88). Resistance to aminoglycosides may be due to one or a combination of the following mechanisms:

- Interference with the transport of aminoglycosides into bacterial cells
- Deletion of receptors on the 30S ribosomal subunit, thus preventing the functioning of aminoglycosides
- The bacterial biotransformation of aminoglycosides to inactive forms

In addition, because the initial transport of aminoglycosides into bacterial cells is an oxygen-dependent process, microorganisms that are able to grow under anaerobic conditions show or develop resistance. Aminoglycosides are poorly absorbed from the gastrointestinal tract, and, for this reason, they are administered intramuscularly. Furthermore, because they do not penetrate the CNS, they may have to be given intrathecally or intraventricularly in the treatment of meningitis. Aminoglycosides are excreted by glomerular filtration, which is greatly reduced in the presence of renal impairment, thus leading to toxic blood levels.

The most serious reactions following aminoglycoside therapy are cochlear damage and vestibular impairment, which lead to vertigo and disturb the ability to maintain postural equilibrium. Aminoglycosides given during pregnancy cause deafness in the newborn. Nephrotoxicity and reversible neuromuscular blockade causing respiratory paralysis have also been seen following the use of high doses.

The neuromuscular blocking effects of depolarizing and nondepolarizing agents are enhanced by aminoglycosides, and prolonged respiratory depression may occur.

CLINDAMYCIN PHOSPHATE
(Cleocin Phosphate, Cleocin T)

Clindamycin, a lincomycin derivative (150 to 450 mg p.o. q. 6 hours), is indicated in infections caused by sensitive organisms.

CLOBAZAM

Clobazam, a 1,5-benzodiazepine derivative, is indicated in the management of ambulant patients with anxiety. Clobazam lacks sedative and amnestic effects, and does not cause impairment of psychomotor skills (see also Table 9).

CLOBETASOL PROPIONATE
(Temovate) (Clobex lotion 0.05%)

Clobetasol is a topical corticosteroid with antiinflammatory, antipruritic, and vasoconstrictive properties. It is thought to act by inducing phospholipase A_2 inhibitory proteins, thus controlling biosynthesis of potent mediators of inflammation. Clobetasol is indicated in the relief of inflammatory and pruritic manifestations of corticosteroid-responsive dermatoses; and moderate to severe plaque-type psoriasis (Olux foam, Clobex lotion, Temovate E cream).

CLOFARABINE
(Clolar solution for injection 1 mg/mL)

Clofarabine is a purine analog that inhibits DNA synthesis by decreasing cellular deoxynucleotide triphosphate pools by an inhibitory action on ribonucleotide reductase, and by terminating DNA chain elongation and inhibiting repair through incorporation into the DNA chain by competitive inhibition of DNA polymerases. Clofarabine is indicated in the treatment of patients 1 to 21 years of age with relapsed or refractory acute lymphoblastic leukemia after at least two prior regimens.

CLOFAZIMINE
(Lamprene)

Clofazimine, a substituted aminophenazine dye with leprostatic properties (50 to 100 mg p.o. once daily), is indicated in the treatment of dapsone-resistant leprosy and erythema nodosum leprosum.

CLOFIBRATE

(Atromid S)

Clofibrate is indicated in the treatment of primary dysbetalipoproteinemia (type III hyperlipidemia) not responding to diet. Clofibrate (Atromid S) reduces VLDL, triglyceride, and cholesterol levels (Figure 34). It does not inhibit cholesterol synthesis. Its primary mechanism of action is activation of lipoprotein lipase. Clofibrate is also considered effective in patients with elevated VLDL levels, especially those who do not respond to dietary restrictions. Because clofibrate displaces coumarin and phenytoin from binding sites, the prothrombin time should be checked on a regular basis in patients who are taking both agents. A flu-like syndrome, characterized by muscular cramps, tenderness, stiffness, and weakness, may occur in some patients.

CLOMIPHENE CITRATE

(Clomid tablets 50 mg)

Clomiphene is an ovulation stimulant that induces ovulation in selected anovulatory women. It is indicated in the treatment of ovulatory failure in women desiring pregnancy when the partner is fertile and potent. **Clomiphene** (Clomid, serophene, others) is approved for the treatment of infertility in anovulatory women, and **fulvestrant** is used for the treatment of breast cancer in women with disease progression after **tamoxifen**.

Clomiphene increases gonadotropin secretion and stimulates ovulation. It increases the amplitude of LH and FSH pulses with changing pulse frequency. This suggests that the drug is acting largely at the pituitary level to block inhibitory actions of estrogen on gonadotropin release from the gland, and and/or is somehow causing the hypothalamus to release larger amounts of GnRH per pulse.

Clomiphene is well absorbed following oral administration, and the drug and its metabolites are eliminated primarily in the feces, and to a lesser extent, in the urine. The long plasma half-life (5 to 7 days) is due largely to plasma-protein binding, enterohepatic circulation, and accumulation in fatty tissues. Other active metabolites with long half-lives also may be produced.

Fulvestrant is administered monthly by intramuscular depot injections. Plasma concentrations reach maximal levels in 7 days and are maintained for a month. Numerous metabolites are formed *in vivo*, possibly by pathways similar to endogenous estrogen metabolism, but the drug is eliminated primarily (90%) via the feces in humans.

Clomiphene is used primarily for treatment of female infertility due to anovulation. By increasing gonadotropin levels, primarily FSH, it enhances follicular recruitment. It is relatively inexpensive, orally active, and requires less extensive monitoring than do other treatment protocols. However, the drug may exhibit untoward effects, including ovarian hyperstimulation, increased incidence of multiple births, ovarian cysts, hot flashes, and blurred vision. In addition, **clomiphene**-induced cycles have a relatively high incidence of luteal phase dysfunction due to inadequate progesterone production, and prolonged use (e.g., 12 or more cycles) may increase the risk of ovarian cancer. The drug should not be administered to pregnant women due to reports of teratogenicity in animals, but there is no evidence of this when the drug has been used to induce ovulation. **Clomiphene** also may be used to evaluate the male reproductive system because testosterone feedback on the hypothalamus and pituitary is mediated to a large degree by estrogens formed from aromatization of the androgen.

CLOMIPHENE CITRATE

(Clomid)

Clomiphene citrate is indicated in the treatment of ovulatory failure. Clomiphene and tamoxifen (Nolvadex) modify or inhibit the actions of estrogens. They accomplish this by binding to the cytoplasmic estrogen receptors that are then translocated to the nucleus. By diminishing the number of estrogen-binding sites, they interfere with the physiologic actions of estrogens. Furthermore, by interfering with the normal hypothalamic and hypophyseal feedback inhibition of estrogen synthesis, these agents cause an increased stimulation of LHRH, follicle-stimulating hormone-releasing hormone (FSHRH), and gonadotropins. This leads to ovarian stimulation and ovulation. Clomiphene has been used successfully in some cases of infertility but causes multiple births. Antiestrogens are able to arrest the growth of estrogen-dependent malignant mammary cells. Clomiphene has been used in certain cases of disseminated breast cancer (see Figure 36).

CLOMIPRAMINE HYDROCHLORIDE

(Anafranil)

Clomipramine is indicated for the treatment of obsessive–compulsive disorder. It mildly blocks the uptake of norepinephrine, but strongly blocks the uptake of serotonin. In addition, clomipramine blocks $alpha_1$-adrenergic, H_1-histamine, and muscarinic cholinergic receptors. It lowers the seizure threshold and should be used cautiously in seizure disorders (see also Tables 5 through 7).

CLONAZEPAM

(Clonopin)

Clonazepam (1.5 mg/day in three divided doses) is used alone or as adjunctive treatment of Lennox–Gastaut syndrome (petit mal variance) and akinetic and myoclonic seizures. It may be used in patients with petit mal (absence) seizures who have failed to respond to succinamides. Clonazepam is actually a broad-spectrum anticonvulsant because it is also effective in tonic–clonic (grand mal) and complex partial (psychomotor-temporal lobe) seizures. Clonazepam causes drowsiness (increased by barbiturate administration) and a dose-dependent ataxia. In addition, behavioral abnormalities such as hypersensitivity, irritability, and aggression may occur, but these are mostly seen in children (see also Figure 50).

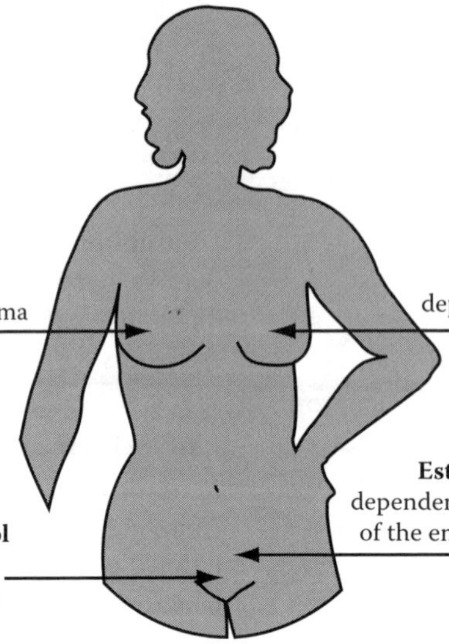

FIGURE 36 Clomiphene, an ovulation stimulant, is a partial estrogen receptor agonist.

CLONAZEPAM

(Klonopin tablets 0.5 mg)

Clonazepam is a benzodiazepine that potentiates action of GABA, inhibitory neurotransmitter, resulting in increased neuronal inhibition and CNS depression, especially in limbic system and reticular formation. It is indicated in the treatment of **Lennox–Gastaut syndrome**; management of akinetic and myoclonic seizures and absence seizures unresponsive to succinimides.

A large number of benzodiazepines have broad antiseizure properties, but only **clonazepam** (Klonopin) and **clorazepate** (Tranxene-SD, others) have been approved in the United States for the long-term treatment of certain types of seizures. **Diazepam** (Valium, Diastat, others) and **lorazepam** (Ativan) have well-defined roles in the management of **status epilepticus**.

The antiseizure actions of the benzodiazepines, as well as other effects that occur at nonsedating doses, result in large part from their ability to enhance GABA-mediated synaptic inhibition. Molecular cloning and study of recombinant receptors have demonstrated that the benzodiazepine receptor is an integral part of the $GABA_A$ receptor. At therapeutically relevant concentrations, benzodiazepines act at subsets of $GABA_A$ receptors and increase the frequency, but not duration, of openings at GABA-activated Cl channels. At higher concentrations, diazepam and many other benzodiazepines can reduce sustained high-frequency firing of neurons, similar to the effects of phenytoin, carbamazepine, and valproate. Although these concentrations correspond to concentrations achieved in patients during treatment of status epilepticus with diazepam, they are considerably higher than those associated with antiseizure or anxiolytic effects in ambulatory patients.

Clonazepam is useful in the therapy of absence seizures as well as myoclonic seizures in children. However, tolerance to its antiseizure effects usually develops after 1 to 6 months of administration, after which some patients will no longer respond to clonazepam at any dosage. The initial dose of **clonazepam** for adults should not exceed 1.5 mg per day, and for children 0.01 to 0.03 mg/µg per day. The dose-dependent side effects are reduced if two or three divided doses are given each day. The dose may be increased every 3 days in amounts of 0.25 to 0.5 mg per day in children and 0.5 to 1 mg per day in adults. The maximal recommended dose is 20 mg per day for adults and 0.2 mg/kg per day for children.

Although diazepam is an effective agent for treatment of status epilepticus, its short duration of action is a disadvantage, leading to the more frequent use of lorazepam. Although diazepam is not useful as an oral agent for the treatment of seizure disorders, clorazepate is effective in combination with certain other drugs in the treatment of partial seizures. The maximal initial dose of clorazepate is 22.6 mg per day in three portions for adults and 15 mg per day in two doses in children. Clorazepate is not recommended for children under the age of 9.

CLONIDINE HYDROCHLORIDE

(Catapress)

Clonidine stimulates $alpha_2$-adrenoreceptors in the brain stem, resulting in a reduced sympathetic outflow and a decrease in peripheral resistance (see Figure 37). Although clonidine is indicated in hypertension, it is being used and/or investigated for alcohol withdrawal, Gilles de la Tourette syndrome, methadone/opiate detoxification, neuralgia, and smoking cessation. Clonidine (0.1 mg b.i.d.) reduces blood pressure within 30 to 60 minutes, has a half-life of 12 to 16 hours, is metabolized partly in the liver, is excreted (50%) unchanged, and its half-life is increased to 30 to 40 hours in renal impairment. Treatment with clonidine should not be stopped abruptly because rebound hypertension occurs, and this effect may be greater in patients receiving beta-adrenergic-blocking agents.

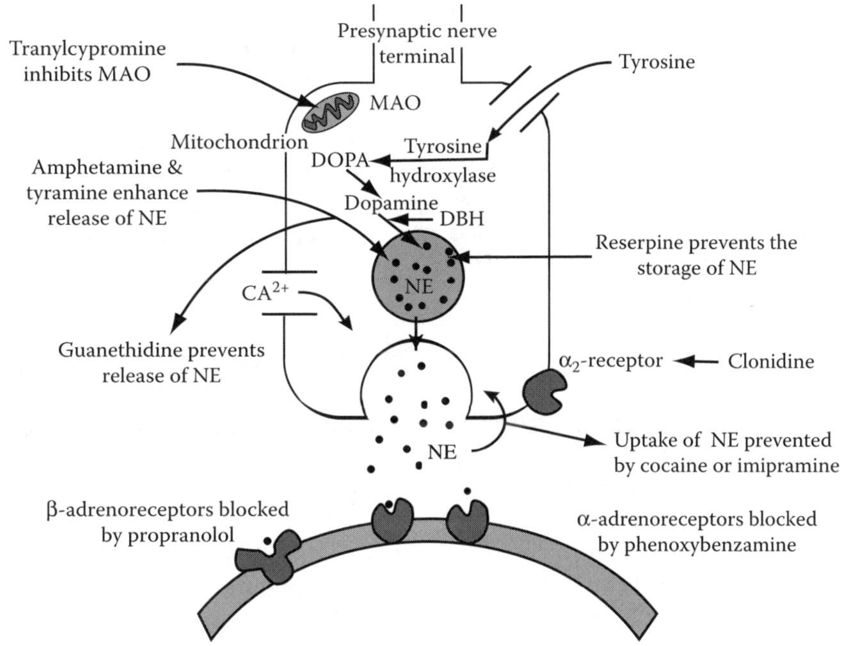

FIGURE 37 Clonidine, a centrally acting antiadrenergic agent, is used in treating hypertension.

Tricyclic antidepressants, which block the uptake sites for biogenic amines, may block the antihypertensive effects of clonidine.

Overdosage with clonidine causes bradycardia, hypotension, CNS depression, respiratory depression, hypothermia, apnea, and hypoventilation. Atropine sulfate is able to reverse bradycardia, and epinephrine, dopamine, or tolazine are effective in combating hypotension.

CLONIDINE HYDROCHLORIDE/ CHLORTHALIDONE

(Clorpres tablets 0.1 mg clonidine and 15 mg chlorthalidone)

Clonidine: stimulates central alpha-adrenergic receptors to inhibit sympathetic cardioaccelerator and vasoconstrictor centers. Chlorthalidone: inhibits reabsorption of the distal convoluted tubules. The combination is used in the treatment of hypertension. The major pharmacological effects of **clonidine** involve changes in blood pressure and heart rate, although the drug has a variety of other important actions. Intravenous infusion of clonidine causes an acute rise in blood pressure, apparently because of activation of postsynaptic α_2 receptors in vascular smooth muscle. The affinity of clonidine for these receptors is high, although the drug is a partial agonist with relatively low efficacy at these sites. The hypertensive response that follows parenteral administration of clonidine generally is not seen when the drug is given orally. However, even after intravenous administration, the transient vasoconstriction is followed by a more prolonged hypotensive response that results from decreased sympathetic outflow from the CNS. The exact mechanism by which clonidine lowers blood pressure is not completely understood. The effect appears to result, at least in part, from activation of α_2-receptors in the lower brain stem region. This central action has been demonstrated by infusing small amounts of the drug into the vertebral arteries or by injecting it directly into the cisterna magna.

The major adverse effects of clonidine are dry mouth and sedation. These responses occur in at least 50% of patients and may require drug discontinuation. However, they may diminish in intensity after several weeks of therapy. Sexual dysfunction also may occur. Marked bradycardia is observed in some patients. These and some of the other adverse effects of clonidine frequently are related to dose, and their incidence may be lower with transdermal administration of clonidine because antihypertensive efficacy may be achieved while avoiding the relatively high peak concentrations that occur after oral administration of the drug. About 15 to 20% of patients develop contact dermatitis when using clonidine in the transdermal system. Withdrawal reactions follow abrupt discontinuation of long-term therapy with clonidine in some hypertensive patients.

The major therapeutic use of clonidine (Catapres, others) is in the treatment of hypertension. **Clonidine** also has apparent efficacy in the off-label treatment of a range of other disorders. Stimulation of α_2-receptors in the GI tract may increase absorption of sodium chloride and fluid and inhibit secretion of bicarbonate. This may explain why clonidine has been found to be useful in reducing diarrhea in some diabetic patients with autonomic neuropathy. **Clonidine** also is useful in treating and preparing addicted subjects for withdrawal from narcotics, alcohol, and tobacco. It may help ameliorate some of the adverse sympathetic nervous activity associated with withdrawal from these agents, as well as decrease craving for the drug. The long-term benefits of clonidine in these settings and in neuropsychiatric disorders remain to be determined. **Clonidine** may be useful in selected patients receiving anesthesia because it may decrease the requirement of the anesthetic and increase hemodynamic stability. Other potential benefits of clonidine and related drugs such as dexmedetomidine (Precedex; a relatively selective α_2-receptor agonist with sedative properties) in anesthesia include preoperative sedation and anxiolysis, drying of secretions, and analgesia. Transdermal administration of clonidine (Catapres) may be useful in reducing the incidence of menopausal hot flashes.

CLOPIDOGREL

(Plavix tablet 75 mg)

Clopidogrel is a thienopyridine derivative, chemically related to ticlopidine, that inhibits platelet aggregation. It acts by irreversibly modifying the platelet ADP receptor. Therefore, platelet aggregation is inhibited for both ADP-mediated and ADP-amplified (by other agonists) platelet activation. Consequently, platelets exposed to clopidogrel are affected for the remainder of their life span. Clopidogrel is indicated in reduction of atherosclerotic events (e.g., MI, stroke, vascular death) in patients with atherosclerosis documented by recent stroke, recent MI, or established peripheral arterial disease; and treatment of acute coronary syndrome (unstable angina/non-Q-wave MI), including patients managed medically and those managed with percutaneous coronary intervention (with or without stent) or coronary artery bypass graft.

Antianginal agents may provide prophylactic or symptomatic treatment, but β-adrenergic-receptor antagonists also reduce mortality apparently by decreasing the incidence of sudden cardiac death associated with myocardial ischemia and infarction. The treatment of cardiac risk factors can reduce the progression or even lead to the regression of atherosclerosis. Aspirin is used routinely in patients with myocardial ischemia, and daily aspirin use reduces the incidence of clinical events. Other antiplatelet agents such as oral **clopidogrel** and intravenous anti-integrin drugs such as **abciximab**, **tirofiban**, and **eptifibatide** have been shown to reduce morbidity in patients with angina who undergo coronary artery stenting; lipid-lowering drugs such as the statins reduce mortality in patients with hypercholesterolemia with or without known coronary artery disease. ACE inhibitors also reduce mortality in patients with coronary disease. Coronary artery bypass surgery and percutaneous coronary interventions such as angioplasty and coronary artery stent deployment can complement pharmacological treatment. In some subsets of patients, percutaneous or surgical revascularization may have a survival advantage over medical treatment alone. Intracoronary drug delivery using drug-eluting coronary stents represents an intersection of mechanical pharmacological approaches in the treatment of coronary artery disease. Novel therapies that modify the expression of vascular or myocardial cell genes eventually may become an important part of the therapy of ischemic heart disease.

CLORAZEPATE DIPOTASSIUM

(Tranxene-SD half strength)

Clorazepate, a benzodiazepine derivative with antianxiety, anticonvulsant, and sedative hypnotic properties (30 mg p.o. initially), is indicated in acute alcohol withdrawal and is used as an adjunct in epilepsy (see also Table 9).

CLORAZEPATE DIPOTASSIUM

(Tranxene T-tab tablets 3.75 mg)

Clorazepate is a benzodiazepine that potentiates action of GABA, an inhibitory neurotransmitter, resulting in increased neuronal inhibition and CNS depression, especially in limbic system and reticular formation. Clorazepate is indicated in the management of anxiety disorders; relief of acute alcohol withdrawal symptoms; and adjunctive therapy in management of partial seizures.

CLOTRIMAZOLE

(Cruex cream 1%, Uese-nex cream 1%, Gyne-Lotrimin 3 vaginal suppositories 200 mg, vaginal cream 2%)

Clotrimazole is an antifungal/mouth and throat product/vaginal antifungal preparation that inhibits yeast growth by increasing cell membrane permeability in susceptible fungi. Clotrimazole has the following uses:

Topical use: Treatment of tinea pedis (athlete's foot), tinea cruris (jock itch), tinea corporis (ringworm), candidiasis, and tinea versicolor

Oral use (troche): Treatment of oropharyngeal candidiasis; prophylaxis of oropharyngeal candidiasis in specific groups of immunocompromised patients

Vaginal use: Treatment of vulvovaginal candidiasis

Topical treatment is useful in many superficial fungal infections—i.e., those confined to the stratum corneum, squamous mucosa, or cornea. Such diseases include dermatophytosis (ringworm), candidiasis, tinea versicolor, piedra, tinea nigra, and fungal keratitis. Topical administration of antifungal agents usually is not successful for mycoses of the nails (onychomycosis) and hair (tinea capitis), and has no place in the treatment of subcutaneous mycoses such as sporotrichosis and chromoblastomycosis. The efficacy of topical agents in the treatment of superficial mycoses depends not only on the type of lesion and the mechanism of action of the drug but also on the viscosity, hydrophobicity, and acidity of the formulation. Regardless of formulation, penetration of topical drugs into hyperkeratotic lesions often is poor. Removal of thick, infected keratin is sometimes a useful adjunct to therapy and is the principal mode of action of Whitfield's ointment.

A plethora of topical agents is available for the treatment of superficial mycoses. Many of the older drugs— including gentian violet, carbol-fuchsin, acrisorcin, triacetin, sulfur, iodine, and aminacrine—are now rarely indicated and are not discussed here. Among the topical agents, the preferred formulation for cutaneous application usually is a cream or solution. Ointments are messy and are too occlusive for macerated or fissured intertriginous lesions. The use of powders, whether applied by shake containers or aerosols, is largely confined to the moist lesions of the groin and other intertriginous lesions. The use of powders, whether applied by shake containers or aerosols, is largely confined to the feet and moist lesions of the groin and other intertriginous areas.

Absorption of **clotrimazole** is less than 0.5% after application to the intact skin; from the vagina, it is 3 to 10%. Fungicidal concentrations remain in the vagina for as long as 3 days after application of the drug. The small amount absorbed is metabolized in the liver and excreted in bile. In adults, an oral dose of 200 mg per day will give rise initially to plasma concentrations of 0.2 to 0.35 μg/mL, followed by a progressive decline.

In a small fraction of recipients, clotrimazole on the skin may cause stinging, erythema, edema, vesication, desquamadon, pruritus, and urticaria. When it is applied to the vagina, about 1.6% of recipients complain of a mild burning sensation, and rarely of lower abdominal cramps, a slight increase in urinary frequency, or skin rash. Occasionally, the sexual partner may experience penile or urethral irritation. By the oral route, clotrimazole can cause gastrointestinal irritation. In patients using troches, the incidence of this side effect is about 5%.

Clotrimazole is available as a 1% cream, lotion, and solution (Lotrimin, Mycelex, others), 1% or 2% vaginal cream or vaginal tablets of 100, 200, or 500 mg (Gyne-lotrimin, Mycelex-G, others), and 10-mg troches (Mycelex, others). On the skin, applications are made twice a day. For the vagina, the standard regimens are one 100-mg tablet once a day at bedtime for 7 days, one 200-mg tablet daily for 3 days, one 500-mg tablet inserted only once, or 5 g of cream once a day for 3 days (2% cream) or 7 days (1% cream). For nonpregnant females, one 200-mg tablet may be used once a day for 3 days. Troches are to be dissolved slowly in the mouth five times a day for 14 days.

Clotrimazole has been reported to cure dermatophyte infections in 60 to 100% of cases. The cure rates in cutaneous candidiasis are 80 to 100%. In vulvovaginal candidiasis, the cure rate is usually above 80% when the 7-day regimen is used. A 3-day regimen of 200 mg once a day appears to be similarly effective, as does single-dose treatment (500 mg). Recurrences are common after all regimens. The cure rate with oral troches for oral and pharyngeal candidiasis may be as high as 100% in the immunocompetent host.

CLOTRIMAZOLE

(Gyne-Lotrimin)

Clotrimazole, an antifungal agent, is used only topically and is available as a 1% cream, lotion, or solution (Lotrimin and Mycelex), as a 1% vaginal cream, as 100-mg or 500-mg vaginal tablets (Gyne-Lotrimin, Mycelex-G), and as 10-mg troches (Mycelex).

CLOXACILLIN SODIUM

(Tegopen)

Cloxacillin (500 mg every 4 to 6 hours for at least 5 days) is indicated in the treatment of infections due to penicillinase-producing staphylococci. Cloxacillin sodium is an acid-stable and penicillinase-resistant penicillin, absorbed orally rapidly but incompletely. It binds to albumin to the extent of 95% and is excreted unchanged in the urine.

Penicillinase-resistant penicillins should be administered cautiously to persons with a history of sensitivity to any penicillins. Tetracycline, a bacteriostatic antibiotic, may antagonize the bactericidal effects of penicillin (see also Table 23).

CLOZAPINE

(Clozaril)

Clozapine, which is associated with higher risk of agranulocytosis and seizures, is indicated (25 mg once or twice daily) only in the management of schizophrenic patients who fail to respond adequately to standard antipsychotic drug treatment. On the other hand, it is relatively free from extrapyramidal side effects such as parkinsonism. Approximately 50% of the administered dose is excreted in the urine and 30% in the feces as inactive demethylated, hydroxylated, and N-oxide derivatives. Clozapine has anticholinergic properties and causes tachycardia, and hence poses a serious risk for a patient with compromised cardiovascular function (see also Table 23).

CLOZAPINE

(Clozapine tablets 12.5 mg)

Clozapine interferes with dopamine binding at D_1, D_2, D_3, and D_5 receptors in CNS; antagonizes adrenergic, cholinergic, histaminergic, and serotonergic neurotransmission. Clozapine is indicated in the management of severely and chronically mentally ill schizophrenic patients who have not responded to or cannot tolerate standard antipsychotic drug treatment; to reduce risk of recurrent suicidal behavior in patients with schizophrenia or schizoaffective disorder who are judged to be at chronic risk for reexperiencing suicidal behavior.

Clozapine (Clozaril), a $5\text{-HT}_{2A/2C}$-receptor antagonist, represents a class of atypical antipsychotic drugs with reduced incidence of extrapyramidal side effects compared to the classical neuroleptics, and possibly a greater efficacy for reducing negative symptoms of schizophrenia. Clozapine also has a high affinity for subtypes of dopamine receptors.

One of the newest strategies for the design of additional atypical antipsychotic drugs is to combine $5\text{-HT}_{2A/2C}$ and dopamine D_2-receptor-blocking actions in the same molecule. **Risperidone** (Risperdal), for example, is a potent 5-HT_{2A}- and D_2-receptor antagonist. Low doses of risperidone have been reported to attenuate negative symptoms of schizophrenia with a low incidence of extrapyramidal side effects. Extrapyramidal effects are commonly seen, however, with doses of risperidone in excess of 6 mg/day. Other atypical antipsychotic agents— **quetiapine** (Seroquel) and **olanzapine** (Zyprexa)—act on multiple receptors, but their antipsychotic properties are thought to be due to antagonism of dopamine and serotonin.

CLUSTERIN

Clusterin is a heterodimeric glycoprotein produced by a wide array of tissues and found in most biological fluids. The proposed physiologic functions of clusterin include complement regulation, lipid transport, sperm maturation, initiation of apoptosis, endocrine secretion, membrane protection, and promotion of cell interactions.

COCCIDIOIDIN

(Spherulin)

Coccidioidin, which is a crude but standardized toluene extract of a mycelial culture filtrate, is used for skin testing. A delayed-type hypersensitivity reaction is elicited, and a positive test is defined as induration exceeding 5 mm in diameter. Another *C. immitis* antigen, prepared from cultured spherules and termed **spherulin**, is more sensitive but less specific than coccidioidin. Skin testing with either antigen does not induce or boost an immune response. The skin test becomes positive within 2 weeks after the onset of symptoms and before the appearance of antibodies and often remains positive indefinitely. A positive reaction has no diagnostic significance without a history of conversion, but a negative test can be used to exclude **coccidioidomycosis**, except in patients with severe disseminated coccidioidomycosis who may have become anergic. Indeed, a negative skin test in confirmed cases is associated with a grave prognosis. Conversely, a positive skin test in healthy subjects implies immunity to symptomatic reinfection.

CODEINE

(Methylmorphine)

Codeine, which is an analgesic and antitussive, is methylmorphine, and pharmacologically resembles morphine, with the following exceptions. The analgesic potency of codeine is approximately one-sixth that of morphine. Codeine raises the pain threshold without altering the patient's reaction to pain and produces very little euphoria. Therefore, 10 mg of morphine is far superior for alleviating pain than 60 mg of codeine.

Unlike morphine, codeine is absorbed orally. The side effects are the same as morphine's but are milder and far less frequent. Codeine produces miosis, respiratory depression, urinary retention, and constipation, but these are not of clinical or toxicological significance (see also Figure 68).

Tolerance to codeine develops very slowly, and the addiction liability is far less than that observed for morphine. Most narcotics such as morphine, codeine, dihydrocodeine, methadone, and levorphanol have antitussive properties. Codeine is used primarily because its addictive liability is low and it is effective orally. The antitussive doses of narcotics are lower than the doses used for analgesic purposes.

CODEINE

(Codeine Contin)

Codeine is an opioid analgesic that stimulates opiate receptors in the CNS; also causes respiratory depression, peripheral vasodilation, inhibition of intestinal perstalsis, stimulation of the chemoreceptors that cause vomiting, increased bladder tone, and suppression of cough reflex. Codeine is indicated in the relief of mild-to-moderate pain; cough suppression.

CODEINE POLISTIREX/CHLORPHENIRAMINE POLISTIREX

(Codeprex suspension, extended-release 20 mg codeine and 4 mg chlorpheniramine maleate per 5 mL)

Codeine: stimulates opiate receptors in the CNS; also causes respiratory depression, peripheral vasodilation, inhibition of intestinal peristalsis, stimulation of chemoreceptors that cause vomiting, increased bladder tone, and suppression of cough reflex. **Chlorpheniramine**: competitively antagonizes histamine at H_1-receptor sites. The combination is indicated in temporary relief of cough; temporary relief of runny nose, sneezing, itching of the nose or throat, and itching watery eyes caused by hay fever, upper respiratory allergies, or allergic rhinitis.

COLCHICINE

Colchicine, an alkaloid obtained from meadow saffron or autumn crocus, may be used both diagnostically to ascertain the presence of gout and prophylactically to prevent its further occurrence. Usually 0.5 mg oral doses of colchicine are given hourly until either the therapeutic effects appear or the side effects develop. In addition to colchicine, phenylbutazone, indomethacin, ACT, and steroid antiinflammatory agents may be used to treat the acute attack of gout.

Colchicine is tolerated well in moderate doses. Nausea, vomiting, diarrhea, and abdominal pain are the most common and earliest untoward effects of overdosage.

In the event of acute poisoning with colchicine, there is hemorrhagic gastroenteritis, extensive vascular damage, nephrotoxicity, muscular depression, and an ascending paralysis of the CNS.

Colchicine produces a leukopenia that is soon replaced by a leukocytosis. The long-term administration of colchicine may lead to myopathy, neuropathy, agranulocytosis, aplastic anemia, alopecia, and azoospermia (see also Figure 13).

COLCHICINE

(Colchicine tablets 0.6 mg, injection 0.5 mg/mL)

Colchicine inhibits inflammation and reduces pain and swelling associated with gouty arthritis. It is indicated in the treatment and relief of pain in attacks of acute gouty arthritis; regular prophylaxis between attacks and is often effective in aborting an attack when taken at the first sign of articular discomfort; colchicine IV is used when rapid response is desired or if GI side effects interfere with oral use. **Colchicine** dramatically relieves acute attacks of gout. It is effective in roughly two-thirds of patients if given within 24 hours of the onset of the attack. Pain, swelling, and redness abate within 12 hours, and are completely gone within 48 to 72 hours. The typical oral dose is 0.6 mg each hour for a total of three doses. This dose should not be exceeded. Treatment with colchicine should not be repeated within 7 days so as to avoid cumulative toxicity.

Colchicine is one of the oldest available therapies for acute gout. Plant extracts containing colchicine were used for joint pain in the 6th century. **Colchicine** now is considered second-line therapy because it has a narrow therapeutic window and a high rate of side effects particularly at higher doses. It exerts a variety of pharmacological effects, but how these occur or how they relate to its activity in gout is not well understood. Colchicine has antimitotic effects, arresting cell division in GI by interfering with microtubule and spindle formation (an effect shared with vinca alkaloids). This effect is greatest on cells with rapid turnover (e.g., neutrophils and GI epithelium). Although somewhat controversial, colchicine may alter neutrophil motility in *ex vivo* assays. It also renders cell membranes more rigid and decreases the secretion of chemotactic factors by activated neutrophils.

Colchicine inhibits the release of histamine-containing granules from mast cells, the secretion of insulin from pancreatic β-cells, and the movement of melanin granules in melanophores. These processes also may involve interference with the microtubular system, but whether this occurs at clinically relevant concentrations is questionable.

Colchicine also exhibits a variety of other pharmacological effects. It lowers body temperature, increases the sensitivity to central depressants, depresses the respiratory center, enhances the response to sympathomimetic agents, constricts blood vessels, and induces hypertension by central vasomotor stimulation. It enhances gastrointestinal activity by neurogenic stimulation but depresses it by a direct effect, and alters neuromuscular function.

The absorption of colchicine is rapid but variable. Peak plasma concentrations occur 0.5 to 2 hours after dosing. In plasma, 50% of **colchicine** is protein-bound. There is significant enterohepatic circulation. The exact metabolism of colchicine is unknown but seems to involve deacetylation by the liver. Only 10 to 20% is excreted in the urine, although this increases in patients with liver disease. The kidney, liver, and spleen also contain high concentrations of **colchicine**, but it apparently is largely excluded from heart skeletal muscle and brain. The plasma half-life of colchicine is approximately 9 hours, but it can be detected in leukocytes and in the urine for at least 9 days after a single intravenous dose.

Exposure of the GI tract to large amounts of colchicine and its metabolites via enterohepatic circulation, and the rapid rate of turnover of the gastrointestinal mucosa, may explain why the GI tract is particularly susceptible to colchicine toxicity. Nausea, vomiting, diarrhea, and abdominal pain are the most common untoward effects of **colchicine** and the earliest signs of impending toxicity. Drug administration should be discontinued as soon as these symptoms occur. There is a latent period, which is not altered by dose or route of administration, of several hours or more between the administration of the drug and the onset of symptoms. For this reason, adverse effects are common during initial dosing for acute gout. However, because patients often remain relatively consistent in their response to a given dose of the drug, toxicity can be reduced or avoided during subsequent courses of therapy by reducing the dose. Acute intoxication causes hemorrhagic gastropathy. Intravenous **colchicine** sometimes is used to treat acute gouty arthritis when other medications are not effective, when the patient is unable to take oral medications, or when rapid therapeutic intervention is necessary. The narrow margin of safety for colchicine is even further diminished by intravenous administration because this route obviates early gastrointestinal side effects that can be a harbinger of serious systemic toxicity. Indiscriminate use of intravenous colchicine has been associated with preventable fatalities. Due to the high rate of serious bone marrow and renal complications (including death from sepsis), this route, although occasionally used, is not generally recommended.

Colchicine toxicity is associated with bone marrow suppression, particularly from the third to eighth days. There is a tendency toward leukocytosis with appearance of less mature forms. Chronic colchicine use may lead to agranulocytosis. Thrombocytopenia also can occur, and disseminated intravascular coagulation has been reported in cases of severe poisoning.

Chronic use is associated with a proximal myopathy. The associated weakness may go unrecognized, and creatine kinase levels should be monitored in those receiving chronic therapy. Ascending paralysis of the CNS has been reported with acute poisoning.

Proteinuria, hematuria, and acute tubular necrosis have been reported in severely intoxicated patients. Gouty nephropathy may occur in chronically treated patients. Azoospermia has been reported with chronic use.

There is no specific therapy for acute colchicine poisoning. Supportive measures should be used, particularly fluid repletion. Activated charcoal may decrease total colchicine exposure. Hemodialysis does not remove colchicine but may be required as part of supportive care. **Colchicine** antibodies and the use of granulocyte colony-stimulating factor to treat the leukopenia are under investigation.

COLESEVELAM HYDROCHLORIDE
(Welchol tablets 625 mg)

Colesevelam is a bile acid sequestrant that increases removal of bile acids from the body by binding them in the intestine, impeding their reabsorption. As the bile acid pool becomes depleted, the conversion of cholesterol to bile acids is increased, which decreases serum cholesterol. Colesevelam is indicated as an adjunctive therapy to diet and exercise given alone or with an HMG-CoA reductase inhibitor for the reduction of elevated LDL cholesterol in patients with primary hypercholesterolemia (Fredrickson type IIa).

The bile–acid sequestrants are highly positively charged and bind negatively charged bile acids. Because of their large size, the resins are not absorbed, and the bound bile acids are excreted in the stool. Because over 95% of bile acids are normally reabsorbed, interruption of this process depletes the pool of bile acids, and hepatic bile–acid synthesis increases. As a result, hepatic cholesterol content declines, stimulating the production of LDL receptors, an effect similar to that of statins. The increase in hepatic LDL receptors increases LDL clearance and lowers LDL-C levels, but this effect is partially offset by the enhanced cholesterol synthesis caused by upregulation of HMG-CoA reductase. Inhibition of activity by a statin substantially increases the effectiveness of the resins. Patients taking cholestyramine and colestipol complain of bloating and dyspepsia. These symptoms can be substantially reduced if the drug is completely suspended in liquid several hours before ingestion (e.g., evening doses can be mixed in the morning and refrigerated; morning doses can be mixed the previous evening and refrigerated). Constipation may occur but sometimes can be prevented by adequate daily water intake and psyllium, if necessary. Colesevelam may be less likely to cause the dyspepsia, bloating, and constipation observed in patients treated with cholestyramine or colestipol.

COLESTIPOL HYDROCHLORIDE

(Colested)

Colestipol (5 to 30 g/day given once or in divided doses) is indicated as adjunctive therapy to diet for the reduction of elevated serum total and LDL and cholesterol in patients with primary hypocholesterolemia who do not respond adequately to diet.

Colestipol and cholestyramine are very large polymeric cationic exchange resins that are insoluble in water. They bind bile acids in the intestinal lumen and prevent their reabsorption (see Figure 34). Chloride is released from cationic quaternary ammonium-binding sites in exchange for bile acids, but the resin itself is not absorbed.

Colestipol causes constipation and a bloating sensation. The absorption of fat-soluble vitamins and certain drugs such as digitalis, thiazides, tetracycline, and phenylbutazone may be altered. Therefore, medications are given either 1 hour before or 2 hours after colestipol.

COLESTIPOL HYDROCHLORIDE

(Colestid tablets 1 g)

Colestipol is a bile acid sequestrant that increases removal of bile acids from the body by forming insoluble complexes in intestine, which are then excreted in feces. As the body loses bile acids, it converts cholesterol from blood to bile acids, thus lowering serum cholesterol. Colestipol is indicated in the reduction of cholesterol in patients with primary hypercholesterolemia who do not respond adequately to diet. Unlabeled uses: treatment of digitalis toxicity.

COLISTIN SULFATE/NEOMYCIN SULFATE/ THONZONIUM BR/HYDROCORTISONE

(Coly-Mysin S Otic suspension 1% hydrocortisone, 4.71 mg neomycin sulfate (equiv. to 3.3 mg neomycin base), 3 mg colistin (as sulfate), and 0.05% thonzonium Br/mL)

Colistin is a steroid and antibiotic combination. **Colistin**: is a bactericidal agent against most Gram-negative organisms, particularly, *P. aeruginosa*. **Neomycin**: inhibits protein synthesis by binding to ribosomal RNA, causing bacterial genetic code misreading. **Thonzonium**: is a surface-active agent that promotes tissue contact by dispersion and penetration of the cellular debris and exudates. **Hydrocortisone**: depresses formation, release, and activity of endogenous mediators of inflammation as well as modifying the body's immune response. The combination is indicated in the treatment of superficial bacterial infections of the external auditory canal caused by susceptible organisms; and treatment of infection of mastoidectomy and fenestration cavities caused by susceptible organisms.

COLLAGENASE

(Collagenase Santyl ointment 250 units of collagenase enzyme/g)

Collagenase contributes to the formation of granulation tissue and subsequent epithelialization of dermal ulcers and severely burned areas. It is indicated in the debriding chronic dermal ulcers and severely burned areas.

COLLAGENASE

(Santyl)

Collagenase, an enzyme concentrate derived from *Clostridium histolytica*, is used to promote debridement of necrotic tissue in dermal ulcers and severe burns.

CONGESTIVE HEART FAILURE: Treatment of

Overt congestive heart failure (CHF) has a prevalence of 1% of the population. The predominant symptoms of patients with CHF are fatigue and dyspnea. Fatigue is thought to result from changes in peripheral muscle metabolism secondary to decreased vasodilative capacity and physical inactivity. An increase of peripheral perfusion by vasodilator therapy and physical activity are therefore recommended. Beside overt decompensation, where dyspnea results from acute pulmonary congestion due to backward failure, increased physiological dead space ventilation caused by pulmonary ventilation/perfusion mismatch accounts, to a large degree, for dyspnea, and can be improved by vasodilator therapy.

According to the pathophysiology of CHF, normalization of loading conditions and myocardial inotropy are the parameters addressed by various pharmacological agents in order to alleviate symptoms and slow progression of the disease. Diuretics are rapid-acting and effective agents to improve congestion and decrease filling pressures. Digitalis improves hemodynamics and symptomatology by increasing inotropy and slowing resting heart rate in atrial fibrillation; however, prognostic effects have yet to be proved. The introduction of vasodilators has significantly improved the prognosis of the disease, and the administration of ACE inhibitors in particular has been shown to slow progression of CHF. This results in a substantial decrease in morbidity and mortality.

CONSTIPATION: Drug-induced

Antacids Containing Calcium Carbonate or Aluminum Hydroxide
Barium sulfate
Clonidine
Diuretics (non-potassium-sparing)
Drugs Possessing Anticholinergic Properties
Antihistamines
Antiparkinsonian agents (e.g., benztropine or trihexyphenidyl)
Phenothiazines
Tricyclic antidepressants
Ganglionic Blocking Agents
Inhibitors of prostaglandin synthesis
Iron preparations
Narcotic Analgesics (Opiates)
Polystyrene sodium sulfonate
Skeletal Muscle Blocking Agents
d-Tubocurarine
Succinylcholine

CONTRACEPTIVES, ORAL COMBINATION PRODUCTS

(Alesse tablets 20 mcg ethinyl estradiol/0.1 mg levonorgestrel, others)

Oral contraceptive medication inhibits ovulation by suppressing gonadotropins, follicle-stimulating hormone, and luteinizing hormone. They prevent pregnancy. Estrogens are highly efficacious, but they do carry a number of risks as well. Many concerns arose initially from studies of early oral contraceptives, which contained high doses of estrogens, but the amount of estrogens (and progestins) in **oral contraceptives** has been markedly decreased, which has significantly diminished the risks associated with their use. Nevertheless, major concerns about the use of estrogens remain today, especially regarding cancer, thromboembolic disease, increased risk of cardiovascular disease, altered cognition, changes in carbohydrate and lipid metabolism, hypertension, gallbladder disease, nausea, migraine, changes in mood, and several lesser side effects.

CONTRACEPTIVES, ORAL (PROGESTIN-ONLY PRODUCTS)

(Micronor tablets 0.35 mg norethindrone)

Alter cervical mucus, interfere with implantation, and may suppress ovulation. They are indicated in the prevention of pregnancy.

CORTICOSTEROIDS

Corticosteroids (Table 11) are synthetic adrenocortical steroids with antiinflammatory actions and effects, and are used in numerous disorders including bronchial asthma. For example, beclomethasone dipropionate (Beclovent, 85 mcg 3 to 4 times daily), dexamethasone sodium phosphate (Decadron phosphate), and triamcinolone acetonide (Azmacort), which are not bronchodilators and are not indicated for rapid relief of acute asthma, are used in bronchospastic states intractable to an adequate trial of conventional therapy.

CORTICOSTEROIDS: Uses for (see also Table 11)

Replacement Therapy
Congenital adrenal hyperplasia
Primary adrenal insufficiency
Secondary adrenal insufficiency
Selective aldosterone deficiency
Musculoskeletal Diseases
Mixed connective tissue syndromes
Polymyalgia rheumatica
Polymyositis
Rheumatoid arthritis
Systemic lupus erythematosus deficiency
Pulmonary Diseases
Aspiration pneumonitis
Bronchoconstrictive diseases
  Acute asthma
  Chronic asthmatic bronchitis
Interstitial diseases
  Hypersensitivity pneumonitis
  Idiopathic pulmonary fibrosis
  Sarcoidosis
Pulmonary vasculitides
Hematologic and Neoplastic Diseases
Aplastic anemias (some forms)
Complications of malignancy
  Hypercalcemia
Hematologic malignancies
  Acute lymphoblastic leukemia
  Lymphomas
  Multiple myeloma
Immune hemolytic anemia
Immune thrombocytopenia
Inflammatory bowel disease
Transfusion reactions
Allergic and Immune Diseases
Acute hypersensitivity reactions
Allergic rhinitis
Anaphylaxis
Angioedema and urticaria
Insect venom allergy
Serum sickness
Some drug allergies
Transplantation rejection
Cardiovascular Diseases
Giant cell arteritis
Myocarditis
Pericarditis
Temporal arteritis
Gastrointestinal Diseases
Chronic active hepatitis
Crohn's disease
Nontropical sprue
Ulcerative colitis
Neurologic Conditions
Acute cerebral edema
Multiple sclerosis
Myasthenia gravis
Eye Diseases
Allergic conjunctivitis
Exophthalmos
Optic neuritis
Scleritis
Uveitis
Skin Diseases
Atopic dermatitis
Contact dermatitis
Erythema multiform
Mycosis fungoides
Pemphigus
Seborrheic dermatitis

TABLE 11
Preparations of Adrenocortical Steroids and Their Synthetic Analogs

Nonproprietary and Proprietary Names	Oral Forms	Injectable Forms
Fludrocortisones acetate (Florinef Acetate)	0.1 mg	—
Cortisol (hydrocortisone) (Cortef, Hydrocortone, others)	5–20 mg	25, 50 mg/mL (susp.)
Beclomethasone dipropionate (Beclovent, Vanceril, others)	Inhalation aerosol	—
Betamethasone	0.6 mg	—
(Celestone)	0.6 mg/5mL syrup	—
Betamethasone benzoate	Topical	—
(Benisone, Uticort)		
Betamethasone dipropionate (Diprosone, others)	Topical	—
Betamethasone sodium phosphate (Celestone Phosphate, others)	—	4 mg/mL
Betamethasone sodium phosphate and acetate (Celestone Soluspan)	—	6 mg/mL (susp.)
Betamethasone valerate (Beta-Val, Valisone, others)	Topical	—
Cortisone acetate (Cortone Acetate)	5–25 mg	25, 50 mg/mL (susp.)
Dexamethasone	0.25–6.0 mg	—
(Decadron, others)	0.5 mg/0.5 mL (elixir, soln.)	
	0.5 mg/0.5 mL (soln.)	
Dexamethasone acetate (Decadron-LA, others)	—	8, 16 mg/mL (susp.)
Dexamethasone sodium phosphate (Decadron Phosphate, Hexadrol Phosphate, others)	—	4–24 mg/mL
Methylprednisolone (Medrol)	2–32 mg	—
Methylprednisolone acetate (Depo-Medrol, Medrol Acetate, others)	—	20–80 mg/mL (susp.)
Paramethasone acetate (Haldrone)	1.2 mg	—
Prednisolone	5mg	—
(Delta-Cortef)	3 mg/mL (syrup)	—
Prednisolone acetate (Econopred, others)	—	25–100 mg/mL (susp.)
Prednisolone tebutate (HYDELTRA-T.B.A., others)	mg/mL (liquid)	—
Prednisone	1–50 mg	—
(Deltasone, others)	1 mg/mL (syrup)	—
	1,5 mg/mL (soln.)	—
Triamcinolone (Aristocort, Kenacort)	1–8 mg	—
Triamcinolone acetonide (Kenalog, others)	—	3,10,40 mg/mL (susp.)
Triamcinolone diacetate	2,4 mg/5mL (syrup)	25,40 mg/mL (susp.)
(Aristocort, Kenacort Diacetate, others)	—	
Triamcinolone hexacetonide (Aristospan)		5, 20 mg/mL (susp.)

Note: Susp. = suspension; soln. = solution.

CORTICOTROPIN (ADRENOCORTICOTROPIC HORMONE; ACTH)

(ACTH powder for injection 40 units/vial)

ACTH stimulates adrenal cortex to produce and secrete adrenocortical hormones (e.g., corticosteroids, glucocorticoids). It is indicated in the diagnostic testing of adrenocortical function; including diuresis or remission of proteinuria in the nephrotic syndrome without uremia of the idiopathic type or that caused by lupus erythematosus; treatment of nonsuppurative thyroiditis, hypercalcemia associated with cancer, acute exacerbations of multiple sclerosis, tuberculous meningitis when accompanied by antituberculous chemotherapy, trichinosis with neurologic or myocardial involvement, and treatment of glucocorticoid responsive rheumatic, collagenous, dermatologic, allergic, ophthalmic, respiratory, hematologic, neoplastic, and GI diseases. Adrenocorticotropic hormone (ACTH, also called **corticotropin**) and the steroid hormone products of the adrenal cortex are considered together because the major physiological and pharmacological effects of ACTH result from its action to increase the circulating levels of adrenocortical steroids. Synthetic derivatives of ACTH are used principally in the diagnostic assessment of adrenocortical function. Because all known therapeutic effects of ACTH can be achieved with corticosteroids, synthetic steroid hormones generally are used therapeutically instead of **ACTH**.

Corticosteroids and their biologically active synthetic derivatives differ in their metabolic (glucocorticoid) and electrolyte-regulating (mineralocorticoid) activities. These agents are employed at physiological doses for replacement therapy when endogenous production is impaired. In addition, glucocorticoids potently suppress inflammation, and their use in a variety of inflammatory and autoimmune diseases makes them among the most frequently prescribed classes of drugs. Because they exert effects on almost every organ system, the clinical use of and withdrawal from corticosteroids are complicated by a number of serious side effects, some of which are life threatening. Therefore, the decision to institute therapy with corticosteroids always requires careful consideration of the relative risks and benefits in each patient.

Agents that inhibit steps in the steroidogenic pathway and thus alter the biosynthesis of adrenocortical steroids are discussed, as are synthetic steroids that inhibit glucocorticoid action. The effects of corticosteroids are numerous and widespread, and include alterations in carbohydrate, protein, and lipid metabolism; maintenance of fluid and electrolyte balance; and preservation of normal function of the cardiovascular system, the immune system, the kidney, skeletal muscle, the endocrine system, and the nervous system.

CORTICOTROPIN

(Adrenocorticotropic Hormone, ACTH, Acthar, ACTHGel, Cortigel-40, Cortigel 80, Cortrophin Gel, Cortrophin-Zinc, HP Acthar Gel)

Corticotropin, an anterior pituitary hormone, is indicated as a diagnostic test of adrenocortical function, as a replacement hormone, in the treatment of multiple sclerosis, in the treatment of severe allergic reactions, collagen disorders, dermatologic disorders, inflammation, and of infantile spasm.

CORTICOTROPIN-RELEASING FACTOR

Corticotropin-releasing factor and arginine vasopressin, which are released predominantly by the paraventricular nucleus of the hypothalamus, are important regulators of corticotropin (ACTH) release, which in turn triggers the release of cortisol and other steroids by the adrenal gland. Both the administration of certain psychoactive agents and emotional arousal originating from the limbic system are able to modify the functions of the pituitary–adrenal axis and to stimulate the synthesis of cortisol. ACTH elicits the following effects. It enhances the synthesis of pregnenolone, activates adenylate cyclase and elevates the cyclic adenosine monophosphate level, enhances the level of adrenal steroids, especially cortisol, and reduces the level of ascorbic acid.

The level of cortisol is thought to directly control the secretion of ACTH through a negative feedback mechanism that may be directed at both the hypothalamus and the anterior pituitary gland. Conversely, a reduced concentration of cortisol or cortisol-like substances eliminates the negative effect and enhances the release of ACTH (see Figure 38).

The metyrapone test may be used diagnostically to evaluate the proper functioning of the anterior pituitary gland. When administered orally, metyrapone inhibits the activity of 11-beta-hydroxylase, which is necessary for the synthesis of cortisol, corticosterone, and aldosterone, promotes the release of corticotropin, which in turn increases production of the precursors (11-deoxycortisol and 11-deoxycorticosterone), and enhances the appearance of 17-hydroxycorticosteroids and 17-ketogenic steroids.

In the event that the pituitary gland is nonfunctional, and therefore cannot stimulate ACTH secretion, the levels of these urinary metabolites will not increase.

CORTISONE (CORTISONE ACETATE)

(Cortone Acetate tablets 25 mg)

Cortisone is a short-acting glucocorticoid; depresses formation, release and activity of endogenous mediators of inflammation; has some slat-retaining properties. It is indicated in the treatment of primary or secondary adrenal cortex insufficiency; rheumatic disorders; collagen diseases; dermatologic diseases; allergic states; allergic and inflammatory ophthalmic processes; respiratory diseases; hematologic disorders; neoplastic diseases; edematous states (caused by nephritic syndrome); GI disease; multiple sclerosis; tuberculous meningitis; and trichninosis with neurologic or myocardial involvement.

CORTISONE

Cortisone (25 to 300 mg/day) is insoluble in water. Cortisone acetate (Bioline) is available in a 25-mg tablet. Hydrocortisone (cortisol, 20 to 240 mg/day) exists in suspension and is insoluble in water. Hydrocortisone cypionate (Cortef, 20 to 240 mg/day) is available in an oral suspension. Hydrocortisone sodium phosphate, a water-soluble salt with a rapid onset but short duration of action, is available for IV, IM, or SC injection. Hydrocortisone sodium succinate (Solu-Cortef) in an initial dose of 100 to 500 mg may be administered IV or IM. The antiinflammatory effect of cortisol is relatively weak (Table 11).

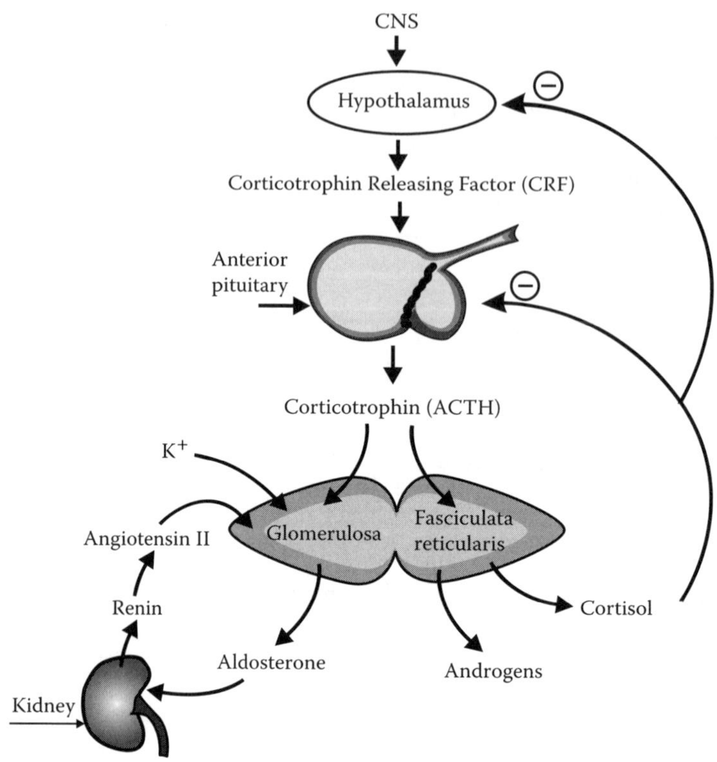

FIGURE 38 Corticotropin (adrenocorticotropic hormone), originating from the anterior pituitary gland, has been used in the treatment of multiple sclerosis and nonsuppurative thyroiditis.

CORTISONE ACETATE

(Cortone)

Cortisone, a substance with glucocorticoid and mineralocorticoid properties (25 to 300 mg p.o. or IM daily on an alternate-day schedule), is indicated in the treatment of adrenal insufficiency, allergy, and inflammation.

COSYNTROPIN

(Cortrosyn)

Cosyntropin, an anterior pituitary hormone (0.25 to 1 mg IM or IV), is used as a diagnostic test of adrenocortical function.

CO-TRIMOXAZOLE (TRIMETHOPRIM-SULFAMETHOXAZOLE)

(Bactrim, Bactrim DS, Bactrim I.V. Infusion, Cotrim, Septra, Septra DS, Septra IV Infusion, SMZ-TMP, Sulfatrim, UroPlus SS, UroPlus OS)

Co-trimoxazole, a sulfonamide and folate antagonist agent with antibiotic properties, is used in urinary tract infections and shigellosis, in otitis media, in *Pneumocystis carinii* pneumonitis, in chronic bronchitis, and in traveler's diarrhea (see Figure 90).

COUMARIN ANTICOAGULANTS

The coumarin anticoagulants, which are orally active, include dicumarol, warfarin sodium (coumadin sodium), warfarin potassium (Athrombokin-K), acenocoumarol (Sintrom), and phenopromcouman (Liquamar).

CROMOLYN SODIUM

(Disodium Cromoglycate)

Cromolyn sodium (inhalation 20 mg/2 mL), Intal in capsules (20 mg for inhalation only), solution (20 mg per amp for nebulizer only), and aerosol spray (delivers 800 mcg), Nasalcrom (nasal solution in 40 mg/mL), and Gastrocom (100 mg capsule for oral administration) are used for prophylactic management of severe bronchial asthma. As an antiasthmatic, antiallergic, and mast cell stabilizer, cromolyn has no bronchodilating, antiinflammatory, anticholinergic, or vasoconstricting properties.

Cromolyn sodium is given by inhalation as an aerosol powder four times a day only as a prophylactic medication (see also Figure 39). Because it is not a bronchodilator, it is not used in the management of status asthmaticus. Because it can inhibit the immediate response to allergen or exercise, it is thought that it suppresses the release of the mediator from mast cells. Cromolyn also prevents the late response and the subsequent hypersecretion, and this suggests it acts on other inflammatory cells such as macrophages or eosinophils. Cromolyn is not effective in all patients. It is the preferred antiinflammatory agent for use in children. The drug is well tolerated and, with the exception of causing minor throat irritation, has no side effects. Nedocromil sodium has biologic and chemical properties similar to those of cromolyn sodium (Figure 39).

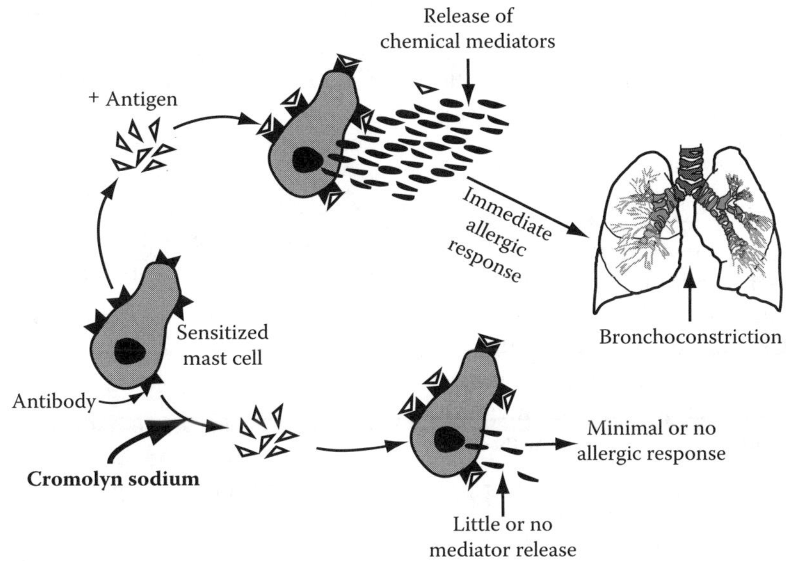

FIGURE 39 Cromolyn sodium, an antiasthmatic preparation, prevents the release of the mediators of type I allergic reactions.

CROHN'S DISEASE: Treatment of

Crohn's disease is an indolent, chronic inflammatory disorder capable of involving the entire alimentary tract from mouth to anus. The etiology and pathogenesis remain unknown, and Crohn's disease might represent more than one etiologically distinct entity. The term "Crohn's disease" is preferable to "granulomatous enteritis" because granulomas are not required for diagnosis and because other inflammatory disorders can affect "regions" of the bowel. Inflammation extends through all layers of the gut wall and involves the adjacent mesentery and lymph nodes. Distal ileum and colon are the most common sites, and the inflammatory process is characteristically discontinuous. The disease is characterized by its prolonged and variable course, by its diversity of clinical manifestation, by its perianal and systemic complications, and by its remarkable tendency to recur after surgical resection of involved gut.

Development of specific therapies for Crohn's disease has been hampered by the incomplete understanding of the underlying etiology and pathogenesis of this disease. In addition, the great variability in its location, extent, and behavior, as well as the imperfect correlation between clinical status and findings on endoscopy and histology, has made the design and interpretation of clinical trials difficult. Considering the dramatically variable natural history of the disease and frequent spontaneous improvement seen in patients on no therapy, the frequent reporting of uncontrolled trials only adds to the confusion.

Traditional medical therapies for Crohn's disease include sulfasalazine and corticosteroids. These are pluripotent, reducing the production of inflammatory mediators and cytokines, although the complex and multiple mechanisms remain incompletely understood. Novel therapies related to newer aminosalicylate preparations such as balsalazide (colazide) or olsalazine (dipentum); newer corticosteroids such as budesonide; immunomodulators such as azathioprine, 6-mercaptopurine, or methotrexate; and antibiotics such as metronidazole are aimed at more specific delivery of active compounds to the site of disease, reduction of systemic absorption and side effects, and modulation of more focal targets within the immune response and the action of specific proinflammatory cytokines.

CROTALINE (CROTALIDAE) ANTIVENIN, POLYVALENT

Crotaline, a snake antivenin, is indicated in the treatment of crotalid (pit viper) bites, including those from rattlesnakes, copperheads, and cottonmouth moccasins.

CROTAMITON

(Eurax)

Crotamiton, a synthetic chloroformate salt possessing scabicide and antipruritic properties (10% cream or lotion), is used for its antipruritic efficacy.

CROTAMITON

(Eurax Cream 10%, lotion 10%)

Crotamiton is a scabicide/pediculicide preparation that causes eradication of scabies (*Sarcoptes scabiei*) and symptomatic treatment of pruritic skin.

CYANOCOBALAMIN (VITAMIN B_{12})

(Berubigen, Betalin 12, Cabadon-M, Cobex, Crystimin-1000, Cyanoject, Cyomin, Kaybovite-1000, Redisol, Rubesol-1000, Rubramin PC, Sytobex, Big Shot B-12 tablets 5000 mcg, Crystamine injection 1000 mcg/mL, Crysti 1000 injection 1000 mcg/mL, Cyanoject injection 1000 mcg/mL, Cyomin injection 1000 mcg/mL, Nascobal gel, intranasal 500 mcg/ 0.1 mL, Rubesol-1000 injection 1000 mcg/mL)

Cyanocobalamin is involved in protein synthesis; essential to growth, cell reproduction, hematopoiesis, and nucleoprotein and ravelin synthesis. Cyanocobalamin is indicated in the treatment of vitamin B_{12} deficiency caused by inadequate utilization of vitamin B_{12}; dietary deficiency of vitamin B_{12} occurring in strict vegetarians, malabsorption syndrome of various causes (e.g., pernicious anemia, GI pathology, fish tapeworm infestation, malignancy of pancreas or bowel, gluten enteropathy, small bowel bacterial overgrowth, gastrectomy, accompanying folic acid deficiency); supplementation because of increased requirements (e.g., associated with pregnancy, thyrotoxicosis, hemolytic anemia, hemorrhage, malignancy, hepatic and renal disease); vitamin B_{12} absorption test (e.g., Schilling test).

Vitamin B_{12} and folic acid are dietary essentials. A deficiency of either vitamin impairs DNA synthesis in any cell in which chromosomal replication and division are taking place. Because tissues with the greatest rate of cell turnover show the most dramatic changes, the hematopoietic system is especially sensitive to deficiencies of these vitamins. An early sign of deficiency is megaloblastic anemia. Abnormal macrocytic red blood cells are produced, and the patient becomes severely anemic. Recognized in the 19th century, this pattern of abnormal hematopoiesis, termed pernicious anemia, spurred investigations that ultimately led to the discovery of vitamin B_{12} and folic acid. Even today, the characteristic abnormality in red blood cell morphology is important for diagnosis and as a therapeutic guide following administration of the vitamins.

HYDROXOCOBALAMIN (VITAMIN B_{12A})

(Alphamin, AlphaRedisol, Codroxomin, Droxomin, Hybalamin, Hydrobexan, Hydro-Cobex, Hydroxo-12, LA-12)

Cyanocobalamin, a water-soluble vitamin (25 mcg p.o. daily as a dietary supplement), is indicated in vitamin B_{12} deficiency resulting from any cause except malabsorption related to pernicious anemia or other GI disease (see Figure 106).

CYCLIZINE HYDROCHLORIDE

(Marezine)

Cyclizine (50 mg taken one-half hour before departure and then every 4 to 6 hours as needed) has antihistaminic, anticholinergic, and antiemetic properties, and is used in the prevention and treatment of nausea, vomiting, and dizziness associated with motion sickness. The side effects of cyclizine are drowsiness, dry nose and throat, urinary retention, tachycardia, and constipation.

CYCLOBENZAPRINE HYDROCHLORIDE

(Flexeril)

Cyclobenzaprine (10 mg t.i.d.) is a centrally acting skeletal muscle relaxant and is indicated as an adjunct to rest and physical therapy for relief of muscular spasm associated with injury related to painful musculoskeletal conditions. However, cyclobenzaprine is not effective in spasticity associated with cerebral or spinal cord injury. Cyclobenzaprine is structurally related to tricyclic antidepressants possessing sedative and anticholinergic properties. Therefore, cyclobenzaprine should be used cautiously in individuals with angle-closure glaucoma and urinary retention due to obstruction or prostatic hypertrophy. Because it causes drowsiness and blurred vision, it should be used carefully when alertness is required.

CYCLOBENZAPRINE HYDROCHLORIDE

(Flexeril tablets 5 mg)

Cyclobenzaprine is a centrally acting skeletal muscle relaxant that relieves skeletal muscle spasms of local origin without interfering with muscle function by acting within the CNS at the brain stem. Structurally and pharmacologically related to tricyclic antidepressants, cyclobenzaprine is indicated in the relief of muscle spasms associated with acute painful musculoskeletal conditions.

CYCLOPENTOLATE HYDROCHLORIDE/ PHENYLEPHRINE HYDROCHLORIDE

(Cyclomydril solution 0.2% cyclopentolate hydrochloride, 1% phenylephrine hydrochloride)

Cyclopentolate: inhibits action of acetylcholine at muscarinic receptors. **Phenylephrine:** stimulates postsynaptic alpha-receptors resulting in vasoconstriction. They are used to cause mydriasis.

CYCLOPENTOLATE HYDROCHLORIDE

(AK-Pentolate, Cyclogyl, I-Pentolate, Pentolair)

Cyclopentolate, an anticholinergic agent with mydriatic and cycloplegic properties (2 drops of 0.5% solution), is used in diagnostic procedures requiring mydriasis and cycloplegia (see also Figure 69).

CYCLOPHOSPHAMIDE

(Cytoxan, Endoxan)

Cyclophosphamide, which is chemically related to nitrogen-mustard, is indicated for multiple myeloma including malignant lymphomas, Hodgkin's disease, lymphocytic lymphoma, mixed-cell type lymphoma, histiocytic lymphoma, Burkitt's lymphoma, and for leukemia including chronic lymphocytic leukemia, chronic granulocytic leukemia, acute myelogenous and monocytic leukemia, and acute lymphoblastic leukemia in children, and in mycosis fungoides, neuroblastoma, carcinoma of the ovary, retinoblastoma, and carcinoma of the breast.

Cyclophosphamide is hydroxylated to 4-hydroxycyclophosphamide and aldophosphamide, which in turn are oxidized to the active antineoplastic alkylating agents, non-nitrogen mustard, and phosphoramide mustard. These agents cross-link cell DNA interfering with the growth of rapidly dividing normal and neoplastic cells (see Figure 28). Cyclophosphamide interferes with normal wound healing and impairs oogenesis and spermatogenesis, and hence may cause sterility and infertility.

Cyclophosphamide causes immunosuppression and may cause secondary neoplasm especially when taken with radiation therapy. The side effects of cyclophosphamide are anorexia, nausea, vomiting, diarrhea, stomatitis, and alopecia. Leukopenia, interstitial pulmonary fibrosis, and hemorrhagic cardiac necrosis occur with large doses.

CYCLOPROPANE

Cyclopropane, an inflammable gas capable of explosion when improperly mixed with oxygen, is a general anesthetic that is rarely used.

Cyclopropane increases the irritability of the heart by acting on its autonomic tissue and has a tendency to induce irregularities that may terminate in fatal fibrillation. The use of epinephrine is contraindicated in cyclopropane anesthesia because this drug tends to induce ventricular fibrillation (see Table 16).

The advantages of cyclopropane are that it is nonirritating, not unpleasant to the patient, and has little effect on the respiration. It differs from the other gaseous anesthetics in that a high concentration of oxygen (85%) is used in conjunction with a relatively low concentration (15%) of cyclopropane, thus providing an adequate supply of oxygen. There is also less pulmonary irritation than with ether (except in asthma, where it is poorly tolerated) and less excitement during induction. Its disadvantages are explosiveness, lack of respiratory stimulation, difficulty in detecting the planes of anesthesia, and the tendency to produce cardiac arrhythmias and postanesthetic headache.

CYCLOSERINE

(Seromycin)

Cycloserine, an isoxizolidone, d-alanine analog (250 mg p.o. q. 12 hours), is indicated as an adjunctive treatment in pulmonary or extrapulmonary tuberculosis.

CYCLOSPORIN

(Cyclosporin A)

Cyclosporin (Sandimmune) is an immunosuppressant that in combination with corticosteroids, is indicated in prophylaxis of organ rejection in kidney, liver, and heart allogenic transplants. Cyclosporin exerts its effects by inhibition of immunocompetent lymphocytes in the G_0- or G_1-phase of the cell cycle. T-lymphocytes are preferentially inhibited. The T-helper cell is the main target, but the T-suppressor cell may also be suppressed. Cyclosporin also inhibits lymphokine production and release including interleukin-2 or T-cell growth factor (TCGF). It does not cause bone marrow suppression. Cyclosporin has caused nephrotoxicity, hepatotoxicity, thrombocytopenia, microangiopathic hemolytic anemia syndrome, hyperkalemia, hyperuricemia, and hypertensive and convulsion seizures. It should not be used with potassium-sparing diuretics. Because hypertension is a common side effect, cyclosporin should be used along with an antihypertensive medication.

CYCLOSPORIN (CYCLOSPORIN A)

(Gengraf capsules 25 mg)

Cyclosporin suppresses cell-mediated immune reactions and some humoral immunity. It is indicated in the prophylaxis of organ rejection in kidney, liver, and heart allogeneic transplants in conjunction with adrenal corticosteroid therapy; treatment of chronic rejection in patients previously treated with other immunosuppressive agents; increased tear production in patients whose tear production is presumed to be suppressed because of ocular inflammation associated with keratoconjunctivitis sicca (ophthalmic emulsion). Gengraf, Neorai: Used for treatment of severe active rheumatoid arthritis (RA) where disease is not adequately responsive to methotrexare; treatment of adult, non-immunocompromised patients with severe, recalcitrant, plaque psoriasis who have failed to respond to a least one systemic therapy or in patients for whom other systemic therapies are contraindicated, or cannot be tolerated.

CYCRIMINE

(Pagitane)

In parkinsonian patients, the deficiency of dopamine causes the cholinergic receptors to be hyperactive. Therefore, anticholinergic drugs may be used to mitigate some of the symptoms. These agents include trihexyphenidyl (Artane), cycrimine (Pagitane), procyclidine (Kemadrin), biperiden (Akineton), orphenadrine (Disipal), and benztropine (Cogentin).

Contraindications to the use of anticholinergic drugs in treating parkinsonism are the same as those for atropine: glaucoma, prostatic hypertrophy, myasthenia gravis, stenosing peptic ulcer, and duodenal or pyloric obstruction. Urinary retention and tachycardia should be heeded and regarded as signs of impending toxicity.

CYPROHEPTADINE

(Periactin)

Cyproheptadine, a serotonin and $histamine_1$-receptor and muscarinic cholinergic receptor-blocking agent, has been used in the treatment of the postgastrectomy dumping syndrome and the intestinal hypermotility seen with carcinoids.

CYPROHEPTADINE HYDROCHLORIDE

(Cyproheptadine Hydrochloride tablets 4 mg)

Cyproheptadine competitively antagonizes histamine at H_1-receptor sites. It also exhibits antiserotonin activity. Cyproheptadine is indicated in the symptomatic relief of perennial and seasonal allergic rhinitis, vasomotor rhinitis, allergic conjunctivitis; amelioration of allergic reactions to blood or plasma; management of allergic pruritic symptoms, mild skin manifestations of uncomplicated urticaria and angioedema, and cold urticaria; dermographism; and adjunctive anaphylactic therapy.

CYPROTERONE ACETATE

(Androcur)

Cyproterone, a substance with antiandrogenic properties, is being investigated for the treatment of severe hirsutism (see Figure 95).

CYTARABINE

(Cytarabine, Cytosar, ARAC)

Cytarabine is an analog of deoxycytidine, differing only in its substitution of sugar arabinose for deoxyribose. It is converted to Ara-CTP, and thereby inhibits DNA-polymerase according to the following reactions:

$$\text{Ara-C} \xrightarrow{\text{Deoxycytidine kinase}} \text{Ara-CMP} \xrightarrow{\text{dCMP kinase}} \text{Ara} - \text{CDP}$$

$$\text{Ara} - \text{CDP} \xrightarrow{\text{NDP kinase}} \text{Ara} - \text{CTP}$$

$$\text{Deoxynucleotides} \xrightarrow[\text{DNA-polymerase}]{} \text{DNA}$$

Cytosine arabinoside is used in the treatment of acute granulocytic leukemia. Doxorubicin, daunorubicin and cytarabine; cytarabine and thioguanine; or cytarabine, vincristine, and prednisone are the combinations of agents employed. Resistance to cytosine arabinoside may stem from the deletion of deoxycytidine kinase, an increased intracellular pool of dCTP, a nucleotide that competes with Arp-CTP, or increased cytidine deaminase activity, converting Ara-C to inactive Ara-U.

The toxic effects of cytosine arabinoside are myelosuppression and injury to the gastrointestinal epithelium, which cause nausea, vomiting, and diarrhea.

CYTARABINE LIPOSOMAL

(DepoCyt suspension equivalent to 10 mg/mL)

Cytarabine is a pyrimidine analog that exhibits cell-phase specificity, primarily killing cells undergoing DNA synthesis (S-phase) and, under certain conditions, blocking the progression of cells from the G_1-phase to the S-phase. It is indicated in lymphomatous meningitis.

CYTOKINES

Cellular diversity in the nervous system evolves from the concerted processes of cell proliferation, differentiation, migration, survival, and synapse formation. Neural adhesion and extracellular matrix molecules have been shown to play crucial roles in axonal migration, guidance, and growth cone targeting.

Cytokines are a heterogeneous group of polypeptide mediators that have been associated with activation of numerous functions, including the immune system and inflammatory responses. The cytokine families include, but are not limited to, interleukins (IL_1-alpha, IL_1-beta, ILIra, and IL-2 to IL-15), chemokines (IL-8/NAP-1, NAP-2, MIP_1-alpha and beta, MCAF/MCP-1, MGSA, and RANTES), tumor necrosis factors (TNF-alpha and TNF-beta), interferons (IFN-alpha, beta, and gamma), colony stimulating factors (G-CSF, M-CSF, GM-CSF, IL-3, and some of the other ILs), growth factors (EGF, FGF, PDGF, TFG-alpha, TGF-beta, and ECGF), neuropoietins (LIF, CNTF, OM, and IL-6), and neurotrophins (BDNF, NGF, NT-3–NT-6, and GDNF).

The neurotrophins represent a family of survival and differentiation factors that exert profound effects on the central and peripheral nervous system. They are currently under investigation as therapeutic agents for the treatment of neurodegenerative disorders and nerve injury either individually or in combination with other trophic factors such as ciliary neurotrophic factor or fibroblast growth factor. Responsiveness of neurons to a given neurotrophin is governed by the expression of two classes of cell surface receptors. For NGF, these are p75NTR (p75) and p140trk (referred to as trk or trk-A) which binds both BDNF and NT-4/5, and trk C receptor that binds only NT-3. After binding ligand, the neurotrophin-receptor complex is internalized and retrogradely transported in the axon to the soma. Both receptors undergo ligand-induced dimerization that activates multiple signal transduction pathways. These include the *ras*-dependent pathway utilized by trk to mediate neurotrophin effects such as survival and differentiation.

Nerve growth factor and brain-derived neurotrophic factor are important neurotrophic factors that are essential for the differentiation and survival of some neural tissues, especially sympathetic neurons. Proinflammatory cytokines, released by activated macrophages and monocytes during infection, can act on neural targets that control thermogenesis, behavior, and mood. In addition to induction of fever, cytokines induce other biologic functions associated with the acute phase response, including hypophagia and sleep. Cytokine production has been detected within the CNS as a result of brain injury, following stab wounds to the brain, during viral and bacterial infections (AIDS and meningitis), and in neurodegenerative processes (multiple sclerosis and Alzheimer's disease). Novel cytokine therapies, such as anticytokine antibodies or specific receptor antagonists acting on the cytokine network, may provide an optimistic feature for treatment of multiple sclerosis and other diseases in which cytokines have been implicated (see also Figure 63).

CYTOKINES: Their Actions

Cytokine	Select Sources	Select Actions
IL-1	Macrophages	Immunoaugmentation
IL-2	T-lymphocytes and LGL	T- and B-cell growth factor
IL-3	T-lymphocytes	Hematopoietic growth factor
IL-4	TH cells	T- and B-cell growth factor; promotes IgE reactions
IL-5	TH cells	Stimulates B-cells and eosinophils
IL-6	Fibroblasts	Hybridoma growth factor; augments inflammation
IL-7	Stromal cells	Lymphopoietin
IL-8	Macrophages	Chemoattracts neutrophils and T-lymphocytes
G-CSF	Monocytes	Myeloid growth factor
M-CSF	Monocytes	Macrophage growth factor
GM-CSF	T-cells	Monomyelocytic growth factor
IFN-a	Leukocytes	Antiviral, antiproliferative, and immunomodulating
IFN-b	Fibroblasts	Induce cell membrane antigens (e.g., MHC)
IFN-g	T-lymphocytes and NK cells	Vascular thromboses and tumor necrosis
TNFa	Macrophages	Inflammatory, immunoenhancing, and tumoricidal
LT = TNFb	T-lymphocytes	Fibroplasia and immunosuppression
TGFb	Platelets and bone	

CYTOMEGALOVIRUS IMMUNE GLOBULIN

(CMV-IGIV, Cytomegalovirus Immune Serum Intravenous [Human], Cytomune-IV) (Cytogam)

Cytomegalovirus immune globulin (150 mg/kg IV within 75 hours of transplant, and then in reduced dosage 2 to 16 weeks post-transplant), is used to attenuate cytomegalovirus (CMV) disease in seronegative kidney transplant recipients who receive a kidney from a CMV seropositive donor.

D

DACARBAZINE

(DTIC-Dome)

Dacarbazine, a cell-cycle phase nonspecific antineoplastic agent (see Figure 15), is indicated in treatment of metastatic malignant melanoma (3 mg/kg/day for 10 days) and second-line therapy for Hodgkin's disease. Dacarbazine is thought to exert its effects by alkylation of a carbonium ion, inhibition of DNA synthesis by acting as a purine analog, and interaction with sulfhydryl groups in proteins. It is metabolized partly to 5-aminomidazole-4-carboxamide (AIC) and partly is excreted unchanged by active tubular secretion. The half-life of carboxamide is altered in hepatic and renal impairment. Dacarbazine causes nausea, vomiting, flu-like syndrome with fever and myalgia, leukopenia, and thrombocytopenia.

DACLIZUMAB

(Zenapax injection 25 mg per 5 mL)

Daclizumab is an immunosuppressive agent that binds with high affinity to the Tac subunit of the high-affinity interleukin-2 (IL-2) complex and inhibits IL-2 binding, thereby impairing the response of the immune system to antigenic challenges.

Daclizumab is indicated in the prophylaxis of acute organ rejection in patients receiving renal transplants.

Anti-IL-2-receptor (Anti-CD25) antibodies: **Daclizumab** (Zenapax), a humanized murine complementarity-determining region (CDR)/human IgG; chimeric monoclonal antibody, and **basiliximab** (Simulect), a murine-human chimeric monoclonal antibody, have been produced by recombinant DNA technology. The composite **daclizumab** antibody consists of human (90%) constant domains of IgG_1 and variable framework regions of the Eu myeloma antibody and murine (10%) CDR of the anti-Tac antibody.

Mechanism of action: **Daclizumab** has a somewhat lower affinity than does basiliximab, but a longer half-life (20 days). The exact mechanism of action of the anti-CD25 is not completely understood, but probably results from the binding of the anti-CD25 mAbs to the IL-2 receptor on the surface of activated, but not resting, T-cells. Significant depletion of T-cells does not appear to play a major role in the mechanism of action of these mAbs. However, other mechanisms of action may mediate the effect of these antibodies. In a study of daclizumab-treated patients, there was a moderate decrease in circulating lymphocytes staining with 7G7, a fluorescein-conjugated antibody that binds a different α-chain epitope than that recognized and bound by daclizumab. Similar results were obtained in studies with basiliximab. These findings indicate that therapy with the anti-IL-2R mAbs results in a relative decrease of the expression of the α-chain, either from depletion of coated lymphocytes or modulation of the α-chain secondary to decreased expression or increased shedding. There is also recent evidence that the β chain may be downregulated by the anti-CD25 antibody.

Anti-IL-2-receptor monoclonal antibodies are used for prophylaxis of acute organ rejection in adult patients. There are two anti-IL-2R preparations for use in clinical transplantation: **daclizumab** and basiliximab. In phase 3 trials, daclizumab was administered in five doses (1 mg/kg given intravenously over 15 minutes in 50 mL to 100 mL of normal saline) starting immediately preceding surgery, and subsequently at biweekly intervals. The half-life of daclizumab was 20 days, resulting in saturation of the IL-2Rα on circulating lymphocytes for up to 120 days after transplantation. In these trials, daclizumab was used with maintenance immunosuppression regimens (cyclosporine, azathioprine, and steroids; cyclosporine and steroids). Subsequently, **daclizumab** was successfully used with a maintenance triple-therapy regimen—either with cyclosporine or tacrolimus, steroids, and mycophenolate mofetil (MMF) substituting for azathioprine. In phase 3 trials, basiliximab was administered in a fixed dose of 20 mg preoperatively and on days 0 and 4 after transplantation. This regimen of basiliximab resulted in a concentration of ≥ 0.2 μg/mL sufficient to saturate IL-2R on circulating lymphocytes for 25 to 35 days after transplantation. The half-life of basiliximab was 7 days. In the phase 3 trials, basiliximab was used with a maintenance regimen consisting of cyclosporine and prednisone. In one randomized trial, basiliximab was safe and effective when used in a maintenance regimen consisting of cyclosporine, MMF, and prednisone.

DACTINOMYCIN

(Actinomycin D, ACT, Cosmegen)

Dactinomycin is an antineoplastic agent that is the principal component of the mixture of actinomycins produced by *Streptomyces parvullus*. It inhibits messenger RNA synthesis. Dactinomycin (0.5 mg/day IV for 5 days), in combination with vincristine, radiotherapy, and surgery, is used in Wilms' tumor; in conjunction with vincristine, cyclophosphamide, and doxorubicin, it is used in choriocarcinoma; in combination with methotrexate, it is used in testicular carcinoma; and in combination with cyclophosphamide and radiotherapy, it is used in Ewing's sarcoma. Dactinomycin inhibits messenger RNA synthesis by anchoring to a purine–pyrimidine (DNA) base pair by intercalation (see Figure 15). The toxicity of dactinomycin increases when combined with radiation therapy.

Adverse effects of dactinomycin, which begin 3 to 4 days after initiation of therapy, include cheilitis, dysphagia, esophagitis, ulcerative stomatitis, pharyngitis, anorexia, abdominal pain, diarrhea, gastrointestinal (GI) ulceration, proctitis, hepatic toxicity, anemia, leukopenia, thrombocytopenia, alopecia, erythema, fatigue, malaise, and lethargy. Many of these adverse effects will continue after cessation of therapy.

The capacity of actinomycins to bind with double-helical DNA is responsible for their biological activity and cytotoxicity. X-ray studies of a crystalline complex between dactinomycin and deoxyguanosine permitted formulation of a model that appears to explain the binding of the drug to DNA. The planar phenoxazone ring intercalates between adjacent guanine–cytosine base pairs of DNA, whereas the polypeptide chains extend along the minor groove of the helix. The summation of these interactions provides great stability to the dactinomycin-DNA complex, and as a result of the binding of dactinomycin, the transcription of DNA by RNA polymerase is blocked. The DNA-dependent RNA polymerases are much more sensitive to the effects of dactinomycin than are the DNA polymerases. In addition, dactinomycin causes single-strand breaks in DNA, possibly through a free-radical intermediate or as a result of the action of topoisomerase II.

Dactinomycin inhibits rapidly proliferating cells of normal and neoplastic origin and, on a molar basis, is among the most potent antitumor agents known. The drug may produce alopecia and, when extravasated subcutaneously, causes marked local inflammation. Erythema, sometimes progressing to necrosis, has been noted in areas of the skin exposed to x-ray radiation before, during, or after administration of dactinomycin.

Dactinomycin is administered by intravenous injection. The drug is excreted both in bile and in the urine, and disappears from plasma with a terminal half-life of 36 hours. Metabolism of the drug is minimal. Dactinomycin does not cross the blood–brain barrier.

The usual daily dose of **dactinomycin** (Actinomycin D, Cosmegen) is 10 to 15 μg/kg; this is given intravenously for 5 days; if no manifestations of toxicity are encountered, additional courses may be given at intervals of 2 to 4 weeks. In other regimens, 3 to 6 μg/kg per day for a total of 125 μg/kg and weekly maintenance doses of 7.5 μg/kg have been used. If infiltrated during administration, the drug is extremely corrosive to soft tissues.

The most important clinical use of dactinomycin is in the treatment of rhabdomyosarcoma and Wilms' tumor in children, where it is curative in combination with primary surgery, radiotherapy, and other drugs, particularly vincristine and cyclophosphamide. Antineoplastic activity has been noted in Ewing's tumor, Kaposi's sarcoma, and soft-tissue sarcomas. **Dactinomycin** can be effective in women with advanced cases of choriocarcinoma in combination with methotrexate. Dactinomycin also has been used as an immunosuppressant in renal transplants.

Toxic manifestations include anorexia, nausea, and vomiting, usually beginning a few hours after administration. Hematopoietic suppression with pancytopenia may occur in the first week after completion of therapy. Proctitis, diarrhea, glossitis, cheilitis, and ulcerations of the oral mucosa are common; dermatological manifestations include alopecia, as well as erythema, desquamation, and increased inflammation and pigmentation in areas previously or concomitantly subjected to x-ray radiation. Severe injury may occur as a result of local toxic extravasation.

DALTEPARIN SODIUM

(Fragmin injection 2500 IU (16 mg/0.2 mL))

Dalteparin is a low-molecular-weight heparin that inhibits reactions that lead to clotting. Dalteparin sodium is indicated in the prophylaxis of deep vein thrombosis (DVT), which may lead to pulmonary embolism in patients undergoing hip replacement surgery or in patients undergoing abdominal surgery who are at risk for thromboembolic complications; and prophylaxis of ischemic complications in unstable angina and non-Q-wave myocardial infarction (MI) in patients on aspirin therapy.

Low-molecular-weight heparin preparations: **Enoxaparin** (Lovenox), **dalteparin** (Fragmin), **tinzaparin** (Innohep, others), **ardeparin** (Normiflo), nadroparin (Fraxiparine, others), and **reviparin** (Clivarine) differ considerably in composition, and it cannot be assumed that two preparations that have similar anti-factor-Xa activity produce equivalent antithrombotic effects. The more predictable pharmacokinetic properties of low-molecular-weight heparins, however, permit administration in a fixed or weight-adjusted dosage regimen once or twice daily by subcutaneous injection. As they have a minimal effect on tests of clotting *in vitro*, monitoring is not done routinely. Patients with end-stage renal failure may require monitoring with an anti-factor-Xa assay because this condition may prolong the half-life of low-molecular-weight heparin. Specific dosage recommendations for various low-molecular-weight heparins may be obtained from the manufacturer's literature. Nadroparin and reviparin are not currently available in the United States.

DANAZOL

(Danocrine capsules 50 mg)

Danazol is a sex hormone that suppresses the pituitary-ovarian axis by inhibiting output of pituitary gonadotropins; has weak, dose-related androgenic activity with no estrogenic or progestational activity. Danazol is indicated in treatment of endometriosis; symptomatic treatment of fibrocystic breast disease; and in prevention of attacks of hereditary angioedema.

DANTROLENE SODIUM

(Dantrium)

Dantrolene sodium is a skeletal muscle relaxant that affects contraction of muscle at a site beyond the myoneural junction and directly on the muscle itself; it is believed to interfere with calcium release from sarcoplasmic reticulum;

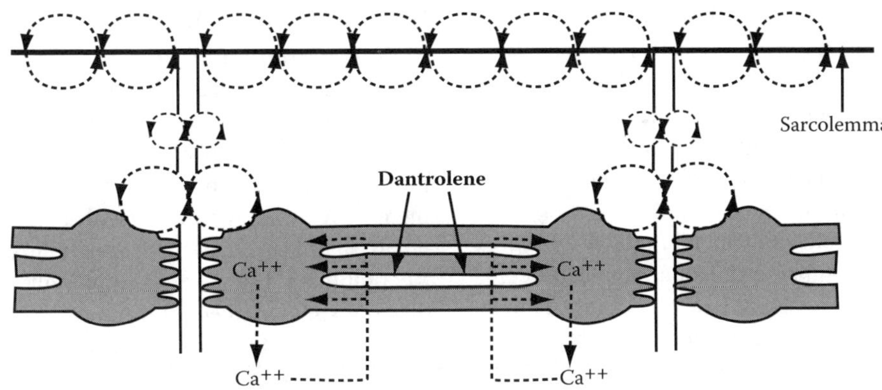

FIGURE 40 Dantrolene, a skeletal muscle relaxant, interferes with the release of calcium ion from the sarcoplasmic reticulum, resulting in decreased muscle contraction.

and affects the central nervous system (CNS), causing drowsiness, dizziness, and generalized weakness. Dantrolene, which has a high risk for causing hepatic toxicity, is indicated in management of spasticity resulting from upper motor neuron disorders such as spinal cord injury, stroke, cerebral palsy, or multiple sclerosis. In addition, it is used in malignant hyperthermia, neuroleptic malignant syndrome, and heat stroke causing painful muscular contraction and rigidity. Dantrolene does not influence the myoneural function but exerts its effects directly on the muscle by interfering with the release of Ca++ from the sarcoplasmic reticulum and dissociating the excitation–contraction coupling (see Figure 40).

The reported side effects of dantrolene are drowsiness, dizziness, weakness, hepatitis, constipation, increased urinary frequency, crystalluria, seizures, visual disturbances, pruritis, urticaria, acne, and skin eruption.

DAPSONE

(DDS)

Dapsone is a leprostatic agent that is indicated in treatment of dermatitis herpetiformis and leprosy. Leprosy (Hansen's disease) is a chronic granulomatous disease that attacks superficial tissues such as the skin, nasal mucosa, and peripheral nerves. There are two types of leprosy: lepromatous and tuberculoid. The sulfones, which are derivatives of 4,4′-diaminodiphenylsulfone, are bacteriostatic. Dapsone (DDS) and sulfoxone sodium are the most useful and effective agents currently available. They should be given in low doses initially, and then the dosage should be gradually increased until a full dose of 300 to 400 mg per week is reached. During this period, the patient must be monitored carefully. With adequate precautions and appropriate doses, sulfones may be used safely for years. Nevertheless, side effects such as anorexia, nervousness, insomnia, blurred vision, paresthesia, and peripheral neuropathy do occur. Hemolysis is common, especially in patients with glucose 6-phosphate dehydrogenase deficiency. A fatal exacerbation of lepromatous leprosy and an infectious mononucleosis-like syndrome rarely occur. Clofazimine (Lamprene) may be effective in patients who show resistance to the sulfones and may also dramatically reduce an exacerbation of leprosy. Red discoloration of the skin and eosinophilic enteritis have occurred following clofazimine therapy.

Not all mycobacterial infections are caused by *Mycobacterium tuberculosis* or *Mycobacterium leprae*. These atypical mycobacteria require treatment with secondary medications as well as other chemotherapeutic agents. For example, *Mycobacterium marinum* causes skin granulomas, and effective drugs in the treatment of the infection are rifampin or minocycline. *Mycobacterium fortuitum* causes skin ulcers, and the medications recommended for treatment are ethambutol, cycloserine, and rifampin in combination with amikacin.

DAPTOMYCIN

(Cubicin powder for injection)

Daptomycin is a lipopeptide that binds to bacterial membranes and causes a rapid depolarization of membrane potential, which inhibits protein, DNA, and RNA synthesis, resulting in bacterial cell death. Daptomycin is indicated in treatment of complicated skin and skin structure infections caused by susceptible strains of Gram-positive microorganisms.

Daptomycin (Cubicin) is a cyclic lipopeptide antibiotic derived from *Streptomyces roseosporus*. Discovered more than 20 years ago, its clinical development has been resumed in response to the increasing need for bactericidal antibiotics effective against vancomycin-resistant Gram-positive bacteria. **Daptomycin** is a bactericidal antibiotic selectively active against aerobic, facultative and anaerobic Gram-positive bacteria. The minimal inhibitory concentration (MIC) susceptibility breakpoint for staphylococci and streptococci is 1 μg/mL; for enterococci it is 4 μg/mL. Approximately 90% of strains of staphylococci and streptococci are inhibited at concentrations of 0.25 to 0.5 μg/mL; the corresponding values for *Enterococcus faecalis* and *E. faecium* are 0.5 to 1 and 2 to 4 μg/mL, respectively. Daptomycin may be active against vancomycin-resistant strains, although MICs tend to be higher for these organisms than for their vancomycin-susceptible counterparts. MICs of *Corynebacterium* spp., *Peptostreptococcus*, *Propionibacterium*, and *Clostridium perfringens* are ≤ 0.5 to 1 μg/mL. *Actinomyces* spp. are inhibited over the concentration range of 4 to 32 μg/mL. *In vitro* activity of daptomycin is Ca^{2+} dependent, and MIC tests should be performed in a medium containing 50 mg/L calcium.

Daptomycin binds to bacterial membranes resulting in depolarization, loss of membrane potential, and cell death. It has concentration-dependent bactericidal activity. Due to its unique mechanism of action, cross-resistance with other antibiotic classes seems not to occur, and there are no known resistance mechanisms. There were two cases (one *S. aureus* and the other *E. faecalis*) among more than 1000 cases treated in which resistance emerged during therapy. Staphylococci with decreased susceptibility to vancomycin have higher daptomycin MICs than fully susceptible strains.

Daptomycin is poorly absorbed orally and should only be administered intravenously. Direct toxicity to muscle precludes intramuscular injection. The steady-state peak serum concentration following intravenous administration of 4 mg/kg in healthy volunteers is approximately 58 μg/mL. Daptomycin displays linear pharmacokinetics at doses up to 8 mg/kg. It is reversibly bound to albumin; protein binding is 92%. The serum half-life is 8 to 9 hours in normal subjects, permitting once-daily dosing. Approximately 80% of the administered dose is recovered in urine; a small amount is excreted in feces. Dosage adjustment is required for creatinine clearance below 30 mL/minute; this is accomplished by administering the recommended dose every 48 hours. For hemodialysis patients, the dose should be administered immediately after dialysis.

Daptomycin neither inhibits nor induces CYPs, and there are no important drug–drug interactions. However, caution is recommended when administering daptomycin in conjunction with aminoglycosides or statins because of potential risks of nephrotoxicity and myopathy, respectively.

Daptomycin is indicated in treatment of complicated skin and skin-structure infections caused by methicillin-susceptible and methicillin-resistant strains of *S. aureus*, hemolytic streptococci, and vancomycin-susceptible *E. faecalis*. Its efficacy is comparable to that of vancomycin. Efficacy in more serious infections, such as endocarditis or complicated bacteremia, has not been demonstrated, although clinical trials are under way. Daptomycin was inferior to comparators for treatment of community-acquired pneumonia and is not indicated for this infection.

Skeletal muscle damage occurs in dogs given daptomycin at doses above 10 mg/kg. Peripheral neuropathic effects with axonal degeneration occurred at higher doses. In humans, elevations of creatine kinase may occur; this does not require discontinuation of the drug unless there are findings of an otherwise unexplained myopathy. In phase 1 and 2 clinical trials, a few patients had evidence of possible neuropathy, although this was not observed in phase 3 studies.

DARBEPOETIN ALFA

(Aranesp solution for injection 25 mcg/mL)

Darbepoetin is a recombinant human erythropoietin that stimulates red blood cell production. Darbepoetin is indicated in treatment of anemia associated with chronic renal failure, whether or not the patient is on dialysis; and treatment of anemia in patients with nonmyeloid malignancies where anemia is caused by coadministered chemotherapy. Recombinant human erythropoietin (**epoetin alfa**), produced using engineered Chinese hamster ovary cells, is nearly identical to the endogenous hormone except for two subtle differences. First, the carbohydrate modification, pattern of epoetin alfa differs slightly from the native protein, but this difference apparently does not alter kineticpotency, or immunoreactivity of the drug. However, modern assays can detect these differences, which is of significance in detecting athletes who use the recombinant product for "blood doping." The second difference probably is related to the manufacturing process, as one commercially available form of the drug was recently associated with the development of antirecombinant erythropoietin antibodies that cross-react with the patient's own erythropoietin, potentially causing pure red cell aplasia. Most of these cases were caused by one preparation of the drug shortly after albumin was removed from the formulation.

Available preparations of epoetin alfa include Epogen, Procrit, and Exprex, supplied in single-use vials of from 2,000 to 40,000 units/mL for intravenous or subcutaneous administration. When injected intravenously, epoetin alfa is cleared from plasma with a half-life of 4 to 8 hours. However, the effect on marrow progenitors is sufficiently sustained that it need only be given three times a week to achieve an adequate response. Combination of the weekly dose into a single injection also can achieve virtually identical results. No significant allergic reactions have been associated with the intravenous or subcutaneous administration of epoetin alfa, and—except as noted previously—antibodies have not been detected even after prolonged administration.

More recently, novel erythropoiesis-stimulating-protein (Nesp) or **darbapoetin alfa** (Aranesp) has been approved for clinical use in patients with indications similar to those for epoetin alfa. It is a genetically modified form of erythropoietin in which four amino acids have been mutated such that additional carbohydrate side chains are added during its synthesis, prolonging the circulatory survival of the drug to 24 to 26 hours.

Recombinant erythropoietin therapy, in conjunction with adequate iron intake, can be highly effective in a number of anemias, especially those associated with a poor erythropoietic response. There is a clear dose–response relationship between the epoetin alfa dose and the rise in hematocrit in anephric patients, with eradication of their anemia at higher doses. Epoetin alfa is also effective in the treatment of anemias associated with surgery, acquired immunodeficiency syndrome (AIDS), cancer chemotherapy, prematurity, and certain chronic inflammatory conditions. **Darbapoetin alfa** also has been approved for use in patients with anemia associated with chronic kidney disease and is under review for several other indications.

During erythropoietin therapy, absolute or functional iron deficiency may develop. Functional iron deficiency (i.e., normal ferritin levels but low transferrin saturation) presumably results from the inability to mobilize iron stores rapidly enough to support the increased erythropoiesis. Virtually all patients eventually will require supplemental iron to increase or maintain transferrin saturation to levels that will adequately support stimulated erythropoiesis. Supplemental iron therapy is recommended for all patients whose serum ferritin is below 100 μg/L or whose serum transferrin saturation is less than 20%.

During initial therapy and after any dosage adjustment, the hematocrit is determined once a week (HIV-infected and cancer patients) or twice a week (renal failure patients) until it has stabilized in the target range and the maintenance dose has been established; the hematocrit then is monitored at regular intervals. If the hematocrit increases by more than 4 points in any 2-week period, the dose should be decreased. Due to the time required for erythropoiesis and the erythrocyte half-life, hematocrit changes lag behind dosage adjustments by 2 to 6 weeks. The dose of **darbepoetin** should be decreased if the hemoglobin increase exceeds 1 g/dl in any two-week period because of the association of excessive rate of rise of hemoglobin with adverse cardiovascular events.

During hemodialysis, patients receiving epoetin alfa or darbepoetin may require increased anticoagulation. Serious thromboembolic events have been reported, including migratory thrombophlebitis, microvascular thrombosis, pulmonary embolism, and thrombosis of the retinal artery and temporal and renal veins. The risk of thrombotic events, including vascular access thromboses, was higher in adults with ischemic heart disease or congestive heart failure (CHF) receiving epoetin alfa therapy with the goal of reaching a normal hematocrit level (42%) than in those with a lower target hematocrit level of 30%. The higher risk of cardiovascular events from erythropoietic therapies may be associated with higher hemoglobin or higher rates of rise of hemoglobin. The hemoglobin level should be managed to avoid exceeding a target level of 12 g/dL. Although epoetin alfa is not associated with direct pressor effects, blood pressure may rise, especially during the early phases of therapy when the hematocrit is increasing. Erythropoietins should be withheld in patients with preexisting uncontrolled hypertension. Patients may require initiation of, or increases in, antihypertensive therapy. Hypertensive encephalopathy and seizures have occurred in chronic renal failure patients treated with epoetin alfa. The incidence of seizures appears to be higher during the first 90 days of therapy with epoetin alfa in patients on dialysis (occurring in about 2.5% of patients) when compared with subsequent 90-day periods. Headache, tachycardia, edema, shortness of breath, nausea, vomiting, diarrhea, injection site stinging, and flu-like symptoms (e.g., arthralgias and myalgias) also have been reported in conjunction with epoetin alfa therapy. Pure red cell aplasia in association with neutralizing antibodies to native erythropoietin has been observed in patients treated with recombinant erythropoietins and in underlying infectious, inflammatory or malignant processes; occult blood loss; underlying hematologic diseases (e.g., thalassemia, refractory anemia, or other myelodysplastic disorders); folic acid or vitamin B_{12} deficiency; hemolysis; aluminum intoxication; bone marrow fibrosis; and osteitis fibrosa cystica.

Patients with anemia secondary to chronic kidney disease are ideal candidates for epoetin alfa therapy. The response in predialysis, peritoneal dialysis, and hemodialysis patients is dependent on the severity of renal failure, erythropoietin dose and route of administration, and iron availability. The subcutaneous route of administration is preferred to the intravenous route because absorption is slower and the amount of drug required is reduced by 20 to 40%.

The dose of epoetin alfa should be adjusted to obtain a gradual rise in the hematocrit over a 2- to 4-month period to a final hematocrit of 33 to 36%. Treatment to hematocrit levels greater than 36% is not recommended because patients treated to a hematocrit level above 40% showed a higher incidence of MI and death. The drug should not be used to replace emergency transfusion in patients who need immediate correction of a life-threatening anemia.

Patients are started on doses of 80 to 120 units/kg of epoetin alfa, given subcutaneously, three times a week. It can be given on a once-a-week schedule, but somewhat more drug is required for an equivalent effect. If the response is poor, the dose should be progressively increased. The final maintenance dose of epoetin alfa can vary from as little as 10 units/kg to more than 300 units/kg, with an average dose of 75 units/kg, three times a week. Children younger than 5 years generally require a higher dose. Resistance to therapy is common in patients who develop an inflammatory illness or become iron deficient, so close monitoring of general health and iron status is essential. Less common causes of resistance include occult blood loss, folic acid deficiency, camitine deficiency, inadequate dialysis, aluminum toxicity, and osteitis fibrosa cystica secondary to hyperparathyroidism.

The most common side effect of epoetin alfa therapy is aggravation of hypertension, which occurs in 20 to 30% of patients and most often is associated with a rapid rise in hematocrit. Blood pressure usually can be controlled either by increasing antihypertensive therapy or ultrafiltration in dialysis patients or by reducing the epoetin alfa dose to slow the hematocrit response.

Darbapoetin alfa is also approved for use in patients who are anemic secondary to chronic kidney disease. The recommended starting dose is 0.45 μg/kg administered intravenously or subcutaneously once weekly, with dose adjustments depending on the response. Similar to epoetin alfa, side effects tend to occur when patients experience a rapid rise in hemoglobin concentration; a rise of less than 1 g/dL every 2 weeks generally has been considered safe.

Epoetin alfa therapy has been approved for the treatment of HIV-infected patients, especially those on zidovudine therapy. Excellent responses to doses of 100 to 300 units/kg, given subcutaneously three times a week, generally are seen in patients with zidovudine-induced anemia. In the face of advanced disease, marrow damage, and elevated serum erythropoietin levels (greater than 500 international units [IU]/L), therapy is less effective.

Epoetin alfa therapy, 150 units/kg three times a week or 450 to 600 units/kg once a week can reduce the transfusion requirement in cancer patients undergoing chemotherapy. Evidence-based guidelines for the therapeutic use of recombinant erythropoietin in patients with cancer have been published. Briefly, the guidelines recommend the use of epoetin alfa in patients with chemotherapy-associated anemia when hemoglobin levels fall below 10 g/dL, basing the decision to treat less severe anemia (hemoglobin between 10 and 12 g/dL) on clinical circumstances. For anemia associated with hematologic malignancies, the guidelines support the use of recombinant erythropoietin in patients with low-grade myelodysplastic syndrome, although the evidence that the drug is effective in anemic patients with multiple myeloma, non-Hodgkin's lymphoma, or chronic lymphocytic elukemia not receiving chemotherapy is less robust. A baseline serum erythropoietin level may help predict the response; most patients with blood levels of more than 500 IU/L are unlikely to respond to any dose of the drug. Most patients treated with epoetin alfa experienced an improvement in their anemia, sense of well-being, and quality of life. This improved sense of well-being, particularly in cancer patients, may not be solely due to the rise in the hematocrit. Erythropoietin receptors have been demonstrated in cells of the CNS, and erythropoietin has been found to act as a cytoprotectant in several models Thus, high levels of the hormone may directly affect cancer patients' sense of well-being.

Darbopoetin alfa also has been tested in cancer patients undergoing chemotherapy, and preliminary studies appear promising. However, recent case reports have suggested a direct effect of both epoetin alfa and darbopoetin alfa in stimulation of tumor cells. For example, patients with cancer of the head and neck randomized to receive recombinant erythropoietin had a statistically significant increase in the likelihood of tumor progression during the duration of the study. This finding is being evaluated and warrants serious attention.

Epoetin alfa has been used perioperatively to treat anemia and reduce the need for transfusion. Patients undergoing elective orthopedic and cardiac procedures have been treated with 150 to 300 units/kg of epoetin alfa once daily for 10 days preceding surgery, on the day of surgery, and for 4 days after surgery. As an alternative, 600 units/kg can be given 21, 14, and 7 days before surgery, with an additional dose on the day of surgery. This can correct a moderately severe preoperative anemia (i.e., hematocrit of 30 to 36%) and reduce the need for transfusion. Epoetin alfa also has been used to improve autologous blood donation. However, the potential benefit generally is small, and the expense is considerable. Patients treated for 3 to 4 weeks with epoetin alfa (300 to 600 units/kg twice a week) are able to donate only one or two more units than untreated patients, and most of the time this goes unused. Still, the ability to stimulate erythropoiesis for blood storage can be invaluable in the patient with multiple alloantibodies to red blood cells.

DARIFENACIN

(Enablex tablets, extended-release 7.5 mg)

Darifenacin is an anticholinergic agent that blocks muscarinic cholinergic receptors. Darifenacin is indicated in treatment of overactive bladder with symptoms of urge urinary incontinence, urgency, and frequency.

Newer muscarinic agonists, **pirenzepine** for M_1, **tripitramine** for M_2, and **darifenacin** for M_3, show selectivity as muscarinic blocking agents. Several muscarinic antagonists show sufficient selectivity in the clinical setting to minimize the bothersome side effects seen with the nonselective agents at therapeutic doses. The basis for the selectivity of these agonists is unclear, as there is limited evidence that agonists discriminate appreciably among the subtypes of muscarinic receptors. However, subsequent radioligand binding studies definitively revealed distinct populations of antagonist binding sites. In particular, the muscarinic antagonist pirenzepine was shown to bind with high affinity to sites in the cerebral cortex and sympathetic ganglia (M_1) but to have lower affinity for sites in cardiac muscle, smooth muscle, and various glands. These data explain the ability of pirenzepine to block agonist-induced responses that are mediated by muscarinic receptors in sympathetic and myenteric ganglia at concentrations considerably lower than those required to block responses that result from direct stimulation of receptors in various effector organs. Antagonists that can further discriminate among various subtypes of muscarinic receptors are now available. For example, tripitramine displays selectivity for cardiac M_2 relative to M_3 muscarinic receptors, whereas darifenacin is relatively selective for antagonizing glandular and smooth-muscle M_3 relative to M_2 receptors.

The cloning of cDNAs that encode muscarinic receptors identified five distinct gene products now designated as M_1 through M_5. All of the known muscarinic receptor subtypes interact with members of a group of heterotrimeric guanine nucleotide-binding regulatory proteins (G-proteins) that in turn are linked to various cellular effectors. Regions within the receptor responsible for the specificity of G-protein coupling have been defined primarily by receptor mutants and chimeras formed between receptor subtypes. In particular, one region at the carboxyl-terminal end of the third intracellular loop of the receptor has been implicated in the specificity of G-protein coupling and shows extensive homology within M_1, M_3, and M_5 receptors and between M_2 and M_4 receptors. Conserved regions in the second intracellular loop also confer specificity for proper G-protein recognition. Although selectivity is not absolute, stimulation of M_1 or M_3 receptors causes hydrolysis of polyphosphoinositides and mobilization of intracellular Ca^{2+} as a consequence of activation of the G_q–PLC pathway; this effect in turn results in a variety of Ca^{2+}-mediated events, either directly or as a consequence of the phosphorylation of target proteins. In contrast, M_2 and M_4 muscarinic receptors inhibit adenylyl cyclase and regulate specific ion channels (e.g., enhancement of K^+ conductance in cardiac atrial tissue) through subunits released from pertussis-toxin-sensitive G-proteins (G_i and G_0), which are distinct from the G-proteins used by M_1 and M_3 receptors.

Studies using muscarinic receptor-subtype-specific antibodies and ligands demonstrate discrete localization of the muscarinic receptor subtypes, for example, within brain regions and in different populations of smooth muscle cells. Subtypes M_1 through M_5 have been disrupted through gene targeting to create null alleles for each of these genes. All of the muscarinic receptor subtype deletions yield mice that are viable and fertile. Studies using these mice indicate that pilocarpine-induced seizures are mediated through M_1, oxotremorine-induced tremors through M_2, analgesia through M_2 and M_4, and hypothermia through M_2 and other subtypes. Carbachol and vagally induced bradycardia are lost in M_2-receptor knockout mice, whereas mice lacking the M_3 receptor show loss of cholinergic bronchoconstriction and urinary bladder contraction. Full abolition of cholinergic bronchoconstriction, salivation, pupillary constriction, and bladder contraction generally requires deletion of more than a single receptor subtype. The minimal phenotypic alteration that accompanies deletion of a single receptor subtype suggests functional redundancy between receptor subtypes in various tissues.

DAUNORUBICIN

(Cerubidine, Daunomycin)

Daunorubicin and doxorubicin (Adriamycin) bind to and cause the intercalation of the DNA molecule, thereby inhibiting DNA template function. They also provoke DNA chain scission and chromosomal damage.

Daunorubicin is useful in treating patients with acute lymphocytic or acute granulocytic leukemia. Adriamycin is useful in cases of solid tumors such as sarcoma, metastatic breast cancer, and thyroid cancer. These agents cause stomatitis, alopecia, myelosuppression, and cardiac abnormalities ranging from arrhythmias to cardiomyopathy (see also Figure 15).

DAUNORUBICIN CITRATE LIPOSOMAL

(DaunoXome solution for injection 2 mg/mL)

Daunorubicin is an anthracycline antibiotic formulated to increase selectivity for solid tumors in site. It is indicated in advanced HIV-associated Kaposi's sarcoma. **Daunorubicin, Doxorubicin, Epirubicin, Idarubicin, and Mitoxantrone** anthracycline antibiotics are among the most important antitumor agents. They are derived from the fungus *Streptococcus peucetius* var. *caesius*. **Idarubicin** and **epirubicin** are analogs of the naturally produced anthracyclines, differing only slightly in chemical structure, but having somewhat distinct patterns of clinical activity. Daunorubicin and idarubicin have been used primarily in acute leukemias, whereas doxorubicin and epirubicin display broader activity against human solid tumors. These agents, all possessing the potential for generating free radicals, cause an unusual and often irreversible cardiomyopathy, the occurrence of which is related to the total dose of the drug. The structurally similar agent mitoxantrone has useful activity against prostate cancer and acute myelocytic leukemia (AML), and is used in high-dose chemotherapy. Mitoxantrone, an anthracenedione, has significantly less cardiotoxicity than do the anthracyclines.

Absorption, fate, and excretion: Daunorubicin, doxorubicin, epirubicin, and idarubicin usually are administered intravenously and cleared by a complex pattern of hepatic metabolism and biliary excretion. The plasma disappearance curve for doxorubicin is multiphasic, with elimination half-lives of 3 hours and about 30 hours. All anthracyclines are converted to an active alcohol intermediate that plays a variable role in their therapeutic activity. Idarubicin has a half-life of about 15 hours, and its active metabolite, idarubicinol, has a half-life of about 40 hours. There is rapid uptake of the drugs in the heart, kidneys, lungs, liver, and spleen. They do not cross the blood–brain barrier.

Daunorubicin and doxorubicin are eliminated by metabolic conversion to a variety of aglycones and other inactive products. Idarubicin is primarily metabolized to idarubicinol, which accumulates in plasma and likely contributes significantly to its activity. Clearance is delayed in the presence of hepatic dysfunction, and at least a 50% initial reduction in dose should be considered in patients with abnormal serum bilirubin levels.

The recommended dosage for idarubicin (Idamycin) is 12 mg/m^2 daily for 3 days by intravenous injection in combination with cytarabine. Slow injection with care over 10 to 15 minutes is recommended to avoid extravasation, as with other anthracyclines.

Daunorubicin (daunomycin, rubidomycin; Cerubidine, others) is available for intravenous use. The recommended dosage is 30 to 60 mg/m^2 daily for 3 days. The agent is administered with appropriate care to prevent extravasation, as severe local vesicant action may result. Total doses greater than 1000 mg/m^2 are associated with a high risk of cardiotoxicity. A daunorubicin citrate liposomal product (Daunoxome) is indicated in the treatment of AIDS-related Kaposi's sarcoma. It is given in a dose of 40 mg/m^2 infused over 60 minutes and repeated every 2 weeks. Patients should be advised that the drug may impart a red color to the urine.

Daunorubicin is primarily used in the treatment of AML in combination with Ara-C and has largely been replaced by idarubicin. The toxic manifestations of daunorubicin as well as idarubicin include bone marrow depression, stomatitis, alopecia, GI disturbances, and dermatological manifestations. Cardiac toxicity is a peculiar adverse effect observed with these agents. It is characterized by tachycardia, arrhythmias, dyspnea, hypotension, pericardial effusion, and CHF that is poorly responsive to digitalis.

Doxorubicin is effective in malignant lymphomas; however, in contrast to **daunorubicin**, it also is active in a number of solid tumors, particularly breast cancer. Used in combination with cyclophosphamide, vinca alkaloids, and other agents, it is an important ingredient for the successful treatment of lymphomas. It is a valuable component of various regimens of chemotherapy for adjuvant and metastatic carcinoma of the breast and small-cell carcinoma of the lung. The drug also is particularly beneficial in a wide range of pediatric and adult sarcomas, including osteogenic, Ewing's, and soft-tissue sarcomas.

The toxic manifestations of doxorubicin are similar to those of **daunorubicin**. Myelosuppression is a major dose-limiting complication, with leukopenia usually reaching a nadir during the second week of therapy and recovering by the fourth week; thrombocytopenia and anemia follow a similar pattern but usually are less pronounced. Stomatitis, GI disturbances, and alopecia are common but reversible. Erythematous streaking near the site of infusion ("adriamycin flare") is a benign local allergic reaction and should not be confused with extravasation. Facial flushing, conjunctivitis, and lacrimation may occur rarely. The drug may produce severe local toxicity in irradiated tissues (e.g., the skin, heart, lung, esophagus, and GI mucosa). Such actions may occur even when the two therapies are not administered concomitantly. Cardiomyopathy is the most important long-term toxicity.

Newer analogs of doxorubicin: valrubicin (Valstar) was approved in 1998 for intravesical therapy of bacille Calmette–Guérin-refractory urinary bladder carcinoma *in situ* in patients for whom immediate cystectomy would be associated with unacceptable morbidity or mortality; epirubicin (4′-epidoxorubicin, Ellence) was approved by the FDA in 1999 as a component of adjuvant therapy following resection of early lymph-node-positive breast cancer.

DEBRISOQUIN

Debrisoquin is an antihypertensive medication. Bethanidine is a short-acting adrenergic neuron blocker; debrisoquin and guanadrel are medium-acting adrenergic neuron blockers, whereas guanethidine is a long-acting adrenergic neuron blocker and also depletes axonal stores of norepinephrine. Debrisoquin causes postural hypotension, fluid retention, failure of ejaculation, and depression. Debrisoquin should be avoided with tyramine-containing substances such as cheese. Debrisoquin and other adrenergic neuron-blocking drugs may interact with amphetamines, ephedrine, phenylephrine, tricyclic antidepressants, and chlorpromazine.

DECAMETHONIUM

Acetylcholine receptors are classified as either muscarinic or nicotinic. The alkaloid muscarine mimics the effects produced by stimulation of the parasympathetic system. These effects are postganglionic and are exerted on exocrine glands, cardiac muscle, and smooth muscle. The alkaloid nicotine mimics the actions of acetylcholine, which include stimulation of all autonomic ganglia, stimulation of the adrenal medulla, and contraction of skeletal muscle (see Figure 12).

Dimethylphenylpiperazinium stimulates the autonomic ganglia; tetraethylammonium and hexamethonium block the autonomic ganglia; phenyltrimethylammonium stimulates skeletal motor muscle end plates; decamethonium produces neuromuscular blockade; and d-tubocurarine blocks both the autonomic ganglia and the motor fiber end plates.

Among the agents cited, only *d*-tubocurarine (see Figure 99) is useful as a drug (skeletal muscle relaxant); the rest are useful only as research tools.

DEFEROXAMINE

(Desferal)

A lethal dose of iron consists of 12 g of an iron preparation containing 1 or 2 g of elemental iron. Therefore, iron toxicity rarely occurs in adults but is frequently seen in children. The mortality rate among untreated children is high (45%). The initial signs and symptoms of iron poisoning are gastrointestinal and usually consist of nausea, vomiting, and diarrhea. If untreated, acidosis, cyanosis, and circulatory collapse may ensue. If the patient survives, there may be gastric scarring and pyloric stenosis resulting from the corrosive action of the iron preparation. Treatment should include induced vomiting and lavage if the poisoning is discovered early, catharsis to hasten evacuation, sodium bicarbonate therapy to combat the acidosis, and the administration of deferoxamine, a specific iron-chelating agent.

One hundred milligrams (100 mg) of deferoxamine is able to bind 8.5 mg of iron. The chelating effects of deferoxamine are maximum at an acidic pH; therefore, when given orally, deferoxamine must be administered before sodium bicarbonate. In the event of iron poisoning, deferoxamine may also be administered intramuscularly. Besides its usefulness in counteracting the effects of iron poisoning, deferoxamine has been used in disorders that involve iron overload, such as ocular hemosiderosis or hemochromatosis.

DELAVIRDINE MESYLATE

(Rescriptor tablets 100 mg)

Delavirdine is an antiretroviral/nonnucleoside reverse transcriptase inhibitor that inhibits replication of HIV-1 infection by interfering with DNA synthesis. Delavirdine is indicated in treatment of HIV-1 infection in combination with appropriate antiretroviral agents when therapy is warranted.

Nonnucleoside reverse transcriptase inhibitors (NNRTIs) include a variety of chemical substrates that bind to the hydrophobic pocket in the p66 subunit of the HIV-1 reverse transcriptase. The NNRTI-binding pocket is not essential for the function of the enzyme and is distant from the active site. These compounds induce a conformational change in the three-dimensional structure of the enzyme that greatly reduces its activity, and thus they act as non-competitive inhibitors. Unlike nucleoside and nucleotide reverse transcriptase inhibitors, these compounds do not require intracellular phosphorylation to attain activity. Because the binding site for NNRTIs is virus strain specific, the approved agents are active against HIV-1 but not HIV-2 or other retroviruses and should not be used to treat HIV-2 infection. These compounds also have no activity against host-cell DNA polymerases. The two most commonly used agents in this category, efavirenz and nevirapine, are quite potent and transiently decrease plasma HIV RNA concentrations by two orders of magnitude or more when used as sole agents.

All three approved NNRTIs are eliminated from the body by hepatic metabolism. **Nevirapine** and **delavirdine** are primarily substrates for the CYP3A4 isoform, whereas **efavirenz** is a substrate for CYP2B6 and CYP3A4. The steady-state elimination half-lives of efavirenz and nevirapine range from 24 to 72 hours, allowing daily dosing. Efavirenz and nevirapine are moderately potent inducers of hepatic drug-metabolizing enzymes including CYP3A4, whereas delavirdine is a CYP3A4 inhibitor. Pharmacokinetic drug interactions are thus an important consideration with this class of compounds and represent a potential source of toxicity.

The NNRTIs are more susceptible to high-level drug resistance than other classes of antiretroviral drugs because a single-amino-acid change in the NNRTI-binding pocket (usually in codons 103 or 181) renders the virus resistant to all available drugs in the class. Unlike nucleoside analogs or protease inhibitors, NNRTIs can induce resistance and virologic relapse within a few days or weeks if given as monotherapy. Exposure to even a single dose of nevirapine in the absence of other antiretroviral drugs is associated with resistance mutations in up to one-third of patients. These agents are potent and highly effective but must be combined with at least two other active agents to avoid resistance.

The use of efavirenz or nevirapine in combination with other antiretroviral drugs is associated with favorable long-term suppression of viremia and elevation of CD4+ lymphocyte counts. Efavirenz in particular is a common component of first regimens for treatment-naive patients in recognition of its convenience, tolerability, and potency. Rashes occur frequently with all NNRTIs, usually during the first 4 weeks of therapy. These generally are mild and self-limited, although rare cases of potentially fatal Stevens–Johnson syndrome have been reported with nevirapine and efavirenz. Fat accumulation can be seen after long-term use of NNRTIs, and fatal hepatitis has been associated with nevirapine use.

As with all drugs in this class, the most common side effect of delavirdine is rash, which occurs in 18 to 36% of subjects. Rash usually is seen in the first few weeks of treatment and often resolves despite continued therapy. The rash may be macular, papular, erythematous, or pruritic and usually involves the trunk and extremities. Fewer than 5% of patients discontinue **delavirdine** because of rash. Severe dermatitis, including erythema multiforme and Stevens–Johnson syndrome, has been reported but is rare. Elevated hepatic transaminases also have been reported, but delavirdine use is not associated with fatal hepatitis. Neutropenia also may occur rarely.

Delavirdine is both a substrate for and an inhibitor of CYP3A4 and can alter the metabolism of other CYP3A4 substrates. Therefore, it should be avoided with certain CYP3A4 substrates with a low therapeutic index, including amiodarone, propafenone, ergot derivatives, pimozide, triazolam, and midazolam. Delavirdine is a weak inhibitor of CYP2C9, CYP2D6, and CYP2C19 *in vitro*. Potent inducers of CYP3A4, such as carbamazepine, phenobarbital, phenytoin, rifabutin, and rifampin, may decrease delavirdine concentrations and should be avoided. Delavirdine increases the plasma concentrations of most HIV protease inhibitors and could be used to modestly enhance the pharmacokinetic profile or reduce the dose of these agents.

DEMECLOCYCLINE

(Declomycin tablets 150 mg)

Demeclocycline inhibits bacterial protein synthesis and is indicated in treatment of infections caused by susceptible strains of Gram-positive and Gram-negative microorganisms. **Oxytetracycline** is a natural product elaborated by *Streptomyces rimosus*. Tetracycline is a semisynthetic derivative of chlortetracycline. **Demeclocycline** is the product of a mutant strain of ***Streptomyces aureofaciens***, and **methacycline**, **doxycycline**, and **minocycline** all are semisynthetic derivatives. Tetracyclines are bacteriostatic antibiotics with activity against a wide range of aerobic and anaerobic Gram-positive and Gram-negative bacteria. They also are effective against some microorganisms, such as *Rickettsia, Coxiella burnetii, Mycoplasma pneumoniae, Chlamydia* spp., *Legionella* spp., *Ureaplasma*, some atypical mycobacteria, and *Plasmodium* spp. that are resistant to cell-wall-active antimicrobial agents. They are not active against fungi.

Demeclocycline, **tetracycline**, **oxytetracycline**, **minocycline**, and **doxycycline** are available in the United States for systemic use. **Chlortetracycline** and **oxytetracycline** are used in ophthalmic preparations. Methacycline is not available. Other derivatives are available in other countries. The more lipophilic drugs, minocycline and doxycycline, usually are the most active by weight, followed by tetracycline. Resistance of a bacterial strain to any one member of the class may result in cross-resistance to other tetracyclines. Bacterial strains with tetracycline minimum inhibitory concentrations (MICs) of ≤ 4 μg/mL are considered susceptible except for *Haemophilus influenzae* and *Streptococcus pneumoniae*, whose susceptibility breakpoints (defined as the upper limit of the concentration at which bacteria are still considered susceptible to a given drug) are ≤ 2 μg/mL, and *Neisseria gonorrhoeae*, with a breakpoint of ≤ 0.25 μg/mL.

Oral absorption of most tetracyclines is incomplete. The percentage of an oral dose that is absorbed with an empty stomach is low for chlortetracycline (30%); intermediate for oxytetracycline, demeclocycline, and tetracycline (60 to 80%); and high for doxycycline (95%) and minocycline (100%). The percentage of unabsorbed drug rises as the dose increases. Absorption mostly takes place in the stomach and upper small intestine and is greater in the fasting state. Absorption of tetracyclines is impaired by the concurrent ingestion of dairy products; aluminum hydroxide gels; calcium, magnesium, and iron or zinc salts; and bismuth subsalicylate. Thus, milk, milk products, antacids, Pepto-Bismol, and dietary Fe and Zn supplements will interfere with tetracycline absorption. The decreased absorption apparently results from chelation of divalent and trivalent cations. With the exception of doxycycline, the primary route of elimination for most tetracyclines is the kidney, although they are also concentrated in the liver and excreted in bile. After biliary excretion, they are partially reabsorbed via enterohepatic recirculation. Elimination via the intestinal tract occurs even when the drugs are given parenterally. Minocycline is an exception and is significantly metabolized by the liver. Comparable amounts of tetracycline (i.e., 20 to 60%) are excreted in the urine within 24 hours following oral or intravenous administration. Approximately 10 to 35% of a dose of oxytetracycline is excreted in active form in the urine, where it can be detected within 30 minutes and reaches a peak concentration about 5 hours after administration. The rate of renal clearance of demeclocycline is less than half that of tetracycline. Decreased hepatic function or obstruction of the common bile duct reduces the biliary excretion of these agents, resulting in longer half-lives and higher plasma concentrations. Because of their enterohepatic circulation, these drugs may remain in the body for a long time after cessation of therapy.

Minocycline is recovered from urine and feces in significantly lower amounts than are the other tetracyclines, and it appears to be metabolized to a considerable extent. Renal clearance of minocycline is low. The drug persists in the body long after its administration is stopped, possibly due to retention in fatty tissues. Nonetheless, the half-life of minocycline is not prolonged in patients with hepatic failure.

Doxycycline at recommended doses does not accumulate significantly in patients with renal failure and thus is one of the safest of the tetracyclines for use in patients with renal impairment. The drug is excreted in the feces. Its half-life may be significantly shortened by concurrent therapy with barbiturates, phenytoin, rifampin, or other inducers of hepatic microsomal enzymes.

DEMECLOCYCLINE HYDROCHLORIDE

(Declomycin, Ledermycin)

Demeclocycline, a tetracycline antibiotic (600 mg p.o. q. 6 hours), is indicated in the treatment of infections caused by susceptible organisms, gonorrhea, and uncomplicated urethral, endocervical, or rectal infection (see also Figure 88).

DENILEUKIN DIFTITOX

(Ontak frozen, solution for injection 150 mcg/mL)

Denileukin, a recombinant-DNA-derived cytotoxic protein fused to diphtheria toxin fragments A and B, is designed to direct the cytocidal action of diphtheria toxin to cells that express the IL-2 receptor. Denileukin is indicated in treatment of cutaneous T-cell lymphoma.

DEOXYNIVALENOL

Deoxynivalenol, also called vomitoxin, is a naturally occurring trichotecene mycotoxin produced by several species of *Fusarium* fungi on a variety of cereal grains. Reports of contaminated grain are not uncommon. Feed refusal and emesis are the major symptoms in individuals fed diets containing deoxynivalenol. Deoxynivalenol delays gastric emptying through serotonin 3-receptors (5HT3) (see also Figure 73).

DERMATAN SULFATE

(DS)

Dermatan sulfate (DS) is a member of a family of structurally complex, sulfated, linear polysaccharides called glycosaminoglycans. The other members of this family of molecules are heparin, heparin sulfate, chondroitin sulfates, and hyaluronic acid. DS and chondroitin sulfates are structurally similar and make up a subfamily of glycosaminoglycans called galactosaminoglycans. Glycosaminoglycans are often found attached to a protein core, resulting in a macromolcule called a proteoglycan. These proteoglycans localize on cell surfaces and in the extracellular matrix. There, they function in the important role of cell–cell interaction, binding a variety of biologically important proteins and localizing these at the cell surface. Glycosaminoglycan DS has been used as an experimental therapeutic agent to modulate a variety of these biological processes.

DERMATOLOGICAL DISORDERS: Treatment with Retinoids

Acne

Cystic acne	Hidradenitis suppurativa
Gram-negative folliculitis	Papular acne

Cutaneous Aging

Disorders of Keratinization

Darier's disease	Pityriasis rubra pilaris
Erythrokeratoderma variabilis	Ichthyoses

Precancerous Conditions

Actinic keratosis
Dysplastic nevus
Leukoplakia

Skin Cancer	
Basal cell cancer	Keratoacanthoma
Cutaneous T-cell lymphoma	Squamous cell cancer
Psoriasis	
Erythrodermic psoriasis	Pustular psoriasis
Psoriasis vulgaris	Pustular psoriasis, palms and soles
Psoriatic arthritis	

DESFLURANE

(Suprane)

Desflurane, a tetrafluorethyl difluoromethyl ether, is used to induce and maintain anesthesia.

DESIPRAMINE

(Norpramin)

Desipramine is a tricyclic antidepressant, inhibits reuptake of norepinephrine and serotonin in CNS, and is indicated in relief of symptoms of depression. Desipramine (75 to 150 mg p.o./day in divided doses) is indicated in endogenous depression; major depression with melancholia or psychotic symptoms; depression associated with organic brain disease, alcoholism, schizophrenia, or mental retardation; and the depressive phase of manic–depressive disorder. Desipramine is absorbed rapidly from the GI tract, distributed widely in the body, and appears also in breast milk. It is bound to plasma proteins to the extent of 90%, undergoes extensive first-pass metabolism, and its metabolites are excreted in urine. Desipramine strongly blocks the norepinephrine uptake mechanism and has no effect on the uptake of serotonin. Desipramine has weak $alpha_1$-adrenergic and muscarinic cholinergic receptor–blocking effects (see also Tables 5 through 7). The concomitant use of desipramine with sympathomimetic amines may cause elevated blood pressure. On the other hand, desipramine, by blocking the uptake sites for norepinephrine may attenuate the antihypertensive effects of guanethidine, guanabenz, guanadrel, clonidine, methyldopa, and reserpine (see Figure 41).

DESIRUDIN

(Iprivask powder for injection)

Desirudin is a thrombin inhibitor that binds to thrombin, blocking the thrombogenic activity of thrombin, thereby prolonging the clotting time of human plasma. Activated partial thromboplastin time (aPTT) is a measure of the anticoagulant activity of desirudin. It is indicated in prophylaxis of deep vein thrombosis, which may lead to pulmonary embolism, in patients undergoing elective hip replacement surgery.

DESLANOSIDE

Among the useful available cardiac glycosides are the following:

Digitalis purpurea	Digitalis lanata	Strophanthus gratus
Digitoxin	Digoxin	Ouabain
Digoxin	Lanatoside C	
Digitalis leaf	Deslanoside	

Of these, only digoxin and digitoxin and, to a certain extent, ouabain are used extensively.

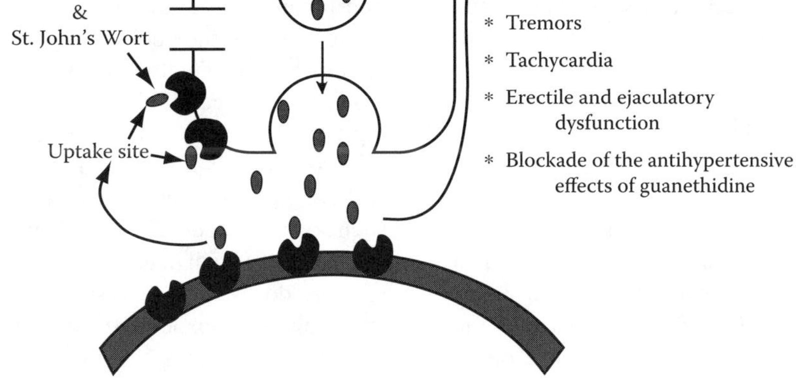

FIGURE 41 Desipramine, a tricyclic antidepressant, causes a strong blockade of the serotonin uptake mechanism. It causes a mild degree of sedation and orthostatic hypotension and has a weak anticholinergic property.

The structures of the cardiac glycosides, including digoxin, have three common components: a steroid nucleus (aglycones or genins), a series of sugar residues in the C_3 position, and a five- or six-membered lactone ring in the C_{17} position.

DESLORATADINE

(Clarinex tablets 5 mg)

Desloratadine is a long-acting histamine antagonist with selective H_1-receptor histamine-antagonist activity. Desloratadine is indicated in relief of nasal and nonnasal symptoms of seasonal and perennial allergic rhinitis; in chronic idiopathic urticaria for relief of symptoms of pruritus and reduction in number and size of hives. The withdrawal of **terfenadine** prompted the development of its active metabolite, **fexofenadine**, as a replacement. This compound lacks the toxic side effects of terfenadine, is not sedating, and retains the antiallergic properties of the parent compound. Another antihistamine developed using this strategy is **desloratidine**, an active metabolite of loratidine. Cetirizine, loratadine, and fexofenadine are all well absorbed and are excreted mainly in the unmetabolized form. Cetirizine and loratadine are excreted primarily into the urine, whereas fexofenadine is excreted primarily in the feces.

Desloratadine, is selective for H_1 receptors, lacks significant anticholinergic actions, and penetrates poorly into the CNS. Taken together, these properties appear to account for the low incidence of side effects of piperidine antihistamines. Second-generation H_1-receptor antagonists lack anticholinergic side effects and are described as nonsedating largely because they do not cross the blood–brain barrier. They include **cetirizine** (Zyrtec), **loratadine** (Claritin), **desloratidine** (Clarinex), and **fexofenadine hydrochloride** (Allegra). Although second-generation nonsedating H_1-receptor blockers are as effective as the first-generation H_1 blockers, they are metabolized by CYP3A4 and, to a lesser extent, by CYP2D6 and should not be coadministered with medications that inhibit these enzymes (e.g., imidazole antifungals and macrolide antibiotics).

H_2-receptor blockers include **cimetidine** (Tagamet), **ranitidine** (Zantac), **famotidine** (Pepcid), and **nizatidine** (Axid). Besides their use in combination with H_1-receptor blockers for pruritus, the H_2-receptor blockers have immunomodulating effects, and this property has been exploited in children to treat warts.

DESMOPRESSIN ACETATE

(1-Deamino-8-D-Arginine Vasopressin) (DDAVP tablets 0.1 mg)

Desmopressin, a synthetic analog of arginine vasopressin, is indicated in nocturnal enuresis; neurogenic diabetes insipidus; polyuria following surgery or trauma in the pituitary region; in combination with factor VIII in the treatment of hemophilia A and von Willebrand's disease. Because desmopressin may be used intranasally, changes in nasal mucosa, including scarring, edema, discharge, blockage, congestion, and atrophic rhinitis, may occur.

Many agents alter the secretion or action of vasopressin; these are cited in Figure 102.

Desmopressin is a posterior pituitary hormone that has antidiuretic effects that decrease urinary volume and increase urine osmolality. It is indicated in control of primary nocturnal enuresis; control of central cranial diabetes insipidus; and maintenance of hemostasis in patients with hemophilia A and type I von Willebrand disease during surgery and postoperatively.

Diabetes insipidus (DI): DI is a disease of impaired renal conservation of water owing either to an inadequate secretion of vasopressin from the neurohypophysis (central DI) or to an insufficient renal response to vasopressin (nephrogenic DI). Very rarely, DI can be caused by an abnormally high rate of degradation of vasopressin by circulating vasopressinases. Pregnancy may accentuate or reveal central and/or nephrogenic DI by increasing plasma levels of vasopressinase and by reducing the renal sensitivity to vasopressin. Patients with DI excrete large volumes (more than 30 mL/kg per day) of dilute (less than 200 mOsm/kg) urine and, if their thirst mechanism is functioning normally, are polydipsic. In contrast to the sweet urine excreted by patients with diabetes mellitus, urine from patients with DI is tasteless; hence the name insipidus. The urinary taste test for DI has been supplanted by the approach of observing whether the patient is able to reduce urine volume and increase urine osmolality after a period of carefully observed fluid deprivation. Central DI can be distinguished from nephrogenic DI by administration of desmopressin, which will increase urine osmolality in patients with central DI but have little or no effect in patients with nephrogenic DI. DI can be differentiated from primary polydipsia by measuring plasma osmolality, which will be low to low-normal in patients with primary polydipsia and high to high-normal in patients with DI.

Only two antidiuretic peptides are available for clinical use in the United States: (1) Vasopressin (synthetic 8-L-arginine vasopressin; Pitressin) is available as a sterile aqueous solution; it may be administered subcutaneously, intramuscularly, or intranasally. (2) **Desmopressin acetate** (synthetic 1-deamino-8-D-arginine vasopressin; DDAVP, others) is available as a sterile aqueous solution packaged for intravenous or subcutaneous injection, in a nasal solution for intranasal administration with either a nasal spray pump or rhinal tube delivery system, and in tablets for oral administration. The therapeutic uses of vasopressin and its congeners can be divided into two main categories according to the type of vasopressin receptor involved.

Most adverse effects are mediated through the V_1 receptor acting on vascular and GI smooth muscle; consequently, such adverse effects are much less common, and less severe, with desmopressin than with vasopressin. After the injection of large doses of vasopressin, marked facial pallor owing to cutaneous vasoconstriction is observed commonly. Increased intestinal activity is likely to cause nausea, belching, cramps, and an urge to defecate. Most serious, however, is the effect on the coronary circulation. Vasopressin should be administered only at low doses and with extreme caution in individuals suffering from vascular disease, especially coronary artery disease. Other cardiac complications include arrhythmia and decreased cardiac output. Peripheral vasoconstriction and gangrene have been encountered in patients receiving large doses of vasopressin.

The major V_2-receptor-mediated adverse effect is water intoxication, which can occur with **desmopressin** or vasopressin. In this regard, many drugs, including carbamazepine, chlorpropamide, morphine, tricyclic antidepressants, and nonsteroidal antiinflammatory drugs (NSAIDs), can potentiate the antidiuretic effects of these peptides. Several drugs such as lithium demeclocycline and ethanol can attenuate the antidiuretic response to desmopressin. **Desmopressin** and vasopressin must be employed cautiously in disease states in which a rapid increase in extracellular water may impose risks (e.g., in angina, hypertension, and heart failure), and should not be used in patients with acute renal failure. Patients receiving **desmopressin** to maintain hemostasis should be advised to reduce fluid intake. Also, it is imperative that these peptides not be administered to patients with primary or psychogenic polydipsia because severe hypotonic hyponatremia will ensue.

Mild facial flushing and headache are the most common adverse effects associated with desmopressin. Allergic reactions ranging from urticaria to anaphylaxis may occur with **desmopressin** or vasopressin. Intranasal administration may cause local adverse effects in the nasal passages, such as edema, rhinorrhea, congestion, irritation, pruritus, and ulceration.

DESONIDE
(DesOwen, Tridesilon)

Desonide, a topical adrenocorticoid with antiinflammatory properties (0.05% cream, lotion, and ointment), is used as an adjunctive therapy for inflammation in acute and chronic corticosteroid-responsive dermatoses (see also Table 14).

DEXAMETHASONE
(Aeroseb-Dex aerosol 0.01%)

Dexamethasone is a topical corticosteroid/glucocorticoid/ corticosteroid. Synthetic long-acting glucocorticoid depresses formation, release, and activity of endogenous mediators of inflammation, including prostaglandins, kinins, histamine, liposomal enzymes, and the complement system. It also modifies the body's immune response. Dexamethasone is indicated in the testing of adrenal cortical hyperfunction and management of primary or secondary adrenal cortex insufficiency, rheumatic disorders, collagen diseases, dermatologic diseases, allergic states, allergic and inflammatory ophthalmic processes, respiratory diseases, hematologic disorders, neoplastic diseases, cerebral edema associated with primary or metastatic brain tumor, craniotomy or head injury, edematous states (caused by nephrotic syndrome), GI diseases, multiple sclerosis, tuberculous meningitis, and trichinosis with neurologic or myocardial involvement. Intralesional administration: used as treatment for such conditions as keloids, psoriatic plaques, discoid lupus erythematosus, alopecia areata. Intra-articular or soft-tissue administration: used in short-term adjunctive treatment for such conditions as synovitis of osteoarthritis, rheumatoid arthritis, acute gouty arthritis, and posttraumatic osteoarthritis. Topical: used for treatment of inflammatory' and pruritic manifestations of corticosteroid-responsive dermatoses. Oral inhalation: used for treatment of corticosteroid-responsive and bronchial asthma bronchospastic states. Intranasal: used for treatment of allergic or inflammatory nasal conditions, nasal polyps (excluding those originating within sinuses). Ophthalmic: used for treatment of steroid-responsive inflammatory conditions of the palpebral and bulbar conjunctiva, lid cornea, and anterior segment of globe.

DEXAMETHASONE (OPHTHALMIC SUSPENSION)
(Maxidex)

DEXAMETHASONE (SYSTEMIC)
(Decadron, Dexone, Hexadrol, SK-Dexamethasone)

DEXAMETHASONE (TOPICAL)
(Aeroseb-Dex, Decaderm, Decaspray)

DEXAMETHASONE/TOBRAMYCIN
(TobraDex ointment 0.1%)

Dexamethasone is a steroid antibiotic combination. Tobramycin inhibits bacterial protein synthesis, causing death; dexamethasone suppresses the inflammatory response. The combination is indicated in superficial bacterial ocular infection or risk of bacterial ocular infection; inflammatory conditions of palpebral and bulbar conjunctiva, cornea, and anterior segments of globe where inherent risk of steroid use in certain infective conjunctivitis is accepted to obtain a diminution of edema and inflammation; chronic anterior uveitis and corneal injury from chemical, radiation, or thermal burns, or penetration of foreign bodies, where risk of superficial ocular infection is high, or an expectation, or when potentially dangerous numbers of bacteria will be present in the eye.

DEXAMETHASONE ACETATE
(Dalalone D.P., Decadron L.A., Decaject L.A., Decameth L.A., Dexacen, Dexasone L.A., Dexone L.A., Solurex L.A.)

DEXAMETHASONE SODIUM PHOSPHATE
(AK-Dex, Dalalone, Decadrol, Decadron, Decaject, Decameth, Dexacen, Dexasone, Dexon, Dexone, Hexadrol Phosphate, Solurex)

Systemic dexamethasone is used in shock (other than adrenal crisis), the dexamethasone suppression test, and adrenal insufficiency.

DEXAMETHASONE SODIUM PHOSPHATE
(AK-Dex, Decadron, Dexair, 1-Methasone, Maxidex, Ocu-Dex)

Dexamethasone, a corticosteroid with ophthalmic antiinflammatory properties (0.1% solution), is used in the treatment of uveitis; iridocyclitis; inflammation of eyelids, conjunctiva, cornea, anterior segment of the globe; and corneal injury from burns or penetration by foreign bodies (see also Table 14).

DEXAMETHASONE SODIUM PHOSPHATE

(Decadron Cream)

Topical dexamethasone (gel and cream 0.1%) is indicated in inflammation of corticosteroid-responsive dermatoses.

DEXAMETHASONE SODIUM PHOSPHATE

(Decadron Phosphate, Hexadrol Phosphate)

Dexamethasone sodium phosphate, an antiinflammatory corticosteroid, is available as a nasal aerosol (84 mcg/metered spray) and is used in the management of perennial or seasonal rhinitis and prevention of recurrence of nasal polyps after surgical removal. It is also used as an oral inhalant to treat bronchial asthma in patients who require corticosteroids to control symptoms. The nasal inhalations may cause itchy nose, dryness, burning, irritation, sneezing, epistaxis, and bloody mucus; oral inhalation may cause flushing, rash, dry mouth, hoarseness, irritation of the tongue or throat, and an impaired sense of taste. Prolonged and inappropriate usage of dexamethasone in a higher-than-therapeutic dosage may result in suppression of the immune mechanism and fungal overgrowth (see Table 14).

DEXAMETHASONE SODIUM PHOSPHATE

(Inhalant)

Dexamethasone (100 mcg/metered spray) is indicated in control of bronchial asthma in patients with steroid-dependent asthma and for relief of symptoms of perennial or seasonal rhinitis; and in prevention of recurrence of nasal polyps after surgical removal.

DEXCHLORPHENIRAMINE MALEATE

(Dexchlorpheniramine Maleate tablets)

Dexchlorpheniramine competitively antagonizes histamine H_1 at receptor sites. It is indicated in treatment of perennial and seasonal allergic rhinitis; vasomotor rhinitis; allergic conjunctivitis; mild, uncomplicated allergic skin manifestations of urticaria and angioedema; amelioration of allergic reactions to blood or plasma; dermographism; and adjunctive anaphylactic therapy.

DEXFENFLURAMINE

Dexfenfluramine, the dextroisomer of fenfluramine, altering serotoninergic transmission, (15 mg b.i.d.) causes weight loss and enhances adherence to weight-lowering programs such as counseling, following dietary advice, behavioral modification, and physical exercise.

DEXMETHYLPHENIDATE HYDROCHLORIDE

(Focalin tablets 2.5 mg)

Dexmethylphenidate is a CNS stimulant that blocks the reuptake of norepinephrine and dopamine into presynaptic neurons and increases release of these monoamines into extraneuronal spaces. It is indicated in treatment of attention-deficit hyperactivity disorder (ADHD).

DEXRAZOXANE

(Zinecard powder for injection)

Dexrazoxane is a cardioprotective agent that reduces the incidence and severity of cardiomyopathy in female breast cancer patients who have received a cumulative doxorubicin dose of 300 mg/m^2 and who may benefit from additional doxorubicin therapy. It is not recommended for use with the initiation of doxorubicin therapy.

DEXTRAN

(Dextran 40 and 70)

Dextran, a branched polysaccharide plasma volume expander, may be used as a supportive measure to treat shock resulting from hemorrhage, burns, surgery, or other trauma. Low-molecular-weight dextran (Dextran 40) has an average molecular weight of 40,000, and its 2.5% solution is equivalent in colloid osmotic pressure to normal plasma. High-molecular-weight dextran (Dextran 70) has an average molecular weight of 70,000. Dextran is excreted gradually by the kidneys, 50% of it within 3 hours, 60% within 6 hours, and 75% within 24 hours. Dextran is used as a prophylaxis against venous thrombosis and thromboembolism as it inhibits vascular stasis, platelet adhesion, and fibrous clot formation. Dextrans are antigenic, and those with the smallest molecular weights are least antigenic.

DEXTRIFERRON

The parenteral iron medications available include iron dextran (ferric hydroxide and high-molecular-weight dextran) for intramuscular use, dextriferron (a complex of ferric hydroxide and partially hydrolyzed dextran) for intravenous use, and saccharated iron oxide (a complex of ferric hydroxide and sucrose) for intravenous use. These preparations are reserved for those cases in which oral preparations are not tolerated, absorbed, or rapid enough in their onset of action, or are otherwise not suitable for noncompliant patients.

DEXTROAMPHETAMINE

(Dexedrine)

Dextroamphetamine is a sympathomimetic amine that is used in narcolepsy and in attention-deficit disorder (ADD) in children. Dextroamphetamine releases norepinephrine and, in high doses, also dopamine. It is absorbed from the GI tract, metabolized in the liver, and excreted unchanged in the urine. Acidification of urine shortens amphetamine's half-life, whereas alkalinization of urine prolongs it. The accumulation of hydroxy metabolite of amphetamine has been thought to cause amphetamine-induced psychosis. Therapeutic doses of amphetamine may cause insomnia, tremor, and restlessness, and toxic doses of amphetamine may cause mydriasis, hypertension, and arrhythmia. Chlorpromazine is an excellent antidote in amphetamine toxicity.

The continuous use of amphetamine causes tolerance, requiring higher doses, and hence there exists a high potential for its abuse. Amphetamine should not be used with a monoamine oxidase A inhibitor such as tranylcypromine, because the chance of inducing hypertension becomes magnified.

Similar caution should be exercised with biogenic amine uptake blockers such as tricyclic antidepressants. Amphetamine is contraindicated in advanced arteriosclerosis; symptomatic cardiovascular disease; moderate to severe hypertension; hyperthyroidism; hypersensitivity or idiosyncrasy to the sympathomimetic amines; glaucoma; agitated states; history of drug abuse; and during or within 14 days following administration of monoamine oxidase (MAO) inhibitors.

DEXTROAMPHETAMINE SACCHARATE/AMPHETAMINE ASPARTATE MONOHYDRATE/DEXTROAMPHETAMINE SULFATE/AMPHETAMINE SULFATE

(Adderall tablets 5 mg)

Dextroamphetamine saccharate activates nonadrenergic neurons, causing CNS and respiratory stimulation. It stimulates the satiety center in the brain, causing appetite suppression; is indicated in narcolepsy (Adderall), and in treatment of ADHD.

Subjective effects similar to those of cocaine are produced by **amphetamine**, **dextroamphetamine**, **methamphetamine**, **phenmetrazine**, **methylphenidate**, and **diethylpropion**. Amphetamines increase synaptic dopamine primarily by stimulating presynaptic release rather than by blockade of reuptake, as is the case with cocaine. Intravenous or smoked methamphetamine produces an abuse/dependence syndrome similar to that seen with cocaine use, although clinical deterioration may progress more rapidly. In animal studies, methamphetamine in doses comparable with those used by human abusers produces neurotoxic effects in dopamine and serotonin neurons. Methamphetamine can be produced in small, clandestine laboratories starting with ephedrine, a widely available nonprescription stimulant. Oral stimulants, such as those prescribed in a weight-reduction program, have short-term efficacy because of tolerance development. Only a small proportion of patients introduced to these appetite suppressants subsequently exhibit dose escalation or drug seeking from various physicians; such patients may meet diagnostic criteria for abuse or addiction. **Fenfluramine** and **phenylpropanolamine** reduce appetite with no evidence of significant abuse potential. **Mazindol** also reduces appetite, with less stimulant properties than amphetamine.

Khat is a plant material widely chewed in East Africa and Yemen for its stimulant properties; these are due to the alkaloidal **cathinone**, a compound similar to amphetamine. Methcathinone, a congener with similar effects, has been synthesized in clandestine laboratories, but widespread use in North America has not been reported. MDMA ("**ecstasy**") also has stimulant properties.

DEXTROMETHORPHAN

(Romilar)

Dextromethorphan (Romilar) is the dextroisomer of the methyl ether of levorphanol. Unlike its levorotatory congener, it possesses no significant analgesic property, exerts no depressant effects on respiration, and lacks addiction liability. It is an antitussive agent with a potency approximately one half that of codeine.

Therapeutic doses of dextromethorphan (15 to 30 mg) produce few or no side effects, whereas excessively high doses (300 to 1500 mg) have been reported to produce a state resembling intoxication accompanied by euphoria.

Besides its antitussive property, recent studies have shown that dextromethorphan has anticonvulsant and neuroprotective properties. Because dextromethorphan interacts with N-methyl-D-aspartate (NMDA) or sigma receptors, it may become important in ameliorating the cerebrovascular and functional consequences of global cerebral ischemia.

DEXTROMETHORPHAN HYDROBROMIDE/ BENZOCAINE

(Cough-X lozenges 5 mg dextromethorphan and 2 mg benzocaine)

Dextromethorphan is a nonnarcotic antitussive agent, which suppresses cough by central action. It is used for temporary relief of minor sore throat and temporary reduction in cough caused by minor throat and bronchial irritation.

DEXTROMETHORPHAN HBR/PHENYLEPHRINE HYDROCHLORIDE/CHLORPHENIRAMINE MALEATE

(Alka-Seltzer Plus Cold)

Dextromethorphan: suppresses cough by central action on the cough center in the medulla. **Phenylephrine**: stimulates postsynaptic alphareceptors, resulting in vasoconstriction, which reduces nasal congestion. **Chlorpheniramine**: competitively antagonizes histamine at H_1-receptor sites. The combination is indicated for temporary relief of coughs and upper respiratory symptoms, including nasal congestion, associated with allergy or common cold.

DEXTROPROPOXYPHENE

(Darvon)

Propoxyphene is structurally very similar to methadone and possesses four stereoisomers. Dextropropoxyphene is an analgesic with a potency two thirds that of codeine. Levopropoxyphene is an antitussive, but lacks analgesic properties.

Adverse reactions to dextropropoxyphene include nausea, vomiting, sedation, dizziness, constipation, and skin rash, with a frequency of incidence somewhat less than that seen with codeine use. Although respiratory depression is a cardinal sign of acute dextropropoxyphene poisoning, the drug apparently does not affect respiration in the usual therapeutic doses of 32 to 65 mg.

DEXTROSE

(D-Glucose)

Dextrose, a carbohydrate, is used in fluid replacement and caloric supplementation in patients who cannot maintain adequate oral intake or are restricted from doing so.

DEXTROTHYROXINE SODIUM

(Choloxin)

Dextrothyroxine, a thyroid hormone with antilipemic effect (1 to 2 mg daily), is used primarily in type II hyperlipoproteinemia.

DEZOCINE

(Dalgan)

Dezocine, an opiate receptor agonist–antagonist, possessing an analgesic property (5 to 20 mg IM q. 3 to 6 hours), is used in the management of moderate to severe pain.

DIABETES MELLITUS: Treatment for Non-Insulin-Dependent Cases

Drugs for NIDDM	Usual Daily Dosage
Sulfonylureas	
First Generation	
Acetohexamide	500 to 750 mg once or divided
Chlorpropamide	250 to 375 mg once
Tolazamide	250 to 500 mg once or divided
Tolbutamide	1000 to 2000 mg once or divided
Second Generation	
Glimepiride	4 mg once
Glipizide	10 to 20 mg once or divided
Glucotrol	
Glucotrol XL sustained-release tablets	5 to 10 mg once
Glyburide	5 to 10 mg once or divided
DiaBeta	
Micronase	
Glynase micronized tablets	3 to 12 mg once or divided
Biguanide	
Metformin	850 mg b.i.d.
Alpha-glucosidase inhibitor	
Acarbose	50 to 100 mg t.i.d.

DIACETYLMORPHINE

(Heroin)

Heroin, a synthetic alkaloid formed from morphine by substituting acetyl for its two hydroxyl groups, resembles morphine in its general effects but acts more strongly on both cerebrum and medulla than does morphine, and is therefore more poisonous, the usual dose being about one fourth that of morphine (see Figure 36). Heroin is a highly addictive substance, and the social danger from it, moreover, seems to be greater than with morphine in that it produces a change in the personality as shown by an utter disregard for the conventions and morals of civilization. Degenerative changes in the individual progress faster than with any of the other narcotic drugs, and all the higher faculties of the mind, such as judgment, self-control, and attention, are weakened, and the addict rapidly becomes a mental and moral degenerate. The heroin habit is most difficult to cure, not only in the active withdrawal period but also in the convalescent stage, and relapse is frequent. Habitues take it either by snuffing or by hypodermic injection. Because of its marked tendency to addiction and its minor therapeutic value, the manufacture and importation of heroin has been outlawed in the United States.

DIAMIDINES

(Pentamidine)

Trypanosomiasis is produced by protozoa of the genus *Trypanosoma* and leads to Gambian or mid-African sleeping sickness (*T. gambiense*), Rhodesian or East African sleeping sickness (*T. rhodesiense*), and Chagas' disease, which is seen in the populations of Central and South America (*T. cruzi*).

Agents effective in the treatment of trypanosomiasis are the aromatic diamidines (pentamidine, stilbamidine, and propamidine). Pentamidine is the preferred drug for the prevention and early treatment of *T. gambiense* infections; however, it cannot penetrate the CNS. Melarsoprol is the drug recommended for *T. gambiense* infections that do not respond to pentamidine or for managing the late meningoencephalitic stages of infection. It does reach the CNS. Nifurtimox (Lampit) is the drug of choice for treating the acute form of Chagas' disease. Suramin (Naphuride) is effective only as therapy for African sleeping sickness.

DIARRHEA: Drug-induced

Antacids (magnesium-containing agents)

Antibiotics	
Any broad-spectrum antibiotic	Sulfonamides
Clindamycin	Tetracyclines
Antihypertensives	
Guanabenz	Methyldopa
Guanadrel	Reserpine
Guanethidine	
Cholinesterase Inhibitors	
Metaclopramide	
Cholinomimetics	
Bethanechol	
Cardiac Agents	
Digitalis	
Digoxin	
Quinidine	

DIAZEPAM

(Valium)

Diazepam is a lipid-soluble but water-insoluble substance. The solvent for parenteral diazepam, it consists of 40% propylene glycol, 10% ethyl alcohol, 5% sodium benzoate, and 1.5% benzyl alcohol. Injection site complications such as phlebitis may result from the injudicious administration of these compounds. As in the case of chlordiazepoxide, diazepam should be given either orally or intravenously. The peak plasma concentration of orally administered diazepam is reached in 2 hours. The short duration of action of diazepam when given intravenously is caused by its tissue redistribution and not by metabolism. In this case, diazepam behaves identically to the ultra-short-acting barbiturates such as thiopental. As a matter of fact, diazepam is metabolized slowly, with the reported half-life varying from 50 to 75 hours. Because some of the metabolites are also active pharmacologically, steady-state concentrations develop slowly, usually 7 to 10 days after the initiation of oral therapy.

When compared to oxazepam, diazepam is absorbed more rapidly and produces discernible sedative effects. Such rapid absorption (peak levels attained in 1 hour) could account for its vast popularity, but could also predispose patients to abuse it. When alcohol in small concentrations (10% by volume) is taken at the same time as an oral dose of diazepam, the rate of absorption is decreased, but not the amount absorbed; a higher concentration of alcohol (50% by volume) may increase diazepam absorption (see also Table 13).

As with chlordiazepoxide, the dosage of diazepam should be lower in the elderly (initial dose, about half the usual), not only because of the pharmacokinetic differences but also because accumulation of the parent drug and active metabolites is more likely to lead to confusion and muscle weakness in the elderly. Furthermore, the elderly seem to be more sensitive to the depressant effects of diazepam than are younger patients.

The plasma protein binding of diazepam is about 97 to 99% in adults, regardless of age, but the distribution volume of around 1 L/kg is higher in the elderly and females. Hypoalbuminemia leads to an increase in the fraction of unbound drug in plasma and a faster rate of elimination, as more drug is available for metabolism.

Diazepam readily crosses the placenta, particularly in the later stages of pregnancy and during labor; its pathways of metabolism are altered in the fetus and newborn, and this prolongs the elimination of both diazepam and desmethyldiazepam. Diazepam must therefore be used judiciously in patients who are pregnant and in labor. Diazepam and desmethyldiazepam appear in breast milk and in the plasma of breast-fed infants (see also Figure 50).

DIAZOXIDE

(Hyperstat)

Diazoxide, which is administered intravenously, is used exclusively in the management of malignant hypertension or a hypertensive crisis. It brings about reflex cardiac acceleration and increased cardiac output. However, it can cause hyperglycemia due to its inhibition of insulin release from the beta cells. Because diazoxide also produces sodium and water retention, it should be given with a diuretic such as furosemide or ethacrynic acid.

DIAZOXIDE, ORAL

(Proglycem oral suspension 50 mg/mL)

Diazoxide is a glucose-elevating agent that produces a prompt dose-related increase in blood glucose by inhibiting pancreatic insulin release. It is indicated in the management of hypoglycemia caused by hyperinsulinism in adults with inoperable islet cell adenoma or carcinoma or extrapancreatic malignancy, in infants and children with leucine sensitivity, islet cell hyperplasia, nesidioblastosis, extrapancreatic malignancy, islet cell adenoma or adenomatosis.

DIAZOXIDE, PARENTERAL

(Hyperstat IV injection 15 mg/mL)

Diazoxide is an agent for hypertensive emergencies. It relaxes smooth muscle in peripheral arterioles, thus reducing BP. Diazoxide is indicated in short-term emergency reduction of BP in severe, nonmalignant, and malignant hypertension in hospitalized patients.

DIBENZAPINE DERIVATIVES

Antidepressants are divided into the following classes: the dibenzapine derivatives are called tricyclic antidepressants and include imipramine (Tofranil), desipramine (Norpramin), amitriptyline (Elavil), nortriptyline (Aventyl), protriptyline (Vivactil), and doxepin (Adapin). The monoamine oxidase inhibitors are used occasionally to treat depression. The hydrazine derivatives consist of isocarboxazid (Marplan) and phenelzine sulfate (Nardil). The nonhydrazine derivatives include tranylcypromine (Parnate). L-Tryptophan is the only member of the monoamine precursors used to treat depression. The newer and second-generation antidepressants include amoxapine, doxepin, fluoxetine, maprotiline, trazodone, mianserin, alprazolam, and bupropion (see also Tables 5 through 7).

DIBUCAINE

(Nupercainal)

Dibucaine, an amine local anesthetic (1% ointment, 0.5% cream), is used topically for temporary relief of pain and itching associated with abrasions, sunburn, minor burns, hemorrhoids, and other minor skin conditions (see also Figure 31).

DICHLORPHENAMIDE

(Daranide)

The carbonic anhydrase inhibitors consist of acetazolamide (Diamox), ethoxzolamide (Cardrase), and dichlorphenamide (Daranide). Acetazolamide is an old agent, whereas ethoxzolamide and dichlorphenamide are newer preparations. Dichlorphenamide is the most potent carbonic anhydrase inhibitor in use today. The presence of SO_2NH_2 (sulfonamide) causes such compounds to inhibit carbonic anhydrase (CA), which catalyzes the hydration of carbon dioxide as follows:

$$CO_2 + H_2O \xrightarrow{CA} H_2CO_3 \rightleftharpoons H^+ + HCO_3^-$$

These agents inhibit carbonic anhydrase in the renal tubular cells in both the proximal and distal tubules. When the rate of hydrogen generation is reduced, HCO^-_3 is lost in urine and the patient tends to become acidotic. However, the plasma concentration of HCO^-_3 is lowered and less is filtered, so the diuresis becomes less effective. In addition, the sodium output is increased because its resorption in exchange for hydrogen is limited by the decreased availability of hydrogen. With less hydrogen available, the exchange of sodium for potassium predominates, and this fosters the loss of potassium. Chloride excretion is not altered significantly. Because the aqueous humor has a high concentration of bicarbonate, carbonic anhydrase inhibitors are primarily used in the treatment of glaucoma. They are no longer used as diuretics or as antiepileptic agents.

DICLOFENAC

(Cataflam tablets 50 mg (as potassium))

Diclofenac decreases inflammation, pain, and fever, probably through inhibition of cyclooxygenase activity and prostaglandin synthesis. It is indicated in the treatment of rheumatoid arthritis, ankylosing spondylitis, and osteoarthritis. Potassium salt is approved for management of mild to moderate pain and primary dysmenorrhea when prompt pain relief is needed. Ophthalmic: used for treatment of postoperative inflammation after cataract removal; temporary relief of pain and photophobia following corneal refractive surgery. Topical: used for treatment of actinic keratosis.

Placebo-controlled trials have now established that at least three selective inhibitors of COX-2—**rofecoxib**, **valdecoxib**, and **celecoxib**—confer an increased risk of heart attack and stroke. This would be expected to complicate treatment with newer, highly selective agents, such as **lumiracoxib** and **etoricoxib**, although definitive information is not yet available. However, of more immediate concern are some NSAIDs, such as **meloxicam** and **diclofenac**, which resemble celecoxib in terms of their selectivity. Evidence for hazards with both drugs has been suggested from observational studies, but controlled trials to address this hypothesis have not been performed. The cardiovascular hazard from both celecoxib and rofecoxib—the two inhibitors for which data are available from placebo-controlled trials lasting more than 1 year—increased with chronicity of dosing. This is consistent with a mechanism-based acceleration of atherogenesis directly via inhibition of PGI_2 and indirectly due to the rise in blood pressure consequent to inhibition of COX-2-derived PGE_2 and PGI_2.

If COX-2 inhibitors are selected, they should be used at the lowest possible dose for the shortest period of time, and patients at risk of cardiovascular disease or prone to thrombosis should not be treated with these drugs. Small absolute risks of thrombosis attributable to these drugs may interact geometrically with small absolute risks from genetic variants such as factor V Leiden, or concomitant therapies such as the anovulant pill.

DICLOFENAC SODIUM

(Voltaren)

Diclofenac has analgesic and antiinflammatory properties and, in a dose of 150 to 250 mg/day, is indicated in acute and chronic treatment of the signs and symptoms of rheumatoid arthritis, osteoarthritis, and ankylosing spondylitis. In addition, it is effective in a dose of 50 mg t.i.d. in the management of pain primarily associated with dysmenorrhea (see also Table 3).

DICLOXACILLIN SODIUM

(Dicloxacillin sodium capsules 250 mg)

Dicloxacillin is a penicillinase-resistant penicillin that inhibits bacterial cell-wall mucopeptide synthesis. It is indicated in the treatment of infections caused by penicillinase-producing staphylococcal infection; and in initial therapy of suspected staphylococcal infection.

DICLOXACILLIN SODIUM

(Pathocil)

Dicloxacillin is indicated in treatment of infections resulting from penicillinase-producing staphylococci. Penicillins, which are the safest of the antibiotics, produce few direct toxic reactions, and most of the serious side effects are hypersensitivity reactions. Penicillins and their by-products, penicilloic acid and penicilloylpolylysine, are antigenic in susceptible individuals who develop immunoglobulin G antibodies to them. Furthermore, all penicillins cross-sensitize and cross-react. Allergic reactions, including anaphylactoid shock, occur in sensitized patients following the repeated administration of penicillin. Anaphylactoid reactions, which are more common following the parenteral administration of penicillin, may be reversed by the administration of corticosteroids (see Figure 74).

The direct toxicity of penicillin following the administration of large doses may include phlebitis if it is given intravenously, injection site inflammatory reactions when given intramuscularly, degeneration of nerve tissue if injected into a nerve, and CNS excitability if given intrathecally.

The broad-spectrum penicillins, such as ampicillin and amoxicillin, may cause GI irritation. Occasionally, the overgrowth of staphylococci, *Pseudomonas*, *Proteus*, or yeasts may be responsible for causing enteritis. Methicillin and nafcillin may precipitate granulocytopenia, and methicillin has been known to cause nephritis. Carbenicillin may cause hypokalemic alkalosis. The properties of the various penicillins are shown in Table 23.

DICUMAROL

The coumarin anticoagulants include dicumarol, warfarin sodium (coumadin sodium), warfarin potassium (Athrombin-K), acenocoumarol (Sintrom), and phenprocouman (Liquamar).

Phytonadisone (vitamin K_1; phylloquinone) is identical to naturally occurring vitamin K_1, which is required for the synthesis of blood coagulation factors such as prothrombin (II), proconvertin (VII), Christmas factor or plasma thromboplastin component (IX), and Stuart–Prower factor (X) in the liver. Dicumarol and ethylbiscoumacetate act as competitive antagonists of vitamin K and interfere with the synthesis of these factors in the liver. Similarly, hypoprothrombinemic-induced bleeding can be rectified by the administration of vitamin K.

DICYCLOMINE HYDROCHLORIDE

(Antispas injection 10 mg/mL)

Dicyclomine is an antispasmodic agent that relieves smooth-muscle spasm of the GI tract through anticholinergic effects and direct action on GI smooth muscle. It is indicated in the treatment of functional bowel/irritable bowel syndrome (e.g., irritable colon, spastic colon, and mucous colitis).

Dicyclomine hydrochloride (Bentyl, others), **flavoxate hydrochloride** (Urispas, others), **oxybutynin chloride** (Ditropan, others), and **tolterodine tartrate** (Detrol) are tertiary amines and **trospium chloride** (Sanctura) is a quaternary amine; all are used for their antispasmodic properties. These agents appear to exert some nonspecific direct relaxant effect on smooth muscle. In therapeutic doses, they decrease spasm of the GI tract, biliary tract, ureter, and uterus.

Anticholinergic agents ("spasmolytics" or "antispasmodics") are often used in patients with irritable bowel syndrome. The most common agents of this class available in the United States are nonspecific antagonists of the muscarinic receptor and include the tertiary amines **dicyclomine** (Bentyl) and hyoscyamine (Levsin, others) and the quaternary ammonium compounds **glycopyrrolate** (Robinul) and **methscopolamine** (Pamine). The advantage of the latter two compounds is that they have a limited propensity to cross the blood–brain barrier and hence a lower risk for neurological side effects such as light-headedness, drowsiness, or nervousness. These agents typically are given either on an as-needed basis (with the onset of pain) or before meals to prevent the pain and fecal urgency that predictably occur in some patients with irritable bowel syndrome (IBS) (with presumed exaggerated gastrocolic reflex).

Analgesic, anticholinergic, and antidiarrheal agents play supportive roles in reducing symptoms and improving quality of life. These drugs should be individualized based on a patient's symptoms and are supplementary to antiinflammatory medications. Oral iron, folate, and vitamin B_{12} should be administered as indicated. **Loperamide** or **diphenoxylate** can be used to reduce the frequency of bowel movements and relieve rectal urgency in patients with mild disease; these agents are contraindicated in patients with severe disease because they may predispose to the development of toxic megacolon. Cholestyramine can be used to prevent bile-salt-induced colonic secretion in patients who have undergone limited ileocolic resections. Anticholinergic agents (dicyclomine hydrochloride, etc.) are used to reduce abdominal cramps, pain, and rectal urgency. As with the antidiarrheal agents, they are contraindicated in severe disease or when obstruction is suspected. Care should be taken to differentiate exacerbation of IBS from symptoms that may be related to coexistent functional bowel disease.

DICYCLOMINE HYDROCHLORIDE

(Bentyl)

Dicyclomine (80 to 160 mg in four equally divided doses) is indicated in the treatment of irritable colon, spastic colon, and mucous colitis. Dicyclomine is an antispasmodic–anticholinergic agent that relieves smooth-muscle spasm of the GI tract. Dicyclomine is contraindicated in obstructive uropathy, obstructive disease of the GI tract, severe ulcerative colitis, reflux esophagitis, unstable cardiovascular status in acute hemorrhage, glaucoma, and myasthenia gravis. The side effects of dicyclomine include dry mouth, dizziness, and blurred vision.

DIDANOSIDE

(ddI) (Videx)

Didanoside, a purine analog with antiviral effects (75 mg/kg p.o. q. 12 hours), is used in advanced human immunodeficiency virus (HIV) infection in patients who cannot tolerate or no longer respond to zidovudine therapy (see also Figure 107).

DIDANOSINE

(Videx tablets)

Didanosine is a nucleoside reverse transcriptase inhibitor that inhibits replication of HIV by interfering with DNA synthesis. **Didanosine** (Videx): is used for treatment of HIV-1 infection in combination with other antiretrovirals. **Didanosine EC** (Videx EC): is used in combination with other antiretroviral agents for the treatment of HIV-1 infection in adults who require once-daily administration of didanosine or an alternative didanosine formulation.

Current treatment assumes that all aspects of the disease derive from the direct toxic effects of HIV on host cells, mainly CD4+ T-lymphocytes. This viewpoint is based on studies demonstrating the importance of high plasma HIV RNA concentration and low CD4+ lymphocyte count as predictors of disease progression and mortality. Validation has come from evidence that treatment regimens associated with long-term suppression of HIV replication (as measured by decreased plasma HIV RNA) and repletion of peripheral CD4 cells are clinically beneficial. The goal of therapy is to suppress virus replication as much as possible for as long as possible. The HIV-encoded, RNA-dependent DNA polymerase, also called reverse transcriptase, converts viral RNA into proviral DNA that is then incorporated into a host cell chromosome. Available inhibitors of this enzyme are either nucleoside/nucleotide analogs or nonnucleoside inhibitors.

Similar to all available antiretroviral drugs, nucleoside and nucleotide reverse-transcriptase inhibitors prevent infection of susceptible cells but have no impact on cells that already harbor HIV. Nucleoside and nucleotide analogs must enter cells and undergo phosphorylation to generate synthetic substrates for the enzyme. The fully phosphorylated analogs block replication of the viral genome both by competitively inhibiting incorporation of native nucleotides and by terminating elongation of nascent proviral DNA because they lack a 3-hydroxyl group. **Didanosine** (2′,3′-deoxyinosme) is a purine nucleoside analog active against HIV-1, HIV-2, and other retroviruses, including HTLV-1. Its IC_{50} against HIV-1 ranges from 10 nM in monocytes-macrophage cells to 10 μM in lymphoblast cell lines. **Didanosine** is acid labile and is degraded at low gastric pH. An antacid buffer is used in most formulations to improve bioavailability. Chewable tablets contain calcium carbonate and magnesium hydroxide, whereas the powder form contains a citrate-phosphate buffer.

Peak concentrations of didanosine are seen approximately 1 hour after oral administration of the chewable tablets or powder formulations and 2 hours after delayed-release capsules. The plasma elimination half-life of the parent drug is approximately 1.5 hours, but the estimated intracellular half-life of dideoxyadenosine 5′-triphosphate is substantially longer, 25 to 40 hours. As a result, **didanosine** can be administered once daily. Didanosine is excreted by both glomerular filtration and tubular secretion, and does not undergo metabolism to a significant degree. Drug doses therefore must be adjusted in patients with renal insufficiency or renal failure.

Didanosine is not protein bound to a significant degree. The cerebrospinal penetration of didanosine is less than that of zidovudine, with a cerebrospinal fluid (CSF)-plasma ratio of 0.2, but the clinical significance of this is unclear. Didanosine has been detected in placental and fetal circulation at a small fraction of concentrations in maternal circulation.

The most serious toxicities associated with didanosine include peripheral neuropathy and pancreatitis, both of which are thought to be a consequence of mitochondrial toxicity. Up to 20% of patients reported peripheral neuropathy in early clinical trials. As with other dideoxynucleosides, peripheral neuropathy is more common with higher doses or concentrations of didanosine and is more prevalent in patients with underlying HIV-related neuropathy or in those receiving other neurotoxic drugs. Typically, this is a symmetrical distal sensory neuropathy that begins in the feet and lower extremities but may involve the hands as it progresses (stocking/glove distribution). Patients complain of pain, numbness, and tingling in the affected extremities. If the drug is stopped as soon as symptoms appear, the neuropathy will stabilize and should improve or resolve. Retinal changes and optic neuritis also have been reported with didanosine, and patients should undergo periodic retinal examinations.

Acute pancreatitis is a rare but potentially fatal complication of didanosine. Acute pancreatitis is associated with higher doses and concentrations of didanosine but has occurred in up to 7% of patients using the recommended dose of 200 mg twice daily. Pancreatitis is more common with advanced HIV disease; other risk factors include a previous history of pancreatitis, alcohol or illicit drug use, and hypertriglyceridemia. Combining didanosine with stavudine, which is also associated with peripheral neuropathy and pancreatitis, increases the risk and severity of both toxicities.

As with other dideoxynucleosides and zidovudine, serious hepatic toxicity—with or without steatosis, hepatomegaly, and lactic acidosis—occurs very rarely but can be fatal. Risk factors for the lactic acidosis-steatosis syndrome include female sex, obesity, and prolonged exposure to the drug.

Other reported adverse effects include elevated hepatic transaminases, headache, and asymptomatic hyperuricemia. Diarrhea is reported more frequently with didanosine than with other nucleoside analogs and has been attributed to the antacid in the buffered oral preparations.

DIENESTROL

(Estraguard)

Dienestrol cream is indicated in the treatment of atrophic vaginitis and kraurosis vulvae. As with all estrogens, dienestrol is contraindicated in known or suspected cancer of the breast, known or suspected estrogen-dependent neoplasia, undiagnosed abnormal genital bleeding, active thrombophlebitis or thromboembolic disorders, and a history of thrombophlebitis, thrombosis, or thromboembolic disorders associated with previous estrogen use (see also Figure 36).

DIETHYLDITHIOCARBAMATE

(Imuthiol)

Diethyldithiocarbamate is under investigation for its possible effectiveness in the treatment of AIDS, caused by HIV, which impairs both cellular and humoral immune functions. This results in increased susceptibility to opportunistic infection and certain malignancies.

DIETHYLPROPION HYDROCHLORIDE

(Nobesine, Nu-Dispoz, Regibon, Ro-Diet, Tenuate, Tepanil)

Diethylpropion, a sympathomimetic agent resembling amphetamine (25 mg p.o. t.i.d.), is used for a short period of time in the treatment of obesity.

DIETHYLPROPION HYDROCHLORIDE

(Tenuate tablets 25 mg)

Diethylpropion is an anorexiant that stimulates the satiety center in brain, causing appetite suppression. It is indicated as a short-term (few weeks) adjunct to a diet plan to reduce weight.

DIETHYLSTILBESTROL

(Stilbestrol)

Diethylstilbestrol is indicated in female hypogonadism, ovariectomy, or primary ovarian failure (0.2 to 0.5 mg p.o. daily in cycles of 3 weeks on and 1 week off); moderate-to-severe vasomotor symptoms of menopause, atrophic vaginitis or kraurosis vulvae (0.2 to 2 mg p.o. daily in cycles of 3 weeks on and 1 week off); in postcoital contraception as a morning-after pill (25 mg p.o. b.i.d. for 5 days); for prostatic cancer (1 to 3 mg p.o. daily); and for breast cancer in postmenopausal women (15 mg daily p.o.). Diethylstilbestrol mimics the action of estrogen in treating female hypogonadism, menopausal symptoms, and atrophic vaginitis. Diethylstilbestrol inhibits the growth of hormone sensitive tissues in advanced inoperable prostatic cancer. Diethylstilbestrol is contraindicated in patients with thrombophlebitis, thromboembolism or history of thromboembolism associated with estrogen use, estrogen-responsive carcinoma, or undiagnosed abnormal genital bleeding, and in pregnant and breast-feeding women. Diethylstilbestrol, when it was given to pregnant women, occasionally caused immediate nausea and vomiting. The slow toxicity included fluid retention and uterine bleeding. The delayed toxicities, which appear many years later in the female offspring when they reach puberty, are vaginal adenosis and clear-cell vaginal adenocarcinoma (see also Figure 36).

DIFENOXIN HYDROCHLORIDE

(with Atropine Sulfate) (Motofen)

Difenoxin, an opiate receptor agonist with antidiarrheal properties (2 mg p.o.), is indicated as an adjunctive treatment of acute nonspecific exacerbations of chronic functional diarrhea.

DIFLORASONE DIACETATE

(Florone, Florone E, Maxiflor, Psorcon)

Diflorasone, a topical adrenocorticoid with antiinflammatory properties (0.05% cream or ointment), is used in inflammation of corticosteroid-responsive dermatoses (see also Table 11).

DIFLUNISAL

(Dolobid)

Diflunisal (initially 1 g followed by 500 mg every 8 to 12 hours) is indicated for acute or long-term symptomatic treatment of mild to moderate pain associated with rheumatoid arthritis and osteoarthritis. Similar to aspirin, diflunisal inhibits prostaglandin synthetase and platelet functions (see Figures 13 and 14). Diflunisal is eliminated primarily by the kidneys, and its plasma half-life of 8 to 12 hours is lengthened in renal impairment. Diflunisal increases the plasma level of acetaminophen; displaces coumarins from protein-binding sites, and enhances the hypoprothrombinemic effects of anticoagulant; and as a uricosuric agent, antagonizes the hyperuricemic effects of hydrochlorothiazide (see also Table 3).

DIGITALIS

(Cardiac Glycosides)

In CHF, the patient's cardiac compensatory mechanism becomes fully activated. This consists of cardiac dilatation and hypertrophy—taking advantage of the Frank–Starling relationship to utilize more contractile elements; sympathetic stimulation—increasing the heart rate to maintain contractility and cardiac output, increasing oxygen consumption through the arterial and venous oxygen difference—increasing extraction of oxygen from limited blood flow; and production of aldosterone—increasing sodium and fluid retention, which may not be advantageous to the organism (see Figure 42). Agents with positive inotropic actions that

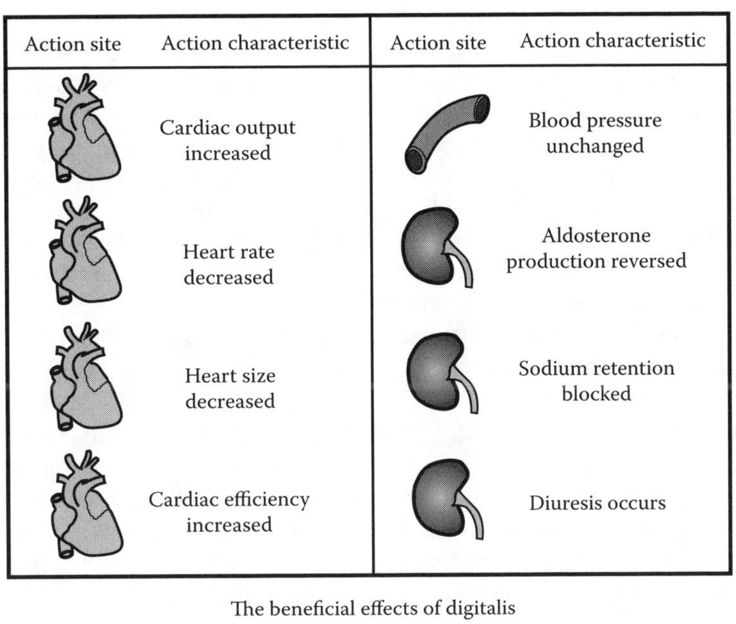

FIGURE 42 The mode of action of digitalis.

may be used in the management of CHF include the cardiac glycosides (e.g., digoxin and digitoxin), dopaminergic analogs (e.g., dobutamine), phosphodiesterase inhibitors (e.g., amrinone and milrinone), angiotensin antagonists (e.g., captopril, enalapril, and lisinopril), and vasodilators (nitrates and hydralazine).

The most important and often-used drugs in the treatment of CHF are the cardiac glycosides, which may exist and occur naturally in the body. Unfortunately, the margin of safety for these drugs is very narrow (therapeutic index, 3.0). Toxicity can develop readily, and careful attention to pharmacokinetic principles is absolutely crucial (see Table 12).

Cardiac glycosides (digitalis) potentiate the coupling of electrical excitation with mechanical contraction and, by augmenting the myoplasmic concentration of calcium, provoke a more forceful contraction. It is thought that digitalis inhibits sodium–calcium exchanges by inhibiting Na^+K^+ATPase. This results in an enhanced intracellular concentration of sodium, which in turn leads to greater sodium influx that then elicits stronger systolic contraction.

The cardiac glycosides increase cardiac output through their positive inotropic effect. They slow heart rate by relieving the sympathetic tone and through their vagotonic effects. They reduce the heart size by relieving the Frank–Starling relationship. They increase cardiac efficiency by increasing cardiac output and decreasing oxygen consumption (decreased heart size and rate).

Blood pressure remains unchanged following the administration of cardiac glycosides. In CHF, the cardiac output is reduced but the total peripheral resistance is increased, and these effects are reversed by cardiac glycosides.

Cardiac glycosides bring about diuresis by increasing both cardiac output and renal blood flow; the latter in turn reverses the renal compensatory mechanism activated in CHF. Consequently, the production of aldosterone is reduced, sodium retention is reversed, and the excretion of edematous fluid is enhanced (see Figure 42).

Cardiac glycosides have a vagotonic effect and may decrease impulse formation in the sinoatrial node. Although automaticity is not directly influenced by digitalis, conduction velocity is decreased. This effect of digitalis on the atrioventricular node is more prominent in the context of CHF, where the vagal tone is low and the adrenergic tone is high. Digitalis shortens the refractory period, in part due to enhanced intracellular calcium levels, decreasing membrane resistance, and increasing membrane potassium conductance, which lead to shortening of the action potential and contribute to shortening of atrial and ventricular refractoriness. The electrophysiologic properties of digitalis make it a useful compound in the treatment of atrial arrhythmias (for its vagotonic effect), atrial flutter (for its depressant effect on atrioventricular conduction), and atrial fibrillation (also for its vagotonic effect).

The toxic effects of digitalis are frequent and may be fatal. Toxicity may result from overdosage, decreased metabolism and excretion, and hypokalemia stemming from the use of thiazide diuretics, diarrhea, and vomiting. Digitalis toxicity has several manifestations and includes any arrhythmia occurring *de novo*, renal insufficiency, electrolyte disturbances, hypothyroidism, visual symptoms, headache, psychotic symptoms, pulmonary disease, and anorexia.

Digitalis toxicity should also be closely watched in elderly patients and those who have had a recent MI, as these predispose to toxic reactions. The most commonly reported signs of toxicity are dysrhythmia such as ventricular ectopic depolarization, second- and third-degree heart block, junctional tachycardia, atrial tachycardia with block, ventricular tachycardia, sinoatrial block, and sinus arrest. Anorexia is seen as a GI complication of cardiac glycoside use, and is followed by nausea and vomiting. The most common visual side effects are blurring, dimness of vision, flickering or flashing lights, color vision (yellow, green, red, and white), cycloplegia, and diplopia. A few of the neuropsychiatric symptoms that have been reported in conjunction with cardiac glycoside use are agitation, apathy, aphasia, ataxia, belligerence, changes in affect or personality, confusion, delirium, delusions, depression, disorientation, dizziness, drowsiness, euphoria, excitement, fatigue, hallucinations, headache, insomnia, irritability, mania, muscle pain, nervousness, neuralgias, nightmares, paresthesia, vertigo, violence, and weakness.

Once digitalis toxicity is diagnosed, digitalis and diuretic use should be stopped. Furthermore, the patient should be monitored closely for any alteration in the pharmacokinetic profile of the cardiac glycoside being used. Treatment with potassium and magnesium may be indicated. Potassium is recommended for patients with digitalis-induced ectopic beat or tachycardia, provided the patient is neither hyperkalemic, uremic, or oliguric. It is the drug of choice if the patient is hypokalemic. To manage digitalis-induced arrhythmia, lidocaine, with its fast onset and short duration of action, is the drug of choice. Because lidocaine is metabolized, it should be used cautiously in patients with liver disease. Phenytoin may be used if potassium or lidocaine prove ineffective. Propranolol is effective in treating ventricular tachycardia. Atropine is effective if digitalis-induced conduction delay is at the atrioventricular node and is mediated via the vagus. Calcium-channel-blocking agents such as verapamil are effective if the arrhythmia is due to reentry, increased diastolic depolarization in the Purkinje fibers, or oscillatory after-potential. In addition to these drugs, a temporary pacemaker may be indicated. The following interventions are contraindicated: quinidine should not be used because it displaces digoxin from binding sites, and bretylium should not be used because it releases norepinephrine. Carotid sinus stimulation should be discouraged, as it may precipitate ventricular fibrillation. The antidigitoxin or the antidigoxin antibodies (Digibind) have been used to control digitalis intoxication. The antibody mobilizes depot digoxin and is excreted by the kidney as an antibody–digoxin complex.

DIGITOXIN
(Crystodigin)

DIGOXIN
(Lanoxin)

The structures of the cardiac glycosides, including digoxin and digitoxin, have three common components, which include a steroid nucleus (aglycones or genins), a series of sugar residues in the C_3 position, and a five- or six-membered lactone ring in the C_{17} position.

The sugar residue in digoxin and digitoxin is -*O*-digitoxose-digitoxose-digitoxose. Digoxin varies from digitoxin in having a hydroxy group at C_{12}. Glycosides possess both lipophilic residues (a steroid nucleus) and hydrophilic residues (a lactone ring and OH group). These residues and other factors strongly influence the pharmacokinetic profiles of these cardiac glycosides. Digitoxin is more lipid soluble than digoxin, is absorbed better when given orally, has a longer half-life, depicts a higher protein binding, and is more extensively metabolized by the liver. Digoxin is excreted primarily unchanged by the kidney. Renal insufficiency alters its half-life and safety. An elevated blood urea nitrogen (BUN) level signals the diminished capacity to eliminate digoxin. A direct relationship exists between the clearance of digoxin and that of creatine, which, in addition to BUN, may be used to assess a patient's ability to excrete digoxin. Table 12 compares the pharmacokinetic profiles of digoxin and digitoxin. Because a drug may require four to five half-lives before attaining a steady-state (maintenance) level, it is logical to assume that it will take digoxin approximately 1 week and digitoxin 4 weeks to reach their maintenance levels (see Digitalis).

DIGOXIN IMMUNE FAB
(Ovine) (Digibind)

Digoxin immune fab, an antibody fragment, is used in potentially life-threatening digoxin or digitoxin intoxication.

DIHYDRALAZINE

Hydralazine and nitrates have been used in patients with CHF. An ACE inhibitor such as lisinopril increases the left-ventricular ejection fraction in patients with CHF, and the drug's effectiveness is not diminished in the presence of impaired renal function. In addition, a vasodilator in combination with an angiotensin-converting enzyme inhibitor has been used in CHF. The vasodilators may be classified as venodilators, arterial dilators, or balanced-type vasodilators (see Table 24). The rationale for vasodilation in the management of CHF is based on the increased arteriolar vasotone that occurs. This initiates a vicious circle in which cardiac function is further depressed by an increase in afterload and in resistance to ejection.

DIHYDROCODEINONE

Most narcotics such as morphine, codeine, dihydrocodeinone, methadone, and levorphanol have antitussive properties. Codeine is used primarily because its addictive liability is low and it is effective orally. The antitussive doses of narcotics are lower than the doses used for analgesic purposes.

DIHYDROCYCLOSPORIN C

This group consists of cyclosporin A and dihydrocyclosporin C. Cyclosporin A, a fungal metabolite, is a cyclic polypeptide that consists of 11 amino acids. It has a biologic half-life of 4 to 6 hours and displays a preferential T-cell cytotoxic property, in that it inhibits the factors that stimulate T-lymphocyte proliferation. Cyclosporin A has been used as the sole immunosuppressant (without prednisone or other drugs) for cadaveric transplants of the kidney, pancreas, and liver. Cyclosporin A has been observed to cause reversible hepatic toxicity and nephrotoxicity. Another fungal metabolite, dihydrocyclosporin C is even more selective than cyclosporin A, in that it suppresses T-lymphocyte production with only marginal effects on the antibody response.

DIHYDROEMETINE

Dihydroemetine is given for 5 days and effects rapid relief of the symptoms of acute amebic dysentery. The patient is then switched to metronidazole. If the response to metronidazole is not satisfactory, dihydroemetine plus tetracycline or dihydroemetine plus paromomycin are given along with the metronidazole.

TABLE 12
Comparison of the Pharmacokinetic Profiles of Digoxin and Digitoxin

Properties	Digoxin	Digitoxin
Lipid solubility	Low	High
Gastrointestinal absorption	Good	Excellent
Protein binding	Low (25%)	High (90%)
Half-life	Short (1–2 days)	Long (6–9 days)
Enterohepatic recycling	Minimal	High
Liver metabolism	Low	High
Excretion	Active drug	Inactive metabolites
Onset of action after intravenous administration	Fast (5–30 minutes)	Slow (4–8 hours)

DIHYDROERGOTAMINE MESYLATE

(DHE 45)

Dihydroergotamine, an ergot alkaloid with vasoconstricting properties (1 mg IM or IV), is used to prevent or abort vascular headaches, including migraine and cluster headaches (see also Figure 93).

DIHYDROMORPHINONE

(Numorphan)

Dihydromorphinone (1 mg IM SC) is a semisynthetic narcotic analgesic, which is far more potent than morphine and has a duration of action of 4 to 6 hours.

DIHYDROMORPHINONE HYDROCHLORIDE

(Dilaudid)

Dilaudid is 5 to 10 times as potent as, and more toxic than, morphine, but its duration of action is shorter, and its effects on the GI tract are less. Chemically, it differs from morphine in that the alcoholic hydroxyl group of that alkaloid is replaced by ketonic oxygen and the adjacent double bond is removed by hydrogenation. Dihydromorphinone produces analgesia and narcosis and acts upon the respiration in a manner similar to morphine, with the difference that it is effective in about one quarter of the dosage. Dihydromorphinone is powerfully analgesic and also markedly depressing to the respiration, although nausea, vomiting, and constipation are not so marked as with morphine. Tolerance and addiction occur readily and the same care should be exercised in prescribing it as is used in the case of natural opium alkaloids.

Dihydromorphinone is used in the same manner as morphine for the relief of pain but in much smaller doses—usually 1 to 2 mg. For cough, a dose about half that size is used. Administered orally, dihydromorphinone is more effective than morphine, and it may also be administered in a rectal suppository. Its principal indication is in acute pain of short duration (see also Figure 68).

DIHYDROPYRIDINE

When calcium homeostasis fails, as occurs in the presence of anoxia, cell viability is threatened by the uncontrolled influx of calcium through the plasma membrane or by the massive release of calcium from intracellular binding and sequestration sites. Agents that affect calcium movements consist of calcium-entry blockers and calcium antagonists (see Table 21 and Figures 84 and 103).

Calcium-entry blockers include those agents that are selective for slow calcium channels in the myocardium (slow channel blockers) and consist of the following categories of substances: benzothiazepines (diltiazem and dihydropyridines)—nifedipine, nicardipine, niludipine, nimodipine, nisoldipine, nitrendipine, ryosidine, amlodipine, azodipine, dazodipine, felodipine, flordipine, iodipine, isradipine, mesudipine, oxodipine, and riodipine; and, phenylalkylamines—verapamil, gallopamil, anipamil, desmethoxyverapamil, emopamil, falipamil, and ronipamil.

DIHYDROTACHYSTEROL

(DHT, DHT Intensol, Hytakerol)

Dihydrotachysterol, a vitamin-D analog with antihypocalcemic properties, is indicated in the treatment of familial hypophosphatemia; hypocalcemia associated with hypoparathyroidism and pseudohypoparathyroidism; and renal osteodystrophy in chronic uremia (see also Figure 66).

DIIODOTYROSINE

(DIT)

The steps involved in the synthesis of thyroid hormones are depicted in Figure 66. First the ingested iodide (100 to 150 μg/day) is actively transported (iodide trapping) and then accumulated in the thyroid gland. Following this, the trapped iodide is oxidized by a peroxidase system to active iodine, which iodinates the tyrosine residue of glycoprotein to yield monoiodotyrosine (MIT) and diiodotyrosine (DIT). This process is called iodide organification. The MIT and DIT combine to form T_3, whereas two molecules of DIT combine to form T_4. T_3 and T_4 are released from thyroglobulin through the actions of pinocytosis and the proteolysis of thyroglobulin by lysosomal enzymes. In the circulation, 75% of T_4 is bound to thyroxine-binding globulin (TBG), and the remainder is bound mostly to thyroxine-binding prealbumin (TBPA). Approximately 0.05% of T_4 remains free. T_3 is similarly bound to TBG, allowing only 0.5% of it to remain in the free form.

DILEVALOL

Dilevalol, a noncardioselective beta-adrenergic-blocking agent, is an isomer of labetalol, has no alpha$_1$-adrenergic-blocking action, but has a potent vasodilating effect, which appears to be mediated via its beta$_2$-agonist effect, and this effect is blocked by propranolol, but not metoprolol (see Figures 37 and 43). Dilevalol decreases peripheral vascular resistance without influencing cardiac output. Dilevalol in a daily dose of 100 to 800 mg is effective in the treatment of mild to moderate hypertension. The plasma concentration of

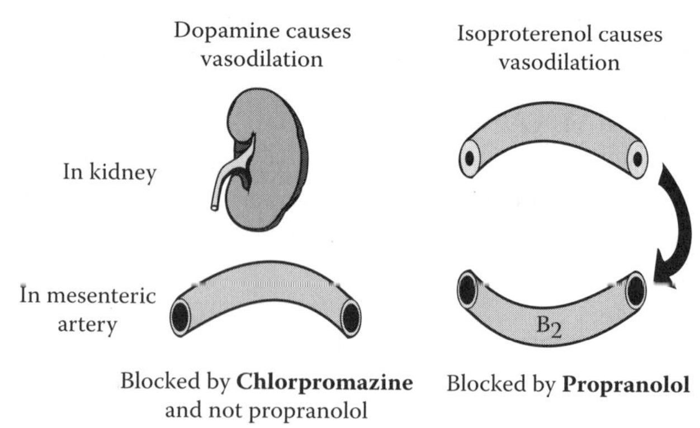

FIGURE 43 Stimulation of the **dopamine receptors** in renal and mesenteric arteries causes vasodilation, which is not blocked by propranolol (beta antagonist) but is blocked by a dopamine-receptor-blocking agent such as **chlorpromazine**.

dilevalol is not altered in renal impairment, and only 3% of the drug is excreted unchanged.

DILTIAZEM HYDROCHLORIDE

(Cardizem)

Diltiazem, a calcium-channel-blocking agent, is indicated in angina pectoris due to coronary artery spasm, chronic stable angina, and essential hypertension (Cardizem CD sustained-release preparation). Diltiazem dilates systemic arteries, decreases total peripheral resistance and afterload. It also decreases myocardial oxygen demand and cardiac work by reducing heart rate, relieving coronary artery spasm, and dilating peripheral vessels. Diltiazem is absorbed from the GI tract rapidly, subjected to massive first-pass effect in the liver, bound to plasma proteins to the extent of 70 to 85%, metabolized in the liver, and partly (35%) excreted unchanged by the kidneys. Overdosage with diltiazem may cause heart block, asystole, and hypotension (see Table 9 and Figure 50).

DIMENHYDRINATE

(Dramamine)

Dimenhydrinate consists of diphenhydramine and chlorotheophylline. It is indicated (50 to 100 mg every 4 to 6 hours) in the prevention and treatment of nausea, vomiting, dizziness, or vertigo of motion sickness. Dimenhydrinate, possessing an anticholinergic action, should be used cautiously in prostatic hypertrophy, stenosing peptic ulcer, pyloroduodenal obstruction, bladder neck obstruction, narrow angle glaucoma, bronchial asthma, cardiac arrhythmias, and any other conditions in which atropine-like compounds are contraindicated. Dimenhydrinate may mask the ototoxic symptoms of aminoglycosides, when used concomitantly. The side effects of dimenhydrinate are drowsiness, diplopia, tachycardia, thickening of bronchial secretions, and dryness of mouth, nose, and throat.

DIMERCAPROL

(BAL in oil)

Dimercaprol, a metal-chelating agent (30 mg/kg IM), is used to treat severe arsenic or gold poisoning.

DIMETHOXANATE

(Cothera)

Noscapine (Nectadon) is a naturally occurring opium alkaloid with a structure and function similar to papaverine. It is antitussive and has no analgesic or addictive properties. Diphenhydramine and chlorcyclizine are antihistaminic agents that also have antitussive properties. Dimethoxanate and pipazethate (Theratuss) are phenothiazine derivatives without analgesic but with weak antitussive and local anesthetic properties.

DINOPROSTONE TROMETHAMINE

(Prostin F2S)

Prostaglandins are mostly used as abortifacients. They may be administered by vaginal suppository (Dinoprostone, which contains prostaglandin E_2), by intramuscular injection (carboprost and tromethamine, which contain 15-methyl prostaglandin F_{2a}), or by intra-amnionic administration (dinoprost and tromethamine, which contain prostaglandin F_{2a}). Other possible uses of prostaglandins may include the treatment of ductus arteriosus (prostaglandin E_1), in the management of peripheral vascular diseases. High levels of prostaglandin F_{2a} may cause dysmenorrhea, and substances such as indomethacin and ibuprofen are effective in relieving these symptoms.

DINOPROSTONE

(Prostin E_2)

Dinoprostone is used to "ripen" an unfavorable cervix in pregnant woman near term. Dinoprostone is the naturally occurring form of prostaglandin E_2 (PGE_2). When administered endocervically, it will stimulate the gravid uterus to contract. In addition to its oxytoxic effect, dinoprostone has a local effect in softening and dilating the cervix. Dinoprostone is contraindicated in fetal distress where delivery is not imminent or where vaginal delivery should not take place, for example, in cases of active herpes genitalia. Dinoprostone is metabolized in the lung, liver, and kidney, and the metabolite is eliminated by the kidneys; and hence, it should be used cautiously in renal and hepatic dysfunction.

DINOPROSTONE (PROSTAGLANDIN E2)

(Cervidil vaginal insert 10 mg)

Dinoprostone is a prostaglandin/agent for cervical ripening. It stimulates gravid uterus to contract; it also stimulates smooth muscle of the GI tract. **Gel**: used for cervical ripening in pregnant women at or near term with a need for labor induction. **Vaginal suppositories**: used for termination of pregnancy from week 12 to 20.

DIPHENADIONE

(Dipaxin)

The coumarin anticoagulants include dicumarol, warfarin sodium (coumadin sodium), warfarin potassium (Athrombin-K), acenocoumarol (Sintrom), and phenprocouman (Liquamar). The inanedione derivatives are phenidione (Hedulin), diphenadione (Dipaxin), and anisindione (Miradon). The pharmacologic properties of oral anticoagulants are identical qualitatively, but their pharmacokinetic parameters and their toxicities vary. Racemic warfarin sodium is the most widely used anticoagulant (see Tables 17 and 18).

DIPHENHYDRAMINE HYDROCHLORIDE

(Benadryl)

Diphenhydramine is an H_1-antihistaminic agent with anticholinergic and sedative properties. Diphenhydramine (25 to 50 mg t.i.d.) is indicated in allergic conjunctivitis, urticaria, and angioedema resulting from food, blood, or plasma; in combination with epinephrine in anaphylactic reactions; in active and prophylactic treatment of motion sickness; and in neuroleptic-induced dystonic reactions. Diphenhydramine has potent anticholinergic effects, and hence should be used cautiously in prostatic hypertrophy, stenosing peptic ulcer, pyloroduodenal obstruction, bladder-neck obstruction, narrow angle glaucoma, bronchial asthma, or cardiac arrhythmias. The sedative properties of diphenhydramine become potentiated by alcohol, sedative-hypnotics, neuroleptics, and tricyclic antidepressants. Monoamine oxidase inhibitors prolong and intensify the anticholinergic effects of diphenhydramine. Overdosage with diphenhydramine may cause profound CNS depression in adults or CNS excitation in children (see also Figures 34 and 37).

DIPHENIDOL

(Vontrol)

Diphenidol (25 mg every 4 hours as needed) is indicated in vertigo and associated nausea and vomiting seen in labyrinthitis and Meniere's disease, and in controlling nausea and vomiting due to malignant neoplasms. Diphenidol may cause auditory and visual hallucination, disorientation, or confusion and hence should be used under careful supervision. Because 90% of diphenidol is excreted in the urine, it should be used cautiously in renal impairment. The antiemetic effects of diphenidol may mask nausea and vomiting associated with a toxic dosage of digitalis (see also Figure 73).

DIPHENOXYLATE HYDROCHLORIDE WITH ATROPINE SULFATE

(Lomotil)

Diphenoxylate is an opiate (schedule V) with antidiarrheal properties. It is usually dispensed with atropine and sold as Lomotil. The atropine is added to discourage the abuse of diphenoxylate by narcotic addicts who are tolerant to massive doses of narcotic but not to the CNS stimulant effects of atropine. Diphenoxylate should be used cautiously in patients with obstructive jaundice because of its potential for hepatic coma, and in patients with diarrhea caused by pseudomembranous colitis because of its potential for toxic megacolon. In addition, it should be used cautiously in the treatment of diarrhea caused by poisoning or by infection by *Shigella*, *Salmonella*, and some strains of *E. coli* because expulsion of intestinal contents may be a protective mechanism. Diphenoxylate should be used with extreme caution in patients with impaired hepatic function, cirrhosis, advanced hepatorenal disease, or abnormal liver function test results, because the drug may precipitate hepatic coma. Because diphenoxylate is structurally related to meperidine, it may cause hypertension when combined with monoamine oxidase inhibitors. As a narcotic, it will augment the CNS depressant effects of alcohol, hypnotic-sedatives, and numerous other drugs, such as neuroleptics or antidepressants that cause sedation.

DIPHENOXYLATE HYDROCHLORIDE/ ATROPINE SULFATE

(Logen tablets 2.5 mg diphenoxylate hydrochloride and 0.025 mg atropine sulfate)

Diphenoxylate is an antidiarrheal agent. **Diphenoxylate**, related to meperidine, decreases motility of the GI tract. **Atropine** discourages deliberate overdosage of diphenoxylate. The combination is indicated as adjunctive therapy in the treatment of diarrhea.

DIPHTHERIA AND TETANUS TOXOIDS, ABSORBED, COMBINED

(TD)

Diphtheria, a diphtheria and tetanus prophylaxis agent, is used for primary immunization.

DIPHTHERIA AND TETANUS TOXOIDS AND PERTUSSIS VACCINE, ABSORBED

(DTP) (Tri-Immunol)

This combination, toxoid and vaccine, is used for primary immunization and booster immunization.

DIPHTHERIA ANTITOXIN, EQUINE

This diphtheria antitoxin is used to prevent or treat diphtheria.

DIPHTHERIA TOXOID, ABSORBED

(For pediatric use)

This diphtheria prophylaxis agent is used in diphtheria immunization.

DIPHTHERIA AND TETANUS TOXOIDS AND ACELLULAR PERTUSSIS ADSORBED, HEPATITIS B (RECOMBINANT) AND INACTIVATED POLIOVIRUS VACCINE COMBINED

(Pediarix injection 25 Lf diphtheria toxoid, 10 Lf tetanus toxoid, 25 mcg inactivated pertussis toxin (PT), 25 mcg filamentous hemagglutinin (FHA), 8 mcg pertactin, 10 mcg hepatitis B surface antigen (HBsAg), 40 D-antigen units (DU) type 1 poliovirus, 8 DU type 2 poliovirus, and 32 DU type 3 poliovirus per 0.5 mL)

Diphtheria and tetanus toxoids induce antibodies against toxins made by *Corynebacterium diphtheriae* and *Clostridium tetani*; pertussis vaccine protects against *Bordetella pertussis*; hepatitis B vaccine induces specific antibodies against hepatitis B virus; poliovirus vaccine induces protective antipoliovirus antibodies, reducing pharyngeal excretion of poliovirus types 1, 2, and 3. It is indicated in active immunization against diphtheria, tetanus, pertussis, all known types of hepatitis B virus and poliomyelitis (caused by types 1, 2, and 3).

DIPIVEFRIN HYDROCHLORIDE

(Propine solution 0.1%)

Dipivefrin is a prodrug of epinephrine and is converted to epinephrine in the eye by hydrolysis. It exerts its action by decreasing aqueous production and enhancing outflow facility. It is indicated in controlling intraocular pressure in chronic open-angle glaucoma.

DIPYRIDAMOLE

(Persantine)

Dipyridamole is indicated as an adjunct to therapy with coumarin anticoagulant in the prevention of postoperative thromboembolic complications of cardiac valve replacement; as an alternative to exercise in thallium myocardial perfusion imaging for the evaluation of coronary artery disease in patients who are unable to exercise; and in long-term therapy for angina pectoris. Dipyridamole inhibits platelet adhesion and is a coronary vasodilator. Inappropriate use of dipyridamole has caused MI, ventricular fibrillation, tachycardia, bronchospasm, and transient cerebral ischemia (see also Figures 14 and 92).

DIPYRONE

Dipyrone is a water-soluble pyrazolone derivative available in oral, rectal, and injectable forms. It has been recognized as an effective analgesic, antipyretic, and antispasmodic drug. Some antiinflammatory properties have also been recognized in pharmacological models, although it is still questionable whether this is of any clinical relevance. Dipyrone is indicated in severe pain, particularly, pain associated with smooth-muscle spasm or colic affecting the GI, biliary, or urinary tract. It is also useful in fever that is refractory to other treatment.

DISOPYRAMIDE PHOSPHATE

(Norpace)

Disopyramide, a type 1 antiarrhythmic agent, in a dose of 100 mg every 6 hours, is indicated in treatment of life-threatening ventricular arrhythmias. Disopyramide depresses automaticity, primarily in the ventricular conducting system. It depresses conduction velocity throughout the heart, but has less effect at the AV node than either quinidine or procainamide. It does not have a vagolytic effect in the heart. Disopyramide terminates reentry by producing bidirectional block. It does not greatly depress blood pressure (BP). Contractility and cardiac output are mildly depressed with its use, but, because the compound is not a vasodilator, a reflex increase in peripheral resistance tends to offset the decline in cardiac output. Similar to quinidine and procainamide, 50% is excreted unmetabolized in the urine. Disopyramide's side effects are primarily gastrointestinal in nature due to its peripheral anticholinergic action, which causes dry mouth and urinary hesitancy. Disopyramide's major therapeutic use is for treating premature ventricular contractions and ventricular tachycardia. It does not appear to be particularly useful in controlling atrial arrhythmias (see also Figure 84).

DISOPYRAMIDE PHOSPHATE

Norpace capsules 100 mg)

Disopyramide is an antiarrhythmic agent that decreases the rate of diastolic depolarization; decreases upstroke velocity; increases action potential duration; and prolongs refractory period. It is indicated in suppression and documented prevention of ventricular arrhythmias considered to be life threatening.

Disopyramide (Norpace, others) exerts electrophysiological effects very similar to those of quinidine, but the drugs have different adverse effect profiles. **Disopyramide** is used to maintain sinus rhythm in patients with atrial flutter or atrial fibrillation and to prevent recurrence of ventricular tachycardia or ventricular fibrillation. It is prescribed as a racemate. The *in vitro* electrophysiological actions of S-(+)-disopyramide are similar to those of quinidine. The R-(–)-enantiomer produces similar Na^+-channel block but does not prolong cardiac action potentials. Unlike quinidine, racemic **disopyramide** is not an α-adrenergic receptor antagonist, but it does exert prominent anticholinergic actions that account for many of its adverse effects. These include precipitation of glaucoma, constipation, dry mouth, and urinary retention; the latter is most common in males with prostatism but can occur in females. **Disopyramide** commonly depresses contractility, which can precipitate heart failure, and can also cause torsade de pointes.

Disopyramide is well absorbed. Binding to plasma proteins is concentration dependent, so a small increase in total concentration may represent a disproportionately larger increase in free drug concentration. **Disopyramide** is eliminated by both hepatic metabolism (to a weakly active metabolite) and renal excretion of unchanged drug. The dose should be reduced in patients with renal dysfunction. Higher than usual dosages may be required in patients receiving drugs that induce hepatic metabolism, such as phenytoin.

DISULFIRAM

(Anabuse)

Disulfiram (tetraethylthiuram disulfied; Antabuse) was taken in the course of an investigation of its potential anthelminthic efficacy by two Danish physicians, who became ill at a cocktail party and were quick to realize that the compound had altered their responses to alcohol. They initiated a series of pharmacological and clinical studies that provided the basis for the use of disulfiram as an adjunct in the treatment of chronic alcoholism. Similar responses to alcohol ingestion are produced by various congeners of disulfiram, namely, **cyanamide,** the fungus ***Coprinus atramentarius***, the hypoglycemic **sulfonylureas, metronidazole,** certain **cephalosporins,** and animal charcoal.

DIURETICS

Carbonic anhydrase inhibitor
Acetazolamide
Osmotic agent
Mannitol

Loop Diuretics

Azosemide	Furosemide	Torsemide
Bumetanide	Muzolimine	Tripamide
Ethacrynic acid	Piretanide	

Thiazide Diuretics

Bendroflumethiazide	Cyclothiazide	Metolazone
Benzthiazide	Hydrochlorothiazide	Polythiazide
Chlorothiazide	Hydroflumethiazide	Quinethazone
Chlorthalidone	Indapamide	Trichlormethiazide
Clopamide	Methyclothiazide	

Potassium-Retaining Diuretics

Amiloride
Spironolactone
Triamterene

TABLE 13
Actions of Adrenergic and Dopaminergic Agents on Their Receptors

Sympathetic Amines Prolactin	$Beta_1$ Positive Inotropy Positive Chronotropy Positive Dromotropy	$Beta_2$ Vasodilation	$Alpha_1$ Vasoconstriction	$Alpha_2$ Vasoconstriction	DA_1 Vasodilation	DA_2 Vasodilation Emesis
Norepinephrine	+++	—	+++	+++	—	—
Dopamine	+++	±	++	++	±	±
Dobutamine	+++	+	+	—	—	—
Ibopamine	++	+	—	—	—	+
Propylbutyldopamine	—	—	+	+	+	+++
Fenoldopam	—	—	—	—	+++	—

Note: DA = dopamine receptor; +++ = major action; ++ = moderate action; + = minimal action; — = actions absent.

DOBUTAMINE HYDROCHLORIDE

(Dobutrex)

Dobutamine (infusion of 2.5 to 10 mcg/kg/minute) is indicated in the short-term treatment of adults with cardiac decompensation due to decreased contractility, resulting from either organic heart disease or surgical procedures involving the heart. Often, digitalis is used prior to infusing dobutamine in patients with atrial fibrillation. The actions of dobutamine on various adrenergic and dopaminergic receptors are summarized in Table 13. In patients with depressed cardiac output, dobutamine increases cardiac output without increasing cardiac rate, and is contraindicated in patients with idiopathic hypertrophic subaortic stenosis. Dobutamine exerts its effects within 1 to 2 minutes, has a half-life of 2 minutes, and is metabolized to 3-0-methyldobutamine,which is then excreted in the urine (see also Figure 49).

DOCETAXEL

(Taxotere)

Docetaxel is the second representative of the new entity of drugs that have a unique taxane ring in common, such as the one seen in paclitaxel. Being more efficacious than paclitaxel, docetaxel is used in ovarian cancer. Paclitaxel and docetaxel inhibit microtubule depolymerization, thereby reducing the formation of stable microtubule bundles (see also Figure 15).

DOCETAXEL

(Taxotere injection 20 mg)

Docetaxel acts by disrupting cells' microtubular network, which is essential for mitotic and interphase cellular functions. Docetaxel binds to free tubulin and promotes the assembly of tubulin into stable microtubules while simultaneously inhibiting their disassembly. Docetaxel is indicated in locally advanced or metastatic breast cancer; locally advanced or metastatic non-small-cell lung cancer. The first compound of this series, paclitaxel (Taxol), was isolated from the bark of the Western yew tree in 1971. Paclitaxel and its congenic, the semisynthetic docetaxel (Taxotere), exhibit unique pharmacological actions as inhibitors of mitosis, differing from the vinca alkaloids and colchicine derivatives in that they bind to a different site on β-tubulin and promote rather than inhibit microtubule formation. The drugs have a central role in the therapy of ovarian, breast, lung, esophageal, bladder, and head and neck cancers. Their optimal dose, schedule, and use in drug combinations are still evolving.

Interest in docetaxel and paclitaxel was stimulated by the finding that the drug possessed the unique ability to promote microtubule formation at cold temperatures and in the absence of GTP. It binds specifically to the β-tubulin subunit of microtubules and antagonizes the disassembly of this key cytoskeletal protein. Schedules for optimal use, alone or in combination with other drugs, including **doxorubicin** and **cisplatin**, are still evolving. Drug interactions have been noted; the sequence of cisplatin preceding paclitaxel decreases paclitaxel clearance and produces greater toxicity than the opposite schedule. **Paclitaxel** decreases doxorubicin clearance and enhances cardiotoxicity, whereas docetaxel has no apparent effect on anthracycline pharmacokinetics.

Docetaxel and paclitaxel have become central components of regimens for treating metastatic ovarian, breast, lung, and head and neck cancers. **Docetaxel** has significant activity with **estramustine** for treatment of hormone-refractory prostate cancer. In current regimens, either drug is administered once weekly or once every 3 weeks, with comparable response rates and somewhat different patterns of toxicity. **Docetaxel** produces greater leukopenia and peripheral edema, whereas paclitaxel causes a higher incidence of hypersensitivity, muscle aching, and neuropathy (particularly when used in combination with a platinum analog). The optimal schedule of taxane administration, alone or in combination with other drugs, is still under evaluation.

DOCUSATE

(Docusate sodium)

Docusate is a fecal softener/sulfactant, which facilitates stool softening by detergent activity. Docusate is indicated in short-term treatment of constipation; prophylaxis in patients who should not strain during defecation (e.g., after anorectal surgery, MI); in evacuation of the colon for rectal and bowel examinations; and prevention of dry, hard stools.

Docusate salts are anionic surfactants that lower the surface tension of the stool to allow mixing of aqueous and fatty substances, softening the stool and permitting easier defecation. However, these agents also stimulate intestinal fluid and electrolyte secretion (possibly by increasing mucosal cyclic AMP) and alter intestinal mucosal permeability. **Docusate sodium** (dioctyl sodium sulfosuccinate; Colace, Doxinate, others) and docusate calcium (dioctyl calcium sulfosuccinate; Surfak, others), are available in several dosage forms. Despite their widespread use, these agents have marginal, if any, efficacy in most cases of constipation.

DOCUSATE CALCIUM
(D-C-S, PRO-CAL-SOF, SURFAK)

DOCUSATE POTASSIUM
(Dialose, Diocto-K, Kasof)

DOCUSATE SODIUM
(Colace, Diocto, Dioeze, Diosuccin, Disonate, Di-Sosul, DOS, Doxinate, D.S.S., Duosol, Modane Soft, Pro-Sof, Regulax SS, Regutol, Theravac-SB)

Docusate salts (50 to 300 mg p.o. daily) are used as stool softeners.

DOFETILIDE
(Tikosyn capsules 125 mcg)

Dofetilide is an antiarrhythmic agent that causes blockade of the cardiac ion channel carrying the rapid component of the delayed rectifier potassium currents. Dofetilide is indicated in maintenance of normal sinus rhythm (delay in time to recurrence of atrial fibrillation/atrial flutter [AF/AFl]) in patients with AF/AFl of more than 1 week duration who have been converted to normal sinus rhythm; and in conversion of AF/AFl to normal sinus rhythm.

Dofetilide (Tikosyn) is a potent and "pure" I_{Kr} blocker. As a result of this specificity, it has virtually no extracardiac pharmacological effects. **Dofetilide** is effective in maintaining sinus rhythm in patients with atrial fibrillation. **Dofetilide** currently is available through a restricted distribution system that includes only physicians, hospitals, and other institutions that have received special educational programs covering proper dosing and treatment initiation. Most of a dose of **dofetilide** is excreted unchanged by the kidneys. In patients with mild to moderate renal failure, decreases in dosage based on creatinine clearance are required to minimize the risk of torsade de pointes. The drug should not be used in patients with advanced renal failure or with inhibitors of renal cation transport. **Dofetilide** also undergoes minor hepatic metabolism. **Torsade de pointes** occurred in 1 to 3% of patients in clinical trials where strict exclusion criteria (e.g., hypokalemia) were applied and continuous ECG monitoring was used to detect marked QT prolongation in the hospital.

DOLASETRON MESYLATE
(Anzemet injection 20 mg/mL)

Dolasetron is a 5-HT_3-receptor antagonist that inhibits serotonin receptors in the tract and chemoreceptor zone. Parenteral or oral used: for prevention of nausea and vomiting associated with initial and repeat courses of emetogenic chemotherapy and prevention of postoperative nausea and vomiting in patients at risk. Parenteral use only: for treatment of postoperative nausea and vomiting. **Ondansetron** (Zofran) is the prototypical drug in this class. Since their introduction in the early 1990s, the 5-HT_3-receptor antagonists have become the most widely used drugs for chemotherapy-induced emesis. Other agents in this class include **granisetron** (Kytril), **dolasetron** (Anzemet) **palonosetron** (Aloxi; intravenous use only) and **tropisetron** (available in some countries but not in the United States). The differences among these agents are related mainly to their chemical structures, 5-HT_3-receptor affinities, and pharmacokinetic profiles.

There is evidence that effects at peripheral and central sites contribute to the efficacy of these agents. 5-HT_3 receptors are present in several critical sites involved in emesis, including vagal afferents, the solitary tract nucleus (STN) (which receives signals from vagal afferents), and the area postrema itself. Serotonin is released by the entero-chromaffin cells of the small intestine in response to chemotherapeutic agents and may stimulate vagal afferents (via 5-HT_3 receptors) to initiate the vomiting reflex. Experimentally, vagotomy has been shown to prevent cisplatin-induced emesis. However, the highest concentrations of 5-HT_3 receptors in the CNS are found in the STN and chemoreceptor trigger zone (CTZ), and antagonists of 5-HT_3 receptors also may suppress nausea and vomiting by acting on these sites. The antiemetic effects of these drugs persist long after they disappear from circulation, suggesting their continuing interaction at the receptor level. In fact, all of these drugs can be administered effectively just once a day.

These agents are absorbed well from the GI tract. Ondansetron is extensively metabolized in the liver by CYP1A2, CYP2D6, and CYP3A4, followed by glucuronide or sulfate conjugation. Patients with hepatic dysfunction have reduced plasma clearance, and some adjustment in the dosage is advisable. These agents are most effective in treating chemotherapy-induced nausea and nausea secondary to upper abdominal irradiation, where all three agents appear to be equally efficacious. They also are effective against hyperemesis of pregnancy and, to a lesser degree, postoperative nausea, but not against motion sickness. Unlike other agents in this class, **palonosetron** may also be helpful in delayed emesis, perhaps a reflection of its long half-life.

These agents are available as tablets, oral solution, and intravenous preparations for injection. For patients on cancer chemotherapy, these drugs can be given in a single intravenous dose infused over 15 minutes, beginning 30 minutes before chemotherapy, or in two to three divided doses, with the first usually given 30 minutes before and subsequent doses at various intervals after chemotherapy. The drugs also can be used intramuscularly or orally.

In general, these drugs are very well tolerated, with the most common adverse effects being constipation or diarrhea, headache, and light-headedness. As a class, these agents have been shown experimentally to induce minor electrocardiographic changes, but these are not expected to be clinically significant in most cases. Phenothiazines such as **prochlorperazine**, **thiethylperazine**, and **chlorpromazine** are among the most commonly used "general purpose" antinauseants and antiemetics. Their effects in this regard are complex, but their principal mechanism of action is dopamine D_2-receptor antagonism at the CTZ. Compared to **metoclopramide** or **ondansetron**, these drugs do not appear to be as uniformly effective in cancer-chemotherapy-induced emesis. On the other hand, they also possess antihistaminc and anticholinergic activities, which are of value in other forms of nausea, such as motion sickness.

Histamine H_1-receptor antagonists are primarily useful for motion sickness and postoperative emesis. They act on vestibular afferents and within the brain stem. **Cyclizine**, **hydroxyzine**, **promethazine**, and **diphenhydramine** are examples of this class of agents. Cyclizine has additional anticholinergic effects that may be useful for patients with abdominal cancer.

The most commonly used muscarinic receptor antagonist is **scopolamine** (hyoscine), which can be injected as the hydrobromide, but usually is administered as the free base in the form of a **transdermal patch** (Transderm-scop). Its principal utility is in the prevention and treatment of motion sickness, although it has been shown to have some activity in postoperative nausea and vomiting, as well. In general, anticholinergic agents have no role in chemotherapy-induced nausea. **Dronabinol** (delta-9-tetrahydrocannabinol; Marinol) is a naturally occurring cannabinoid that can be synthesized chemically or extracted from the marijuana plant, *Cannabis sativa*. The exact mechanism of the antiemetic action of dronabinol is unknown but probably relates to stimulation of the CB_1 subtype of cannabinoid receptors on neurons in and around the vomiting center.

DONEPEZIL

(Aricept tablets 5 mg)

Donepezil is a cholinesterase inhibitor which increases acetylcholine by inhibiting acetylcholinesterase, thereby increasing cholinergic function. It is indicated in the treatment of mild to moderate dementia of the Alzheimer type. A deficiency of intact cholinergic neurons, particularly those extending from subcortical areas such as the nucleus basalis of Meynert, has been observed in patients with progressive dementia of the Alzheimer type. Using a rationale similar to that in other CNS degenerative diseases, therapy for enhancing concentrations of cholinergic neurotransmitters in the CNS was investigated. In 1993 the PDA approved **tacrine** (tetrahydroaminoacridine) for use in mild to moderate Alzheimer's disease, but a high incidence of hepatotoxicity limits the utility of this drug. About 30% of the patients receiving low doses of tacrine within 3 months have alanine aminotransferase values three times normal; upon discontinuing the drug, liver function values return to normal in 90% of the patients. Other side effects are typical of AChE inhibitors.

More recently, **donepezil** was approved for clinical use. At 5- and 10-mg daily oral doses, improved cognition and global clinical function were seen in the 21- to 81-week intervals studied. In long-term studies, the drug delayed symptomatic progression of the disease for periods up to 55 weeks. Side effects are largely attributable to excessive cholinergic stimulation, with nausea, diarrhea, and vomiting being most frequently reported. The drug is well tolerated in single daily doses. Usually, 5-mg doses are administered at night for 4 to 6 weeks; if this is well tolerated, the dose can be increased to 10 mg daily.

Rivastigmine, a long-acting carbamoylating inhibitor, has recently been approved for use in the United States and Europe. Although fewer studies have been conducted, its efficacy, tolerability, and side effects are similar to those of **donepezil**. **Eptastigmine**, another carbamoylating inhibitor, was associated with adverse hematologic effects in two studies, resulting in suspension of clinical trials. Galantamine is another AChE inhibitor recently approved by the PDA. It has a side-effect profile similar to those of donepezil and rivastigmine.

Four inhibitors of AChE currently are approved by the FDA for treatment of Alzheimer's disease: **tacrine** (1,2,3,4-tetrahydro-9-aminoacridine; Cognex), **donepezil** (Aricept), **rivastigmine** (Excelon), and **galantamine** (Razadyne). Tacrine is a potent centrally acting inhibitor of AChE. Studies of oral tacrine in combination with lecithin have confirmed that there is indeed an effect of tacrine on some measures of memory performance, but the magnitude of improvement observed with the combination of lecithin and tacrine is modest at best. The side effects of tacrine often are significant and dose limiting; abdominal cramping, anorexia, nausea, vomiting, and diarrhea are observed in up to one-third of patients receiving therapeutic doses, and elevations of serum transaminases are observed in up to 50% of those treated. Because of significant side effects, tacrine is not used widely, clinically. **Donepezil** is a selective inhibitor of AChE in the CNS with little effect on AChE in peripheral tissues. It produces modest improvements in cognitive scores in Alzheimer's disease patients and has a long half-life, allowing once-daily dosing. Rivastigmine and galantamine are dosed twice daily and produce a similar degree of cognitive improvement. Adverse effects associated with **donepezil**, rivastigmine, and galantamine are similar in character but generally less frequent and less severe than those observed with tacrine; they include nausea, diarrhea, vomiting, and insomnia. **Donepezil**, rivastigmine, and galantamine are not associated with the hepatotoxicity that limits the use of tacrine.

DOMPERIDONE

Domperidone (100 mg p.o.) is an antiemetic agent that blocks selectively peripheral dopamine receptors in the chemoreceptor trigger zone for emesis, as well as those in the GI tract. Unlike metoclopramide, domperidone does not pass across the blood–brain barrier, and hence it is thought to be devoid of any extrapyramidal side effects. Clinical evidence indicates that domperidone, by blocking dopamine receptors in the wall of the GI tract, enhances normal synchronized GI peristalsis and motility in the proximal portion of the GI tract (see also Figure 73).

DOPAMINE HYDROCHLORIDE

(Intropin)

Peripheral dopaminergic receptor agents are useful in the treatment of CHF. Two distinct subtypes of dopamine receptors have been identified. The dopamine$_2$ (DA_2) receptors are located at various sites within the sympathetic nervous system, and their activation results in inhibition of the sympathetic nervous system. In contrast, activation of the postsynaptic dopamine$_1$ (DA_1) receptors, which are located on vascular smooth muscles, causes vasodilation in the renal, mesentery, cerebral, and coronary vascular beds. Thus, the pharmacologic response to the activation of DA_2 and DA_1 receptors is hypotension, bradycardia, diuresis, and natriuresis (see Figure 49 and Table 13). Dopamine stimulates dopamine, alpha-, and beta-adrenergic receptors. The use of dopamine in CHF is limited because it causes nausea and vomiting, becomes inactive when given orally, increases afterload (alpha-adrenergic-receptor-mediated peripheral vasoconstriction), and enhances oxygen demand on the left ventricle (see also Figure 49).

DOPAMINE HYDROCHLORIDE

(Dopamine hydrochloride injection 40 mg/mL)

Dopamine hydrochloride is a vasopressor that stimulates beta$_1$ receptors in the heart, causing more complete and forceful contractions (inotropy). It also acts on alpha receptors (dose-dependent) and has dopaminergic effects. Dopamine hydrochloride is indicated in the correction of hemodynamic imbalances present in shock syndrome after MI, trauma, endotoxic septicemia, surgery, and renal failure or imbalances in conditions of chronic refractory cardiac decompensation (e.g., CHF).

The cardiovascular effects of **dopamine** are mediated by several distinct types of receptors that vary in their affinity to dopamine. At low concentrations, the primary interaction of dopamine is with vascular D_1 receptors, especially in the renal, mesenteric, and coronary beds. By activating adenylyl cyclase and raising intracellular concentrations of cAMP, D_1-receptor stimulation leads to vasodilation. Infusion of low doses of dopamine causes an increase in glomerular filtration rate, renal blood flow, and Na^+ excretion. Activation of D_1 receptors on renal tubular cells decreases sodium transport by cAMP-dependent and cAMP-independent mechanisms. Increasing cAMP production in the proximal tubular cells and the medullary part of the thick ascending limb of the loop of Henle inhibits the Na^+-H^+ exchanger and the Na^+K^+-ATPase pump. The renal tubular actions of dopamine that cause natriuresis may be augmented by the increase in renal blood flow and the small increase in the glomerular filtration rate that follow its administration. The resulting increase in hydrostatic pressure in the peritubular capillaries and reduction in oncotic pressure may contribute to diminished reabsorption of sodium by the proximal tubular cells. As a consequence, dopamine has pharmacologically appropriate effects in the management of states of low cardiac output associated with compromised renal function, such as severe CHF.

At somewhat higher concentrations, dopamine exerts a positive inotropic effect on the myocardium, acting on β_1-adrenergic receptors. Dopamine also causes the release of norepinephrine from nerve terminals, which contributes to its effects on the heart. Tachycardia is less prominent during infusion of dopamine than of isoproterenol. **Dopamine** usually increases systolic blood pressure and pulse pressure and either has no effect on diastolic blood pressure or increases it slightly. Total peripheral resistance usually is unchanged when low or intermediate doses of dopamine are given, probably because of the ability of dopamine to reduce regional arterial resistance in some vascular beds, such as mesenteric and renal, while causing only minor increases in others. At high concentrations, dopamine activates vascular α_1 receptors, leading to more general vasoconstriction.

Although there are specific **dopamine** receptors in the CNS, injected dopamine usually has no central effects because it does not readily cross the blood–brain barrier.

Before dopamine is administered to patients in shock, hypovolemia should be corrected by transfusion of whole blood, plasma, or other appropriate fluids. Untoward effects due to overdosage generally are attributable to excessive sympathomimetic activity (although this also may be the response to worsening shock). Nausea, vomiting, tachycardia, anginal pain, arrhythmias, headache, hypertension, and peripheral vasoconstriction may be encountered during dopamine infusion. Extravasation of large amounts of **dopamine** during infusion may cause ischemic necrosis and sloughing. Rarely, gangrene of the fingers or toes has followed prolonged infusion of the drug.

Dopamine should be avoided or used at a much reduced dosage (one-tenth or less) if the patient has received a MAO inhibitor. Careful adjustment of dosage also is necessary in patients who are taking tricyclic antidepressants. **Dopamine** (Intropin, others) is used in the treatment of severe CHF, particularly in patients with oliguria and low or normal peripheral vascular resistance. The drug also may improve physiological parameters in the treatment of cardiogenic and septic shock. Although **dopamine** may acutely improve cardiac and renal function in severely ill patients with chronic heart disease or renal failure, there is relatively little evidence supporting long-term benefits in clinical outcome.

Dopamine hydrochloride is used only intravenously. The drug initially is administered at a rate of 2 to 5 μg/kg per minute; this rate may be increased gradually up to 20 to 50 μg/kg per minute or more, as the clinical situation dictates. During the infusion, patients require clinical assessment of myocardial function, perfusion of vital organs such as the brain, and the production of urine. Most patients should receive intensive care, with monitoring of arterial and venous pressures and the ECG. Reduction in urine flow, tachycardia, or the development of arrhythmias may be indications to slow or terminate the infusion. The duration of action of dopamine is brief, and hence the rate of administration can be used to control the intensity of effect.

Related drugs include **fenoldopam** and **dopexamine**. Fenoldopam (Corlopam), a benzodiazepine derivative, is a rapidly acting vasodilator used for control of severe hypertension (e.g., malignant hypertension with end-organ damage) in hospitalized patients for not more than 48 hours. Fenoldopam is an agonist for D_1 peripheral dopamine receptors and binds with moderate affinity to α_2-adrenergic receptors; it has no significant affinity to D_2 receptors or α_1- or β-adrenergic receptors. Fenoldopam is a racemic mixture; the R-isomer is the active component. It dilates a variety of blood vessels, including coronary arteries, afferent and efferent arterioles in the kidney, and mesenteric arteries.

Less than 6% of an orally administered dose is absorbed because of extensive first-pass formation of sulfate, methyl, and glucuronide conjugates. The elimination half-life of intravenously infused fenoldopam, estimated from the decline in plasma concentration in hypertensive patients after the cessation of a 2-hour infusion, is 10 minutes. Adverse effects are related to the vasodilation and include headache, flushing, dizziness, and tachycardia or bradycardia.

Dopexamine (Dopacard) is a synthetic analog related to dopamine with intrinsic activity at **dopamine D_1** and D_2 receptors as well as at β_2 receptors; it may have other effects such as inhibition of catecholamine uptake. It appears to have favorable hemodynamic actions in patients with severe CHF, sepsis, and shock. In patients with low cardiac output, dopexamine infusion significantly increases stroke volume with a decrease in systemic vascular resistance Tachycardia and hypotension can occur, but usually only at high infusion rates.

DORNASE ALFA (DNASE)

(Pulmozyme solution for inhalation 1 mg/mL)

Dornase alfa is a mucolytic agent that cleaves DNA released by neutrophils that are mobilized to respiratory tract in response to infection, reducing viscoelasticity of purulent lung secretions, increasing airflow, and decreasing risk of infection. It is used in the treatment of cystic fibrosis.

DORNASE ALFA RECOMBINANT

(Pulmozyme)

Dornase alpha, a recombinant human deoxyribonuclease I, a mucolytic enzyme with respiratory stimulant properties, is used to improve pulmonary function and reduce the frequency of moderate to severe respiratory infections in patients with cystic fibrosis.

DORZOLAMIDE

(Trusopt solution 2%)

Dorzolamide is a carbonic anhydrase inhibitor that inhibits carbonic anhydrase enzyme, reducing the rate of aqueous humor formation and thus lowering intraocular pressure (IOP). It is indicated in the treatment of elevated IOP in patients with ocular hypertension or open-angle glaucoma.

The development of a topical carbonic anhydrase inhibitor took many years but was an important event because of the poor side-effect profile of oral carbonic anhydrase inhibitors (CAIs). **Dorzolamide** (Trusopt) and **brinzolamide** (Azopt) both work by inhibiting carbonic anhydrase (isoenzyme II), which is found in the ciliary body epithelium. This reduces the formation of bicarbonate ions, which reduces fluid transport and thus IOP.

Any of these four drug classes can be used as additive second- or third-line therapy. In fact, the β-receptor antagonist timolol has been combined with the carbonic anhydrase inhibitor **dorzolamide** in a single medication (**Cosopt**).

Such combinations reduce the number of drops needed and may improve compliance. Other combination products involving prostaglandin analogs and β-blockers are in development.

Topical **miotic agents** are historically important glaucoma medications but are less commonly used today. Miotics lower IOP by causing muscarinic-induced contraction of the ciliary muscle, which facilitates aqueous outflow. They do not affect aqueous production. Multiple miotic agents have been developed. **Pilocarpine** and **carbachol** are cholinomimetics that stimulate muscarinic receptors. **Echothiophate** (Phospholine iodide) is an organophosphate inhibitor of acetylcholinesterase; it is relatively stable in aqueous solution and, by virtue of its quaternary ammonium structure, is positively charged and poorly absorbed. The usefulness of these medicines is lessened by their numerous side effects and the need to use them three to four times a day.

If combined topical therapy fails to achieve the target IOP or fails to halt glaucomatous optic nerve damage, then systemic therapy with carbonic anhydrase inhibitors is a final medication option before resorting to laser or incisional surgical treatment. The best-tolerated oral preparation is **acetazolamide** in sustained-release capsules, followed by **methazolamide**. The least well-tolerated are acetazolamide tablets.

Toxicity of agents in treatment of glaucoma: Ciliary body spasm is a muscarinic cholinergic effect that can lead to induced myopia and a changing refraction due to iris and ciliary body contraction as the drug effect waxes and wanes between doses. Headaches can occur from the iris and ciliary body contraction. Epinephrine-related compounds, effective in IOP reduction, can cause a vasoconstriction–vasodilation rebound phenomenon leading to a red eye. Ocular and skin allergies from topical epinephrine, related prodrug formulations, apraclonidine, and brimonidine are common. Brimonidine is less likely to cause ocular allergy and is therefore more commonly used. These agents can cause CNS depression and apnea in neonates and are contraindicated in children under 2 years of age.

DORZOLAMIDE HYDROCHLORIDE/TIMOLOL MALEATE

(Cosopt solution 2% dorzolamide, 0.5% timolol)

Dorzolamide is an agent for glaucoma. It inhibits carbonic anhydrase enzyme, reducing the rate of aqueous humor formation thus lowering IOP (dorzolamide); reduces elevated and normal IOP via decreasing production of aqueous humor or increasing flow (timolol).

The combination is indicated in reduction of IOP in patients with ocular hypertension or open-angle glaucoma. **Timolol** (Blocadren, others) is a potent, non-subtype-selective β-receptor antagonist. It has no intrinsic sympathomimetic or membrane-stabilizing activity. It is used to treat hypertension, CHF, migraine prophylaxis, and has been widely used for treatment of open-angle glaucoma and intraocular hypertension.

Timolol is well absorbed from the GI tract. It is metabolized extensively by CYP2D6 in the liver and undergoes first-pass metabolism. Only a small amount of unchanged drug appears in the urine. The half-life in plasma is about 4 hours. Interestingly, the ocular formulation of **timolol** (Timoptic, others), used for treatment of glaucoma, may be extensively absorbed systemically; adverse effects can occur in susceptible patients, such as those with asthma or CHF. The systemic administration of cimetidine with topical ocular **timolol** increases the degree of β_1-blockade, resulting in a reduction of resting heart rate, IOP, and exercise tolerance.

DOXACURIUM

(Nuromax)

Doxacurium is indicated as an adjunct to general anesthesia to produce skeletal muscle relaxation; and in facilitating endotracheal intubation. Doxacurium is a long-acting nondepolarizing skeletal muscle relaxant, which binds to cholinergic receptors on the motor end plate, and its action is antagonized by neostigmine, an inhibitor of acetylcholinesterase. Doxacurium, which is 3 and 10 times more potent than pancuronium and metocurine, respectively, does not alter heart or blood pressure in therapeutic doses. Doxacurium should be used cautiously in patients with neuromuscular diseases such as myasthenia gravis and the myasthenic syndrome. The action of doxacurium, similar to other skeletal muscle-relaxing agents, is altered in conditions where electrolytes and/or acid–base balance have been disturbed. For example, the action of doxacurium is altered by magnesium salts used in the management of eclampsia or preeclampsia. Carbamazepine delays the onset and shortness of action of doxacurium. Isoflurane, enflurane, and halothane decrease the ED_{50} and prolong the duration of neuromuscular blockade (see also Figure 99).

DOXAPRAM HYDROCHLORIDE

(Dopram)

Doxapram (0.5 to 1 mg/kg) is used as a postanesthesia respiratory stimulation, in drug-induced CNS depression, and in acute hypercapnia associated with chronic obstructive pulmonary disease.

DOXAPRAM HYDROCHLORIDE

(Dopram injection 20 mg/mL)

Doxapram is an analeptic that increases the depth of respirations (tidal volume) by stimulating the respiratory center in CNS; respiratory rate may increase slightly. It may elevate BP by increasing cardiac output. Respiratory depression from opiates is reversed without affecting pain relief. It is indicated when one requires the stimulation of deep breathing in postoperative patients; for reversal of respiratory depression caused by anesthesia (other than muscle relaxants) or drug overdose; and as a temporary measure in acute respiratory failure in patients with chronic obstructive pulmonary disease (COPD) who are not undergoing mechanical ventilation.

DOXAZOSIN MESYLATE

(Cardura)

Doxazosin, an alpha-adrenergic-blocking agent (1 mg p.o. daily), is used in the treatment of essential hypertension.

DOXAZOSIN MESYLATE

(Cardura tablets 1 mg)

Doxazosin is an $alpha_1$-adrenergic-receptor blocker that selectively blocks postsynaptic $alpha_1$-adrenergic receptors, resulting in dilation of arterioles and veins. Doxazosin is indicated in the treatment of hypertension, alone or in combination with other agents, and in benign prostatic hyperplasia (BPH).

DOXEPIN HYDROCHLORIDE

(Adapin)

Doxepin (75 mg p.o. daily) is indicated in psychoneurotic patients with depression or anxiety; depression and/or anxiety of chronic alcoholism; depression and/or anxiety associated with organic disease; and in manic–depressive disorders. Doxepin blocks the uptake sites for norepinephrine and, to a lesser extent, that of serotonin. Doxepin blocks $alpha_1$-adrenergic receptors, H_1-histaminergic receptors, and muscarinic cholinergic receptors. It causes heavy sedation and marked orthostatic hypotension. Because of its anticholinergic properties, it should be used cautiously in prostatic hypertrophy, stenosing peptic ulcer, pyloroduodenal obstruction, bladder-neck obstruction, narrow angle glaucoma, bronchial asthma, and cardiac arrhythmias (see Tables 5 through 7).

DOXORUBICIN

(Adriamycin)

Daunorubicin (daunomycin and cerubidine) and doxorubicin bind to and cause the intercalation of the DNA molecule, thereby inhibiting DNA template function. They also provoke DNA chain scission and chromosomal damage. Daunorubicin is useful in treating patients with acute lymphocytic or acute granulocytic leukemia. Adriamycin is useful in cases of solid tumors such as sarcoma, metastatic breast cancer, and thyroid cancer. These agents cause stomatitis, alopecia, myelosuppression, and cardiac abnormalities ranging from arrhythmias to cardiomyopathy (see also Figure 15).

DOXORUBICIN, CONVENTIONAL

(Adriamycin RDF preservative-free solution for injection 2 mg/mL)

Doxorubicin is an anthracycline antibiotic. Cells treated with doxorubicin have been shown to manifest the characteristic morphologic changes associated with apoptosis or programmed cell death. Doxorubicin-induced apoptosis may be an integral component of the cellular mechanism of action relating to therapeutic effects, toxicities, or both.

Indications—adults: leukemias, lymphomas, soft-tissue and bone sarcomas; breast, ovarian, transitional cell bladder, thyroid, bronchogenic, and gastric carcinoma; **children**: leukemias, lymphomas, Wilms' tumor, neuroblastoma, and bone sarcomas.

DOXORUBICIN, LIPOSOMAL

(Doxil solution for injection equivalent to 2 mg/mL doxorubicin hydrochloride liposomal in single-use 10 or 30 mLvials)

Doxorubicin is an antineoplastic/anthracycline antibiotic. It binds DNA and inhibits nucleic acid synthesis. Cell structure studies have demonstrated rapid cell penetration and perinuclear chromatin binding, rapid inhibition of mitotic activity and nucleic acid synthesis, and induction of mutagenesis and chromosomal aberrations. It is indicated in treatment of ovarian cancer in patients whose disease has progressed or recurred after platinum-based chemotherapy; and in treatment of AIDS-related Kaposi's sarcoma in patients whose disease has progressed on prior combination chemotherapy or who are intolerant to such therapy.

Daunorubicin, doxorubicin, epirubicin, idarubicin, and mitoxantrone are among the most important antitumor agents. They are derived from the fungus *S. peucetius* var. *caesius*. Idarubicin and epirubicin are analogs of the naturally produced anthracyclines, differing only slightly in chemical structure, but having somewhat distinct patterns of clinical activity. Daunorubicin and idarubicin have been used primarily in acute leukemias, whereas **doxorubicin** and epirubicin display broader activity against human solid tumors. These agents, all of which possess the potential for generating free radicals, cause an unusual and often irreversible cardiomyopathy, the occurrence of which is related to the total dose of the drug. The structurally similar agent **mitoxantrone** has a useful activity against prostate cancer and AML, and is used in high-dose chemotherapy. Mitoxantrone, an anthracenedione, has significantly less cardiotoxicity than do the anthracyclines.

The anthracycline antibiotics have a tetracyclic ring structure attached to an unusual sugar, daunosamine. All cytotoxic agents of this class have quinone and hydroquinone moieties on adjacent rings that permit the gain and loss of electrons. Although there are marked differences in the clinical use of daunorubicin and doxorubicin, their chemical structures differ only by a single hydroxyl group on C14. Idarubicin is 4-demethoxydaunorubicin, a synthetic derivative of daunorubicin, whereas epirubicin is an epimer at the 4′-position of the sugar. Mitoxantrone lacks a glycosidic side group.

A number of important biochemical effects have been described for the anthracyclines and anthracenediones, all of which could contribute to their therapeutic and toxic effects. These compounds can intercalate with DNA, directly affecting transcription and replication. A more important action is the ability of these drugs to form a tripartite complex with topoisomerase II and DNA. Topoisomerase II is an ATP-dependent enzyme that binds to DNA and produces double-strand breaks at the 3′ phosphate backbone, allowing strand passage and uncoiling of supercoiled DNA. Following strand passage, topoisomerase II religates the DNA strands. This enzymatic function is essential for DNA replication and repair. Formation of the tripartite complex with anthracyclines and with etoposide inhibits the religation of the broken DNA strands, leading to apoptosis. Defects in DNA double-strand break repairs sensitize cells to damage by these drugs, whereas overexpression of transcription-linked DNA repair may contribute to resistance. Anthracyclines, by virtue of their quinone groups, also generate free radicals in solution, and in both normal and malignant tissues. Anthracyclines can form semiquinone radical intermediates, which in turn can react with oxygen to produce superoxide anion radicals. These can generate both hydrogen peroxide and hydroxyl radicals (•OH), which attack DNA and oxidize DNA bases. The production of free radicals is significantly stimulated by the interaction of doxorubicin with iron. Enzymatic defenses such as superoxide dismutase and catalase are believed to have an important role in protecting cells against the toxicity of the anthracyclines, and these defenses can be augmented by exogenous antioxidants such as alpha tocopherol or by an iron chelator, dexrazoxane (Zinecard), which protects against cardiac toxicity.

Exposure of cells to anthracyclines leads to apoptosis; mediators of this process include the p53 DNA-damage sensor and activated caspases (proteases), although ceramide, a lipid breakdown product, and the fas receptor–ligand system also have been implicated in selected tumor cells. Daunorubicin, **doxorubicin**, epirubicin, and idarubicin usually are administered intravenously and are cleared by a complex pattern of hepatic metabolism and biliary excretion. All anthracyclines are converted to an active metabolite, indarubicinol, which has a half-life of about 40 hours. There is rapid uptake of the drugs in the heart, kidneys, lungs, liver, and spleen. They do not cross the blood–brain barrier.

Daunorubicin and doxorubicin are eliminated by metabolic conversion to a variety of aglycones and other inactive products. Idarubicin is primarily metabolized to idarubicinol, which accumulates in plasma and likely contributes significantly to its activity. Clearance is delayed in the presence of hepatic dysfunction, and at least a 50% initial reduction in dose should be considered in patients with abnormal serum bilirubin levels.

The recommended dosage for **idarubicin** (idamycin) is 12 mg/m^2 daily for 3 days by intravenous injection in combination with cytarabine. Slow injection with care over 10 to 15 minutes is recommended to avoid extravasation, as with other anthracyclines.

Daunorubicin—therapeutic uses: Daunorubicin (daunomycin, rubidomycin, cerubidine, others) is available for intravenous use. The recommended dosage is 30 to 60 mg/m^2 daily for 3 days. The agent is administered with appropriate care to prevent extravasation, because severe local vesicant action may result. Total doses of greater than 1000 mg/m^2 are associated with a high risk of cardiotoxicity. A daunorubicin citrate liposomal product (Daunoxome) is indicated for the treatment of AIDS-related Kaposi's sarcoma. It is given in a dose of 40 mg/m^2 infused over 60 minutes and repeated every 2 weeks. Patients should be advised that the drug may impart a red color to the urine.

Daunorubicin is primarily used in the treatment of AML in combination with Ara-C and has largely been replaced by idarubicin.

The toxic manifestations of daunorubicin as well as idarubicin include bone marrow depression, stomatitis. alopecia, GI disturbances, and dermatological manifestations. Cardiac toxicity is a peculiar adverse effect observed with these agents. It is characterized by tachycardia, arrhythmias, dyspnea, hypotension, pericardial effusion, and CHF that is poorly responsive to digitalis.

Therapeutic uses—**doxorubicin** (Adriamycin, others) is available for intravenous use. The recommended dose is 50 to 75 mg/m^2, administered as a single rapid intravenous infusion repeated after 21 days. Care should be taken to avoid extravasation as severe local vesicant action and tissue necrosis may result. A **doxorubicin** liposomal product (Doxil) is available for treatment of AIDS-related Kaposi's sarcoma and is given intravenously in a dose of 20 mg/m^2 over 30 minutes and repeated every 3 weeks.

Newer analogs of **doxorubicin**: Valrubicin (Valstar) was approved in 1998 for intravesical therapy of bacille Calmette-Guérin-refractory urinary bladder carcinoma *in situ* in patients for whom immediate cystectomy would be associated with unacceptable morbidity or mortality. **Epirubicin** (4′-epidoxorubicin, Ellence) was approved by the PDA in 1999 as a component of adjuvant therapy following resection of early lymph-node-positive breast cancer.

A related anthracenedione, mitoxantrone, has been approved for use in AML. Mitoxantrone has limited ability to produce quinone-type free radicals and causes less cardiac toxicity than does doxorubicin. It produces acute myelosuppression, cardiac toxicity, and mucositis as its major toxicities; the drug causes less nausea and vomiting and alopecia than does doxorubicin. It is also used as a component of experimental high-dose chemotherapy regimens, with uncertain efficacy.

Mitoxantrone (Novantrone) is supplied for intravenous infusion. To induce remission in acute nonlymphocytic leukemia in adults, the drug is given in a daily dose of 12 mg/m^2 for 3 days as a component of a regimen that also includes cytosine arabinoside. Mitoxantrone also is used in advanced hormone-resistant prostate cancer in a dose of 12 to 14 mg/m^2 every 21 days. Mitoxantrone has been approved by the FDA for the treatment of late-stage, secondary progressive multiple sclerosis.

DOXYCYCLINE

(Adoxa tablets 50 mg)

Doxycycline is an antimalarial preparation/mouth-and-throat product/tetracycline. It inhibits bacterial protein synthesis and is indicated in treatment of infections caused by susceptible strains of Gram-positive and Gram-negative bacteria (e.g., *Rickettsia, M. pneumoniae*); trachoma and susceptible infections when penicillins are contraindicated; acute intestinal amebiasis; uncomplicated gonorrhea in adults; prophylaxis of malaria caused by *Plasmodium falciparum*; anthrax (including inhalational anthrax); and severe acne. Periodontitis: use for tablet–adjunct treatment to scaling and root planing to promote attachment-level gain and reduce pocket depth. Subgingival injection: use for chronic adult periodontitis for a gain in clinical attachment, reduction in probing depth, and reduction in bleeding on probing.

DOXYCYCLINE HYCLATE

(Vibramycin)

Doxycycline is indicated in gonorrhea in patients allergic to penicillin; primary or secondary syphilis in patients allergic to penicillin; *Chlamydia trachomatis*, nongonococcal urethritis, and uncomplicated urethral, endocervical, or rectal infections and prophylaxis for rape victims; and in prevention of "traveler's diarrhea," commonly caused by enterotoxigenic *E. coli*. Doxycycline, which is absorbed well (90 to 100%), has the least affinity to calcium, and hence its absorption is not altered by milk products. Doxycycline is excreted primarily unchanged by the kidneys, and its half-life is prolonged in renal impairment. Doxycycline is contraindicated in pregnancy, and in young children because it discolors teeth permanently. When doxycycline is used with digoxin or oral anticoagulant, the dosage for digoxin and anticoagulant should be reduced (see also Table 21 and Figures 84 and 103).

DROLOXIFENE

The new antiestrogen droloxifene has a 10- to 60-fold higher binding affinity to the estrogen receptor compared to the related compound tamoxifen. A similar relationship was found in growth inhibition studies, which showed that droloxifene inhibited human breast cancer cells more effectively than tamoxifen, predominantly in drug concentrations that are found in humans during therapy. Therefore, it can be assumed that droloxifene may represent an important step forward in the treatment of mammary carcinomas in women through its better tolerability and increased efficacy compared with tamoxifen. For long-term adjuvant or preventative treatment of breast cancer, droloxifene may well be the safer choice (see also Figures 36 and 48).

DRONABINOL

(Marinol) (THC)

Dronabinol is a cannabinoid with antiemetic effects and is used in a dosage of 5 mg/m^2 p.o. 1 to 3 hours prior to administration of antineoplastic agents. Dronabinol is excreted primarily in feces via the biliary tract. Dronabinol may cause euphoria, drowsiness, altered thinking, hallucination, confusion, and impaired coordination (see also Figures 73 and 81). In addition, dronabinol is used to stimulate appetite in anorexia associated with AIDS-related weight loss.

DRONABINOL

(Marinol capsules)

Dronabinol is an antiemetic/antivertigo agent, which is indicated in the control of chemotherapy-induced nausea and vomiting unresponsive to other antiemetics; and appetite stimulation in AIDS cachexia.

Dronabinol (delta-9-tetrahydrocannabinol; marinol) is a naturally occurring cannabinoid that can be synthesized chemically or extracted from the marijuana plant, *Cannabis sativa*. The exact mechanism of the antiemetic action of dronabinol is unknown but probably relates to stimulation of the cannabinoid, the subtype of cannabinoid receptors on neurons in and around the vomiting center. **Dronabinol** is a highly lipid-soluble compound that is absorbed readily after oral administration; its onset of action occurs within an hour, and peak levels are achieved within 2 to 4 hours. It undergoes extensive first-pass metabolism with limited systemic bioavailability after single doses (only 10 to 20%). Active and inactive metabolites are formed in the liver; the principal active metabolite is 11-OH-delta-9-tetrahydrocannabinol. These metabolites are excreted primarily via the biliary-fecal route, with only 10 to 15% excreted in the urine. Both dronabinol and its metabolites are highly bound (>95%) to plasma proteins. Because of its large volume of distribution a single dose of dronabinol can result in detectable levels of metabolites for several weeks.

Dronabinol is a useful prophylactic agent in patients receiving cancer chemotherapy when other antiemetic medications are not effective. It can also stimulate appetite and has been used in patients with AIDS and anorexia. As an antiemetic agent, it is administered at an initial dose of 5 mg/m^2 given 1 to 3 hours before chemotherapy and then every 2 to 4 hours afterward for a total of four to six doses. If this is not adequate, incremental increases in dose can be made up to a maximum of 15 mg/m^2. For other indications, the usual starting dose is 2.5 mg twice a day; this can be titrated up to 20 mg a day.

Dronabinol has complex effects on the CNS, including a prominent central sympathomimetic activity. This can lead to palpitations, tachycardia, vasodilation, hypotension, and conjunctival injection (bloodshot eyes). Patient supervision is necessary because marijuana-like "highs" (e.g., euphoria, somnolence, detachment, dizziness, anxiety, nervousness, panic, etc.) can occur, as can more disturbing effects such as paranoid reactions and thinking abnormalities. After abrupt withdrawal of dronabinol, an abstinence syndrome manifested by irritability, insomnia, and restlessness can occur. Because of its high affinity for plasma proteins, dronabinol can displace other plasma-protein-bound drugs, whose doses may have to be adjusted as a consequence. Dronabinol should be prescribed with great caution to persons with a history of substance abuse (alcohol and drugs) because it also may be abused by these patients.

DROPERIDOL

(Inapsine)

Droperidol is used as an adjunct for induction and maintenance of general anesthesia and as an anesthetic in diagnostic procedures. Droperidol, which has antiemetic properties, causes marked sedation and potentiates the CNS depressant effects of alcohol, hypnotic–sedatives, and numerous psychoactive agents. Droperidol is absorbed well through an IM injection—sedation begins in 3 minutes, peaks at 30 minutes, and lasts for 2 to 4 hours. Droperidol is metabolized by the liver to *p*-fluoro-phenylacetic acid and *p*-hydroxypiperidine, and its metabolites are excreted in urine and feces.

DROTRECOGIN ALFA (ACTIVATED)

(Xigris powder for infusion, lyophilized 5 mg, powder for infusion, lyophilized 20 mg)

Drotrecogin is a recombinant human activated protein C that exerts an antithrombotic effect by inhibiting factor Va and factor VIIIa. It is indicated in the reduction of mortality in adult patients with severe sepsis who have a high risk of death. **Drotrecogin alfa**: Drotrecogin alfa (Xigris) is a recombinant form of human activated protein C that inhibits coagulation by proteolytic inactivation of factor Va and factor VIIIa. It also has antiinflammatory effects. A 96-hour continuous infusion of drotrecogin alfa decreases mortality in adult patients who are at high risk of death from severe sepsis if given within 48 hours of the onset of organ dysfunction (e.g., shock, hypoxemia, and oliguria). The major adverse effect is bleeding.

DULOXETINE HYDROCHLORIDE

(Cymbalta capsule 22.4 mg)

Duloxetine is a serotonin and norepinephrine reuptake inhibitor, which causes potentiation of serotonergic and noradrenergic activity in the CNS. It is used in depression. In addition to the wide use of modern antidepressants to treat depression associated with general medical illnesses, several psychosomatic disorders may respond at least partly to treatment with tricyclic antidepressants, MAO (monoamine oxidase) inhibitors, or SSRIs (selective serotonin reuptake inhibitors). These include chronic pain disorders, such as diabetic and other peripheral neuropathic syndromes (for which tertiary-amine tricyclics probably are superior to fluoxetine and both **duloxetine** and **venlafaxine** also may be effective), fibromyalgia, peptic ulcer and irritable bowel syndrome, hot flashes of menopause, chronic fatigue, cataplexy, tics, migraine, and sleep apnea. These disorders may have some psychobiological relationship to mood or anxiety disorders.

DUTASTERIDE

(Avodart capsules 0.5 mg)

Dutasteride is an androgen hormone inhibitor, which inhibits the conversion of testosterone to 5-alpha-dihydrotestosterone, a potent androgen. It is indicated in treatment of symptomatic benign prostatic hyperplasia (BPH) in men with an enlarged prostate.

Benign prostatic hyperplasia: BPH produces symptomatic urethral obstruction in a significant percentage of older men, leading to weak stream, urinary frequency, and nocturia. These symptoms are due to a combination of mechanical pressure on the urethra due to the increase in smooth-muscle mass and the α_1-receptor-mediated increase in smooth-muscle tone in the prostate and neck of the bladder. Alpha$_1$-receptors in the trigone muscle of the bladder and urethra contribute to the resistance to outflow of urine. **Prazosin** reduces this resistance in some patients with impaired bladder emptying caused by prostatic obstruction or parasympathetic decentralization from spinal injury. The efficacy and importance of α-receptor antagonists in the medical treatment of BPH have been demonstrated in multiple controlled clinical trials. Transurethral resection of the prostate is the accepted surgical treatment for symptoms of urinary obstruction in men with BPH; however, there are some serious potential complications (e.g., risk of impotence), and improvement may not be permanent. Other less invasive procedures also are available. Medical therapy has utilized α-receptor antagonists for many years. Finasteride (Propecia) and **dutasteride** (Avodart), two drugs that inhibit conversion of testosterone to dihydrotestosterone and can reduce prostate volume in some patients, are approved for this indication. However, the overall efficacy appears less than that observed with α_1-receptor antagonists. **Finasteride** (Proscar) is an antagonist of 5α-reductase, especially type II; **dutasteride** (Avodart) is an antagonist of types I and II; both drugs block the conversion of testosterone to dihydrotestosterone, especially in the male external genitalia. These agents were developed to treat BPH and are approved in the United States and many other countries for this purpose. When they are administered to men with moderately severe symptoms due to obstruction of urinary tract outflow, serum and prostatic concentrations of dihydrotestosterone decrease, prostatic volume decreases, and urine flow rate increases. Impotence is a well-documented, albeit infrequent, side effect of this use, although the mechanism is not understood. Finasteride also is approved for use in the treatment of male pattern baldness under the trade name **Propecia**, even though that effect is presumably mediated via type I 5α-reductase. Finasteride appears to be as effective as flutamide and the combination of estrogen and cyproterone in the treatment of **hirsutism**.

DUODENAL ULCERS: Treatment of Histamine$_2$ (H_2) Receptor Antagonists

Cimetidine	Nizatidine
Famotidine	Ranitidine

Proton-Pump Inhibitors

Omeprazole

Aluminum Hydroxide Complex of Sucrose-Enhancing Mucosal Defense Mechanism

Sucralfate

Prostaglandin Analog

Misoprostol

Antacids

Aluminum hydroxide
Magnesium hydroxide
Simethicone antacids

DYCLONINE HYDROCHLORIDE

(Dyclone, Sucrets)

Dyclonine, a topical local anesthetic, is indicated in the relief of pain and itching from minor burns, insect bites, or irritations, or episiotomy or anogenital lesion; and in anesthetizing mucous membranes before endoscopic procedures such as laryngoscopy and bronchoscopy, or endotracheal procedures. For example, for bronchoscopy, dyclonine (1% solution) is sprayed into the larynx and trachea every 5 minutes until laryngeal reflex is abolished. Dyclonine blocks conduction of impulses at the sensory nerve endings by altering cell membrane permeability to ionic transfer.

DYPHYLLINE

(Dylline)

Dyphylline (200 to 800 mg p.o. every 6 hours) is indicated in the relief of acute and chronic bronchial asthma and reversible bronchospasm associated with chronic bronchitis and emphysema. It should be used cautiously in patients with compromised cardiac or circulatory function, diabetes, glaucoma, hypertension, hyperthyroidism, peptic ulcer, or gastroesophageal reflux, because the drug may worsen these symptoms or conditions. Sympathomimetic agents act synergistically with dyphylline, and probenecid enhances the half-life of dyphylline by blocking its renal tubular secretion (see also Figure 94).

DYPHYLLINE
(Lufyllin tablets 200 mg)

Dyphylline is a xanthine derivative related to **theophylline**. It relaxes bronchial smooth muscle and stimulates central respiratory drive. It is indicated in the relief of acute bronchial asthma and reversible bronchospasm associated with chronic bronchitis and emphysema. A large number of derivatives of the methylxanthines have been prepared and examined for their ability to inhibit cyclic nucleotide phosphodiesterases (PDEs) and antagonize receptor-mediated actions of adenosine, the two best characterized cellular actions of the methylxanthines. Although certain modifications dissociate these two activities to some degree, these compounds are not used therapeutically.

Dyphylline [l,3-dimethyl-7-(2′,3-dihydroxypropyl)xanthine] and theophylline inhibit cyclic nucletide PDEs, thereby preventing breakdown of cyclic AMP and cyclic GMP to 5′-AMP and 5′-GMP, respectively. Inhibition of PDEs will lead to an accumulation of cAMP and cGMP, thereby increasing signal transduction through these pathways. The cyclic nucleotide PDEs are members of a superfamily of genetically distinct enzymes. Theophylline and related methylxanthines are relatively nonselective in the PDE subtypes they inhibit.

Cyclic nucleotide production is regulated by endogenous receptor–ligand interactions leading to activation of adenylyl cyclase and guanylyl cyclase. Inhibitors of PDEs therefore can be thought of as drugs that enhance the activity of endogenous autacoids, hormones, and neurotransmitters that signal via cyclic nucleotide messengers. This may explain why the *in vivo* potency often exceeds that observed *in vitro*.

Theophylline is a competitive antagonist at adenosine receptors. Adenosine can act as an autacoid and transmitter with myriad biological actions. Of particular relevance to asthma are the observations that adenosine can cause bronchoconstriction in asthmatics and potentiate immunologically induced mediator release from human-lung mast cells. Inhibition of the actions of adenosine therefore also must be considered when attempting to explain the mechanism of action of theophylline.

Theophylline may also owe part of its antiinflammatory action to its ability to activate histone deacetylases in the nucleus. In theory, the deacetylation of histones could decrease the transcription of several proinflammatory genes and potentiate the effect of corticosteroids.

Dyphylline and theophylline effectively relax airway smooth muscle; this bronchodilation likely contributes to their acute therapeutic efficacy in asthma. Both adenosine receptor antagonism and PDE inhibition are likely involved in the bronchodilating effect of theophylline. Adenosine does not contract isolated human bronchial smooth muscle directly, but when it is inhaled, it acts as a potent bronchoconstrictor in asthmatic subjects. Therefore, inhibition of this function of adenosine may contribute to theophylline-induced bronchodilation in some asthmatic subjects. Inhibition of PDE4 and PDE5 effectively relaxes human isolated bronchial smooth muscle. It thus seems likely that inhibition of PDEs also contributes to the bronchodilating effect of theophylline. Studies with the related methylxanthine **enprofylline** (3-propylxanthine), which has been investigated extensively for treatment of asthma in Europe, also support a mechanistic role for PDE inhibition in the bronchodilator actions of theophylline. Enprofylline is more potent than theophylline as a bronchodilator but is much less potent in inhibiting most types of adenosine receptors. The latter point, however, must be interpreted cautiously. Activation of the A_{2B} subtypes of adenosine receptor causes several proinflammatory effects, and both theophylline and enprofylline are potent competitive antagonists of A_{2B} adenosine receptors.

Theophylline also inhibits synthesis and secretion of inflammatory mediators from numerous cell types, including mast cells and basophils. This effect of theophylline is likely due to PDE inhibition and can be mimicked in large part with drugs that selectively inhibit PDE4 isozyme. At therapeutic concentrations, the antiinflammatory effect of theophylline may be more relevant to the drug's therapeutic actions than direct bronchodilation, but this remains unproven.

Consistent with an important role of PDE4 in obstructive lung disease, selective PDE4 inhibitors have been evaluated in clinical trials for the treatment of asthma and COPD. In one study, **cilomilast** (Ariflo, 15 mg twice daily for 10 weeks) decreased inflammatory cell infiltration significantly in bronchial biopsies of patients with COPD. Further studies are needed to define the role of PDE4 inhibitors in asthma and COPD, but these drugs are promising candidates for new approaches to asthma therapy.

Theophylline, a methylxanthine, is among the least expensive drugs used to treat asthma, and consequently, it remains a commonly used drug for this indication in many countries. In industrialized countries, the advent of inhaled glucocorticoids, β-adrenergic-receptor agonists, and leukotriene- modifying drugs has diminished theophylline use significantly, and it has been relegated to a third- or fourth-line treatment in patients whose asthma is otherwise difficult to control.

E

EBASTINE

Histamine$_1$ (H_1) receptors mediate such actions as bronchoconstriction and the contraction of smooth muscles in the gastrointestinal tract. Ebastine is a histamine$_1$-receptor blocker. Terfenadine, astemizole, loratadine, and certirizine are second-generation antihistamine agents that are relatively nonsedating. Other H_1-receptor antagonists currently undergoing clinical trials are azelastine, ebastine, and levocabastine (see also Figures 34 and 59).

ECHOTHIOPHATE IODIDE

(Phospholine Iodide powder for reconstitution 6.25 mg to make 0.125%)

Echothiophate is a cholinesterase inhibitor that causes miosis, increase in facility of outflow of aqueous humor, a fall in IOP, and potentiation of accommodation by enhancing the effect of endogenously liberated acetylcholine in the iris, ciliary muscle, and other parasympathetic innervated structures of the eye. It is indicated in the treatment of chronic open-angle glaucoma; and treatment of accommodative esotropia (see also Figure 12).

ECONAZOLE NITRATE

(Spectazole cream 1%)

Econazole nitrate is a topical/antifungal agent. It increases cell membrane permeability in susceptible fungi. It is indicated in the treatment of tinea pedis (athlete's foot), tinea cruris (jock itch), tinea corporis (ringworm), cutaneous candidiasis, and tinea versicolor. **Econazole** is the deschloro derivative of **miconazole**. Econazole readily penetrates the stratum corneum and is found in effective concentrations down to the mid-dermis. However, less than 1% of an applied dose appears to be absorbed into the blood. Approximately 3% of recipients have local erythema, burning, stinging, or itching. Econazole nitrate (Spectazole, others) is available as a water-miscible cream (1%) to be applied twice a day.

Miconazole, a very close chemical congener of econazole, readily penetrates the stratum corneum of the skin, and persists there for more than 4 days after application. Less than 1% is absorbed into the blood. Absorption is no more than 1.3% from the vagina.

Adverse effects from topical application to the vagina include burning, itching, or irritation in 7% of recipients and, infrequently, pelvic cramps (0.2%), headache, hives, or skin rash. Irritation, burning, and maceration are rare after cutaneous application. Miconazole is considered safe for use during pregnancy, although some authors recommend avoiding its vaginal use during the first trimester. Miconazole nitrate is available as a dermatologic ointment, cream, solution, spray, or powder (Micatin, Monistat-derm, others). To avoid maceration, only the lotion should be applied to intertriginous areas. It is available as a 2% and 4% vaginal cream, and as 100-mg, 200-mg, or 1200-mg vaginal suppositories (Monistat 7, Monistat 3, others), to be applied high in the vagina at bedtime for 7, 3, or 1 (days), respectively.

In the treatment of tinea pedis, tinea cruris, and tinea versicolor the cure rate may be over 90%. In the treatment of vulvovaginal candidiasis, the mycologic cure rate at the end of 1 month is about 80 to 95%. Pruritus sometimes is relieved after a single application. Some vaginal infections caused by *Candida glabrata* also respond.

Terconazole and **butoconazole:** Terconazole is a ketal triazole with structural similarities to ketoconazole. The mechanism of action of terconazole is similar to that of the imidazoles. The 80-mg vaginal suppository is inserted at bedtime for 3 days, whereas the 0.4% vaginal cream is used for 7 days, and the 0.8% cream for 3 days. Clinical efficacy and patient acceptance of both preparations are at least as good as for clotrimazole in patients with vaginal candidiasis. **Butoconazole** is an imidazole that is pharmacologically quite comparable to clotrimazole.

Butoconazole nitrate (Mycelex 3, others) is available as a 2% vaginal cream; it is used at bedtime in nonpregnant females.

Fungal infections are among the most common causes of skin disease in the United States, and numerous effective topical and oral antifungal agents have been developed. Griseofulvin, topical and oral imidazoles, triazoles, and allylamines are the most effective agents available

The azoles **miconazole** (Micatin, others) and **econazole** (Spectrazole, others) and the allylamines **naftifine** (Naftin) and **terbinafine** (Lamisil, others) are effective topical agents for the treatment of localized tinea corporis and uncomplicated tinea pedis. Topical therapy with the azoles is preferred for localized cutaneous candidiasis and tinea versicolor.

Systemic therapy is necessary for the treatment of tinea capitis. Oral griseofulvin (fulvicin V/F, P/G, others) has been the traditional medication for treatment of tinea capitis. Oral terbinafine is a safe and effective alternative to griseofulvin in treating tinea capitis in children.

Topical therapy with the azoles and allylamines is effective for tinea pedis. Macerated toe web disease may require the addition of antibacterial therapy. **Econazole nitrate**, which has a limited antibacterial spectrum, can be useful in this situation. Systemic therapy with **griseofulvin**, **terbinafine**, or **itraconazole** (Sporanox, others) is used for more extensive tinea pedis. It should be recognized that long-term topical therapy may be necessary in some patients after courses of systemic antifungal therapy.

Onychomycosis: Fungal infection of the nails is caused most frequently by dermatophytes and *Candida*. Mixed infections are common. The nail must be cultured or clipped for histological examination before initiating therapy because up to a third of dystrophic nails that appear clinically to be onychomycosis are actually due to psoriasis or other conditions.

Systemic therapy is necessary for effective management of onychomycosis. Treatment of onychomycosis of toenails with **griseofulvin** for 12 to 18 months produces a cure rate of 50% and a relapse rate of 50% after 1 year. Terbinafine and itraconazole offer significant potential advantages. They quickly produce high drug levels in the nail, which persist after therapy is discontinued. Additional advantages include a broader spectrum of coverage with **itraconazole** and few drug interactions with **terbinafine**. Treatment of toenail onychomycosis requires 3 months with terbinafine (250 mg/day) or itraconazole (pulsed dosing 1 week per month for 3 months). Cure rates of 75% or greater have been achieved with both drugs.

Ciclopirox topical (Penlac) solution is a nail lacquer that is PDA approved for the treatment of onychomycosis but demonstrates low complete cure rates.

EDETATE CALCIUM DISODIUM

(Calcium EDTA) (Calcium Disodium Versenate)

Edetate calcium disodium, a metal-chelating agent, is indicated in the treatment of symptomatic lead poisoning without encephalopathy and blood lead concentrations less than 100 mcg/dL, or in the treatment of severe lead poisoning with symptoms of encephalopathy and/or blood lead concentrations greater than 100 mcg/dL.

EDETATE DISODIUM

(EDTA) (Chealamide, Disotate, Endrate)

Edetate disodium, a heavy metal antagonist, is indicated in hypercalcemia (500 mg/kg daily by slow IV infusion) and in digitalis-induced cardiac arrhythmias (15 mg/kg/hour by IV infusion). Ethylenediaminetetraacetic acid (EDTA) will lower serum levels of calcium, magnesium, and zinc. It should not be used in anuria, and renal excretory functions (BUN and creatinine) should be monitored carefully. EDTA should be used cautiously in hypokalemia and in patients with limited cardiac reserve.

EDTA, its sodium salt (edetate disodium, Na_2EDTA), and a number of closely related compounds chelate many divalent and trivalent metals. The cation used to make a water-soluble salt of EDTA has an important role in the toxicity of the chelator. Na_2EDTA causes hypocalcemic tetany. However, **edetate calcium disodium** ($CaNa_2EDTA$) can be used for treatment of poisoning by metals that have higher affinity for the chelating agent than does Ca^{2+}.

The pharmacological effects of $CaNa_2EDTA$ result from formation of chelates with divalent and trivalent metals in the body. Accessible metal ions (both exogenous and endogenous) with a higher affinity for $CaNa_2EDTA$ than Ca_{2+} will be chelated, mobilized, and usually excreted. Because EDTA is charged at physiological pH, it does not significantly penetrate cells; its volume of distribution approximates extracellular fluid space. Experimental studies in mice have shown that administration of $CaNa_2EDTA$ mobilizes several endogenous metallic cations, including those of zinc, manganese, and iron. The main therapeutic use of $CaNa_2EDTA$ is in the treatment of metal intoxications, especially lead intoxication.

$CaNa_2EDTA$ is available as edetate calcium disodium (calcium disodium versenate). Intramuscular administration of $CaNa_2EDTA$ results in good absorption, but pain occurs at the injection site; consequently, the chelator injection often is mixed with a local anesthetic or administered intravenously. For intravenous use, $CaNa_2EDTA$ is diluted in either 5% dextrose or 0.9% saline and is administered slowly by intravenous drip. A dilute solution is necessary to avoid thrombophlebitis. To minimize nephrotoxicity, adequate urine production should be established prior to and during treatment with $CaNa_2EDTA$. However, in patients with lead encephalopathy and increased intracranial pressure, excess fluids must be avoided. In such cases, conservative replacement of fluid is advised, and intramuscular administration of $CaNa_2EDTA$ is recommended.

The successful use of $CaNa_2EDTA$ in the treatment of **lead poisoning** is due, in part, to the capacity of lead to displace calcium from the chelate. Enhanced mobilization and excretion of lead indicate that the metal is accessible to **EDTA**. Bone provides the primary source of lead that is chelated by $CaNa_2EDTA$. After such chelation, lead is redistributed from soft tissues to the skeleton.

Mercury poisoning, by contrast, does not respond to the drug although mercury displaces calcium from $CaNa_2EDTA$ *in vitro*. Mercury is unavailable to the chelate perhaps because it is too tightly bound by sulfhydryl groups or sequestered in body compartments that are not penetrated by $CaNa_2EDTA$.

Corneal band keratopathy: **Edetate disodium** (disodium EDTA; Endrate) is a chelating agent that can be used to remove a band keratopathy (i.e., a calcium deposit at the level of Bowman's membrane on the cornea). After the overlying corneal epithelium is removed, it is applied topically to chelate the calcium deposits from the cornea.

EDROPHONIUM CHLORIDE

(Enlon injection 10 mg/mL)

Edrophonium is an anticholinesterase muscle stimulant that facilitates myoneural junction impulse transmission by inhibiting acetylcholine destruction by cholinesterase. It is indicated in differential diagnosis of myasthenia gravis; as an adjunct in evaluating treatment of myasthenia gravis; in evaluation of emergency treatment of myasthenic crises; in reversal of neuromuscular blockade by curare gallamine or tubo-curarine; and in treatment of respiratory depression caused by curare overdose.

Current use of anti-AChE agents is limited to four conditions in the periphery: atony of the smooth muscle of the intestinal tract and urinary bladder, glaucoma, myasthenia gravis, and reversal of the paralysis of competitive neuromuscular blocking drugs. Long-acting and hydrophobic

ChE inhibitors are the only inhibitors with well-documented efficacy, albeit limited, in the treatment of dementia symptoms of Alzheimer's disease. Physostigmine, with its shorter duration of action, is useful in the treatment of intoxication by atropine and several drugs with anticholinergic side effects; it also is indicated for the treatment of Friedreich's or other inherited ataxias. **Edrophonium** has been used for terminating attacks of paroxysmal supraventricular tachycardia.

Edrophonium chloride, a cholinesterase inhibitor (10 mg IV given over 30 to 45 seconds), may be used as a curare antagonist (to reverse neuromuscular blocking action), and for reversal of nondepolarizing muscle relaxants (see also Figures 17 and 79).

EFALIZUMAB

(Raptiva powder for injection)

Efalizumab is an immunosuppressive agent that inhibits binding of leukocyte function antigen-1 to intercellular adhesion molecule-1, thereby interfering with the adhesion of leukocytes to other cell types. Efalizumab is indicated in the treatment of chronic moderate to severe plaque psoriasis in adult patients who are candidates for systemic therapy or phototherapy. **Efalizumab** (Raptiva) is a humanized monoclonal antibody against the CD11a molecule of LFA-1. By binding to CD11a on T-cells, **efalizumab** prevents binding of LFA-1 to intercellular adhesion molecule 1 (ICAM-1) on the surface of antigen-presenting cells, vascular endothelial cells, and cells in the dermis and epidermis, thereby interfering with T-cell activation and migration and cytotoxic T-cell function. **Efalizumab** is FDA approved for the treatment of moderate to severe psoriasis in patients who are candidates for systemic therapy.

Etanercept (Enbrel) is FDA approved for the treatment of psoriasis, psoriatic arthritis, rheumatoid arthritis, juvenile rheumatoid arthritis, and ankylosing spondylitis. Etanercept is a soluble, recombinant, fully human tumor necrosis factor (TNF) receptor fusion protein consisting of two molecules of the ligand-binding portion of the TNF receptor fused to the Fc portion of IgGl. As a dimeric molecule, it can bind two molecules of TNF. Etanercept binds soluble and membrane-bound TNF, thereby inhibiting the action of TNF.

Infliximab (Remicade) is a mouse–human chimeric monoclonal antibody that binds to soluble and membrane-bound TNF-α and inhibits binding with its receptors. Infliximab is a complement-fixing antibody that induces complement-dependent and cell-mediated lysis when bound to cell-surface-bound TNF-α. It also induces proinflammatory cytokines, such as IL-1 and IL-6, and enhances leukocyte migration. Infliximab is FDA approved for the treatment of Crohn's disease and rheumatoid arthritis, but it is also in phase trials for the treatment of psoriasis.

EFAVIRENZ

(Sustiva capsules 50 mg)

Efavirenz is a nonnucleoside reverse transcriptase inhibitor that causes noncompetitive inhibition of HIV-1 reverse transcriptase. It is indicated in the treatment of HIV-1 infection in combination with other antiretroviral agents. Efavirenz is a 1,4-dihydro-2H-3,1-benzoxazin-2-one NNRTI with potent activity against HIV-1. The *in vitro* IC_{50} of this drug ranges from 3 to 9 nM. Like other compounds in this class, **efavirenz** does not have significant activity against HTV-2 or other retroviruses.

Efavirenz is a noncompetitive inhibitor that binds to a site on the HIV-1 reverse transcriptase that is distant from the active site, thus inducing a conformational change that disrupts catalytic activity. Because the target site is HIV-1-specific and is not essential for the enzyme, resistance can develop rapidly. The most common resistance mutation seen clinically is at codon 103 of reverse transcriptase (K103N), and this decreases susceptibility up to one-hundredfold or greater. Additional resistance mutations have been seen at codons 100, 106, 108, 181, 188, 190, and 225, but either the K103N or Y181C mutation is sufficient to produce clinical treatment failure. Cross-resistance extends to all PDA-approved NNRTIs.

Efavirenz is well absorbed from the gastrointestinal tract and reaches peak plasma concentrations within 5 hours. There is diminished absorption of the drug with increasing doses. Bioavailability (AUC) is increased by 22% with a high-fat meal. Efavirenz is more than 99% bound to plasma proteins and, as a consequence, has a low CSF-plasma ratio of 0.01. The clinical significance of this low CNS penetration is unclear, especially because the major toxicities of efavirenz involve the CNS. It is recommended that the drug be taken initially on an empty stomach at bedtime to reduce side effects.

Efavirenz is cleared via oxidative metabolism, mainly by CYP2B6 and, to a lesser extent, by CYP3A4. The parent drug is not excreted renally to a significant degree. Efavirenz is cleared slowly, with an elimination half-life of 40 to 55 hours at steady state. This safely allows once-daily dosing.

Rash occurs frequently with **efavirenz**, in up to 27% of adult patients. It usually occurs within the first few weeks of treatment and rarely requires drug discontinuation. Life-threatening skin eruptions, such as **Stevens–Johnson syndrome**, have been reported during postmarketing experience with efavirenz but are rare.

The most important adverse effects of efavirenz involve the CNS. Up to 53% of patients report some CNS or psychiatric side effects, but fewer than 5% discontinue the drug for this reason. CNS symptoms may occur with the first dose and may last for hours. More severe symptoms may require weeks to resolve. Patients commonly report dizziness, impaired concentration, dysphoria, vivid or disturbing dreams, and insomnia. Episodes of frank psychosis (depression, hallucinations, and/or mania) have been associated with initiating efavirenz. Fortunately, CNS side effects generally become more tolerable and resolve within the first 4 weeks of therapy.

Other side effects reported with efavirenz include headache, increased hepatic transaminases, and elevated serum cholesterol. False-positive urine screening tests for marijuana metabolites also can occur depending on the assay used.

Efavirenz is the only antiretroviral drug that is unequivocally teratogenic in primates. When efavirenz was administered to pregnant cynomolgus monkeys, 25% of fetuses developed malformations. In six cases where women were exposed to efavirenz during the first trimester of pregnancy, fetuses or infants had significant malformations, mainly of the brain and spinal cord. Women of child-bearing potential, therefore, should use two methods of birth control and avoid pregnancy while taking efavirenz.

Efavirenz is a moderate inducer of hepatic enzymes, especially CYP3A4. It undergoes limited auto-induction, but because of its long half-life, there is no need to alter drug dose during the first few weeks of treatment. It decreases concentrations of phenobarbital, phenytoin, and carbamazepine; the methadone AUC is reduced by 33 to 66% at steady state. Rifampin concentrations are unchanged by concurrent efavirenz use, but rifampin may reduce efavirenz concentrations. Efavirenz reduces the rifabutin AUC by 38% on average. **Efavirenz** has a variable effect on HIV protease inhibitors. Indinavir, saquinavir, and amprenavir concentrations are reduced, but ritonavir and nelfinavir concentrations are increased. Drugs that induce CYP2B6 or CYP3A4 (e.g., **phenobarbital**, **phenytoin**, and **carbamazepine**) would be expected to increase the clearance of efavirenz, and should be avoided.

Efavirenz was the first antiretroviral agent approved by the FDA for once-daily administration. Initial short-term monotherapy studies showed substantial decreases in plasma HIV RNA, but the drug should only be used in combination with other effective agents, and should not be added as the sole new agent to a failing regimen. In antiretroviral-naïve patients receiving efavirenz, zidovudine, and lamivudine, 70% achieved undetectable plasma HIV-1 RNA compared with 48% of those receiving indinavir plus zidovudine and lamivudine. Much of this difference appeared to be the consequence of improved patient adherence to the efavirenz regimen. **Efavirenz** also has been used effectively in patients who have failed previous antiretroviral therapy in combination with other active drugs. In pediatric HIV infection, 60% of children failing prior therapy with a nucleoside reverse-transcriptase inhibitor had sustained virologic benefit after 48 weeks of treatment with efavirenz, nelfinavir, and a nucleoside analog.

Efavirenz is used widely in the developed world because of its convenience, effectiveness, and long-term tolerability. To date, no antiretroviral regimen has produced better long-term treatment responses than any efavirenz-containing regimen in randomized, prospective clinical trials. As a result, **efavirenz** plus two nucleoside reverse-transcriptase inhibitors was one of two regimens preferred in 2004 for treatment-naïve patients.

EFLORNITHINE HYDROCHLORIDE (DFM0) (Ornidyl)

Eflornithine, an ornithine decarboxylase inhibitor with antiprotozoal activity (100 mg/kg q. 6 hours), is used in the treatment of the meningoencephalitic stage of *Trypanosoma brucei gambiense* infection (sleeping sickness) and in treatment of *Pneumocystis carinii* pneumonia in AIDS patients.

ELECTROLYTES AND SKELETAL MUSCLE RELAXANTS

The generation of action potentials by muscle and nerve results from changes in the conductance of their membranes to sodium and potassium, and normal neuromuscular function depends on the maintenance of the correct ratio between intracellular and extracellular ionic concentrations. An acute decrease in the extracellular potassium concentration tends to elevate the end plate transmembrane potential, causing hyperpolarization together with a greater sensitivity to the nondepolarizing muscle relaxants. Conversely, an increased extracellular potassium concentration lowers the resting end plate transmembrane potential and thereby partially depolarizes the membrane, which should augment the effects of the depolarizing agents and oppose the action of the nondepolarizing drugs. Diuretic-induced chronic hypokalemia reduces the pancuronium requirements for neuromuscular blockade, and thus, more neostigmine is required to achieve antagonism. The release of acetylcholine from the motor nerve terminal is also affected by calcium and magnesium ion concentrations, which have opposing effects. Calcium increases the quantal release of the postjunctional membrane to transmitter and enhances the excitation–contraction coupling mechanisms of muscle. In contrast, magnesium decreases acetylcholine release and reduces the sensitivity of the postjunctional membrane to acetylcholine. Consequently, the action of the nondepolarizing muscle relaxants can be accentuated by low calcium and high magnesium levels. In addition, magnesium augments the block produced by depolarizing relaxants. Therefore, the dose of a muscle relaxant should be reduced in patients who have toxemia associated with pregnancy and are undergoing magnesium replacement therapy (see also Figures 32 and 99).

ELETRIPTAN HYDROBROMIDE (Relpax tablets 24.2 mg)

Eletriptan is a serotonin 5-HT_1-receptor agonist with selective agonist for the vascular serotonin (5-HT_1)-receptor subtype, causing vasoconstriction of cranial arteries. It is indicated in the acute treatment of migraine with or without aura.

EMEDASTINE

The most common symptoms of allergic conjunctivitis treated by ophthalmologists include ocular pruritis, erythema, edema, and tearing. The traditional drugs of choice to treat these symptoms of allergic conjunctivitis have been antihistamines alone or in combination with vasoconstrictors. Antihistamines currently employed in this area as topical solutions include pheniramine, antazoline, pyrilamine, and levocabastine. However, these drugs have some disadvantages such as low potency (antazoline), slow onset of action (levocabastine), short duration of action (antazoline, pyrilamine, pheniramine), discomfort/tolerance (ketotifen, levocabastine), and significant side effects (e.g., they can raise intraocular pressure and cause mydriasis and ocular dryness) due to other receptor-binding activities. Emedastine is a novel antihistaminic/antiallergic drug that potentially inhibits histamine-induced vascular permeability in the conjunctiva and blocks the allergic response in a model of passive conjunctival anaphylaxis. In addition, emedastine potently inhibits histamine-induced airway resistance and skin vascular permeability (see also Figure 39).

EMETICS

Ipecac is a mixture of the alcohol-soluble alkaloid that is obtained from the South American plant *Cephaelis ipecacuanha* and is used solely in the form of syrup of ipecac. Apomorphine hydrochloride and copper sulfate are also emetics. Syrup of ipecac and copper sulfate cause emesis by locally irritating the stomach, whereas apomorphine stimulates the chemoreceptor trigger zone for emesis located in the caudal portion of the fourth ventricle (area postrema), which in turn stimulates the vomiting center in the lateral reticular formation of the medulla (see also Figure 73).

EMLA

(Astra)

Emla is a topical anesthetic ointment containing a mixture of lidocaine (2 to 5%) and prilocaine (2 to 5%), which is useful in reducing the pain associated with venipuncture.

EMTRICITABINE/TENOFOVIR DISOPROXIL FUMARATE

(Truvada tablets 200 mg emtricitabine/300 mg tenofovir disoproxil fumarate disoproxil)

Emtricitabine is a nonnucleoside analog reverse-transcriptase inhibitor combination. **Emtricitabine**: inhibits activity of HIV-1 reverse transcriptase by competing with the natural substrate deoxycytidine 5-triphosphate and by being incorporated into nascent viral DNA, resulting in chain termination. **Tenofovir disoproxil fumarate**: is a prodrug of tenofovir that inhibits the activity of HIV-1 reverse transcriptase by competing with deoxyadenosine 5-triphosphate and by DNA chain termination after incorporation into DNA. The combination is indicated in the treatment of HIV-1 infection in combination with other antiretroviral agents.

Emtricitabine is a cytosine analog that is chemically related to **lamivudine** and shares many of that drug's pharmacodynamic properties. Like lamivudine, it has two chiral centers and is manufactured as the enantiomerically pure (2*R*,5*S*)-5-fluoro-l-[2-(hydroxymethyl)-l,3-oxathiolan-5-yl]cytosine (FTC). **Emtricitabine** is active against HIV-1, HIV-2, and HBV. The IC_{50} of emtricitabine against laboratory strains of HIV-1 ranges from 2 to 530 nM, although, on average, the drug is about 10 times more active *in vitro* than lamivudine.

Emtricitabine enters cells by passive diffusion and is phosphorylated by deoxycytidine kinase and cellular kinases to its active metabolite, **emtricitabine 5′-triphosphate**. The intracellular triphosphate acts as a competitive inhibitor of reverse transcriptase and is incorporated into HIV DNA to cause chain termination. Like lamivudine, emtricitabine has low affinity for human DNA polymerases, explaining its low toxicity to the host.

High-level resistance to **emtricitabine** occurs with the same mutation (methionine-to-valine substitution at codon 184) affecting lamivudine, although this appears to occur less frequently with emtricitabine. In three studies, M184V occurred about half as frequently with emtricitabine-containing regimens as with lamivudine, and patients presenting with virologic failure were two to three times as likely to have wild-type virus at the time of failure as compared with lamivudine. The M184V mutation restores zidovudine susceptibility to zidovudine-resistant HIV and also partially restores tenofovir susceptibility to tenofovir-resistant HIV harboring the K65R mutation. The same K65R mutation confers resistance to emtricitabine and the other cytosine analogs lamivudine and zalcitabine, as well as didanosine, stavudine, and abacavir.

Emtricitabine is absorbed rapidly and has an oral bioavailability of 93%. Food reduces the C_{max} but does not affect the AUC, and the drug can be taken without regard to meals. **Emtricitabine** is not bound significantly to plasma proteins. Compared with other nucleoside analogs, the drug has a slow systemic clearance and long elimination half-life of 8 to 10 hours. In addition, the estimated half-life of the intracellular triphosphate is very long, up to 39 hours in one report. This provides the pharmacokinetic rationale for once-daily dosing of this drug. Emtricitabine is excreted primarily unchanged in the urine, undergoing glomerular filtration and active tubular secretion.

Emtricitabine is one of the least toxic antiretroviral drugs and, like its chemical relative lamivudine, has few significant adverse effects and no effect on mitochondrial DNA *in vitro*. Prolonged exposure has been associated with hyperpigmentation of the skin, especially in sun-exposed areas. Elevated hepatic transaminases, hepatitis, and pancreatitis have been reported, but these have occurred in association with other drugs known to cause these toxicities. Because emtricitabine also has *in vitro* activity against HBV, caution is warranted in using this drug in patients coinfected with hepatitis B virus (HBV); discontinuation of lamivudine, which is closely related to emtricitabine, has been associated with a rebound of HBV replication and exacerbation of hepatitis.

Emtricitabine is not metabolized to a significant extent by CYPs, and it is not susceptible to any known metabolic drug interactions. The possibility of a pharmacokinetic interaction involving renal tubular secretion, such as that between trimethoprim and lamivudine, has not been investigated for emtricitabine, although the drug does not alter the pharmacokinetics of tenofovir.

Emtricitabine is PDA approved for treating HIV infection in adults in combination with other antiretroviral agents. Two small monotherapy trials showed that the maximal antiviral effect of emtricitabine (mean 1.9 log unit decrease in plasma HIV RNA concentration) was achieved with a dose of 200 mg/day. Several large trials have confirmed the antiretroviral activity of emtricitabine in three-drug regimens with other agents including nucleoside or nucleotide analogs, protease inhibitors, and/or NNRTIs. In two randomized comparison studies, emtricitabine- and lamivudine-based triple-combination regimens had similar efficacy.

ENALAPRIL MALEATE

(Vasotec tablets 2.5 mg)

Enalapril is an ACE inhibitor that competitively inhibits angiotensin I-converting enzyme, preventing conversion of angiotensin I to angiotensin II, a potent vasoconstrictor that also stimulates release of aldosterone. It results in decreases in BP, reduced sodium absorption, and potassium retention. Enalapril is indicated in the treatment of hypertension and symptomatic congestive heart failure (CHF) in combination with diuretics and digitalis and asymptomatic left ventricular dysfunction.

Enalapril is indicated in the treatment of hypertension either by itself or in combination with thiazide-like diuretics; and in the symptomatic treatment of CHF, usually in combination with a diuretic and digitalis. Enalapril becomes hydrolyzed to enalaprilat, which in turn inhibits angiotensin-converting enzyme (ACE). The beneficial effects of enalapril in hypertension or heart failure appear to result primarily from suppression of the renin angiotensin-aldosterone system. The lower plasma level of angiotensin II leads to decreased vasopressor activity and to decreased aldosterone secretion. Because enalapril lowers blood pressure in low renin hypertension, it may exert its effects also by increasing the level of bradykinin. Enalapril is known to have caused angioedema of the face, extremities, lips, tongue, glottis, and/or larynx. Antihistaminics are effective in relieving the symptoms.

Many ACE inhibitors have been synthesized. These drugs can be classified into three broad groups based on chemical structure: (1) sulfhydryl-containing ACE inhibitors structurally related to **captopril** (e.g., **fentiapril**, **pivalopril**, **zofenopril**, and **alacepril**); (2) dicarboxyl-containing ACE inhibitors structurally related to **enalapril** (e.g., **lisinopril**, **benazepril**, **quinapril**, **moexipril**, **ramipril**, **trandolapril**, **spirapril**, **perindopril**, **pentopril**, and **cilazapril**); and (3) phosphorus-containing ACE inhibitors structurally related to fosinopril. Many ACE inhibitors are ester-containing prodrugs that are 100 to 1000 times less potent but have a much better oral bioavailability than the active molecules. Currently, 11 ACE inhibitors are available for clinical use in the United States. In general, ACE inhibitors differ with regard to three properties: (1) potency, (2) whether ACE inhibition is primarily a direct effect of the drug itself or the effect of an active metabolite, and (3) pharmacokinetics (i.e., extent of absorption, effect of food on absorption, plasma half-life, tissue distribution, and mechanisms of elimination).

There is no compelling reason to favor one ACE inhibitor over another because all ACE inhibitors effectively block the conversion of angiotensin I to angiotensin II, and all have similar therapeutic indications, adverse-effect profiles, and contraindications. However, the Quality-of-Life Hypertension Study Group reported that although captopril and enalapril are indistinguishable with regard to antihypertensive efficacy and safety, captopril may have a more favorable effect on quality of life. Because hypertension usually requires lifelong treatment, quality-of-life issues are an important consideration in comparing antihypertensive drugs. ACE inhibitors differ markedly in tissue distribution, and it is possible that this difference could be exploited to inhibit some local renin-angiotensin systems while leaving others relatively intact. Whether site-specific inhibition actually confers therapeutic advantages remains to be established.

With the notable exceptions of fosinopril and spirapril (which display balanced elimination by the liver and kidneys), ACE inhibitors are cleared predominantly by the kidneys. Therefore, impaired renal function significantly diminishes the plasma clearance of most ACE inhibitors, and dosages of these drugs should be reduced in patients with renal impairment. Elevated plasma renin activity (PRA) renders patients hyperresponsive to ACE inhibitor-induced hypotension, and initial dosages of all ACE inhibitors should be reduced in patients with high plasma levels of renin (e.g., patients with heart failure and salt-depleted patients).

Enalapril maleate, the second ACE inhibitor approved in the United States, is a prodrug that is hydrolyzed by esterases in the liver to produce the active dicarboxylic acid, enalaprilat. Enalaprilat is a highly potent inhibitor of ACE with a K_i of 0.2 nM. Although it also contains a "proline surrogate," enalaprilat differs from captopril in that it is an analog of a tripeptide rather than of a dipeptide. Enalapril is absorbed rapidly when given orally and has an oral bioavailability of about 60% (not reduced by food). Although peak concentrations of **enalapril** in plasma occur within an hour, enalaprilat concentrations peak only after 3 to 4 hours. **Enalapril** has a half-life of only 1.3 hours, but enalaprilat, because of tight binding to ACE, has a plasma half-life of about 11 hours. Nearly all the drug is eliminated by the kidneys as either intact enalapril or enalaprilat. The oral dosage of enalapril ranges from 2.5 to 40 mg daily (single or divided dosage), with 2.5 and 5 mg daily being appropriate for the initiation of therapy for heart failure and hypertension, respectively. The initial dose for hypertensive patients who are taking diuretics, are water- or Na^+-depleted, or have heart failure, is 2.5 mg daily.

ENALAPRIL MALEATE/ HYDROCHLOROTHIAZIDE

(Vaseretic 5-12.5 tablets 12.5 mg hydrochlorothiazide 5 mg enalapril maleate)

Enalapril is an antihypertensive combination. **Enalapril** causes vasodilation and decreased BP; **hydrochlorothiazide** causes loss of body water and increases urine output. The combination is indicated in the treatment of hypertension.

ENCAINIDE HYDROCHLORIDE

Encainide, a class IC antiarrhythmic agent, is available on a limited basis only to patients with life-threatening ventricular arrhythmias. Encainide slows conduction velocity, inhibits automaticity, and increases the ratio of the effective refractory period to action potential duration. It blocks the sodium channel of Purkinje fibers and the myocardium. Encainide is absorbed well, reaches peak plasma level in 30 to 90 minutes, becomes metabolized to *O*-demethyl encainide (ODE) and 3-methoxy-*O*-demethyl encainide (MODE), which are active antiarrhythmic agents, and the metabolites are excreted by the kidneys. In renal impairment, the clearance of ODE and MODE is decreased, and hence the dosage should be reduced. Encainide may either worsen or create new arrhythmias, especially in electrolyte-imbalanced patients. Encainide is known to have caused sinus bradycardia, sinus pause, or sinus arrest (see also Figure 84).

ENDORPHINS

For many years, pharmacologists considered the possibility that opioids mimic a naturally ongoing process. Investigations isolated opiate-like peptides from the brain that consisted of two similar pentapeptides with the following sequences:

Try-Gly-Gly-Phe-Met (met-enkephalin)
Try-Gly-Gly-Phe-Leu (leu-enkephalin)

Both peptides behave as agonists and inhibit opiate receptor binding, with affinities comparable to the affinity of morphine. The effects of met-enkephalin and leu-enkephalin are reversed by naloxone. Three distinct families of peptides have been identified thus far: the enkephalins, the endorphins, and the dynorphins.

ENDOTHELINS

Endothelial cells synthesize and release substances that cause vasoconstriction or vasorelaxation. Endothelin is a potent, slow-acting, and long-lasting vasoconstrictor peptide that exerts a wide variety of effects, which include constriction of airway, intestinal, and uterine smooth muscle; positive inotropic and chronotropic actions plus stimulation of atrial natriuretic peptide release; inhibition of renin release from isolated glomeruli; and inhibition of ouabain-sensitive Na^+K^+ATPase in the inner medullary collecting duct cells. It also blocks the antidiuretic effect of vasopressin *in vivo*, modulates catecholamine release from the sympathetic termini and adrenomedullary chromaffin cells, stimulates aldosterone release in adrenocortical glomerular cells, and stimulates CNS effects, including a potent pressor action that is mediated by increased sympathetic outflow and the stimulation of substance P release from the spinal cord (see Figure 44).

The currently available data suggest that the signal transduction at the endothelium receptor in vascular smooth muscle may be similar to that of angiotensin II and vasopressin.

ENFLURANE

(Enthrane)

Enflurane is indicated to provide analgesia for vaginal delivery, and in combination with other anesthetic agents, it is used for delivery by cesarean section. It does provide adequate muscular relaxation. Enflurane, an inhalation anesthetic, produces rapid induction and recovery. It obtunds pharyngeal and laryngeal reflexes and causes salivary

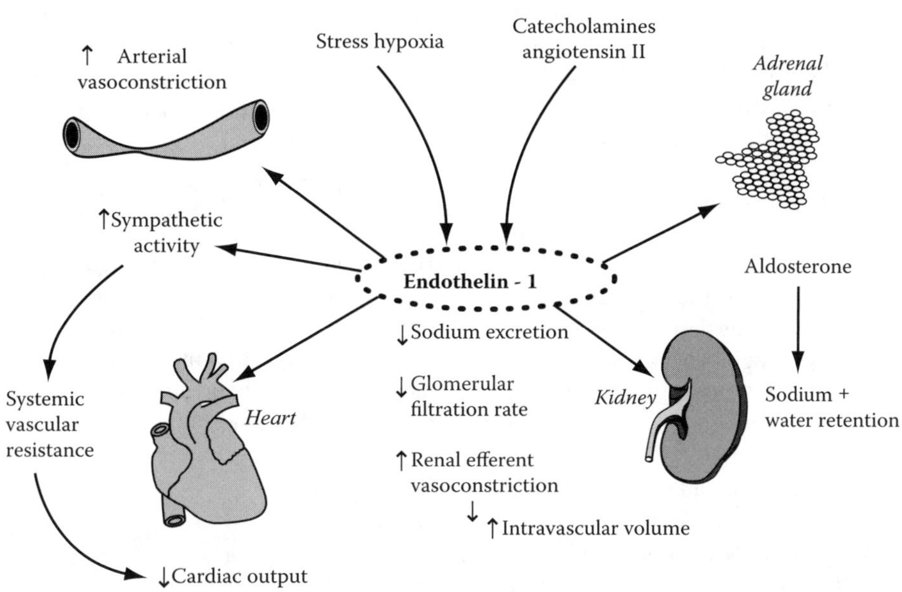

FIGURE 44 Endothelial cells synthesize and release substances that cause vasoconstriction or vasorelaxation. **Endothelin** is a potent, slow-acting and long-lasting vasoconstrictor peptide that exerts a wide variety of effects.

secretion. Because it releases fluoride ion, it may cause renal failure in susceptible individuals (see also Table 16).

ENFUVIRTIDE

(Fuzeon injection 90 mg/mL)

Enfuvirtide is a fusion inhibitor that interferes with entry of HIV-1 into cells by inhibiting fusion of viral and cellular membranes. It is indicated in combination with other antiretroviral agents for the treatment of HIV-1 infection in treatment-experienced patients with evidence of HIV-1 replication despite ongoing antiretroviral therapy.

Enfuvirtide is the only available HIV entry inhibitor, although there are a number of investigational drugs in this class. **Enfuvirtide** is a large, synthetic HIV-derived peptide that was investigated originally as a possible vaccine component in part because of a high degree of sequence conservation among HIV-1 strains. This peptide turned out to have potent anti-HIV activity *in vitro*, a property eventually attributed to selective inhibition of HIV-mediated membrane fusion. **Enfuvirtide** is expensive to manufacture and must be administered by subcutaneous injection twice daily. Thus cost and route of administration may limit its use. In contrast, most investigational entry inhibitors are orally available small molecules. Enfuvirtide is a 36-ammo-acid synthetic peptide whose sequence is derived from a part of the transmembrane gp41 region of HIV-1 that is involved in fusion of the virus membrane lipid bilayer with that of the host cell. **Enfuvirtide** is not active against HIV-2 but has a broad range of potencies against HIV-1 laboratory and clinical isolates. The reported *in vitro* IC_{50} is from 0.1 nM to 1.7 μM, depending on the HIV-1 strain and testing method employed.

Enfuvirtide has a unique mechanism of antiretroviral action. The peptide blocks the interaction between the N36 and C34 sequences of the gp41 glycoprotein by binding to a hydrophobic groove in the N36 coil. This prevents formation of a six-helix bundle critical for membrane fusion and viral entry into the host cell. **Enfuvirtide** inhibits infection of CD4+ cells by free virus particles, as well as cell-to-cell transmission of HIV *in vitro*. It retains activity against viruses that have become resistant to antiretroviral agents of other classes because of its unique mechanism of action.

HIV can develop resistance to this drug through specific mutations in the enfuvirtide-binding domain of gp41. Of the patients experiencing virologic failure during enfuvirtide treatment, 94% had mutations in the gp41 region associated with enfuvirtide resistance *in vitro*. The most common mutations involve a V38A or N43D substitution. Single-amino-acid substitutions can confer up to 450 times resistance *in vitro*, although high-level clinical resistance is usually associated with two or more ammo acid changes.

The most prominent adverse effects of enfuvirtide are injection-site reactions. In 98% of patients, one or more local side effects including pain, erythema, and induration at the site of injection are seen; 80% of patients develop nodules or cysts. Between 4 and 5% of patients discontinue treatment because of local reactions. Use of **enfuvirtide** has been associated with a higher incidence of lymphadenopathy and pneumonia in at least one study. Whether these are direct drug effects, a secondary consequence of drug-related immune dysfunction, or effects from another mechanism is currently the subject of investigation. **Enfuvirtide** suppresses interleukin 12 production *in vitro* by more than 90% at concentrations equal to or less than those required to inhibit HIV replication, although the role this might play in clinical immunosuppression is unclear.

Enfuvirtide is not metabolized to a significant extent and is not known to alter the concentrations of any coadministered drugs. Ritonavir, rifampin, or ritonavir plus saquinavir did not alter enfuvirtide concentrations.

Enfuvirtide is approved by the FDA for use only in treatment-experienced adults who have evidence of HIV replication despite ongoing antiretroviral therapy. In phase III clinical trials involving patients with documented multidrug-resistant HIV-1, the administration of **enfuvirtide** (90 mg subcutaneously twice daily) in combination with an optimized background regimen was associated with undetectable (<50 copies/ml) plasma HIV-1 RNA concentrations after 24 weeks of treatment in twice as many patients as those who used the optimized background regimen alone (12.2 to 19.6% versus 5.3 to 7.3%). Treatment response appears to be much more likely in patients with at least two other active drugs in the regimen, based on history and HIV genotype. Given the cost, inconvenience, and cutaneous toxicity of this drug, enfuvirtide generally is reserved for patients who have failed all other feasible antiretroviral regimens.

ENKEPHALINS

For many years, pharmacologists considered the possibility that opioids mimic a naturally ongoing process. Investigations isolated opiate-like peptides from the brain that consisted of two similar pentapeptides with the following sequences:

Try-Gly-Gly-Phe-Met (met-enkephalin)
Try-Gly-Gly-Phe-Leu (leu-enkephalin)

Both peptides behave as agonists and inhibit opiate receptor binding, with affinities comparable to the affinity of morphine. The effects of met-enkephalin and leu-enkephalin are reversed by naloxone. Three distinct families of peptides have been identified thus far: the enkephalins, the endorphins, and the dynorphins.

ENOXACIN

(Penetrex)

Enoxacin (single dose of 400 mg) is indicated in the treatment of uncomplicated urethral or cervical gonorrhea due to *Neisseria gonorrhoeae*; or uncomplicated cystitis (200 mg q. 12 hours/7 days) due to *Escherichia coli, Staphylococcus epidermidis*, or *S. saprophyticus*; complicated due to *E. coli, Klebsiella pneumoniae, Proteus mirabilis, Pseudomonas aeruginosa, S. epidermidis*, or *Enterobacter cloacae*. Enoxacin diffuses into cervix, fallopian tube, and myometrium at levels approximately one to two times those achieved in plasma, and into kidney and prostate at levels approximately two to four times those achieved in plasma. Enoxacin becomes bound to the extent of 40%, and this is decreased to 15% in patients with renal impairment requiring a reduction in total dosage. Bismuth subsalicylate decreases the availability of enoxacin. The activity of cytochrome P450 isoenzyme responsible for metabolism of methylxanthines (caffeine, theophylline, and theobromine) is inhibited by enoxacin prolonging their actions. Quinolones, including enoxacin, reduce the clearance of warfarin. The side effects of enoxacin may include headache, dizziness, somnolence, gastrointestinal pain, skin rash, and vaginal moniliasis. The quinolones and fluoroquinolones may produce arthropathy, and hence should not be used in pregnant women (see also Figure 74).

ENOXAPARIN SODIUM

(Lovenox injection 30 mg/0.3 mL)

Enoxaparin is a low-molecular-weight heparin that causes a higher anti-factor Xa to antithrombin activities (anti-factor IIa) ratio than heparin, which may prevent thrombosis. Enoxaparin is indicated in prevention of deep vein thrombosis (DVT), which may lead to pulmonary embolism (PE) in patients undergoing hip or knee replacement surgery or abdominal surgery; in conjunction with warfarin sodium for inpatient treatment of acute DVT with and without PE or outpatient treatment of acute DVT without PE; prevention of ischemic complications of unstable and non-Q-wave MI when coadministered with aspirin; and in medical patients who are at risk for thromboembolic complications due to severely restricted mobility during acute illness. Enoxaparin (30 mg b.i.d. SC) is indicated in the prevention of DVT, which may lead to pulmonary embolism, following hip replacement surgery. Enoxaparin is contraindicated in a patient with active major bleeding or with thrombocytopenia. Furthermore, it should be used cautiously in conditions with increased risk of hemorrhage such as bacterial endocarditis, congenital or acquired bleeding disorders, active ulceration, hemorrhagic stroke, or shortly after brain, spinal, or ophthalmological surgery. Protamine sulfate (1% solution) is able to antidote the overdosage of enoxaparin (see also Tables 17 and 18).

Enoxaparin (Lovenox), **dalteparin** (Fragmin), **tinzaparin** (Innohep, others), **ardeparin** (Normilfo), **nadroparin** (Fraxiparine, others), and **reviparin** (Clivarine) differ considerably in composition, and it cannot be assumed that two preparations that have similar anti-factor Xa activity will produce equivalent antithrombotic effects. The more predictable pharmacokinetic properties of low-molecular-weight heparins, however, permit administration in a fixed or weight-adjusted dosage regimen once or twice daily by subcutaneous injection. Because they have a minimal effect on tests of clotting *in vitro*, monitoring is not done routinely. Patients with end-stage renal failure may require monitoring with an anti-factor Xa assay because this condition may prolong the half-life of low-molecular-weight heparin. Specific dosage recommendations for various low-molecular-weight heparins may be obtained from the manufacturer's literature.

ENOXIMONE

Amrinone, milrinone, and enoximone differ from aminophylline in that they exhibit a certain degree of selectivity for peak III phosphodiesterase (Figure 23), which is found predominantly in myocardial and vascular tissues. These agents exert both positive inotropic and direct vasodilating actions. Circulating catecholamines released from adrenergic nerve terminals, and exogenous sympathomimetic drugs act on beta-adrenergic and alpha-adrenergic receptors, respectively. Simulation of beta-adrenergic receptors activates adenylate cyclase, resulting in increased cyclic adenosine monophosphate (cyclic AMP) production, which in turn augments calcium influx through the slow calcium channels, presumably due to the activation of protein kinases that phosphorylate the slow calcium channel (see Figure 84). The mechanism by which the stimulation of alpha-adrenergic receptors increases myocardial contractility is not fully understood, but it may also involve an action on the slow calcium channel. Tyramine acts on adrenergic nerve terminals to release catecholamines, which then act on adrenergic receptors. Calcium-channel agonists act directly on the calcium channel to increase calcium influx, intracellular cyclic AMP is degraded by phosphodiesterase, and the subsequent inhibition of cardiac phosphodiesterases results in increased intracellular cyclic AMP levels. This mechanism appears to be largely responsible for the actions of several of the newer positive inotropic agents. The cyclic AMP concentration can also be increased independently of beta-adrenergic receptors through the direct stimulation of adenylate cyclase with forskolin (see also Figure 52).

ENPROFYLLINE

Enprofylline is a methylxanthine bronchodilator that may be used in the treatment of bronchial asthma. The methylxanthines consist of aminophylline, dyphylline, enprofylline, and pentoxifylline. Aminophylline (theophylline ethylenediamine) is the most widely used of the soluble theophyllines. Its main therapeutic effect is bronchodilation. In addition, it causes CNS stimulation, cardiac acceleration, diuresis, and gastric secretion. Aminophylline is available in an oral, rectal (pediatric), or intravenous solution, which is used in the treatment of status asthmaticus. Although aminophylline is a less effective bronchodilator than beta-adrenergic agonists, it is particularly useful in preventing nocturnal asthma (see also Figure 94).

ENTACAPONE

Entacapone, a peripherally acting inhibitor of catechol-*O*-methyltransferase, is a valuable adjunct to levodopa in parkinsonian patients.

ENTACAPONE

(Comtan tablets 200 mg)

Entacapone inhibits catechol-*O*-methyltransferase (COMT), thus blocking the degradation of catechols including dopamine and levodopa. This may lead to more sustained levels of dopamine and consequently a more prolonged antiparkinson effect. Entacapone is indicated as an adjunct to levodopa/carbidopa for the treatment of idiopathic Parkinson's disease in patients who experience signs and symptoms of end-of-dose "wearing-off" effects. **Entacapone** and **tolcapone** are nitrocatechol-type COMT inhibitors. Entacapone is a peripherally acting COMT inhibitor, whereas tolcapone also inhibits COMT activity in the brain. COMT inhibition has been shown to attenuate levodopa toxicity on dopamine neurons and enhance dopamine action in the brain of patients with Parkinson's disease. On the other hand, nonselective monoamine oxidase (MAO) inhibitors, such as tranylcypromine, potentiate the effects of tyramine and may potentiate effects of neurotransmitters. While most MAO inhibitors used as antidepressants inhibit both MAO-A and MAO-B, selective MAO-A and MAO-B inhibitors are available. **Selegiline** is a selective and irreversible MAO-B inhibitor that also has been used as an adjunct in the treatment of Parkinson's disease.

Two COMT inhibitors presently are available for this use in the United States: tolcapone (Tasmar) and **entacapone** (Comtan). Both these agents have been shown in double-blind trials to reduce the clinical symptoms of "wearing off" in patients treated with levodopa/carbidopa. Although the magnitude of their clinical effects and mechanisms of action are similar, they differ with respect to pharmacokinetic properties and adverse effects. Tolcapone has a relatively long duration of action, allowing for administration two to three times a day, and appears to act by both central and peripheral inhibition of COMT. The duration of action of **entacapone** is short, around 2 hours, so it usually is administered simultaneously with each dose of levodopa/carbidopa. The action of entacapone is attributable principally to peripheral inhibition of COMT. The common adverse effects of these agents are similar to those observed in patients treated with levodopa/carbidopa alone, and include nausea, orthostatic hypotension, vivid dreams, confusion, and hallucination. An important adverse effect associated with tolcapone is hepatotoxicity. In clinical trials, up to 2% of the patients treated had increases in serum alanine aminotransferase and aspartate transaminase; after marketing, three fatal cases of fulminant hepatic failure in patients taking tolcapone were observed, leading to addition of a warning to the label. At present, tolcapone should be used only in patients who have not responded to other therapies and with appropriate monitoring for hepatic injury. Entacapone has not been associated with hepatotoxicity and requires no special monitoring. It also is available in fixed-dose combinations with levodopa/carbidopa (**Stalevo**).

ENTECAVIR

(Baraclude tablets 0.5 mg)

Entecavir is an antiviral agent that inhibits HBV polymerase (reverse transcriptase) by competing with the natural substrate deoxyguanosine triphosphate. It is indicated in the treatment of chronic HBV in adults with evidence of active viral replication and either evidence of persistent elevations in serum aminotransferases (ALT or AST) or histologically active disease.

ENZYMES AND HORMONES OF THE GASTROINTESTINAL TRACT: Actions of

Enzymes/ Hormones	Sites of Secretion	Main Actions
Amylase	Parotid and submandibular glands	Converts carbohydrates, starch, and glycogen to simple disaccharides
Cholecystokinin	Duodenum, jejunum	Stimulates pancreatic enzyme secretion and gallbladder contraction
Chymotrypsinogen	Pancreas	Breaks down proteins into proteases and peptides
Enteroglucagon	Duodenum	Inhibits pancreatic enzyme secretion and bowel motility
Gastric inhibitory peptide	Small intestine	Decreases gastric motility and stimulates insulin secretion
Gastrin	Stomach, duodenum	Stimulates gastric acid secretion and mucosal growth
Glucagon	Pancreas	Stimulates hepatic glycogenolysis and inhibits motility
Lipase	Pancreas	Hydrolyzes short-chain and medium-chain triglycerides, involved in fat absorption
Pancreatic polypeptide	Pancreas	Inhibits gallbladder contraction and pancreatic and biliary secretion
Pepsinogen	Stomach	Converts large proteins into polypeptides
Secretin	Small intestine	Stimulates hepatic and pancreatic water and bicarbonate secretion
Trypsinogen	Pancreas	Breaks down proteins into proteases and peptides
Vasoactive inhibitory peptide	Small intestine, pancreas	Vasodilator; stimulates water and bicarbonate secretion, release of insulin and glucagon, and production of small-intestinal juice

EPHEDRINE

(Bofedrol)

EPHEDRINE HYDROCHLORIDE

(Efedron)

EPHEDRINE SULFATE

(Ectasule Minus, Ephed II, Slo-Fedrin, Vicks Va-tro-nol)

Ephedrine, a sympathomimetic amine, is used to correct hypotensive states (25 to 50 mg IM or SC), to treat orthostatic hypotension (25 mg p.o. once daily to q.i.d.), and as a bronchodilator or nasal congestant (see also Table 24).

Ephedrine (25 to 50 mg p.o. t.i.d.) is indicated in the treatment of allergic disorders such as bronchial asthma; nasal congestion in acute coryza; vasomotor rhinitis, acute sinusitis, and hay fever. Ephedrine (25 to 30 mg slowly SC, IM, or IV) has been used to relieve acute bronchospasm, but epinephrine is more effective. Ephedrine is also used in shock. It is a naturally occurring sympathomimetic agent that stimulates alpha and beta receptors and CNS. It is less potent than epinephrine but has a longer duration of action (see also Figure 37).

Ephedrine is both an α- and a β-receptor agonist; in addition, it enhances release of norepinephrine from sympathetic neurons and therefore is a mixed-acting sympathomimetic drug. It contains two asymmetrical carbon atoms; only *l*-ephedrine and racemic ephedrine are used clinically.

Ephedrine does not contain a catechol moiety and is effective after oral administration. The drug stimulates heart rate and cardiac output and variably increases peripheral resistance; as a result, ephedrine usually increases blood pressure. Stimulation of the α receptors of smooth-muscle cells in the bladder base may increase the resistance to the outflow of urine. Activation of β receptors in the lungs promotes bronchodilation. Ephedrine is a potent CNS stimulant. After oral administration, effects of the drug may persist for several hours. It is eliminated in the urine largely as unchanged drug, with a half-life of about 3 to 6 hours.

In the past, **ephedrine** was used to treat Stokes–Adams attacks with complete heart block and as a CNS stimulant in narcolepsy and depressive states. It has been replaced by alternate treatments in each of these disorders. In addition, its use as a bronchodilator in patients with asthma has become much less extensive with the development of β_2-selective agonists. **Ephedrine** has been used to promote urinary continence, although its efficacy is not clear. Indeed, the drug may cause urinary retention, particularly in men with benign prostatic hyperplasia. Ephedrine also has been used to treat the hypotension that may occur with spinal anesthesia.

Untoward effects of ephedrine include hypertension, particularly after parenteral administration or with higher-than-recommended oral dosing. Insomnia is a common CNS adverse effect. Tachyphylaxis may occur with repetitive dosing. Concerns have been raised about the safety of ephedrine. Usual or higher-than-recommended doses may cause important adverse effects in susceptible individuals, and are especially of concern in patients with underlying cardiovascular disease that might be unrecognized. Of potentially greater cause for concern, large amounts of herbal preparations containing ephedrine (**ma huang**, **ephedra**) are utilized around the world. There can be considerable variability in the content of ephedrine in these preparations, which may lead to inadvertent consumption of higher-than-usual doses of ephedrine and its isomers. Because of this, the FDA has banned the sale of dietary supplements containing ephedra effective April, 2004.

Although barbiturates largely have been replaced by benzodiazepines and other compounds for sedation, **phenobarbital** and **butabarbital** are still available as "sedatives" in a host of combinations of questionable efficacy for the treatment of functional gastrointestinal disorders and asthma. They also are included in analgesic combinations, possibly counterproductively. Barbiturates, especially butabarbital and phenobarbital, are used sometimes to antagonize unwanted CNS-stimulant effects of various drugs such as **ephedrine**, **dextroamphetamine**, and **theophylline**, although a preferred approach is adjustment of dosage or substitution of alternative therapy for the primary agents. Phenobarbital still is used to treat hypnosedative withdrawal.

EPILEPTIC SEIZURES: Treatment of

Seizure Type	Drug of Choice	Alternate
	Partial Seizures	
Simple partial	Carbamazepine, phenytoin, phenobarbital, primidone, valproate	Gabapentin, lamotrigine
Complex partial	Carbamazepine, phenobarbital, phenytoin, primidone, valproate	Gabapentin, lamotrigine
Partial with secondarily generalized tonic–clonic seizure	Carbamazepine, phenobarbital, phenytoin, primidone, valproate	Gabapentin, lamotrigine
	Generalized Seizures	
Absence seizure	Clonazepam, ethosuximide, valproate	Lamotrigine
Myoclonic seizure	Valproate	
Tonic–clonic seizure	Carbamazepine, phenobarbital, phenytoin, primidone, valproate	

EPINASTINE HYDROCHLORIDE (Elestat Ophthalmic solution 0.05%)

Epinastine is an ophthalmic antihistaminic agent with direct H_1-receptor antagonist activity that inhibits the release of histamine from the mast cell. It is indicated in prevention of itching associated with allergic conjunctivits. Topical antihistamines include emedastine difumarate (Emadine) and levocabastine hydrochloride (Livostin). **Cromolyn sodium** (Crolom), which prevents the release of histamine and other autacoids from mast cells, has found limited use in treating conjunctivitis that is thought to be allergen-mediated, such as vernal conjunctivitis. **Lodoxamide tromethamine** (Alomide) and **pemirolast** (Alamast), mast-cell stabilizers, also are available for ophthalmic use. **Nedocromil** (Alocril) also is primarily a mast-cell stabilizer with some antihistamine properties. **Olopatadine hydrochloride** (Patanol), **ketotifen fumarate** (Zaditor), and **azelastine** (Optivar) are H_1 antagonists with mast-cell-stabilizing properties. **Epinastine** (Elestat) antagonizes H_1 and H_2 receptors and exhibits mast-cell-stabilizing activity.

EPINEPHRINE

(Bronkaid Mist, EpiPen, EpiPen Jr, Primatene Mist Solution, Sus-Phrine)

EPINEPHRINE BITARTRATE

(AsthmaHaler, Bronitin Mist, Bronkaid Mist Suspension, Epitrate, Medihaler-Epi, Primatene Mist Suspension)

EPINEPHRINE HYDROCHLORIDE

(Adrenalin Chloride, AsthmaNefrin, Epifrin, Glaucon, microNefrin, S-2 Inhalant, Vaponefrin)

EPINEPHRYL BORATE

(Epinal, Eppy/N)

Epinephrine, a sympathomimetic amine, is used as a bronchodilator (one inhalation per metered aerosol); to restore cardiac rhythm in cardiac arrest (0.5 to 1 mg IV bolus); to treat open-angle glaucoma (1 to 2 drops of 1 to 2% solution), and to prolong the effect of local anesthetics. Epinephrine is a sympathomimetic drug that activates an adrenergic receptor mechanism on effector cells and initiates cell actions of the sympathetic nervous system except on the arteries of the face and sweat glands (see Figure 37). It acts on both alpha and beta receptors, but the beta effect may predominate. The functions associated with alpha receptors are vasoconstriction, mydriasis, and intestinal relaxation. The functions associated with beta receptors are vasodilation, cardioacceleration, bronchial relaxation, positive inotropic effect, intestinal relaxation, and glycogenolysis and fatty acid release. The $beta_1$ receptors are responsible for cardiac stimulation and vasodepression. $Beta_2$ agonists are especially useful in the treatment of asthma because they produce bronchodilation without causing much cardiac acceleration.

The actions of norepinephrine and epinephrine on the cardiovascular system may be quite different when both drugs are administered in small doses (0.1 to 0.4 μg/kg/min in a slow intravenous infusion), but are essentially the same when given in large doses. The following are the effects of small doses of norepinephrine in humans: systolic pressure—increased; diastolic pressure—increased; mean pressure—increased; heart rate—slightly decreased; cardiac output—slightly decreased; and peripheral resistance—increased.

The effects of small doses of epinephrine in humans are: systolic pressure—increased; diastolic pressure—decreased (increased by larger dose); mean pressure—unchanged; cardiac output—increased; and peripheral resistance—decreased. Epinephrine increases the heart rate, force of contraction, irritability, and coronary blood flow. The inherent chronotropic effect of norepinephrine is opposed by reflex slowing that is secondary to vasoconstriction and elevated blood pressure. Epinephrine is a dilator of bronchial smooth muscle ($beta_2$ receptor), whereas norepinephrine is a weak dilator. Isoproterenol is more active than epinephrine. Both epinephrine and isoproterenol elevate the blood glucose level by stimulating glycogenolysis and by inhibiting glucose utilization. The therapeutic uses of epinephrine and its related drugs are as a bronchodilator ($beta_2$-receptor activation in asthma), as a mydriatic (contracts radial muscle), in glaucoma (lowers intraocular pressure [IOP]), for allergic reactions (prevents antigen-induced histamine releases), in hypotension (increases the mean pressure), as a nasal decongestant (mephentermine), as a local anesthesia (produces a bloodless field of operation, delays absorption and yields a longer duration of anesthetic action, and protects the brain and heart against the toxic effects of local anesthetics), and as cardiac stimulants (epinephrine or isoproterenol may be injected in heart block to improve atrioventricular conduction velocity and stimulate ventricular automaticity) (see also Figure 80).

EPIRUBICIN HYDROCHLORIDE

(Ellence solution for injection 2 mg/mL)

Epirubicin is a cell-cycle-phase, nonspecific anthracycline. It forms a complex with DNA by intercalation of its planar rings between nucleotide base pairs, with consequent inhibition of nucleic acid (DNA and RNA) and protein synthesis. It is indicated in breast cancer with axillary node. Epirubicin is a new anthracycline that has activity similar to doxorubicin (Adriamycin) in a variety of solid neoplasms and hematologic malignancies. Importantly, epirubicin causes less cardiotoxicity than doxorubicin (see also Figure 15).

Daunorubicin, **Doxorubicin**, **Epirubicin**, **Idarubicin**, and **Mitoxantrone** are anthracycline antibiotics that are among the most important antitumor agents. They are derived from the fungus *Streptococcus peucetius* var. *caesius*. Idarubicin and **epirubicin** are analogs of the naturally produced anthracyclines, differing only slightly in chemical structure, but having somewhat distinct patterns of clinical activity. Daunorubicin and idarubicin have been used primarily in the acute leukemias, whereas doxorubicin and epirubicin display broader activity against human solid tumors. These agents, which all possess potential for generating free radicals, cause an unusual and often irreversible cardiomyopathy, the occurrence of which is related to the total dose of the drug. The structurally similar agent mitoxantrone has useful activity against prostate cancer and acute myelogenous leukemia (AML), and is used in high-dose chemotherapy. Mitoxantrone, an anthracenedione, has significantly less cardiotoxicity than the anthracyclines.

Valrubicin (Valstar) was approved in 1998 for intravesical therapy of bacille Calmette–Guérin-refractory urinary bladder carcinoma *in situ* in patients for whom immediate cystectomy would be associated with unacceptable morbidity or mortality. **Epirubicin** (4′-epidoxorubicin, Ellence) was approved by the FDA in 1999 as a component of adjuvant therapy following resection of early lymph-node-positive breast cancer.

EPLERENONE

(Inspra tablets 25 mg)

Eplerenone is a selective aldosterone receptor antagonist that binds to the mineralocorticoid receptor (MR), blocking the binding of aldosterone. It is indicated in the treatment of hypertension; improves survival of stable patients with left ventricular systolic dysfunction and clinical evidence of CHF after an acute myocardial infarction (MI). Currently, two MR antagonists are available in the United States, **spironolactone** (a 17-spirolactone) and **eplerenone**.

Drugs such as spironolactone and **eplerenone** competitively inhibit the binding of aldosterone to the MR. Unlike the MR-aldosterone complex, the MR-spironolactone complex is not able to induce the synthesis of MPs. Because spironolactone and **eplerenone** block the biological effects of aldosterone, these agents also are referred to as aldosterone antagonists. MR antagonists are the only diuretics that do not require access to the tubular lumen to induce diuresis.

As with other K^+-sparing diuretics, spironolactone often is coadministered with thiazide or loop diuretics in the treatment of edema and hypertension. Such combinations result in increased mobilization of edema fluid while causing lesser perturbations of K^+ homeostasis. Spironolactone is particularly useful in the treatment of primary hyperaldosteronism (adrenal adenomas or bilateral adrenal hyperplasia) and of refractory edema associated with secondary aldosteronism (cardiac failure, hepatic cirrhosis, nephrotic syndrome, and severe ascites). Spironolactone is considered the diuretic of choice in patients with hepatic cirrhosis. Added to standard therapy, spironolactone substantially reduces morbidity and mortality and ventricular arrhythmias in patients with heart failure.

Clinical experience with **eplerenone** is limited. Nonetheless, eplerenone appears to be a safe and effective antihypertensive drug. In patients with acute myocardial infarction complicated by left ventricular systolic dysfunction, addition of eplerenone to optimal medical therapy significantly reduces morbidity and mortality.

As with other K^+-sparing diuretics, MR antagonists may cause life-threatening hyperkalemia. Indeed, hyperkalemia is the principal risk of MR antagonists. Therefore, these drugs are contraindicated in patients with hyperkalemia and in those at increased risk of developing hyperkalemia either because of disease or because of administration of other medications. MR antagonists also can induce metabolic acidosis in cirrhotic patients.

Salicylates may reduce the tubular secretion of canrenone and decrease the diuretic efficacy of spironolactone, and spironolactone may alter the clearance of digitalis glycosides. Owing to its affinity for other steroid receptors, spironolactone may cause gynecomastia, impotence, decreased libido, hirsutism, deepening of the voice, and menstrual irregularities. It also may induce diarrhea, gastritis, gastric bleeding, and peptic ulcers (the drug is contraindicated in patients with peptic ulcers). CNS adverse effects include drowsiness, lethargy, ataxia, confusion, and headache. Spironolactone may cause skin rashes and, rarely, blood dyscrasias. Breast cancer has occurred in patients taking spironolactone chronically (cause and effect not established), and high doses of spironolactone have been associated with malignant tumors in rats. Whether or not therapeutic doses of spironolactone can induce malignancies remains an open question. Strong inhibitors of CYP3A4 may increase plasma levels of eplerenone, and such drugs should not be administered to patients taking **eplerenone**, and vice versa. Other than hyperkalemia and gastrointestinal disorders, the rate of adverse events for **eplerenone** is similar to that of placebo.

EPOETIN ALFA (EPO)

(Epogen injection 2000 units/mL, injection)

Epoetin Alfa (EPO) is a recombinant human erythropoietin that stimulates red blood cell production. It is indicated in the treatment of anemia related to chronic renal failure (CRF), zidovudine therapy in HIV-infected patients and nonmyeloid malignancies, and reduction of allogenic blood transfusions in surgery patients. Recombinant human erythropoietin (**epoetin alfa**), produced using engineered Chinese hamster ovary cells, is nearly identical to the endogenous hormone except for two subtle differences. First, the carbohydrate modification pattern of epoetin alfa differs slightly from the native protein, but this difference apparently does not alter kinetics potency, or immunoreactivity of the drug. However, modern assays can detect these differences, which is of significance for detecting athletes who use the recombinant product for "blood doping." The second difference probably is related to the manufacturing process, as one commercially available form of the drug was recently associated with the development of anti-recombinant erythropoietin antibodies that cross-react with the patient's own erythropoietin, potentially causing pure red cell aplasia. Most of these cases were caused by one preparation of the drug shortly after albumin was removed from the formulation.

Available preparations of epoetin alfa include Epogen, Procrit, and Exprex, supplied in single-use vials of from 2,000 to 40,000 units/mL for intravenous or subcutaneous administration. When injected intravenously, epoetin alfa cleared from plasma with a half-life of 4 to 8 hours. However, the effect on marrow progenitors is sufficiently sustained that it need only be given three times a week to achieve an adequate response. Combination of the weekly dose into a single injection also can achieve virtually identical results. No significant allergic reactions have been associated with the intravenous or subcutaneous administration of epoetin alfa, and—except as noted earlier—antibodies have not been detected even after prolonged administration.

More recently, novel erythropoiesis-stimulating protein (NESP) or darbapoetin alfa (Aranesp) has been approved for clinical use in patients with indications similar to those for epoetin alfa. It is a genetically modified form of erythropoietin in which four amino acids have been mutated such that additional carbohydrate side chains are added during its synthesis, prolonging the circulatory survival of the drug to 24 to 26 hours. Recombinant erythropoietin therapy, in conjunction with adequate iron intake, can be highly effective in a number of anemias, especially those associated with a poor erythropoietic response. There is a clear dose-response relationship between the **epoetin alfa** dose and the rise in hematocrit in anephric patients, with eradication of their anemia at higher doses. **Epoetin alfa** also is effective in the treatment of anemias associated with surgery, AIDS, cancer chemotherapy, prematurity, and certain chronic inflammatory conditions. **Darbapoetin alfa** also has been approved for use in patients with anemia associated with chronic kidney disease, and is under review for several other indications.

During erythropoietin therapy, absolute or functional iron deficiency may develop. Functional iron deficiency (i.e., normal ferritin levels but low transferrin saturation) presumably results from the inability to mobilize iron stores rapidly enough to support the increased erythropoiesis. Virtually all patients eventually will require supplemental iron to increase or maintain transferrin saturation to levels that will adequately support stimulated erythropoiesis. Supplemental iron therapy is recommended for all patients whose serum ferritin is below 100 μg/L or whose serum transferrin saturation is less than 20%.

During initial therapy and after any dosage adjustment, the hematocrit is determined once a week (HIV-infected and cancer patients) or twice a week (renal failure patients) until it has stabilized in the target range and the maintenance dose has been established; the hematocrit then is monitored at regular intervals. If the hematocrit increases by more than four points in any 2-week period, the dose should be decreased. Due to the time required for erythropoiesis and the erythrocyte half-life, hematocrit changes lag behind dosage adjustments by 2 to 6 weeks. The dose of darbepoetin should be decreased if the hemoglobin increase exceeds 1 g/dL in any 2-week period because of the association of an excessive rate of rise of hemoglobin with adverse cardiovascular events.

During hemodialysis, patients receiving epoetin alfa or darbepoetin may require increased anticoagulation. Serious thromboembolic events have been reported, including migratory thrombophlebitis, microvascular thrombosis, pulmonary embolism, and thrombosis of the retinal artery and temporal and renal veins. The risk of thrombotic events, including vascular access thromboses, was higher in adults with ischemic heart disease or CHF receiving epoetin alfa therapy with the goal of reaching a normal hematocrit (42%) than in those with a lower-target hematocrit of 30%. The higher risk of cardiovascular events from erythropoietic therapies may be associated with higher hemoglobin or higher rates of rise of hemoglobin. The hemoglobin level should be managed to avoid exceeding a target level of 12 g/dL. Although epoetin alfa is not associated with direct pressor effects, blood pressure may rise, especially during the early phases of therapy when the hematocrit is increasing. Erythropoietins should be withheld in patients with preexisting uncontrolled hypertension. Patients may require initiation of, or increases in, antihypertensive therapy. Hypertensive encephalopathy and seizures have occurred in chronic renal failure patients treated with epoetin alfa. The incidence of seizures appears to be higher during the first 90 days of therapy with **epoetin alfa** in patients on dialysis (occurring in about 2.5% of patients) when compared with subsequent 90-day periods. Headache, tachycardia, edema, shortness of breath, nausea, vomiting, diarrhea, injection site stinging, and flu-like symptoms (e.g., arthralgias and myalgias) also have been reported in conjunction with epoetin alfa therapy. Pure red-cell aplasia in association with neutralizing antibodies to native erythropoietin has been observed in patients treated with recombinant erythropoietins; underlying infectious, inflammatory or malignant processes; occult blood loss; underlying hematologic diseases (e.g., thalassemia, refractory anemia, or other myelodysplastic disorders); folic acid or vitamin B_{12} deficiency; hemolysis; aluminum intoxication; bone marrow fibrosis; and osteitis fibrosa cystica.

Patients with anemia secondary to chronic kidney disease are ideal candidates for epoetin alfa therapy. The response in predialysis, peritoneal dialysis, and hemodialysis patients is dependent on severity of the renal failure, the erythropoietin dose and route of administration, and iron availability. The subcutaneous route of administration is preferred over the intravenous route because absorption is slower and the amount of drug required is reduced by 20 to 40%.

The dose of **epoetin alfa** should be adjusted to obtain a gradual rise in the hematocrit over a 2- to 4-month period to a final hematocrit of 33 to 36%. Treatment to hematocrit levels greater than 36% is not recommended, as patients treated to a hematocrit above 40% showed a higher incidence of myocardial infarction and death. The drug should not be used to replace emergency transfusion in patients who need immediate correction of a life-threatening anemia.

Patients are started on doses of 80 to 120 units/kg of epoetin alfa, given subcutaneously three times a week. It can be given on a once-a-week schedule, but somewhat more drug is required for an equivalent effect. If the response is poor, the dose should be progressively increased. The final maintenance dose of epoetin alfa can vary from as little as 10 units/kg to more than 300 units/kg, with an average dose of 75 units/kg, three times a week. Children younger than 5 years generally require a higher dose. Resistance to therapy is common in patients who develop an inflammatory illness or become iron deficient, so close monitoring of general health and iron status is essential. Less common causes of resistance include occult blood loss, folic acid deficiency, carnitine deficiency, inadequate dialysis, aluminum toxicity, and osteitis fibrosa cystica secondary to hyperparathyroidism.

The most common side effect of **epoetin alfa** therapy is aggravation of hypertension, which occurs in 20 to 30% of patients and most often is associated with a rapid rise in hematocrit. Blood pressure usually can be controlled either by increasing antihypertensive therapy or ultrafiltration in dialysis patients or by reducing the epoetin alfa dose to slow the hematocrit response.

Darbapoetin alfa also is approved for use in patients who are anemic secondary to chronic kidney disease. The recommended starting dose is 0.45 μg/kg administered intravenously or subcutaneously once weekly, with dose adjustments depending on the response. Like epoetin alfa, side effects tend to occur when patients experience a rapid rise in hemoglobin concentration; a rise of less than 1 g/dL every 2 weeks generally has been considered safe.

Epoetin alfa therapy has been approved for the treatment of HIV-infected patients, especially those on zidovudine therapy. Excellent responses to doses of 100 to 300 units/kg, given subcutaneously three times a week, generally are seen in patients with zidovudine-induced anemia. In the face of advanced disease, marrow damage, and elevated serum erythropoietin levels (greater than 500 IU/L), therapy is less effective.

Epoetin alfa therapy, 150 units/kg three times a week or 450 to 600 units/kg once a week, can reduce the transfusion requirement in cancer patients undergoing chemotherapy. Evidence-based guidelines for the therapeutic use of recombinant erythropoietin in patients with cancer have been published. Briefly, the guidelines recommend the use of epoetin alfa in patients with chemotherapy-associated anemia when hemoglobin levels fall below 10 g/dL, basing the decision to treat less severe anemia (hemoglobin between 10 and 12 g/dL) on clinical circumstances. For anemia associated with hematologic malignancies, the guidelines support the use of recombinant erythropoietin in patients with low-grade myelodysplastic syndrome, although the evidence that the drug is effective in anemic patients with multiple myeloma, non-Hodgkin's lymphoma, or chronic lymphocytic leukemia not receiving chemotherapy is less robust. A baseline serum erythropoietin level may help to predict the response; most patients with blood levels of more than 500 IU/L are unlikely to respond to any dose of the drug. Most patients treated with epoetin alfa experienced an improvement in their anemia, sense of well-being, and quality of life. This improved sense of well-being, particularly in cancer patients, may not be solely due to the rise in the hematocrit. Erythropoietin receptors have been demonstrated in cells of the CNS, and erythropoietin has been found to act as a cytoprotectant in several models of CNS ischemia. Thus, high levels of the hormone may directly affect cancer patients' sense of well-being.

Darbopoetin alfa also has been tested in cancer patients undergoing chemotherapy, and preliminary studies appear promising. However, recent case reports have suggested a direct effect of both epoetin alfa and darbopoetin alfa in the stimulation of tumor cells. For example, patients with cancer of the head and neck randomized to receive recombinant erythropoietin had a statistically significant increase in likelihood of tumor progression during the duration of the study. This finding is being evaluated by the FDA and warrants serious attention.

Epoetin alfa has been used perioperatively to treat anemia and reduce the need for transfusion. Patients undergoing elective orthopedic and cardiac procedures have been treated with 150 to 300 units/kg of epoetin alfa once daily for the 10 days preceding surgery, on the day of surgery, and for 4 days after surgery. As an alternative, 600 units/kg can be given on days 21, 14, and 7 before surgery, with an additional dose on the day of surgery. This can correct a moderately severe preoperative anemia (i.e., hematocrit 30 to 36%) and reduce the need for transfusion. Epoetin alfa also has been used to improve autologous blood donation. However, the potential benefit generally is small, and the expense is considerable. Patients treated for 3 to 4 weeks with epoetin alfa (300 to 600 units/kg twice a week) are able to donate only one or two more units than untreated patients, and most of the time this goes unused. Still, the ability to stimulate erythropoiesis for blood storage can be invaluable in the patient with multiple alloantibodies to red blood cells.

Epoetin alfa has received orphan drug status from the FDA for the treatment of the anemia of prematurity, HIV infection, and myelodysplasia. In the latter case, even very high doses or more than 1000 units/kg two to three times a week have had limited success. The utility of very high-dose therapy in other hematological disorders, such as sickle cell anemia, still is under study. Highly competitive athletes have used **epoetin alfa** to increase their hemoglobin levels ("**blood doping**") and improve performance.

EPOETIN ALFA

(Erythropoietin) (Epogen, Procrit)

Epoetin alfa, a glycoprotein with antianemic effects (50 to 100 units/kg three times weekly), is used to treat anemia associated with chronic renal failure and anemia related to zidovudine therapy in patients infected with HIV (see Figures 46 and 47).

EPOPROSTENOL SODIUM

(Flolan powder for reconstitution)

Epoprostenol is a peripheral vasodilator, with a direct vasodilation of pulmonary and systemic arterial vascular beds; and inhibition of platelet aggregation. It is indicated in long-term IV treatment of primary pulmonary hypertension.

EPROSARTAN MESYLATE

(Teveten tablets 400 mg)

Eprosartan is an angiotensin II-receptor antagonist, which antagonizes the effect of angiotensin II (vasoconstriction and aldosterone secretion) by blocking the angiotensin II receptor (AT_1 receptor) in vascular smooth muscle and the adrenal gland, producing decreased BP.

Pulmonary hypertension is a rare idiopathic disease that mainly affects young adults. It leads to right-sided heart failure and frequently is fatal. Long-term therapy with PGI_2 (**epoprostenol**, Flolan) has either delayed or precluded the need for lung or heart–lung transplantation in a number of patients. In addition, many affected individuals have had a marked improvement in symptoms after receiving treatment

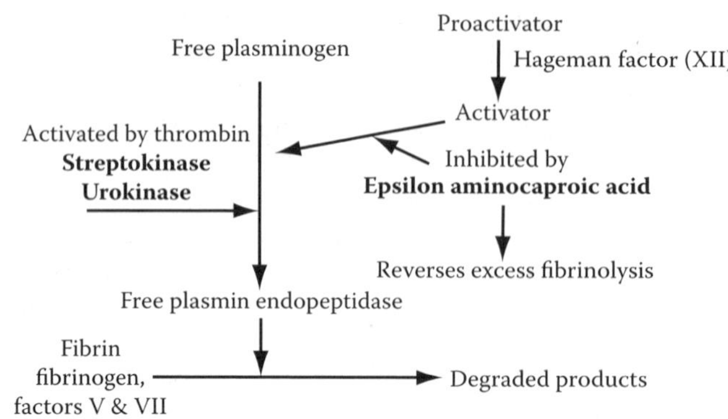

FIGURE 45 The effects of streptokinase or urokinase may be counteracted by **epsilon-aminocaproic acid**.

with PGI_2. **Epoprostenol** also has been used successfully to treat portopulmonary hypertension that arises secondary to liver disease, again with a goal of facilitating ultimate transplantation. The angiotensin II-receptor blockers (ARBs) available for clinical use bind to the AT_1 receptor with high affinity and generally are more selective for the AT_1 receptor. The rank-order affinity of the AT_1 receptor for ARBs is **candesartan** = **omesartan** > **irbesartan** = **eprosartan** > **telmisartan** = **valsartan** = EXP 3174 (the active metabolite of losartan) > **losartan**. Although binding of ARBs to the AT_1 receptor is competitive, the inhibition by ARBs of biological responses to angiotensin II often is insurmountable; i.e., the maximal response to angiotensin II cannot be restored in the presence of the ARB regardless of the concentration of angiotensin II added to the experimental preparation. Of the currently available ARBs, candesartan suppresses the maximal response to angiotensin II the most, whereas insurmountable blockade by irbesartan, **eprosartan**, telmisartan, and valsartan is less. Although losartan antagonism is surmountable, its active metabolite, EXP 3174, causes some degree of insurmountable blockade. The mechanism of insurmountable antagonism by ARBs may be due to slow dissociation kinetics of the compounds from the AT_1 receptor; however, a number of other factors may contribute, such as ARB-induced receptor internalization and alternative binding sites for ARBs on the AT_1 receptor. Regardless of the mechanism, insurmountable antagonism has the theoretical advantage of sustained receptor blockade even with increased levels of endogenous ligand and with missed doses of drug. Whether this theoretical advantage translates into an enhanced clinical performance remains to be determined.

Eprosartan (Teveten): Peak plasma levels are obtained approximately 1 to 2 hours after oral administration, and the plasma half-life ranges from 5 to 9 hours. **Eprosartan** is metabolized in part to the glucuronide conjugate, and the parent compound and its glucuronide conjugate are cleared by renal elimination and biliary excretion. The plasma clearance of **eprosartan** is affected by both renal insufficiency and hepatic insufficiency. The recommended dosage of eprosartan is 400 to 800 mg/day in one or two doses.

EPSILON-AMINOCAPROIC ACID

Fibrinolysis takes place according to the scheme depicted in Figure 45. Plasmin, an endopeptide that is converted from plasminogen by an activator, hydrolyzes fibrin, fibrinogen, factor V, and factor VIII to their inactive products. Hageman factor (factor XII) converts a proactivator to the active activator. Agents such as thrombin, streptokinase, and urokinase therefore enhance the formation of plasmin and hence have fibrinolytic properties. Epsilon-aminocaproic acid inhibits the activator-mediated formation of plasmin and hence may be used as an antidote to streptokinase-urokinase, or in a defibrination syndrome when bleeding from a mucous membrane occurs (Figure 45).

EPTIFIBATIDE

(Integrilin injection for solution 0.75 mg/mL)

Eptifibatide is a glycoprotein IIb/IIIa inhibitor that inhibits platelet aggregation by preventing the binding of fibrinogen, von Willebrand factor, and other adhesive ligands to glycoprotein IIb/IIIa. It is indicated in the treatment of acute coronary syndrome, including patients managed medically and those undergoing percutaneous coronary intervention (PCI); treatment of PCI, including patients undergoing intracoronary stenting.

Antianginal agents may provide prophylactic or symptomatic treatment, but β-adrenergic-receptor antagonists also reduce mortality apparently by decreasing the incidence of sudden cardiac death associated with myocardial ischemia and infarction. The treatment of cardiac risk factors can reduce the progression or even lead to the regression of atherosclerosis. Aspirin is used routinely in patients with myocardial ischemia, and daily aspirin use reduces the incidence of clinical events. Other antiplatelet agents such as oral **clopidogrel** and intravenous antiintegrin drugs such as **abciximab**, **tirofiban**, and **eptifibatide** have been shown to reduce morbidity in patients with angina who undergo coronary artery stenting. Lipid-lowering drugs such as the statins reduce mortality in patients with hypercholesterolemia with or without known coronary artery disease. ACE inhibitors also reduce mortality in patients with coronary disease. Coronary artery bypass surgery and percutaneous coronary interventions such as angioplasty and coronary artery stent deployment can complement pharmacological treatment. In some subsets of patients, percutaneous or surgical revascularization may have a survival advantage over medical treatment alone. Intracoronary drug delivery using drug-eluting coronary stents represents an intersection of mechanical and pharmacological approaches in the treatment of coronary artery disease. Novel therapies that modify the expression of vascular or myocardial cell genes eventually may become an important part of the therapy of ischemic heart disease.

Eptifibatide: Eptifibatide (integrilin) is a cyclic peptide inhibitor of the fibrinogen binding site on $\alpha_{IIB}\beta_3$. It blocks platelet aggregation *in vitro* after intravenous infusion into patients. Eptifibatide is given as a bolus of 180 μg/kg followed by 2 μg/kg per minute for up to 96 hours. It is used to treat acute coronary syndrome and for angioplastic coronary interventions. In the latter case, myocardial infarction and death have been reduced by about 20%. Although the drug has not been compared directly to abciximab, it appears that its benefit is somewhat less than that obtained with the antibody, perhaps because eptifibatide is specific for $\alpha_{IIB}\beta_3$ and does not react with the vitronectin receptor. The duration of action of the drug is relatively short, and platelet aggregation is restored within 6 to 12 hours after cessation of infusion. **Eptifibatide** generally is administered in conjunction with aspirin and heparin.

The major side effect is bleeding, as is the case with abciximab. The frequency of major bleeding in trials was about 10%, compared with about 9% in a placebo group, which included heparin. Thrombocytopenia has been seen in 0.5 to 1% of patients.

Tirofiban: Tirofiban (Aggrastat), a nonpeptide, small-molecule inhibitor of $\alpha_{IIB}\beta_3$, appears to have a similar mechanism of action as **eptifibatide**. Tirofiban has a short duration of action and has efficacy in non-Q-wave myocardial infarction and unstable angina. Reductions in death and myocardial infarction have been about 20% compared to placebo, results similar to those with eptifibatide. Side effects also are similar to those of **eptifibatide**. The agent is specific to $\alpha_{IIB}\beta_3$ and does not react with the vitronectin receptor. Metaanalysis of trials using $\alpha_{IIB}\beta_3$ inhibitors suggests that their value in antiplatelet therapy after acute myocardial infarction is limited. Tirofiban is administered intravenously at an initial rate of 0.4 μg/kg per minute for 30 minutes, and then continued at 0.1 mg/kg per minute for 12 to 24 hours after angioplasty or atherectomy. It is used in conjunction with heparin.

ERECTILE DYSFUNCTION: Treatment of

Erectile dysfunction (ED) is a condition defined by the inability to attain or maintain penile erection sufficient for satisfactory sexual intercourse. In 1995, it was estimated that approximately 152 million men worldwide suffered from ED, with projections for 2025 growing to a prevalence of 322 million affected men. In the past, ED was believed to be caused by nonspecific psychological causes; however, in the past two decades, the majority of cases have been attributed to an organic etiology. Although ED patients can have a number of medical conditions, organic ED is usually associated with vascular risk factors such as arteriosclerosis, hypertension, diabetes mellitus, Peyronie's disease, and renal disease. In addition, pelvic trauma and pelvic surgery (radical prostatectomy or radical cystectomy) can cause ED by either vascular or nerve damage.

Since the early 1980s, understanding about the pharmacology of the erectile mechanism has advanced significantly. Basic research in corporal cavernosal smooth-muscle (CCSM) physiology and identification of the central mediators involved in the erectile process has contributed to the development of pharmacological agents that can effectively treat ED patients. At present, the diagnosis and treatment of ED has evolved to the point where virtually every patient suffering from ED can be successfully treated. Vacuum erection devices, intracavernosal injection therapy, intraurethral suppositories, oral medications, penile vascular procedures, and surgical implantation of prosthetic devices offer most men a viable option to correct their ED. However, despite the overall success and efficacy of the aforementioned therapies, there are implicit side effects, complications, and contraindications. Therefore, the development of future therapeutic options for the treatment of ED should focus on those strategies with fewer adverse effects and an absence of contraindications. Gene therapy for the treatment of ED may become a viable and relatively noninvasive therapeutic option.

Impotence—A variety of endocrine, vascular, neurological, and psychiatric diseases disrupt normal sexual and

Neurologic diseases causing erectile dysfunction are:

Alzheimer's disease	Primary autonomic insufficiency
Amyloidosis	Primary and metastatic tumors
Cerebrovascular accidents	Spinal arachnoiditis
Cervical spondylosis	Spinal cord trauma
Multiple sclerosis	Syphilis
Parkinson's disease	Temporal lobe epilepsy
Pelvic trauma	

Surgical or traumatic causes of erectile dysfunctions are:

Abdominoperineal resection	Penectomy
Aortoiliac surgery	Proctocolectomy
Bilateral orchiectomy	Prostate biopsy
Cystectomy	Prostatectomy; radical or simple
Genital trauma	Renal transplantation
Inguinoscrotal surgery	Retroperitoneal lymphadenectomy
Internal urethrotomy; sphincterotomy	Spinal cord injury
Pelvic fractures	Sympathectomy
Pelvic radiation therapy	

Pharmacological Management of Erectile Dysfunction

Drugs used for intracavernous vasoactive injection therapy

Alprostadil (prostaglandin E_1)	Moxisylyte
Atropine	Multiple-drug mixtures
Calcitonin gene-related peptide	Papaverine
Linsidomine	Phentolamine

Oral pharmacological therapy

Apomorphine	Pentoxifylline (oxpentifylline)
Arginine	Phentolamine
Bromocriptine	Testosterone replacement therapy
Fluoxetine	Trazodone
Naltrexone	Yohimbine

Topical pharmacological therapy

Alprostadil and dinoprostone (prostaglandin E_2)	Nitroglycerin (glyceryl trinitrate)
	Papaverine

Minoxidil

Phosphodiesterase inhibitors (sildenafil, Viagra)

Viagra (sildenafil)—In March 1998, the FDA announced that Viagra®, a new drug from Pfizer, Inc., has been approved as treatment for male sexual dysfunction

Cialis (tadalafil)—Works fast, within 30 min in some patients, and can work up to 36 hours

Vardenafil (Levitra)—This is an FDA-approval oral prescription medication for the treatment of ED in men

Cyclic AMP activators (vasoactive intestinal polypeptide)

reproductive function in men. Furthermore, sexual dysfunction may be the presenting symptom of systemic disease. Cells in the corpus cavernosum produce NO (nitrous oxide) during sexual arousal in response to nonadrenergic, noncholinergic neurotransmission. NO stimulates the formation of cyclic GMP, which leads to relaxation of smooth muscle of the corpus cavernosum and penile arteries, engorgement of the corpus cavernosum, and erection. The accumulation of cyclic GMP can be enhanced by inhibition of the cyclic GMP-specific phosphodiestrase PDE5 family. **Sildenafil** (**Viagra**) and congeners inhibit PDE5 and have been demonstrated to improve erectile function in patients with erectile dysfunction. Not surprisingly, PDE5 inhibitors have assumed the status of widely used recreational drugs. Since the introduction of sildenafil, two additional PDE5 inhibitors have been developed for use in therapy of erectile dysfunction. **Tadalafil** (Cialis) and **vardenafil** (**Levitra**) share similar therapeutic efficacy and side-effect profiles with sildenafil; tadalafil has a longer time to onset of action and a longer therapeutic half-life than the other PDE5 inhibitors. Sildenafil has been the most thoroughly characterized of these compounds, but all three PDE5 inhibitors are contraindicated for patients taking organic nitrate vasodilators or adrenergic-receptor antagonists.

The side effects of **sildenafil** and other **PDE5 inhibitors** are largely predictable on the basis of their effects on PDE5. Headache, flushing, and rhinitis may be observed, as may dyspepsia owing to relaxation of the lower esophageal sphincter. **Sildenafil** and vardenafil also weakly inhibit PDE6, the enzyme involved in photoreceptor signal transduction, and can produce visual disturbances, most notably changes in the perception of color hue or brightness. **Tadalafil** inhibits PDE11, a widely distributed phosphodiesterase isoform, but the clinical importance of this effect is not clear. The most important toxicity of all these PDE5 inhibitors is hemodynamic. When given alone to men with severe coronary artery disease, these drugs have modest effects on blood pressure, producing less than a 10% fall in systolic, diastolic, and mean systemic pressures, and in pulmonary artery systolic and mean pressures. However, sildenafil, tadalafil, and vardenafil all have a significant and potentially dangerous interaction with organic nitrates, the therapeutic actions of which are mediated via their conversion to NO with resulting increases in cyclic GMP. In the presence of a PDE5 inhibitor, nitrates cause profound increases in cyclic GMP and can produce dramatic reductions in blood pressure. Compared with controls, healthy male subjects pretreated with sildenafil or the other PDE5 inhibitors exhibit a much greater decrease in systolic blood pressure when treated with sublingual **glyceryl trinitrate**, and in many subjects a fall of more than 25 mmHg was detected. This drug class toxicity is the basis for the warning that PDE5 inhibitors should not be prescribed to patients receiving any form of nitrate, and dictates that patients should be questioned about the use of PDE5 inhibitors within 24 hours before nitrates are administered. A period of longer than 24 hours may be needed following administration of a PDE5 inhibitor for safe use of nitrates, especially with tadalafil because of its prolonged half-life. In the event that patients develop significant hypotension following combined administration of sildenafil and a nitrate, fluids and α-adrenergic-receptor agonists, if needed, should be used for support.

Sildenafil, tadalafil, and vardenafil are metabolized via cytochrome P450 (CYP3A4), and their toxicity may be enhanced in patients who receive other substrates of this enzyme, including macrolide and imidazole antibiotics, some statins, and antiretroviral agents. PDE5 inhibitors also may prolong cardiac repolarization by blocking the I_{Kr}. Although these interactions and effects are important clinically, the overall incidence and profile of adverse events observed with PDE5 inhibitors, when used without nitrates, are consistent with the expected background frequency of the same events in the treated population. In patients with coronary artery disease whose exercise capacity indicates that sexual activity is unlikely to precipitate angina and who are not currently taking nitrates, the use of PDE5 inhibitors can be considered. Such therapy needs to be individualized, and appropriate warnings must be given about the risk of toxicity if nitrates are taken subsequently for angina; this drug interaction may persist for approximately 24 hours for sildenafil and vardenafil, and for considerably longer with tadalafil. Alternative nonnitrate antianginal therapy, such as β-adrenergic-receptor antagonists, should be used during these time periods.

ERGOCALCIFEROL

(Vitamin D) (Calciferol, Deltalin, Gelseals, Drisdol, Vitamin D capsules)

Ergocalciferol, a vitamin with antihypocalcemic properties, is indicated in nutritional rickets or osteomalacia (25 to 125 mcg p.o. daily), in familial hypophosphatemia (250 mcg to 1.5 mg p.o. daily), in vitamin D-dependent rickets (250 mcg to 1.5 mg p.o. daily), and in hypoparathyroidism (625 mcg to 5 mg p.o. daily) (see also Figure 105).

ERGOLOID MESYLATES (DIHYDROERGOTOXINE)

(Gerimal tablets, oral 1 mg)

Ergoloid is a psychotherapeutic that enhances cerebral blood flow. It is indicated in the treatment of age-related decline in mental capacity, primary progressive dementia, Alzheimer dementia, multi-infarct dementia, and senile onset.

ERGONOVINE MALEATE

(Ergotrate tablets 0.2 mg)

Ergonovine is a uterine stimulant that increases strength, duration, and frequency of uterine contractions and decreases uterine bleeding. It is indicated in prevention and treatment of postpartum and postabortal hemorrhage caused by uterine atony.

The ergot alkaloids can all be considered to be derivatives of the tetracyclic compound 6-methylergoline. The naturally occurring alkaloids contain a substituent in the beta configurations at position 8 and a double bond in ring D. The natural alkaloids of therapeutic interest are amide derivatives of *d*-lysergic acid. The first pure ergot alkaloid, ergotamine, was obtained in 1920, followed by the isolation of ergonovine in 1932. Numerous semisynthetic derivatives of the ergot alkaloids have been prepared by catalytic hydrogenation of the natural alkaloids, e.g., dihydroergotamine. Another synthetic derivative, bromocriptine (2-bromo-α-ergocryptine), is used to control the secretion of prolactin, a property derived from its dopamine agonist effect. Other products of this series include lysergic acid diethylamide (LSD), a potent hallucinogenic drug, and methysergide, a serotonin antagonist.

The oral administration of ergotamine by itself generally results in low or undetectable systemic drug concentrations because of extensive first-pass metabolism. Bioavailability after sublingual administration probably is less than 1% and is inadequate for therapeutic purposes. The bioavailability after administration of rectal suppositories is greater. Ergotamine is metabolized in the liver by largely undefined pathways, and 90% of the metabolites are excreted in the bile. Only traces of unmetabolized drug are found in urine and feces. Despite a plasma half-life of approximately 2 hours, ergotamine produces vasoconstriction that lasts for 24 hours or longer. Dihydroergotamine is eliminated more rapidly than ergotamine, presumably due to its rapid hepatic clearance.

Ergonovine and methylergonovine are rapidly absorbed after oral administration and reach peak concentrations in plasma within 60 to 90 minutes that are more than tenfold those achieved with an equivalent dose of ergotamine. A uterotonic effect in postpartum women can be observed within 10 minutes after oral administration of 0.2 mg of ergonovine. Judging from the relative durations of action, ergonovine is metabolized and/or eliminated more rapidly than ergotamine. The half-life of methylergonovine in plasma ranges between 0.5 and 2 hours.

The multiple pharmacological effects of ergot alkaloids have complicated the determination of their precise mechanism of action in the acute treatment of migraine. Based on the mechanism of action of sumatriptan and other $5\text{-HT}_{1B/1D}$-receptor agonists, the actions of ergot alkaloids at $5\text{-HT}_{1B/1D}$ receptors likely mediate their acute antimigraine effects. The ergot derivative methysergide, which acts more commonly as a 5-HT-receptor antagonist, has been used for the prophylactic treatment of migraine headaches and is discussed in the following text, in the section on 5-HT-receptor antagonists.

The use of ergot alkaloids for migraine should be restricted to patients having frequent, moderate migraine or infrequent, severe migraine attacks. As with other medications used to abort an attack, the patient should be advised to take ergot preparations as soon as possible after the onset of a headache. Gastrointestinal absorption of ergot alkaloids is erratic, perhaps contributing to the large variation in patient response to these drugs. Accordingly, available preparations currently in the United States include sublingual tablets of **ergotamine tartrate** (Ergomar) and a nasal spray and solution for injection of **dihydroergotamine mesylate** (Migranal and D.H.E. 45, respectively). The recommended dose for ergotamine tartrate is 2 mg sublingually, which can be repeated at 30-minute intervals if necessary up to a total dose of 6 mg in a 24-hour period, or 10 mg a week. Dihydroergotamine mesylate injections can be given intravenously, subcutaneously, or intramuscularly. The recommended dose is 1 mg, which can be repeated after 1 hour if necessary up to a total dose of 2 mg (intravenously) or 3 mg (subcutaneously or intramuscularly) in a 24-hour period, or 6 mg in a week. The dose of dihydroergotamine mesylate administered as a nasal spray is 0.5 mg (one spray) in each nostril, repeated after 15 minutes for a total dose of 2 mg (4 sprays). The safety of more than 3 mg over 24 hours or 4 mg over 7 days has not been established.

Nausea and vomiting, due to a direct effect on CNS emetic centers, occur in approximately 10% of patients after oral administration of ergotamine, and in about twice that number after parenteral administration. This side effect is problematic because nausea and sometimes vomiting are part of the symptomatology of a migraine headache. Leg weakness is common, and muscle pains that occasionally are severe may occur in the extremities. Numbness and tingling of fingers and toes are other reminders of the ergotism that this alkaloid may cause. Precordial distress and pain suggestive of angina pectoris, as well as transient tachycardia or bradycardia, also have been noted, presumably as a result of coronary vasospasm induced by ergotamine. Localized edema and itching may occur in an occasional hypersensitive patient, but usually do not necessitate interruption of ergotamine therapy. In the event of acute or chronic poisoning (ergotism), treatment consists of complete withdrawal of the offending drug and symptomatic measures. The latter include attempts to maintain adequate circulation by agents such as anticoagulants, low-molecular-weight dextran, and potent vasodilator drugs, such as intravenous sodium nitroprusside. Dihydroergotamine has lower potency than ergotamine as an emetic and as a vasoconstrictor and oxytocic.

Ergot alkaloids are contraindicated in women who are or may become pregnant, because the drugs may cause fetal distress and miscarriage. Ergot alkaloids also are contraindicated in patients with peripheral vascular disease, coronary artery disease, hypertension, impaired hepatic or renal function, and sepsis. Ergot alkaloids should not be taken within 24 hours of the use of the triptans, and should not be used concurrently with other drugs that can cause vasoconstriction.

All of the natural ergot alkaloids markedly increase the motor activity of the uterus. After small doses, contractions are increased in force or frequency, or both, but are followed by a normal degree of relaxation. As the dose is increased, contractions become more forceful and prolonged, resting tone is dramatically increased, and sustained contracture can result. Although this characteristic precludes their use for induction or facilitation of labor, it is quite compatible with their use postpartum or after abortion to control bleeding and maintain uterine contraction. The gravid uterus is very sensitive, and small doses of ergot alkaloids can be given immediately postpartum to obtain a marked uterine response, usually without significant side effects. In current obstetric practice, ergot alkaloids are used primarily to prevent postpartum hemorrhage. Although all natural ergot alkaloids have qualitatively the same effect on the uterus, **ergonovine** is the most active, and also is less toxic than ergotamine. For these reasons, ergonovine and its semisynthetic derivative methylergonovine have replaced other ergot preparations as uterine-stimulating agents in obstetrics.

ERGONOVINE MALEATE

(Ergotrate)

Ergonovine (0.2 mg IM) is indicated in prevention and treatment of postpartum and postabortal hemorrhage. It exerts its effects by acting as a partial agonist or antagonist at alpha-adrenergic, dopaminergic, or tryptaminergic receptors. The onset of action of ergonovine is 40 seconds, and 7 to 8 minutes when given intravenously or intramuscularly. Inappropriate uses of ergonovine in higher-than-therapeutic concentrations may cause impairment of the uteroplacental blood flow, uterine rupture, cervical and perineal laceration, and trauma to the infant.

ERGOT ALKALOIDS

Bromocriptine, used in Parkinson's disease
Dihydroergotamine
Ergotamine
Methylergonovine
Methysergide, used in headaches

Ergot alkaloids have complex and diverse actions. For example, the marked effects of ergotamine on the cardiovascular system are due to vasoconstriction, depression of vasomotor centers, and peripheral adrenergic blockade.

ERGOTAMINE TARTRATE

(Ergomar, Ergostat, Medihaler-Ergotamine, Wigrettes)

Ergotamine, an ergot alkaloid (2 mg sublingually), is used to prevent or abort vascular headache, including migraine and cluster headaches (see also Figure 93).

ERLOTINIB

(Tarceva tablets 25 mg)

Erlotinib is an epidermal growth factor receptor inhibitor that inhibits intracellular phosphorylation of tyrosine kinase associated with the epidermal growth factor receptor. It is indicated in the treatment of locally advanced or metastatic non-small-cell lung cancer after failure of at least 1 prior chemotherapy regimen. **Erlotinib** (Tarceva) is a human HER1/EGFR tyrosine kinase inhibitor with the following chemical formula: *N*-(3-ethynylphenyl)-6,7-bis(2-methoxyethoxy)-4-quinazolinamine. It is indicated in treatment of patients with locally advanced or metastatic non-small-cell lung cancer.

Erlotinib is about 60% absorbed after oral administration, and its bioavailability is substantially increased to almost 100% by food. Peak plasma levels occur 4 hours after an oral dose. Following absorption, erlotinib is approximately 93% protein-bound to albumin and α_1-acid glycoprotein. Its half-life is ~36 hours. **Erlotinib** is metabolized primarily by CYP3A4 and, to a lesser extent, by CYP1A2 and CYP1A1.

The most common adverse reactions in patients receiving **erlotinib** were diarrhea and rash. Serious interstitial lung disease also has been reported. Other adverse effects include elevated liver enzymes and bleeding, especially in patients receiving warfarin. Coadministration of CYP3A4 inhibitors is expected to increase toxicity to **erlotinib**.

ERTAPENEM

(Invanz powder, lyophilized 1.046 g ertapenem sodium (equivalent to 1 g ertapenem))

Ertapenem is a carbapenem that inhibits cell wall synthesis. It is indicated in the treatment of moderate to severe complicated intra-abdominal infections, complicated skin and skin structure infections, community-acquired pneumonia, complicated urinary tract infections (UTIs) (including pyelonephritis), and acute pelvic infections (including postpartum endomyometritis, septic abortion, and postsurgical gynecologic infections) caused by susceptible microorganisms.

Aztreonam (Azactam) is a monocyclic β-lactam compound (a monobactam) isolated from *Chromobacterium violaceum*.

Ertapenem (Invanz) differs from imipenem and meropenem by having a larger serum half-life that allows once-daily dosing and by having inferior activity against *P. aeruginosa* and *Acinetobacter* spp. Its spectrum of activity against Gram-positive organisms, Enterobacteriaceae, and anaerobes makes it attractive for use in intra-abdominal and pelvic infections.

Aztreonam interacts with penicillin-binding proteins of susceptible microorganisms and induces the formation of long filamentous bacterial structures. The compound is resistant to many of the β-lactamases that are elaborated by most Gram-negative bacteria. The antimicrobial activity of aztreonam differs from those of other β-lactam antibiotics and more closely resembles that of an aminoglycoside. Aztreonam has activity only against Gram-negative bacteria; it has no activity against Gram-positive bacteria and anaerobic organisms. However, activity against Enterobacteriaceae is excellent, as is that against *P. aeruginosa*. It is also highly active *in vitro* against *H. influenzae* and gonococci.

ERYTHRITYL TETRANITRATE

(Cardilate)

Erythrityl tetranitrate (5 to 10 mg sublingually) is used for prophylaxis and long-term treatment of frequent or recurrent angina pain and in reduced exercise tolerance associated with angina pectoris (see Nitroglycerin) (see Figures 69 and 70).

ERYTHROMYCIN

(Akne-mycin ointment 2%, E.E.S. 200 suspension 200 mg per 5 mL as ethylsuccinate, E.E.S. 400 tablets 400 mg as ethylsuccinate)

Erythromycin is a macrolide/ophthalmic/otic/topical antibiotic that interferes with microbial protein synthesis.

Indications

Oral/IV use: for treatment of infections of the respiratory tract, skin and skin structure, and STDs caused by susceptible organisms; treatment of pertussis, diphtheria, erythrasima, intestinal amebiasis, conjunctivitis of the newborn, Legionnaires' disease, listeriosis, nongonococcal urethritis, pneumonia of infancy, urogenital infections during pregnancy; treatment of acute pelvic inflammatory disease, syphilis, uncomplicated urethral, endocervical, or rectal infections in adults; prevention of attacks of rheumatic fever; prevention of bacterial endocarditis.

Ophthalmic use: for treatment of superficial ocular infections caused by strains of susceptible organisms; and prophylaxis of neonatal conjunctivitis.

Topical use: for treatment of acne vulgaris.

Motilin is a 22-amino acid peptide hormone found in the gastrointestinal (GI) M cells, as well as in some enterochromaffin cells of the upper small bowel. Motilin is a potent contractile agent of the upper GI tract. Its levels fluctuate in association with the migrating motor complex and appear to be responsible for the amplification, if not the actual induction, of phase III activity. In addition, motilin receptors are found on smooth-muscle cells and enteric neurons. The effects of motilin can be mimicked by **erythromycin**, a discovery that arose from the frequent occurrence of GI side effects with the use of this antibiotic. This property is shared to varying extents by other macrolide antibiotics, including **oleandomycin**, **azithromycin**, and **clarithromycin**. In addition to its motilin-like effects, which are most pronounced at higher doses (250 to 500 mg), **erythromycin** at lower doses (e.g., 40 to 80 mg) also may act by other poorly defined mechanisms that may involve cholinergic facilitation.

Erythromycin induces phase III migrating motor complex activity in dogs and increases smooth-muscle contractility. It has multiple effects on upper GI motility, increasing lower esophageal pressure and stimulating gastric and small-bowel contractility. By contrast, it has little or no effect on colonic motility. At doses higher than 3 mg/kg, it can produce a spastic type of contraction in the small bowel, resulting in cramps, impairment of transit, and vomiting.

The best-established use of **erythromycin** as a prokinetic agent is in patients with diabetic gastroparesis, where it can improve gastric emptying in the short term. **Erythromycin**-stimulated gastric contractions can be intense and result in "dumping" of relatively undigested food into the small bowel. This potential disadvantage can be exploited clinically to clear the stomach of undigestible residue such as plastic tubes or bezoars. Anecdotally, erythromycin also has been of benefit in patients with small-bowel dysmotility such as that seen in scleroderma, ileus, or pseudo-obstruction. Rapid development of tolerance to **erythromycin**, possibly by downregulation of the motilin receptor, and undesirable (in this context) antibiotic effects have limited the use of this drug as a prokinetic agent. Several nonantibiotic synthetic analogs of erythromycin and peptide analogs of motilin have been developed; to date, the clinical results have been disappointing.

A standard dose of **erythromycin** for gastric stimulation is 3 μg/kg intravenously or 200 to 250 mg orally every 8 hours. For small-bowel stimulation, a smaller dose (e.g., 40 mg intravenously) may be more useful, as higher doses may actually retard motility of this organ.

Erythromycin was discovered in 1952 in the metabolic products of a strain of *Streptomyces erythreus*. **Clarithromycin** and **azithromycin** are semisynthetic derivatives of erythromycin. Macrolide antibiotics contain a many-membered lactone ring (14-membered rings for **erythromycin** and clarithromycin, and a 15-membered ring for azithromycin) to which are attached one or more deoxy sugars. Clarithromycin differs from erythromycin only by methylation of the hydroxyl group at the 6 position, and azithromycin differs by the addition of a methyl-substituted nitrogen atom into the lactone ring. These structural modifications improve acid stability and tissue penetration and broaden the spectrum of activity.

Erythromycin usually is bacteriostatic but may be bactericidal in high concentrations against very susceptible organisms. The antibiotic is most active *in vitro* against aerobic Gram-positive cocci and bacilli. Susceptible strains of *S. pyogenes, S. pneumoniae*, and viridans streptococci have MICs that range from 0.015 to 1 μg/mL. Macrolide resistance is common among streptococci. Because the mechanisms producing resistance to erythromycin affect all macrolides, cross-resistance among them is complete. The prevalence of macrolide resistance among group A streptococcal isolates, which can be as high as 40%, is related to consumption of macrolide antibiotics within the population. Macrolide resistance among *S. pneumoniae* often coexists with penicillin resistance. Only 5% of penicillin-susceptible strains are macrolide resistant, whereas 50% or more of penicillin-resistant strains may be macrolide resistant. Staphylococci are not reliably sensitive to **erythromycin**.

Macrolide antibiotics are bacteriostatic agents that inhibit protein synthesis by binding reversibly to 50S ribosomal subunits of sensitive microorganisms at or very near the site that binds chloramphenicol (Figure 88). **Erythromycin** does not inhibit peptide bond formation *per se*, but rather inhibits the translocation step wherein a newly synthesized peptidyl tRNA molecule moves from the acceptor site on the ribosome to the peptidyl donor site. Gram-positive bacteria accumulate about 100 times more **erythromycin** than do Gram-negative bacteria. Cells are considerably more permeable to the unionized form of the drug, which probably explains the increased antimicrobial activity at alkaline pH.

Erythromycin is cross resistant to clindamycin and streptogramin B (quinupristin). Gram-positive bacilli also are sensitive to erythromycin; typical MICs are 1 μg/mL for *Clostridium perfringens*, from 0.2 to 3 μg/mL for *Corynebacterium diphtheriae*, and from 0.25 to 4 μg/mL for *Listeria monocytogenes.*

Erythromycin is inactive against most aerobic enteric Gram-negative bacilli. It has modest activity *in vitro* against other Gram-negative organisms, including *H. influenzae* (MIC, 1 to 32 μg/mL) and *N. meningitidis* (MIC, 0.4 to 1.6 μg/mL), and good activity against most strains of *N. gonorrhoeae* (MIC, 0.12 to 2 μg/mL). Useful antibacterial activity also is observed against *Pasteurella multocida, Borrelia* spp., and *Bordetella pertussis*. Resistance is common for *B. fragilis* (the MIC ranging from 2 to 32 μg/mL). Macrolides are usually active against *Campylobacter jejuni* (MIC, 0.5 to 4 μg/mL). **Erythromycin** is active against *M. pneumoniae* (MIC, 0.004 to 0.02 μg/mL) and *Legionella pneumophila* (MIC, 0.01 to 2 μg/mL). Most strains of *C. trachomatis* are inhibited by 0.06 to 2 μg/mL of **erythromycin**. Some of the atypical mycobacteria, including *M. scrofulaceum*, are sensitive to erythromycin *in vitro*; *M. kansasii* and *M. avium-intracellulare* vary in sensitivity. *M. fortuitum* is resistant. Macrolides have no effect on viruses, yeasts, or fungi.

Clarithromycin is slightly more potent than erythromycin against sensitive strains of streptococci and staphylococci, and has modest activity against *H. influenzae* and *N. gonorrhoeae*. It has good activity against *M. catarrhalis, Chlamydia* spp., *L. pneumophila, B. burgdorferi, Mycoplasma pneumoniae*, and *H. pylori.*

Azithromycin generally is less active than **erythromycin** against Gram-positive organisms, and slightly more active than either erythromycin or clarithromycin against *H. influenzae* and *Campylobacter* spp. Azithromycin is very active against *M. catarrhalis, P. multocida, Chlamydia* spp., *M. pneumoniae, L. pneumophila, B. burgdorferi, Fusobacterium* spp., and *N. gonorrhoeae.*

In general, organisms are considered susceptible to clarithromycin and azithromycin at MICs ≤ 2 μg/mL. An exception is *H. influenzae*, with MIC breakpoints of ≤ 8 μg/mL and ≤ 4 μg/mL for clarithromycin and azithromycin, respectively.

Azithromycin and clarithromycin have enhanced activity against *M. avium-intracellulare*, as well as against some protozoa (e.g., *Toxoplasma gondii*, *Cryptosporidium*, and *Plasmodium* spp.). Clarithromycin has good activity against *Mycobacterium leprae.*

Erythromycin diffuses readily into intracellular fluids, achieving antibacterial activity in essentially all sites except the brain and CSF. Erythromycin penetrates into prostatic fluid, achieving concentrations approximately 40% of those in plasma. Concentrations in middle ear exudate reach only 50% of serum concentrations, and thus may be inadequate for the treatment of otitis media caused by *H. influenzae.* Protein binding is approximately 70 to 80% for erythromycin base and even higher, 96%, for the estolate. **Erythromycin** traverses the placenta, and drug concentrations in fetal plasma are about 5 to 20% of those in the maternal circulation. Concentrations in breast milk are 50% of those in serum.

Clarithromycin and its active metabolite, 14-hydroxyclarithromycin, distribute widely and achieve high intracellular concentrations throughout the body. Tissue concentrations generally exceed serum concentrations. Concentrations in middle-ear fluid are 50% higher than simultaneous serum concentrations for clarithromycin and the active metabolite. Protein binding of clarithromycin ranges from 40 to 70% and is concentration dependent.

Azithromycin's unique pharmacokinetic properties include extensive tissue distribution and high drug concentrations within cells (including phagocytes), resulting in much greater concentrations of drugs in tissue or secretions compared to simultaneous serum concentrations Tissue fibroblasts act as the natural reservoir for the drug *in vivo.* Protein binding is 50% at very low plasma concentrations and less at higher concentrations. Only 2 to 5% of orally administered erythromycin is excreted in active form in the urine; this value is from 12 to 15% after intravenous infusion. The antibiotic is concentrated in the liver and is excreted in the bile, which may contain as much as 250 μg/mL when serum concentrations are very high. The serum elimination half-life of erythromycin is approximately 1.6 hours. Although the half-life may be prolonged in patients with anuria, dosage reduction is not routinely recommended in renal-failure patients. The drug is not removed significantly by either peritoneal dialysis or hemodialysis.

Depending on the nature and severity of the infection, the usual oral dose of erythromycin (erythromycin base; E-Mycin, others) for adults ranges from 1 to 2 g per day, in equally divided and spaced amounts, usually given every 6 hours. Daily doses of erythromycin as large as 8 g orally, given for 3 months, have been well tolerated. Food should not be taken concurrently, if possible, with erythromycin base or the stearate formulations, but this is not necessary with **erythromycin estolate** or **erythromycin ethylsuccinate** (E.E.S., others). The oral dose of erythromycin for children is 30 to 50 mg/kg per day, divided into four portions; this dose may be doubled for severe infections. Intramuscular administration of erythromycin is not recom-mended because of pain upon injection. Intravenous administration is generally reserved for the therapy of severe infections, such as legionellosis. The usual dose is 0.5 to 1 g every 6 hours; 1 g of erythromycin gluceptate has been given intravenously every 6 hours for as long as 4 weeks with no adverse effects except for thrombophlebitis at the site of injection. **Erythromycin lactobionate** (Erythromycin lactobionate-IV) is available for intravenous injection.

A macrolide or tetracycline is the drug of choice for mycoplasma infections. **Erythromycin** reduces the duration of fever caused by *M. pneumoniae* and accelerates the rate of clearing of the chest radiographs. It has been considered as the drug of choice for treatment of pneumonia caused by *L. pneumophila, L. micdadei*, or other *Legionella* spp. Because of excellent *in vitro* activity, superior tissue concentration, the ease of administration as a single daily dose, and better tolerability compared to erythromycin, azithromycin (or a fluoroquinolone) has supplanted erythromycin as the first-line agent for treatment of legionellosis. The recommended dose is 500 mg daily, intravenously or orally, for a total of 10 to 14 days.

Chlamydial infections can be treated effectively with any of the macrolides. A single 1-g dose of azithromycin is recommended for patients with uncomplicated urethral, endocervical, rectal, or epididymal infections because of the ease of compliance. During pregnancy, **erythromycin** base, 500 mg four times daily for 7 days, is recommended as first-line therapy for chlamydial urogenital infections. Azithromycin, 1 g orally as a single dose, is a suitable alternative. **Erythromycin** base is preferred for chlamydial pneumonia of infancy and ophthalmia neonatorum (50 mg/kg per day in four divided doses for 10 to 14 days). Azithromycin, 1 g a week for 3 weeks, may be effective for lymphogranuloma venereum.

Pneumonia caused by *Chlamydia pneumoniae* responds to macrolides, fluoroquinolones, and tetracyclines in standard doses for community-acquired pneumonia. No comparative trials have been conducted to determine which agent, if any, is most efficacious. Duration of therapy also is ill defined. In practice, a specific etiological diagnosis rarely is made, and length of treatment, typically 7 to 10 days, often is determined empirically based on clinical response.

Erythromycin 250 mg four times daily for 7 days is very effective for acute infections or for eradicating the carrier state. The other macrolides also are likely to be effective; because clinical experience with them is lacking, they are not FDA approved for this indication. The presence of an antibiotic does not alter the course of an acute infection with the diphtheria bacillus or the risk of complications. Antitoxin is indicated in the treatment of acute infection.

Erythromycin is the drug of choice for treating persons with *B. pertussis* disease and for postexposure prophylaxis of household members and close contacts. A 7-day regimen of erythromycin estolate (40 mg/kg per day, maximum 1 g/day) is as effective as the 14-day regimens traditionally recommended. Clarithromycin and azithromycin also are effective. If administered early in the course of whooping cough, erythromycin may shorten the duration of illness; it has little influence on the disease once the paroxysmal stage is reached, although it may eliminate the microorganisms from the nasopharynx. Nasopharyngeal cultures should be obtained from people with pertussis who do not improve with erythromycin therapy because resistance has been reported.

Pharyngitis, scarlet fever, erysipelas, and cellulitis caused by *S. pyogenes* and pneumonia caused by *S. pneumoniae* respond to macrolides. They are valuable alternatives for treatment of patients who have a serious allergy to penicillin. Unfortunately, macrolide-resistant strains are increasingly encountered. Penicillin-resistant strains of *S. pneumoniae* also are very likely to be resistant to macrolides.

Erythromycin has been an alternative agent for the treatment of relatively minor infections caused by either penicillin-sensitive or penicillin-resistant *S. aureus*. However, many strains of *S. aureus* are resistant to macrolides, and they no longer can be relied upon unless *in vitro* susceptibility has been documented.

The treatment of gastroenteritis caused by *C. jejuni* with erythromycin (250 to 500 mg orally four times a day for 7 days) hastens eradication of the microorganism from the stools and reduces the duration of symptoms. Availability of fluoroquinolones, which are highly active against *Campylobacter* species and other enteric pathogens, largely has replaced the use of erythromycin for this disease in adults. Erythromycin remains useful for treatment of *Campylobacter* gastroenteritis in children.

Clarithromycin, 500 mg, in combination with omeprazole, 20 mg, and amoxicillin, 1 g, each administered twice daily for 10 to 14 days, is effective for treatment of peptic ulcer disease caused by *H. pylori*. Numerous other regimens, some effective as 7-day treatments, have been studied and also are effective. The more effective regimens generally include three agents, one of which usually is clarithromycin.

Erythromycin (500 mg orally every 6 hours for 10 days) may be given to eradicate *Clostridium tetani* in patients with tetanus who are allergic to penicillin. However, the mainstays of therapy are débridement, physiological support, tetanus antitoxin, and drug control of convulsions.

Erythromycin has been used in the treatment of early syphilis in patients who are allergic to penicillin, but it no longer is recommended. Tetracyclines are the recommended alternative in penicillin-allergic patients. During pregnancy, it is recommended that patients be desensitized to penicillin.

Clarithromycin or azithromycin is recommended as first-line therapy for prophylaxis and treatment of disseminated infection caused by *M. avium-intracellulare* in AIDS patients and for treatment of pulmonary disease in non-HIV-infected patients. Azithromycin (1.2 g once weekly) or clarithromycin (500 mg twice daily) is recommended for primary prevention for AIDS patients with fewer than 50 CD cells per mm^3. Single-agent therapy should not be used for treatment of active disease or for secondary prevention in AIDS patients. Clarithromycin (500 mg twice daily) plus ethambutol (15 mg/kg once daily) with or without rifabutin is an effective combination regimen. Azithromycin (500 mg once daily) may be used instead of clarithromycin, but clarithromycin appears to be slightly more efficacious. Clarithromycin also has been used with minocycline for the treatment of *Mycobacterium leprae* in lepromatous leprosy.

Clarithromycin and azithromycin have been used in the treatment of toxoplasmosis encephalitis and diarrhea due to *Cryptosporidium* in AIDS patients. Rigorous clinical trials demonstrating efficacy of macrolides for these infections are lacking.

Penicillin is the drug of choice for the prophylaxis of recurrences of rheumatic fever. Erythromycin is an effective alternative for individuals who are allergic to penicillin.

Erythromycin has been recommended as an alternative to penicillin in allergic patients for prevention of bacterial endocarditis after dental or respiratory-tract procedures. Clindamycin has replaced erythromycin for use in penicillin-allergic patients. Clarithromycin or azithromycin as a single 500-mg dose also may be used.

Serious untoward effects are rarely caused by erythromycin. Among the allergic reactions observed are fever, eosinophilia, and skin eruptions, which may occur alone or in combination; each disappears shortly after therapy is stopped. Cholestatic hepatitis is the most striking side effect. It is caused primarily by erythromycin estolate and rarely by the ethylsuccinate or the stearate. The illness starts after about 10 to 20 days of treatment and is characterized initially by nausea, vomiting, and abdominal cramps. The pain often mimics that of acute cholecystitis. These symptoms are followed shortly thereafter by jaundice, which may be accompanied by fever, leukocytosis, eosinophilia, and elevated transaminases in plasma. Biopsy of the liver reveals cholestasis, periportal infiltration by neutrophils, lymphocytes, and eosinophils, and occasionally, necrosis of neighboring parenchymal cells. Findings usually resolve within a few days after cessation of drug therapy and rarely are prolonged. The syndrome may represent a hypersensitivity reaction to the estolate ester.

Erythromycin and clarithromycin inhibit CYP3A4 and are associated with clinically significant drug interactions. Erythromycin potentiates the effects of carbamazepine, corticosteroids, cyclosporine, digoxin, ergot alkaloids, theophylline, triazolam, valproate, and warfarin, probably by interfering with CYP-mediated metabolism of these drugs. Clarithromycin, which is structurally related to erythromycin, has a similar drug interaction profile. Azithromycin, which differs from erythromycin and clarithromycin because of its 15-membered lactone 1-g structure, and dirithromycin, which is a longer-acting 14-membered lactone ring analog of **erythromycin** analog, appear to be free of these drug interactions. Caution is advised, nevertheless, when using azithromycin in conjunction with drugs known to interact with erythromycin.

ERYTHROMYCIN/BENZOYL PEROXIDE

(Benzamycin gel 5% benzoyl peroxide, 3% erythromycin)

Erythromycin is a topical treatment of acne vulgaris. Resistant strains of *P. acnes* are emerging that may respond to judicious use of **retinoids** in combination with antibiotics. Commonly used topical antimicrobials in acne include erythromycin, clindamycin (Cleocin-t), and **benzoyl peroxide** and antibiotic-benzoyl peroxide combinations (Benzamycin, Benzaclin, others). Other antimicrobials used in treating acne include sulfacetamide (Klaron), sulfacetamide/sulfur combinations (Sulfacet-R), metronidazole (Metrocream, Metrogel, Noritate), and azelaic acid (Azelex). Systemic therapy is prescribed for patients with more extensive disease and acne that is resistant to topical therapy. Effective agents include tetracycline (Sumycin, others), minocycline (Minocin, others), erythromycin (Eryc, others), clindamycin (Cleocin), and trimethoprim-sulfamethoxazole (Bactrim, others). Antibiotics usually are administered twice daily, and doses are tapered after control is achieved. Tetracycline is the most commonly employed antibiotic because it is inexpensive, safe, and effective. The initial daily dose is usually 1 g in divided doses. Although tetracycline is an antimicrobial agent, its efficacy in acne may be more dependent on its antiinflammatory activity.

ERYTHROMYCIN ETHYLSUCCINATE/SULFISOXAZOLE

(Eryzole granules for oral suspension)

Erythromycin suppresses bacterial protein synthesis; **sulfonamides** interfere with bacterial folic-acid synthesis. This combination is indicated in the treatment of acute otitis media in children caused by susceptible strains of *H. influenzae.*

The sulfonamides may be classified into three groups on the basis of the rapidity with which they are absorbed and excreted: (1) agents that are absorbed and excreted rapidly, such as **sulfisoxazole** and sulfadiazine; (2) agents that are absorbed very poorly when administered orally and hence are active in the bowel lumen, such as sulfasalazine; (3) agents that are used mainly topically, such as sulfacetamide, mafenide, and silver sulfadiazine; and (4) long-acting sulfonamides, such as sulfadoxine, that are absorbed rapidly but excreted slowly.

Sulfisoxazole acetyl is tasteless and hence preferred for oral use in children. **Sulfisoxazole** acetyl is marketed in combination with erythromycin ethylsuccinate (Pediazole, others) for use in children with otitis media. The urine becomes orange-red soon after ingestion of this mixture because of the presence of **phenazopyridine**, an orange-red dye.

Fewer than 0.1% of patients receiving **sulfisoxazole** suffer serious toxic reactions. The untoward effects produced by this agent are similar to those that follow the administration of other sulfonamides. Because of its relatively high solubility in the urine as compared with sulfadiazine, **sulfisoxazole** only infrequently produces hematuria or crystalluria (0.2 to 0.3%). Despite this, patients taking this drug should ingest an adequate quantity of water. **Sulfisoxazole** and all sulfonamides that are absorbed must be used with caution in patients with impaired renal function. Like all sulfonamides, **sulfisoxazole** may produce hypersensitivity reactions, some of which are potentially lethal. Sulfisoxazole currently is preferred over other sulfonamides by most clinicians when a rapidly absorbed and rapidly excreted sulfonamide is indicated.

Sulfamethoxazole is a close congener of sulfisoxazole, but its rates of enteric absorption and urinary excretion are slower. It is administered orally and employed for both systemic and urinary tract infections. Precautions must be observed to avoid sulfamethoxazole crystalluria because of the high percentage of the acetylated, relatively insoluble form of the drug in the urine. The clinical uses of sulfamethoxazole are the same as those for sulfisoxazole. It also is marketed in fixed-dose combinations with trimethoprim.

ERYTHROMYCIN

(Erythocin)

Erythromycin, as a penicillin alternative, is a medium- to broad-spectrum antibiotic. It possesses both bactericidal and bacteriostatic properties, depending on the concentration of the drug being used and the microorganisms being treated. Erythromycin is effective against Gram-positive organisms such as *Streptococcus pyogenes* and *pneumoniae*. In larger doses, it is effective against *Staphylococcus epidermidis* and *aureus*. In addition, Gram-positive bacilli such as *Clostridium perfringens*, *Corynebacterium diphtheriae*, and *Listeria monocytogenes* are also susceptible to erythromycin. It is also effective against *Mycoplasma pneumoniae* and *Legionella pneumophilia*, which causes Legionnaires' disease. Erythromycin exerts its effect by binding to a 23S ribosomal RNA on the 50S ribosomal subunit, and this inhibits protein synthesis. Aminoacyl translocation reactions and elongation of the peptide chain are then blocked (see Figure 88). Resistance occurs from the methylation of ribosomal RNA receptors, preventing the attachment of erythomycin to 50S ribosomes. Erythromycin, which is destroyed by gastric secretions, is supplied as enteric-coated tablets, which are absorbed well from the upper part of the small intestine. Erythromycin stearate is acid resistant. Erythromycin is largely excreted in the bile, and the urinary excretion is negligible. Erythromycin, and especially erythromycin estolate, can cause cholestatic hepatitis.

ERYTHROMYCIN BASE

(E-Mycin, ERYC, Eryfed, Ethril 500, Erythrocin, Erythromycin Base Filmtabs, Robimycin)

ERYTHROMYCIN ESTOLATE

(Ilosone)

ERYTHROMYCIN ETHYLSUCCINATE

(E.E.S., E-Mycin E, EryPed, Pediamycin, Pediazole, Wyamycin E)

ERYTHROMYCIN STEARATE

(Erypar Filmseal, Erythrocin Stearate, Ethril, Wyamycin S)

ERYTHROMYCIN (TOPICAL)

(Akne-Mycin, A/T/S, EryDerm, Erymax, Eryvette, Staticin, T-Stat)

Erythromycin, an antibiotic, is indicated in acute pelvic inflammatory disease caused by *Neisseria gonorrhoeae*; in endocarditis prophylaxis for dental procedures in patients allergic to penicillin, erythromycin base, estolate, or stearate; and in the treatment of intestinal amebiasis in patients who cannot receive metronidazole, erythromycin base, estolate, or stearate. It is used as treatment for mild to moderate severe respiratory tract, skin, and soft-tissue infections caused by susceptible organisms, as well as for syphilis, Legionnaires' disease, uncomplicated urethral, endocervical, or rectal infections when tetracyclines are contraindicated, urogenital *Chlamydia trachomatis* infections during pregnancy, conjunctivitis caused by *C. trachomatis* in neonates, pneumonia of infancy caused by *C. trachomatis*, and topical treatment of acne vulgaris.

ERYTHROPOIETIN

(Procrit)

Hematopoietic stem cells and progenitor cells undergo extensive proliferation and differentiation *in vitro* under the influence of at least eleven hematopoietic growth factors. These include interleukin-1, -3, and -6; interferon alpha, beta, and gamma; and erythropoietin.

Erythropoietin is produced primarily by peritubular cells in the proximal tubule of the kidney. These cells not only produce erythropoietin but also the oxygen sensor that stimulates erythropoietin production (Figure 46). Erythropoietin, which consists of 193 amino acid residues, has a molecular weight of 34,000 and is glycosylated. Its synthesis increases in the presence of anemia and hypoxia.

Erythropoietin is effective in the treatment of anemia associated with chronic renal failure (Figure 47). It is also effective

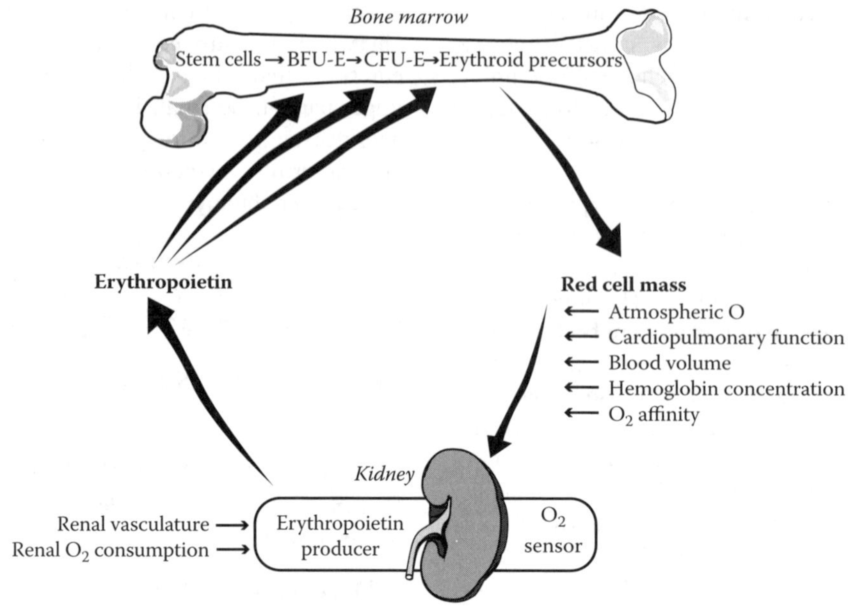

FIGURE 46 Erythropoietin is produced primarily by **peritubular cells** in proximal tubule of the kidney. These cells not only produce erythropoietin but also the **oxygen sensor** that stimulates erythropoietin production.

in managing the anemia seen in patients with AIDS who are being treated with zidovudine (AZT) and the anemia associated with cancer chemotherapy. Patients who are to undergo elective surgery may receive erythropoietin preoperatively to increase red cell production, thus permitting the storage of large volumes of blood for autologous transfusion (see Figure 47).

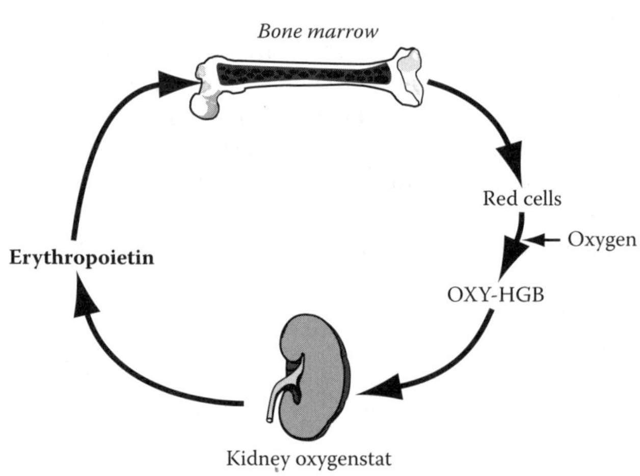

FIGURE 47 Erythropoietin is effective for the treatment of anemia associated with **chronic renal failure**.

ESCITALOPRAM OXALATE

(Lexapro tablets 5 mg)

Escitalopram is a selective serotonin reuptake inhibitor that inhibits the CNS neuronal uptake of serotonin, potentiating serotonergic activity. It is indicated in the major depressive disorders and generalized anxiety.

ESMOLOL

(Brevibloc)

Esmolol is an ultra-short-acting intravenous cardioselective beta-adrenergic-receptor antagonist with a short elimination half-life of 9 minutes. It is used in situations where a brief duration of adrenergic block is required, such as tracheal intubation and stressful surgical stimuli. Esmolol causes hypotension, which is accompanied by diaphoresis (see also Figures 37, 49, 67, and 83). Esmolol, a β_1-adrenergic-blocking agent with antiarrhythmic properties (50 to 200 mcg/kg/min), is indicated in the treatment of intraoperative tachycardia and/or hypertension.

ESMOLOL HYDROCHLORIDE

(Brevibloc injection 10 mg/mL)

Esmolol blocks beta receptors primarily affecting cardiovascular system (e.g., decreases heart rate, contractility, BP) and lungs (promoting bronchospasm). It is indicated in the short-term management of supraventricular tachyarrhythmias and noncompensatory sinus tachycardia.

Esmolol (Brevibloc, others) is a β_1-selective antagonist with a very short duration of action. It has little if any intrinsic sympathomimetic activity, and it lacks membrane-stabilizing actions. **Esmolol** is administered intravenously and is used when β-blockade of short duration is desired, or in critically ill patients in whom adverse effects of bradycardia, heart failure, or hypotension may necessitate rapid withdrawal of the drug.

Esmolol has a half-life of about 8 minutes and an apparent volume of distribution of approximately 2 L/kg. The drug contains an ester linkage, and it is hydrolyzed rapidly by esterases in erythrocytes. The half-life of the carboxylic acid metabolite of **esmolol** is far longer (4 hours), and it accumulates during prolonged infusion of esmolol. However, this metabolite has very low potency as a β-receptor antagonist (1/500 of the potency of esmolol); it is excreted in the urine.

The onset and cessation of β-receptor blockade with esmolol are rapid; peak hemodynamic effects occur within 6 to 10 minutes of administration of a loading dose, and there is substantial attenuation of β-blockade within 20 minutes of stopping an infusion. Esmolol may have striking hypotensive effects in normal subjects, although the mechanism of this effect is unclear.

Because **esmolol** is used in urgent settings where immediate onset of β-blockade is warranted, a partial loading dose typically is administered, followed by a continuous infusion of the drug. If an adequate therapeutic effect is not observed within 5 minutes, the same loading dose is repeated, followed by a maintenance infusion at a higher rate. This process, including progressively greater infusion rates, may need to be repeated until the desired end point (e.g., lowered heart rate or blood pressure) is approached.

ESMOLOL HYDROCHLORIDE

(Brevibloc)

Esmolol is a class II antiarrhythmic agent with ultra-short-acting beta-adrenergic-blocking activity that is used (50 to 200 mcg/kg/minute) to treat supraventricular tachycardia such as atrial fibrillation or atrial flutter. It is rapidly metabolized by erythrocyte esterases via hydrolysis of the methyl ester. Unlike succinylcholine, esmolol is not metabolized by plasma cholinesterase (see also Figures 67 and 83).

ESOMEPRAZOLE

(Nexium capsules, delayed-release 20 mg)

Esomeprazole is a proton-pump inhibitor that suppresses gastric acid secretion by blocking the proton pump within gastric parietal cells. Oral use: for treatment of heartburn and other symptoms of gastroesophageal reflux disease (GERD); short-term treatment in healing and symptomatic resolution of erosive esophagitis; to maintain symptom resolution and healing of erosive esophagitis; in combination with amoxicillin and clarithromycin for treatment of *H. pylori* infection and duodenal ulcer disease to eradicate *H. pylori*, reduction in occurrence of gastric ulcers associated with continuous nonsteroidal antiinflammatory drugs (NSAIDs) therapy in patients at risk of developing gastric ulcers. IV use: as an alternative to oral therapy when oral therapy with esomeprazole delayed-release capsules is not possible or appropriate for the short-term treatment (up to 10 days) of gastroesophageal reflux disease (GERD) in patients with history of erosive esophagitis.

The most potent suppressors of gastric acid secretion are inhibitors of the gastric H^+K^+-ATPase (proton pump). In typical doses, these drugs diminish the daily production of acid (basal and stimulated) by 80 to 95%. Five proton-pump inhibitors are available for clinical use: omeprazole (Prilosec, Rapinex, Zegerid) and its S-isomer, **esomeprazole** (Nexium), **lansoprazole** (Prevacid), **rabeprazole** (Aciphex), and **pantoprazole** (Protonix). These drugs have different substitutions on their pyridine and/or benzimidazole groups but are remarkably similar in their pharmacological properties. Omeprazole is a racemic mixture of R- and S-isomers; the S-isomer, esomeprazole (S-omeprazole), is eliminated less rapidly than R-omeprazole, which theoretically provides a therapeutic advantage because of the increased half-life. Despite claims to the contrary, all proton-pump inhibitors have equivalent efficacy at comparable doses.

Proton-pump inhibitors are prodrugs that require activation in an acid environment. After absorption into the systemic circulation, the prodrug diffuses into the parietal cells of the stomach and accumulates in the acidic secretory canaliculi. Here, it is activated by proton-catalyzed formation of a tetracyclic sulfonamide, trapping the drug so that it cannot diffuse back across the canalicular membrane. The activated form then binds covalently with sulfhydryl groups of cysteines in the H^+K^+-ATPase, irreversibly inactivating the pump molecule. Acid secretion resumes only after new pump molecules are synthesized and inserted into the luminal membrane, providing a prolonged (up to 24- to 48-hour) suppression of acid secretion, despite the much shorter plasma half-lives (0.5 to 2 hours) of the parent compounds. Because they block the final step in acid production, the proton-pump inhibitors are effective in acid suppression regardless of other stimulating factors.

To prevent degradation of proton-pump inhibitors by acid in the gastric lumen, oral dosage forms are supplied in different formulations: (1) enteric-coated drugs contained inside gelatin capsules (omeprazole, **esomeprazole**, and lansoprazole); (2) enteric-coated granules supplied as a powder for suspension (lansoprazole); (3) enteric-coated tablets (pantoprazole, rabeprazole, and omeprazole); and (4) powdered drug combined with sodium bicarbonate (omeprazole). The delayed-release and enteric-coated tablets dissolve only at alkaline pH, whereas the admixture of omeprazole with sodium bicarbonate simply neutralizes stomach acid; both strategies substantially improve the oral bioavailability of these acid-labile drugs. Until recently, the requirement for enteric coating posed a challenge to the administration of proton-pump inhibitors in patients for whom the oral route of administration is not available. These patients and those requiring immediate acid suppression now can be treated parenterally with pantoprazole or lansoprazole, both of which are approved for intravenous administration in the United States. A single intravenous bolus of 80 mg of pantoprazole inhibits acid production by 80 to 90% within an hour, and this inhibition persists for up to 21 hours, permitting once-daily dosing to achieve the desired degree of hypochlorhydria. The PDA-approved dose of intravenous pantoprazole for gastroesophageal reflux disease is 40 mg daily for up to 10 days. Higher doses (e.g., 160 to 240 mg in divided doses) are used to manage hypersecretory conditions such as the **Zollinger–Ellison syndrome**.

An intravenous formulation of esomeprazole is available in Europe but not in the United States.

Proton-pump inhibitors generally cause remarkably few adverse effects. The most common side effects are nausea, abdominal pain, constipation, flatulence, and diarrhea. Subacute myopathy, arthralgias, headaches, and skin rashes also have been reported. As noted previously, proton-pump inhibitors are metabolized by hepatic CYPs and therefore may interfere with the elimination of other drugs cleared by this route. Proton-pump inhibitors have been observed to interact with warfarin (**esomeprazole**, lansoprazole, omeprazole, and rabeprazole), diazepam (esomeprazole and omeprazole), and cyclosporine (omeprazole and rabeprazole). Among the proton-pump inhibitors, only omeprazole inhibits CYP2C19 (thereby decreasing the clearance of disulfiram, phenytoin, and other drugs) and induces the expression of CYP1A2 (thereby increasing the clearance of imipramine, several antipsychotic drugs, tacrine, and theophylline).

Chronic treatment with omeprazole decreases the absorption of vitamin B_{12}, but the clinical relevance of this effect is not clear. Loss of gastric acidity also may affect the bioavailability of such drugs as ketoconazole, ampicillin esters, and iron salts.

Hypergastrinemia is more frequent and more severe with proton-pump inhibitors than with H_2-receptor antagonists, and gastrin levels of >500 ng/L occur in approximately 5 to 10% of users with chronic omeprazole administration. This hypersecretion may predispose patients to rebound hypersecretion of gastric acid upon discontinuation of therapy.

The control of acid-peptic disease represents a major triumph for modern pharmacology. Proton-pump inhibitors are considered superior for acid suppression in most clinically significant acid-peptic diseases, including gastroesophageal reflux disease, peptic ulcers, and NSAID-induced ulcers. Proton-pump inhibitors also are employed in combination with antibiotics to eradicate infection with *H. pylori*, and thereby play a role in preventing recurrent peptic ulcers These agents largely have replaced the use of misoprostol and sucralfate, although the latter still is a low-cost alternative for prophylaxis against stress ulcers. The delay in maximal inhibition of acid secretion with proton-pump inhibitors (3 to 5 days) makes them less suited for use on an as-needed basis for symptom relief. In this setting, H_1-receptor antagonists, while less effective than proton-pump inhibitors in suppressing acid secretion, have a more rapid onset of action that makes them useful for patient-directed management of mild or infrequent symptoms.

ESTAZOLAM

(ProSom tablets 1 mg)

Estazolam is a benzodiazepine that potentiates action of GABA, an inhibitory neurotransmitter, resulting in increased neuronal inhibition and CNS depression, especially in limbic system and reticular formation. It is indicated for the short-term management of insomnia characterized by difficulty in falling asleep, frequent nocturnal awakenings, and/or early-morning awakenings.

The benzodiazepine derivative includes the (1) ultra-short-acting benzodiazepines, (2) short-acting agents, with half-lives less than 6 hours, including **triazolam**, the non-benzodiazepine **zolpidem** (half-life approximately 2 hours), and zopiclone (half-life 5 to 6 hours), (3) intermediate-acting agents, with half-lives of 6 to 24 hours, including **estazolam** and **temazepam**, and (4) long-acting agents, with half-lives greater than 24 hours, including **flurazepam**, **diazepam**, and **quazepam**.

Estazolam (1 mg at bedtime) is indicated for the short-term management of insomnia characterized by difficulty in falling asleep, frequent nocturnal awakening, or early-morning awakenings. Estazolam may cause fetal damage and hence is contraindicated in pregnancy. It causes CNS depression and potentiates the CNS depressant effects of alcohol, and other CNS drugs should be used cautiously whenever alertness and vigilance are required (see also Table 9).

ESTERIFIED ESTROGENS/ METHYLTESTOSTERONE

(Estratest tablets 1.25 mg esterified estrogens and 2.5 mg methyltestosterone)

This is estrogen and androgen combined. **Esterified estrogens**: promote growth and development of female reproductive system and secondary sex characteristics; affect release of pituitary gonadotropins; inhibit ovulation and prevent postpartum breast engorgement; conserve calcium and phosphorous and encourage bone formation; and override stimulatory effects of testosterone. **Methyltestosterone**: promotes growth and development of male reproductive organs; maintains secondary sex characteristics; increases protein anabolism; decreases protein catabolism.

The combination is indicated in the treatment of moderate to severe vasomotor symptoms associated with the menopause in patients not improved by estrogens alone.

ESTERIFIED ESTROGENS

(Estratab, Menest)

Esterified estrogen is used in prostatic cancer (1.25 to 2.5 mg p.o. t.i.d.); in female hypogonadism, ovariectomy, and primary ovarian failure (2.5 mg daily p.o. in a cycle of three weeks on medication and one week medication-free); and in menopausal symptoms (Figure 48).

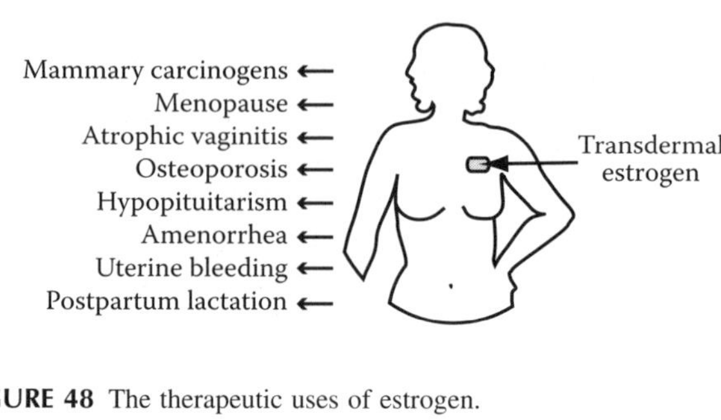

FIGURE 48 The therapeutic uses of estrogen.

ESTRADIOL

(Estrace, Estrace vaginal cream, Estraderm)

ESTRADIOL

(Estraderm)

The estradiol transdermal system is indicated in the treatment of vasomotor symptoms associated with menopause. It is also used to treat female hypogonadism, primary ovarian failure, atrophic conditions (atrophic vaginitis or kraurosis vulvae), and in the prevention of osteoporosis (see Estrogen and Figure 48).

ESTRADIOL CYPIONATE

(Depestro, DepGynogen, Depo-Estradiol Cypionate, Depogen, Dura-Estrin, Estra-D, Estro-cyp, Estrofem, Estroject-L.A., Estronol-L.A., Hormogen Depot)

ESTRADIOL VALERATE

(Dioval, Dioval XX, Dioval 40, Duragen, Estradiol L.A., Estradiol L.A. 20, Estradiol L.A. 40, Estraval Gynogen L.A. 10, Gynogen L.A. 20, L.A.E. 20, Valergen-10, Valergen-20, Valergen-40)

POLYESTRADIOL PHOSPHATE

(Estradurin)

These various estradiol preparations, available in oral, injectable, and cream forms, are used in atrophic vaginitis, atrophic dystrophy of the vulva, menopausal symptoms, hypogonadism, ovariectomy, primary ovarian failure; postpartum breast engorgement; female hypogonadism; inoperable breast cancer; inoperable prostatic cancer; and in advancing prostatic carcinoma deemed inoperable (see also Figure 48).

ESTRADIOL

(Alora transdermal system 0.77 mg)

Estradiol is an estrogen that promotes growth and development of the female reproductive system and secondary sex characteristics; affects release of pituitary gonadotropins; inhibits ovulation and prevents postpartum breast engorgement; conserves calcium and phosphorous and encourages bone formation; overrides stimulatory effects of testosterone.

Estradiol is indicated in the management of moderate to severe vasomotor symptoms associated with menopause, female hypogonadism, female castration, primary ovarian failure, postpartum breast engorgement, and atrophic conditions caused by deficient endogenous estrogen production; atrophic urethritis; palliative treatment of metastatic breast or prostate cancer in selected women and men; prevention and treatment of osteoporosis; abnormal uterine bleeding caused by hormonal imbalance in the absence of organic pathology and only when associated with a hypoplastic or atrophic endometrium.

ESTRADIOL/LEVONORGESTREL

(ClimaraPro transdermal patch estradiol 0.045 mg and levonorgestrel 0.015 mg per day)

Estradiol is estrogen and progestin combined. **Estrogens** are essential in developing and maintaining the female reproductive system and secondary sex characteristics. **Progestins** transform proliferative endometrium into secretory endometrium. The combination is indicated in treatment of moderate to severe vasomotor symptoms associated with menopause.

Conjugated estrogens and medroxyprogesterone acetate (MPA) historically have been used most commonly in menopausal hormone regimens, although estradiol, estrone, and estriol have been used as estrogens, and **norethindrone**, **norgestimate**, **levonorgestrel**, **norethisterone**, and **progesterone** also have been widely used. Various "continuous" or "cyclic" regimens have been used; the latter regimens include drug-free days. An example of a cyclic regimen is as follows: (1) administration of an estrogen for 25 days; (2) the addition of MPA for the last 12 to 14 days of estrogen treatment; and (3) 5 to 6 days with no hormone treatment, during which withdrawal bleeding normally occurs due to breakdown and shedding of the endometrium. Continuous administration of combined estrogen plus progestin does not lead to regular, recurrent endometrial shedding, but may cause intermittent spotting or bleeding, especially in the first year of use. Other regimens include a progestin intermittently (e.g., every third month), but the long-term endometrial safety of these regimens remains to be firmly established. Prempro (conjugated estrogens plus MPA given as a fixed dose daily) and premphase (conjugated estrogens given for 28 days plus MPA given for 14 out of 28 days) are widely used combination formulations. Other combination products available in the United States are ethinyl estradiol plus norethindrone acetate, Activella (estradiol plus norethindrone), and Prefest (estradiol and norgestimate). Doses and regimens are usually adjusted empirically based on control of symptoms, patient acceptance of bleeding patterns, and/or other untoward effects.

Another pharmacological consideration is the route of effects administration. Oral administration exposes the liver to higher concentrations of estrogens than transdermal administration. Either route effectively relieves vasomotor symptoms and protects against bone loss. Oral, but not transdermal estrogen, may increase sex hormone-binding globulin (SHBG), other binding globulins, and angiotensinogen; the oral route might be expected to cause greater increases in the cholesterol content of the bile. Transdermal estrogen appears to cause smaller beneficial changes in LDL and HDL profiles (approximately 50% of those seen with the oral route), but may be preferred in women with hypertriglyceridemia.

Tibolone (Livial) is widely used in treatment of vasomotor symptoms and prevention of osteoporosis. The parent compound itself is devoid of activity, but it is metabolized in a tissue-selective manner to three metabolites that have predominantly estrogenic, progestogenic, and androgenic activities. The drug appears to increase bone mineral density and decrease vasomotor symptoms without stimulating the endometrium, but its effects on fractures, breast cancer, and long-term outcomes remain to be established.

Regardless of the specific agent or regimen, menopausal hormone therapy with estrogens should use the lowest dose and shortest duration necessary to achieve an appropriate therapeutic goal.

ESTRADIOL/NORETHINDRONE ACETATE

(CombiPatch transdermal patch 0.05 mg estradiol/0.14 mg norethindrone acetate/day, transdermal patch 0.05 mg estradiol/0.25 mg norethindrone acetate/day)

Estradiol is estrogen and progestin combined. **Estrogens** are essential in developing and maintaining the female reproductive system and secondary sex characteristics. **Progestins** transform proliferative endometrium into secretory endometrium. The combination is indicated in treatment of moderate to severe vasomotor symptoms associated with menopause; vulvar and vaginal atrophy; hypoestrogenism caused by hypogonadism, castration, or primary ovarian failure.

ESTRAMUSTINE PHOSPHATE SODIUM

(Emcyt capsules for oral use 140 mg estramustine phosphate)

Estramustine appears to act as a relatively weak alkylating agent and imparts a weak estrogenic activity. The estrogenic portion of the molecule acts as a carrier to facilitate selective uptake of the drug into estrogen-receptor-positive cells. Because of the selective steroidal uptake, the alkylating effect of the nitrogen mustard is enhanced in these cells. Estramustine phosphate is readily dephosphorylated during absorption, and the major metabolites in plasma are estromustine, the estrone analog, estradiol, and estrone. Terminal half-life of estramustine phosphate is approximately 20 hours, and it is mainly excreted in the stool. Estramustine is indicated as a palliative therapy of metastatic or progressive prostate cancer.

Estramustine (Emcyt) is a combination of estradiol coupled to normustine (nornitrogen mustard) by a carbamate link. **Estramustine** has weaker estrogenic and antineoplastic activity than estradiol and other alkylating agents. Although the intent of the combination was to enhance the uptake of the alkylating agent into estradiol-sensitive prostate cancer cells, **estramustine** does not appear to function *in vivo* as an alkylating agent. Rather, estramustine binds to β-tubulin and microtubule-associated proteins, causing microtubule disassembly and antimitotic actions.

Resistance to **estramustine** has been described. It is used for the treatment of metastatic or progressive prostate cancer at a usual initial dose of 10 to 16 mg/kg daily in three or four divided doses.

Following oral administration, at least 75% of a dose of **estramustine** is absorbed from the gastrointestinal tract and rapidly dephosphorylated. **Estramustine** is found in the body mainly as its oxidized 17-keto analog isomer, estromustine; both forms accumulate in the prostate. Some hydrolysis of the carbamate linkage occurs in the liver, releasing estradiol, estrone, and the normustine group. **Estramustine** and estromustine have plasma half-lives of 10 to 20 hours, respectively, and are excreted with their metabolites, mainly in the feces.

In addition to myelosuppression, **estramustine** also possesses estrogenic side effects (gynecomastia, impotence, and elevated risk of thrombosis, and fluid retention) and is associated with hypercalcemia, acute attacks of porphyria, impaired glucose tolerance, and hypersensitivity reactions including angioedema.

Docetaxel and **paclitaxel** have become central components of regimens for treating metastatic ovarian, breast, lung, and head and neck cancers. Docetaxel has significant activity with **estramustine** for treatment of hormone-refractory prostate cancer. In current regimens, either drug is administered once weekly or once every 3 weeks, with comparable response rates and somewhat different patterns of toxicity. Docetaxel produces greater leukopenia and peripheral edema, whereas paclitaxel causes a higher incidence of hypersensitivity, muscle aching, and neuropathy (particularly when used in combination with a platinum analog). The optimal schedule of taxane administration, alone or in combination with other drugs, is still under evaluation.

ESTROGEN, CONJUGATED OR ESTERIFIED

(Menest tablets 0.3 mg)

Conjugated estrogen promotes growth and development of the female reproductive system and secondary sex characteristics; affects release of pituitary gonadotropins; inhibits ovulation and prevents postpartum breast engorgement; conserves calcium and phosphorous and encourages bone formation; overrides stimulatory effects of testosterone.

It is indicated in the management of moderate to severe vasomotor symptoms associated with menopause; treatment of atrophic vaginitis, kraurosis vulvae, female hypogonadism, symptoms of female castration, and primary ovarian failure; prevention and treatment of osteoporosis (conjugated estrogens); palliative treatment of metastatic breast or prostate cancer in selected women and men; treatment of postpartum breast engorgement and abnormal uterine bleeding.

ESTROGEN, CONJUGATED/MEDROXYPROGESTERONE ACETATE

(Premphase tablets 0.625 mg conjugated estrogens and 0.625 mg conjugated estrogens/5 mg medroxyprogesterone acetate)

Conjugated estrogen is estrogens and progestins combined. **Conjugated estrogens**: promote growth and development of the female reproductive system and secondary sex characteristics; affect release of pituitary gonadotropins; inhibit ovulation and prevent postpartum breast engorgement; conserve calcium and phosphorous and encourage bone formation; override stimulatory effects of testosterone; **progesterone**: inhibits secretion of pituitary gonadotropins, thereby preventing follicular maturation and ovulation (contraceptive effect); inhibits spontaneous uterine contraction; transforms proliferative endometrium into secretory endometrium.

The combination is indicated in the treatment of moderate to severe vasomotor symptoms associated with menopause; treatment of vulval and vaginal atrophy; and osteoporosis prevention.

The established benefits of estrogen therapy in postmenopausal women include amelioration of vasomotor symptoms and the prevention of bone fractures and urogenital atrophy.

The decline in ovarian function at menopause is associated with vasomotor symptoms in most women. The characteristic hot flashes may alternate with chilly sensations, inappropriate sweating, and (less commonly) paresthesias. Treatment with estrogen is specific and is the most efficacious pharmacotherapy for these symptoms. If estrogen is contraindicated or otherwise undesirable, other options may be considered.

Medroxyprogesterone acetate may provide some relief of vasomotor symptoms for certain patients, and the α_2-adrenergic agonist **clonidine** diminishes vasomotor symptoms in some women, presumably by blocking the CNS outflow that regulates blood flow to cutaneous vessels. In many women, hot flashes diminish within several years; when prescribed for this purpose, the dose and duration of estrogen use should thus be the minimum necessary to provide relief.

Osteoporosis is a disorder of the skeleton associated with the loss of bone mass. The result is thinning and weakening of the bones and an increased incidence of fractures, particularly compression fractures of the vertebrae and minimal-trauma fractures of the hip and wrist. The frequency and severity of these fractures and their associated complications (e.g., death and permanent disability) are a major public health problem, especially as the population continues to age. Osteoporosis is an indication for estrogen therapy, which clearly is efficacious in decreasing the incidence of fractures. However, because of the risks associated with estrogen use, first-line use of other drugs should be carefully considered. Nevertheless, it is important to note that the majority of fractures in the postmenopausal period occur in women without a prior history of osteoporosis, and estrogens are the most efficacious agents available for prevention of fractures at all sites in such women.

The primary mechanism by which estrogens act is to decrease bone resorption; consequently, estrogens are more effective at preventing rather than restoring bone loss. They are most effective if treatment is initiated before significant bone loss occurs, and their maximal beneficial effects require continuous use; bone loss resumes when treatment is discontinued. An appropriate diet with adequate intake of Ca^{2+} and vitamin D, and weight-bearing exercise enhance the effects of estrogen treatment. Public health efforts to improve diet and exercise patterns in girls and young women also are rational approaches to increasing bone mass.

Loss of tissue lining in the vagina or bladder leads to a variety of symptoms in many postmenopausal women. These include dryness and itching of the vagina, dyspareunia, swelling of tissues in the genital region, pain during urination, a need to urinate urgently or often, and sudden or unexpected urinary incontinence. When estrogens are being used solely for relief of vulvar and vaginal atrophy, local administration as a vaginal cream, ring device, or tablets may be considered.

The incidence of cardiovascular disease is low in premenopausal women, rising rapidly after menopause, and epidemiological studies consistently showed an association between estrogen use and reduced cardiovascular disease in postmenopausal women. Furthermore, estrogens produce a favorable lipoprotein profile, promote vasodilation, inhibit the response to vascular injury, and reduce atherosclerosis. Studies such as these led to the widespread use of estrogen for prevention of cardiovascular disease in postmenopausal women.

ESTROGEN AND PROGESTIN

(Brevicon 21-day, Brevicon 28-day, Demulen 1/35-21, Demulen 1/35-28, Enovid 5 mg, Enovid E-21, Loestrin 21 1/20, Loestrin 21 1.5/30, Loestrin Fe 1/20, Loestrin Fe 1.5/30, Lo/Ovral, Lo/Ovral-28, Modicon 21, Modicon 28, Nordette-21, Nordette-28, Norinyl 1+35 21day, Norinyl 1+50 28-day, Norinyl 1+80 21-day, Norinyl 1+80 28-day, Norinyl 2 mg, Norlestrin 21 1/50, Norlestrin 21 2.5/50, Norlestrin 28 1/50, Norlestrin Fe 1/50, Norlestrin Fe 2.5/50, Ortho-Novum 1/35 21, Ortho-Novum 1/35 28, Ortho Novum 1/50 21, Ortho-Novum 1/50 28, Ortho-Novum 1/80 21, Ortho-Novum 1/80 28, Ortho Novum 2 mg 21, Ortho-Novum 7/7/7-21, Ortho-Novum 7/7/7-28, Ortho-Novum 10/11-21, Ortho-Novum 10/11-28, Ovcon-35, Ovcon-50, Ovral, Ovral-28, Ovulen-21, Ovulen-28, Tri-Norinyl-21, Tri-Norinyl-28, Triphasil-21, Triphasil-28)

Estrogen and progestin hormonal combinations are used as oral contraceptive medication.

ESTROGENIC PREPARATIONS

	Estrone
Injectable	Estrone aqueous suspension and estrogenic substance or estrogens aqueous suspension (primarily estrone)
Oral	Conjugated estrogens (50–65% sodium estrone sulfate and 20–35% sodium equilin sulfate)
	Esterified estrogens (75–85% estrone sulfate and 6–15% sodium equilin)
Vaginal creams	Estropiate
	Conjugated estrogens
	Estradiol
Injectable	Estradiol valerate (in oil)
	Estradiol cypionate (in oil)
Oral	Micronized estradiol
Vaginal creams	Micronized estradiol
Transdermal	Estradiol
	Others
Oral	Ethinyl estradiol
	Quinestrol
	Chlorotrianisene
Vaginal creams	Dienestrol

ESTROGENIC SUBSTANCES, CONJUGATED

(Estracon, Premarin, Progen Tabs)

Estrogen, possessing antineoplastic and antiosteoporotic properties, is indicated in abnormal uterine bleeding (hormonal imbalance), in castration, primary ovarian failure, and osteoporosis, in female hypogonadism, in menopausal symptoms, atrophic vaginitis, or kraurosis vulvae, in prostatic cancer, and in breast cancer (see also Figure 48).

ESTROGENS

Estrogens are synthesized mainly in the ovaries, the placenta, and the adrenal glands. A minute amount of estradiol is synthesized in the testes. Estrogens are synthesized according to the following scheme:

Cholesterol → pregnenolone → progesterone → androstenedione → estradiol 17 beta → estrone → estriol

Estrogen dramatically influences the growth and development of the female reproductive organs. The uterus and vagina are sensitive to the biochemical actions of estrogens, which are as follows: early events—release of histamine, synthesis of cyclic adenosine monophosphate (cyclic AMP), stimulation of RNA polymerase, and increased excitability of the myometrium; intermediate events—synthesis of RNA and DNA, inhibition of water, and stimulation of certain enzymes; late events—increased secretory activity, morphologic changes, increased protein synthesis, stimulation of lipid and carbohydrate metabolism, and increased gravimetric responses.

Estrogens are used extensively in the treatment of endocrine and nonendocrine disease, a few of which are cited: menopause—as a replacement therapy; atrophic vaginitis—to thicken epithelial cells and to cause mucosal cells to proliferate; hypopituitarism—to correct vaginal mucosal atrophy, maintain breast development, and minimize calcium loss from bone; cancer—used in postmenopausal mammary carcinoma; primary hypogonadism—to correct ovarian failure; osteoporosis—estrogen by itself or with a hypercalcemic steroid is used in the treatment of osteoporosis; primary amenorrhea—to cause endometrium to proliferate; uterine bleeding—to reverse estrogen deficiency (in this case, oral contraceptives containing 80 to 100 μg of estrogen are recommended); postpartum lactation—to relieve postpartum painful breast engorgement and prevent postpartum lactation; bromocriptine is also effective; control of height—to cause closure of the epiphyses in unusually tall young girls; and dermatologic problems—used with some success in the treatment of acne. Low-dose estrogens are safe only when taken for a limited period. The most-often-reported side effects are breakthrough bleeding, breast tenderness and, very infrequently, gastrointestinal upsets. When estrogens are used in large doses or injudiciously, they may cause thromboembolic disorders, hypertension in susceptible individuals, and cholestasis. Estrogens are contraindicated in patients with estrogen-dependent neoplasms such as carcinoma of the breast or endometrium. Vaginal adenocarcinoma has been reported in young women whose mothers were treated with diethylstilbestrol in an effort to prevent miscarriage (see also Figure 48).

ESTROGENS, SYNTHETIC CONJUGATED, A OR B

(Cenestin tablets 0.3 mg)

Estrogen, synthetic conjugated, A or B, is an estrogen. Estrogens are responsible for the development and maintenance of the female reproductive system and secondary sexual characteristics. Circulating estrogens modulate the pituitary secretion of the gonadotropins: luteinizing hormone (LH) and follicle-stimulating hormone (FSH) through a negative feedback mechanism, and estrogen replacement therapy acts to reduce the elevated levels of these hormones seen in postmenopausal women.

Estrogen is indicated in the treatment of moderate to severe symptoms associated with menopause (synthetic conjugated estrogens, A or B); moderate to severe symptoms of vulvar and vaginal atrophy (synthetic conjugated estrogens A, 0.3 mg only).

ESTRONE

(Bestrone, Estrone-A, Estronol, Kestrone-5, Theelin Aqueous)

ESTROPIPATE

(Ogen)

Estrone or estropipate is used in the treatment of atrophic vaginitis and menopausal symptoms, female hypogonadism, primary ovarian failure, after castration, or in prostatic cancer (see also Figure 48).

ESTROPIPATE (PIPERAZINE ESTRONE SULFATE)

(Ogen tablets 0.625 mg)

Estropipate is an estrogen that promotes growth and development of the female reproductive system and secondary sex characteristics; affects release of ovulation and prevents postpartum breast engorgement; conserves calcium and phosphorous and encourages bone formation; overrides stimulatory effects of testosterone.

Estropipate is indicated in the management of moderate to severe vasomotor symptoms associated with menopause; female hypogonadism, female castration, primary ovarian failure, and atrophic conditions caused by deficient endogenous estrogen production; prevention and treatment of osteoporosis.

Oral administration is common and may utilize estradiol, conjugated estrogens, esters of estrone and other estrogens, and ethinyl estradiol. A special micronized preparation of estradiol (Estrace, others) that yields a large surface for rapid absorption is required for oral administration, although high doses must be used because absolute bioavailability remains low due to first-pass metabolism. Ethinyl estradiol is used orally, as the ethinyl substitution in the C17 position inhibits first-pass hepatic metabolism. Other common oral preparations contain conjugated equine estrogens (Premarin), which are primarily the sulfate esters of estrone, equilin, and other naturally occurring compounds; esterified esters; or mixtures of conjugated estrogens prepared from plant-derived sources (Cenestin). These are hydrolyzed by enzymes present in the lower gut that remove the charged sulfate groups and allow absorption of estrogen across the intestinal epithelium. In another oral preparation, **estropipate** (Ortho-est, ogen), estrone is solubilized as the sulfate and stabilized with piperazine. Due largely to differences in metabolism, the potencies of various oral preparations differ widely; ethinyl estradiol, for example, is much more potent than conjugated estrogens.

A number of foodstuffs and plant-derived products, largely from soy, are available as nonprescription items and often are touted as providing benefits similar to those from compounds with established estrogenic activity. These products may contain flavonoids such as **genistein**, which display estrogenic activity in laboratory tests, albeit generally much less than that of estradiol. In theory, these preparations could produce appreciable estrogenic effects, but their efficacy at relevant doses has not been established in human trials.

ESZOPICLONE

(Lunesta tablets 1 mg)

Eszopiclone is a nonbarbiturate sedative and hypnotic that binds to GABA-receptor complexes located close to or allosterically coupled to benzodiazepine receptors. It is indicated in the treatment of insomnia.

ETANERCEPT

(Enbrel injection 50 mg/mL, powder for injection, lyophilized 25 mg)

Etanercept is an immunomodulator that binds specifically to tumor necrosis factor (TNF), blocks its interaction with cell surface TNF receptors, and modulates biological responses that are induced or regulated by TNF. It is indicated in reducing signs and symptoms and inciting the progression of structural damage in moderately to severely active rheumatoid arthritis; reducing signs and symptoms of moderately to severely active polyarticular-course **juvenile rheumatoid arthritis** (JRA) in patients responding inadequately to one or more disease-modifying antirheumatic drugs; reducing signs and symptoms of psoriatic arthritis; reducing signs and symptoms in patients with active ankylosing spondylitis. It may be used in combination with **methotrexate** (MTX) in patients who do not respond adequately to MTX alone in the treatment of rheumatoid or psoriatic arthritis, and in treatment of patients with chronic moderate to severe plaque psoriasis who are candidates for systemic therapy or phototherapy.

Although not a monoclonal antibody, **etanercept** (Enbrel) is mechanistically related to infliximab because it also targets TNF-α. Etanercept contains the ligand-binding portion of a human TNF-α receptor fused to the Fc portion of human IgG_1, and binds to TNF-α and prevents it from interacting with its receptors. It is approved in the United States for treatment of the symptoms of rheumatoid arthritis in patients who have not responded to other treatments. **Etanercept** can be used in combination with methotrexate in patients who have not responded adequately to methotrexate alone. As with infliximab, serious infections have occurred after treatment with etanercept. Injection-site reactions (erythema, itching, pain, or swelling) have occurred in more than one-third of etanercept-treated patients.

Adalimimab (Humira) is another anti-TNF product for intravenous use. This recombinant human IgG_1 monoclonal antibody was created by phage display technology and is approved for use in rheumatoid arthritis.

Etanercept (Enbrel) is FDA approved for the treatment of psoriasis, psoriatic arthritis, rheumatoid arthritis, juvenile rheumatoid arthritis, and ankylosing spondylitis. **Etanercept** is a soluble, recombinant, fully human TNF receptor fusion protein consisting of two molecules of the ligand-binding portion of the TNF receptor fused to the Fc portion of IgG_1. As a dimeric molecule, it can bind two molecules of TNF. **Etanercept** binds soluble and membrane-bound TNF, thereby inhibiting the action of TNF.

Etanercept is administered by subcutaneous injection at doses of either 25 or 50 mg twice a week. In a phase III, placebo-controlled, double-blind, parallel-group study, 34 and 44% of patients receiving the 25-mg dose reached PASI reductions of 75% at 12 and 24 weeks, respectively, and 58 and 70% of patients achieved PASI reductions of 50% at 12 and 24 weeks, respectively. At the 50-mg dose, 49 and 59% reached PASI reduction of 75% at 12 and 24 weeks, respectively, and 74 and 77% reached PASI reductions of 50% at 12 and 24 weeks, respectively. Except for injection-site reactions, the drug is well tolerated. Monthly complete blood counts with a differential should be monitored for the first 3 months of treatment. Potential side effects include aplastic anemia, increased risk of infection, and exacerbation of CHF and demyelinating disorders. The risk of malignancy is unknown but may be increased with the use of **etanercept**.

ETHACRYNIC ACID

(Edecrin)

The major loop diuretics are furosemide (Lasix) and ethacrynic acid. Furosemide is chemically related to the thiazide diuretics, but ethacrynic acid is not. These agents inhibit the active resorption of chloride (and sodium) in the thick, ascending medullary portion of the loop of Henle and also in the cortical portion of the loop or the distal tubule. The diuresis they produce, which is similar to that seen with the thiazides, predominantly causes a loss of chloride, sodium, and potassium, but HCO_3 excretion is not increased. Although large volumes of fluid can be excreted with the use of these agents, the ability of the kidney to produce either a dilute or concentrated urine is greatly diminished. These agents are most efficacious with about a 20% loss in the filtered load of sodium (furosemide, 15 to 30%; ethacrynic acid, 17 to 23%). Loop diuretics are ordinarily taken orally, but can be given intravenously if a rapid onset of action is sought, as when used in combination with antihypertensive medications in the management of hypertensive crisis. Furosemide and ethacrynic acid undergo some active renal tubular secretion as well as glomerular filtration. A minor portion is excreted by the liver. Loop diuretics are used for treating the following conditions: in edema of cardiac, hepatic, or renal origin, including acute pulmonary edema and hypertensive crisis; in acute renal failure, to maintain urine flow, though an excessive loss of extracellular fluid volume can cause a decrease in the glomerular filtration rate (GFR); and in hyperkalemia (see Figure 17).

Excessive volume depletion, hyponatremia, and hypotension are major risks associated with the use of loop diuretics, and the side effects of hypokalemia, hyperuricemia, and hyperglycemia are always present. Loop diuretics should not be used concurrently with ototoxic aminoglycoside antibiotics (i.e., streptomycin, gentamicin, kanamycin, tobramycin) (see also Table 25).

ETHACRYNIC ACID (ETHACRYNATE (Edecrin tablets 25 mg)

Ethacrynic acid is a loop diuretic that inhibits reabsorption of sodium and chloride in proximal and distal tubules and in the loop of Henle. Drugs in this group of diuretics inhibit the activity of the N^+-K^+-$2Cl^-$ symporter in the thick ascending limb of the loop of Henle; hence, these diuretics also are referred to as loop diuretics. Although the proximal tubule reabsorbs approximately 65% of the filtered Na^+, diuretics acting only in the proximal tubule have limited efficacy because the thick ascending limb has a great reabsorptive capacity and reabsorbs most of the rejectate from the proximal tubule. Diuretics acting predominantly at sites past the thick ascending limb also have limited efficacy because only a small percentage of the filtered Na^+ load reaches these more distal sites. In contrast, inhibitors of N^+-K^+-$2Cl^-$ symport in the thick ascending limb are highly efficacious, and for this reason, they sometimes are called **high-ceiling diuretics**. The efficacy of inhibitors of N^+-K^+-$2Cl^-$ symport in the thick ascending limb of the loop of Henle is due to a combination of two factors: (1) Approximately 25% of the filtered Na^+ load normally is reabsorbed by the thick ascending limb, and (2) nephron segments past the thick ascending limb do not possess the reabsorptive capacity to rescue the flood of rejectate exiting the thick ascending limb.

Inhibitors of N^+-K^+-$2Cl^-$ symport are a chemically diverse group. Only **furosemide** (Lasix), **bumetanide** (Bumex), **ethacrynic acid** (Edecrin), and **torsemide** (Demadex) are available. Furosemide and bumetanide contain a sulfonamide moiety. Ethacrynic acid is a phenoxyacetic acid derivative and torsemide is a sulfonylurea.

Because furosemide, bumetanide, **ethacrynic acid**, and torsemide are bound extensively to plasma proteins, delivery of these drugs to the tubules by filtration is limited. However, they are secreted efficiently by the organic acid transport system in the proximal tubule and thereby gain access to their binding sites on the N^+-K^+-$2Cl^-$ symport in the luminal membrane of the thick ascending limb. Probenecid shifts the plasma concentration-response curve to furosemide to the right by competitively inhibiting furosemide secretion by the organic acid transport system.

Approximately 65% of furosemide is excreted unchanged in the urine, and the remainder is conjugated to glucuronic acid in the kidney. Accordingly, in patients with renal, but not liver, disease, the elimination half-life of furosemide is prolonged. In contrast, bumetanide and torsemide have significant hepatic metabolism, so the elimination half-lives of these loop diuretics are prolonged by liver, but not renal, disease.

Although the average oral availability of furosemide is approximately 60%, oral availability of furosemide varies from 10 to 100%. In contrast, oral availabilities of bumetanide and torsemide are reliably high. Heart failure patients have fewer hospitalizations and better quality of life with torsemide than with furosemide, perhaps because of the more reliable absorption of torsemide.

As a class, loop diuretics have short elimination half-lives, and prolonged-release preparations are not available. Consequently, often the dosing interval is too short to maintain adequate levels of loop diuretics in the tubular lumen. Note that torsemide has a longer $t_{1/2}$ than other agents available in the United States. As the concentration of loop diuretics in the tubular lumen declines, nephrons begin to avidly reabsorb Na^+, which often nullifies the overall effect of the loop diuretic on total-body Na^+. This phenomenon of "postdiuretic Na^+ retention" can be overcome by restricting dietary Na^+ intake or by more frequent administration of the loop diuretic.

A major use of loop diuretics is in the treatment of acute pulmonary edema. A rapid increase in venous capacitance in conjunction with a brisk natriuresis reduces left ventricular filling pressures and thereby rapidly relieves pulmonary edema. Loop diuretics are also used widely for the treatment of chronic CHF when diminution of extracellular fluid volume is desirable to minimize venous and pulmonary congestion. In this regard, a metaanalysis of randomized clinical trials demonstrates that diuretics cause a significant reduction in mortality and the risk of worsening heart failure, as well as an improvement.

Diuretics are used widely for the treatment of hypertension, and controlled clinical trials demonstrating reduced morbidity and mortality have been conducted with N^+- Cl^- symport (thiazides and thiazide-like diuretics) but not N^+-K^+-$2Cl^-$ symport inhibitors. Nonetheless, N^+-K^+-$2Cl^-$ symport inhibitors appear to lower blood pressure as effectively as N^+-Cl^- symport inhibitors while causing smaller perturbations in the lipid profile. However, the short elimination half-lives of loop diuretics render them less useful for hypertension than thiazide-type diuretics. The edema of nephrotic syndrome often is refractory to other classes of diuretics, and loop diuretics often are the only drugs capable of reducing the massive edema associated with this renal disease. Loop diuretics also are employed in the treatment of edema and ascites of liver cirrhosis; however, care must be taken not to induce **encephalopathy** or **hepatorenal syndrome**. In patients with a drug overdose, loop diuretics can be used to induce a forced diuresis to facilitate more rapid renal elimination of the offending drug. Loop diuretics, combined with isotonic saline administration to prevent volume depletion, are used to treat hypercalcemia. They interfere with the kidneys' capacity to produce a concentrated urine. Consequently, loop diuretics combined with hypertonic saline are useful for the treatment of life-threatening hyponatremia. They also are used to treat edema associated with chronic renal insufficiency.

Loop diuretics can cause ototoxicity that manifests as tinnitus, hearing impairment, deafness, vertigo, and a sense of fullness in the ears. Hearing impairment and deafness are usually, but not always, reversible. Ototoxicity occurs most frequently with rapid intravenous administration and least frequently with oral administration. **Ethacrynic acid** appears to induce ototoxicity more often than other loop diuretics, and should be used only in patients who cannot tolerate the other loop diuretics. Loop diuretics also can cause hyperuricemia (occasionally leading to gout) and hyperglycemia (infrequently precipitating diabetes mellitus), and can increase plasma levels of LDL cholesterol and triglycerides while decreasing plasma levels of HDL cholesterol. Other adverse effects include skin rashes, photosensitivity, paresthesias, bone marrow depression, and gastrointestinal disturbances.

Contraindications to the use of loop diuretics include severe Na^+ and volume depletion, hypersensitivity to sulfonamides (for sulfonamide-based loop diuretics), and anuria unresponsive to a trial dose of loop diuretic.

Drug interactions may occur when loop diuretics are coadministered with (1) aminoglycosides (synergism of ototoxicity caused by both drugs), (2) anticoagulants (increased anticoagulant activity), (3) digitalis glycosides (increased digitalis-induced arrhythmias), (4) lithium (increased plasma levels of lithium), (5) propranolol (increased plasma levels of propranolol), (6) sulfonylureas (hyperglycemia), (7) cisplatin (increased risk of diuretic-induced ototoxicity), (8) NSAIDs (blunted diuretic response and salicylate toxicity when given with high doses of salicylates), (9) probenecid (blunted diuretic response), (10) thiazide diuretics (synergism of diuretic activity of both drugs leading to profound diuresis), and (11) amphotericin B (increased potential for nephrotoxicity and toxicity and intensification of electrolyte imbalance).

Loop diuretics may cause direct vascular effects. They, particularly furosemide, acutely increase systemic venous capacitance and thereby decrease left ventricular filling pressure. This effect, which may be mediated by prostaglandins and requires intact kidneys, benefits patients with pulmonary edema even before diuresis ensues. Furosemide and emacrynic acid can inhibit N^+-K^+ ATPase, glycolysis, mitochondrial respiration, the microsomal Ca^{2+}-pump, adenylyl cyclase, phosphodiesterase, and prostaglandin dehydrogenase; however, these effects do not have therapeutic implications. *In vitro*, high doses of inhibitors of N^+-K^+-$2Cl^-$ symport can inhibit electrolyte transport in many tissues. Only in the inner ear, where alterations in the electrolyte composition of endolymph may contribute to drug-induced ototoxicity, is this effect important clinically.

ETHAMBUTOL HYDROCHLORIDE

(Myambutol tablets 100 mg)

Ethambutol inhibits synthesis of one or more metabolites, causing impairment of cell metabolism, arrest of multiplication, and cell death. It is indicated in the treatment of tuberculosis, in combination with other agents in patients with *Mycobacterium tuberculosis* resistant to isoniazid or rifampin, or when there is intolerance to other antituberculous agents.

Drugs used in the treatment of tuberculosis can be divided into two major categories. "First-line" agents combine the greatest level of efficacy with an acceptable degree of toxicity; these include **isoniazid**, **rifampin**, **ethambutol**, **streptomycin**, and **pyrazinamide**. The large majority of patients with tuberculosis can be treated successfully with these drugs. Excellent results for patients with non-drug-resistant tuberculosis can be obtained with a 6-month course of treatment; for the first 2 months, isoniazid, rifampin, **ethambutol**, and pyrazinamide are given, followed by isoniazid and rifampin for the remaining 4 months. Administration of rifampin in combination with isoniazid for 9 months also is effective therapy for all forms of disease caused by strains of *M. tuberculosis* susceptible to both agents. Occasionally, because of microbial resistance, it may be necessary to resort to "second-line" drugs in addition; thus, treatment may be initiated with 5 to 6 drugs. This category of agents includes **moxifloxacin** or **gatifloxacin**, **ethionamide**, **aminosalicylic acid**, **cycloserine**, **amikacin**, **kanamycin**, **capreomycin**, and **linezolid**. In HIV-infected patients receiving protease inhibitors and/or nonnucleoside reverse-transcriptase inhibitors, drug interactions with the rifamycins (rifampin, rifapentine, rifabutin) are an important concern. Directly observed therapy, in which a health care worker actually witnesses the ingestion of medications, improves the outcome of tuberculosis treatment regimens.

Isoniazid is ineffective in the treatment of leprosy or *M. avium* complex infection. Lepromatous (multibacillary) leprosy is treated with **dapsone**, **clofazimine**, and rifampin for a minimum of 2 years, whereas tuberculoid (paucibacillary) leprosy is treated with dapsone and rifampin for 6 months.

Ethambutol is a water-soluble and heat-stable compound. Nearly all strains of *M. tuberculosis* and *M. kansasii* as well as a number of strains of MAC are sensitive to **ethambutol**. The sensitivities of other nontuberculous organisms are variable. Ethambutol has no effect on other bacteria.

It suppresses the growth of most isoniazid- and streptomycin-resistant tubercle bacilli. Resistance to ethambutol develops very slowly *in vitro*.

Mycobacteria take up **ethambutol** rapidly when the drug is added to cultures that are in the exponential growth phase. However, growth is not significantly inhibited before about 24 hours. **Ethambutol** inhibits **arabinosyl transferases** involved in cell-wall biosynthesis. Bacterial resistance to the drug develops *in vivo* via single amino acid mutations in the embA gene when ethambutol is given in the absence of other effective agents.

About 75 to 80% of an orally administered dose of **ethambutol** is absorbed from the gastrointestinal tract. Concentrations in plasma are maximal in humans 2 to 4 hours after the drug is taken and are proportional to the dose. A single dose of 25 mg/kg produces a plasma concentration of 2 to 5 pg/mL at 2 to 4 hours. The drug has a half-life of 3 to 4 hours. Within 24 hours, 75% of an ingested dose of **ethambutol** is excreted unchanged in the urine; up to 15% is excreted in the form of two metabolites—an aldehyde and a dicarboxylic acid derivative. Renal clearance of **ethambutol** is approximately 7 $mL{\cdot}min^{-1}{\cdot}kg^{-1}$; thus it is evident that the drug is excreted by tubular secretion in addition to glomerular filtration.

Ethambutol (ethambutol hydrochloride; Myambutol) has been used with notable success in the therapy of tuberculosis of various forms when given concurrently with isoniazid. Because of a lower incidence of toxic effects and better acceptance by patients, **ethambutol** has essentially replaced **aminosalicylic acid**.

Ethambutol is available for oral administration in tablets containing the D isomer. The usual adult dose of ethambutol is 15 mg/kg given once a day. Some physicians prefer to treat with 25 mg/kg per day for the first 60 days and then to reduce the dose to 15 mg/kg per day, particularly for those who have received previous therapy. **Ethambutol** accumulates in patients with impaired renal function and adjustment of dosage is necessary.

Ethambutol is not recommended for children under 5 years of age, in part because of concern about the ability to test their visual acuity. Children from ages 6 to 12 years should receive 10 to 15 mg/kg per day.

The use of ethambutol in the chemotherapy of tuberculosis is described in the following text. The most important side effect is optic neuritis, resulting in decreased visual acuity and loss of ability to differentiate red from green. The incidence of this reaction is proportional to the dose of ethambutol and is observed in 15% of patients receiving 50 mg/kg day, in 5% of patients receiving 25 mg/kg per day, and fewer than 1% of patients receiving daily doses of 15 mg/kg (the recommended dose for treatment of tuberculosis). The intensity of the visual difficulty is related to the duration of therapy after the decreased visual acuity first becomes apparent, and may be unilateral or bilateral. Tests of visual acuity and red–green discrimination prior to the start of therapy and periodically thereafter are thus recommended. Recovery usually occurs when ethambutol is withdrawn; the time required is a function of the degree of visual impairment.

Ethambutol produces very few untoward reactions. Fewer than 2% of nearly 2000 patients who received daily doses of 15 mg/kg of ethambutol had adverse reactions: 0.8% experienced diminished visual acuity, 0.5% had a rash, and 0.3% developed drug fever. Other side effects that have been observed are pruritus, joint pain, gastrointestinal upset, abdominal pain, malaise, headache, dizziness, mental confusion, disorientation, and possible hallucinations. Numbness and tingling of the fingers owing to peripheral neuritis are infrequent. Anaphylaxis and leukopenia are rare.

Therapy with ethambutol results in an increased concentration of urate in the blood in about 50% of patients, owing to decreased renal excretion of uric acid. The effect may be detectable as early as 24 hours after a single dose or as late as 90 days after treatment is started. This untoward effect is possibly enhanced by isoniazid and pyridoxine.

ETHAMBUTOL HYDROCHLORIDE

(Myambutol)

Ethambutol (15 to 25 mg/kg/day) is used in conjunction with other antituberculosis drugs in pulmonary tuberculosis. It is effective against strains of *M. tuberculosis* but does not seem to be active against fungi, viruses, or other bacteria. Ethambutol is metabolized in the liver (20%), and a significant portion of it (50%) is excreted unchanged in the urine, and hence the dosage should be reduced in renal impairment. Ethambutol may cause retrobulbar neuritis, and patients treated for a prolonged period of time should have vision examination including visual fields. Most visual effects are reversible following discontinuation of the drug. In addition, ethambutol has caused dermatitis, pruritis, anorexia, headache, dizziness, vomiting, fever, and joint pain. Aluminum salts delay and reduce the absorption of ethambutol.

ETHANOLAMINE OLEATE

(Ethamolin)

Ethanolamine, a sclerosing agent, is indicated in the treatment of patients with esophageal varices that have recently bled, with the intention of preventing rebleeding. When injected IV, it acts primarily by irritation of the intimal endothelium of the vein and produces a sterile dose-related inflammatory response. This results in fibrosis and occlusion of the vein. The adverse reactions following ethanolamine include pleural effusion, infiltration, esophageal ulcer, esophageal stricture, pneumonia, pyrexia, and retrosternal pain.

ETHAPROPRAZINE HYDROCHLORIDE

(Parsidol)

Ethapropazine is used as an adjunct in the treatment of Parkinson's disease or in neuroleptic-induced parkinsonism. Most phenothiazine neuroleptics have weak anticholinergic properties. However, the anticholinergic effects of thioridazine or ethapropazine are pronounced, and all the cautions cited for atropine apply to these agents as well. Indeed, fatal tachyarrhythmias and other electrocardiographic changes, such as blunting and notching of T waves, prolongation of the QT interval, increased convexity of the ST segment, and appearance of V waves have been caused through the injudicious use of thioridazine (1500 to 3600 mg/day), especially in elderly patients.

ETHAVERINE HYDROCHLORIDE

(Circubid, Ethaquin, Ethatab, Ethavex-100, Isovex, Pavaspan)

Ethaverine, an isoquinoline derivative with peripheral vasodilating properties (100 to 200 mg p.o. t.i.d. q. 12 hours), is indicated in peripheral and cerebrovascular insufficiency associated with arterial spasm and in spastic conditions of the gastrointestinal and genitourinary tracts.

ETHCHLORVYNOL

(Placidyl)

Ethchlorvynol (500 mg at bedtime), which has sedative–hypnotic, anticonvulsant, and muscle relaxant properties, is indicated in the management of insomnia. The onset and duration of action are 15 minutes and 6 hours, respectively. Ethchlorvynol, which should not be used for more than one week, causes psychological and physical dependence when used for a prolonged period of time, and its sudden discontinuation will produce abstinence syndromes characterized by convulsions, delirium, schizoid reaction, perceptual distortions, memory loss, ataxia, insomnia, slurring of speech, unusual anxiety, irritability, agitation, tremors, anorexia, nausea, vomiting, weakness, dizziness, sweating, muscle twitching, or weight loss.

Ethchlorvynol or phenobarbital may be used in the management of withdrawal symptoms. The CNS depressant effects of ethchlorvynol will be enhanced by alcohol, barbiturates, narcotics, and numerous other drugs. Ethchlorvynol will reduce the hypoprothrombinemic effects of anticoagulants requiring dose adjustment of the anticoagulant.

ETHER

The pharmacology of nitrous oxide, cyclopropane, halothane, and ether is summarized in Table 16. Ether and cyclopropane are seldom used in anesthesiology.

ETHINYL ESTRADIOL

(Estinyl)

Ethinyl tablets are indicated in the treatment of vasomotor symptoms associated with menopause; in female hypogonadism; in prostatic carcinoma; and in breast cancer. For additional information, see Estrogen and Figure 48.

ETHINYL ESTRADIOL-ETHYNODIOL DIACETATE

(Demulen)

Demulen contains 1 mg of ethynodiol diacetate and 35 mcg of ethinyl estradiol. Demulen 1/35 and Demulen 1/50 are indicated for prevention of pregnancy and are used as oral contraceptive medications (see Figure 56). They act by suppression of gonadotropins. Oral contraceptive medications should be used cautiously in thrombophlebitis, thromboembolic disorders, cerebral vascular disease, myocardial infarction, coronary artery disease, carcinoma of the breast, carcinoma of any section of the reproductive tract, abnormal genital bleeding, suspected pregnancy, and history of cholestatic jaundice. Ethinyl estradiol-levonorgestrel (Nordette), ethinyl estradiol-norethindrone (Ortho-Novum), ethinyl estradiol-norethindrone acetate-ferrous fumarate (Loestrin Fe), and ethinyl estradiol-norgestrel (Lo/Ovral) are all oral contraceptive medications with the same indication or contraindications as cited for Demulen.

ETHIONAMIDE

(Trecator-SC)

Ethionamide, which has bacteriostatic actions against *M. tuberculosis* (0.5 to 1 g/day in divided doses) is indicated in the treatment of tuberculosis where first-line drugs such as isoniazid and rifampin have failed. The side effects of ethionamide may include nausea and vomiting, diarrhea, metallic taste, hepatitis, jaundice, stomatitis, depression, drowsiness, asthenia, peripheral neuritis, olfactory disturbances, diplopia, blurred vision, optic neuritis, convulsions, postural hypotension, thrombocytopenia, gynecomastia, impotence, menorrhagia, or diabetes mellitus.

ETHIONAMIDE

(Trecator-SC tablets 250 mg)

Ethionamide is an antituberculosis agent that causes inhibition of peptide synthesis in susceptible organisms. It is indicated in the treatment of tuberculosis, in combination with other agents, in patients with *M. tuberculosis* resistant to isoniazid or **rifampin**, or when there is intolerance to other antituberculous agents.

ETHOSUXIMIDE

(Zarotin)

Ethosuximide, methsuximide (Celontin), and phensuximide (Milontin) are indicated for control of absence (petit mal) seizures. These agents suppress the paroxysmal three-cycle-per-second spike and wave activity associated with lapses of consciousness common in absence seizures. Ethosuximide is extensively metabolized in the liver to inactive metabolites, and 20% of it is excreted unchanged by the kidneys. Ethosuximide is not effective in grand mal seizures, and may increase their frequency. Ethosuximide is known to have caused systemic lupus erythematosus, blood dyscrasias, and impairment of hepatic and renal function. The most frequent side effects of ethosuximide are nausea, vomiting, gastric upset, cramps, anorexia, diarrhea, weight loss, epigastric and abdominal pain, and constipation.

ETHOTOIN

(Peganone)

Ethotoin (250 mg p.o. q.i.d.) is indicated in the management of generalized tonic–clonic (grand mal) or complex partial (psychomotor) seizures. Similar to phenytoin, ethotoin stabilizes neuronal membrane, increases the efflux of sodium, and prevents the spread of the seizure process. Unlike phenytoin, ethotoin has no antiarrhythmic activity. The side effects of ethotoin may include fatigue, insomnia, dizziness, headache, numbness, chest pain, rash, diplopia, nystagmus, gingival hyperplasia, and blood dyscrasias (see also Figures 32 and 76).

ETHOXZOLAMIDE

(Cadrase, Ethamide)

The carbonic anhydrase inhibitors consist of acetazolamide (Diamox), ethoxzolamide, and dichlorphenamide (Daranide). Acetazolamide is an old agent, whereas ethoxzolamide and dichlorphenamide are newer preparations. Dichlorphenamide is the most potent carbonic anhydrase inhibitor in use today. The presence of SO_2NH_2 (sulfonamide) causes such compounds to inhibit carbonic anhydrase (CA), which catalyzes the hydration of carbon dioxide as follows:

$$CO_2 + H_2O \xrightarrow{CA} H_2CO_3 \rightleftharpoons H^+ + HCO^-_3$$

These agents inhibit carbonic anhydrase in the renal tubular cells in both the proximal and distal tubules. When the rate of hydrogen generation is reduced, HCO^-_3 is lost in urine and the patient tends to become acidotic. However, the plasma concentration of HCO^-_3 is lowered and less is filtered, so the diuresis becomes less effective. In addition, the sodium output is increased because its resorption in exchange for hydrogen is limited by the decreased availability of hydrogen. With less hydrogen available, the exchange of sodium for potassium predominates, and this fosters the loss of potassium. Chloride excretion is not altered significantly. Because the aqueous humor has a high concentration of bicarbonate, carbonic anhydrase inhibitors are primarily used in the treatment of glaucoma. They are no longer used as diuretics or as antiepileptic agents.

ETHYL ALCOHOL

As a CNS depressant, ethyl alcohol (ethanol) obeys the law of descending depression, in that it first inhibits the cerebral cortex, then the cerebellum, spinal cord, and medullary center. Taken in small quantities, alcohol brings about a feeling of well-being. When consumed in large quantities, alcohol produces more boisterous behavior. Self-control is lost and judgment is impaired. Alcohol works by depressing the inhibitory control mechanism and the reticular activating system. If a large amount of alcohol is consumed within a short time, unconsciousness and general anesthesia ensue. Death is due to respiratory and cardiac failure. Because numerous drugs in toxic doses can produce ataxia and slurred speech (e.g., phenytoin), for medicolegal purposes, the only acceptable means of proving intoxication is by determining the level of alcohol in any biologic fluid or in expired air. Alcohol produces dilation of the skin vessels, flushing, and a sensation of warmth. Alcohol also interferes with the normal cutaneous vasoconstriction in response to cold. The body heat is therefore lost very rapidly, and the internal temperature consequently falls. At toxic alcohol levels, the hypothalamic temperature-regulating mechanism becomes depressed, and the fall in body temperature becomes pronounced. For these reasons, consuming alcoholic beverages for the purpose of keeping warm in cold weather is obviously irrational. As a gastric secretagogue, alcohol stimulates the secretion of gastric juice, which is rich in acid and pepsin. Therefore, the consumption of alcohol is contraindicated in subjects with untreated acid-pepsin disease. In addition, alcohol releases histamine, which in turn releases gastric juice. This effect is not blocked by atropine. In toxic doses (20%), gastric secretion is inhibited and peptic activity is depressed. From this, it is easy to deduce that small amounts of alcohol stimulate appetite and aid digestion, but large amounts may produce indigestion.

Alcohol is also a carminative substance in that it facilitates the expulsion of gas from the stomach. It enhances the accumulation of fat in the liver. In alcoholics, this fat accumulation continues, and cirrhosis of the liver may ensue; however, the two phenomena are not related. Alcohol may release epinephrine, which leads to transient hyperglycemia and hyperlipemia. Therefore, alcohol consumption is contraindicated in diabetics. It causes diuresis by increasing fluid intake and by inhibiting the secretion of antidiuretic hormone elaborated by the posterior pituitary gland. Alcohol has teratogenic effects that are manifested by CNS dysfunction (such as low IQ and microencephaly), slow growth, a characteristic cluster of facial abnormalities (such as short palpebral fissures, hypoplastic upper lip, and short nose), and a variable set of major and minor malformations. Alcohol is absorbed from the stomach, and very rapidly from the small intestine. Patients who have undergone gastrectomy may therefore become intoxicated relatively quickly. The absorption that takes place through unbroken skin is negligible. As a water-soluble substance with a low molecular weight, alcohol is distributed uniformly throughout all tissues and tissue fluids. It passes across the placental barrier, is found in spinal fluid, and accumulates in the brain. Consequently, any physiologic fluids (urine, blood, spinal fluid, breast milk, or saliva) are suitable for determining the concentration of alcohol. The metabolism of ethanol, which shows genetic polymorphism, is catalyzed primarily by alcohol dehydrogenase with zero-order kinetics, according to the following scheme.

$$\text{Ethanol} \xrightarrow{\text{Alcohol dehydrogenase}} \text{acetaldehyde} \xrightarrow{\text{Acetaldehyde dehydrogenase}} \text{acetic acid}$$

NAD⁺ NADH NAD⁺ NADH

The rate-limiting factor in the metabolism of ethanol is the availability of NAD^+.

Ethanol is not metabolized by cytochrome P-450 enzymes (microsomal drug-metabolizing systems [MEDS]). However, it is metabolized to a certain extent by the microsomal ethanol-oxidizing system (MEDS).

Although ethanol is not metabolized by the microsomal drug-metabolizing system, it inhibits it and increases the rate of its synthesis. This effect may create a significant alcohol–drug interaction in both nonalcoholics and alcoholics who are taking medications.

Poisoning may be characterized by inebriation, muscular incoordination, blurred vision, impaired reaction time, excitement due to loss of inhibitions, impairment of consciousness, coma, tachycardia, and slow respiration. A blood alcohol level of 80 mg/dL can produce recognizable features of drunkenness; a level above 300 mg/dL is life-threatening. In children, severe hypoglycemia and convulsions may also occur.

Acute poisoning is treated with gastric aspiration and lavage combined with intensive supportive therapy, including thorough assessment of the patient plus measures to prevent respiratory failure. In cases of very severe poisoning, peritoneal dialysis or hemodialysis may be necessary.

Chronic alcoholism produces pathologic changes such as chronic gastritis, cirrhosis of the liver, alcoholic cardiomyopathy, Korsakoff's syndrome, bloatedness, flabby muscles, fine tremors, impaired physical capacity and stamina, diminished will power, and impaired memory. Accompanying malnutrition may contribute to alcohol-induced tissue injury.

Delirium tremens usually arises in a chronic alcoholic. The clinical features may include hallucinations, intense fear, sleeplessness, restlessness, agitation, delirium, and sometimes grand mal convulsions. In addition, tachycardia, hypotension, and clover-shaped ST changes in the electrocardiogram are evident.

The treatment of patients during a delirium tremens episode includes the intravenous administration of another CNS depressant (usually diazepam) during the acute phase, followed by the oral administration of chlordiazepoxide or oxazepam. In addition, other medications plus dietary management may become essential.

ETHYL CHLORIDE

(Chloroethane) (Ethyl Chloride Spray)

Ethyl chloride, a halogenated hydrocarbon with local anesthetic and counterirritant properties, is used as a local anesthetic in minor operative procedures and to relieve pain caused by insect stings and burns; and as a counterirritant to relieve myofascial and visceral pain syndromes.

ETHYLENEDIAMINETETRAACETIC ACID

(EDTA)

Ethylenediaminetetraacetic acid, by chelating calcium ions, is a direct anticoagulant in an *in vitro* system. EDTA is poorly administered from the gastrointestinal tract. The rapid intravenous administration of sodium EDTA causes hypocalcemic tetany. In addition, ethylene glycolbis (beta-aminoethyl ether)-*N*, *N*, *N′*, *N′*-tetraacetic acid (EGTA), potassium fluoride, and potassium citrate are calcium-binding agents. Fluoride poisoning causes gastrointestinal disturbances, clonic convulsions, and hypotension, as well as respiratory and cardiac failure.

ETHYLESTRENOL

(Maxibolin)

Ethylestrenol (4 mg p.o. daily) is an anabolic steroid that is used to promote weight gain; to combat tissue depletion, anemia; and to overcome the catabolic effects of corticosteroids, osteoporosis, immobilization, and debilitation. Ethylestrenol enhances the production of erythropoietin by the kidneys and hence increases the red blood cell mass and volume (see Figure 95). Ethylestrenol may retain electrolytes and fluid and hence may become detrimental in patients with severe cardiac and renal diseases. Ethylestrenol is contraindicated in prostatic hypertrophy with obstruction and severe types of cancer (see also Table 8).

ETIDOCAINE HYDROCHLORIDE

(Duranest)

Etidocaine is a long-acting derivative of lidocaine but is far more potent. It is effective for filtration anesthesia, peripheral nerve block, and epidural and caudal blockade (see also Figure 31).

ETIDRONATE DISODIUM

(Didronel tablets 200 mg)

Etidronate is a bisphosphonate that inhibits normal and abnormal bone resorption; and reduces bone formation. It is indicated in the treatment of symptomatic Paget's disease; prevention and treatment of heterotopic ossification following total hip replacement or caused by spinal cord injury.

Medronate, **clodronate**, and **etidronate** contain a chlorophenyl group (**tiludronate**). They are the least potent and, in some instances, cause bone demineralization. Second-generation aminobisphosphonates (e.g., **alendronate** and **pamidronate**) contain a nitrogen group in the side chain. They are 10 to 100 times more potent than first-generation compounds. Third-generation bisphosphonates (e.g.. **risedronate** and **zoledronate**) contain a nitrogen atom within a heterocyclic ring and are up to 10,000 times more potent than first-generation agents.

Bisphosphonates concentrate at sites of active remodeling. Because they are highly negatively charged, bisphosphonates are membrane impermeable but are incorporated into the bone matrix by fluid-phase endocytosis. Bisphosphonates remain in the matrix until the bone is remodeled and then are released in the acid environment of the resorption lacunae beneath the osteoclast as the overlying mineral matrix is dissolved. The importance of this process for the antiresorptive effect of bisphosphonates is evidenced by the fact that calcitonin blocks the antiresorptive action.

Although bisphosphonates prevent hydroxyapatite dissolution, their antiresorptive action is due to direct inhibitory effects on osteoclasts rather than strictly physiochemical effects. The antiresorptive activity apparently involves two primary mechanisms: osteoclast apoptosis and inhibition of components of the cholesterol biosynthetic pathway.

ETINTIDINE

Stimulation of the H_2 receptors elicits a variety of responses, the most widely studied of which is gastric acid secretion from the parietal cells of the gastric glands. However, many other effects mediated by H_2 receptors are manifested in peripheral tissues. These include the positive chronotropic action in the auricular muscle, the inotropic action in the ventricular muscle, and the lipolytic effect in fat cells. In addition, the extensive use of cimetidine has led to the synthesis and marketing of more specific and efficacious analogs (see also Figure 34).

Examples of the various H_2-receptor blocking agents are:

Imidazole derivatives
Cimetidine and etintidine
Furan derivatives
Ranitidine and nizatidine
Guanidinothiazole derivatives
Famotidine
Piperidinomethylphenoxy derivatives
Roxatidine acetate and roxatidine

The pharmacological properties of cimetidine, ranitidine, and famotidine are outlined in Table 10.

ETODOLAC

(Lodine capsules 200 mg)

Etodolac is a nonsteroidal antiinflammatory drug (NSAID) that decreases inflammation, pain and fever, probably through inhibition of cyclooxygenase activity and prostaglandin synthesis.

Etodolac is another acetic acid derivative with some degree of COX-2 selectivity. Thus, at antiinflammatory doses, the frequency of gastric irritation may be less than with other tNSAIDs.

Etodolac is rapidly and well absorbed orally. It is highly bound to plasma protein and undergoes hepatic metabolism and renal excretion. The drug may undergo enterohepatic circulation in humans; its half-life in plasma is about 7 hours.

A single oral dose (200 to 400 mg) of **etodolac** (Lodine) provides postoperative analgesia that typically lasts for 6 to 8 hours. **Etodolac** also is effective in the treatment of osteoarthritis and rheumatoid arthritis, and the drug appears to be uricosuric. A sustained-release preparation (Lodine XL) is available, allowing once-a-day administration.

ETODOLAC

(Lodine)

Etodolac, which inhibits prostaglandin biosynthesis (see Figure 13), is indicated in acute and long-term use in the management of the signs and symptoms of osteoarthritis. It is a nonsteroidal antiinflammatory agent that possesses analgesic, antipyretic, and antiinflammatory properties. The most common side effects of etodolac are dyspepsia, abdominal pain, diarrhea, flatulence, nausea, vomiting, gastritis, or constipation (see also Table 3).

ETOMIDATE

(Amidate)

Etomidate is a nonbarbiturate hypnotic without analgesic activity and is used for induction of general anesthesia, for supplementing subpotent anesthetics such as nitrous oxide in oxygen, and for maintenance of anesthesia for short operative procedures. Etomidate lowers cerebral blood flow, and similar to ketamine, methohexital, or thiopental, also reduces cerebral oxygen consumption (see also Table 16).

The onset of action of etomidate, when given intravenously (0.2 to 0.6 mg/kg), is 1 minute, and duration of its action is 3 to 6 minutes. The addition of 0.1 mg of IV fentanyl will hasten recovery, in part because less etomidate will be required to induce anesthesia.

ETOPOSIDE

(VePesid concentrate for injection 20 mg/mL, liquid-filled capsules for oral use 50 mg, Toposar concentrate for injection 20 mg/mL, liquid-filled capsules for oral use 50 mg, Etopophos powder for injection 100 mg vial)

Etoposide is a podophyllotoxin derivative. Its main effect appears to be at the G_2 portion of the cell cycle. At high concentrations (10 mcg/mL or more), lysis of cells entering mitosis is seen; at low concentrations (0.3 to 10 mcg/ mL), cells are inhibited from entering prophase. Predominant macromolecular effect appears to be DNA synthesis inhibition. Etoposide is indicated in refractory testicular tumors, and small-cell lung cancer.

Etoposide and **teniposide** are similar in their actions and in the spectrum of human tumors affected. Unlike podophyllotoxin, but like the anthracyclines, they form a ternary complex with topoisomerase II and DNA and prevent resealing of the break that normally follows topoisomerase binding to DNA. The enzyme remains bound to the free end of the broken DNA strand, leading to an accumulation of DNA breaks and cell death. Cells in the S and G_2 phases of the cell cycle are most sensitive to etoposide and teniposide. Resistant cells demonstrate amplification of the mdr-l gene that encodes the *P*-glycoprotein drug efflux transporter, mutation or decreased expression of topoisomerase II, or mutations of the p53 tumor suppressor gene, a required component of the apoptotic pathway.

Oral administration of etoposide results in variable absorption that averages about 50%. After intravenous injection, peak plasma concentrations of 30 μg/mL are achieved; there is a biphasic pattern of clearance with a terminal half-life of about 6 to 8 hours in patients with normal renal function. Approximately 40% of an administered dose is excreted intact in the urine. In patients with compromised renal function, dosage should be reduced in proportion to the reduction in creatinine clearance. In patients with advanced liver disease, low serum albumin and elevated bilirubin (which displaces etoposide from albumin) tend to increase the unbound fraction of the drug, increasing the toxicity of any given dose. However, guidelines for dose reduction in this circumstance have not been defined. Drug concentrations in the cerebrospinal fluid average 1 to 10% of those in plasma.

The intravenous dose (Vepesid, Toposar, Etopophos) for testicular cancer in combination therapy is 50 to 100 mg/m^2 for 5 days, or 100 mg/m^2 on alternate days for three doses. For small-cell carcinoma of the lung, the dose in combination therapy is 50 to 120 mo/m^2 per day intravenously for 3 days, or 50 mg per day orally for 21 days. Cycles of therapy usually are repeated every 3 to 4 weeks. When given intravenously, the drug should be administered slowly during a 30- to 60-minute infusion to avoid hypotension and bronchospasm, which likely result from the additives used to dissolve etoposide, a relatively insoluble compound.

A disturbing complication of **etoposide** therapy has emerged—long-term follow-up of patients with childhood acute lymphoblastic leukemia, who develop an unusual form of acute nonlymphocytic leukemia with a translocation in chromosome 11 at 11q23. At this locus is found a gene or genes (the MLL or mixed-lineage leukemia gene) that regulates the proliferation of pluripotent stem cells. The leukemic cells have the cytological appearance of acute monocytic or monomyelocytic leukemia. Another distinguishing feature of etoposide-related leukemia is the short time interval between the end of treatment and onset of leukemia (1 to 3 years), as compared to the 4- to 5-year interval for secondary leukemias related to alkylating agents, and the absence of a myelodysplastic period preceding leukemia. Patients receiving weekly or twice-weekly doses of etoposide, with cumulative doses above 2000 mg/m^2, seem to be at higher risk of leukemia.

Etoposide is used primarily in treatment of testicular tumors in combination with **bleomycin** and **cisplatin**, and in combination with cisplatin and **ifosfamide** for small-cell carcinoma of the lung. It also is active against non-Hodgkin's lymphomas, acute nonlymphocytic leukemia, and Kaposi's sarcoma associated with AIDS. **Etoposide** has a favorable toxicity profile for dose escalation in that its primary acute toxicity is myelosuppression. In combination with ifosfamide and carboplatin, it is frequently used for high-dose chemotherapy in total doses of 1500 to 2000 mg/m^2.

The dose-limiting toxicity of **etoposide** is leukopenia, with a nadir at 10 to 14 days and recovery by 3 weeks. Thrombocytopenia occurs less often and usually is not severe. Nausea, vomiting, stomatitis, and diarrhea occur in approximately 15% of patients treated intravenously and in about 55% of patients who receive the drug orally. Alopecia is common but reversible. Fever, phlebitis, dermatitis, and allergic reactions including anaphylaxis have been observed. Hepatic toxicity is particularly evident after high-dose treatment. For both etoposide and teniposide, toxicity is increased in patients with decreased serum albumin, an effect related to decreased protein binding of the drug.

ETOPOSIDE
(Vepesid)

Etoposide (70 mg/m^2/day p.o.) is an antineoplastic agent that is indicated in small-cell carcinoma of the lung and testicular carcinoma. Etoposide exerts its cytotoxic action by arresting cells in the metaphase portion of cell division. The drug also inhibits cells from entering mitosis and depresses DNA and RNA synthesis (see also Figure 15).

Etoposide is mostly excreted unchanged by the kidneys. The adverse effects of etoposide include nausea and vomiting, headache, weakness, paresthesia, hypotension, palpitation, tachycardia, bone marrow depression, leukopenia, thrombocytopenia, and reversible alopecia.

EUCATROPINE

Eucatropine is a synthetic muscarinic cholinergic receptor antagonist. The various applications of synthetic muscarinic receptor antagonists are listed below:

Ophthalmology
- Homatropine
  - Produces mydriasis and cycloplegia
- Eucatropine
  - Produces only mydriasis

Preoperative uses
- Atropine
  - To prevent excess salivation and bradycardia
- Scopolamine
  - In obstetrics, to produce sedation and amnesia

Cardiac uses
- Atropine
  - To reduce severe bradycardia in hyperactive carotid sinus reflex
  - Diagnostically in Wolff–Parkinson–White syndrome to restore the PRS complex to normal duration

Gastrointestinal disorders
- In peptic ulcer
  - To diminish vagally mediated secretion of gastric juices and slow gastric emptying (propantheline, oxyphenonium, pirenzepine)
- In diarrhea associated with dysenteries and diverticulitis
- In excess salivation associated with heavy-metal poisoning or in parkinsonism

Neurologic diseases
- In parkinsonism (trihexyphenidyl or benztropine)
- In drug-induced pseudoparkinsonism (trihexyphenidyl or benztropine)
- In vestibular disorders such as motion sickness (scopolamine)

Methantheline and propantheline are synthetic derivatives that, besides their antimuscarinic effects, are ganglionic blocking agents and block the skeletal neuromuscular junction. Propantheline and oxyphenonium reduce gastric secretion, whereas pirenzepine, in addition to reducing gastric secretion, also reduces gastric motility (see Figure 37).

EXEMESTANE

(Aromasin tablets for oral use 25 mg)

Exemestane is an aromatase inhibitor (AI), which causes an irreversible, steroidal aromatase inactivation. It lowers circulating estrogen concentrations in postmenopausal women. Exemestane is 90% bound to plasma proteins. It is extensively metabolized. Exemestane is indicated in advanced breast cancer in postmenopausal women with disease progression following tamoxifen therapy. Unlabeled uses: are for prevention of prostate cancer.

Aminoglutethimide (Cytadren; AG), a first-generation type 2 AI, originally was developed as an anticonvulsant but was subsequently found to inhibit the synthesis of adrenocortical steroids. AG is a nonspecific weak AI, administered as a 250-mg dose four times daily with hydrocortisone supplementation because of unwanted adrenal suppression. Because of significant toxicities related to its anticonvulsant structure and its relatively weak inhibition of aromatase, its use has declined considerably with the advent of newer AIs.

Second-generation AIs include **formestane** (4-hydroxyandrostenedione; Lentaron), a type 1 steroidal inactivator; **fadrozole**, a type 2 **imidazole**; and **rogletimide** (pyridoglutethimide), a type 2 inhibitor structurally similar to aminoglutethimide. Formestane was the first steroidal aromatase inactivator widely used for the treatment of breast cancer patients. Because of better aromatase inhibition *in vivo* following parenteral administration, it is administered as an intramuscular depot injection. However, formestane has also been shown to be active when given orally. It suppresses plasma sex-hormone-binding globulin (SHBG), which is interpreted as an androgenic side effect. The response rates in phase II and III trials were about 25 to 40%. Due to the introduction of novel compounds, especially **exemestane**, formestane is not widely used today.

The third-generation inhibitors, developed in the 1990s, include the type 1 steroidal agent exemestane and the type 2 nonsteroidal imidazoles **anastrozole** and **letrozole**. Currently, third-generation AIs are most commonly used for the treatment of early-stage and advanced breast cancer.

Anastrozole is a potent and selective triazole AI. It, like letrozole, binds competitively and specifically to the heme of the CYP19. Anastrozole 1 or 10 mg administered once daily for 28 days reduces total body aromatization by 96.7 and 98.1%, respectively. In addition, anastrozole reduces local aromatization in large, ER-positive breast tumors.

Exemestane (Aromasin) is a more potent, orally administered analog natural substrate androstenedione that lowers estrogen levels more effectively than formestane. In contrast to the reversible competitive inhibitors anastrozole and letrozole, **exemestane** irreversibly inactivates the enzyme, and, therefore is referred to as a "suicide substrate." Doses of 25 mg per day inhibit aromatase activity by 98%, and lower plasma estrone and estradiol levels by about 90%. It has less androgenic activity than formestane, but otherwise has a similar toxicity profile.

Exemestane is rapidly absorbed from the gastrointestinal tract, reaching maximum plasma levels after 2 hours. Its absorption is increased by 40% after a high-fat meal. **Exemestane** is extensively protein-bound in plasma and has a terminal half-life of approximately 24 hours. It is extensively metabolized in the liver to inactive metabolites. A key metabolite, **17-β-hydroxyexemestane**, which is formed by reduction of the 17-oxo group via 17-β-hydroxysteroid dehydrogenase, has weak androgenic activity, which also could contribute to antitumor activity. Excretion is distributed almost equally between the urine and feces. Because significant quantities of active metabolites are excreted in the urine, exemestane doses should be adjusted in patients with renal dysfunction.

Exemestane has been tested in a randomized clinical trial in postmenopausal women with estrogen-receptor-positive breast cancer. Women who had completed 2 to 3 years of adjuvant tamoxifen were randomized to complete a total of 5 years of adjuvant treatment with tamoxifen or **exemestane**. The unadjusted hazard ratio in the exemestane group versus the tamoxifen group was 0.68, representing a 32% reduction in risk and corresponding to an absolute benefit in terms of disease-free survival of 4.7% at 3 years after randomization. Overall survival was not significantly different in the two groups.

In advanced breast cancer, exemestane has been evaluated in a phase III trial against megestrol in women with disease progressing on prior antiestrogen therapy. Patients receiving **exemestane** had a similar response rate but improved time to disease progression, time to treatment failure, and longer duration of survival compared with those taking megestrol acetate. Responses to treatment also have been shown in women with disease progressing on prior nonsteroidal aromatase inhibitors.

Exemestane generally is well tolerated. Discontinuations due to toxicity are not common (2.8%). Hot flashes, nausea, fatigue, increased sweating, peripheral edema, and increased appetite have been reported. In the trial comparing exemestane to tamoxifen in early-stage breast cancer, exemestane was associated with more frequent arthralgia and diarrhea, but gynecologic symptoms, vaginal bleeding, and muscle cramps were more frequent with tamoxifen. Visual disturbances and clinical fractures were more common with exemestane.

EXENATIDE

(Byetta subcutaneous injection 5 mcg/dose)

Exenatide is an antidiabetic agent/incretin mimetic agent that mimics antihyperglycemic actions of incretins, including enhancing glucose-dependent insulin secretion, suppressing inappropriately elevated glucagon secretion, slowing gastric emptying, and reducing food intake. It is indicated as an adjunctive therapy to improve glycemic control in patients with type 2 diabetes mellitus who are taking metformin, a sulfonylurea, or a combination of metformin and a sulfonylurea but who have not achieved adequate glycemic control.

EXPECTORANTS: Drugs that Increase Respiratory Tract Fluid

Classes of Expectorant	Examples	Mechanism of Action
Mucolytics compounds with free thiol group	*N*-acetylcysteine Ethylcysteine Mercaptoethane sodium sulfonate Mecysteine	Destroy disulfide bonds of proteins and glycoproteins
Proteolytic enzymes	Trypsin, chymotrypsin	Hydrolyze peptide bonds of proteins or glycoproteins
Deoxyribonuclease	Deoxyribonuclease	Destroys deoxyribonucleic acid fibers
Mucoregulators	Bromhexine Ambroxol Carbocysteine	Alter the secretory activity of the bronchial mucosa Activate sialomucin synthesis
"Hydrating" agents	Sodium chloride Sodium bicarbonate, water	Correct water and electrolyte disorders in secretions
Tensio-active agents	Tyloxapol	Make secretions less adhesive
Other compounds	Eprazinone	Modify fibrillate structures

Expectorants may have a demulcent (soothing and irritation-allaying) effect on the cells of the respiratory tract and assist in repelling invasion through providing a medium for the upward propulsion of foreign particles by ciliary action.

EZETIMIBE

(Zetia tablets 10 mg)

Ezetimibe is an antihyperlipidemic agent that inhibits absorption of cholesterol by the small intestine. It is indicated to be administered alone or with HMG-CoA reductase inhibitors as adjunctive therapy to diet for reduction of elevated total cholesterol, LDL, and apolipoprotein (Apo) in patients with primary hypercholesterolemia; with atorvastatin or simvastatin for the reduction of elevated total cholesterol and LDL levels in patients with homozygous familial hypercholesterolemia as an adjunct to other lipid-lowering treatments or if such treatments are unavailable; and as adjunctive therapy to diet for the reduction of elevated sitosterol and campesterol levels in patients with homozygous familial sitosterolemia.

EZETIMIBE/SIMVASTATIN

(Vytorin 10/10 tablets 10 mg ezetimibe/ 10 mg simvastatin)

Ezetimibe is an antihyperlipidemic combination. **Ezetimibe**: inhibits absorption of cholesterol by the small intestine. **Simvastatin**: increases the rate at which the body removes cholesterol from blood and reduces production of cholesterol by inhibiting enzyme that catalyzes an early rate-limiting step in cholesterol synthesis. The combination is indicated as an adjunctive treatment to diet for reduction of elevated total cholesterol, LDL cholesterol, triglycerides, non-HDL cholesterol, and Apo B, and to increase HDL cholesterol in patients with primary hypercholesterolemia or mixed hyperlipidemia; and as an adjunct to other lipid-lowering treatment for the reduction of total cholesterol and LDL cholesterol in patients with homozygous familial hypercholesterolemia.

Ezetimibe is the first of a new class of drugs that specifically reduces the intestinal absorption of cholesterol. The drug is absorbed into the intestinal epithelial cell, where it is believed to interfere with the sterol transporter system. This prevents both free cholesterol and plant sterols (phytosterols) from being transported into the cell from the intestinal lumen. The drug is absorbed rapidly and glucuronidated in the intestinal cell before secretion into the blood. **Ezetimibe** is avidly taken up by the liver from the portal blood and excreted into the bile, resulting in low peripheral blood concentrations. The glucuronide conjugate is hydrolyzed and absorbed, and is equally effective in inhibiting sterol absorption. This enterohepatic recycling is responsible for a half-life in the body of more than 20 hours. The principal benefit is a reduction in low-density cholesterol (LDL-C).

Recent data indicate that ezetimibe inhibits a specific transport process in jejunal enterocytes, which take up cholesterol from the lumen. The putative transport protein is Niemann-Pick C1-like 1 protein (NPC1L1). In wild-type mice, ezetimibe inhibits cholesterol absorption by about 70%; in NPC1L1 knockout mice, cholesterol absorption is 86% lower than in wild-type mice, and ezetimibe has no effect on cholesterol absorption. **Ezetimibe** does not affect intestinal triglyceride absorption. In human subjects, ezetimibe reduced cholesterol absorption by 54%, precipitating a compensatory increase in cholesterol synthesis, which can be inhibited with a cholesterol synthesis inhibitor such as a statin. There is also a substantial reduction of plasma levels of plant sterols (campesterol and sitosterol concentrations are reduced by 48 and 41%, respectively), indicating that **ezetimibe** also inhibits intestinal absorption of plant sterols.

The consequence of inhibiting intestinal cholesterol absorption is a reduction in the incorporation of cholesterol into chylomicrons. The reduced cholesterol content of chylomicrons diminishes the delivery of cholesterol to the liver by chylomicron remnants. The diminished remnant cholesterol content may decrease atherogenesis directly, as chylomicron remnants are very atherogenic lipoproteins. In experimental animal models of remnant dyslipidemia, ezetimibe profoundly diminished diet-induced atherosclerosis.

Reduced delivery of intestinal cholesterol to the liver by chylomicron remnants stimulates expression of the hepatic genes regulating LDL-receptor expression and cholesterol biosynthesis. The greater expression of hepatic LDL receptors enhances LDL-C clearance from the plasma.

Indeed, ezetimibe reduces LDL-C levels by 15% to 20%. Fasting triglyceride levels decrease about 5%, and HDL-C levels increase about 1 to 2%.

The maximal efficacy of ezetimibe for lowering LDL-C is between 15 and 20% when used as monotherapy. This reduction is equivalent to, or less than, that attained with 10- to 20-mg doses of most statins. Consequently, the role of ezetimibe as monotherapy of patients with elevated LDL-C levels appears to be limited to the small group of statin-intolerant patients.

The actions of ezetimibe are complementary to those of statins. Statins, which inhibit cholesterol biosynthesis, increase intestinal cholesterol absorption. **Ezetimibe**, which inhibits intestinal cholesterol absorption, enhances cholesterol biosynthesis by as much as 3.5 times in experimental animals. Dual therapy with these two classes of drugs prevents the enhanced cholesterol synthesis induced by ezetimibe and the increase in cholesterol absorption induced by statins. This combination provides additive reductions in LDL-C levels irrespective of the statin employed. There is a further reduction of 15 to 20% in LDL-C when **ezetimibe** is combined with any statin at any dose. Increasing statin dosages from the usual starting dose of 20 mg to 80 mg normally yields only an additional 12% reduction in LDL-C, whereas adding ezetimibe, 10 mg daily, to 20 mg of a statin will reduce LDL-C by an additional 18 to 20%.

A combination tablet containing ezetimibe, 10 mg, and various doses of simvastatin (10, 20, 40, and 80 mg) has been approved (**Vytorin**). At the highest simvastatin dose (80 mg), plus ezetimibe (10 mg), average LDL-C reduction was 60%, which is greater than can be attained with any statin as monotherapy.

Statins are cholesterol-lowering agents that reversibly inhibit HMG-CoA reductase, which catalyzes a rate-limiting step in cholesterol biosynthesis. Statins affect serum cholesterol by inhibiting cholesterol biosynthesis in the liver, and this organ is their main target. On the other hand, exposure of extrahepatic cells in smooth muscle to these drugs may cause adverse effects. Among the statins, **pravastatin**, **fluvastatin**, **cerivastatin**, **atorvastatin**, **rosuvastatin**, and **pitavastatin** are given in a biologically active open-acid form, whereas **simvastatin** and **lovastatin** are administered as inactive prodrugs with lactone rings. The open-acid statins are relatively hydrophilic and have low membrane permeabilities. However, most of the statins in the acid form are substrates of uptake transporters, so they are taken up efficiently by the liver and undergo enterohepatic circulation.

Statins, in combination with the bile-acid-binding resins **cholestyramine** and **colestipol** produce 20 to 30% greater reductions in LDL-C than can be achieved with statins alone. Preliminary data indicate that colesevelam hydrochloride plus a statin lowers LDL-C by 8 to 16% more than statins alone. Niacin also can enhance the effect of statins, but the occurrence of myopathy increases when statin doses greater than 25% of maximum (e.g., 20 mg of **simvastatin** or atorvastatin) are used with niacin. The combination of a fibrate (**clofibrate**, **gemfibrozil**, or fenofibrate) with a statin is particularly useful in patients with hypertriglyceridemia and high LDL-C levels. This combination increases the risk of myopathy but usually is safe with a fibrate at its usual maximal dose and a statin at no more than 25% of its maximal dose. Fenofibrate, which is least likely to interfere with statin metabolism, appears to be the safest fibrate to use with statins. Triple therapy with resins, niacin, and statins can reduce LDL-C by up to 70%. **Vytorin**, a fixed combination of simvastatin (10, 20, 40 or 80 mg) and ezetimibe (10mg), decreased LDL-C levels by up to 60% at 24 weeks.

F

FACTOR IX COMPLEX

(AlphaNine SD, Bebulin VH Immuno Konyne 80, Monanine, Profilinine Heat-Treated, Proplex SX-T, Proplex T)

Factor IX complex, a blood derivative with hemostatic properties, is used in factor IX deficiency (hemophilia B or Christmas disease) in patients with factor VIII inhibition, in factor VII deficiency, and in overdosage with anticoagulant (see also Tables 17 and 18 and Figure 92).

FACTOR IX CONCENTRATES

(AlphaNine SO powder for injection, dried plasma fraction of Factor IX, BeneFix powder for injection, nonpyrogenic lyophilized, purified protein produced by recombinant DNA, Monorune powder for injection lyophilized concentrate of Factor IX, plasma-derived, Profilnine SD powder for injection, lyophilized concentrate of Factor IX, plasma-derived, Proplex T powder for injection, plasma derived concentrate of clotting Factors II, VII, IX, and X, Bebulin VH powder for injection, purified freeze-dried concentrate of coagulation Factor IX, II, X, and VII (low amounts), heat-treated)

Factor IX is an antihemophilic agent that restores hemostasis in patients with factor IX deficiency. It is indicated in the control and prevention of hemorrhagic episodes in patients with hemophilia B (factor IX deficiency) (Proplex T only); bleeding episodes in patients with inhibitors to factor VIII, and prevention or control of bleeding episodes in patients with factor VII deficiency.

FAMCICLOVIR

(Famvir tablets 250 mg)

Famciclovir is an antiherpes virus agent that converts to penciclovir, which inhibits viral DNA replication by interfering with viral DNA polymerase. It is indicated in the treatment of acute herpes zoster; treatment or suppression of recurrent genital herpes in immunocompetent patients; and treatment of recurrent mucocutaneous herpes simplex infections in HIV-infected patients.

Famciclovir, the oral formulation of penciclovir, is a new antiherpes agent that is well absorbed following oral administration with little intersubject variability, and is rapidly converted to penciclovir with a bioavailability of 77%. Furthermore, although the activities of penciclovir and acyclovir against varicella-zoster virus (VZV) in infected cell lines appear to be comparable, penciclovir-triphosphate persists in virus-infected cells far longer than acyclovir-triphosphate, resulting in more prolonged antiviral activity. The intracellular half-life of penciclovir-triphosphate in VZV-infected cells is reported to be 9 hours, whereas that of acyclovir-triphosphate is 0.8 hour. These findings indicate that famciclovir has the potential to be administered without compromising therapeutic efficacy (see also Figure 16).

Viral infections of the skin are very common and include verrucae [human papillomavirus (HPV)], herpes simplex (HSV), condyloma acuminatum (HPV), molluscum contagiosum (poxvirus), and chicken pox [varicella-zoster virus (VZV)]. **Acyclovir** (Zovirax), **famciclovir** (Famvir), and **valacyclovir** (Valtrex) frequently are used systemically to treat herpes simplex and varicella infections. **Cidofovir** (Vistide) may be useful in treating acyclovir-resistant HSV or VZV and other cutaneous viral infections. Topically, acyclovir, docosanol (Abreva), and penciclovir (Denavir) are available for treating mucocutaneous HSV. **Podophyllin** (25% solution) and **podofilox** (condylox; 0.5% solution) are used to treat condylomata. Interferons α-2b (Intron-A), α-nl, and α-n3 (Alferon N) may be useful for treating refractory or recurrent warts.

Famciclovir is the diacetyl ester prodrug of 6-deoxy penciclovir and lacks intrinsic antiviral activity. Penciclovir (9-[4-hydroxy-3-hydroxymethylbut-l-yl] guanine) is an acyclic guanine nucleoside analog. The side chain differs structurally in that the oxygen has been replaced by a carbon and an additional hydroxymethyl group is present.

Penciclovir is similar to acyclovir in its spectrum of activity and potency against HSV and VZV. The inhibitory concentrations of penciclovir depend on cell type but are usually within twofold of those of acyclovir for HSV and VZV. It also is inhibitory for hepatitis B virus (HBV).

Penciclovir is an inhibitor of viral DNA synthesis. In HSV- or VZV-infected cells, penciclovir is phosphorylated initially by viral thymidine kinase. Penciclovir triphosphate serves as a competitive inhibitor of viral DNA polymerase. Although penciclovir triphosphate is approximately one-hundred times as potent as acyclovir triphosphate in inhibiting viral DNA polymerase, it is present in much higher concentrations and for more prolonged periods in infected cells than acyclovir triphosphate. The prolonged intracellular $t_{1/2}$ of penciclovir triphosphate, 7 to 20 hours, is associated with prolonged antiviral effects. Because penciclovir has a 3′-hydroxyl group, it is not an obligate chain terminator but does inhibit DNA elongation.

Resistant variants owing to thymidine kinase or DNA polymerase mutations can be selected by passage *in vitro*, but the occurrence of resistance during clinical use is currently low. Thymidine kinase-deficient, acyclovir-resistant herpes viruses are cross-resistant to penciclovir.

Oral penciclovir has low (5%) bioavailability. In contrast, **famciclovir** is well absorbed orally and converted rapidly to penciclovir by deacetylation of the side chain and oxidation of the purine ring during and following absorption from the intestine. The bioavailability of penciclovir is 65 to 77% following oral administration of **famciclovir**. Food slows absorption but does not reduce overall bioavailability. After single 250- or 500-mg doses of famciclovir, the peak plasma concentration of penciclovir averages 1.6 and 3.3 μg/mL, respectively. A small quantity of the 6-deoxy precursor but no **famciclovir** is detectable in plasma. After intravenous infusion of penciclovir at 10 mg/kg, peak plasma levels average 12 μg/mL. The volume of distribution is about twice the volume of total body water. The plasma $t_{1/2}$ of elimination of penciclovir averages about 2 hours, and over 90% is excreted unchanged in the urine, probably by both filtration and active tubular secretion. Following oral **famciclovir** administration, nonrenal clearance accounts for about 10% of each dose, primarily through fecal excretion, but penciclovir (60% of dose) and its 6-deoxy precursor (<10% of dose) are eliminated primarily in the urine. The plasma half-life averages 9.9 hours in renal insufficiency (Cl_{cr} < 30 mL/min); hemodialysis efficiently removes penciclovir. Lower peak plasma concentrations of penciclovir but no reduction in overall bioavailability occur in compensated chronic hepatic insufficiency.

Oral famciclovir is well tolerated but may be associated with headache, diarrhea, and nausea. Urticaria, rash, and hallucinations or confusional states (predominantly in the elderly) have been reported. Topical penciclovir, which is formulated in 40% propylene glycol and a cetomacrogol base, is associated infrequently with application-site reactions (~1%). The short-term tolerance of famciclovir is comparable with that of acyclovir.

Penciclovir is mutagenic at high concentrations *in vitro*; studies in laboratory animals indicate that chronic **famciclovir** administration is tumorigenic and decreases spermatogenesis and fertility in rodents and dogs; long-term administration (1 year) does not affect spermatogenesis in men. No teratogenic effects have been observed in animals, but safety during pregnancy has not been identified to date with famciclover or penciclover.

Oral **famciclovir**, topical penciclovir, and intravenous penciclovir are approved for managing HSV and VZV infections in various countries. Oral famciclovir (250 mg three times a day for 7 to 10 days) is as effective as acyclovir in treating first-episode genital herpes. In patients with recurrent genital HSV, patient-initiated famciclovir treatment (125 or 250 mg twice a day for 5 days) reduces healing time and symptoms by about one day. **Famciclovir** (250 mg twice a day for up to 1 year) is effective for suppression of recurrent genital HSV, but single daily doses are less effective. Higher doses (500 mg twice a day) reduce HSV recurrences in HIV-infected persons. Intravenous penciclovir (5 mg/kg every 8 or 12 hours for 7 days) is comparable with intravenous acyclovir for treating mucocutaneous HSV infections in immunocompromised hosts. In immunocompetent persons with recurrent orolabial HSV, topical 1% penciclovir cream (applied every 2 hours while awake for 4 days) shortens healing time and symptoms by about one day.

In immunocompetent adults with herpes zoster of 3 days' duration or less, **famciclovir** (500 mg three times a day for 10 days) is at least as effective as acyclovir (800 mg five times daily) in reducing healing time and zoster-associated pain, particularly in those 50 years of age and older. **Famciclovir** is comparable with valacyclovir in treating zoster and reducing associated pain in older adults. **Famciclovir** (500 mg three times a day for 7 to 10 days) also is comparable with high-dose oral acyclovir in treating zoster in immunocompromised patients and in those with ophthalmic zoster.

Famciclovir is associated with dose-related reductions in HBV DNA and transaminase levels in patients with chronic HBV hepatitis but is less effective than lamivudine. Famciclovir is also ineffective in treating lamivudine-resistant HBV infection owing to emergence of multiply resistant variants.

FAMOTIDINE

(Pepcid tablets 20 mg)

Famotidine is a histamine H_2 antagonist, which competitively blocks histamine at H_2 receptors, particularly those in gastric parietal cells, leading to inhibition of gastric acid secretion. It is indicated in short-term treatment of active duodenal ulcer; maintenance therapy for duodenal ulcer patients at reduced dosage after healing of an active ulcer and in short-term treatment of active benign gastric ulcer.

Famotidine (40 mg once a day at bedtime) is indicated for the short-term (4 weeks) treatment of active duodenal ulcer; as maintenance therapy for duodenal ulcer at reduced dosage after healing has taken place; for short-term treatment of gastroesophageal reflux disease; and in the treatment of hypersecretory conditions such as Zollinger–Ellison syndrome or multiple endocrine adenoma. Famotidine, which is a competitive inhibitor of H_2 receptors, inhibits gastric secretion. It is absorbed incompletely (40 to 50%), metabolized partly to an S-oxide metabolite, and partly is excreted unchanged in the urine (see also Table 10 and Figure 23).

The description of selective histamine$_1$-receptor blockade was a landmark in the treatment of acid-peptic disease. Before the availability of the H_2-receptor antagonists, the standard of care was simply acid neutralization in the stomach lumen, generally with inadequate results. The long history of safety and efficacy with the preceptor antagonists eventually led to their availability without a prescription. Increasingly, however, proton-pump inhibitors are replacing the H_2-receptor antagonists in clinical practice.

The H_2-receptor antagonists inhibit acid production by reversibly competing with histamine for binding to H_2 receptors on the basolateral membrane of parietal cells. Four different H_2-receptor antagonists, which differ mainly in their pharmacokinetics and propensity to cause drug interactions, are available in the United States: **cimetidine** (Tagamet), **ranitidine** (Zantac), **famotidine** (Pepcid), and **nizatidine** (Axid). These drugs are less potent than proton-pump inhibitors but still suppress 24-hour gastric acid secretion by about 70%. The H_2-receptor antagonists predominantly inhibit basal acid secretion, which accounts for their efficacy in suppressing nocturnal acid secretion. Because the most important determinant of duodenal ulcer healing is the level of nocturnal acidity, evening dosing of H_2-receptor antagonists is adequate therapy in most instances. Ranitidine and nizatidine also may stimulate GI motility, but the clinical importance of this effect is unknown.

All four H_2-receptor antagonists are available as prescription and over-the-counter formulations for oral administration. Intravenous and intramuscular preparations of cimetidine, ranitidine, and famotidine also are available. When the oral or nasogastric routes are not an option, these drugs can be given in intermittent intravenous boluses or by continuous intravenous infusion. The latter provides better control of gastric pH, but is not proven to be more effective in preventing clinically significant bleeding in critically ill patients.

The H_2-receptor antagonists are rapidly absorbed after oral administration, with peak serum concentrations within 3 hours. Absorption may be enhanced by food or decreased by antacids, but these effects probably are unimportant clinically. Therapeutic levels are achieved rapidly after intravenous dosing and are maintained for 4 to 5 hours (cimetidine), 6 to 8 hours (ranitidine), or 10 to 12 hours (**famotidine**). Unlike proton-pump inhibitors, only a small percentage of H_2-receptor antagonists are protein bound. Small amounts (from <10 to 35%) of these drugs undergo metabolism in the liver, but liver disease *per se* is not an indication for dose adjustment. The kidneys excrete these drugs and their metabolites by filtration and renal tubular secretion, and it is important to reduce doses of H_2-receptor antagonists in patients with decreased creatinine clearance. Neither hemodialysis nor peritoneal dialysis clears significant amounts of the drugs.

Like the proton-pump inhibitors, the H_2-receptor antagonists generally are well tolerated, with a low (3%) incidence of adverse effects. Side effects usually are minor and include diarrhea, headache, drowsiness, fatigue, muscular pain, and constipation. Less common side effects include those affecting the CNS (confusion, delirium, hallucinations, slurred speech, and headaches), which occur primarily with intravenous (IV) administration of the drugs or in elderly subjects. Long-term use of cimetidine at high doses—seldom used clinically today—decreases testosterone binding to the androgen receptor and inhibits a CYP that hydroxylates estradiol. Clinically, these effects can cause galactorrhea in women and gynecomastia, reduced sperm count, and impotence in men. Several reports have associated H_2-receptor antagonists with various blood dyscrasias, including thrombocytopenia. H_2-receptor antagonists cross the placenta and are excreted in breast milk. Although no major teratogenic risk has been associated with these agents, caution nevertheless is warranted when they are used in pregnancy.

The control of acid-peptic disease represents a major triumph for modern pharmacology. Proton-pump inhibitors are considered superior for acid suppression in most clinically significant acid-peptic diseases, including gastroesophageal reflux disease, peptic ulcers, and nonsteroidal antiinflammatory drug (NSAID)-induced ulcers. Proton-pump inhibitors also are employed in combination with antibiotics to eradicate infection with *H. pylori*, thereby playing a role in preventing recurrent peptic ulcers. These agents largely have replaced the use of miroprostol and sucralfate, although the latter still is a low-cost alternative for prophylaxis against stress ulcers. The delay in maximal inhibition of acid secretion with the proton-pump inhibitors (3 to 5 days) makes them less suited for use on an as-needed basis for symptom relief. In this setting H_2-receptor antagonists, although less effective than proton-pump inhibitors in suppressing acid secretion, have a more rapid onset of action that makes them useful for patient-directed management of mild or infrequent symptoms.

FASUDIL HYDROCHLORIDE

Fasudil, a novel intracellular calcium antagonist, dilates the spastic cerebral arteries in the chronic stage of an experimental model of subarachnoid hemorrhage. Fasudil increases cerebral blood flow and does not change systemic blood pressure (see also Table 20 and Figures 84 and 103).

FAT EMULSIONS

(Intralipid 10%, Intralipid 20%, Liposyn 10%, Liposyn 20%, Liposyn II 10%, Liposyn II 20%, Liposyn III 10% and 20%, Nutrilipid 10% and 20%, Soyacal 10%, Soyacal 20%, Travamulsion 10%, Travamulsion 20%)

Fat emulsions are used as a source of calories adjunctive to total parenteral nutrition.

FAZADINIUM

Fazadinium, similar to *d*-tubocurarine chloride, is a nondepolarizing or competitive blocking skeletal muscle relaxant. Fazadium, which is slightly less potent than *d*-tubocurarine, has a rapid onset and a long duration of action. It has anticholinergic properties and raises heart rate and cardiac output (see also Figure 79).

FELBAMATE

(Felbatol tablets 400 mg)

Felbamate is an anticonvulsant that reduces seizure spread in generalized tonic–clonic or partial seizures and may increase seizure threshold in absence seizures. Felbamate is indicated as a monotherapy or adjunctive therapy in treatment of partial seizures with and without generalization in epileptic adults, and as adjunctive therapy in treatment of partial and generalized seizures associated with **Lennox–Gastaut syndrome** in children.

Felbamate (1200 mg/day) is indicated in partial seizures and in Lennox–Gastaut syndrome. Felbamate increases the seizure threshold and prevents the spread of the seizure process. It is absorbed well, becomes bound to plasma proteins to the extent of 90%, is metabolized to parahydroxyfelbamate, and 2-hydroxyfelbamate, and 30 to 40% of the dosage is excreted unchanged in the urine. Felbamate causes aplastic anemia and hence should be used cautiously. It increases the level of phenytoin and valproic acid, and decreases the level of carbamazepine (see also Figure 33).

Felbamate (Felbatol) is a dicarbamate that was approved by the FDA for partial seizures in 1993. An association between **felbamate** and aplastic anemia in at least 10 cases resulted in a recommendation by the FDA and the manufacturer for the immediate withdrawal of most patients from treatment with this drug.

Felbamate is effective in both the maximal electroshock and pentylenetetrazol seizure models. Clinically relevant concentrations of felbamate inhibit N-methyl-D-aspartate (NMDA)-evoked responses and potentiate gamma-aminobutyric acid (GABA)-evoked responses in whole-cell, voltage-clamp recordings of cultured rat hippocampal neurons. This dual action on excitatory and inhibitory transmitter response may contribute to the wide spectrum of action of the drug in seizure models.

An active controlled, randomized, double-blind protocol demonstrated the efficacy of **felbamate** in patients with poorly control partial and secondarily generalized seizures. **Felbamate** also was found to be efficacious against seizures in patients with Lennox–Gastaut syndrome. The clinical efficacy of this compound, which inhibited responses to NMDA and potentiated those to GABA, underscores the potential value of additional antiseizure agents with similar mechanisms of action.

The Lennox–Gastaut syndrome is a severe form of epilepsy that usually begins in childhood and is characterized by cognitive impairments and multiple types of seizures including tonic-clonic, tonic, atonic, myoclonic, and atypical absence seizures. Addition of **lamotrigine** to other antiseizure drugs resulted in improved seizure control in comparison to placebo in a double-blind trial, demonstrating lamotrigine to be an effective and well-tolerated drug for this treatment-resistant form of epilepsy. **Felbamate** also was found to be effective for seizures in this syndrome, but the occasional occurrence of aplastic anemia has limited its use. **Topiramate** has also been demonstrated to be effective for Lennox–Gastaut syndrome.

FELODIPINE

(Plendil tablets, extended release 2.5 mg)

Felodipine is a calcium-channel-blocking agent, which inhibits movement of calcium ions across cell membrane in systemic and coronary vascular smooth muscle, altering contractile process.

Felodipine, a calcium-channel antagonist, is indicated in the treatment of hypertension. Following administration of felodipine, a reduction in blood pressure (BP) occurs within two hours, the heart rate increases during the first week, and the renal vascular resistance is decreased whereas the glomerular filtration rate remains unchanged. The reported adverse effects in descending order of occurrence are: peripheral edema (20%), headache, flushing, dizziness, upper respiratory infection, asthenia, cough, paraesthesia, dyspepsia, chest pain, nausea, muscle cramps, palpitation, abdominal pain, constipation, diarrhea, pharyngitis, rhinorrhea, back pain, and rash (2%) (see also Table 21 and Figure 84).

Voltage-sensitive Ca^{2+} channels (L-type or slow channels) mediate the entry of extracellular Ca^{2+} into smooth muscle and cardiac myocytes, and sinoatrial (SA) and atrioventricular (AV) nodal cells, in response to electrical depolarization. In both smooth muscle and cardiac myocytes, Ca^{2+} is a trigger for contraction, albeit by different mechanisms. Ca^{2+}-channel antagonists, also called Ca^{2+}-entry mockers, inhibit Ca^{2+}-channel function. In vascular smooth muscle, this leads to relaxation, especially in arterial beds. These drugs also may produce negative inotronic and chronotropic effects in the heart.

The 10 Ca^{2+}-channel antagonists that are in clinical use in the United States have diverse chemical structures. Five classes of compounds have been examined: **phenylalkylamines**, **dihydropyridines**, **benzothiazepines**, **diphenylpiperazines**, and a **diarylaminopropylamine**. At present, **verapamil** (a phenylalkylamine); **diltiazpem** (a benzothiazepine); **nifedipine**, **amlodipine**, **felodipine**, **isradipine**, **nicardipine**, **nisoldipine**, and **nimodipine** (dihydropyridines); and **bepridil** (a diarylaminopropylarmine ether used only for refractory angina) are approved for clinical use in the United States. Although these agents are commonly grouped together as "calcium-channel blockers," there are fundamental differences among verapamil, diltiazem, and the dihydropyridines, especially with respect to pharmacologic characteristics, drug interactions, and toxicities.

An increased concentration of cytosolic Ca^{2+} causes increased contraction in cardiac and vascular smooth muscle cells. The entry of extracellular Ca^{2+} is more important in initiating the contraction of cardiac myocytes (Ca^{2+}-induced Ca^{2+} release). The release of Ca^{2+} from intracellular storage sites also contributes to contraction of vascular smooth muscle, particularly in some vascular beds. Cytosolic Ca^{2+} concentrations may be increased by various contractile stimuli. Thus, many hormones and neurohormones increase Ca^{2+} influx through so-called receptor-operated channels, whereas high external concentrations of $K^{+\prime}$ and depolarizing electrical stimuli increase Ca^{2+} influx through voltage-sensitive, or "potential operated," channels. The Ca^{2+}-channel antagonists produce their effects by binding to the o^ subunit of the L-type Ca^{2+} channels and reducing Ca^{2+} flux through the channel.

Although the absorption of these agents is nearly complete after oral administration, their bioavailability is reduced, in some cases markedly, by first-pass hepatic metabolism. The effects of these drugs are evident within 30 to 60 minutes of an oral dose, with the exception of the more slowly absorbed and longer-acting agents amiodipine, isradipine, and **felodipine**. For comparison, peak effects of verapamil occur within 15 minutes of its intravenous administration. These agents all are bound extensively to plasma proteins (70 to 98%); their elimination half-lives vary widely and range from 1.3 to 64 hours. During repeated oral administration, bioavailability and half-life may increase because of saturation of hepatic metabolism. A major metabolite of diltiazem is desacetyldiltiazem, which has about one-half of diltiazem's potency as a vasodilator. *N*-Demethylation of verapamil results in production of norverapamil, which is biologically active but much less potent than the parent compound. The half-life of norverapamil is about 10 hours. The metabolites of the dihydropyridines are inactive or weakly active. In patients with hepatic cirrhosis, the bioavailabilities and half-lives of the Ca^{2+}-channel blockers may be increased, and dosage should be decreased accordingly. The half-lives of these agents also may be longer in older patients. Except for diltiazem and nifedipine, all the Ca^{2+}-channel blockers are administered as racemic mixtures.

FENFLURAMINE HYDROCHLORIDE (Pondimin)

Fenfluramine (20 mg t.i.d. before meals), an amphetamine-like drug, is an anorexic drug. The antiappetite effect of fenfluramine is blocked by agents that lower the level of serotonin receptor in the brain. Fenfluramine also enhances the utilization of glucose. Fenfluramine is de-ethylated to norfenfluramine, which is subsequently oxidized to *M*-trifluoromethylhippuric acid. Fenfluramine and norfenfluramine are also excreted unchanged in the urine. A greater amount of fenfluramine is excreted when urine is acidic. The half-lives of amphetamine and fenfluramine are 5 and 20 hours, respectively. Fenfluramine is contraindicated in glaucoma or psychosis, and should not be coadministered with a monoamine oxidase inhibitor (see also Figure 37).

FENOFIBRATE (Lofibra capsules 67 mg)

Fenofibrate is an antihyperlipidemic agent that decreases plasma levels of triglycerides by decreasing their synthesis. It also reduces plasma levels of very-low-density lipoprotein (VLDL) cholesterol by reducing their release into the circulation and increasing catabolism; and reduces serum uric acid levels by increasing urinary excretion of uric acid. It is indicated as an adjunctive therapy to diet for treatment of hypertriglyceridemia in adult patients with type 4 or 5 hyperlipidemia; as adjunctive therapy to diet for the reduction of low-density lipoprotein cholesterol (LDL-C), total cholesterol, triglycerides, and apolipoprotein B, and to increase high-density lipoprotein cholesterol (HDL-C) in adults with primary hypercholesterolemia or mixed dyslipidemia (Fredrickson types IIa and IIb).

In patients with mild hypertriglyceridemia (e.g., triglycerides <400 mg/dL), fibrate treatment decreases triglyceride levels by up to 50% and increases HDL-C concentrations about 15%; LDL-C levels may be unchanged or increase. The second-generation agents, such as **fenofibrate**, **bezafibrate**, and **ciprofibrate**, lower VLDL levels to a degree similar to that produced by gemfibrozil, but they also are more likely to decrease LDL levels by 15 to 20%. In patients with more marked hypertriglyceridemia (e.g., 400 to 1000 mg/dL), a similar fall in triglycerides occurs, but LDL increases of 10 to 30% are seen frequently. Normotriglyceridemic patients with heterozygous familial hypercholesterolemia usually experience little change in LDL levels with **gemfibrozil**; with the other fibric acid agents, reductions as great as 20% may occur in some patients.

Fibrates usually are the drugs of choice for treating severe hypertriglyceridemia and the chylomicronemia syndrome. Although the primary therapy is to remove alcohol and as much fat from the diet as possible, fibrates help both by increasing triglyceride clearance and by decreasing hepatic triglyceride synthesis. In patients with chylomicronemia syndrome, fibrate maintenance therapy and a low-fat diet keep triglyceride levels well below 1000 mg/dL and thus prevent episodes of pancreatitis.

In a 5-year study of hyperlipidemic men, gemfibrozil reduced total cholesterol by 10% and LDL-C by 11%, raised HDL-C levels by 11%, and decreased triglycerides by 35%. Overall, there was a 34% decrease in the sum of fatal plus nonfatal cardiovascular events without any effect on total mortality. No increased incidence of gallstones or cancers was observed. Subgroup analysis suggested that the greatest benefit occurred in the subjects with the highest levels of VLDL or combined VLDL and LDL and in those with the lowest HDL-C levels (<35 mg/dL). Gemfibrozil may have affected the outcome by influencing platelet function, coagulation factor synthesis, or LDL size. In a recent secondary prevention trial, gemfibrozil reduced fatal and nonfatal CHD events by 22% despite a lack of effect on LDL-C levels. HDL-C levels increased by 6%, which may have contributed to the favorable outcome.

All of the fibrate drugs are absorbed rapidly and efficiently (>90%) when given with a meal but less efficiently when taken on an empty stomach. The ester bond is hydrolyzed rapidly, and peak plasma concentrations are attained within 1 to 4 hours. More than 95% of these drugs in plasma are bound to protein, nearly exclusively to albumin. The half-lives of fibrates differ significantly ranging from 1.1 hours (gemfibrozil) to 20 hours (**fenofibrate**). The drugs are widely distributed throughout the body, and concentrations in liver, kidney, and intestine exceed the plasma level. Gemfibrozil is transferred across the placenta. The fibrate drugs are excreted predominantly as glucuronide conjugates; 60 to 90% of an oral dose is excreted in the urine, with smaller amounts appearing in the feces. Excretion of these drugs is impaired in renal failure, though excretion of gemfibrozil is less severely compromised in renal insufficiency than is excretion of other fibrates. Nevertheless, the use of fibrate is contraindicated in patients with renal failure.

Fibric acid is well tolerated. Side effects may occur in 5 to 10% of patients but most often are not sufficient to cause discontinuation of the drug. Gastrointestinal (GI) side effects occur in up to 5% of patients. Other side effects are reported infrequently and include rash, urticaria, hair loss, myalgias, fatigue, headache, impotence, and anemia. Minor increases in liver transaminases and alkaline phosphatase have been reported. Clofibrate, bezafibrate, and fenofibrate have been reported to potentiate the action of oral anticoagulants, in part by displacing them from their binding sites on albumin. Careful monitoring of the prothrombin time and reduction in dosage of the anticoagulant may be appropriate when treatment with a fibrate is begun.

A myopathy syndrome occasionally occurs in subjects taking clofibrate, gemfibrozil, or **fenofibrate**, and may occur in up to 5% of patients treated with a combination of gemfibrozil and higher doses of statins. To diminish the risk of myopathy, statin doses should be reduced when combination therapy of a statin plus a fibrate is employed. Several drug interactions may contribute to this adverse response. Gemfibrozil inhibits hepatic uptake of statins by OATP2. Gemfibrozil also competes for the same glucuronosyl transferases that metabolize most statins. As a consequence, levels of both drugs may be increased when they are coadministered. Patients taking this combination should be instructed to be aware of the potential symptoms and should be followed at 3-month intervals with careful history and determination of CK values until a stable pattern is established. Patients taking fibrates with rosuvastatin should be followed especially closely even if low doses (5 to 10 mg) of rosuvastatin are employed until there is more experience with and knowledge of the safety of this specific combination. **Fenofibrate** is glucuronidated by enzymes that are not involved in statin glucuronidation. Thus, feno-fibrate-statin combinations are less likely to cause myopathy than combination therapy with gemfibrozil and statins.

All of the fibrates increase the lithogenicity of bile. Clofibrate use has been associated with increased risk of gallstone formation; gemfibrozil and fenofibrate reportedly do not increase biliary tract disease.

Renal failure is a relative contraindication to the use of fibric acid agents, as is hepatic dysfunction. Combined statin-fibrate therapy should be avoided in patients with compromised renal function. Gemfibrozil should be used with caution and at a reduced dosage to treat the hyperlipidemia of renal failure. Fibrates should not be used by children or pregnant women.

FENOLDOPAM

Peripheral dopaminergic receptor agents are useful in the treatment of congestive heart failure (CHF). Two distinct subtypes of dopamine receptors have been identified. The dopamine (DA_1) receptors, which are located on vascular smooth muscles, cause vasodilation in the renal, mesentery, cerebral, and coronary vascular beds (see Figure 49). Thus, the pharmacologic response to activation of the DA_2- and DA_1-receptor receptors is hypotension, bradycardia, diuresis, and natriuresis. Fenoldopam is an orally active DA_1-receptor agonist. It is more potent than dopamine in causing

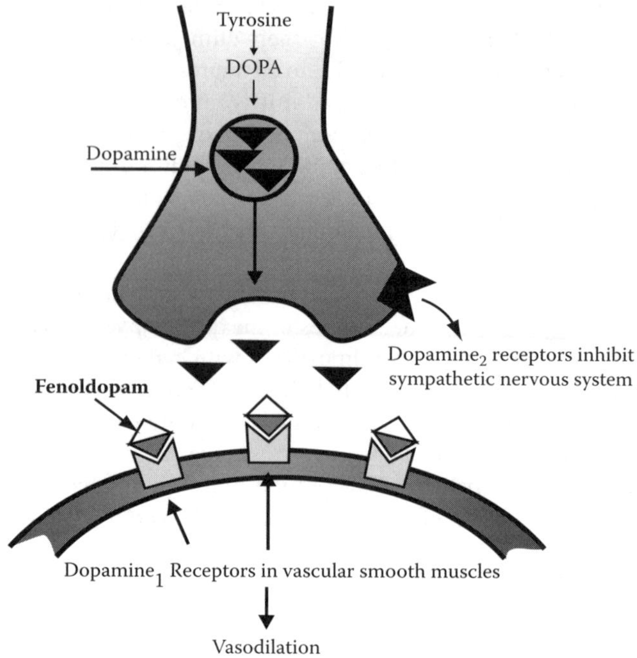

FIGURE 49 **Fenoldopam**, an oral drug, is more potent than dopamine in causing renal vasodilation without having adrenergic, cholinergic, or histaminergic properties.

renal vasodilation without having adrenergic, cholinergic, or histaminergic properties. The comparative actions of norepinephrine, dopamine, dobutamine, ibopamine, propylbutyldopamine, and fenoldopam are shown in Table 13.

FENOPROFEN CALCIUM (Ansaid)

Fenoprofen (200 to 300 mg in divided doses b.i.d. or t.i.d.) is indicated for acute or long-term treatment of the signs and symptoms of rheumatoid arthritis and osteoarthritis. Fenoprofen is a propionic acid derivative and, similar to ibuprofen, naproxen, flurbiprofen, or ketoprofen, has analgesic, antipyretic, and antiinflammatory properties (see also Table 3).

FENOPROFEN CALCIUM (Fenoprofen tablets 600 mg)

Fenoprofen is a NSAID agent, which decreases inflammation, pain, and fever, probably through inhibition of cyclooxygenase activity and prostaglandin synthesis. It is indicated in the symptomatic relief for rheumatoid arthritis, osteoarthritis, and mild to moderate pain.

The pharmacodynamics properties of the propionic acid derivatives (**ibuprofen**, **naproxen**, **flurbiprofen**, **fenoprofen**, **ketoprofen**, and **oxaprozin**) do not differ significantly. All are nonselective cyclooxygenase inhibitors with the effects and side effects common to other tNSAIDs. Although there is considerable variation in their potency as COX inhibitors, this is not of obvious clinical consequence. Some of the propionic acid derivatives, particularly naproxen, have prominent inhibitory effects on leukocyte function, and some data suggest that naproxen may have slightly better efficacy with regard to analgesia and relief of morning stiffness. Epidemiological studies suggest that while the relative risk of myocardial infarction is unaltered by ibuprofen, it is reduced by around 10% by naproxen, compared to a reduction of 20 to 25% by aspirin. This suggestion of benefit accords with the clinical pharmacology of naproxen that suggests that some but not all individuals dosed with 500 mg twice daily sustain platelet inhibition throughout the dosing interval.

Oral doses of **fenoprofen** are readily but incompletely (85%) absorbed. The presence of food in the stomach retards absorption and lowers peak concentrations in plasma, which usually are achieved within 2 hours. The concomitant administration of antacids does not seem to alter the concentrations that are achieved.

After absorption, **fenoprofen** binds avidly to protein, is extensively metabolized, and is excreted in the urine with a half-life of approximately 3 hours.

The GI side effects of fenoprofen are similar to those of ibuprofen or naproxen and occur in approximately 15% of patients.

FENOTEROL HYDROBROMIDE

Fenoterol (200 to 400 mcg by inhalation), a $beta_2$-adrenergic receptor agonist, is being used in patients with moderate to severe asthma, with chronic obstructive pulmonary disease, in protection against exercise-induced asthma, and for acute treatment of asthma attack. However, no apparent advantage of fenoterol over equipotent doses of albuterol or terbutaline has been demonstrated in clinical trials (see also Figure 94).

FENTANYL CITRATE

(Sublimaze injection 0.05 mg base)

Fentanyl is an opioid analgesic that is a potent, short-acting, rapid-onset opiate agonist that relieves pain by stimulating opiate receptors in the CNS; also causes respiratory depression, peripheral vasodilation, inhibition of intestinal peristalsis, sphincter of Oddi spasm, stimulation of chemoreceptors that cause vomiting, and increased bladder tone.

It is indicated in short-term analgesia before, during, and after anesthesia; as a supplement to general or regional anesthesia; for administration with a neuroleptic during anesthesia; and as anesthesia with oxygen for high-risk patients. Fentanyl (0.05 to 0.1 mg IM) is an opioid analgesic that is used as an analgesic of short duration during anesthesia, is used in combination with a neuroleptic such as droperidol to produce dissociative anesthesia; and as an anesthetic agent in combination with oxygen in high-risk surgery such as open heart surgery. Fentanyl interacts predominantly with the opioid μ receptors that are distributed in the spinal cord and brain. Fentanyl produces analgesia, miosis, sedation, and respiratory depression which lasts longer than its analgesic effects. Like morphine, fentanyl raises the pain threshold and alters the patient's reactions to pain (see also Figure 68). Fentanyl increases the tone and decreases the propulsive contractions of the smooth muscles in the GI tract and hence causes constipation. Duragesic is a transdermal system providing continuous system delivery of fentanyl for 72 hours. It causes life-threatening hypoventilation and is contraindicated in the management of acute or postoperative pain.

Fentanyl (Sublimaze), **sufentanil** (Sufenta), **alfentanil** (Alfenta), **remifentanil** (Ultiva), **meperidine** (Demerol), and **morphine** are the major parenteral opioids used in the perioperative period. The primary analgesic activity of each of these drugs is produced by agonist activity at μ-opioid receptors. Their order of potency (relative to morphine) is: sufentanil (l000x) > remifentanil (300x) > **fentanyl** (l00x) > alfentanil (15x) > morphine (1x) > meperidine (0.lx).

The choice of a perioperative opioid is based primarily on duration of action, given that at appropriate doses, all produce similar analgesia and side effects. Remifentanil has an ultra-short duration of action (~10 minutes) and accumulates minimally with repeated doses or infusion; it is particularly well suited for procedures that are briefly painful, but for which little analgesia is required postoperatively. Single doses of **fentanyl**, alfentanil an sufentanil all have similar intermediate durations of action (30, 20, and 15 minutes, respectively), but recovery after prolonged administration varies considerably. **Fentanyl's** action lengthens most with infusion, sufentanil's much less so, and alfentanil's the least. Except for remifentanil, all of the aforementioned opioids are metabolized in the liver, followed by renal and biliary excretion of the metabolites. Remifentanil is hydrolyzed by tissue and plasma esterases. After prolonged administration, morphine metabolites have significant analgesic and hypnotic activity.

Very large doses of morphine can be used to produce anesthesia—however, decreased peripheral resistance and blood pressure are troublesome. **Fentanyl** and sufentanil, which are potent and selective μ agonists, are less likely to cause hemodynamic instability during surgery, in part because they do not cause the release of histamine.

Morphine-like opioids should be used with caution in patients who have a decreased blood volume because these agents can aggravate hypovolemic shock. Morphine should be used with great care in patients with cor pulmonale because deaths after ordinary therapeutic doses have been reported. The concurrent use of certain phenothiazines may increase the risk of morphine-induced hypotension.

Cerebral circulation is not affected directly by therapeutic doses of morphine. However, opioid-induced respiratory depression and CO_2 retention can result in cerebral vasodilation and an increase in cerebrospinal fluid pressure; the pressure increase does not occur when Pco_2 is maintained at normal levels by artificial ventilation.

FENTANYL TRANSDERMAL SYSTEM

(Duragesic-12 transdermal system 1.25 mg)

Fentanyl is an opioid analgesic that is a potent opiate agonist that relieves pain by stimulating opiate receptors in the

CNS; it also causes respiratory depression, peripheral vasodilation, inhibition of intestinal peristalsis, sphincter of Oddi spasm, stimulation of chemoreceptors that cause vomiting, and increased bladder tone. It is indicated in the management of persistent moderate to severe chronic pain that requires continuous opioid administration for a prolonged period of time and that cannot be managed by other means. **Fentanyl** is a synthetic opioid related to the phenylpiperidines. The actions of **fentanyl** and its congeners, **sufentanil**, **remifentanil**, and **alfentanil**, are similar to those of other receptor agonists. **Fentanyl** is a popular drug in anesthetic practice because of its relatively shorter time to peak analgesic effect, rapid termination of effect after small bolus doses, and relative cardiovascular stability.

Pharmacological properties—analgesia: The analgesic effects of **Fentanyl** and sufentanil are similar to those of morphine and other μ opioids. Fentanyl is approximately 100 times more potent than morphine, and sufentanil is approximately 1000 times more potent than morphine. These drugs are most commonly administered intravenously, although both also are commonly administered epidurally and intrathecally for acute postoperative and chronic pain management. **Fentanyl** and sufentanil are far more lipid soluble than morphine; thus the risk of delayed respiratory depression from rostral spread of intraspinally administered narcotic to respiratory centers is greatly reduced. The time to peak analgesic effect after intravenous administration of fentanyl and sufentanil is less than that for morphine and meperidine. Recovery from analgesic effects also occurs more quickly. However, with larger doses or prolonged infusions, the effects of these drugs become more lasting, with durations of action becoming similar to those of longer-acting opioids.

Other CNS effects: As with other μ opioids, nausea, vomiting, and itching can be observed with **fentanyl**. Muscle rigidity, although possible with all narcotics, appears to be more common after administration of bolus doses of **fentanyl** or its congeners. This effect is felt to be centrally mediated and may be due in part to their increased potency relative to morphine. Rigidity can be mitigated by increased bolus dosing, slower administration of boluses, and pretreatment with a nonopioid anesthetic induction agent. Rigidity can be treated with depolarizing or nondepolarizing neuromuscular-blocking agents while controlling the patient's ventilation. Care must be taken to make sure that the patient is not simply immobilized but aware. Respiratory depression is similar to that observed with other μ receptor agonists, but the onset is more rapid.

Fentanyl and its derivatives decrease the heart rate and can mildly decrease BP. However, these drugs do not release histamine and, in general, provide a marked degree of cardiovascular stability. Direct depressant effects on the myocardium are minimal. For this reason, high doses of fentanyl or sufentanil are commonly used as the primary anesthetic for patients undergoing cardiovascular surgery or for patients with poor cardiac function.

These agents are highly lipid soluble and rapidly cross the blood–brain barrier. This is reflected in the half-life for equilibration between the plasma and cerebrospinal fluid of approximately 5 minutes for **fentanyl** and sufentanil. The levels in plasma and cerebrospinal fluid decline rapidly owing to redistribution of fentanyl from highly perfused tissue groups to other tissues, such as muscle and fat. As saturation of less well-perfused tissue occurs, the duration of effect of fentanyl and sufentanil approaches the length of their elimination half-lives of between 3 and 4 hours. Fentanyl and sufentanil undergo hepatic metabolism and renal excretion. Therefore, with the use of higher doses or prolonged infusions, fentanyl and sufentanil become longer acting.

Fentanyl citrate (Sublimaze) and sufentanil citrate (Sufenta) have gained widespread popularity as anesthetic adjuvants. They are used commonly either intravenously, epidurally, or intrathecally. Epidural use of fentanyl and sufentanil for postoperative or labor analgesia has gained increasing popularity. A combination of epidural opioids with local anesthetics permits reduction in the dosage of both components, minimizing the side effects of the local anesthetic (i.e., motor blockade) and the opioid (i.e., urinary retention, itching, and delayed respiratory depression in the case of morphine). Intravenous use of **fentanyl** and sufentanil for postoperative pain has been effective but limited by clinical concerns about muscle rigidity. However, the use of fentanyl and sufentanil in chronic pain treatment has become more widespread. Epidural and intrathecal infusions, both with and without local anesthetic, are used in the management of chronic malignant pain and selected cases of nonmalignant pain. Also, the development of novel, less invasive routes of administration for fentanyl has facilitated the use of these compounds in chronic pain management. Transdermal patches (**Duragesic**) that provide sustained release of fentanyl for 48 hours or more are available

FEPRADINOL

Fepradinol is an antiinflammatory agent which possesses inhibitory activity on acute inflammation, and this effect does not seem to be related to an inhibitory effect on prostaglandin biosynthesis. Therefore, the mechanism of antiinflammatory effects of fepradinol are different from those of indomethacin or piroxicam (see also Table 3 and Figure 13).

FERROUS SALTS

Ferrous sulfate (20% elemental iron) and ferrous gluconate (11.6% elemental iron) are used in iron deficiency anemia. Extensive numbers of oral preparations are available for the treatment of iron deficiency. In general, the ferrous salts (ferrous sulfate, ferrous gluconate, and ferrous fumerate) are better absorbed than the ferric salts (ferric sulfate). Ferrous calcium citrate is mostly used in patients during pregnancy to provide iron as well as calcium. The parenteral iron medications available include iron-dextran (ferric hydroxide and high-molecular-weight dextran) for intramuscular use, dextriferron (a complex of ferric hydroxide and partially hydrolyzed dextran) for intravenous use, and saccharated iron oxide (a complex of ferric hydroxide and sucrose) for intravenous use. These preparations are reserved for those cases in which oral preparations are not tolerated, absorbed, or rapid enough in their onset of action, or are otherwise not suitable for noncompliant patients. A lethal dose of iron consists of 12 g of an iron preparation containing 1 or 2 g of elemental iron. Therefore, iron toxicity rarely occurs in adults but is frequently seen in children. The mortality rate among untreated children is high (45%). The initial signs and symptoms of iron poisoning are gastrointestinal and usually consist of nausea, vomiting, and diarrhea. If untreated, acidosis, cyanosis, and circulatory collapse may ensue. If the patient survives, there may be gastric scarring and pyloric stenosis resulting from the corrosive action of the iron preparation. Treatment should include induced vomiting and lavage if the poisoning is discovered early, catharsis to hasten evacuation, sodium bicarbonate therapy to combat the acidosis, and the administration of deferoxamine (Desferal), a specific iron-chelating agent. One hundred milligrams of deferoxamine is able to bind 8.5 mg of iron. The chelating effects of deferoxamine are maximum at an acidic pH; therefore, when given orally, deferoxamine must be administered before the sodium bicarbonate. In the event of iron poisoning, deferoxamine may also be administered intramuscularly. Besides its usefulness in counteracting the effects of iron poisoning, deferoxamine has been used in disorders that involve iron overload such as ocular hemosiderosis or hemochromatosis.

FEXOFENADINE HYDROCHLORIDE

(Allegra tablets 30 mg)

Fexofenadine is a peripherally selective histamine receptor antagonist that competitively antagonizes histamine at the H_1-receptor site. It is indicated in the symptomatic relief of symptoms (nasal and nonnasal) associated with seasonal allergic rhinitis; and treatment of uncomplicated skin manifestations of chronic idiopathic urticaria.

First-generation piperidines (cyproheptadine, phenindamine): Cyproheptadine uniquely has both antihistamine and antiserotonin activity. Cyproheptadine and phenindamine cause drowsiness and also have significant anticholinergic effects.

Second-generation piperidines (prototype: terfenadine): **Terfenadine** and **astemizole** were withdrawn from the market. Current drugs in this class include **loratadine**, **desloratadine**, and **fexofenadine**. These agents are highly selective for H_1 receptors, lack significant anticholinergic actions, and penetrate poorly into the CNS. Taken together, these properties appear to account for the low incidence of side effects of piperidine antihistamines.

Second-generation H_1-receptor antagonists lack anticholinergic side effects and are described as nonsedating largely because they do not cross the blood–brain barrier. They include cetirizine (Zyrtec), loratadine (Claritin), desloratidine (Clarinex), and **fexofenadine** hydrochloride (Allegra). Although second-generation nonsedating H_1-receptor blockers are as effective as the first-generation H_1 blockers, they are metabolized by CYP3A4 and, to a lesser extent, by CYP2D6 and should not be coadministered with medications that inhibit these enzymes (e.g., imidazole antifungals and macrolide antibiotics).

H_2-receptor blockers include **cimetidine** (Tagament), **ranitidine** (Zantac), **famotidine** (Pepcid), and **nizatidine** (Axid). Besides their use in combination with H_1-receptor blockers for pruritus, the H_2-receptor blockers have immunomodulating effects, and this property has been exploited in children to treat warts.

FEXOFENADINE HYDROCHLORIDE/ PSEUDOEPHEDRINE HYDROCHLORIDE

(Allegra-D tablets 120 mg pseudoephedrine/60 mg fexofenadine)

Fexofenadine is an antihistamine/decongestant. **Fexofenadine**: competitively antagonizes histamine at the H_1-receptor site. **Pseudoephedrine**: causes vasoconstriction and subsequent shrinkage of nasal mucous membranes by alpha-adrenergic stimulation, promoting nasal drainage. They are indicated in relief of symptoms associated with seasonal allergic rhinitis. H_1 antagonists have an established and valued place in symptomatic treatment of various immediate hypersensitivity reactions. In addition, the central properties of some of the series are of therapeutic value for suppressing motion sickness or for sedation.

FIBRINOLYSIN AND DEOXYRIBONUCLEASE, COMBINED (BOVINE)

(Elase)

Fibrinolysin and deoxyribonuclease, a proteolytic enzyme and a topical debriding agent, are used as a topical debridement of inflamed or infected skin lesions and wounds.

FILGRASTIM

(Granulocyte colony stimulating factor, G-CSF) (Neupogen)

Filgrastim, a CSF (5 mcg/kg SC or IV), is used to decrease incidence of infection after cancer chemotherapy for nonmyeloid malignancies (see also Cytokines and Figure 63). Filgrastim is a granulocyte colony-stimulating factor; it stimulates neutrophil production within bone marrow. It is indicated in cancer patients receiving myelosuppressive chemotherapy; patients with acute myeloid leukemia receiving induction or consolidation chemotherapy; cancer patients receiving bone marrow transplant; patients with sever chronic neutropenia; peripheral blood progenitor cell (PBPC) collection and therapy in cancer patients.

Colony-stimulating factor (G-CSF): Recombinant human G-CSF **filgrastim** (Neupogen) is a 175-amino acid glycoprotein produced in *E. coli*. Unlike natural G-CSF, it is not glycosylated and carries an extra N-terminal methionine. The principal action of **filgrastim** is the stimulation of CFU-G to increase neutrophil production. It also enhances the phagocytic and cytotoxic functions of neutrophils.

Filgrastim is effective in the treatment of severe neutropenia after autologous hematopoietic stem cell transplantation and high-dose cancer chemotherapy. Like GM-CSF, filgrastim shortens the period of severe neutropenia and reduces morbidity secondary to bacterial and fungal infections. When used as a part of an intensive chemotherapy regimen, it can decrease the frequency of hospitalization for febrile neutropenia and interruptions in the chemotherapy protocol; a positive impact on patient survival has not been demonstrated. G-CSF also is effective in the treatment of severe congenital neutropenias. In patients with cyclic neutropenia, G-CSF therapy will increase the level of neutrophils and shorten the length of the cycle sufficiently to prevent recurrent bacterial infections. Filgrastim therapy can improve neutrophil counts in some patients with myelodysplasia or marrow damage (moderately severe aplastic anemia or tumor infiltration of the marrow). The neutropenia of AIDS patients receiving zidovudine also can be partially or completely reversed. Filgrastim is routinely used in patients undergoing peripheral blood stem cell (PBSC) collection for stem cell transplantation. It promotes the release of CD34+ progenitor cells from the marrow, reducing the number of collections necessary for transplant. Moreover, **filorastim**-mobilized PBSCs appear more capable of rapid engraftment. PBSC-transplanted patients require fewer days of platelet and red blood cell transfusions and a shorter duration of hospitalization than do patients receiving autologous bone marrow transplants.

Filgrastim is administered by subcutaneous (SC) injection or intravenous (IV) infusion over at least 30 minutes at doses of 1 to 20 μg/kg/day. The usual starting dose in a patient receiving myelosuppressive chemotherapy is 5 μg/kg/day. The distribution and clearance rate from plasma (half-life of 3.5 hours) are similar for both routes of administration. As with GM-CSF therapy, filgrastim given daily after hematopoietic stem cell transplantation or intensive cancer chemotherapy will increase granulocyte production and shorten the period of severe neutropenia. Frequent blood counts should be obtained to determine the effectiveness of the treatment and guide dosage adjustment. In patients who received intensive myelosuppressive cancer chemotherapy, daily administration of G-CSF for 14 to 21 days or longer may be necessary to correct the neutropenia. With less intensive chemotherapy, fewer than 7 days of treatment may suffice. In AIDS patients on zidovudine or patients with cyclic neutropenia, chronic G-CSF therapy often is required.

Adverse reactions to filgrastim include mild to moderate bone pain in patients receiving high doses over a protracted period, local skin reactions following subcutaneous injection, and rare cutaneous necrotizing vasculitis. Patients with a history of hypersensitivity to proteins produced by *E. coli* should not receive the drug. Marked granulocytosis with counts greater than 100,000/μl can occur in patients receiving **filgrastim** over a prolonged period of time. However, this is not associated with any reported clinical morbidity or mortality and rapidly resolves once therapy is discontinued. Mild to moderate splenomegaly has been observed in patients on long-term therapy.

FINASTERIDE

(Propecia tablets 1 mg)

Finasteride is an androgen hormone inhibitor that inhibits conversion of testosterone into 5-alpha-dihydrotestosterone, a potent androgen. Indications: **Propecia**: for treatment of male pattern hair loss (androgenic alopecia) in men only; **Proscar**: for treatment of symptomatic benign prostatic hyperplasia (BPH) in men with enlarged prostate; in combination with **doxazosin** to reduce the risk of symptomatic progression of BPH. Finasteride is a potent 5-alpha-reductase inhibitor that has shown limited success in men treated for benign prostatic hyperplasia. 5-Alpha-reductase is necessary for the prostatic conversion of testosterone to dihydrotestosterone (DHT), the specific steroid that stimulates prostate transitional zone growth. Finasteride reduces the size of the prostate gland by 20%, but this does not correlate well with improvement in symptoms (see also Figure 96).

Finasteride (Proscar) is an antagonist of 5α-reductase, especially type II; **dutasteride** (Avodart) is an antagonist of types I and II; both drugs block the conversion of testosterone to DHT, especially in the male external genitalia. These agents were developed to treat benign prostatic hyperplasia. When they are administered to men with moderately severe symptoms due to obstruction of urinary tract outflow, serum and prostatic concentrations of dihydrotestosterone decrease, prostatic volume decreases, and urine flow rate increases. Impotence is a well documented, albeit infrequent, side effect of this use, although the mechanism is not understood. **Finasteride** also is approved for use in the treatment of male pattern baldness under the trade name Propecia, even though that effect is presumably mediated via type I 5α-reductase. Finasteride appears to be as effective as flutamide and the combination of estrogen and cyproterone in the treatment of hirsutism.

FLAVOCOXID

(Limbrel capsule 250 mg)

Flavocoxid is a nutritional supplement causing an inhibition of prostaglandin synthesis by inhibition of cyclooxygenase. Also, flavocoxid may act as an antioxidant, reducing reactive oxygen species including hydroxyl radical, superoxide anion radical, and hydrogen peroxide. Flavocoxid reduces proinflammatory cytokine interleukin-1-beta and tumor necrosis factor alpha *in vitro*. It is indicated in the dietary management of osteoarthritis, including associated inflammation.

FLAVOXATE

(Urispas tablets 100 mg)

Flavoxate is a urinary tract and spasmodic/alicalinizer, which counteracts smooth-muscle spasms of urinary tract. It is indicated in symptomatic relief of dysuria, urgency, nocturia, suprapubic pain, frequency and incontinence associated with cystitis, prostatitis, urethritis, urethrocystitis/urethrotrigonitis. Flavoxate, a flavone derivative and urinary tract spasmolytic (100 to 200 mg p.o. t.i.d.), is used in the symptomatic relief of dysuria, frequency, urgency, nocturia, incontinence, and suprapubic pain associated with urologic, disorders.

Dicyclomine hydrochloride (Bentyl, others), **flavoxate hydrochloride** (Urispas, others), **oxybutynin chloride** (Ditropan, others), and **tolterodine tartrate** (Detrol) are tertiary amines and **trospium chloride** (Sanctura) is a quaternary amine; all are used for their antispasmodic properties. These agents appear to exert some nonspecific direct relaxant effect on smooth muscle. In therapeutic doses they decrease spasm of the gastrointestinal tract, biliary tract, ureter, and uterus.

FLECAINIDE ACETATE

(Tambocor)

Flecainide, is an antiarrhythmic agent that is indicated for prevention of paroxysmal supraventricular tachycardia including atrioventricular nodal reentrant tachycardia, atrioventricular reentrant tachycardia, and paroxysmal atrial fibrillation and flutter (see also Figure 84).

Flecainide, one of a classic membrane-stabilizing group of antiarrhythmic agents, decreases intracardiac conduction in all parts of the heart with the greatest effects being noted in the His-Purkinje system. Effects upon atrioventricular (AV) nodal conduction time and intra-atrial conduction time, although present, are less pronounced than those on the ventricular conduction system.

Flecainide is absorbed well, has a long half-life of 3 to 5 days, is metabolized to –O-dealkylated flecainide (active antiarrhythmic agent with less potency than flecainide) and to –O-dealkylated lactam of flecainide, which is an inactive metabolite. A portion of flecainide is excreted unchanged. Flecainide, like other antiarrhythmic agents, can cause new or worsen supraventricular or ventricular arrhythmias. Ventricular proarrhythmic effects range from an increase in frequency of premature ventricular complexes (PVCs) to the development of more severe ventricular tachycardia, e.g., tachycardia that is more sustained or more resistant to conversion to sinus rhythm, with potentially fatal consequences.

The noncardiac side effects of flecainide in descending order of occurrence are: dizziness (20%), visual disturbances, dyspnea, headache, nausea, fatigue, palpitation, chest pain, asthenia, tremor, constipation, edema, and abdominal pain (2%).

The effects of **flecainide** (Tambocor) therapy are thought to be attributable to the drug's very long $\tau_{recovery}$ from Na^+ channel block, **flecainide** increased mortality in patients convalescing from myocardial infarction. However, it continues to be approved for the maintenance of sinus rhythm in patients with supraventricular arrhythmias, including atrial fibrillation, in whom structural heart disease is absent.

Flecainide blocks Na^+ current and delayed rectifier K^+ current (I_{Kr}) *in vitro* at similar concentrations, 1 to 2μM. It also blocks Ca^{2+} currents *in vitro*. Action potential duration is shortened in Purkinje cells, probably owing to block of late-opening Na^+ channels, but is prolonged in ventricular cells, probably owing to block of delayed rectifier current. Flecainide does not cause EADs *in vitro* or torsade de pointes. In atrial tissue, flecainide disproportionately prolongs action potentials at fast rates, an especially desirable antiarrhythmic drug effect; this effect contrasts with that of quinidine, which prolongs atrial action potentials to a greater extent at slower rates. **Flecainide** prolongs the duration of PR, QRS, and QT intervals even at normal heart rates.

Flecainide produces few subjective complaints in most patients; dose-related blurred vision is the most common noncardiac adverse effect. It can exacerbate CHF in patients with depressed left-ventricular performance. The most serious adverse effects are provocation or exacerbation of potentially lethal arrhythmias. These include acceleration of ventricular rate in patients with atrial flutter, increased frequency of episodes of reentrant ventricular tachycardia, and increased mortality in patients convalescing from myocardial infarction.

In choosing among available therapeutic options, it is important to establish clear therapeutic goals. For example, three options are available in patients with atrial fibrillation: (1) Reduce the ventricular response using AV nodal blocking agents such as digitalis, verapamil, diltiazem, or β-adrenergic antagonists; (2) restore and maintain normal rhythm using drugs such as **quinidine**, **flecainide**, or **amiodarone**; or (3) decide not to implement antiarrhythmic therapy, especially if the patient truly is asymptomatic. Most patients with atrial fibrillation also benefit from anticoagulation to reduce stroke incidence regardless of symptoms.

FLEROXACIN

(Megalone)

The quinolones include nalidixic acid (NegGram), cinoxacin (Cinobac), norfloxacin (Noroxin), and ciprofloxacin (Cipro). Other members of the quinolone family are pefloxacin, ofloxacin, enoxacin, and fleroxacin (Figure 85). The bacterial enzyme DNA gyrase is responsible for the continuous introduction of negative supercoils into DNA, and the quinolones inhibit this gyrase-mediated DNA supercoiling. Nalidixic acid and cinoxacin are bactericidal against Gram-negative organisms that cause urinary tract infections. The fluoroquinolones are bactericidal and considerably more potent against *E. coli* and various species of *Salmonella*, *Shigella*, *Enterobacter*, *Campylobacter*, and *Neisseria*. Ciprofloxacin also has good activity against staphylococci, including methicillin-resistant strains.

The quinolones and fluoroquinolones may produce arthropathy, and hence should not be used in prepubertal children or pregnant women. Nalidixic acid and cinoxacin are useful only for treating urinary tract infections. Ciprofloxacin is useful for both urinary tract infections and prostatitis (see also Figure 85).

FLESTOLOL

Flestolol is a nonselective, ultra-short-acting beta-adrenergic-receptor-blocking agent. It is 50 times more potent than esmolol, is given by intravenous infusion, and has a half-life of 7.2 minutes. Flestolol contains an ester group (Figure 37) and hence is rapidly metabolized by tissue esterases to inactive metabolites. It has no intrinsic sympathomimetic activity or alpha-adrenergic-receptor-blocking effects, and possesses a weak membrane stabilizing property. Flestolol is able to control heart rate in patients with atrial flutter or fibrillation, improve the hemodynamic status of patients with ischemic heart disease, and relieve chest pain in patients with unstable angina.

FLOSEQUINAN

Flosequinan is a vasodilator. Vasodilators in combination with an angiotensin-converting enzyme (ACE) inhibitor have been used in congestive heart failure. The vasodilators may be classified as venodilators, arterial dilators, or balanced-type vasodilators (Table 26). The rationale for vasodilation in the management of CHF is based on the increased arteriolar vasotone that occurs. This initiates a vicious circle in which cardiac function is further depressed by an increase in afterload and in resistance to ejection.

FLOXURIDINE

(FUDR powder for injection 500 mg)

Floxuridine is a pyrimidine antimetabolite with its primary effect to interfere with the synthesis of deoxyribonucleic acid (DNA) and to a lesser extent inhibit the formation of ribonucleic acid (RNA). It is indicated in palliative management of GI adenocarcinoma metastatic to the liver administered by continuous regional intra-arterial infusion as long as cancer does not extend beyond the area perfused by a single artery. Floxuridine, an antimetabolite and antineoplastic agent (0.1 to 0.6 mg/kg daily by intra-arterial infusion), is used to treat brain, breast, head, neck, liver, gallbladder, and bile duct cancer (see also Figure 15).

Fluorouracil (5-FU) requires enzymatic conversion to the nucleotide (ribosylation and phosphorylation) in order to exert its cytotoxic activity. Several routes are available for the formation of **floxuridine** monophosphate (FUMP). 5-FU may be converted to fluorouridine by uridine phosphorylase and then to FUMP by uridine kinase, or it may react directly with 5-phosphoribosyl-1-pyrophosphate (PRPP), in a reaction catalyzed by orotate phosphoribosyl transferase, to form FUMP. Many metabolic pathways are available to FUMP. As the triphosphate FUTP, it may be incorporated into RNA. An alternative reaction sequence crucial for antineoplastic activity involves reduction of FUDP by ribonucleotide reductase to the deoxynucleotide level and formation of fluorodeoxyuridine monophosphate (FdUMP). 5-FU also may be converted by thymidine phosphorylase to the deoxyriboside fluorodeoxyuridine (FUdR), and then by thymidine kinase to fluorodeoxyuridine monophosphate (FdUMP), a potent inhibitor of thymidylate synthesis. This complex metabolic pathway for the generation of FdUMP may be bypassed through administration of floxuridine (fluorodeoxyuridine; FUdR), which is converted directly to FdUMP by thymidine kinase. FUdR is rarely used in clinical practice.

Floxuridine (FUdR): FUdR (fluorodeoxyuridine; FUDR) is used primarily by continuous infusion into the hepatic artery for treatment of metastatic carcinoma of the colon or following resection of hepatic metastases, the response rate to such infusion is 40 to 50%, or double that observed with intravenous administration. Intrahepatic arterial infusion for 14 to 21 days may be used with minimal systemic toxicity. However, there is a significant risk of biliary sclerosis if this route is used for multiple cycles of therapy. Treatment should be discontinued at the earliest manifestation of toxicity (usually stomatitis or diarrhea) because the maximal effects of bone marrow suppression and gut toxicity will not be evident until days 7 to 14.

FLUCONAZOLE

(Diflucan tablets 50 mg)

Fluconazole is an antiinfective/antifungal agent that interferes with the formation of fungal cell membrane, causing leakage of cellular contents and cell death. It is indicated for oropharyngeal and esophageal candidiasis; vaginal candidiasis; prevention of candidiasis in bone marrow transplant; *Cryptococcal meningitis*.

Fluconazole (50 to 400 mg given daily) is indicated in the treatment of oropharyngeal and esophageal candidiasis. It is employed in the treatment of candidal urinary tract infections, peritonitis, and systemic candidal infections (including candidemia, disseminated candidiasis, and pneumonia), as a prophylactic measure to reduce the incidence of candidiasis in patients undergoing bone marrow transplantation who receive cytotoxic chemotherapy or radiation therapy, and in the treatment of cryptococcal meningitis. Fluconazole, a synthetic broad-spectrum antifungal agent, inhibits fungal cytochrome P-450 and sterol C-14 alpha demethylation. The steady-state concentration of fluconazole is reached in 5 to 10 days, the concentration in cerebrospinal fluid approaches 80% of the corresponding plasma concentration, and 80% of the administered dose is excreted unchanged in the urine. Hence, the dosage in renal impairment should be adjusted downward. Fluconazole is excreted in breast milk, and its use in nursing mothers is discouraged. Most fungi show a higher sensitivity to fluconazole *in vivo* than *in vitro*. Fluconazole interacts with numerous drugs, some of which will be cited here. Cimetidine reduces the plasma level of fluconazole; hydrochlorothiazide enhances the plasma level of fluconazole; rifampin reduces the half-life of fluconazole; fluconazole increases the plasma level of cyclosporin; fluconazole enhances the hypoprothrombinemic effects of warfarin; and fluconazole increases the hypoglycemic effects of the sulfonylureas tolbutamide, glyburide, and glipizide. The reported side effects of fluconazole are dizziness, headache, itching, rash, nausea, vomiting, abdominal pain, diarrhea, thrombocytopenia, elevated transaminase levels, and hypokalemia (see also Figure 21).

Fluconazole is a fluorinated bistriazole. **Fluconazole** is almost completely absorbed from the GI tract. Plasma concentrations are essentially the same whether the drug is given orally or intravenously, and its bioavailability is unaltered by food or gastric acidity. Peak plasma concentrations are 4 to 8 μg/mL after repetitive doses of 100 mg. Renal excretion accounts for over 90% of elimination, and the elimination half-life is 25 to 30 hours. Fluconazole diffuses readily into body fluids, including breast milk, sputum, and saliva; concentrations in CSF can reach 50 to 90% of the simultaneous values in plasma. The dosage interval should be increased from 24 to 48 hours with a creatinine clearance of 21 to 40 mL/min and to 72 hours at 10 to 20 ml/min. A dose of 100 to 200 mg should be given after each hemodialysis. About 11 to 12% of drug in the plasma is protein bound.

Fluconazole is an inhibitor of CYP3A4 and CYP2C9. Fluconazole significantly increases plasma concentrations amprenavir, cisapride, cyclosporine, phenytoin, sulfonylureas (glipizide, tolbutamide, others), tacrolimus, theophylline, telithromycin, and warfarin. Patients who receive more than 400 mg daily or azotemic patients who have elevated fluconazole blood levels may experience drug interactions not otherwise seen. Drugs that decrease gastric acidity do not significantly lower fluconazole blood levels.

Fluconazole, 200 mg on the first day and then 100 mg daily for at least 2 weeks, is effective in oropharyngeal candidiasis. Esophageal candidiasis responds to 100 to 200 mg daily, and this dose also has been used to decrease candiduria in high-risk patients. A single dose of 150 mg is effective in uncomplicated vaginal candidiasis. A dose of 400 mg daily decreases the incidence of deep candidiasis in allogeneic bone marrow transplant recipients and is useful in treating candidemia of nonimmunosuppressed patients. Fluconazole is not proven to be effective treatment for deep candidiasis in profoundly neutropenic patients. In patients who have not been receiving fluconazole prophylaxis, the drug has been used successfully as empirical treatment of febrile neutropenia in patients not responding to antibacterial agents and who are not judged to be at high risk of fungal infections. Based on resistance *in vitro*, *Candida krusei* would not be expected to respond to fluconazole or other azoles.

Cryptococcosis: **Fluconazole**, 400 mg daily, is used for the initial 8 weeks in the treatment of cryptococcal meningitis in patients with AIDS after the patient's clinical condition has been stabilized with intravenous amphotericin B. After 8 weeks, the dose is decreased to 200 mg daily and continued indefinitely. If the patient responds to HAART, has a CD4 count maintained above 100 to 200/mm^3 for at least 6 months, and is asymptomatic from cryptococcal meningitis, it is reasonable to discontinue maintenance fluconazole as long as the CD4 response is maintained. A lumbar CSF with negative culture and no cryptococcal antigen provides additional assurance that the infection is inactive. For AIDS patients with **cryptococcal meningitis** who are alert and oriented and have other favorable prognostic signs, initial therapy with 400 mg daily may be considered. Fluconazole 400 mg daily has been recommended as continuation therapy in non-AIDS patients with cryptococcal meningitis who have responded to an initial course of C-AMB or Ambisome and for patients with pulmonary cryptococcosis.

Fluconazole is the drug of choice for treatment of **coccidioidal meningitis** because of much less morbidity than with intrathecal amphotericin B. In other forms of coccidioidomycosis, fluconazole is comparable to itraconazole. Fluconazole has activity against histoplasmosis, blastomycosis, sporotrichosis, and ringworm, but response is less than with equivalent doses of itraconazole. Fluconazole is not effective in the prevention or treatment of aspergillosis. As with other azoles, with the possible exception of posaconazole, there is no activity in mucormycosis.

Nausea and vomiting may occur at doses above 200 mg daily. Patients receiving 800 mg daily may require parenteral antiemetics. Side effects in patients receiving more than 7 days of drug, regardless of dose, include the following: nausea, 3.7%; headache, 1.9%; skin rash, 1.8%; vomiting, 1.7%; abdominal pain, 1.7%; and diarrhea, 1.5%. Reversible alopecia may occur with prolonged therapy at 400 mg daily. Rare cases of deaths due to hepatic failure or Stevens–Johnson syndrome have been reported. **Fluconazole** is teratogenic in rodents and has been associated with skeletal and cardiac deformities in three infants born to two women taking high doses during pregnancy. Thus, the drug should be avoided during pregnancy.

FLUCYTOSINE

(Ancobon capsules 250 mg)

Flucytosine is an antiinfective/antifungal agent that interferes with DNA and RNA synthesis. It is active against *Candida* and *Cryptococcus*. It is indicated in the treatment of serious infections caused by susceptible strains of *Candida* or *Cryptococcus*.

Flucytosine (5 FC, 5-fluorocytosine) is indicated in the treatment of septicemia, endocarditis, and urinary tract infection (*Candida*), and in meningitis and pulmonary infections (*Cryptococcus*). Flucytosine, which usually is used in combination with amphotericin B, has activity against *Candida* and *Cryptococcus* in both *in vivo* and *in vitro* systems. Flucytosine is absorbed well, distributed throughout the body, exhibits low binding to plasma proteins, and 80 to 90% of the administered dosage is excreted unchanged in the urine. Flucytosine should be used cautiously in patients with a history of bone marrow depression or hematologic disease, and in patients receiving radiation therapy along with drugs known to cause bone marrow depression. The antifungal action of flucytosine may be reduced by cytosine. Flucytosine has caused emesis; abdominal pain; diarrhea; anorexia; dry mouth; duodenal ulcer; GI hemorrhage; hepatic dysfunction; jaundice; ulcerative colitis, bilirubin elevation; elevation of hepatic enzymes; azotemia; creatinine and blood urea nitrogen (BUN) elevation; crystalluria; renal failure; anemia; agranulocytosis; aplastic anemia; eosinophilia; leukopenia; pancytopenia; thrombocytopenia; ataxia; hearing loss; headache; paresthesia; parkinsonism; peripheral neuropathy; pyrexia; vertigo; sedation; confusion; hallucinations; and psychosis. The side effects and toxicity occur at blood levels greater than 100 mcg/mL.

Flucytosine is a fluorinated pyrimidine related to **fluorouracil** and **floxuridine**. It is a 5-fluorocytosine. **Flucytosine** has clinically useful activity against *Cryptococcus neoformans*, *Candida* spp., and the agents of chlomoblastomycosis. Within these species, determination of susceptibility *in vitro* has been extremely dependent on the method employed, and susceptibility testing performed on isolates obtained prior to treatment has not correlated with clinical outcome.

All susceptible fungi are capable of deaminating flucytosine to 5-fluorouracil, a potent antimetabolite that is used in cancer chemotherapy. Fluorouracil is metabolized fast to **5-fluorouracil-ribose monophosphate** (5-FUMP) by the enzyme uracil phosphodbosyi transferase (UPRTase, also called uridine monophosphate pyrophosphorylase). As in mammalian cells, 5-FUMP then is either incorporated into RNA (via synthesis of 5-fluorouridine triphosphate) or metabolized to 5-fluoro-2′-*S* deoxyuridine-5-monophosphate (5-FdUMP), a potent inhibitor of thymidylate synthetase. DNA synthesis is impaired as the ultimate inhibition of this latter reaction. The selective action of flucytosine is due to the lack or low levels of cytosine deaminase in mammalian cells, which prevents metabolism to fluorouracil.

Flucytosine is absorbed rapidly and well from the GI tract. It is widely distributed in the body, with a volume of distribution that approximates total-body water, and is minimally bound to plasma proteins. The peak plasma concentration in patients with normal renal function is approximately 70 to 80 μg/mL, achieved 1 to 2 hours after a dose of 37.5 mg/kg. Approximately 80% of a given dose is excreted unchanged in the urine; concentrations in the urine range from 200 to 500 μg/mL. The half-life of the drag is 3 to 6 hours in normal individuals. In renal failure, the half-life may be as long as 200 hours. The clearance of flucytosine is approximately equivalent to that of creatinine. Because of its obligate renal excretion, modification of dosage is necessary in patients with decreased renal function, and concentrations of drug in plasma should be measured periodically. Peak concentrations should range between 50 and 100 μg/mL. Flucytosine is cleared by hemodialysis, and patients undergoing such treatment should receive a single dose of 37.5 mg/kg after dialysis; the drug also is removed by peritoneal dialysis.

Flucytosine concentration in CSF is about 65 to 90% of that found simultaneously in the plasma. The drug also appears to penetrate into the aqueous humor.

Flucytosine (Ancobon) is given orally at 100 mg/kg/day, in four divided doses at 6-hour intervals. Dosage must be adjusted for decreased renal function. Flucytosine is used predominantly in combination with **amphotericin** B. Flucytosine caused no added toxicity when added to 0.7 mg/kg of amphotericin B for the initial 2 weeks of therapy of cryptococcal meningitis in AIDS patients. Although the CSF colony count diminished more rapidly with combination therapy, there was no apparent impact on mortality or morbidity. An all-oral regimen of flucytosine plus fluconazole also has been advocated for therapy of AIDS patients with cryptococcosis, but the combination has substantial gastrointestinal toxicity with no evidence that **flucytosine** adds benefit to the regimen. In cryptococcal meningitis of non-AIDS patients, the role of flucytosine is more conjectural. The addition of flucytosine to 6 weeks or more of therapy with C-AMB runs the risk of substantial bone marrow suppression or colitis if the flucytosine dose is not promptly adjusted downward as amphotericin B-induced azotemia occurs. It is now common practice in HIV-negative patients with cryptococcal meningitis to begin with C-AMB or ambisome plus flucytosine and change to fluconazole after the patient has improved. Prospective study of this regimen is needed in HIV-negative patients, where the goal is a cure and not just suppression of symptoms.

Flucytosine may depress the bone marrow and lead to leukopenia and thrombocytopenia; patients are more prone to this complication if they have an underlying hematological disorder, are being treated with radiation or drugs that injure the bone marrow, or have a history of treatment with such agents. Other untoward effects—including rash, nausea, vomiting, diarrhea, and severe enterocolitis—have been noted. In approximately 5% of patients, plasma levels of hepatic enzymes are elevated, but this effect reverses when therapy is stopped. Toxicity is more frequent in patients with AIDS or azotemia (including those who are receiving amphotericin B concurrently) and when plasma drug concentrations exceed 100 μg/mL. Toxicity may result from conversion of flucytosine to 5-fluorouracil by the microbial flora in the intestinal tract of the host.

Knowledge of the status of the individual patient's renal and hepatic function also is essential, especially when excessive plasma or tissue concentrations of the drugs may cause serious toxicity. Most antimicrobial agents and their metabolites are eliminated primarily by the kidneys. Nomograms are available to facilitate adjustment of dosage of many such agents in patients with renal insufficiency. One must be particularly careful when using aminoglycosides, vancomycin, or **flucytosine** in patients with impaired renal function because these drugs are eliminated exclusively by renal mechanisms, and their toxicity correlates with their concentration in plasma and tissue.

FLUDARABINE PHOSPHATE

(Fludara powder for injection 50 mg)

Fludarabine is a purine antimetabolite. Fludarabine is a fluorinated nucleotide analog of the antiviral agent vidarabine. Fludarabine's metabolite appears to act by inhibiting DNA polymerase alpha, ribonucleotide reductase, and DNA primase, thus inhibiting DNA synthesis. It is indicated in refactory or progressive chronic B-cell lymphocytic leukemia.

Fludarabine, an antimetabolite with antineoplastic properties, is indicated in the treatment of B-cell chronic lymphocytic leukemia (CLL) in patients who have not responded or responded inadequately to at least one standard alkylating regimen. Fludarabine works primarily by inhibiting DNA synthesis. The compound also possesses lymphocytotoxic activity with preferential activity toward T-lymphocytes (see also Figure 15).

Fludarabine phosphate, a fluorinated deamination-resistant nucleotide analog of the antiviral agent **vidarabine** (9-β-D-arabinofuranosyl-adenine), is active in CLL and low-grade lymphomas. After rapid extracellular dephosphorylation to the nucleoside fludarabine, it is rephosphorylated intracellularly by deoxycytidine kinase to the active triphosphate derivative. This antimetabolite inhibits DNA polymerase, DNA primase DNA ligase, and ribonucleotide reductase, and is incorporated into DNA and RNA. The triphosphate nucleotide is an effective chain terminator when incorporated into DNA, and the incorporation of **fludarabine** into RNA inhibits RNA function, RNA processing, and mRNA translation.

A major effect of this drug may be its activation of apoptosis, which may explain its activity against indolent lymphoproliferative disease, where only a small fraction of cells are in S phase. In experimental tumors, resistance to **fludarabine** is associated with decreased activity of deoxycytidine kinase, the enzyme that phosphorylates the drug.

Fludarabine phosphate is administered intravenously and is rapidly converted to fludarabine in the plasma. The terminal half-life of fludarabine is approximately 10 hours. The compound is primarily eliminated by renal excretion, and approximately 23% appears in the urine as fludarabine because of its relative resistance to deamination by adenosine deaminase.

Fludarabine phosphate (Fludara) is available for intravenous use. The recommended dose of **fludarabine** phosphate is 20 to 30 mg/m^2 daily for 5 days. The drug is admi-nistered intravenously by infusion during a period of 30 minutes to 2 hours. Dosage may need to be reduced in renal impairment. Treatment may be repeated every 4 weeks, and at these doses gradual improvement usually occurs during a period of two to three cycles.

Fludarabine phosphate is used primarily for the treatment of patients with CLL, although experience is accumulating that suggests effectiveness in B-cell lymphomas refractory to standard therapy. In CLL patients previously refractory to a regimen containing a standard alkylating agent, response rates of 32 to 48% have been reported. Activity also has been seen with indolent non-Hodgkin's lymphoma, promyelocytic leukemia, cutaneous T-cell lymphoma, and Waldenstrom's macroglobulinemia. In patients with previously untreated low-grade lymphomas, fludarabine phosphate in combination with either cyclophosphamide or with dexamethasone and mitoxantrone has resulted in a high rate of response. There is growing interest in its use as a potent immunosuppressive agent, with high-dose alkylators, in nonmyeloablative stem-cell transplantation.

FLUDROCORTISONE ACETATE

(Florinef Acetate)

Fludrocortisone (0.1 mg/day) is indicated as a partial replacement therapy for primary and secondary adrenocortical insufficiency in Addison's disease and for the treatment of salt-losing adrenogenital syndrome. Fludrocortisone is an adrenal cortical steroid with both glucocorticoid and pronounced mineralocorticoid activities (Table 11), but it is used primarily for its mineralocorticoid effects. It acts on the renal distal tubules to enhance the reabsorption of sodium and increase the urinary excretion of both potassium and hydrogen ions. Fludrocortisone is readily absorbed from the GI tract, having a plasma half-life of 3.5 hours, and a biological half-life of 18 to 36 hours. The side effects of fludrocortisone, when it is given in larger than therapeutic doses and for a prolonged period of time, are hypokalemia, alkalosis, edema, hypertension, weight gain, enlarged heart, and congestive heart failure. High sodium diets will aggravate and accelerate the side effects. Patients with Addison's disease are more sensitive to the action of fludrocortisone and exhibit these side effects to an exaggerated degree (see also Figure 28).

FLUMAZENIL

(Romazicon)

Flumazenil is an antidote that antagonizes actions of benzodiazepines on the CNS by blocking receptors. It is used for complete or partial reversal of sedative effects of benzodiazepines where general anesthesia is induced or maintained with benzodiazepines, where sedation is produced with benzodiazepines for diagnostic or therapeutic procedures, and for the management of benzodiazepine overdose.

Flumazenil (0.1 to 1.0 mg IV) is indicated for reversal of the sedative effects of benzodiazepine derivatives. Flumazenil is an antagonist at the benzodiazepine receptor in the benzodiazepine–GABA receptor chloride-channel complex. Flumazenil does not antagonize the CNS depressant effects of ethanol, barbiturates, or general anesthetics, although these agents influence GABAergic transmission (see Figure 50).

The pharmacokinetics of flumazenil is not altered by age, gender, or renal failure. Flumazenil may precipitate

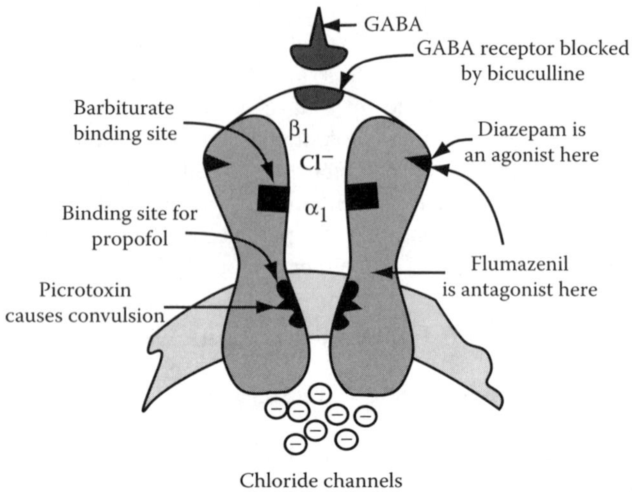

FIGURE 50 Flumazenil, a benzodiazepine receptor antagonist, is used to reverse the sedative effects of benzodiazepines after anesthesia.

benzodiazepine withdrawal syndrome (dizziness, mild confusion, emotional lability, agitation, anxiety) or convulsive seizures, especially in patients who have taken benzodiazepines in large doses and for a long period of time. Following administration of flumazenil, the patient's vital signs should be monitored carefully. Flumazenil does not consistently reverse amnesia.

Flumazenil, a benzodiazepine-receptor antagonist, is an imidazobenzodiazepine that behaves as a specific benzodiazepine antagonist. **Flumazenil** binds with high affinity to specific sites on the $GABA_A$ receptor, where it competitively antagonizes the binding and allosteric effects of benzodiazepines and other ligands. Both the electrophysiological and behavioral effects of agonist or inverse-agonist benzodiazepines and β-carbolines also are antagonized. In animal models, the intrinsic pharmacological actions of **flumazenil** have been subtle; effects resembling those of inverse agonists sometimes have been detected at low doses, whereas slight benzodiazepine-like effects often have been evident at high doses. The evidence for intrinsic activity in human subjects is even more vague, except for modest anticonvulsant effects at high doses. However, anticonvulsant effects cannot be relied on for therapeutic utility because the administration of **flumazenil** may precipitate seizures under certain circumstances.

Flumazenil is available only for IV administration. Although absorbed rapidly after oral administration, less than 25% of the drug reaches the systemic circulation owing to extensive first-pass hepatic metabolism; effective oral doses are apt to cause headache and dizziness. On intravenous administration, flumazenil is eliminated almost entirely by hepatic metabolism to inactive products with a half-life of about 1 hour; the duration of clinical effects usually is only 30 to 60 minutes.

The primary indications for the use of **flumazenil** are the management of suspected benzodiazepine overdose and the reversal of sedative effects produced by benzodiazepines administered during either general anesthesia or diagnostic and/or therapeutic procedures.

The administration of a series of small injections is preferred to a single bolus injection. A total of 1 mg **flumazenil** given over 1 to 3 minutes usually is sufficient to abolish the effects of therapeutic doses of benzodiazepines; patients with suspected benzodiazepine overdose should respond adequately to a cumulative dose of 1 to 5 mg given over 2 to 10 minutes; a lack of response to 5 mg flumazenil strongly suggests that a benzodiazepine is not the major cause of sedation. Additional courses of treatment with **flumazenil** may be needed within 20 to 30 minutes should sedation reappear. Flumazenil is not effective in single-drug overdoses with either barbiturates or tricyclic antidepressants. To the contrary, the administration of **flumazenil** in these settings may be associated with the onset of seizures, especially in patients poisoned with tricyclic antidepressants.

FLUNARIZINE

Flunarizine, which interacts with serotonergic receptors (see Figure 93), is undergoing clinical investigation for its efficacy in migraine headache (see Figure 93). Extensive ligand-binding studies and molecular biologic examination of membrane preparations have revealed that there are at least 14 types of serotonin receptors, including: $5HT_{1A}$, $5HT_{1B}$, $5HT_{1D}$, $5HT_3$, and $5HT_4$. The many actions of Serotonin include:

- Involvement in the neural network that regulates intestinal motility
- Release by a carcinoid
- Release by platelets (also ADP) during aggregation
- Causing vasoconstriction by stimulating $5HT_2$ receptors, and this effect is blocked by ketanserine
- Causing vasodilation by stimulating $5HT_1$ receptors
- Causing positive inotropic and chronotropic effects by interacting with both $5HT_1$ and $5HT_3$ receptors
- Increasing the motility of the stomach as well as small and large intestines
- Causing uterine contractions
- Causing bronchial contractions

Ketanserine, a $5HT_2$ and $alpha_1$-adrenergic-receptor antagonist, lowers BP. Methysergide, a $5HT_{1C}$ antagonist, has been used for the prophylactic treatment of migraine and other vascular headache, including Horton's syndrome. Calcium-entry blockers such as flunarizine have been shown to be effective in treating migraine. Cyproheptadine, a serotonin and $histamine_1$ receptor and muscarinic cholinergic receptor-blocking agent, has been used in the treatment of the postgastrectomy dumping syndrome and the intestinal hypermotility seen with a carcinoid. Sumatriptan, an agonist of the $5HT_1$-like receptor, is highly effective in the treatment of migraine (see also Figure 93). Ondansetron, granisetron, tropisetron, and batanopride are antagonists of the $5HT_3$ receptor, and are considered effective in controlling cancer chemotherapy-induced emesis (see also Figure 73). Clozapine, an effective antipsychotic agent with little or no extrapyramidal side effects, blocks the $5HT_2$ receptor (see Table 2).

FLUNISOLIDE

(Nasalide)

Flunisolide nasal spray is indicated for the topical treatment of the symptoms of seasonal rhinitis. Flunisolide, a potent glucocorticoid but weak mineralocorticoid, possesses local antiinflammatory properties. It stimulates the synthesis of enzymes needed to decrease the inflammatory response. The antiinflammatory and vasoconstrictor potency of topically applied flunisolide is several hundred times greater than that of hydrocortisone and about equal to that of an equal weight of triamcinolone. Flunisolide is contraindicated in patients with acute status asthmaticus; in patients with tuberculosis or viral, fungal, or bacterial respiratory infections; and in patients who are hypersensitive to any component of the preparation. It should be used cautiously in patients receiving systemic corticosteroids because of increased risk of hypothalamic–pituitary–adrenal axis suppression; when substituting inhalant for oral systemic administration (because withdrawal symptoms may occur); and in patients with healing nasal septal ulcers, oral or nasal surgery, or trauma (see also Tables 11 and 14).

FLUNISOLIDE

(Nasal inhalant Nasalide)

Flunisolide, a glucocorticoid with antiinflammatory and antiasthmatic properties (two inhalants b.i.d.) is used in steroid-dependent asthma (see also Table 14).

FLUOCINOLONE ACETONIDE

(Derma-Smoothe/FS, Fluonid, Flurosyn, Neo-Synalar, FS shampoo Synalar, Synalar-HP, Synemol)

Fluocinolone, a topical adrenocorticoid with antiinflammatory properties (0.01% solution; 0.1% shampoo; 0.025% ointment, 0.01 to 0.2% cream), is used in inflammation of corticoid-responsive dermatoses (see also Table 14).

FLUOCINONIDE

(FAPG, Lidex, Lidex-E)

Fluocinonide, a topical adrenocorticoid with antiinflammatory properties (0.05% cream, gel, ointment, solution), is used in inflammation of corticosteroid-responsive dermatoses (see also Table 14).

FLUOCINOLONE ACETONIDE

(Capex shampoo 0.01%)

Fluocinolone is a low- to medium-potency topical corticosteroid with antiinflammatory, antipruritic, and vasoconstrictive properties, thought to act by induction of phospholipase A2 inhibitory proteins (lipocortins). Lipocortins appear to control biosynthesis of potent mediators of inflammation (prostaglandins, leukotrienes) by inhibiting the release of their common precursor, arachidonic acid. Arachidonic acid is released from membrane phospholipids by phospholipase A2. **Capex:** is used for treatment of seborrheic dermatitis of the scalp; **Derma-Smoothe/FS**: is used for treatment of scalp psoriasis; **Retisert intravitreal implant**: is used for treatment of chronic noninfectious uveitis affecting the posterior segment of the eye; **Synalar**: is used for relief of inflammatory and pruritic manifestations of corticosteroid-responsive dermatosis.

FLUORESCEIN SODIUM/PROPARACAINE HYDROCHLORIDE

(Fluoracaine solution 0.5% proparacaine hydrochloride and 0.25% fluorescein sodium)

Fluorescein: is a diagnostic aid (corneal trauma indicator). **Proparacaine**: stabilizes neuronal membranes by inhibiting the ionic fluxes required for the initiation and conduction of impulses, thereby effecting local anesthetic action. They are indicated in procedures requiring a disclosing agent in combination with an anesthetic agent (e.g., tonometry, gonioscopy, removal of corneal foreign bodies and other short corneal or conjunctival procedures).

A number of agents are used in an ocular examination (e.g., mydriatic agents and topical anesthetics, and dyes to evaluate corneal surface integrity) to facilitate intraocular surgery (e.g., mydriatic and miotic agents, topical and local anesthetics) and to help in making a diagnosis in cases of anisocoria and retinal abnormalities (e.g., intravenous contrast agents).

Epiphora (excessive tearing) and surface problems of the cornea and conjunctiva are commonly encountered external ocular disorders. The dyes **fluorescein**, **rose bengal**, and **lissamine green** are used in evaluating these problems. Available both as a 2% alkaline solution and as an impregnated paper strip, fluorescein reveals epithelial defects of the cornea and conjunctiva, and aqueous humor leakage that may occur after trauma or ocular surgery. In the setting of epiphora, **fluorescein** is used to help determine the patency of the nasolacrimal system. In addition, this dye is used as part of the procedure of **applanation tonometry** (intraocular pressure [IOP] measurement) and to assist in determining the proper fit of rigid and semirigid contact lenses. **Fluorescein** in combination with **proparacaine** or **benoxinate** is available for procedures in which a disclosing agent is needed in conjunction with a topical anesthetic. Fluorexon (Fluoresoft), a high-molecular-weight fluorescent solution, is used when **fluorescein** is contraindicated (as when soft contact lenses are in place).

Rose bengal and lissamine green, which also are available as a 1% solution and as saturated paper strips, stain devitalized tissue on the cornea and conjunctiva.

The integrity of the blood-retinal and retinal pigment epithelial barriers may be examined directly by retinal angiography using intravenous administration or either **fluorescein sodium** or **indocyanine green**. These agents commonly cause nausea and may precipitate serious allergic reactions in susceptible individuals.

Verteporfin (Visudyne) is approved for photodynamic therapy of the exudative form of age-related macular degeneration.

FLUORESCEIN SODIUM

(Fluorescite, Fluor-I-Strip, Fluor-I-Strip A.T., Ful-Glo, Funduscein)

Fluorescein, a dye, is used as a diagnostic aid in corneal abrasions and foreign bodies; for fitting hard contact lenses; lacrimal patency; fundus photography; and applanation tonometry.

FLUORMETHOLONE

(Fluor-Op, Ophthalmic FML Liquifilm, Ophthalamic, FML ointment)

Fluorometholone, a corticosteroid with ophthalmic antiinflammatory properties (instill 2 drops in conjunctival sac), is used in inflammatory and allergic conditions of cornea, conjunctiva, sclera, and anterior uvea.

FLUORODEOXYURIDINE

(Floxuridine)

Fluorodeoxyuridine, a pyrimidine analog, is an antineoplastic agent. Fluorouracil and fluorodeoxyuridine inhibit pyrimidine nucleotide biosynthesis and interfere with the synthesis and actions of nucleic acids. To exert its effect, 5-FU must first be converted to nucleotide derivatives such as 5-FdUMP. Similarly, FUdR is also converted to FdUMP.

FdUMP inhibits thymidylate synthetase, and this in turn inhibits the essential formation of dTTP, one of the four precursors of DNA. In addition, 5-fluorouracil is sequentially converted to 5-FUTP, which becomes incorporated into RNA, thus inhibiting its processing and functioning. Fluorouracil is used for the following types of cancer:

Breast carcinoma: Cyclophosphamide, methotrexate, fluorouracil, and prednisone (CMP+P). The alternate drugs are doxorubicin and cyclophosphamide.
Colon carcinoma: Fluorouracil.
Gastric adenocarcinoma: Fluorouracil, doxorubicin (Adriamycin), and mitomycin (FAM), or fluorouracil and semustine.
Hepatocellular carcinoma: Fluorouracil alone or in combination with lomustine.
Pancreatic adenocarcinoma: Fluorouracil.

Resistance to 5-fluorouracil occurs as the result of one or a combination of the following factors:

Deletion of uridine kinase
Deletion of nucleoside phosphorylase
Deletion of orotic acid phosphoribosyltransferase
Increased thymidylate kinase

Because 5-fluorouracil is metabolized rapidly in the liver, it is administered intravenously and not orally. It causes myelosuppression and mucositis.

FLUOROMETHOLONE/SULFACETAMIDE

(FML-S ophthalmic suspension 0.1% fluorometholone and 10% sodium sulfacetamide)

Fluorometholone: depresses formation, release, and activity of endogenous mediators of inflammation as well as modifying the body's immune response. **Sulfacetamide**: competitively antagonizes para-aminobenzoic acid (PABA), an essential component of folic acid synthesis.

It is indicated in the treatment of steroid-responsive inflammatory ocular conditions for which a corticosreroid is indicated and where superficial bacterial ocular infection or a risk of bacterial ocular infection exists. Ocular steroids are indicated in inflammatory conditions of the palpebral and bulbar conjunctiva, cornea, and anterior segment of the globe, where the inherent risk of steroid use in certain infective conjunctivitis is accepted to obtain a diminution in edema and inflammation. They are also indicated in chronic anterior uveitis and corneal injury from chemical, radiation, or thermal burns or penetration of foreign bodies. Use of corticosteroids in combination with an antiinfective agent is indicated where the risk of superficial ocular infection is high or where there is an expectation that potentially dangerous numbers of bacteria will be present.

FLUOROQUINOLONES

The fluoroquinolones are bactericidal and considerably more potent against *E. coli* and various species of *Salmonella*, *Shigella*, *Enterobacter*, *Campylobacter*, and *Neisseria*. Ciprofloxacin also has good activity against staphylococci, including methicillin-resistant strains.

FLUOROURACIL

(Adrucil injection 50 mg/mL, Carac cream 0.5%, Efudex cream 5%, solution 2%, solution 5%, Huoropkx cream 1%, solution 1%)

Fluorouracil is a pyrimidine antimetabolite. The metabolism of fluorouracil in the anabolic pathway blocks the methylation reaction of deoxyuridylic acid to chymidylic acid. In this manner, fluorouracil interferes with the synthesis of DNA and to a lesser extent inhibits the formation of RNA. It is indicated in colon, rectum, breast, gastric, and pancreatic carcinoma (injection); multiple actinic or solar keratoses, and superficial basal-cell carcinoma (topical).

5-Fluorouracil (initially 7 to 12 mg/kg IV for 4 days), a cell-cycle-phase-specific antineoplastic agent, is indicated in colon, rectal, breast, ovarian, cervical, gastric, esophageal, bladder, liver, and pancreatic cancer. Fluorouracil exerts its cytotoxic activity by acting as an antimetabolite, competing for the enzyme that is important in the synthesis of thymidine, an essential substrate for DNA synthesis. Therefore, DNA synthesis is inhibited. The drug also inhibits RNA synthesis to a lesser extent (see also Figure 15).

5-Fluorouracil is absorbed poorly after an oral administration, and hence is given intravenously. It crosses the blood–brain barrier and is distributed widely in the body. 5-Fluorouracil is metabolized in the urine and the metabolites are primarily excreted through the lung as carbon dioxide. The toxicity of fluorouracil is enhanced by leucovorin calcium. 5-Fluorouracil causes stomatitis and esophagopharyngitis leading to ulceration, diarrhea, anorexia, nausea and emesis, leukopenia, and a reversible alopecia.

FLUOXETINE

(Prozac)

Fluoxetine, a selective serotonin uptake inhibitor (SSUI), (20 mg p.o./day) is indicated in the treatment of depression and depressive compulsive disorder (see Figure 51).

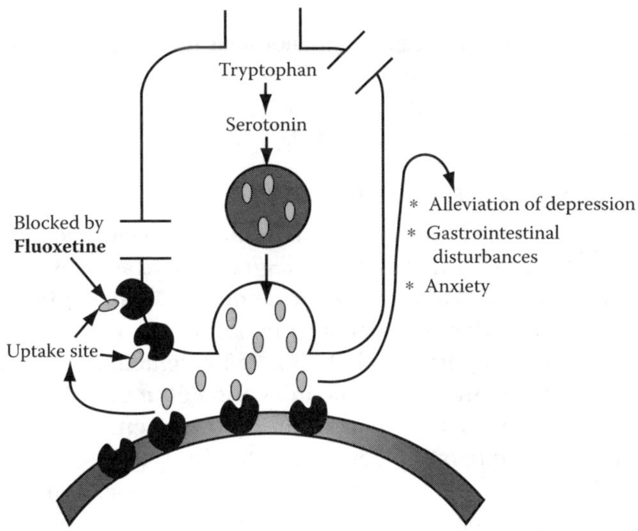

FIGURE 51 Fluoxetine, a specific serotonin uptake site inhibitor, is a second-generation antidepressant which does not cause sedation or orthostatic hypotension and possesses no anticholinergic properties.

It inhibits the neuronal uptake of serotonin but not that of norepinephrine (Figure 86 and Tables 5 through 7).

Fluoxetine is absorbed well from the GI tract, is bound to plasma proteins to the extent of 95%, is metabolized in the liver to norfluoxetine, and is excreted in the urine. Tryptophan is used as an antidepressant. However, the combined use of tryptophan, which increases the level of serotonin, and fluoxetine, which inhibits the neuronal uptake of serotonin, enhances the side effects of fluoxetine such as GI disturbances, anxiety, and insomnia (see Figure 86).

FLUOXYMESTERONE

(Fluoxymesterone tablets 10 mg)

Fluoxymesterone promotes growth and development of male reproductive organs, maintains secondary sex characteristics, increases protein anabolism, and decreases protein catabolism. It is used for replacement therapy in conditions associated with symptoms of deficiency or absence of endogenous testosterone; delayed puberty (men); palliation of androgen-responsive recurrent mammary cancer in women who are more than 1 year but less than 5 years postmenopausal (women).

FLUOXYMESTERONE

(Halotestin)

Fluoxymesterone is a steroid with an androgenic property that is used in primary hypogonadism and testicular failure due to cryptorchidism, vanishing testes syndrome, or orchidectomy; and in hypogonadotrophic hypogonadism and luteinizing hormone-releasing hormone (LHRH) deficiency or pituitary hypothalamic injury from tumors, trauma, or radiation. It mimics the actions of testosterone, which is responsible for normal growth and development of the male sex organs and for the maintenance of secondary sex characteristics. In female postmenopausal patients, fluoxymesterone may be indicated in the palliation of recurrent mammary cancer (see also Table 11 and Figure 95).

Fluoxymesterone is contraindicated in male subjects with known or suspected carcinoma of the prostate gland. Prolonged use of high-dosage 17-alpha-alkyl androgens is known to have caused hypercalcemia, hepatic adenoma, hepatocellular carcinoma, and hepatitis. Fluoxymesterone, which accelerates bone maturation without producing linear growth, should be used cautiously in males with delayed puberty. Edema and CHF may occur in patients with preexisting cardiovascular problems. Androgens cause virilization in female subjects.

FLUPHENAZINE HYDROCHLORIDE

(Prolixin)

Fluphenazine (0.5 to 10 mg p.o. daily in divided doses q. 6 to 8 hours) is indicated in the management of manifestations of psychotic disorders. As depicted in Table 2, its potency equals that of haloperidol. In addition, similar to haloperidol it produces movement disorders such as akathisia, dystonia, parkinsonism, neuroleptic malignant syndrome, and tardive dyskinesia. The drug is available as fluphenazine decanoate and fluphenazine enanthate which are intended for depot injection, with an onset of action of 24 to 72 hours, and a duration of action of two weeks. Neuroleptics are not of any value if patients do not take them at the dosage that has been prescribed, or if their bodies do not absorb the orally administered drug effectively. It has been estimated that 10 to 25% of schizophrenic inpatients somehow fail to ingest the prescribed dosage, and that 25 to 50% of schizophrenic outpatients deviate from or default on their medication regimens. This has obvious consequences in terms of the relapse rate and revolving door syndrome.

The development of long-acting formulations, both injectable and oral, carries the potential to remedy these two treatment liabilities. These new formulations have already made an impact on the treatment of the unreliable drug taker, the poor oral absorbers, and those patients being treated in outpatient settings who are too ill to assume responsibility for their own drug taking. These long-acting psychotropics are remarkably free of side effects when given for extended periods. Full blood counts, urinalysis, and renal function tests are essentially normal, even after years of continuous treatment with these drugs. The only significant hazard that is associated with the continuous, prolonged use of these medications is tardive dyskinesia. There are indications, however, that the injectable psychotropic drugs produce less, or less persistent, tardive dyskinesia than do the orally administered neuroleptics. This is probably due to the fact that the injectable forms can be given in lower dosages. See also Phenothiazine Derivatives.

FLURANDRENOLIDE

(Cordran, Cordran SP)

Flurandrenolide, a topical adrenocorticoid with antiinflammatory properties (cream, lotion, ointment 0.025 to 0.05%), is used in inflammation of corticosteroid-responsive dermatoses (see also Table 11).

FLURAZEPAM HYDROCHLORIDE

(Dalmane)

Flurazepam (15 to 30 mg p.o. at bedtime) is a benzodiazepine derivative sedative–hypnotic that is used in the management of insomnia. Flurazepam depresses the CNS at the limbic and subcortical levels of the brain. It produces a sedative effect by potentiating the effect of the neurotransmitter gamma-amino-butyric acid on its receptor in the ascending reticular activating system, which increases inhibition and blocks both cortical and limbic arousal (see also Figure 50).

When given orally, flurazepam is absorbed rapidly, is bound to plasma proteins to the extent of 97%, exerts its hypnotic effects within 20 minutes, and is metabolized to desalkylflurazepam which is excreted in the urine. Flurazepam potentiates the CNS-depressing effects of alcohol, barbiturates, antihistaminics, antidepressants, and several neuroleptics. Cimetidine inhibits the metabolism of flurazepam and hence its duration of action. On the other hand, heavy smoking accelerates the metabolism of flurazepam. The side effects of flurazepam in higher than therapeutic dosage include confusion, depression, drowsiness, lethargy, daytime sedation, disturbed coordination, hangover effect, ataxia, dizziness, syncope, nightmares, fatigue, slurred speech, tremor, vertigo, and headache. The incidence and severity of these side effects are more pronounced in elderly subjects. As the metabolism and elimination of flurazepam is retarded in elderly subjects, the dosage should be adjusted downward. Flurazepam is excreted in breast milk causing sedation, feeding difficulties, and weight loss in the infants, and hence should be avoided in breast-feeding women (see also Table 9).

FLURBIPROFEN

(Ansaid)

Flurbiprofen is a nonsteroidal antiinflammatory drug of the 2-arylpropionic acid class. The recommended dosages for flurbiprofen are 50 mg q. 4 to 6 hours for analgesia and 100 to 300 mg/day for the treatment of inflammatory conditions (see also Table 3).

Flurbiprofen is indicated for the acute or long-term treatment of rheumatoid arthritis and osteoarthritis. It is a potent inhibitor of prostaglandin synthetase (see Figures 13 and 14). Flurbiprofen is absorbed well orally, is bound to plasma proteins to the extent of 99%, is metabolized in the liver to pharmacologically active metabolites, and the metabolites are excreted in the urine. Flurbiprofen increases the actions of oral anticoagulants and decreases the effectiveness of diuretics. Flurbiprofen is contraindicated in patients who are allergic to aspirin (see also Table 12).

FLUTAMIDE

(Eulexin)

Flutamide, a nonsteroidal antiandrogen (250 mg p.o. q. 8 hours), is indicated in the treatment of metastatic prostatic carcinoma in combination with LHRH analogs, such as leuprolide acetate (see also Table 13).

FLUTICASONE PROPIONATE

(Flonase Nasal spray 50 mcg/actuation, Flovenc aerosol 44 mcg/actuation, aerosol 110 mcg/actuation, aerosol 220 mcg/actuation, Florent disk with powder for inhalation 50 mcg/actuation, powder for inhalation 100 mcg/actuation, powder for inhalation 250 mcg/actuation, Florent rotadisk powder for inhalation 50 mcg/actuation, powder for inhalation 100 mcg/actuation, powder for inhalation 250 mcg/actuation)

Fluticasone is a corticosteroid that exerts potent antiinflammatory effect on nasal passages for management of the nasal symptoms of seasonal and perennial allergic and nonallergic rhinitis in adults and pediatric patients 4 years and older (**Flonaze**); patients requiring oral corticosteroid therapy for asthma (**Flovent**, **Flovent Rotadisk**, **Flovent Diskus**); maintenance treatment of asthma as prophylactic therapy in patients 4 years and older (**Flovent Diskus, Flovent Rotadisk**) and 12 years and older (**Flovent**).

FLUTICASONE PROPIONATE

(Culivate)

Fluticasone, a topical corticosteroid with antiinflammatory properties (0.05% cream, 0.005% ointment), is used in the relief of inflammation and pruritis of corticosteroid-responsive dermatoses.

FLUTICASONE PROPIONATE/SALMETEROL

(Atvair diskus powder for inhalation 100 mcg fluticasone propionate, 50 mcg salmeterol, powder for inhalation 250 mcg fluticasone propionate, 50 mcg salmeterol, powder for inhalation 500 mcg fluticasone propionate, 50 mcg salmeterol)

Fluticasone is a respiratory inhalant combination. **Fluticasone**: inhibits multiple cell types (e.g., mast cells) and mediator production or secretion (e.g., histamine) involved in the asthmatic response. **Salmeterol**: produces bronchodilation by relaxing bronchial smooth muscle through beta-2-receptor stimulation. Indications: they are indicated in long-term maintenance treatment of asthma; and COPD associated with chronic bronchitis.

The use of orally administered β-adrenergic agonists for bronchodilation has not gained wide acceptance largely because of the greater risk of side effects, especially tremulousness, muscle cramps, cardiac tachyarrhythmias, and metabolic disturbances. There are two primary situations in which oral adrenergic agonists are used. First, brief courses of oral therapy (**albuterol** or **metaproterenol syrups**) are well tolerated and effective in young children (<5 years old) who cannot manipulate metered-dose inhalers yet have occasional wheezing with viral upper respiratory infections. Second, in some patients with severe asthma exacerbations, any aerosol, whether delivered via a metered-dose inhaler or a nebulizer, can worsen cough and bronchospasm owing to local irritation. In this setting, oral therapy with β_2-adrenergic agonists (e.g., albuterol, metaproterenol, or terbutaline tablets) can be effective. However, the frequency of adverse systemic side effects with orally administered agents is higher in adults than in children.

Although glucocorticoids are very effective in controlling asthma, treatment with systemic glucocorticoids comes at the cost of considerable adverse effects. A major advance in asthma therapy was the development of inhaled glucocorticoids that targeted the drug directly to the relevant site of inflammation. These formulations greatly enhance the therapeutic index of the drugs, substantially diminishing the number and degree of side effects without sacrificing clinical utility. There are currently five glucocorticoids available in the United States for inhalation therapy: **beclomethasone dipropionate** (Beclovent, Vanceril), **triamcinolone acetonide** (Azmacort), **flunisolide** (Aero-Bid), **budesonide** (Pulmicort), and **fluticasone propionate** (Flovent). Although they differ markedly in their affinities for the glucocorticoid receptor, with fluticasone and budesonide having much higher affinities than beclomethasone, they are all effective in controlling asthma at the appropriate doses. Few studies have directly assessed the relative therapeutic index of the various formulations of inhaled steroids in the treatment of asthma, but available data indicate that none has a clearly superior therapeutic index.

Inhaled glucocorticoids are used prophylactically to control asthma rather than acutely to reverse asthma symptoms. As with all prophylactic therapies, compliance is a significant concern. Issues relating to drug compliance, therefore, become relevant when choosing among the various steroid formulations. The newer, highly potent drugs (e.g., **fluticasone**, **flunisolide**, and **budesonide**) can be effective with as little as one or two puffs administered twice or even once daily. This more convenient dosage regimen may be preferred by patients, providing improved compliance and better asthma control. The appropriate dose of steroid must be determined empirically. Important variables that influence the effective dose include the severity of disease, the particular steroid used, and the device used for drug delivery, which determines the actual quantity of drug delivered to the lungs. When determining the optimal dose, one should keep in mind that maximal improvement in lung function may not occur until after several weeks of treatment.

FLUVASTATIN

(Lescol capsules 20 mg)

Fluvastatin is an antihyperlipidemic/HMG-CoA reductase inhibitor that increases the rate at which the body removes cholesterol from blood and reduces production of cholesterol in the body by inhibiting enzyme that catalyzes an early rate-limiting step in cholesterol synthesis, increases HDL, and reduces LDL, VLDL, and triglycerides.

Atherosclerosis use: to slow the progression of coronary atherosclerosis. **Hypercholesterolemia** use: for reduction of elevated total cholesterol, LDL, apo-B, and triglyceride cholesterol levels and to increase HDL levels. **Secondary prevention of coronary events**: used to reduce the risk of undergoing coronary revascularization procedures in patients with coronary heart disease.

Statins are cholesterol-lowering agents that reversibly inhibit HMG-CoA reductase, which catalyzes a rate-limiting step in cholesterol biosynthesis. Statins affect serum cholesterol by inhibiting cholesterol biosynthesis in the liver, and this organ is their main target. On the other hand, exposure of extrahepatic cells in smooth muscle to these drugs may cause adverse effects. Among the statins, **pravastatin**, **fluvastatin**, **cerivastatin**, **atorvastatin**, **rosuvastatin**, and **pitavastatin** are given in a biologically active open-acid form, whereas simvastatin and lovastatin are administered as inactive prodrugs with lactone rings.

Fluvastatin, a cholesterol-lowering agent that inhibits hydroxy-methylglutaryl-coenzyme A (MHG-CoA) reductase, is effective in the reduction of low-density lipoprotein and total cholesterol levels in patients with primary hypercholesterolemia (types IIa and IIb) when response to diet and other nonpharmacologic measures have been inadequate (see also Figure 35).

FLUVOXAMINE MALEATE

Fluvoxamine, an antidepressant, is a potent and selective serotonin reuptake inhibitor (see Figure 86) which is devoid of anticholinergic, antihistaminic, or cardiotoxic properties. Fluvoxamine offers depressed patients an equivalent level of therapeutic benefit when compared with imipramine (see Tables 5 through 7).

FOLIC ACID

(Folacin; Pteroylglutamic acid; Folate)

Both vitamin B_{12} and folic acid are essential for the synthesis of DNA, and this process is impaired in patients with megaloblastic anemia (see Figure 106). In the absence of adequate DNA synthesis, cells cannot divide but continue to grow. Megaloblastic anemia may also be associated with neurologic disturbances such as paresthesias, diminution of vibration sensation, loss of memory, confusion, irritability, and psychosis, which are due to vitamin B_{12} rather than folic acid deficiency. Folic acid deficiency may result from the following:

- Nutritional deficiency
- Malabsorption syndrome
- Reduced folate-binding protein
- Folic acid antagonists (e.g., methotrexate)
- Drugs reducing the level of folic acid (anticonvulsants and pyrimethamine)
- Agents blocking purine synthesis (e.g., mercaptopurine, thioguanine) or pyrimidine synthesis (5-fluorouracil)
- Hemolytic diseases (accelerated hematopoiesis)
- Proliferative diseases and other conditions
- Folic acid is administered orally and should not be used in the treatment of pernicious anemia

Exogenous folate is required for nucleoprotein synthesis and maintenance of normal erythropoiesis. Folic acid stimulates production of red and white blood cells and platelets in certain megaloblastic anemias. Folic acid is the precursor of tetrahydrofolic acid, which is involved as a cofactor for transformylation reactions in the biosynthesis of purines and thymidylates of nucleic acids. Impairment of thymidylate synthesis in patients with folic acid deficiency is thought to account for the defective DNA synthesis that leads to megaloblast formation and megaloblastic and macrocytic anemias.

Folic acid is found in liver, dried beans, peas, lentils, oranges, whole-wheat products, asparagus, beets, broccoli, brussel sprouts, and spinach as reduced folate polyglutamate, which undergoes hydrolysis reduction and methylation in the GI tract before it is absorbed. Folic acid is metabolized in the liver to 7,8-dihydrofolic acid and eventually to 5,6,7,8-tetrahydrofolic acid. Tetrahydrofolic acid derivatives are distributed to all body tissues but are stored primarily in the liver. Pregnant women are more prone to develop folate deficiency as reflected in larger dosage recommendations. Folate-deficient mothers may be more prone to complications of pregnancy and fetal abnormalities, including fetal anomalies, placental abruption, toxemia, abortions, placenta previa, low birth weight, and premature delivery.

FOLIC ACID/COBALAMIN/PYRIDOXINE HYDROCHLORIDE

(Folix tablets 25 mg vitamin B_6, 1 mg vitamin B_{12}, 2.5 mg folic acid)

Folic acid/cobalamin/pyridoxine hydrochloride are nutritional combinations. **Folic acid and cobalamin**: reduce homocysteine by metabolizing it to methionine. **Pyridoxine**: facilitates breakdown of homocysteine to cysteine and other by-products. They are indicated for nutritional requirement of patients with end-stage renal failure, dialysis, hyperhomocysteinemia, homocystinuria, nutrient malabsorption or inadequate dietary intake, particularly for patients with or at risk for cardiovascular disease, cerebrovascular disease, peripheral vascular disease, arteriosclerotic vascular disease, neurological disorders, Alzheimer's disease, and renal disease.

FOLIC ACID ANTAGONISTS

Methotrexate (Amethopterin) is a folic acid antagonist that binds to dihydrofolate reductase, thus interfering with the synthesis of the active cofactor tetrahydrofolic acid, which is necessary for the synthesis of thymidylate, purine nucleotides, and the amino acids serine and methionine. Methotrexate is used for the following types of cancer:

- Acute lymphoid leukemia: During the initial phase, vincristine and prednisone are used; methotrexate and mercaptopurine are used for maintenance therapy; in addition, methotrexate is given intrathecally, with or without radiotherapy, to prevent meningeal leukemia
- Diffuse histiocyte lymphoma: Cyclophosphamide, vincristine, methotrexate, and cytarabine (COMA)
- Mycosis fungoides: Methotrexate
- Squamous cell, large-cell anaplastic, and adenocarcinoma: Doxorubicin and cyclophosphamide, or methotrexate
- Head-and-neck squamous cell: *Cis*-platinum and bleomycin, or methotrexate
- Choriocarcinoma: Methotrexate

Tumor cells acquire resistance to methotrexate as the result of several factors:

- The deletion of a high-affinity, carrier-mediated transport system for reduced folates
- An increase in the concentration of dihydrofolate reductase
- The formation of a biochemically altered reductase with reduced affinity for methotrexate

To overcome this resistance, higher doses of methotrexate need to be administered.

The effects of methotrexate may be reversed by the administration of leucovorin, the reduced folate. This leucovorin "rescue" prevents or reduces the toxicity of methotrexate, which is expressed as mouth lesions (stomatitis), injury to the GI epithelium (diarrhea), leukopenia, and thrombocytopenia.

FOLINIC ACID

(Leucovorin calcium, Citrovorum factor)

Leucovorin is used to reduce the toxicity ("rescue") of high dose methotrexate in osteosarcoma; to counteract the action of folic-acid antagonists such as pyrimethamine or trimethoprim; and in combination with 4-fluorouracil to prolong survival in patients with advanced colorectal cancer. In this case, leucovorin enhances the toxicity of 5-fluorouracil (5-FU), and the doses of 5-FU should be reduced.

The adverse reactions following treatment with combination leucovorin/5-fluorouracil in descending order of occurrence are: stomatitis (75%), nausea, leukopenia (69%), diarrhea, vomiting, alopecia (42%), dermatitis, anorexia, fatigue, thrombocytopenia, infection, and constipation (3%).

FOLLITROPIN ALFA

(Gonal-f powder for injection, lyophilized 82 units, follicle-stimulating hormone (FSH) activity (to deliver 75 units), powder for injection, lyophilized 600 units FSH activity (to deliver 450 units), powder for injection, lyophilized 1200 units FSH activity (to deliver 1050 units) • Gonol-f RFF Pen injection 415 units FSH activity (to deliver at least 300 units per 0.05 mL), injection 568 units FSH activity (to deliver at least 450 units per 0.75 mL), injection 1026 units FSH activity (to deliver at least 900 units per 1.5 mL))

Follitropin alfa is gonadotropin, which stimulates ovarian follicular growth in women who do not have primary ovarian failure. It is indicated in induction of ovulation and pregnancy in anovulatory infertile patients in whom the cause of infertility is functional and not caused by primary ovarian failure; to stimulate development of multiple follicles in ovulatory patients undergoing assisted reproductive therapy (ART [e.g., *in vitro* fertilization]); and for induction of spermatogenesis in men with primary and secondary hypogonadotropic hypogonadism in whom the cause of infertility is not primary testicular failure (except prefilled pen).

Gonadotropins are purified from human urine or prepared using recombinant DNA technology. Several preparations of urinary gonadotropins have been developed. **Chorionic gonadotropin** (Pregnyl, Novarel, Profasi, others), which mimics the action of LH, is obtained from the urine of pregnant women. Urine from postmenopausal women is the source of **menotropins** (Pergonal, Repronex), which contain roughly equal amounts of FSH and LH, as well as a number of other urinary proteins. Because of their relatively low purity, menotropins are administered intramuscularly to decrease the incidence of hypersensitivity reactions. Urofollitropin (uFSH; Bravelle) is a highly purified FSH prepared by immunoconcentration with monoclonal antibodies and pure enough to be administered subcutaneously.

Recombinant preparations of gonadotropins are assuming an increasing role in clinical practice. Recombinant FSH (rFSH) is prepared by expressing cDNAs encoding the α and β subunits of FSH in a mammalian cell line, yielding products whose glycosylation pattern mimics that of FSH produced by gonadotropes. The two rFSH preparations that are available (**follitropin** α [Gonal-F] and **follitropin** β [Puregon, Follistim) differ slightly in their carbohydrate structures; both exhibit less inter-batch variability than do preparations purified from urine and can be administered subcutaneously because they are considerably purer. The recombinant preparations are more expensive than the naturally derived hormones, and their relative advantages (i.e., efficacy, lower frequency of side effects such as ovarian hyperstimulation) have not been definitively established despite much debate in the published literature.

Recombinant forms of hCG (choriogonadotropin alfa; Ovidrel) and LH (Luveris, Lhadi) also have been developed and are being investigated for the treatment of infertility. Providing that their cost–benefit ratios are favorable, it is likely that these recombinant gonadotropin preparations will have an increasing role in the future, possibly replacing the urinary preparations entirely. In addition, recombinant technology is likely to lead to improved forms of gonadotropins with increased half-lives or higher clinical efficacy.

FOLLITROPIN BETA

(Follistim powder for injection, lyophilized 75 IU IFS activity)

Follitropin beta is a gonadotropin that stimulates ovarian follicular growth in women who do not have primary ovarian failure. It is indicated for development of multiple follicles in ovulatory patients participating in an assisted reproductive technology (ART) program; and for induction of ovulation and pregnancy in anovulatory infertile patients in whom the cause of infertility is functional and not caused by primary ovarian failure.

FONDAPARINUX SODIUM

(Arixtra injection 2.5 mg)

Fondaparinux is a selective inhibitor factor Xa possessing a selective inhibition of antithrombin III (ATIII), which potentiates the innate neutralization of factor Xa by ATIII. Neutralization of factor Xa interrupts the blood coagulation cascade and inhibits thrombin formation and thrombus development. It is indicated for prophylaxis of deep vein thrombosis (DVT) that may lead to pulmonary embolism in patients undergoing hip fracture surgery including extended prophylaxis, hip replacement surgery, or knee replacement surgery. When administered in conjunction with warfarin, fondaparinux is indicated for treatment of acute DVT and acute pulmonary embolism.

FORMOTEROL

Formoterol is a selective beta$_2$-adrenergic-receptor agonist. The selective beta$_2$-adrenergic stimulants cause bronchodilation without cardiac acceleration. Metaproterenol and terbutaline are available in tablet form, and terbutaline is also available for subcutaneous injection. Metaproterenol and albuterol are available in metered-dose inhalers. Inhaled selective beta$_2$-adrenergic-receptor agonists (albuterol, terbutaline, fenoterol, and bitolterol) have a rapid onset of action and are effective for 3 to 6 hours. Formoterol and salmeterol are longer-acting agents (12 hours) and may prove useful in treating nocturnal symptoms. The side effects of beta-adrenergic-receptor agonists are tremor, tachycardia, and palpitations (see also Figure 37).

FORMOTEROL FUMARATE

Foradil Aerolizer inhalation powder in capsules 12 mcg (as fumarate))

Formoterol is a sympathomimetic agent that relaxes bronchial smooth muscles. It is indicated in long-term maintenance treatment of asthma; prevention of bronchospasms; prevention of exercise-induced bronchospasm; concomitant therapy with short-acting beta$_2$-agonists, inhaled or systemic

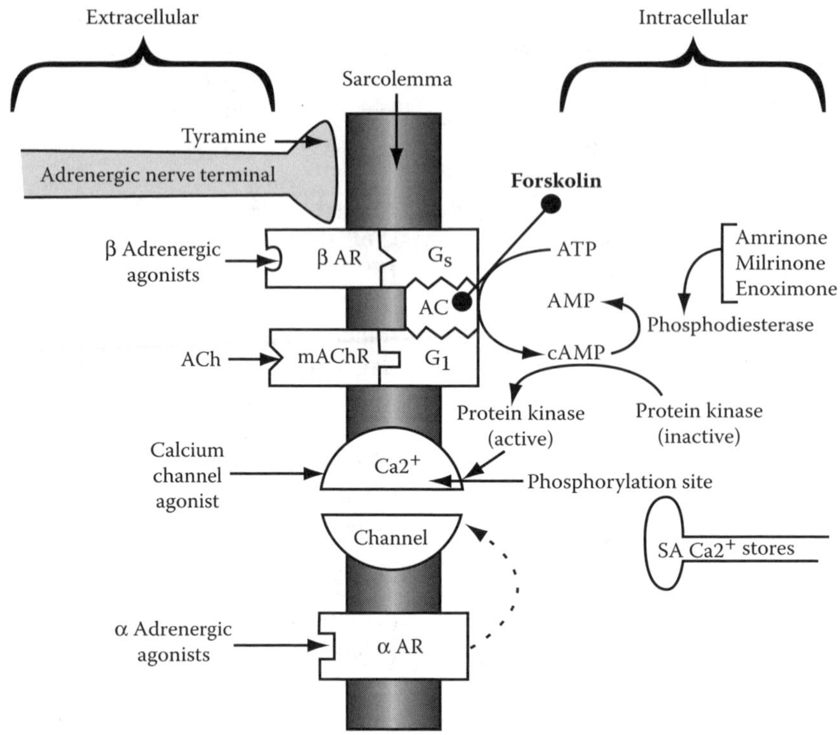

FIGURE 52 **Forskolin**, which is isolated from *Coleus forskohlii*, stimulates adenylate cyclase.

corticosteroids, and theophylline therapy; and long-term administration in the maintenance of bronchoconstriction in patients with chronic obstructive pulmonary disease (COPD), including chronic bronchitis and emphysema.

Formoterol (Foradil) is a long-acting β_2-selective-receptor agonist. Significant bronchodilation occurs within minutes of inhalation of a therapeutic dose, which may persist for up to 12 hours. It is highly lipophilic and has high affinity for β_2 receptors. Its major advantage over many other β_2-selective agonists is this prolonged duration of action, which may be particularly advantageous in settings such as nocturnal asthma. **Formoterol's** sustained action is due to its insertion into the lipid bilayer of the plasma membrane, from which it gradually diffuses to provide prolonged stimulation of β_2 receptors. It is FDA-approved for treatment of asthma, bronchospasm, prophylaxis of exercise-induced bronchospasm, and **COPD**. It can be used concomitantly with short-acting β_2 agonists, glucocorticoids (inhaled or systemic), and theophylline.

Salmeterol xinafoate (Serevent) and **formoterol** (Foradil) are long-lasting adrenergic agents with very high selectivity for the β_2-receptor subtype. Inhalation of salmeterol provides persistent bronchodilation lasting over 12 hours. The mechanism underlying the extended duration of action of salmeterol is not yet fully understood. The extended side chain on salmeterol renders it 10,000 times more lipophilic than albuterol. The lipophilicity regulates the diffusion rate away from the receptor by determining the degree of partitioning in the lipid bilayer of the membrane. Subsequent to binding the receptor, the less lipophilic, short-acting agonists are removed rapidly from the receptor environment by diffusion in the aqueous phase. Unbound salmeterol, by contrast, persists in the membrane and only slowly dissociates from the receptor environment.

FORSKOLIN

Forskolin, which is isolated from *Coleus forskohlii*, stimulates adenylate cyclase (see Figure 52).

FOSAMPRENAVIR CALCIUM

(Lexiva tablets 700 mg)

Fosamprenavir is a protease inhibitor. **Fosamprenavir** is a prodrug of **amprenavir** that inhibits HIV protease, the enzyme required to form functional proteins in HIV-infected patients. It is indicated in the treatment of HIV infections in combination with other antiretroviral agents.

FOSCARNET SODIUM (PHOSPHONOFORMIC ACID)

(Foscavir injection 24 mg/mL)

Foscarnet is an antiviral agent that inhibits replication of all known herpes viruses, including cytomegalovirus (CMV), herpes simplex virus types 1 and 2 (HSV-1, HSV-2), human herpes virus 6 (HHV-6), Epstein–Barr virus (EBV) and varicella-zoster virus (VZV). It is indicated in the treatment of CMV retinitis in patients with AIDS; treatment of acyclovir-resistant mucocutaneous HSV infections in immunocompromised patients; and as combination therapy with ganciclovir for patients who have relapsed after monotherapy with either drug.

Amprenavir is an *N,N*-disubstituted (hydroxyethyl) amino sulfonamide nonpeptide HIV protease inhibitor. Although developed using a sophisticated structure-based drug-design program, the same compound was identified previously using a more traditional high-throughput screen of an available chemical library. Amprenavir is the only available HIV protease inhibitor that contains a sulfonamide moiety, which may play a role in its dermatological side effects. The drug is active against both HIV-1 and HIV-2, with an IC_{90} for wild-type HIV-1 of approximately 80 nM.

Fosamprenavir is a phosphonooxy prodrug of amprenavir that has the advantage of greatly increased water solubility and improved oral bioavailability. This allows reduction in the pill burden from 16 capsules to 4 tablets per day. The original amprenavir formulation contained D-α-tocopheryl polyethylene glycol, which delivered a high daily dose of vitamin E; this excipient is not required with fosamprenavir. **Fosamprenavir** is as effective, more convenient, and generally better tolerated than amprenavir.

Clinical trials have demonstrated long-term virologic benefit in treatment-naive patients receiving amprenavir (1200 mg every 12 hours) in combination with zidovudine and lamivudine. Similar results are seen when amprenavir is combined with ritonavir.

One comparative trial found that an amprenavir-based regimen was less effective than an indinavir-based regimen, with HIV RNA values of less than 400 copies/mL in only 30% of the amprenavir-treated patients compared with 49% of the indinavir-treated patients after 48 weeks. This may reflect poor adherence to amprenavir owing to high pill burden and side effects. Several large randomized trials have established a better track record for **fosamprenavir**, showing equivalent or superior long-term viral RNA effects as nelfinavir in treatment-naive patients. However, in one comparative trial in treatment-experienced patients, **fosamprenavir** combined with ritonavir was marginally inferior to the lopinavir–ritonavir coformulation.

FOSCARNET SODIUM

(Phosphonoformic Acid) (Foscavir)

Foscarnet, a pyrophosphate analog with antiviral activity (60 mg/kg IV, is used in cytomegalovirus (CMV) retinitis in patients with acquired immunodeficiency syndrome (AIDS) (see also Figure 16).

FOSFOMYCIN TROMETHAMINE

(Monurol granules 3 g)

Fosfomycin is antiinfective/antiseptic in nature. It interferes with bacterial cell-wall biosynthesis. It is indicated in the treatment of uncomplicated UTI (acute cystitis) in women caused by susceptible strains of specific microorganisms.

As a significant percentage of urinary tract infections in many parts of the world are caused by sulfonamide-resistant microorganisms, sulfonamides are no longer a therapy of first choice. Trimethoprim-sulfamethoxazole, a quinolone, trimethoprim, **fosfomycin**, or **ampicillin** are the preferred agents. However, sulfisoxazole may be used effectively in areas where the prevalence of resistance is not high or when the organism is known to be sensitive. The usual dosage is 2 to 4 g initially followed by 1 to 2 g, orally four times a day for 5 to 10 days. Patients with acute pyelonephritis with high fever and other severe constitutional manifestations are at risk of bacteremia and shock and should not be treated with a sulfonamide.

Fosfomycin competitively inhibits angiotensin I-converting enzyme, preventing conversion of angiotensin I to angiotensin II, a potent vasoconstrictor that also stimulates release of aldosterone. It results in decrease in BP, reduced sodium reabsorption, and potassium retention, and is indicated in hypertension and heart failure.

FOSINOPRIL SODIUM

(Monopril)

Fosinopril, an ACE inhibitor with antihypertensive properties (10 mg p.o. daily), is used in the treatment of hypertension (see also Figure 24).

FOSPHENYTOIN

(Cerebyx injection 150 mg (100 mg phenytoin sodium))

Fosphenytoin is a hydantoin/anticonvulsant. Fosphenytoin is a prodrug that is converted to the active metabolite phenytoin. It appears to act at the motor cortex by inhibiting spread of seizure activity. It possibly works by promoting sodium efflux from neurons, thereby stabilizing the threshold against hyperexcitability. It is indicated in short-term parenteral administration when other means of phenytoin administration are unavailable, inappropriate, or less advantageous; for treatment of generalized convulsive status epilepticus; prevention and treatment of seizures occurring during neurosurgery; and short-term substitution for oral phenytoin.

FROVATRIPTAN SUCCINATE

(Frova tablets 2.5 mg (as base))

Frovatriptan is a serotonin 5-HT_1-receptor agonist, which selectively agonizes 5-hydroxy-tryptamine$_1$ ($5\text{-HT}_{1B/1D}$) receptor, inhibiting excessive dilation of extracerebral and intracranial arteries in migraine. It is indicated in acute treatment of migraine attacks with or without aura in adults.

FRUCTOSE

(Levulose)

Fructose, a carbohydrate, is used as a source of carbohydrate calories primarily when fluid replacement is also indicated and as a dextrose substitute for patients with diabetes.

FULVESTRANT

(Faslodex solution for injection 50 mg/mL)

Fulvestrant is an antiestrogen. Fulvestrant competitively binds to the estrogen receptor and downregulates the estrogen receptor protein in human breast cancer cells. It is indicated in the treatment of hormone receptor-positive metastatic breast cancer in postmenopausal women with disease progression following antiestrogen therapy.

FUNGAL INFECTIONS: Treatment of

Infections	Drugs of Choice	Alternatives
Aspergillosis	Amphotericin B	Itraconazole
Blastomycosis	Ketoconazole or Amphotericin B	Itraconazole
Candidiasis		
Oropharyngeal	Clotrimazole troches	Fluconazole Ketoconazole
Esophageal	Fluconazole or Ketoconazole	Amphotericin B
Systemic	Amphotericin B or Flucytosine	Fluconazole
Chromomycosis	Flucytosine	Itraconazole
Coccidioidomycosis	Ketoconazole or Amphotericin B	Itraconazole, Fluconazole
Cryptococcosis	Amphotericin B ± Flucytosine	Fluconazole
Chronic suppression		Itraconazole
	Fluconazole	Amphotericin B
Histoplasmosis	Ketoconazole or Amphotericin B	Itraconazole
Chronic suppression	Amphotericin B	Itraconazole
Mucormycosis	Amphotericin B	No dependable alternative
Paracoccidioidomycosis	Ketoconazole or Amphotericin B	Itraconazole, a sulfonamide
Pseudallescheriasis	Ketoconazole or Miconazole	Itraconazole
Sporotrichosis		
Cutaneous	Potassium iodide	Local heat, Itraconazole
Systemic	Amphotericin B	Itraconazole

FUROSEMIDE

(Lasix)

The major loop diuretics are furosemide (Lasix) and ethacrynic acid (Edecrin). Furosemide is chemically related to the thiazide diuretics, but ethacrynic acid is not. These agents inhibit the active resorption of chloride (and sodium) in the thick, ascending medullary portion of the loop of Henle and also in the cortical portion of the loop or the distal tubule. The diuresis they produce, which is similar to that seen with the thiazides, predominantly causes a loss of chloride, sodium, and potassium, but HCO_3 excretion is not increased. Although large volumes of fluid can be excreted with the use of these agents, the ability of the kidney to produce either a dilute or concentrated urine is greatly diminished. These agents are the most efficacious of all the diuretics now on the market, usually producing about a 20% loss in the filtered load of sodium (furosemide, 15 to 30%; ethacrynic acid, 17 to 23%).

Loop diuretics are ordinarily taken orally but can be given intravenously if a very rapid onset of action is sought, as when used in combination with antihypertensive medications in the management of a hypertensive crisis. Furosemide and ethacrynic acid undergo some active renal tubular secretion as well as glomerular filtration. A minor portion is excreted by the liver.

Loop diuretics are used for treating the following conditions:

- In the edema of cardiac, hepatic, or renal origin, including acute pulmonary edema and hypertensive crisis
- In acute renal failure, to maintain urine flow, though an excessive loss of extracellular fluid volume can cause a decrease in the GFR
- In hypercalcemia

Excessive volume depletion, hyponatremia, and hypotension are major risks associated with the use of loop diuretics, and the side effects of hypokalemia, hyperuricemia, and hyperglycemia are always present. Loop diuretics should not be used concurrently with ototoxic aminoglycoside antibiotics (i.e., streptomycin, gentamicin, kanamycin, tobramycin) (see also Table 25 and Figure 17).

G

GABAPENTIN

(Neurotin tablets 600 mg)

Gabapentin, an anticonvulsant that stimulates gamma-aminobutyric acid (GABA) receptors, is used as an adjunctive therapy in treatment of partial seizures with or without secondary generalization in patients older than 12 years of age with epilepsy; adjunctive therapy for partial seizures in children 3 to 12 years of age; and for management of postherpetic neuralgia in adults (see Figure 53).

Gabapentin (Neurontin) is an antiseizure drug that consists of a GABA molecule covalently bound to a lipophilic cyclohexane ring. **Gabapentin** was designed to be a centrally active GABA agonist, with its high lipid solubility aimed at facilitating its transfer across the blood–brain barrier.

Gabapentin inhibits tonic hind limb extension in the electroshock seizure model. Interestingly, gabapentin also inhibits clonic seizures induced by pentylenetetrazol. Its efficacy in both these tests parallels that of valproic acid and distinguishes it from phenytoin and carbamazepine. Despite its design as a GABA agonist, gabapentin does not mimic GABA when iontophoretically applied to neurons in primary culture.

Gabapentin may promote nonvesicular release of GABA through a poorly understood mechanism. **Gabapentin** binds a protein in cortical membranes with an amino acid sequence identical to that of the α2δ subunit of the L type of voltage-sensitive Ca^{2+} channel, yet gabapentin does not affect Ca^{2+} currents of the T, N, or L types of Ca^{2+} channels in dorsal root ganglion cells. Gabapentin has not been found consistently to reduce sustained repetitive firing of action potentials.

Gabapentin is absorbed after oral administration and is not metabolized in humans. It is not bound to plasma proteins. It is excreted unchanged, mainly in the urine. Its half-life, when it is used as monotherapy, is 4 to 6 hours. It has no known interactions with other antiseizure drugs.

Gabapentin is effective for partial seizures, with and without secondary generalization, when used in addition to other antiseizure drugs.

Double-blind placebo-controlled trials of adults with refractory partial seizures demonstrated that addition of **gabapentin** to other antiseizure drugs was superior to placebo. A double-blind study of **gabapentin** (900 or 1800 mg/day) monotherapy disclosed that it was equivalent to carbamazepine (600 mg/day) for newly diagnosed partial or generalized epilepsy. Gabapentin also is being used for the treatment of migraine, chronic pain, and bipolar disorder.

Gabapentin usually is effective in doses of 900 to 1800 mg daily in three doses, although 3600 mg may be required in

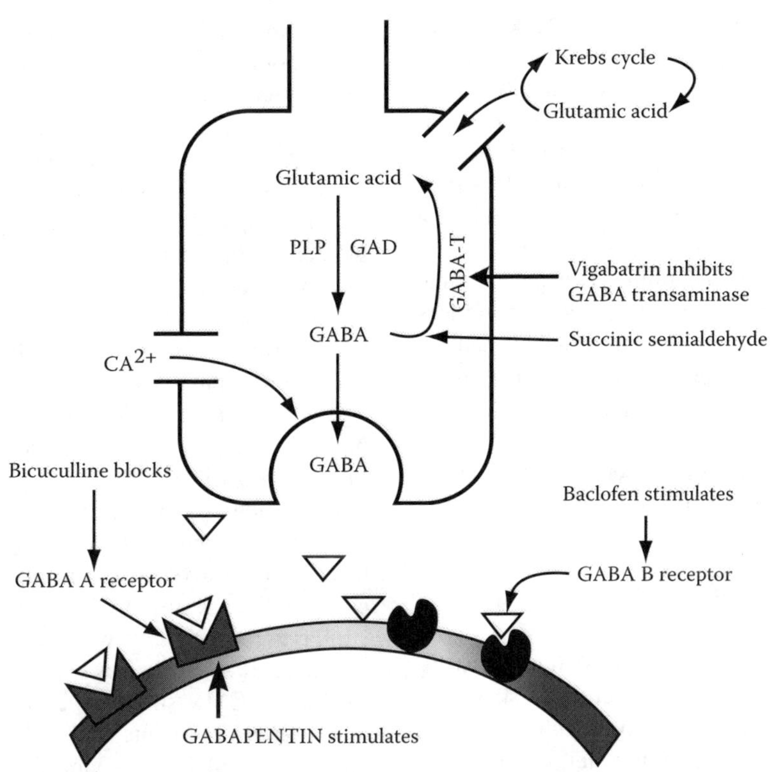

FIGURE 53 GABApentin is used as an adjunctive treatment of partial seizures, with and without secondary generalization.

some patients to achieve reasonable seizure control. Therapy usually is begun with a low dose (300 mg once on the first day), which is increased in daily increments of 300 mg until an effective dose is reached.

Overall, **gabapentin** is well tolerated with the most common adverse effects of somnolence, dizziness, ataxia, and fatigue. These effects usually are mild to moderate in severity but resolve within 2 weeks of onset during continued treatment.

GALANTAMINE HYDROBROMIDE

(Reminyl tablets 4 mg)

Galantamine is a cholinesterase (AChE) that enhances cholinergic function by increasing acetylcholine. It is indicated in the treatment of mild to moderate dementia of the Alzheimer type.

Four inhibitors of AChE currently are approved by the FDA for treatment of Alzheimer's disease (AD): **tacrine** (1,2,3,4-tetrahydro-9-aminoacridine; Cognex), **donepezil** (Aricept), **rivastigmine** (Excelon), and **galantamine** (razadyne). Tacrine is a potent centrally acting inhibitor of AChE. Studies of oral tacrine in combination with lecithin have confirmed that there is indeed an effect of tacrine on some measures of memory performance, but the magnitude of improvement observed with the combination of lecithin and tacrine is modest at best. The side effects of tacrine often are significant and dose-limiting; abdominal cramping, anorexia, nausea, vomiting, and diarrhea are observed in up to one-third of patients receiving therapeutic doses, and elevations of serum transaminases are observed in up to 50% of those treated. Because of significant side effects, tacrine is not used widely clinically. Donepezil is a selective inhibitor of AChE in the central nervous system (CNS) with little effect on AChE in peripheral tissues. It produces modest improvements in cognitive scores in AD patients and has a long half-life, allowing once-daily dosing. Rivastigmine and galantamine are dosed twice daily and produce a similar degree of cognitive improvement. Adverse effects associated with donepezil, rivastigmine, and galantamine are similar in character but generally less frequent and less severe than those observed with tacrine; they include nausea, diarrhea, vomiting, and insomnia. Donepezil, rivastigmine, and galantamine are not associated with the hepatotoxicity that limits the use of tacrine.

An alternative strategy for the treatment of AD is the use of the NMDA glutamate-receptor antagonist **memantine** (Namenda).

GALLAMINE TRIETHIODIDE

(Flaxedil)

Gallamine, a nondepolarizing neuromuscular blocking agent (1 mg/kg IV), is used as an adjunct to anesthesia to induce skeletal muscle relaxation, facilitate intubation and mechanical ventilation, reduce fractures and dislocations, and to weaken muscle contractions in pharmacologically or electrically induced convulsions (see also Figure 99).

GALLIUM NITRATE

(Ganite injection 25 mg/mL)

Gallium exerts a hypocalcemic effect by inhibiting calcium resorption from bone, possibly by stabilizing bone matrix, thereby reducing increased bone turnover. It is indicated in the treatment of symptomatic, cancer-related hypercalcemia unresponsive to adequate hydration.

GALSULFASE

(Naglazyme solution for injection)

Galsulfase is an endocrine and metabolic agent. It is a glycoprotein that is intended to provide an exogenous enzyme that will be taken up into lyosome and increase the catabolism of glycosaminoglycans. This is most likely mediated by the binding of mannose-6-phosphate-terminated oligosaccharide chains of galsulfase to specific mannose-6-phosphate receptors. It is indicated in the treatment of patients with mucopolysaccaridosis (MPS) VI.

GANCICLOVIR SODIUM

(DHPG, Cytovene)

Ganciclovir is indicated in the treatment of cytomegalovirus (CMV) retinitis in immunocompromised patients and for the prevention of cytomegalovirus disease in transplant patients who may be at risk for developing cytomegalovirus disease. Ganciclovir is a synthetic nucleoside analog of 2′-deoxyguanosine with efficacy against CMV, herpes simplex virus 1 and 2, Epstein–Barr virus, and varicella zoster virus. Ganciclovir is converted to ganciclovir triphosphate, which is preferentially accumulated in CMV-inhibiting viral-DNA polymerase and by incorporating into viral DNA terminating viral DNA chain elongation. Ganciclovir, which binds to plasma protein to the extent of 2%, is mostly excreted unchanged in the urine, and hence should be used cautiously in patients with renal impairment. Probenecid reduces the renal clearance of ganciclovir. Ganciclovir has caused granulocytopenia and thrombocytopenia, especially in elderly subjects with reduced glomerular filtration. Cytotoxic drugs that inhibit replication of rapidly dividing cell populations such as bone marrow, spermatogonia, and germinal layers of skin and gastrointestinal (GI) mucosa may have additive toxicity when administered concomitantly with ganciclovir (see also Figure 16).

Ganciclovir (9-[1,3-dihydroxy-2-propoxymethyl] guanine) is an acyclic guanine nucleoside analog that is similar in structure to acyclovir except in having an additional hydroxymethyl group on the acyclic side chain. **Valganciclovir** is the L-valyl ester prodrug of ganciclovir. This agent has inhibitory activity against all herpesviruses, but is especially active against CMV. Inhibitory concentrations are similar to those of acyclovir for herpes simplex virus (HSV) and varicella-zoster virus (VZV) but 10 to 100 times lower for human CMV strains (0.2 to 2.8 μg/mL).

Ganciclovir inhibits viral DNA synthesis. It is monophosphated intracellularly by viral thymidine kinase during HSV infection and by a viral phosphotransferase encoding the UL97 gene during CMV infection. Ganciclovir diphosphate and ganciclovir triphosphate are formed by cellular enzymes. At least tenfold higher concentrations of **ganciclovir** triphosphate are present in CMV-infected than in uninfected cells. The triphosphate competitive inhibitor of deoxyguanosine triphosphate incorporated into DNA preferentially inhibits viral rather than host cellular DNA polymerases. **Ganciclovir** is incorporated into both viral and cellular DNA. Incorporation into viral DNA causes eventual cessation of DNA-chain elongation.

Intracellular **ganciclovir** triphosphate concentrations are tenfold higher than those of acyclovir triphosphate and decline much more slowly with an intracellular $\tau_{1/2}$ of elimination exceeding 24 hours. These differences may account in part for **ganciclovir's** greater anti-CMV activity and provide the rationale for single daily doses in suppressing human CMV infections.

CMV can become resistant to ganciclovir by one of two mechanisms: reduced intracellular ganciclovir phosphorylation owing to mutations in the viral phosphotransferase encoded by the UL97 gene, and mutations in viral DNA polymerase. Resistant CMV clinical isolates have 4 to more than 20 times the increases in inhibitory concentrations. Resistance has been associated primarily with impaired phosphorylation but sometimes only with DNA polymerase mutations. Highly resistant variants with dual UL97 and polymerase mutations are cross-resistant to cidofovir and variably to foscarnet. **Ganciclovir** also is much less active against acyclovir-resistant thymidine-kinase-deficient HSV strains.

The oral bioavailability of **ganciclovir** averages 6 to 9% following ingestion with food. Peak and trough plasma levels are about 0.5 to 1.2, and 0.2 to 0.5 μg/mL, respectively, after 1000-mg doses every 8 hours. Oral valganciclovir is well absorbed and hydrolyzed rapidly to ganciclovir. The bioavailability of ganciclovir averages 61% following valganciclovir. Food increases the bioavailability of ganciclovir by about 25%, and peak **ganciclovir** concentrations average 6.1 μg/mL after 875-mg doses. High oral valganciclovir doses in the fed state provide ganciclovir exposures comparable with intravenous dosing. Following intravenous administration of 5 mg/kg doses of ganciclovir, peak and trough plasma concentrations average 8 to 11 and 0.6 to 1.2 μg/mL, respectively. Following intravenous dosing, vitreous fluid levels are similar to or higher than those in plasma, and average about 1 μg/mL. Vitreous levels decline with a half-life of 23 to 26 hours. Intraocular sustained-release **ganciclovir** implants provide vitreous levels of about 4.1 μg/mL.

The plasma half-life is about 2 to 4 hours in patients with normal renal function. Over 90% of ganciclovir is eliminated unchanged by renal excretion through glomerular filtration and tubular secretion. Consequently, the plasma increases almost linearly as creatinine clearance declines, and may reach 28 to 40 hours in those with severe renal insufficiency.

Myelosuppression is the principal dose-limiting toxicity of ganciclovir. Neutropenia occurs in about 15 to 40% of patients, and thrombocytopenia in 5 to 20%. Neutropenia is observed most commonly during the second week of treatment and usually is reversible within 1 week of drug cessation. Persistent fatal neutropenia has occurred. Oral valganciclovir is associated with headache and gastrointestinal disturbance (nausea, pain, and diarrhea) in addition to the toxicities associated with intravenous ganciclovir, including neutropenia. Recombinant granulocyte colony-stimulating factor (G-CSF, **filgrastim**, lenograstim) may be useful in treating ganciclovir-induced neutropenia.

CNS side effects occur in 5 to 15% of patients, and range in severity from headache to behavioral changes to convulsions and coma. About one-third of patients have had to interrupt or prematurely stop intravenous **ganciclovir** therapy because of bone marrow or CNS toxicity. Infusion-related phlebitis, azotemia, anemia, rash, fever, liver function test abnormalities, nausea or vomiting, and eosinophilia also have been described.

Teratogenicity, embryotoxicity, irreversible reproductive toxicity, and myelotoxicity have been observed in animals at **ganciclovir** dosages comparable with those used in human beings. **Ganciclovir** is classified in pregnancy as category C.

Zidovudine and probably other cytotoxic agents increase the risk of myelosuppression, as do nephrotoxic agents that impair ganciclovir excretion. Probenecid, and possibly acyclovir, reduce renal clearance of ganciclovir. Zalcitabine increases oral **ganciclovir** exposure by an average of 22%. Oral ganciclovir increases the absorption and peak plasma concentrations of didanosine by approximately twofold, and that of zidovudine by about 20%.

Ganciclovir is effective in the treatment and chronic suppression of CMV retinitis in immunocompromised patients and for prevention of CMV disease in transplant patients. In CMV retinitis, initial induction treatment (5 mg/kg intravenously every 12 hours for 10 to 21 days) is associated with improvement or stabilization in about 85% of patients. Reduced viral excretion is usually evident by 1 week, and funduscopic improvement is seen by 2 weeks. Because of the high risk of relapse, AIDS patients with retinitis require suppressive therapy with high doses of ganciclovir (30 to 35 mg/kg per week). Oral ganciclovir (1000 mg three times daily) is effective for suppression of retinitis after initial intravenous treatment. Oral valganciclovir (900 mg twice daily for 21 days initial treatment) is comparable with intravenous dosing for initial control and sustained suppression (900 mg daily) of CMV retinitis.

Intravitreal ganciclovir injections have been used in some patients, and an intraocular sustained-release ganciclovir implant (vitrasert) is more effective than systemic dosing in suppressing retinitis progression.

Ganciclovir therapy (5 mg/kg every 12 hours for 14 to 21 days) may benefit other CMV syndromes in AIDS patients or solid-organ-transplant recipients. Response rates of 67% or higher have been found in combination with a decrease in immunosuppressive therapy. The duration of therapy depends on demonstrating clearance of viremia; an early switch from intravenous ganciclovir to oral valganciclovir is feasible. Recurrent CMV disease occurs commonly after initial treatment. In bone marrow transplant recipients with CMV pneumonia, ganciclovir alone appears ineffective. However, ganciclovir combined with intravenous immunoglobulin or CMV immunoglobulin reduces the mortality of CMV pneumonia by about one-half. Ganciclovir treatment may benefit infants with congential CMV disease, and further studies are in progress.

Ganciclovir has been used for both prophylaxis and preemptive therapy of CMV infections in transplant recipients. In bone marrow transplant recipients, preemptive **ganciclovir** treatment (5 mg/kg every 12 hours for 7 to 14 days followed by 5 mg/kg every day to days 100 to 120 after transplant) starting when CMV is isolated from bronchoalveolar lavage or from other sites is highly effective in preventing CMV pneumonia and appears to reduce mortality in these patients. Initiation of ganciclovir at the time of engraftment also reduces CMV disease rates but does not improve survival in part because of infections owing to **ganciclovir**-related neutropenia.

Intravenous **ganciclovir**, oral ganciclovir, and oral valganciclovir reduce the risk of CMV disease in solid-organ-transplant recipients. Oral ganciclovir (1000 mg three times daily for 3 months) reduces CMV disease risk in liver transplant recipients, including high-risk patients with primary infection or those receiving antilymphocyte antibodies. Oral valganciclovir prophylaxis generally is more effective than high-dose oral acyclovir. Oral valganciclovir (900 mg once daily) provides somewhat greater antiviral effects and similar reductions in CMV disease as oral ganciclovir in mismatched solid-organ-transplant recipients.

In advanced HIV disease, oral **ganciclovir** (1000 mg three times daily) may reduce the risk of CMV disease and possibly mortality in those not receiving didanosine. The addition of oral high-dose **ganciclovir** (1500 mg three times daily) to the intraocular **ganciclovir** implant further delays the time to retinitis progression and reduces the risk of new CMV disease and possibly the risk of Kaposi's sarcoma.

Ganciclovir resistance emerges in a minority of transplant patients, especially mismatched solid-organ recipients, and is associated with poorer prognosis. The use of antithymocyte globulin and prolonged ganciclovir exposure are risk factors. Recovery of ganciclovir-resistant CMV isolates has been associated with progressive CMV disease in AIDS and other immunocompromised patients. Over one-quarter of retinitis patients have resistant isolates by 9 months of therapy, and resistant CMV has been recovered from CSP, vitreous fluid, and visceral sites.

A ganciclovir ophthalmic gel formulation appears to be effective in treating HSV keratitis. Oral **ganciclovir** reduces hepatitis B virus (HBV) DNA levels and aminotransferase levels in chronic hepatitis B.

Systemic **ganciclovir** has been studied in conjunction with suicide gene therapy expressing HSV thymidine kinase for treatment of brain tumors and a variety of other malignancies.

GASTRIN

Histamine, as a normal constituent of the gastric mucosa, controls both microcirculation and gastric secretion. The gastric secretagogues are acetylcholine, histamine, and gastrin. The action of acetylcholine is blocked by atropine, and the action of histamine is blocked by cimetidine, butrimamide, and metiamide. No specific antagonist is available for gastrin (see Figure 34).

GASTROESOPHAGEAL REFLUX DISEASE (GERD): Treatment of

Esophagitis results from excessive reflux of gastric juice rather than excessive gastric secretion. The squamous epithelium of the esophagus is intolerant of repetitive exposure to gastric juice for prolonged periods. Low-grade esophagitis is evident only by histopathological examination. High-grade changes are seen endoscopically as erosions and ulcerations. Peptic strictures and Barrett's metaplasia result from the response that follows ulceration.

The goals of drug therapy of reflux esophagitis are to increase the strength and competence of the antireflux barrier, to enhance esophageal acid clearance, to improve gastric emptying and pyloric sphincter competence, to prevent reflux of duodenal contents, to coat inflamed and denuded tissue, and, above all, to decrease the volume of pH of gastric contents.

Prokinetic Agents

Cisapride is currently considered the drug of choice among the motility-modulating agents to treat GERD. It is more potent and has fewer side effects as compared to the older prokinetics.

Mucosa-Coating Drugs

Sucralfate is a topically active aluminum hydroxide salt of sucrose octasulfate.

Histamine$_2$-Receptor-Blocking Agents

Cimetidine
Famotidine
Nizatidine
Ranitidine
Roxatidine

Proton-Pump Inhibitors

Omeprazole

Although usually a mild condition appropriately treated with episodic self-medication and lifestyle modifications, GERD can also result in severe symptoms or in complications. The complications of GERD can be categorized as those involving the esophagus (principally esophagitis, esophageal stricture, or Barrett's metaplasia and cancer) or organs other than the esophagus (principally asthma and otolaryngological manifestations).

GATIFLOXACIN

(Tequin tablets 200 mg)

Gatifloxacin is a fluoroquinolone/ophthalmic/antibiotic. It is indicated in treatment of bacterial infections, including chronic bronchitis; acute sinusitis; community-acquired pneumonia; uncomplicated and complicated UTIs; pyelonephritis; uncomplicated urethral and cervical gonorrhea; uncomplicated skin and skin-structure infections; uncomplicated rectal infections in women; and bacterial conjunctivitis (ophthalmic). The quinolones (e.g., **ciprofloxacin**, **levofloxacin**, **moxifloxacin**, and **gatifloxacin**) have inhibitory activity against MAC bacteria *in vitro* (at concentrations of ≤100 μg/mL). Minimal inhibitory concentrations for *M. fortuitum* and *M. kansasii* are ≤3 μg/mL for these quinolones, but *M. chelonae* usually are resistant. Single-agent therapy of *M. fortuitum* infection with ciprofloxacin has been associated with the development of resistance. Ciprofloxacin, 750 mg twice daily or 500 mg three times daily, has been used as part of a four-drug regimen (with clarithromycin, rifabutin, and amikacin) as salvage therapy for MAC infections in HIV-infected patients, with improvement in symptoms. Multidrug-resistant tuberculosis has been treated with ofloxacin, 300 or 800 mg each day, in combination with second-line agents. Moxifloxacin and gatifloxacin are more active *in vitro* than the older fluoroquinolones and would be expected to be useful agents clinically.

GEMCITABINE HYDROCHLORIDE

(Gemzar lyophilized powder for injection 200 mg)

Gemcitabine is a pyrimidine analog that exhibits cell-phase specificy, primarily killing cells undergoing DNA synthesis in the S-phase. It also blocks the progression of cells through the G1/S-phase boundary. It is indicated in locally advanced or metastatic pancreatic adenocarcinoma in patients previously treated with 5-fluorouracil; and locally advanced or metastatic non-small-cell lung cancer.

Gemcitabine (2′, 2′ difluorodeoxycytidine; dFdC), a difluoro analog of deoxycytidine, has become an important drug for patients with metastatic pancreatic cancer; non-small-cell lung cancer; and ovarian, bladder, esophageal, and head and neck cancer.

Gemcitabine enters cells via active nucleoside transporters. Intracellularly, deoxycytidine kinase phosphorylates gemcitabine to produce difluorodeoxycytidine monophosphate (dFdCMP), from which point it is converted to difluorodeoxycytidine di- and triphosphate (dFdCDP and dFdCTP). Although its anabolism and effects on DNA in general mimic those of cytarabine, there are differences in kinetics of inhibition, additional sites of action, effects of incorporation into DNA, and spectrum of clinical activity. Unlike cytarabine, the cytotoxicity of **gemcitabine** is not confined to the S-phase of the cell cycle, and the drug is equally effective against confluent cells and cells in logarithmic growth phase. The cytotoxic activity may be a result of several actions on DNA synthesis: dFdCTP competes with dCTP as a weak inhibitor of DNA polymerase; dFdCDP is a potent inhibitor of ribonucleotide reductase, resulting in depletion of deoxyribonucleotide pools necessary for DNA synthesis; and dFdCTP is incorporated into DNA and, after the incorporation of one more additional nucleotide, leads to DNA strand termination. This "extra" nucleotide may be important in hiding the dFdCTP from DNA repair enzymes, as the incorporated dFdCMP appears to be resistant to repair. The ability of cells to incorporate dFdCTP into DNA is critical for gemcitabine-induced apoptosis.

Gemcitabine is administered as an intravenous infusion. The pharmacokinetics of the parent compound are largely determined by deamination, and the predominant urinary elimination product is the inactive metabolite difluorodeoxyuridine (dFdU). **Gemcitabine** has a short plasma half-life of approximately 15 minutes, with women and elderly

---

GAUCHER'S DISEASE: Treatment of

Gaucher's disease is the most prevalent lysosomal storage disorder, caused by an inherited defect in the lysosomal enzyme, glucocerebrosidase, and consequent accumulation of glucocerebrosidase in the cells of the reticuloendothelial system. There is a high incidence of the most common variant, type I, among Ashkenazi Jews. The other two variants, types II and III, are relatively rare and have been described among all ethnic groups.

The earliest sign of Gaucher's disease is generally splenomegaly, which may be massive, but even when not palpable, can be demonstrated by ultrasound. Anemia and thrombocytopenia, resulting in fatigue and bleeding tendencies, respectively, are among the prominent features and are often the initial presenting signs of Gaucher's disease. In type II Gaucher's disease, the neurological signs include the classical triad of trismus, strabismus, and retroflexion of the head, as well as spasticity, hyperreflexia, and seizures during the first year of life. The effective enzyme replacement therapy for Gaucher's disease is the use of a placenta-derived macrophage-targeted glucocerebrosidase.

Of the surgical options available prior to enzyme therapy, splenectomy was most often recommended to combat thrombocytopenia and anemia, mechanical complications, and growth retardation.

It is hoped that, in the future, Gaucher's disease, currently a model of enzyme replacement therapy, will prove to be a model of a curative form of gene transfer therapy for inherited metabolic disorders. In this case CD34 cells from the patient's blood will be genetically corrected *in vitro* and transplanted back into the patient.

---

subjects having slower clearance. Clearance is dose-independent, but can vary widely among individuals.

Similar to that of cytarabine, conversion of gemcitabine to dFdCMP by deoxycytidine kinase is saturated at infusion rates of approximately 10 mg/m^2 per minute, which produce plasma drug concentrations in the range of 15 to 20 μM. In an attempt to increase dFdCTP formation, the duration of infusion at this maximum concentration has been extended to 150 minutes. In contrast to a fixed infusion duration of 30 minutes, the 150-minute infusion produces a higher level of dFdCTP within peripheral blood mononuclear cells and increases the degree of myelosuppression, but has uncertain effects on antitumor activity.

The activity of dFdCTP on DNA repair mechanisms may allow for increased cytotoxicity of other chemotherapeutic agents, particularly platinum compounds. Preclinical studies of tumor cell lines show that cisplatin-DNA adducts are enhanced in the presence of gemcitabine, presumably through suppression of nuclear excision repair. The standard dosing schedule for **gemcitabine** (Gemzar) is a 30-minute intravenous infusion of 1 to 1.2 g/m^2 on days 1, 8, and 15 of each cycle. The principal toxicity of **gemcitabine** is suppression. In general, the longer-duration infusions lead to greater myelosuppression. Nonhematologic toxicities including a flu-like syndrome, asthenia, and mild elevation in liver transaminases may occur in 40% or more of patients. Although severe nonhematologic toxicities are rare, interstitial pneumonitis may occur and is responsive to steroids. Rarely, patients on gemcitabine treatment for many months may develop a slowly progressive hemolytic uremic syndrome, necessitating drug discontinuation. **Gemcitabine** is a very potent radiosensitizer and should not be used with radiotherapy except in closely monitored clinical trials.

GEMFIBROZIL

(Lopid tablets 600 mg)

Gemfibrozil is a fibric-acid derivative that decreases blood levels of triglycerides and VLDL by decreasing their production. It also decreases cholesterol and increases HDL.

Gemfibrozil is indicated in the treatment of hypertriglyceridemia in adult patients with type IV or V hyperlipidemia that presents risk of pancreatitis and does not respond to diet; and reduction of coronary heart disease risk in type IIb patients who have low HDL levels (in addition to elevated LDL and triglycerides) and have not responded to other measures.

Clofibrate, the prototype of the fibric-acid derivatives, is the ethyl ester of *p*-chlorophenoxyisobutyrate. **Gemfibrozil** is a nonhalogenated phenoxypentanoic acid and thus is distinct from the halo-generated number of fibric-acid analogs (e.g., fenofibrate, bezafibrate, and ciprofibrate have been developed and are used).

Clofibrate is available for oral administration. The usual dose is 2 g per day in divided doses. This compound is little used but may be useful in patients who do not tolerate **gemfibrozil** or **fenofibrate**. Gemfibrozil (Lopid) is usually administered as a 600-mg dose taken twice a day, 30 minutes before the morning and evening meals. The Tricor brand of fenofibrate is available in tablets or 48 and 145 mg. The usual daily dose is 145 mg. Generic fenofibrate (Lofibra) is available in capsules containing 67, 134, and 200 mg. Tricor, 145 mg, and Lofibra, 200 mg, are equivalent doses.

A myopathy syndrome occasionally occurs in subjects taking clofibrate, gemfibrozil, or fenofibrate, and may occur in up to 5% of patients treated with a combination of gemfibrozil and higher doses of statins. To diminish the risk of myopathy, statin doses should be reduced when combination therapy of a statin plus a fibrate is employed. Several drug interactions may contribute to this adverse response. **Gemfibrozil** inhibits hepatic uptake of statins by OATP2. It also competes for the same glucuronosyl transferases that metabolize most statins. As a consequence, levels of both drugs may be increased when they are coadministered. Patients taking this combination should be instructed to be aware of the potential symptoms and should be followed at 3-month intervals with careful history and determination of creatine kinase (CK) values until a stable pattern is established. Patients taking fibrates with rosuvastatin should be followed especially closely even if low doses (5 to 10 mg) of rosuvastatin are employed, until there is more experience with and knowledge of the safety of this specific combination. Fenofibrate is glucuronidated by enzymes that are not involved in statin glucuronidation. Thus, feno–fibrate–statin combinations are less likely to cause myopathy than combination therapy with gemfibrozil and statins.

All of the fibrates increase the lithogenicity of bile. Clofibrate use has been associated with increased risk of gallstone formation; gemfibrozil and fenofibrate reportedly do not increase biliary tract disease.

Renal failure is a relative contraindication to the use of fibric-acid agents, as is hepatic dysfunction. Combined statin–fibrate therapy should be avoided in patients with compromised renal function. Gemfibrozil should be used with caution and at a reduced dosage to treat the hyperlipidemia of renal failure. Fibrates should not be used by children or pregnant women.

Gemfibrozil is another cholesterol-lowering agent that acts by a different mechanism and also causes a severe pharmacokinetic interaction with **cerivastatin**. Gemfibrozil glucuronide inhibits the CYP2C8-mediated metabolism and OATP (organic anion transporting polypeptide)-mediated uptake of cerivastatin more potently than gemfibrozil. Laboratory data show that the glucuronide is highly concentrated in the liver versus plasma probably owing to transporter-mediated active uptake and intracellular formation of the conjugate. Therefore, it may be that gemfibrozil glucuronide, concentrated in the hepatocytes, inhibits the CYP2C8-mediated metabolism of cerivastatin. **Gemfibrozil** markedly (four- to fivefold) increases the plasma concentration of cerivastatin but does not greatly increase (1.3 to 2 times) that of unmetabolized statins **pravastatin**, **pitavastatin**, and **rosuvastatin**, a result that also suggests that this interaction is caused by inhibition of metabolism. Thus, when an inhibitor of drug-metabolizing enzymes is highly concentrated in hepatocytes by active transport, extensive inhibition of the drug-metabolizing enzymes may be observed because of the high concentration of the inhibitor in the vicinity of the drug-metabolizing enzymes.

GEMIFLOXACIN MESYLATE

(Factive tablets 320 mg)

Gemifloxacin is a fluoroquinolone that interferes with microbial DNA synthesis. It is indicated in the treatment of acute bacterial exacerbation of chronic bronchitis and community-acquired pneumonia (mild to moderate) caused by susceptible strains of designated microorganisms. The first quinolone, **nalidixic acid**, was isolated as a by-product of the synthesis of chloroquine. It has been available in the treatment of urinary tract infections for many years. The introduction of fluorinated 4-quinolones, such as **ciprofloxacin** (Cipro), **moxifloxacin** (Avelox), and **gatifloxacin** (Tequin) represents a particularly important therapeutic advance because these agents have broad antimicrobial activity and are effective after oral administration for the treatment of a wide variety of infectious diseases. Relatively few side effects appear to accompany the use of these fluoroquinolones, and microbial resistance to their action does not develop rapidly. Rare and potentially fatal side effects, however, have resulted in the withdrawal from the market of temafloxacin (immune hemolytic anemia), trovafloxacin (hepatotoxicity), grepafloxacin (cardiotoxicity), and clinafloxacin (phototoxicity). In all these cases, the side effects were so infrequent as to be missed by prerelease clinical trials and detected only by postmarketing surveillance.

Several of the new fluoroquinolones have activity against anaerobic bacteria, including **garenoxacin** and **gemifloxacin**. The fluoroquinolones are potent bactericidal agents against *E. coli* and various species of *Salmonella*, *Shigella*, *Enterobacter*, *Campylobacter*, and *Neisseria*. Minimal inhibitory concentrations of the fluoroquinolones for 90% of these strains (MIC_{90}) usually are less than 0.2 μg/mL. Ciprofloxacin is more active than norfloxacin (Noroxin) against *P. aeruginosa*; values of MIC_{90} range from 0.5 to 6 μg/mL. Fluoroquinolones also have good activity against staphylococci, but not against methicillin-resistant strains (MIC_{90} = 0.1 to 2 μg/mL).

Activity against streptococci is limited to a subset of the quinolones, including levofloxacin (Levaquin), gatifloxacin (Tequin), and moxifloxacin (Avelox). Several intracellular bacteria are inhibited by fluoroquinolones at concentrations that can be achieved in plasma; these include species of *Chlamydia*, *Mycoplasma*, *Legionella*, *Brucella*, and *Mycobacterium* (including *Mycobacterium tuberculosis*). Ciprofloxacin, ofloxacin (Floxin), and pefloxacin have MIC_{90} values from 0.5 to 3 μg/mL for *M. fortuitum*, *M. kansasii*, and *M. tuberculosis*; ofloxacin and pefloxacin are active in animal models of leprosy. However, clinical experience with these pathogens remains limited.

GEMTUZUMAB OZOGAMICIN

(Mylotarg sterile preservative-free powder for injection)

Gemtuzumab is a monoclonal antibody. It is a chemotherapy agent composed of a recombinant humanized IgG_4 kappa antibody conjugated with a cytotoxic antitumor antibiotic, calicheamicin, isolated from fermentation of a bacterium. The antibody portion of gemtuzumab ozogamicin binds specifically to the CD33 antigen, which is expressed on the surface of leukemic blasts in patients with acute myeloid leukemia (AML), ultimately resulting in DNA double-strand breaks and cell death. CD33-positive AML in first relapse in patients at least 60 years who are not candidates for conventional cytotoxic therapy.

GENE THERAPY (e.g., for acquired immune deficiency syndrome (AIDS))

Gene therapy is defined as the introduction of new genetic material into the cells of an individual that results in a therapeutic benefit. Gene therapy holds considerable potential for the treatment of both hereditary and acquired genetic diseases. Because in its normal life cycle the HIV-1 virus integrates into the host cell's genome, AIDS can be regarded as an acquired genetic disease. Therefore, AIDS may be amenable to treatment by gene therapy approaches.

Gene therapy for HIV-1 infection requires the introduction of genes that will effectively inhibit HIV-1 replication by efficiently inhibiting expression of HIV-1 viral genes or altering the normal function of HIV-1-associated proteins. The ultimate goal of gene therapy is to inhibit HIV-1 viral replication and the resulting AIDS pathogenesis. Anti-HIV-1 gene therapy approaches can be divided into three broad categories: (1) gene therapies based on nucleic acid moieties, including gene vaccines, antisense DNA/RNA, RNA decoys that function by competition for the binding of proteins essential for HIV-1 replication, and catalytic RNA moieties (ribozymes) that inhibit HIV-1 gene expression by cleaving the viral RNA; (2) protein approaches (transdominant negative proteins and single-chain antibodies) that are based on the intracellular expression of protein moieties that interfere or inhibit normal viral replication or function; and (3) immunotherapeutic approaches in which HIV-1-specific lymphocytes are generated and used to inhibit HIV replication.

Some other therapeutic gene therapy trials are:

- Gene Therapy for the Treatment of Recurrent Pediatric Malignant Astrocytomas with *In Vivo* Tumor Transduction with the Herpes Simplex-Thymidine Kinase Gene
- Human MDR Gene Transfer in Patients with Advanced Cancer

- Gene Therapy for Human Brain Tumors Using Episome-Based Antisense cDNA Transcription of Insulin-Like Growth Factor I
- Immunization of Malignant Melanoma Patients with Interleukin-2-Secreting Melanoma Cells Expressing Defined Allogeneic Histocompatibility Antigens
- Genetically Engineered Autologous Tumor Vaccines Producing Interleukin-2 for the Treatment of Metastatic Melanoma
- Intrathecal Gene Therapy for the Treatment of Leptomeningeal Carcinomatosis
- Retrovirus-Mediated Transfer of the cDNA for Human Glucocerebrosidase into Peripheral Blood Repopulating Cells of Patients with Gaucher's Disease
- Adoptive Immunotherapy of Melanoma with Activated Lymph Node Cells Primed *In Vivo* with Autologous Tumor Cells Transduced with the IL-4 Gene
- Gene Therapy for Cystic Fibrosis Using Cationic Liposome Mediated Gene Transfer.
- Gene Therapy of Patients with Advanced Cancer Using Tumor Infiltration Lymphocytes Transduced with the Gene Coding for Tumor Necrosis Factor
- Immunization of Cancer Patients Using Autologous Cancer Cells Modified by Insertion of the Gene for Tumor Necrosis Factor (TNF)
- Immunization of Cancer Patients Using Autologous Cancer Cells Modified by Insertion of the Gene for Interleukin-2 (IL-2)
- Gene Therapy for the Treatment of Recurrent Glioblastoma Multiforme with *In Vivo* Tumor Transduction with the Herpes Simplex–Thymidine Kinase Gene/Ganciclovir System
- Gene Therapy for the Treatment of Brain Tumors Using Intra-Tumoral Transduction with the Thymidine Kinase Gene and Intravenous Ganciclovir
- Immunization with HLA-A2 Matched Allogeneic Melanoma Cells that Secrete Interleukin-2 in Patients with Metastatic Melanoma
- Immunization with IL-2-Secreting Allogeneic HLA-A2 Matched Renal Cell Carcinoma Cells in Patients with Advanced Renal Cell Carcinoma
- Clinical Protocol for Modification of Oncogene and Tumor Suppressor Gene Expression in Non-Small-Cell Lung Cancer (NSCLC)
- Cystic Fibrosis Gene Therapy Using an Adenovirus Vector: *In vivo* Safety and Efficacy in Nasal Epithelium.
- Administration of Neomycin Resistance Gene Marked EBV Specific Cytotoxic T Lymphocytes to Recipients of Mismatched–Related or Phenotypically Similar Unrelated Donor Marrow Grafts
- Retroviral Mediated Gene Transfer of the Fanconi Anemia Complementation Group C Gene to Hematopoietic Progenitors of Group C Patients
- Clinical Protocol for Modification of Tumor Suppressor Gene Expression and Induction of Apoptosis in Non-Small-Cell Lung Cancer (NSCLC) with an Adenovirus Vector Expressing Wildtype p53 and Cisplatin

GENERAL ANESTHETICS

Anesthesia is the controllable and reversible depression of the CNS that is characterized by a lack of perception of all sensations, by analgesia, and by amnesia. An ideal anesthetic is an inexpensive agent that has the following characteristics: it has a fast rate of induction and a rapid rate of emergence; it is nonexplosive and a good muscle relaxant; it has analgesic properties and does not cause respiratory or myocardial depression; it is nontoxic to the liver and kidney; it is inert metabolically and does not interact adversely with other pharmacologic agents used as pre- and postanesthetic medications; and it does not cause any postanesthetic complications. However, the search for this nonexistent ideal anesthetic agent continues.

A patient scheduled for surgery experiences discomfort and much anxiety. This preoperative behavior may be characterized by thoughts of excessive and unrealistic danger of anesthetics or the surgical procedure, and by repetitive and redundant inquiries about the preanesthetic and postoperative events. On the other hand, patients may manifest their anxiety by silence, avoidance of eye contact, lack of interest, or lack of communication. A visit by a caring physician or a nurse is extremely useful and supportive for reassuring and allaying a patient's concerns. A reassured patient sleeps easier, requires less anesthetics and analgesics, and shows fewer postanesthetic complications.

The choice of an anesthetic is always made by an anesthesiologist after consultation with the attending physician or surgeon. The anesthetic is selected based on many factors, including the patient's age, complicating and preexisting disease, the nature of the operation, the patient's previous experience with anesthetics, and the nature of nonanesthetic medications to be taken by the patient.

Because general anesthetics alter the cardiac and respiratory physiology, those agents causing myocardial irritability, hypotension, circulatory depression, or tachyarrhythmia should be used with extreme caution in patients with preexisting cardiovascular problems. Furthermore, agents causing respiratory depression should be used with caution in patients with bronchitis, emphysema, muscular dystrophy, or myasthenia gravis, as well as in those in bronchospastic states. The use of skeletal muscle relaxants should be monitored in conditions of respiratory insufficiency such as kyphoscoliosis. The opioids, which further depress respiration, should also be used with extreme care.

Preexisting endocrine disorders such as hypothyroidism, hyperthyroidism, and diabetes mellitus should also dictate the choice of general anesthetics. In patients with hyperthyroidism, agents causing cardiac acceleration (atropine or sympathomimetic amines) should be used carefully.

Because the release of insulin is reduced by sympathomimetic amines and increased by their appropriate blockers, severe hyperglycemia or hypoglycemia may be caused in susceptible patients who have been given inappropriate anesthetics. Patients who require medications on a permanent basis should be evaluated carefully, and the choice of anesthetics made judiciously.

Antihypertensive medications, diuretics causing hypokalemia that may predispose to cardiac irritability, and anticoagulants may have to be discontinued or their regimens modified in surgical patients.

The foregoing represents only a brief description of the cautions that should be taken into consideration when choosing an anesthetic.

Preanesthetic medications are given for the following reasons:

- To sedate and reduce anxiety (secobarbital, diazepam)
- To relieve pain, if present (opiates)
- To reduce excess salivation (anticholinergics such as atropine)
- To prevent bradycardia during surgery (atropine)
- To facilitate intubation (succinylcholine)

The general anesthetics are classified as either inhalational or intravenous. The inhalational anesthetic agents include:

- Halogenated hydrocarbons
- Halothane
- Anesthetic ethers
- Enflurane
- Isoflurane
- Methoxyflurane
- Anesthetic gases
- Nitrous oxide

The intravenous anesthetic agents include:

- Barbiturates
    - Thiopental
    - Methohexital
- Nonbarbiturates
    - Dissociative anesthetics-ketamine (see also Figure 82)
    - Benzodiazepines—diazepam, midazolam, lorazepam, flumazenil (antagonist)
    - Neuroleptic anesthetics—droperidol, haloperidol
    - Imidazole derivatives—etomidate
    - Phenol derivatives—propofol (see also Figure 82)

Morphine may be used for patients undergoing open-heart surgery. It is given in a dose of 0.5 to 3.0 mg/kg administered intravenously over a 15- to 20-minute period, which produces unconsciousness. Morphine is supplemented with nitrous oxide and a muscle relaxant.

Dantrolene is used for patients who are genetically disposed to malignant hyperthermia. Malignant hyperpyrexia represents an inherited muscular abnormality that presents clinically as a syndrome of life-threatening complications that arise during general anesthesia. The primary defect in malignant hyperpyrexic susceptible muscle resides in the process that regulates myoplasmic calcium concentrations. Recent investigations have also implicated abnormalities in the phosphoinositide cycle and in the sarcoplasmic–reticular calcium-releasing channels. In the event of anesthetic-induced malignant hyperthermia, the offending anesthetics should be discontinued and dantrolene administered in an initial dose of 1 mg/kg (see also Figure 40).

Thiopental is used in patients undergoing carotid endarterectomy for whom the maintenance of oxygen and nutrients to the brain during the temporary period of surgical occlusion of the common, internal, and external carotid arteries is essential. Thiopental, given as a bolus of 4 to 5 mg/kg or as an intravenous infusion of 10 mg/kg over 20 to 30 minutes, protects the brain against ischemia. The general anesthetic may be 0.3 to 0.6% halothane in 50 to 60% nitrous oxide in oxygen.

General anesthetics alter the excitation of the neuronal membrane and modify impulse conduction. Specifically, the general anesthetics have the following common properties:

- They decrease the activity of neurons by increasing their threshold to fire.
- By interfering with sodium influx, they prevent the action potential from rising to a normal rate.

At the present time, the depth of anesthesia is judged by the presence or absence of the eyelash reflex, the respiratory rate, and the response of the heart rate and blood pressure to surgical stimulation.

In the past, the pupillary signs have been used to judge the depth of anesthesia; however, premedication with opiate (causing miosis) or with anticholinergics (causing mydriasis) may make these signs unreliable. If both morphine and atropine have been administered, the miotic effect of morphine dominates. In addition, the reaction to light and pupillary signs are less predictable in patients aged 50 and over, and the reaction to light is absent with halothane and enflurane. Nevertheless, the classic signs of general anesthesia following the administration of diethyl ether, as originally described by Guedel, are still valid for educating students of medicine concerning the dose-dependent actions of general anesthetics (see Table 16).

The various stages of anesthesia seem to be sponsored by the dose-dependent alteration of the physiology of different populations of neurons in the CNS. Furthermore, the various anesthetics do indeed show specificity in this respect.

Stage I (analgesia) is brought about by a decrease in the activity of the dorsal horn of the spinal cord, which interferes with the sensory transmission in the spinothalamic tract.

Stage II (excitement or delirium) represents the period of anesthetic-mediated "disinhibition." It is due to the blockade of inhibitory neurons (Golgi type II cells), which then frees up the actions of excitatory neurotransmitters.

Stage III (muscle relaxation and time of surgery) represents the time when a high concentration of anesthetic is reached in the brain, while the reticular activating system and the spinal reflexes are suppressed. The swallowing, retching, and vomiting reflexes are also diminished. This stage, which is divided into four planes, is the time when surgery is performed.

Stage IV (death) occurs when the medullary neurons in the respiratory and vasomotor centers are completely depressed. General anesthetics depress the respiratory center only when given in higher-than-therapeutic doses; morphine, on the other hand, depresses the respiratory center at a dose that does not cause narcosis.

The states of anesthesia are directly related and dependent on the concentration of an anesthetic in the brain; that is, the higher the concentration, the deeper the state of anesthesia. The administration of general anesthetics is arbitrarily divided into three phases:

Induction—the time from the onset of administration of an anesthetic to a stage where surgery becomes suitable

Maintenance—the duration of time a patient is kept in a state of surgical anesthesia

Emergence—the time between the discontinuation of an anesthetic agent until the patient regains consciousness

The concentrations of general anesthetics in the brain depend on their solubility, their concentration in the inspired air, the rate of pulmonary ventilation, the rate of pulmonary blood flow, and the concentration gradient of the anesthetic between arterial and mixed venous blood.

The blood–gas partition coefficient is an index of the solubility of an anesthetic or its induction time, as depicted by the following examples.

Anesthetic Agents	Blood–Gas	Induction Time (minutes)
Nitrous oxide	0.47	2–3
Isoflurane	1.4	5–10
Enflurane	1.9	5–10
Halothane	2.36	10

Similarly, the amount of an anesthetic needed to produce anesthesia depends on the relative lipid solubility (oil–gas) of the compound, as denoted by the following examples.

Anesthetic Agents	Oil–Gas	Minimal Anesthetic Concentration (vol%)
Nitrous oxide	1.4	101
Enflurane	98	1.68
Isoflurane	99	1.40
Halothane	224	0.76

Furthermore, the greater the lipid solubility of an anesthetic, the lower the anesthetic tension needed to produce anesthesia. At equilibrium, the concentrations of an anesthetic in the brain and fat cells are high, but are low in the blood. Finally, the potency of an anesthetic is inversely related to its minimum anesthetic concentration.

GENTAMICIN

(Garamycin ointment 3 mg/g (ophthalmic), ointment 0.1% (as 1.7 mg sulfate/g), cream 0.1% (as 1.7 mg sulfate/g), solution 3 mg/mL (ophthalmic), injection 40 mg/mL (as sulfate))

Gentamicin is an aminoglycoside/ophthalmic antibiotic that inhibits production of bacterial protein, causing bacterial cell death. It is indicated for short-term treatment of serious infections caused by susceptible strains of microorganisms, especially Gram-negative bacteria; adjunct to systemic gentamicin in serious CNS infections (intrathecal); treatment of superficial ocular infections (ophthalmic); treatment of primary (e.g., impetigo contagiosa) and secondary (e.g., infectious eczemafoid dermatitis) skin infections; skin cysts and superficial skin infections, infection prophylaxis, and aid to healing (topical). The aminoglycoside group includes **gentamicin**, **tobramycin**, **amikacin**, **netilmicin**, **kanamycin**, **streptomycin**, and **neomycin**. These drugs are used primarily to treat infections caused by aerobic Gram-negative bacteria; streptomycin is an important agent for the treatment of tuberculosis. In contrast to most inhibitors of microbial protein synthesis, which are bacteriostatic, the aminoglycosides are bactericidal inhibitors of protein synthesis. Mutations affecting proteins in the bacterial ribosome, the target for these drugs, can confer marked resistance to their action. However, most commonly, resistance is due to acquisition of plasmids or transposon-encoding genes for aminoglycoside-metabolizing enzymes or from impaired transport of drug into the cell. Thus, there can be cross-resistance between members of the class.

These agents contain amino sugars linked to an aminocyclitol ring by glycosidic bonds. They are polycations, and their polarity is responsible in part for pharmacokinetic properties shared by all members of the group. For example, none is absorbed adequately after oral administration, inadequate concentrations are found in cerebrospinal fluid (CSF), and all are excreted relatively rapidly by the normal kidney.

Although aminoglycosides are widely used and important agents, serious toxicity limits their usefulness. All members of the group share the same spectrum of toxicity, most notably nephrotoxicity and ototoxicity, which can involve the auditory and vestibular (AV) functions of the eighth cranial nerve.

The antibacterial activity of **gentamicin**, **tobramycin**, **kanamycin**, **netilmicin**, and **amikacin** is directed primarily against aerobic Gram-negative bacilli. Kanamycin, like streptomycin, has a more limited spectrum compared with other aminoglycosides; in particular, it should not be used to treat infections caused by *Serratia* or *P. aeruginosa.* Aminoglycosides have little activity against anaerobic microorganisms or facultative bacteria under anaerobic condi-tions. Their action against most Gram-positive bacteria is limited, and they should not be used as single agents to treat infections caused by Gram-positive bacteria. In combination with a cell-wall-active agent, such as a penicillin or vancomycin, an aminoglycoside (streptomycin and **gentamicin** have been tested most extensively) produces a synergistic bactericidal effect *in vitro* against enterococci, streptococci, and staphylococci. Clinically, the superiority of aminoglycoside combination regimens over β-lactams alone is not proven except in relatively few infections.

The aerobic Gram-negative bacilli vary in their susceptibility to the aminoglycosides. Tobramycin and gentamicin exhibit similar activity against most Gram-negative bacilli, although tobramycin usually is more active against *P. aeruginosa* and some *Proteus* spp. Many Gram-negative bacilli that are resistant to gentamicin because of plasmid-mediated inactivating enzymes also are resistant to tobramycin. Amikacin and, in some instances, netilmicin retain their activity against gentamicine-resistant strains because they are a poor substrate for many of the aminoglycoside-inactivating enzymes.

All aminoglycosides have the potential to produce reversible and irreversible vestibular, cochlear, and renal toxicity. These side effects complicate the use of these compounds and make their proper administration difficult.

Vestibular and auditory dysfunction can follow the administration of any of the aminoglycosides. Studies of animals and human beings have documented progressive accumulation of these drugs in the perilymph and endolymph of the inner ear. Accumulation occurs predominantly when concentrations in plasma are high. Diffusion back into the bloodstream is slow; the half-lives of the aminoglycosides are five to six times longer in the otic fluids than in plasma. Back-diffusion is concentration dependent and is facilitated at the trough concentration of drug in plasma. Ototoxicity is more likely to occur in patients with persistently elevated concentrations of drug in plasma. However, even a single dose of tobramycin has been reported to produce slight temporary cochlear dysfunction during periods when the concentration in plasma is at its peak. Ototoxicity has been linked to mutations in a mitochondrial ribosomal RNA gene, indicating that a genetic predisposition exists for this side effect. Oxidant stress probably plays a role, and *ras* activation has been implicated. Ototoxicity is largely irreversible and results from progressive destruction of vestibular or cochlear cells, which are highly sensitive to damage by aminoglycosides. Studies in guinea pigs exposed to large doses of gentamicin reveal degeneration of the type I sensory hair cells in the central part of the crista ampullaris (vestibular organ) and fusion of individual sensory hairs into giant hairs. Similar studies with **gentamicin** and tobramycin also demonstrate loss of hair cells in a cochlea of the organ of Corti. With increasing dosage and prolonged exposure, damage progresses from the base of the cochlea, where high-frequency sounds are processed, to the apex, which is necessary for the perception of low frequencies. Although these histological changes correlate with the ability of the cochlea to generate an action potential in response to sound, the biochemical mechanism for ototoxicity is poorly understood.

Early changes induced by aminoglycosides have been shown in experimental ototoxicity to be reversible by Ca^{2+}. Once sensory cells are lost, however, regeneration does not occur; retrograde degeneration of the auditory nerve follows, resulting in irreversible hearing loss. It has been suggested that aminoglycosides interfere with the active transport system essential for the maintenance of the ionic balance of the endolymph. This would lead to alteration in the normal concentrations of ions in the labyrinthine fluids, with impairment of electrical activity and nerve conduction. Eventually, the electrolyte changes, or perhaps the drugs themselves, damage the hair cells irreversibly. The degree of permanent dysfunction correlates with the number of destroyed or altered sensory hair cells, and is thought to be related to sustained exposure to the drug. Interestingly, total dose and duration of aminoglycoside exposure and other risk factors, such as advanced age, bacteremia, liver disease, and renal disease, that reasonably might predispose one to ototoxicity, have not been proven to do so. Repeated courses of aminoglycosides, each probably resulting in the loss of more cells, seem to lead to deafness. Drugs such as **ethacrynic acid** and **furosemide** potentiate the ototoxic effects of the aminoglycosides in animals. Although all aminoglycosides are capable of affecting cochlear and vestibular function, some preferential toxicity is evident. Streptomycin and gentamicin produce predominantly vestibular effects, whereas amikacin, kanamycin, and neomycin primarily affect auditory function; tobramycin affects both equally.

Approximately 8 to 26% of patients who receive an aminoglycoside for more than several days will develop mild renal impairment that is almost always reversible. The toxicity results from accumulation and retention of aminoglycoside in the proximal tubular cells. The initial manifestation of damage at this site is excretion of enzymes of the renal tubular brush border. After several days, there is a defect in renal concentrating ability, mild proteinuria, and the appearance of hyaline and granular casts. The glomerular filtration rate is reduced after several additional days. The nonoliguric phase of renal insufficiency is thought to be due to the effects of aminoglycosides on the distal portion of the nephron with a reduced sensitivity of the collecting-duct epithelium to endogenous antidiuretic hormone. Although severe acute tubular necrosis may occur rarely, the most common significant finding is a mild rise in plasma creatinine (5 to 20 μg/mL; 40 to 175 μM). Hypokalemia, hypocalcemia, and hypophosphatemia are seen very infrequently. The impairment in renal function is almost always reversible because the proximal tubular cells have the capacity to regenerate.

GENTIAN VIOLET

Gentian violet, a triphenylmethane (rosaniline) dye, with topical antibacterial and antifungal activities (12% solution), is used in cutaneous or mucocutaneous infections caused by *Candida albicans*, and other superficial skin infections.

GEPIRONE HYDROCHLORIDE

Gepirone (30 to 60 mg/day), which interacts with serotonergic systems, is an anxioselective agent possessing properties similar to buspirone and ipsapirone. It is an agonist on presynaptic serotonin ($5HT_1A$) autoreceptors inhibiting the release and firing of serotonergic neurons.

Although the benzodiazepines are now viewed as having a direct action at a binding site coupled to the GABA receptor (see Figure 50), this view was predated by the suggestion that serotonergic systems interacted with the benzodiazepines. This view was spawned by the observation that benzodiazepines inhibit the firing of serotonergic neurons in the dorsal raphe nucleus, decrease brain serotonin turnover, and reverse the preconflict effects of direct serotonergic stimulation of the dorsal raphe. As with buspirone, lesions of the serotonergic system abolish diazepam's efficacy in a conflict test. A body of data supports the candidacy of serotonin as a mediator of the anxiolytic effects of benzodiazepines downstream from the GABA receptor. There is a convincing body of evidence that several types of serotonin (5-HT) receptors exist in the mammalian brain, two of which are well characterized: 5-HT_1 and 5-HT_2 sites. The 5-HT_1 sites can be further subdivided into at least three distinct subsets, which differ in their regional distribution and functions and are currently termed 5-HT_{1A}, 5-HT_{1B}, and 5-HT_{1C} sites.

The 5-HT receptors in the hippocampus and other parts of the limbic system are primarily of the 5-HT_{1A} type. It is therefore tempting to speculate that drugs that display a high degree of selectivity for these receptor sites can selectively affect anxiety states. A breakthrough in that direction came with the discovery that buspirone, a drug with anxiolytic activity in humans, can help elucidate the role of 5-HT in anxiety. Buspirone, gepirone, and ipsapirone may therefore offer new therapeutic directions in the treatment of anxiety.

Gepirone is absorbed rapidly when given orally, and undergoes extensive first-pass metabolism to an active metabolite, which is excreted by the kidneys. The most frequently reported adverse effects are dizziness, nausea, headache, drowsiness, and weakness. Gepirone does not impair memory, verbal fluency, or psychomotor performance. Like buspirone, gepirone does not appear to have a potential for causing physical dependence or addiction in humans, and it is expected that gepirone will not interact with alcohol or sedative–hypnotic drugs.

GILLES DE LA TOURETTE'S SYNDROME: Treatment of

Gilles de la Tourette's syndrome is characterized by involuntary movements, echolalia, echopraxia, coprolalia, and strange, uncontrollable sounds. The differential diagnosis includes the various movement disorders that can present in childhood. Other disorders characterized by tics are distinguished by resolution of the tics by early adulthood or by the restricted number of tics.

Wilson's disease can simulate Gilles de la Tourette's syndrome; it must be excluded because it responds well to medical treatment. In addition to a movement disorder, Wilson's disease produces hepatic involvement, Kayser–Fleischer corneal rings, and abnormalities of serum copper and ceruloplasmin, which are absent in Gilles de la Tourette's syndrome.

Sydenham's chorea can be difficult to recognize if there is no recent history of rheumatic fever or polyarthritis and no clinical evidence of cardiac involvement, but this disorder is a self-limiting one, usually clearing in 3 to 6 months.

Bobble-head syndrome, which can be difficult to distinguish from Gilles de la Tourette's syndrome, is characterized by rapid, rhythmic bobbing of the head in children with progressive hydrocephalus. Treatment is symptomatic and, if effective, must be continued indefinitely.

Clonidine has been reported to ameliorate motor or vocal tics in roughly 50% of children so treated. It may act by reducing activity in noradrenergic neurons arising in the locus ceruleus.

Haloperidol is often effective. It is started at a low daily dose (0.25 mg), which is gradually increased by 0.25 mg every 4 or 5 days until there is maximum benefit with a minimum of side effects or until side effects limit further increments.

Phenothiazines such as fluphenazine may help, but patients who are unresponsive to haloperidol usually fail with these drugs as well.

Patients occasionally respond favorably to clonazepam or carbamazepine, but diazepam, barbiturates, tricyclic antidepressants, phenytoin, and cholinergic agonists (such as deanol) are usually not helpful.

GLATIRAMER ACETATE

(Copaxone injection 20 mg)

Glatiramer is an immunosuppressive agent that modifies the immune processes thought to be responsible for multiple sclerosis (MS). It is indicated in reducing the frequency of relapses in patients with relapsing–remitting MS.

Random polymers that contain amino acids commonly used as major histocompatibility complexes (MHC) anchors and T-cell-receptor contact residues have been proposed as possible "universal APLs (altered peptide ligands)." **Glatiramer acetate** (GA) is a random sequence polypeptide consisting of four amino acids (alanine [A], lysine [K], glutamate [E], and tyrosine [Y] at a molar ratio of A:K:E:Y of 4.5:3.6:1.5:1) with an average length of 40 to 100 amino acids. Directly labeled **GA** binds efficiently to different murine H2 I-A molecules, as well as to their human counterparts, the MHC class II DR molecules, but does not bind MHC class II DQ or MHC class I molecules *in vitro*. In clinical trials, **GA**, administered subcutaneously to patients with relapsing–remitting MS, decreased the rate of exacerbations by about 30%. *In vivo* administration of **GA** induces highly cross-reactive $CD4^+$ T-cells that are immune deviated to secrete Th2 cytokines, and prevents the appearance of new lesions detectable by magnetic resonance imaging (MRI). This represents one of the first successful uses of an agent that ameliorates autoimmune disease by altering signals through the T-cell receptor complex.

For relapsing–remitting attacks and for secondary progressive MS, the alkylating agent **cyclophosphamide** and the anthracenedionene-derivative **mitoxantrone** (Novatrone) are currently used in patients refractory to other immunomodulators. These agents, used primarily for cancer chemotherapy, have significant toxicities. Although cyclophosphamide in patients with MS may not be limited by an accumulated dose exposure, mitoxantrone can be tolerated only up to an accumulated dose of 100 to 140 mg/m^2. The utility of **interferon** therapy in patients with secondary progressive MS is unclear. In primary progressive MS, with no discrete attacks and less observed inflammation, suppression of inflammation seems to be less helpful. A minority of patients at this stage will respond to high doses of glucocorticoids.

Each of the agents mentioned previously has side effects and contraindications that may be limiting: infections (for glucocorticoids); hypersensitivity and pregnancy (for immunomodulators); and prior anthracycline/anthracenedione use, mediastinal irradiation, or cardiac disease (mitoxantrone). With all of these agents, it is clear that the earlier they are used, the more effective they are in preventing disease relapses. What is not clear is whether any of these agents will prevent or diminish the later onset of secondary progressive disease, which causes the more severe form of disability. Given the fluctuating nature of this disease, only long-term studies lasting decades will answer this question.

A number of other new immunomodulatory therapies are completing phase III trials. One is a monoclonal antibody, **natalizumab** (Antegren), directed against the adhesion molecule α_4 integrin; natalizumab binds to α_4 integrin and antagonizes interactions with integrin heterodimers containing α_4 integrin, such as $\alpha_4\beta_1$ integrin, that is expressed on the surface of activated lymphocytes and monocytes. Preclinical data suggest that an interaction of $\alpha_4\beta_1$ integrin with VCAM-1 (vascular cellular-adhesion molecule 1) is critical for T-cell trafficking from the periphery into the CNS; thus, blocking this interaction would hypothetically inhibit disease exacerbations. In fact, phase II clinical trials have demonstrated a significant decrease in the number of new lesions as determined by MRI and clinical attacks in MS patients receiving natalizumab. Monoclonal antibodies directed against the IL-2 receptor are also entering phase III clinical trials.

GLAUCOMA: Treatment for

Drugs	Usual Daily Dosage
Adrenergic Agonist	
Dipivefrin hydrochloride	1 drop b.i.d.
Beta-blockers	
Betaxolol	1 drop b.i.d.
Levobunolol	1 drop b.i.d.
	1 drop once
Metipranolol	1 drop b.i.d.
Timolol-Timoptic	1 drop b.i.d.
Timoptic-XE	1 drop once
Carbonic Anhydrase Inhibitor	
Dorzolamide	1 drop t.i.d.
Cholinergic Agent	
Pilocarpine hydrochloride	1 drop q.i.d.
Prostaglandin	
Latanoprost	1 drop once

GLIMEPIRIDE

(Amaryl tablets 1 mg)

Glimepiride is a sulfonylurea that decreases blood glucose by stimulating insulin release from pancreas. It may also decrease hepatic glucose production as well as increase sensitivity to insulin.

GLIPIZIDE

(Glucotrol tablets 5 mg)

Glipizide is a sulfonylurea that decreases blood glucose by stimulating insulin release from pancreas and by increasing tissue sensitivity to insulin. It is indicated as an adjunct to diet to lower blood glucose in patients with non-insulin-dependent diabetes mellitus (type 2) whose hyperglycemia cannot be controlled by diet alone.

It lowers blood glucose levels by stimulating insulin release from functioning beta cells in the pancreas. After

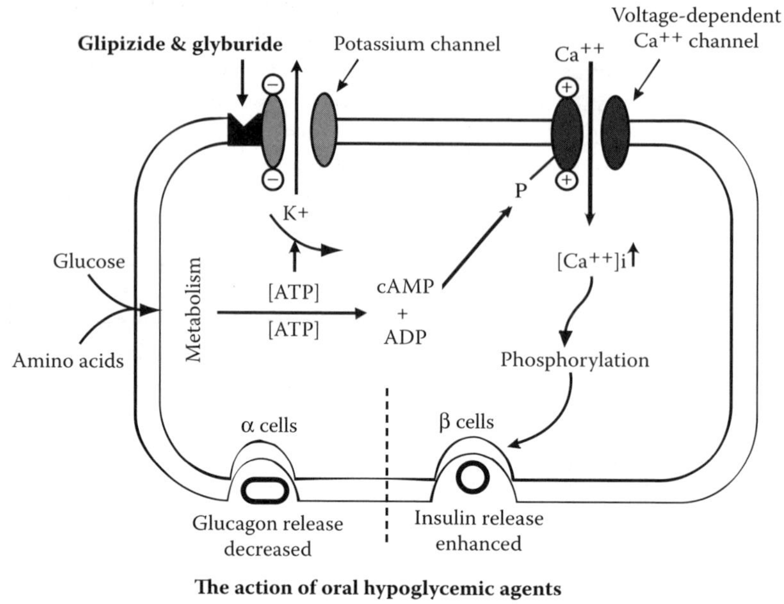

FIGURE 54 Sulfonylureas such as **glyburide** and **glipizide** bind to sulfonylurea receptors located on the surface of beta cells and trigger insulin release.

prolonged administration, the drug's hypoglycemic effects appear to reflect extrapancreatic effects, possibly including reduction of basal hepatal glucose production and enhanced peripheral sensitivity to insulin (see Figure 54). The latter may result either from an increase in the number of insulin receptors or from changes in events subsequent to insulin binding. The properties of glipizide are compared with other hypoglycemic agents in Table 1.

Glipizide is absorbed rapidly, is bound to plasma protein to the extent of 92 to 99%, and is metabolized to inactive metabolites, which are excreted in the urine.

The first-generation sulfonylureas vary considerably in their half-lives and extents of metabolism. The half-life of **acetohexamide** is short, but the drug is reduced to an active compound whose half-life is similar to those of **tolbutamide** and **tolazamide** (4 to 7 hours). It may be necessary to take these drugs in divided daily doses. Chlorpropamide has a long half-life (24 to 48 hours). The second-generation agents are approximately 100 times more potent than those in the first group. Although their half-lives are short (3 to 5 hours), their hypoglycemic effects are evident for 12 to 24 hours, and they often can be administered once daily. The reason for the discrepancies between their half-lives and duration of action is not clear.

All the sulfonylureas are metabolized by the liver, and the metabolites are excreted in the urine. The metabolism of chlorpropamide is incomplete, and about 20% of the drug is excreted unchanged. Therefore, sulfonylureas should be administered with caution to patients with either renal or hepatic insufficiency.

Adverse effects of the sulfonylureas are infrequent, occurring in about 4% of patients taking first-generation drugs, and perhaps slightly less often in patients receiving second-generation agents. Not unexpectedly, sulfonylureas may cause hypoglycemic reactions, including coma. This is a particular problem in elderly patients with impaired hepatic or renal function who are taking longer-acting sulfonylureas. Sulfonylureas can be ranked in order of decreasing risk of causing hypoglycemia. It used to be thought that longer-acting sulfonylureas resulted in a greater prevalence of hypoglycemia. That is certainly the case when comparing the older preparations such as chlorpropamide (long acting) against tolbutamide (short acting). However, more recent second-generation sulfonylureas have very differing incidences of causing hypoglycemia despite similar half-lives. Thus glyburide (glibenclamide) has been reported to result in hypoglycemia in up to 20 to 30% of users, whereas another long-acting sulfonylurea, **glimepiride**, results in hypoglycemia in only 2 to 4% of users. A modified long-acting version of glipizide also results in a lower hypoglycemia frequency relative to gliburide.

Recent studies have provided an insight into the physiological basis for the differing rates of hypoglycemia occurring with these long-acting sulfonylureas. As described earlier for insulin, the ability of the body to inhibit endogenous insulin secretion is central to the homeostatic defense against hypoglycemia. This lucose-dependent inhibition of insulin secretion during hypoglycemia occurs with glimepiride but not with glyburide. Additionally, the major anti-insulin counterregulatory hormone glucagon appears to be reduced by **glyburide** during hypoglycemia but is preserved during glimepiride therapy.

Severe hypoglycemia in the elderly can present as an acute neurological emergency that may mimic a cerebrovascular accident. Thus, it is important to check the plasma glucose level of any elderly patient presenting with acute neurological symptoms. Because of the long half-life of some sulfonylureas, it may be necessary to treat elderly hypoglycemic patients for 24 to 48 hours with an intravenous glucose infusion.

Many other drugs may potentiate the effects of the sulfonylureas, particularly the first-generation agents, by inhibiting their metabolism or excretion. Some drugs also displace the sulfonylureas from binding proteins, thereby transiently increasing the free concentration. These include other sulfonamides, clofibrate, and salicylates. Other drugs, especially ethanol, may enhance the action of sulfonylureas by causing hypoglycemia.

Other side effects of sulfonylureas include nausea and vomiting, cholestatic jaundice, agranulocytosis, aplastic and hemolytic anemias, generalized hypersensitivity reactions, and dermatological reactions.

GLIPIZIDE/METFORMIN HYDROCHLORIDE

(Metaglip tablets 2.5 mg)

Glipizide/metformin is a combination antidiabetic agent. **Glipizide**: decreases blood glucose by stimulating insulin release from the pancreas and by increasing tissue sensitivity to insulin. **Metformin**: decreases blood glucose by reducing hepatic glucose production and may decrease intestinal absorption of glucose and increase response to insulin.

They are indicated in initial treatment as an adjunct to diet and exercise, to improve glycemic control in patients with type 2 diabetes whose hyperglycemia cannot be satisfactorily managed with diet and exercise alone; and as a second-line therapy when diet, exercise, and initial treatment with a sulfonylurea or metformin do not result in adequate glycemic control in patients with type 2 diabetes. **Metformin** (glucophage, others) and **phenformin** were introduced in 1957, and **buformin** was introduced in 1958. The latter was of limited use, but metformin and phenformin were used widely. Phenformin was withdrawn in many countries during the 1970s because of an association with lactic acidosis. **Metformin** has been associated only rarely with that complication, and has been used widely in Europe and Canada; it became available in the United States in 1995. Metformin given alone or in combination with a sulfonylurea improves glycemic control and lipid concentrations in patients who respond poorly to diet or to a sulfonylurea alone.

Metformin is antihyperglycemic, not hypoglycemic. It does not cause insulin release from the pancreas, and generally does not cause hypoglycemia, even in large doses. **Metformin** has no significant secretion of glucagon, cortisol, growth hormone. It reduces glucose levels primarily by decreasing hepatic glucose production and by increasing insulin action in muscle and fat. At a molecular level, these actions are mediated at least in part by activation of the cellular kinase AMP-activated protein kinase (AMP kinase). The mechanism by which metformin reduces hepatic glucose production is controversial, but most data indicate an effect on reducing gluconeogenesis. **Metformin** also may decrease plasma glucose by reducing the absorption of glucose from the intestine, but this action has not been shown to have clinical relevance.

Metformin is absorbed mainly from the small intestine. The drug is stable, does not bind to plasma proteins, and is excreted unchanged in the urine. It has a half-life of about 2 hours. The maximum recommended daily dose of metformin in the United States is 2.5 g given in three doses with meals.

Patients with renal impairment should not receive **metformin**. Other contraindications include hepatic disease, a past history of lactic acidosis, cardiac failure requiring pharmacological therapy, or chronic hypoxic lung disease. The drug also should be discontinued temporarily prior to the administration of intravenous contrast media and prior to any surgical procedure. The drug should not be readministered any sooner than 48 hours after such procedures, and should be withheld until renal function is determined to be normal. These conditions all predispose to increased lactate production and hence to the potentially fatal complication of lactic acidosis. The reported incidence of lactic acidosis during **metformin** treatment is less than 0.1 cases per 1000 patient-years, and the mortality risk is even lower.

Acute side effects of **metformin**, which occur in up to 20% of patients, include diarrhea, abdominal discomfort, nausea, metallic taste, and anorexia. These usually can be minimized by increasing the dosage of the drug slowly and taking it with meals. Intestinal absorption of vitamin B_{12} and folate often is decreased during chronic metformin therapy, and calcium supplements reverse the effect of **metformin** on vitamin B_{12} absorption.

Consideration should be given to stopping treatment with metformin if the plasma lactate level exceeds 3 mM, or in the setting of decreased renal or hepatic function. It also is prudent to stop metformin if a patient is undergoing a prolonged fast or is treated with a very-low-calorie diet. Myocardial infarction (MI) or septicemia mandates immediate drug discontinuation. **Metformin** usually is administered in divided doses two or three times daily. The maximum effective dose is 2.5 g/day. **Metformin** lowers hemoglobin A_{1c} values by about 2%, an effect comparable with that of the sulfonylureas. It does not promote weight gain, and reduces plasma triglycerides by 15 to 20%. There is a strong consensus that reduction in hemoglobin A_{1c} by any therapy (insulin or oral agents) diminishes microvascular complications. **Metformin**, however, is the only therapeutic agent that has been demonstrated to reduce macrovascular events in type 2 diabetes mellitus. It can be administered in combination with sulfonylureas, thiazolizinediones, and/or insulin. Fixed-dose combinations containing **metformin** and glyburide (Glucovance, others), glipizide (Metaglip), and rosiglitazone (Avandamet) are available.

GLUCAGON

(GlucaGen powder for injection 1 mg (1 unit), Glucagon emergency kit powder for injection 1 mg (1 unit), Glucagon diagnostic kit powder for injection 1 mg (1 unit))

Glucagon is a glucose-elevating agent that elevates blood glucose concentrations (by stimulating production from liver glycogen stores), relaxes smooth muscle of the GI tract, decreases gastric and pancreatic secretions in the GI tract, and increases myocardial contractility. It is indicated in treatment of severe hypoglycemic reactions in diabetic patients when glucose administration is not possible, or during insulin shock therapy in psychiatric patients; and as a diagnostic aid in radiologic examination of stomach, duodenum, small bowel, and colon when diminished intestinal motility would be advantageous. **GlucaGen**: is used for treatment of severe hypoglycemic reactions that may occur in patients with diabetes treated with insulin; and as a diagnostic aid during radiologic examinations to temporarily inhibit movement of the GI tract.

Glucagon (0.5 to 1 mg SC 1 hour after coma) is an antihypoglycemic agent that is indicated in coma of insulin shock therapy. Following ingestion of a meal or the administration of glucose (e.g., in a glucose tolerance test), the glucose level rises, causing the release of insulin and inhibiting the release of hyperglycemic glucagon. Excess glucose is transformed into glycogen in the liver and the muscles. The high level of amino acids and fatty free acid fosters the respective formation of proteins in the muscles and triglycerides in the adipose tissues.

In a nondiabetic fasting subject, the ensuing hypoglycemia not only discourages the release of insulin but also activates the homeostatic mechanisms that block the action of insulin and convert the storage forms of fuel into utilizable glucose. Consequently, a number of hormones including glucagon, epinephrine, and glucocorticoid are released, and these convert glycogen into glucose, triglyceride into free fatty acid, and proteins into amino acids (gluconeogenesis), respectively. Furthermore, the uptake and utilization of glucose in the peripheral tissue decrease. The muscles and other tissues utilize amino acids and free fatty acid, thus providing the brain with an adequate supply of glucose.

Glucagon increases plasma glucose levels and causes smooth-muscle relaxation and an inotropic myocardial effect because of the stimulation of adenylate cyclase to produce cyclic 3′,5′-adenosine monophosphate (AMP). Cyclic AMP (cAMP) initiates a series of reactions that leads to the degradation of glycogen to glucose. Hepatic stores of glycogen are necessary for glucagon to exert an antihypoglycemic effect.

Glucagon is a single-chain polypeptide of 29 amino acids. It has significant homology with several other polypeptide hormones, including **secretin**, **vasoactive intestinal peptide**, and **gastrointestinal inhibitory polypeptide**. The primary sequence of glucagon is identical in human beings, cattle, pigs, and rats.

Glucagon is synthesized from preproglucagon, a 180-amino-acid precursor with five separately processed domains. An amino-terminal signal peptide is followed by glicentin-related pancreatic peptide, glucagon, GLP-1, and glucagon-like peptide-2. Processing of the protein is sequential and occurs in a tissue-specific fashion; this results in different secretory peptides in pancreatic α cells and intestinal α-like cells (termed *L* cells). **Glicentin**, a major processing intermediate, consists of glicentin-related pancreatic polypeptide at the amino terminus and glucagon at the carboxyl terminus, with an Arg-Arg pair between. Enteroglucagon (or oxyntomodulin) consists of glucagon and a carboxyl-terminal hexapeptide linked by an Arg-Arg pair.

The highly controlled nature of the processing suggests that these peptides may have distinct biological functions. In the pancreatic cell, the granule consists of a central core of glucagon surrounded by a halo of glicentin. Intestinal L cells contain only glicentin and presumably lack the enzyme required to process this precursor to glucagon. Enteroglucagon binds to hepatic glucagon receptors and stimulates adenylyl cyclase with 10 to 20% of the potency of glucagon. GLP-1 is an extremely potent potentiator of insulin secretion, although it apparently lacks significant hepatic actions. Glicentin, enteroglucagon, and the glucagon-like peptides are found predominantly in the intestine, and their secretion continues after total pancreatectomy.

Glucagon secretion is regulated by dietary glucose, insulin, amino acids, and fatty acids. As in insulin secretion, glucose is a more effective inhibitor of glucagon secretion when taken orally than when administered intravenously, suggesting a possible role for gastrointestinal hormones in the response. The effect of glucose is lost in untreated or undertreated type 1 diabetes mellitus patients and in isolated pancreatic cells, indicating that at least part of the effect is secreted.

Plasma concentrations of **glucagon** are elevated in poorly controlled diabetic patients. Because it enhances gluconeogenesis and glycogenolysis, glucagon exacerbates the hyperglycemia of diabetes. However, this abnormality of glucagon secretion appears to be secondary to the diabetic state and is corrected with improved control of the disease. The importance of the hyperglucagonemia in diabetes has been evaluated by administration of somatostatin. Although somatostatin does not restore glucose metabolism to normal, it significantly slows the rate of development of hyperglycemia and ketonemia in insulin-deficient subjects with type 1 diabetes mellitus. In normal individuals, glucagon secretion increases in response to hypoglycemia, but this important defense mechanism against insulin-induced hypoglycemia is lost in type 1 diabetes mellitus.

Glucagon is degraded extensively in liver, kidney plasma, and other sites of action. Its half-life in plasma is approximately 3 to 6 minutes. Proteolytic removal of the amino-terminal histidine residue leads to loss of biological activity.

Glucagon interacts with a glycoprotein GPCR on the plasma membrane of target cells that signals through G_S. The primary effects of glucagon on the liver are mediated by cAMP. In general, modifications of the amino-terminal region of glucagon (e.g., [Phe^1]glucagon and des-His_1-[Glu^1]glucagon amide) result in molecules that behave as partial agonists that retain some affinity for the glucagon receptor but have a markedly reduced capacity to stimulate adenylyl cyclase.

Glucagon activates phosphorylase, the rate-limiting enzyme in glycogenolysis, via cAMP-stimulated phosphorylation, whereas concurrent phosphorylation of **glycogen** synthase inactivates the enzyme; glycogenolysis is enhanced, and glycogen synthesis is inhibited. cAMP also stimulates transcription of the gene for phosphoenolpyruvate carboxylase, a rate-limiting enzyme in gluconeogenesis. These effects normally are opposed by insulin, and insulin is dominant when maximal concentrations of both hormones are present.

Glucagon exerts effects on tissues other than liver, especially at higher concentrations. In adipose tissue, it stimulates adenylate cyclase and increases lipolysis. In the heart, glucagon increases the force contraction. **Glucagon** has relaxant effects on the GI tract; this has been observed with analogs that apparently do not stimulate adenylylate cyclase. Some tissues (including liver) possess a second type of glucagon receptor that is linked to generation of IP_3, diacylglycerol, and Ca^{2+}. The role of this receptor in metabolic regulation remains uncertain.

Glucagon is used to treat severe hypoglycemia, particularly in diabetic patients when intravenous glucose is available; it also is used by radiologists for its inhibitory effects on the GI tract.

All glucagon used clinically is extracted from bovine and porcine pancreas; its sequence is identical to that of the human hormone. For hypoglycemic reactions, 1 mg is administered intravenously, intramuscularly, or subcutaneously. The first two routes are preferred in an emergency. Clinical improvement is sought within 10 minutes to minimize the risk of neurological damage from hypoglycemia. The hyperglycemic action of glucagon is transient and may be inadequate if hepatic stores of glycogen are depleted. After the initial response to glucagon, patients should be given glucose or urged to eat to prevent recurrent hypoglycemia. Nausea and vomiting are the most frequent adverse effects.

Glucagon also is used to relax the intestinal tract to facilitate radiographic examination of the upper and lower GI tract with barium and retrograde ileography, and in MRI of the GI tract. **Glucagon** has been used to treat the spasm associated with acute diverticulitis and disorders of the biliary tract and sphincter of Oddi, as an adjunct in basket retrieval of biliary calculi, and for impaction of the esophagus and intussusception. Finally, it has been used diagnostically to distinguish obstructive from hepatocellular jaundice.

Glucagon releases catecholamines from **pheochromocytomas** and has been used experimentally as a diagnostic test for this disorder. Based on this effect, **glucagon** therapy is contraindicated in pheochromocytoma. The hormone also has been used as a cardiac inotropic agent for the treatment of shock, particularly when prior administration of a β-adrenergic-receptor antagonist has rendered β-adrenergic-receptor agonists ineffective.

GLUCOCORTICOIDS

The glucocorticoids mainly influence carbohydrate metabolism and, to a certain extent, protein and lipid metabolism (see Table 14 and Figure 55). The main glucocorticoid is cortisol, with a daily secretion of 15 mg. Cortisol is synthesized through the 11-beta-hydroxylation of 11-deoxycortisol. Besides cortisol, the adrenal gland also synthesizes and releases a small amount of corticosterone, whose synthesis from 11-deoxycorticosterone is catalyzed by 11-beta-hydroxylase. A deficiency of 11-beta-hydroxylase causes:

- Diminished secretion of cortisol
- Diminished secretion of corticosterone
- Enhanced compensatory secretion of ACTH
- Enhanced secretion of 11-deoxycortisol and 11-deoxycorticosterone
- Enhanced secretion of androgens

TABLE 14
Actions of Glucocorticoids

Steroids	Antiinflammatory Potency (% compared to cortisol)	Sodium Retention (% compared to cortisol)
Betamethasone	20	0
Dexamethasone	20	0
Fludrocortisone	12	100
Paramethasone	6	0
Triamcinolone	5	0
Methylprednisolone	4	0
Prednisolone	3	0.8
Prednisone	2.5	0.8
Cortisol	1	1

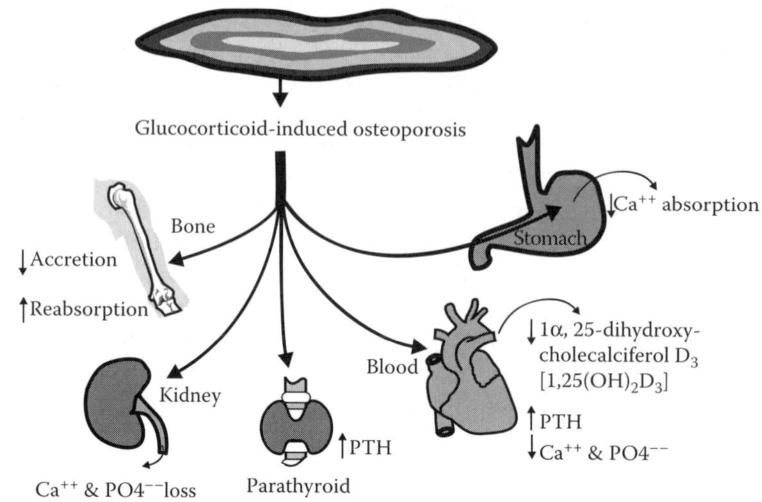

FIGURE 55 The glucocorticoids possess a plethora of physiologic actions, including a role in **differentiation** and **development**. They are vital in the treatment of adrenal insufficiency and are used extensively in large pharmacologic doses as **antiinflammatory** and **immunosuppressive** agents.

The clinical manifestations of 11-beta-hydroxylase deficiency are virilization, resulting from the overproduction of androgen, and hypertension, stemming from the overproduction of deoxycorticosteroids.

The glucocorticoids work by binding to specific intracellular receptors in target tissues. The receptor hormone complex is then transported into the nucleus where the complex interacts with the DNA, thus augmenting the synthesis of specific RNAs.

Cortisol, corticosterone, aldosterone, and the synthetic steroids used in steroid therapy (e.g., prednisolone, dexamethasone, and triamcinolone) are glucocorticoid agonists and therefore elicit glucocorticoid responses. A number of other steroids bind to the glucocorticoid receptor and thus suppress glucocorticoid responses (see Tables 11 and 14).

GLUTETHIMIDE

(Doriden)

Glutethimide (250 to 500 mg at bedtime) is indicated in short-term (a few days) relief of insomnia. It exhibits pronounced atropine-like effects including mydriasis and inhibition of secretion and motility of the GI tract. Similar to barbiturates, glutethimide depresses the CNS and has addictive effects with alcohol and other CNS drugs. It depresses rapid-eye-movement (REM) sleep and is associated with REM rebound. Glutethimide induces the activity of hepatic microsomal enzyme and accelerates the metabolism of anticoagulants, and hence reduces their effectiveness, thus requiring dose adjustment.

Overdosage with glutethimide (10 to 20 g) produces symptoms that are identical to those produced by barbiturates, which include profound CNS depression, hypothermia, altered deep-tendon reflexes, absence of corneal and papillary reflexes, absence of response to painful stimulation, hypoventilation, cyanosis, and apnea. Because the absorption of glutethimide from the GI tract is erratic, a fluctuating level of alertness may be observed. Glutethimide is a lipid-soluble substance, accumulates in adipose tissues, and is released steadily, which requires careful monitoring of the victim's vital signs even when consciousness has been regained. Glutethimide has been replaced by safer hypnotic–sedative medications.

GLYBURIDE

(DiaBeta tablets 1.25 mg)

Glyburide is a sulfonylurea that decreases blood glucose by stimulating insulin release from the pancreas. It may also decrease hepatic glucose production or increase response to insulin. Glyburide is indicated as an adjunct to diet to lower blood glucose in patients with non-insulin-dependent diabetes mellitus (type 2) whose hyperglycemia cannot be controlled by diet alone; and in combination with metformin when diet and glyburide or diet and metformin alone do not result in adequate glycemic control.

The release of insulin is enhanced by certain physiologic substances (glucose, leucine, arginine, gastrin, secretin, and pancreozymin) and by certain pharmacologic agents (oral hypoglycemic agents). The release of insulin is also inhibited by some physiologic substances (epinephrine and norepinephrine) as well as by some pharmacologic substances (thiazide diuretics, diazoxide, and chlorpromazine).

Oral hypoglycemic agents have advantages over insulin because, by releasing insulin and by decreasing the release of glucagon, they mimic physiologic processes and cause fewer allergic reactions. Furthermore, they are effective in an oral form, thus eliminating the need for daily injections. The properties of these agents are described in Table 1 and Figure 54.

Sulfonylureas such as glyburide and glipizide bind to sulfonylurea receptors located on the surface of beta cells and trigger insulin releases at nanomolar concentrations (Figure 54). Sulfonylureas bind to ATP-sensitive potassium channels and inhibit potassium efflux through these channels. The inhibition of ATP-sensitive potassium channels then leads to depolarization of the beta cell; this opens voltage-dependent calcium channels and allows the entry of extracellular calcium. The rising level of cytosolic free calcium next triggers the release of insulin. An increase in the cAMP levels in the cells can also open the voltage-dependent calcium channels, thus increasing calcium influx into the cells. Glyburide lowers blood glucose levels by stimulating the insulin release from functioning beta cells in the pancreas. After prolonged administration, the drug's hypoglycemic effects appear to be related to extrapancreatic effects, possibly including reduction of basal hepatic glucose production and enhanced peripheral sensitivity to insulin. The latter may result either from an increase in the number of insulin receptors or from changes in events subsequent to insulin binding.

The sulfonylureas have similar spectra of activities; thus, their pharmacokinetic properties are their most distinctive characteristics. Although the rates of absorption of the different sulfonylureas vary, all are effectively absorbed from the GI tract. However, food and hyperglycemia can reduce the absorption of sulfonylureas. Hyperglycemia *per se* inhibits gastric and intestinal motility and thus can retard the absorption of many drugs. In view of the time required to reach an optimal concentration in plasma, sulfonylureas with short half-lives may be more effective when given 30 minutes before eating. Sulfonylureas in plasma are largely (90 to 99%) bound to protein, especially albumin; plasma protein binding is least for chlorpropamide and greatest for **glyburide**. The volume of distribution of most of the sulfonylureas is about 0.2 L/kg.

The first-generation sulfonylureas vary considerably in their half-lives and extents of metabolism. The half-life of **acetohexamide** is short, but the drug is reduced to an active compound whose half-life is similar to those of **tolbutamide** and **tolazamide** (4 to 7 hours). It may be necessary to take these drugs in divided daily doses. **Chlorpropamide** has a long half-life (24 to 48 hours). The second-generation agents are approximately 100 times more potent than those in the first group. Although their half-lives are short (3 to 5 hours), their hypoglycemic effects are evident for 12 to 24 hours, and they often can be administered once daily. The reason for the discrepancies between their half-lives and duration of action is not clear.

All the sulfonylureas are metabolized by the liver, and the metabolites are excreted in the urine. Metabolism of chlorpropamide is incomplete, and about 20% of the drug is excreted unchanged. Thus sulfonylureas should be administered with caution to patients with either renal or hepatic insufficiency.

Adverse effects of the sulfonylureas are infrequent, occurring in about 4% of patients taking first-generation drugs, and perhaps slightly less often in patients receiving second-generation agents. Not unexpectedly, sulfonylureas may cause hypoglycemic reactions, including coma. This is a particular problem in elderly patients with impaired hepatic or renal function who are taking longer-acting sulfonylureas. Sulfonylureas can be ranked in order of decreasing risk of causing hypoglycemia. It used to be thought that longer-acting sulfonylureas resulted in a greater prevalence of hypoglycemia. That is certainly the case when comparing the older preparations such as chlorpropamide (long acting) against tolbutamide (short acting). However, more recent second-generation sulfonylureas have very differing incidences of causing hypoglycemia despite similar half-lives. Thus, **glyburide** (glibenclamide) has been reported to result in hypoglycemia in up to 20 to 30% of users, whereas another long-acting sulfonylurea, glimepiride, results in hypoglycemia in only 2 to 4% of users. A modified long-acting version of glipizide also results in a lower hypoglycemia frequency relative to glyburide.

Recent studies have provided an insight into the physiological basis for the differing rates of hypoglycemia occurring with these long-acting sulfonylureas. As described earlier for insulin, the ability of the body to inhibit endogenous insulin secretion is central to the homeostatic defense against hypoglycemia. This glucose-dependent inhibition of insulin secretion during hypoglycemia occurs with glimepiride but not with **glyburide**. Additionally, the major anti-insulin counterregulatory hormone glucagon appears to be reduced by **glyburide** during hypoglycemia but is preserved during glimepiride therapy.

Severe hypoglycemia in the elderly can present an acute neurological emergency that may mimic a cerebrovascular accident. Thus, it is important to check the plasma glucose level of any elderly patient presenting with acute neurological symptoms. Because of the long half-life of some sulfonylureas, it may be necessary to treat elderly hypoglycemic patients for 24 to 48 hours with an intravenous glucose infusion.

Many other drugs may potentiate the effects of the sulfonylureas, particularly the first-generation agents, by inhibiting their metabolism or excretion. Some drugs also displace the sulfonylureas from binding proteins, thereby transiently increasing the free concentration. These include other sulfonamides, clofibrate, and salicylates. Other drugs, especially ethanol, may enhance the action of sulfonylureas by causing hypoglycemia.

Other side effects of sulfonylureas include nausea and vomiting, cholestatic jaundice, agranulocytosis, aplastic and hemolytic anemias, generalized hypersensitivity reactions, and dermatological reactions.

GLYCERIN (GLYCEROL)

(Colace suppositories glycerin, Fleet Babylax liquid 4 mL/applicator, Ophthalgan solution (ophthalmic) glycerin, Osmoglyn solution 50% (0.6 g glycerin/mL), Sani-Supp suppositories glycerin)

Glycerin is a hyperosmotic/osmotic diuretic/ophthalmic agent that reduces intraocular pressure (IOP) by creating an osmotic gradient between plasma and ocular fluids (**oral form**); promotes bowel evacuation by local irritation and hyperosmotic actions (**rectal form**); reduces edema and clears corneal haze by attracting water through semipermeable corneal epithelium (**ophthalmic form**). **Oral**: used for control of acute attack of glaucoma; reduction of IOP prior to and after ocular surgery. **Rectal**: used for short-term treatment of constipation; to evacuate the colon for rectal and bowel examinations. **Ophthalmic**: used for clearance of edematous corneas to facilitate ophthalmoscopic and gonioscopic examination in acute glaucoma, bullous keratitis, and Fuchs' endothelial dystrophy.

The osmotic diuretics and related agents consist of mannitol (Osmitrol), urea (Ureaphil), glycerin (Glycerol, Osmoglyn), and isosorbide (Hydronol). Mannitol and urea are nonelectrolytes that are freely filterable, and undergo very little or no metabolism or renal tubular resorption. When given in sufficient quantities, these drugs increase the osmolarity of plasma and the amount of both the glomerular filtrate and the renal tubular fluid. The presence of such a drug in the lumen prevents the resorption of sodium from the tubular fluid, but some additional sodium is excreted as a normal constituent of the increased volume of urine. Osmotic diuretics are not effective in removing the edematous fluid caused by sodium retention but can maintain the flow of urine even when the glomerular filtration rate (GFR) is decreased. Osmotic diuretics are given by intravenous infusion in a hypertonic solution, and they are excreted by glomerular filtration (see Figure 17 and Table 25).

Enemas commonly are employed either by themselves or as adjuncts to bowel preparation regimens to empty the distal colon or rectum of retained solid material. Bowel distention by any means will produce an evacuation reflex in most people, and almost any form of enema, including normal saline solution, can achieve this. Specialized enemas contain additional substances that either are osmotically active or irritant; however, their safety and efficacy have not been studied in a rigorous manner. Repeated enemas with tap water or other hypotonic solutions can cause hyponatremia; repeated enemas with sodium phosphate-containing solution can cause hypocalcemia. Phosphate-containing enemas also are known to alter the appearance of rectal mucosa.

Glycerine is a trihydroxy alcohol that is absorbed orally but acts as a hygroscopic agent and lubricant when given rectally. The resultant water retention stimulates peristalsis and usually produces a bowel movement in less than an hour. **Glycerin** is for rectal use only and is given in a single daily dose as a 2- or 3-g rectal suppository or as 5 to 15 ml of an 80% solution in enema form. Rectal glycerin may cause local discomfort, burning, or hyperemia and (minimal) bleeding. Some glycerin suppositories contain sodium stearate, which can cause local irritation.

The current management of dry eyes usually includes instilling artificial tears and ophthalmic lubricants. In general, tear substitutes are hypotonic or isotonic solutions composed of electrolytes, surfactants, preservatives, and some viscosity-increasing agent that prolongs the residence time in the cul-de-sac and precorneal tear film. Common viscosity agents include cellulose polymers (e.g., **carboxymethylcellulose**, **hydroxyethyl cellulose**, **hydroxypropyl cellulose**, **hydroxypropyl methylcellulose**, and **methylcellulose**), polyvinyl alcohol, polyethylene glycol, polysorbate, mineral oil, **glycerin**, and dextran. The tear substitutes are available as preservative-containing or preservative-free preparations. The viscosity of the tear substitute depends on its exact formulation and can range from watery to gel-like. Some tear formulations also are combined with a vasoconstrictor, such as **naphazoline**, **phenylephrine**, or **tetrahydrozoline**. In other countries, hyaluronic acid sometimes is used as a viscous agent.

The lubricating ointments are composed of a mixture of white petrolatum, mineral oil, liquid or alcohol lanolin, and sometimes a preservative. These highly viscous formulations cause considerable blurring of vision, and consequently they are used primarily at bedtime, in critically ill patients, or in very severe dry-eye conditions. Such aqueous and ointment formulations are only fair substitutes for the precorneal tear film, which is truly a poorly understood lipid, aqueous, and mucin trilaminar barrier.

Many local eye conditions and systemic diseases may affect the precorneal tear film. Local eye disease, such as blepharitis, ocular rosacea, ocular pemphigoid, chemical burns, or corneal dystrophies, may alter the ocular surface and change the tear composition. Appropriate treatment of the symptomatic dry eye includes treating the accompanying disease and possibly the addition of tear substitutes. There also are a number of systemic conditions that may manifest themselves with symptomatic dry eyes, including Sjögren's syndrome, rheumatoid arthritis, vitamin A deficiency, Stevens–Johnson syndrome, and trachoma. Treating the systemic disease may not eliminate the symptomatic dry-eye complaints; chronic therapy with tear substitutes or surgical occlusion of the lacrimal drainage system may be indicated.

The main osmotic drugs for ocular use include **glycerin**, **mannitol**, and **hypertonic saline**. With the availability of these agents, the use of urea for management of acutely elevated IOP is nearly obsolete.

Ophthalmologists occasionally use glycerin and mannitol for short-term management of acute rises in IOP. Sporadically, these agents are used intraoperatively to dehydrate the vitreous prior to anterior segment surgical procedures. Many patients with acute glaucoma do not tolerate oral medications because of nausea; therefore, intravenous administration of mannitol and/or **acetazolamide** may be preferred over oral administration of glycerin. These agents should be used with caution in patients with CHF or renal failure.

Corneal edema is a clinical sign of corneal endothelial dysfunction, and topical osmotic agents may effectively dehydrate the cornea. Identifying the cause of corneal edema will guide therapy, and topical osmotic agents, such as hypertonic saline, may temporize the need for surgical intervention in the form of a corneal transplant. Sodium chloride is available in either aqueous or ointment formulations. Topical glycerin also is available; however, because it causes pain upon contact with the cornea and conjunctiva, its use is limited to urgent evaluation of filtration-angle structures. In general, when corneal edema occurs secondary to acute glaucoma, the use of an oral osmotic agent to help reduce IOP is preferred to topical glycerin, which simply clears the cornea temporarily. Reducing the IOP will help clear the cornea more permanently to allow both a view of the filtration angle by gonioscopy and a clear view of the iris as required to perform **laser iridotomy**.

GLYCOPYRROLATE

(Robinul tablets 1 mg)

Glycopyrrolate is an antispasmodic agent that exerts anticholinergic effects, resulting in GI smooth-muscle relaxation; diminished volume and acidity of GI secretions; and reduced pharyngeal, tracheal, and bronchial secretions. **Oral** use: adjunctive treatment of peptic ulcer. **Parenteral** use: preoperative administration for reduction of salivary, tracheobronchial, and pharyngeal secretions, reduction of volume and acidity of gastric secretions, and blockade of cardiac vagal inhibitory reflexes before and during induction of anesthesia and intubation; intraoperatively for counteraction of drug-induced or vagal traction reflexes with associated arrhythmias.

Glycopyrrolate (Robinul, others) is employed orally to inhibit GI motility and also is used parenterally to block the effects of vagal stimulation during anesthesia and surgery.

Dicyclomine hydrochloride (Bentyl, others), flavoxate hydrochloride (Urispas, others), **oxybutynin chloride** (Ditropan, others), and **tolterodine tartrate** (Detrol) are tertiary amines, and **trospium chloride** (Sanctura) is a quaternary amine; all are used for their antispasmodic properties. These agents appear to exert some nonspecific direct relaxant effect on smooth muscle. In therapeutic doses, they decrease spasm of the GI tract, biliary tract, ureter, and uterus.

Anticholinergic agents (spasmolytics or antispasmodics) often are used in patients with irritable bowel syndrome (IBS). The most common agents of this class available in the United States are nonspecific antagonists of the muscarinic receptor and include the tertiary amines **dicyclomine** (Bentyl) and **hyoscyamine** (Levsin, others), and the quaternary ammonium compounds **glycopyrrolate** (Robinul) and **methscopolamine** (Pamine). The advantage of the latter two compounds is that they have a limited propensity to cross the blood–brain barrier and hence are a lower risk for neurological side effects such as light-headedness, drowsiness, or nervousness. These agents typically are given either on an as-needed basis (with the onset of pain) or before meals to prevent the pain and fecal urgency that predictably occur in some patients with IBS (with presumed exaggerated gastrocolic reflex).

Dicyclomine is given in doses of 10 to 20 mg orally every 4 to 6 hours as necessary. Hyoscyamine is available in many forms, including oral capsules, tablets, elixir, drops, a nonaerosol spray (0.125 to 0.25 mg every 4 hours as needed), and an extended-release form for oral use (0.375 mg every 12 hours as needed). **Glycopyrrolate** also comes in extended-release tablets (2 mg once or twice a day), in addition to a standard-release form (1 mg up to three times a day). Methscopolamine is provided as 2.5-mg tablets, and the dose is 1 or 2 tablets, three to four times a day.

Clidinium bromide, another quaternary ammonium compound with antimuscarinic activity, is used in a fixed combination with **chlordiazepoxide hydrochloride** (2.5 mg of clidinium and 5 mg of chlordiazepoxide; Librax); however, such combinations are of limited value in patients with IBS because of the risk of habituation and rebound withdrawal. **Cimetropium** is another antimuscarinic compound that reportedly is effective in patients with IBS. **Otilonium bromide** has been used extensively for patients with IBS in other parts of the world. It is an ammonium salt with antimuscarinic effects that also appears to block Ca^{2+} channels and neurokinin NK-2 receptors. **Mebeverine hydrochloride** is a derivative of hydroxybenzamide that appears to have a direct effect on the smooth-muscle cell, blocking K^+ and Ca^{2+} channels. It is widely used outside of the United States as an antispasmodic agent for patients with IBS.

GOLD SALTS

Drugs used in the treatment of arthritis are:

- Aurothioglucose (Solganal)
- Gold sodium thiomalate (Myochrysine)
- Auranofin (Ridaura)

Gold salt therapy is reserved for patients with progressive disease who do not obtain satisfactory relief from therapy with aspirin-like drugs (see Table 3). The principle that underlies this therapy is that gold, which accumulates in lysosomes, decreases the migration and phagocytic activity of macrophages. Aurothioglucose, gold sodium thiomalate, or auranofin may cause toxic effects such as cutaneous reactions (from erythema to exfoliative dermatitis) as well as albuminuria, hematuria, and thrombocytopenia.

Besides the nonsteroidal antiinflammatory agents and gold, other drugs are also used for the treatment of rheumatoid arthritis. These include immunosuppressive agents, glucocorticoids (see Table 14), penicillamine, and hydroxychloroquine. With the exception of glucocorticoids, these drugs resemble gold salts in that they do not possess antiinflammatory or analgesic properties, and their therapeutic effects become evident only after several weeks or months of treatment (see also Table 3).

GOLD SODIUM THIOMALATE (MYOCHRYSINE)

(Aurolate injection 50 mg/mL)

Gold sodium thiomalate is a gold compound that suppresses symptoms of rheumatoid arthritis, and may slow progression of this disease. It is indicated in the symptomatic relief of active adult and juvenile rheumatoid arthritis not adequately controlled by other therapies. Gold sodium thiomalate (10 mg IM initially) is indicated in the management of rheumatoid arthritis.

GONADORELIN ACETATE

(Lutrepulse)

Gonadorelin, a GnRH with fertility-inducing properties (5 mcg IV q. 90 minutes for 21 days), is used to induce ovulation in women with primary hypothalamic amenorrhea (see Table 15).

TABLE 15
GnRH Analogs with Agonist Activity

Structures	Generic Names
9-Amino acid analogs:	
[D-Trp^6,Pro^{9}Net]GnRH	Deslorelin
[D-Trp^6,NMeLeu^7,Pro^{9}Net]GnRH	Lutrelin
[D-Leu^6,Pro^{9}Net]GnRH	Leuprolide
D-His(Bzl)^6,Pro^{9}Net]GnRH	Histrelin
[D-Ser(t-But)^6,Pro^{9}Net]GnRH	Buserelin
10-Amino acid analogs:	
Native GnRH	Gonadorelin, Lutrepulse
[D-Naphthyl-Ala(2)^6]GnRH	Nafarelin
[D-Ser(t-But)^6,AzaGly^{10}]GnRH	Goserelin
[D-Trp^6]GnRH	Tryptorelin

Note: GnRH = gonadotropin-releasing hormone.

GONADORELIN HYDROCHLORIDE

(Factrel)

Gonadorelin, a LHRH (100 mcg SC), is used in the diagnosis of hypogonadism (see Table 15).

GONADOTROPIN-RELEASING HORMONE

The pituitary hormones responsible for regulating gonadal function are LH and FSH (see Figure 56). In males, LH stimulates the Leydig's cells to synthesize testosterone; FSH stimulates the Sertoli's cells to synthesize inhibin and androgen-binding protein and, in conjunction with high intratesticular concentrations of testosterone, initiates and maintains spermatogenesis. In females, LH stimulates androgen synthesis, and FSH increases estrogen and inhibin synthesis in the granulosa cells. Both LH and FSH are released from the gonadotroph cells of the anterior pituitary in response to the hypothalamic GnRH, also known as LHRH.

GnRH is a decapeptide with the following structure: pyro Glu-His-Trp-Ser-Tyr-Gly-Leu-Arg-Pro-Gly-NH_2 (see Table 15).

GnRH is used to induce puberty in males with idiopathic hypogonadotropic hypogonadism (IHH). GnRH (15 to 150 ng/kg/hour) is administered by an infusion pump that

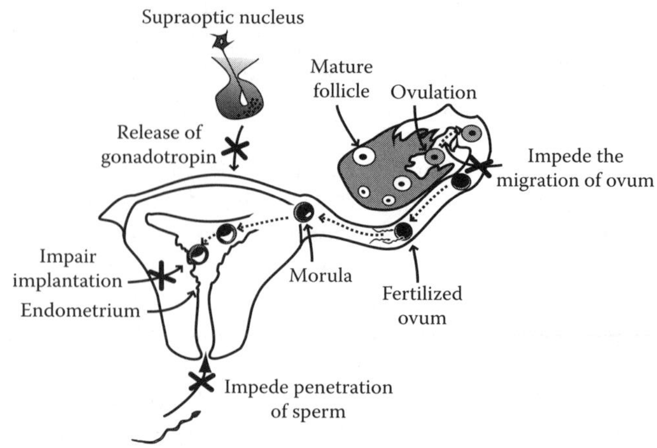

FIGURE 56 The antifertility agents suppress ovulation by inhibiting the release of hypophyseal ovulation-regulating gonadotropin, producing thick mucus from the cervical glands and hence impeding the penetration of sperm cells into the uterus, impeding the transfer of the ovum from the oviduct to the uterus, and preventing implantation of the fertilized ovum should fertilization take place.

delivers GnRH as a bolus, but in a pulsatile fashion. This induces the secretion of LH and FSH, the level of testosterone rises, the size of the testes increases, and spermatogenesis commences.

GnRH is used in females to treat hypothalamic amenorrhea. A deficit in the synthesis of GnRH has been implicated as the source of menstrual disturbances, hypoprolactinemia, anorexia nervosa, stress- and weight-loss-associated amenorrhea, athletes' amenorrhea, some forms of the polycystic ovarian disease syndrome, and infertility associated with hypothalamic tumors (see Table 15).

The GnRH analogs (Table 15) are administered subcutaneously, by nasal spray, or by long-acting depots, and may be used to (1) desensitize the gonadotrophs in patients with idiopathic precocious puberty, (2) treat prostate cancer and benign prostatic hypertrophy (androgen-dependent tumor), replacing the old methods of treating patients with castration or with high-dose estrogen therapy, and (3) to ameliorate gynecological diseases such as endometriosis.

The long-term use of GnRH analogs may foster hot flashes, osteoporosis, vaginal dryness, and dyspareunia (difficult coitus). These side effects may result from the prolonged hypoestrogenemia brought about by GnRH use.

GONORRHEA: Treatment of

Types of Infections	Regimen of Choice
Uncomplicated urethral, endocervical, rectal, proctitis, or epididymitis infection	Ceftriaxone 250 mg IM once; or ciprofloxacin 500 mg p.o. once; or norfloxacin 800 mg p.o. or cefuroxime axetil 1 g p.o. once plus probenecid 1 g; or cefotaxime 1 g IM once or ceftizoxime 500 mg IM once **plus** Doxycycline 100 mg two times daily for 7 days or tetracycline 500 mg four times daily for 7 days

Types of Infections	Regimen of Choice
Gonococcal infections in pregnancy	Ceftriaxone 250 mg IM **once** plus Erythromycin base 500 mg PO four times daily for 7 days
Disseminated gonococcal infection	Ceftriaxone 1 g IM or IV every 24 hours or ceftizoxime 1 g IV every 8 hours **or** cefotaxime 1 g IV every 8 hours until all symptoms resolve
Gonococcal ophthalmia	Ceftriaxone 1.0 g IM as a single dose
Adults and children (>20 kg) Neonates	Ceftriaxone 25–50 mg/kg IV or IM in a single daily dose for 7 days **or** cefotaxime 25 mg/kg IV or IM two times daily for 7 days
Infants born to mothers with gonococcal infection	Ceftriaxone 50 mg/kg IV or IM, not to exceed 125 mg

GOSERELIN ACETATE
(Zoladex implant 3.6 mg, implant 10.8 mg)

Goserelin is a GnRH analog that acts as a potent inhibitor of pituitary gonadotropin secretion. Goserelin 3.6 mg is used as an implant for palliative treatment of advanced breast cancer in pre- and perimenopausal women and as an endometrial thinning agent prior to endometrial ablation for dysfunctional uterine bleeding. Goserelin 3.6 and 10.8 mg implants are used for palliative treatment of advanced carcinoma of the prostate; and in combination with flutamide for management of locally confined stage T2b-T4 (stage B2-C) carcinoma of the prostate.

The most common form of **androgen deprivation therapy** (ADT) involves chemical suppression of the pituitary with GnRH agonists. These cause an initial surge in levels of LH and FSH, followed by inhibition of gonadotropin release. This results in reduction of testicular production of testosterone to castration levels. GnRH agonists in common use include **leuprolide** (Lupron, others), **goserelin** (Zoladex), **triptorelin** (Trelstar), and **buserelin** (Suprefact).

Until recently, synthetic GnRH (gonadorelin acetate, Lutrepulse) was used to treat patients with reproductive disorders secondary to disordered secretion of GnRH or GnRH deficiency. In women, it was administered either intravenously or subcutaneously by a pump in pulses that promoted a physiological cycle, with a starting dose of 2.5 μg per pulse every 120 minutes. If necessary, the dose was increased to 10 to 20 μg per pulse until ovulation was induced. Advantages over gonadotropin therapy included a lower risk of multiple pregnancies and a decreased need to monitor plasma estrogen levels or follicle size by ovarian ultrasonography. Side effects generally were minimal; the most common was local irritation due to the infusion device. In women, normal cycling levels of ovarian steroids could be achieved, leading to ovulation and menstruation. Because of its complexity, this regimen was previously available only in specialized centers of reproductive endocrinology. Production was discontinued by the United States manufacturer in 2003, and GnRH is no longer available.

Two GnRH antagonists, **ganirelix** (Antagon) and **cetrorelix** (Cetrotide), have been used to suppress the LH surge and thus prevent premature follicular luteinization in ovarian-stimulation protocols that are part of assisted reproduction techniques. The GnRH antagonist is given either in the follicular phase (termed the "short protocol") or in the midluteal phase (termed the "long protocol")—in conjunction with gonadotropins—to induce follicular maturation. Ovulation is then induced with human chorionic gonadotrophin (hCG) or luteinizing hormone (LH). Because they lack the initial stimulation of gonadotropin secretion seen with GnRH agonists, the GnRH antagonists provide a more rapid effect and are likely to become the preferred drugs in this setting.

GOSSYPOL

Cyproterone inhibits the action of androgens (see Figure 95), and gossypol prevents spermatogenesis without altering the other endocrine functions of the testis (Figure 57).

GOUT: Treatment of

Gout results from the deposition of urate crystals (monosodium urate monohydrate) in joints, leading to an acute inflammatory response, or in soft tissues, such as cartilage, causing no inflammation. Most cases of gout are characterized by the sudden onset of severe acute monarticular arthritis in a peripheral joint in the leg.

Three treatments are available for patients with acute gouty arthritis. Colchicine is less favored now than in the past because its onset of action is slow and it invariably causes diarrhea. Nonsteroidal antiinflammatory drugs, which are currently favored, are rapidly effective but may have serious side effects. Corticosteroids, administered either intraarticularly or parenterally, are used increasingly in patients with monarticular gout, especially if oral drug therapy is not feasible.

Drugs used in the management of gout are:

To treat acute gouty arthritis
Colchicine
Corticosteroids
NSAIDs

To prevent acute attacks
Colchicine
NSAIDs

To lower serum urate concentrations
Allopurinol
Benzbromarone
Diflunisal
Probenecid
Salicylate
Sulfinpyrazone

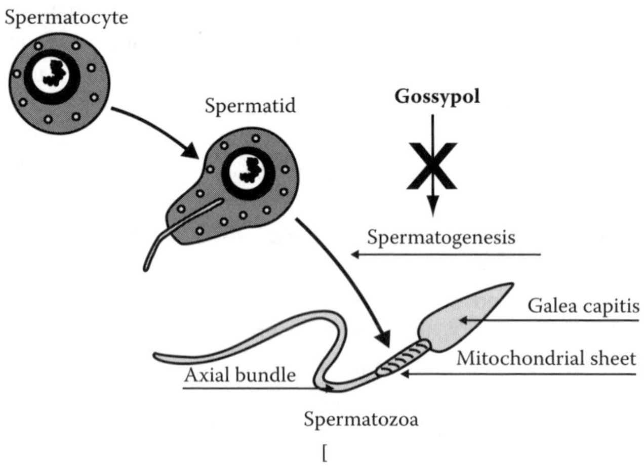

FIGURE 57 **Cyproterone** inhibits the action of androgens, and **gossypol** prevents spermatogenesis without altering the other endocrine functions of the testis.

GRANISETRON

A new class of antiemetic agents, the serotonin antagonists, has been identified. These agents could be clinically useful in a wide range of areas. Selective antagonists of the serotonin (5-hydroxytryptamine) type 3 (5-HT_3) receptor such as batanopride, granisetron, ondansetron, or zancopride have proved in early clinical trials to be potent antiemetic agents in patients undergoing cytotoxic chemotherapy. Their efficacy has been shown to be comparable or superior to that of conventional phenothiazine antiemetics. The toxic effects observed so far with these agents have been modest, and include headache (14%); asthenia, somnolence, and diarrhea (4%) (see Figure 73).

GRANISETRON HYDROCHLORIDE

(Kytril injection 1 mg/mL, tablets 1 mg)

Granisetron hydrochloride is a 5-HT_3-receptor antagonist. Serotonin receptors of the 5-HT_3 type are located peripherally on vagal nerve terminals, enteric neurons in the GI tract, and centrally in the chemoreceptor trigger zone. During chemotherapy, mucosal enterochromaffin cells from the small intestine release serotonin, which stimulates the 5-HT_3 receptors. This evokes vagal afferent discharge, inducing vomiting. Clearance is predominantly by hepatic metabolism, and plasma protein binding is approximately 65%.

Indications: Adults—used for prevention of chemotherapy-induced nausea and vomiting; prevention of radiation-induced nausea and vomiting (oral only); postoperative nausea and vomiting (injection only). **Pediatric** (2 to 16 years)—used for prevention of chemotherapy-induced nausea and vomiting (injection only). Safety and efficacy are not established in patients younger than 2 years.

Granisetron is indicated in prevention of nausea and vomiting associated with cancer chemotherapy. The recommended dose is 10 mcg/kg infused IV over 5 minutes beginning within 30 minutes before initiation of chemotherapy and only when chemotherapy is given (see Figure 73).

Ondansetron (Zofran) is the prototypical drug in this class. Since their introduction in the early 1990s, the 5-HT_3-receptor antagonists have become the most widely used drugs for chemotherapy-induced emesis. Other agents in this class include **granisetron** (Kytril), **dolasetron** (Anzemet), **palonosetron** (Aloxi; intravenous use only), and **tropisetron**.

There is evidence that effects at peripheral and central sites contribute to the efficacy of these agents. 5-HT_3 receptors are present in several critical sites involved in emesis, including vagal afferents, the STN (which receives signals from vagal afferents), and the area postrema itself. Serotonin is released by the enterochromaffin cells of the small intestine in response to chemotherapeutic agents and may stimulate vagal afferents (via 5-HT_3 receptors) to initiate the vomiting reflex. Experimentally, vagotomy has been shown to prevent cisplatin-induced emesis. However, the highest concentrations of 5-HT_3 receptors in the CNS are found in the solitary tract nucleus (STN) and chemoreceptor trigger zone (CTZ), and antagonists of 5-HT_3 receptors also may suppress nausea and vomiting by acting at these sites.

GRISEOFULVIN

(Grifulvin V tablets 250 mg (as microsize))

Griseofulvin is an antifungal agent that is deposited preferentially into infected skin, which gradually sloughs off and is replaced by noninfected tissue; and binds tightly to new keratin, which becomes highly resistant to fungal invasions. It is indicated in the treatment of ringworm infections of skin, hair, and nails caused by susceptible fungi.

Griseofulvin, a fungistatic agent, is effective against various dermatophytes, including *Microsporum*, *Epidermophyton*, and *Trichophyton*, that produce diseases of the skin, hair, and nails. It exerts its effect by inhibiting fungal mitosis. It is effective in the treatment of ringworm infections of the skin and nails, namely tinea corporis, tinea pedis, tinea cruris, tinea barbae, tinea capitis, and tinea unguium, when caused by one or more of the following genera of fungi: *Trichophyton rubrum, T tonsurans, T. mentagrophytes, T. interdigitalis, T. verrucosum, T. mengini, T. gallinae, T. crateriform, T. sulphureum, T. schoenleini, Microsporum audouini, M. canis, M. gypseum*, and *Epidermophyton floccosum*.

Prior to therapy, the types of fungi responsible for the infection must be identified. The use of this drug is not justified in minor or trivial infections that will respond to topical agents alone.

Griseofulvin is deposited in the keratin precursor cells that are gradually replaced by healthy tissue. Griseofulvin has caused skin rashes, urticaria, angioneurotic edema, lupus-like syndrome, photosensitivity, and proteinuria. The serum level of griseofulvin is reduced by barbiturates; and griseofulvin reduces the hypoprothrombinemic effects of warfarin and actions of oral contraceptive medications.

GRISEOFULVIN MICROSIZE (Fulvicin-U/F, Grifulvin V, Grisactin)

GRISEOFULVIN ULTRAMICROSIZE

(Fulvicin P/G, Gris-Peg, Grisactin Ultra)

Griseofulvin, a penicillium antibiotic (330 to 375 mg p.o. daily), is indicated in the treatment of tinea corporis, tinea capitis, or tinea cruris infections.

GROWTH HORMONE-RELEASING HORMONE (GHRH)

Growth hormone is secreted in a pulsatile fashion during sleep by the somatotrophs of the anterior pituitary gland. Two hypothalamic peptides, GHRH and somatostatin (somatotropin release-inhibiting hormone), are the principal stimulatory and inhibitory factors of GHRH, respectively. Growth hormone deficiency in children causes short stature, which will respond to GHRH replacement therapy (see also Table 15).

GUAIFENESIN (GLYCERYL GUAIACOLATE)

(Allfen Jr tablets 400 mg, Anti-Tuss syrup 100 mg per 5 mL, Breonesin capsules 200 mg, Diabetic Tussin EX liquid 100 mg per 5 mL, Duracuss-G tablets 1200 mg)

Guaifenesin is an expectorant that enhances the output of respiratory tract fluid by reducing adhesiveness and surface tension, thus facilitating removal of viscous mucus and making nonproductive coughs more productive and less frequent. Efficacy is not well documented. Guaifenesin is indicated in the temporary relief of cough associated with respiratory tract infections and related conditions such as sinusitis, pharyngitis, bronchitis, and asthma when these conditions are complicated by tenacious mucus or mucus plugs and congestion; is effective for productive as well as nonproductive cough, particularly dry, nonproductive cough that tends to injure mucous membranes of the air passages; and helps loosen phlegm and thin bronchial secretions in patients with stable chronic bronchitis.

GUAIFENESIN/CODEINE PHOSPHATE

(Guaitussin AC syrup 10 mg codeine phosphate and 100 mg guaifenesin per 5 mL)

An antitussive with expectorant, **guaifenesin** may enhance output of respiratory tract fluid by reducing adhesiveness and surface tension, enhancing removal of viscous mucus, and making nonproductive coughs more productive and less frequent. **Codeine** stimulates opiate receptors in CNS, and also causes suppression of cough. They are indicated in temporary control of cough caused by minor throat and bronchial irritation as occurs with common cold or inhaled irritants; assist in loosening phlegm (mucus) and thinning bronchial secretions to make cough more productive.

GUANABENZ

Guanabenz (8 to 64 mg given in divided doses) is an orally active central alpha$_2$-adrenergic agonist, which is structurally similar to clonidine and lowers BP. The major advantages of guanabenz are lack of fluid retention and a beneficial effect on serum lipids (Figure 58).

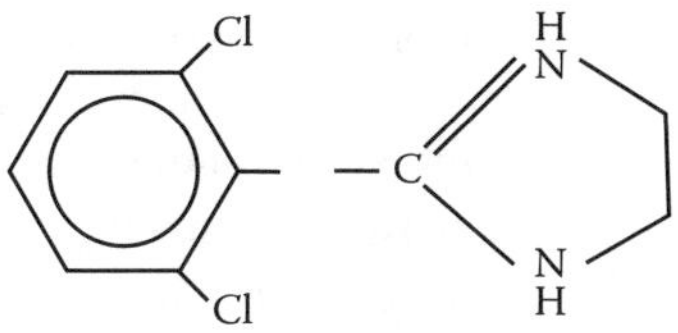

Clonidine

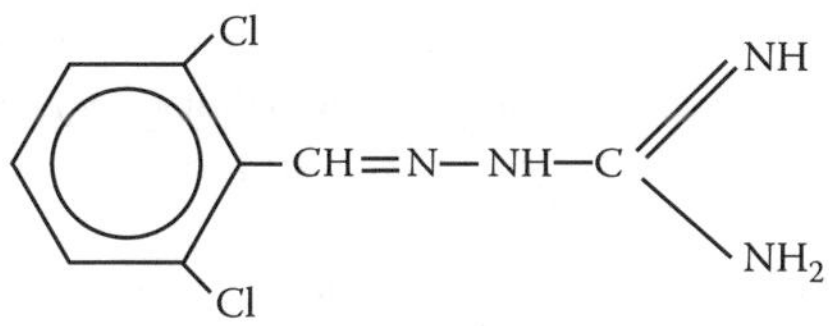

Guanabenz

FIGURE 58 Guanabenz lowers blood pressure by stimulating the central alpha$_2$-adrenergic receptor, decreasing central sympathetic outflow, and thus decreasing peripheral vascular resistance.

Guanabenz is rapidly and completely absorbed from the GI tract, exerts its effects within 2 hours, has a duration of action of 10 hours, is metabolized in the liver by hydroxylation followed by glucuronidation, and 2% of it is excreted unchanged by the liver.

Guanabenz has been shown to reduce heart rate and myocardial contractility in animals. However, in hypertensive patients, BP appears to be lowered via a reduction in peripheral resistance with minimal effects on heart rate and contractility. Fluid and electrolyte homeostasis and GFR are not affected by guanabenz. The most noteworthy metabolic action of guanabenz is a reduction in total cholesterol level. In contrast to the other two available alpha-adrenergic agonists, clonidine and methyldopa, glucose intolerance has not been associated with chronic treatment with guanabenz.

Guanabenz is used in the treatment of essential hypertension, and its efficacy compares well with that of methyldopa, clonidine, propranolol, and hydrochlorothiazide. Similar to other centrally acting alpha$_2$-adrenergic agonists (clonidine, guanfacine, methyldopa), it produces sedation and dry mouth, which occur within the first 2 weeks of therapy and tend to dissipate with long-term administration.

Abrupt cessation of guanabenz therapy may be associated with a discontinuation syndrome similar to that seen with clonidine, where the blood pressure may rise 5 to 20 mmHg above pretreatment values. During abrupt withdrawal of guanabenz from patients taking beta-blocking agents, increases in plasma catecholamines may induce marked vasoconstriction because peripheral alpha receptors are unopposed by peripheral vasodilatory beta receptors. Consequently, the use of guanabenz in combination with beta-blockers should probably be restricted to patients who are well informed and reliable.

GUANABENZ ACETATE

(Wytensin tablets 4 mg)

Guanabenz is a centerally acting antiadrenergic agent that stimulates central alpha$_2$-adrenergic receptors, inhibiting sympathetic outflow from brain to peripheral circulation. It is indicated in the treatment of hypertension alone or with a thiazide diuretic. **Guanabenz** and **guanfacine** are closely related chemically and pharmacologically.

Guanabenz (Wytensin, others) is a centrally acting α_2 agonist that decreases BP by a mechanism similar to those of clonidine and guanfacine. **Guanabenz** has a half-life of 4 to 6 hours and is extensively metabolized by the liver. Dosage adjustment may be necessary in patients with hepatic cirrhosis. The adverse effects caused by **guanabenz** (e.g., dry mouth and sedation) are similar to those seen with **clonidine**.

Clonidine (Catapres), **guanabenz** (Wytensin), and **guanfacine** (Tenex) stimulate the α_{2A} subtype of α_2-adrenergic receptors in the brain stem, resulting in a reduction in sympathetic outflow from the CNS. The decrease in plasma concentrations of norepinephrine is correlated directly with the hypotensive effect. Patients who have had a spinal cord transection above the level of the sympathetic outflow tracts do not display a hypotensive response to clonidine. At doses higher than those required to stimulate central α_2 receptors, these drugs can activate α_2 receptors of the α_2 subtype on vascular smooth-muscle cells. This effect accounts for the initial vasoconstriction that is seen when overdoses of these drugs are taken, and it has been postulated to be responsible for the loss of therapeutic effect that is observed with high doses. A major limitation in the use of these drugs is the paucity of information about their efficacy in reducing the risk of cardiovascular consequences of hypertension.

The α_2-adrenergic agonists lower arterial pressure by an effect on both cardiac output and peripheral resistance. In the supine position, when the sympathetic tone to the vasculature is low, the major effect is to reduce both heart rate and stroke volume; however, in the upright position, when sympathetic outflow to the vasculature is normally increased, these drugs reduce vascular resistance. This action may lead to postural hypotension. The decrease in cardiac sympathetic tone leads to a reduction in myocardial contractility and heart rate; this could promote CHF in susceptible patients.

Many patients experience annoying and sometimes intolerable adverse effects with these drugs. Sedation and **xerostomia** are prominent adverse effects. The xerostomia may be accompanied by dry nasal mucosa, dry eyes, and parotid gland swelling and pain. Postural hypotension and erectile dysfunction may be prominent in some patients. Clonidine may produce a lower incidence of dry mouth and sedation when given transdermally, perhaps because high peak concentrations are avoided. Less common CNS side effects include sleep disturbances with vivid dreams or nightmares, restlessness, and depression. Cardiac effects related to the sympatholytic action of these drugs include symptomatic bradycardia and sinus arrest in patients with dysfunction of the sinoatrial node, and AV block in patients with AV nodal disease or in patients taking other drugs that depress AV conduction. Some 15 to 20% of patients who receive transdermal clonidine may develop contact dermatitis.

GUANADREL

(Hylorel tablets 10 mg)

Guanadrel a peripherally acting antiadrenergic agent that inhibits vasoconstriction by restraining norepinephrine release from nerve storage sites; depletion of norepinephrine causes relaxation of vascular smooth muscle, decreasing total peripheral resistance, and venous return. It is indicated in the treatment of hypertension in patients not responding adequately to thiazide-type diuretics.

Guanethidine, guanadrel, debrisoquin, and bethanidine are all adrenergic neuron blockers with antihypertensive properties. Guanadrel (5 mg twice a day) is transported to presynaptic terminals by the catecholamine uptake mechanism, and then slowly displaces norepinephrine from its storage sites to be metabolized presynaptically. The reduction in neurotransmitter release in response to sympathetic nerve stimulation leads to reduced arteriolar vasoconstriction, especially the reflex increase in sympathetic tone that occurs with a change in position. Guanadrel is absorbed rapidly from the GI tract, has an onset of action of 2 hours, a duration of action of 10 hours, is metabolized by the liver, and partly excreted unchanged by the kidneys. Morning orthostatic hypotension is less frequent with guanadrel than with guanethidine (see also Figure 37).

Guanadrel (Hylorel) specifically inhibits the function of peripheral postganglionic adrenergic neurons. It is an exogenous **false neurotransmitter** that is accumulated, stored, and released like norepinephrine but is inactive at adrenergic receptors. The drug reaches its site of action by active transport into the neuron by the same transporter that is responsible for the reuptake of norepinephrine. In the neuron, **guanadrel** is concentrated within the adrenergic storage vesicle, where it replaces norepinephrine. During chronic administration, **guanadrel** acts as a "false neurotransmitter": it is present in storage vesicles, depletes the normal transmitter, can be released by stimuli that normally release norepinephrine, but is inactive at adrenergic receptors. This replacement of norepinephrine with an inactive transmitter is probably the principal mechanism of action of **guanadrel**.

When given intravenously, guanadrel initially releases norepinephrine in an amount sufficient to increase arterial blood pressure. This is not noticeable with oral administration because norepinephrine is released only slowly from the vesicles under this circumstance and is degraded within the neuron by monoamine oxidase. Nonetheless, because of the potential for norepinephrine release, **guanadrel** is contraindicated in patients with pheochromocytoma.

During adrenergic neuron blockade with **guanadrel**, effector cells become supersensitive to norepinephrine. The supersensitivity is similar to that produced by postganglionic sympathetic denervation.

Essentially, all of the therapeutic and adverse effects of guanadrel result from functional sympathetic blockade. The antihypertensive effect is achieved by a reduction in peripheral vascular resistance that results from inhibition of a receptor-mediated vasoconstriction. Consequently, arterial pressure is reduced modestly in the supine position when sympathetic activity is usually low, but the pressure can fall to a greater extent during situations in which reflex sympathetic activation is a mechanism for maintaining arterial pressure, such as assumption of the upright posture, exercise, and depletion of plasma volume. Plasma volume often expands, which may diminish the antihypertensive efficacy of guanadrel and require administration of diuretic to restore the antihypertensive effect.

Guanadrel is rapidly absorbed, leading to maximal levels in plasma at 1 to 2 hours. Because it must be transported into and must accumulate in adrenergic neurons, the maximum effect on BP is not seen until 4 to 5 hours. Although the β phase of its elimination has an estimated half-life of 5 to 10 hours, this almost certainly does not reflect the longer half-life of the drug stored at its site of action in the secretory vesicles of adrenergic neurons. The half-life of the pharmacological effect of guanadrel is determined by the drug's persistence in this neuronal pool, and is probably at least 10 hours. **Guanadrel** is administered in a regimen of twice-daily doses.

Guanadrel is cleared from the body by both renal and nonrenal disposition. Its elimination is impaired in patients with renal insufficiency; total-body clearance was reduced by four- to fivefold in a group of patients with a creatinine clearance averaging 13 mL per minute.

Guanadrel produces undesirable effects that are related entirely to sympathetic blockade. Symptomatic hypotension during standing, exercise, ingestion of alcohol, or hot weather is the result of the lack of sympathetic compensation for these stresses. A general feeling of fatigue and lassitude is partially, but not entirely, related to postural hypotension. Sexual dysfunction usually presents as delayed or retrograde ejaculation. Diarrhea also may occur.

Because guanadrel is actively transported to its site of action, drugs that block or compete for the catecholamine transporter on the presynaptic membrane will inhibit the effect of **guanadrel**. Such drugs include the tricyclic antidepressants, cocaine, chlorpromazine, ephedrine, phenylpropanolamine, and amphetamine.

Because of the availability of a number of drugs that lower BP without producing this degree of orthostatic hypotension, **guanadrel** is not employed in the monotherapy of hypertension, and is used chiefly as an additional agent in patients who have not achieved a satisfactory antihypertensive effect on multiple other agents. The need to use this drug arises very rarely. The usual starting dose is 10 mg daily, and side effects can be minimized by not exceeding 20 mg daily.

GUANETHIDINE MONOSULFATE

(Ismelin)

Guanethidine monosulfate is a peripherally acting antiadrenergic agent that interferes with release or distribution of norepinephrine from nerve endings, resulting in reduction in total peripheral resistance and diastolic and systolic BP. It is indicated in the treatment of moderate and severe hypertension and renal hypertension, including that secondary to pyelonephritis, renal amyloidosis, and renal artery stenosis.

α-Methyltyrosine (metyrosine) blocks the synthesis of norepinephrine by inhibiting tyrosine hydroxylase, the enzyme that catalyzes the rate-limiting step in catecholamine synthesis. This drug occasionally may be useful in treating selected patients with pheochromocytoma. On the other hand, **methyldopa**, an inhibitor of aromatic L-amino acid decarboxylase, is—like dopa itself—successively decarboxylated and hydroxylated in its side chain to form the putative "false neurotransmitter" α-methylnorepinephrine. **Bretylium**, **guanadrel**, and **guanethidine** act by preventing the release of norepinephrine by the nerve impulse. However, such agents can transiently stimulate the release of norepinephrine because of their capacity to displace the amine from storage sites.

Guanethidine (initial dose 10 mg daily) is indicated in the management of moderate to severe hypertension. It is transported to presynaptic terminals by the catecholamine uptake mechanism, and then slowly displaces norepinephrine from its storage sites to be metabolized presynaptically.

In contrast to the actions of ganglionic blocking agents, guanethidine suppresses equally the responses mediated by alpha- and beta-adrenergic receptors but does not produce parasympathetic blockade. It reduces both the systolic and diastolic pressures, and the effect is especially pronounced when the patient is standing.

Guanethidine is absorbed to the extent of 30 to 50%, is metabolized in the liver to a less active compound, and is excreted slowly in the urine. Guanethidine has a half-life of 4 to 8 days, requiring 10 to 14 days to evaluate its antihypertensive effects. It causes pronounced orthostatic hypotension. In order to minimize sodium retention, guanethidine is used along with a diuretic. Substances that inhibit the biogenic amine uptake mechanism such as imipramine reduce the antihypertensive effects of guanethidine (see also Figure 37).

GUANFACINE HYDROCHLORIDE

(Tenex)

Guanfacine (1 mg/day at bedtime) is indicated in the management of hypertension. Clonidine, guanfacine, guanabenz, and methyldopa are centrally acting $alpha_2$-adrenergic-receptor agonists. Guanfacine reduces sympathetic nerve impulses from the vasomotor center to the heart and blood vessels, resulting in a decrease in peripheral vascular resistance and a reduction in heart rate.

Guanfacine is absorbed orally, is bound to plasma proteins to the extent of 70%, metabolized in the liver, and 50% of it is excreted unchanged in the urine. The half-life of guanfacine is lengthened in renal impairment. Similar to other centrally acting $alpha_2$-adrenergic-receptor agonists, guanfacine causes sedation, especially during the first week, and hence should be given at bedtime.

Similar to clonidine, an abrupt cessation of therapy with guanfacine causes an increase in plasma and urinary catecholamines, nervousness, and rebound hypertension after 2 to 4 days, which is delayed when compared to that of clonidine. The adverse effects of guanfacine are dry mouth (30%), and somnolence, anesthesia, and dizziness (11%).

GUANIDINE

(Guanidine hydrochloride tablets 125 mg)

Guanidine is a cholinergic muscle stimulant that enhances release of acetylcholine following a nerve impulse and appears to slow rates of depolarization and repolarization of muscle-cell membranes. It is indicated in reducing symptoms of muscle weakness and easy fatigability associated with **Lambert–Eaton syndrome**.

H

HAEMOPHILUS B CONJUGATE VACCINE

(ActHIB powder for injection, lyophilized 10 mcg purified capsular polysaccharide)

Haemophilus b is a bacterial vaccine that induces specific protective antibodies against *Haemophilus influenzae* type b (Hib). It is indicated for induction of active immunity against Hib infection. Routine immunization of all infants beginning at age 2 months is recommended.

HAEMOPHILUS B VACCINES

(Haemophilus b vaccines)

HAEMOPHILUS B CONJUGATE VACCINE, DIPHTHERIA CRM_{197} PROTEIN CONJUGATE (HBOC)

(HibTITER)

HAEMOPHILUS B CONJUGATE VACCINE, DIPHTHERIA TOXOID CONJUGATE

(PRP-D) (ProHIBIT)

HAEMOPHILUS B CONJUGATE VACCINE, MENINGOCOCCAL PROTEIN CONJUGATE (PRP-OMP)

(PedvaxHIB)

Haemophilus vaccine is indicated for routine immunization.

HALAZEPAM

(Paxipam)

Halazepam (20 to 40 mg p.o. t.i.d.) is used as an antianxiety agent. It depresses the CNS by enhancing the effects of gamma-aminobutyric acid (GABA) in the ascending reticular activating system and hence causing inhibition of cortical and limbic arousal (see Figure 50). Halazepam (half-life of 14 hours) is absorbed orally, distributed widely throughout the body, bound to proteins to the extent of 85 to 90%, metabolized to desmethyldiazepam (an active metabolite with a half-life of 150 hours), and is excreted as glucuronide conjugate in the urine. Halazepam potentiates the CNS-depressant effects of neuroleptics, antidepressants, narcotic analgesics, barbiturates, and ethanol. Disulfiram inhibits the metabolism of halazepam, and heavy smoking accelerates it. Clinical manifestations of overdose include somnolence, confusion, coma, hypoactive reflexes, dyspnea, labored breathing, hypotension, bradycardia, slurred speech, and unsteady gait or impaired coordination. Because of decreased elimination and greater sensitivity to the CNS-depressing effects, the dosage of halazepam in elderly subjects should be lower (see also Table 9).

HALCINONIDE

(Halog ointment 0.1%, cream 0.1%, solution 0.1%)

Halcinonide is a topical corticosteroid that produces antiinflammatory, antipruritic, and vasoconstrictive effects. It is indicated in the relief of inflammation and pruritus caused by corticosteroid-responsive dermatoses. Halcinonide, a topical adrenocorticoid with antiinflammatory properties (cream, ointment, solution 0.025 to 0.1%), is indicated in inflammation of acute and chronic corticosteroid-responsive dermatoses (see also Table 11).

HALOBETASOL PROPIONATE

(Ultravate cream 0.05%, ointment 0.05%)

Halobetasol is a topical corticosteroid that is a very high-potency topical glucocorticoid with antiinflammatory, antipruritic, and vasoconstrictive properties. It is thought to act by inducing phospholipase A_2 inhibitory proteins, thus controlling biosynthesis of potent mediators of inflammation. It provides relief of inflammatory and pruritic manifestations of corticosteroid-responsive dermatoses. Halobetasol, a topical corticosteroid with antiinflammatory properties (0.05% cream and ointment), is used in the relief of inflammation and pruritus of corticosteroid-responsive dermatoses (see also Table 11).

HALOPERIDOL

(Haldol tablets 0.5mg)

Haloperidol is a phenylbutylpiperadine derivative antipsychotic, apparently caused by dopamine-receptor blockage in CNS. It is indicated in the management of psychotic disorders; control of Tourette's disorder in children and adults; management of severe behavioral problems in children; short-term treatment of hyperactive children; and long-term antipsychotic therapy (haloperidol decanoate).

Haloperidol is a butyrophenone derivative with antipsychotic action similar to that of piperazine phenothiazines such as fluphenazine. Haloperidol (0.5 to 2 mg t.i.d.) is indicated in the management of psychotic disorders; in Tourette's disorder for the control of tics and vocal utterances; in severe behavioral problems of children with combative and explosive nature; in hyperactive impulse disorder in children associated with aggression, low frustration tolerance, and impulsive behavior, and in elderly subjects with senile dementia (see also Table 9).

Haloperidol blocks dopamine receptors in the brain and hence produces a very high incidence of movement disorders such as parkinsonism (see phenothiazine derivatives). Its mechanism of action in Gilles de la Tourette's syndrome is unknown. In addition to blocking dopamine receptors, haloperidol has many other central and peripheral effects; it has weak peripheral anticholinergic and antiemetic effects, produces both alpha and ganglionic blockade, and counteracts histamine- and serotonin-mediated activities.

Haloperidol is absorbed well orally and intramuscularly (haloperidol decanoate), distributed widely in the body while accumulating in adipose tissue, binds to protein heavily (90 to 99%), and is metabolized in the liver. Haloperidol is eliminated unchanged in the feces and urine to the extent of 15 and 40%, respectively.

The highest incidence of adverse effects of haloperidol include the CNS-involving extrapyramidal symptoms such as dystonia, akathisia, parkinsonism, tardive dyskinesia, and neuroleptic malignant syndrome. Overdose with haloperidol causes CNS depression characterized by deep, unarousable sleep and possible coma, hypotension or hypertension, extrapyramidal symptoms, dystonia, abnormal involuntary movements, agitation, seizures, arrhythmias, ECG changes (may show QT prolongation and torsade de pointes), hypothermia or hyperthermia, and autonomic nervous system dysfunction. Overdose with long-acting decanoate requires prolonged recovery time. Treatment is symptomatic and supportive in nature (see also Table 2).

HALOPROGIN

(Halotex)

Haloprogin is available as a 1% cream or solution that is applied topically. It is applied twice a day for 2 to 4 weeks. It is used principally in the treatment of tinea pedis, tinea cruris, tinea corporis, tinea manuum, and tinea versicolor. Haloprogin's mechanisms of action in yeast cells are thought to be inhibition of respiration and disruption of yeast cell membranes. Its mechanism of action in dermatophytes is unknown.

HALOTHANE

(Fluothane)

Halothane is 2-bromo-2-chloro-1,1,1-trifluoroethane:

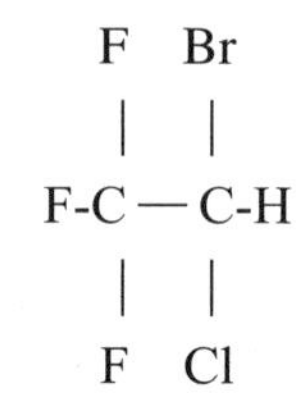

Mixtures of halothane with air or oxygen are not flammable or explosive.

Halothane is a potent anesthetic agent with properties that allow a smooth and rather rapid loss of consciousness that progresses to anesthesia. Thiopental is used for induction of anesthesia, and halothane is used for its maintenance (see Table 16).

TABLE 16
Summary Pharmacology of Nitrous Oxide, Cyclopropane, Halothane, and Ether

Nature and Effects	N_2O	Cyclopropane	Halothane	Ether
Volatile anesthetic	No	No	Yes	Yes
Rate of induction	Fast (2–3 min)	Fast (1–2 min)	Slow (10 min)	Slow (10–20 min)
Potentially explosive anesthetic	No	Yes	No	Yes
Respiration	NC	Depressed	Depressed	Stimulates indirectly, depresses directly
Myocardial depression	NC	Yes	Yes	Yes
Myocardioal depression compensated by increased sympathetic activity	—	Yes	No	Yes
Sensitizes heart to catecholamines	No	Yes	Yes	No
Produces excessive salivation and respiratory secretions	No	No	No	Yes
Potentiates neuromuscular blocking agents	No	Yes	Yes	Yes
Nausea and vomiting during emergence	Low	Frequent	Low	Frequent
Liver damage	No	No	Moderate	No
Kidney damage	No	No	No	No
Heat regulatory center	NC	Depressed	Depressed	Depressed
Release of epinephrine from the adrenal gland	No	Increased	Decreased	Increased
Analgesia	Good	Good	Poor	Good
Muscle relaxation	NC	Adequate	Minimal	Good

Note: NC = no change. Nitrous oxide (N_2O) is a nonexplosive and nonflammable gas.

The signs of depth of anesthesia achieved with halothane that are of the most practical value are blood pressure, which is progressively depressed, and response to surgical stimulation (e.g., pulse rate, blood pressure, movement, or even awakening). Hypotension results from two main effects. First, the myocardium is depressed directly, and cardiac output is decreased; second, the normal baroreceptor-mediated tachycardia in response to hypotension is obtunded.

If the patient anesthetized with halothane is allowed to breathe spontaneously, an increased partial pressure of carbon dioxide in the arterial blood is common and is indicative of ventilatory depression. There also is an increased difference between the partial pressure of oxygen in the alveolar gas and in the arterial blood, indicating less efficient exchange of gas. Halothane thus influences both ventilatory control and the efficiency of oxygen transfer. To compensate for these effects, ventilation frequently is assisted or controlled by manual or mechanical means, and the concentration of inspired oxygen is increased.

Because cerebral blood flow generally increases during halothane anesthesia, cerebrospinal fluid pressure increases. Halothane thus may aggravate conditions in which the intracranial pressure is elevated. The cerebral metabolic consumption of oxygen is reduced. Recovery of mental function after even brief anesthesia with halothane is not complete for several hours, but this phenomenon probably contributes little to the more prolonged impairment of psychological performance that has been reported after major surgery. Shivering during recovery is common and represents both a response to heat loss and an expression of neurological recovery.

Anesthesia with halothane causes some relaxation by central depression; in addition, the duration and magnitude of the muscular relaxation induced by nondepolarizing skeletal muscle relaxants such as tubocurarine or pancuronium are increased (see also Figure 99).

Inhibition of natural or induced uterine contractions by halothane during parturition may prolong the process of delivery, as well as increase blood loss. Thus, other agents or techniques may be preferred for the relief of obstetrical pain.

Halothane causes dose-dependent reductions of renal blood flow and the rate of glomerular filtration.

Halothane-induced hepatitis that occurs in the postoperative period most often is due to transmission of hepatitis virus (e.g., in transfused blood), involvement of the liver by disease processes, or damage by known hepatotoxic drugs. Hepatic necrosis, although rare, does occur with halothane.

Approximately 60 to 80% of absorbed halothane is eliminated unchanged in the exhaled gas in the first 24 hours after its administration, and smaller amounts continue to be exhaled for several days or even weeks. Of the fraction not exhaled, as much as 50% undergoes biotransformation, and the rest is eliminated unchanged by other routes.

In conclusion, the introduction of enflurane, isoflurane, and desflurane and the availability of a variety of intravenous agents have dramatically reduced the use of halothane in more recent years (see Table 16).

HEART FAILURE: Treatment of

ACE Inhibitors	
Captopril	Quinapril
Enalapril	Lisinopril
Enalaprilat	Ramipril
Angiotensin-Receptor Antagonist	
Losartan	
Adrenergic-Receptor Antagonists	
Bucindolol	Phentolamine
Carvedilol	Prazosin
Labetalol	Quinazoline
Ca^{2+}-Channel-Blocking Drugs	
Amlodipine	
Nifedipine	
"Direct" Vasodilators	
Hydralazine	
Nicorandil	
Nitrovasodilators	
Isosorbide dinitrate	
Nitroglycerin	
Sodium nitroprusside	
Phosphodiesterase Inhibitors	
Amrinone	
Milrinone	
Vesnarinone	
Sympathomimetics	
Dobutamine	

HEMICHOLINIUM

Acetylcholine receptors are classified as either muscarinic or nicotinic. The alkaloid muscarine mimics the effects produced by stimulation of the parasympathetic system. These effects are postganglionic and are exerted on exocrine glands, cardiac muscles, and smooth muscle. The alkaloid nicotine mimics the actions of acetylcholine, which include stimulation of all autonomic ganglia, stimulation of the adrenal medulla, and contraction of skeletal muscle.

Dimethylphenylpipazinium stimulates the autonomic ganglia; tetraethylammonium and hexamethonium block the autonomic ganglia; phenyltrimethylammonium stimulates skeletal muscle end plates; decamethonium produces neuromuscular blockage; and d-tubocurarine blocks the autonomic ganglia and the motor fiber end plates.

Among the agents cited, only *d*-tubocurarine is useful as a drug (skeletal muscle relaxant); the rest are useful only as research tools (see Figure 99).

HEMOSTATIC MECHANISMS AND DRUGS INFLUENCING THEM

Drugs Affecting Platelet Functions

Antiplatelet Agents
Cyclooxygenase inhibitors
- Aspirin
- Sulfinpyrazone
- Other nonsteroidal antiinflammatory agents

Phosphodiesterase inhibitors (dipyridamole)
Ticlopidine
Phospholipase inhibitors
Thromboxane synthetase inhibitors
Prostacyclin
Thromboxane receptor blockers

Platelet-Promoting Agents
Desmopressin
Estrogens

Drugs Affecting Coagulation

Anticoagulant Agents
Heparin
Vitamin K antagonists
- Coumarins (warfarin and dicoumarol)
- Indanediones

Ancrod

Procoagulant agents
Vitamin K
Desmopressin
Danazol

Drugs Affecting Fibrinolysis

Antifibrinolytic agents
Lysine analogs
Epsilon amino caproic acid
Tranexamic acid

Profibrinolytic Agents
Urinary plasminogen activator
Urokinase
Streptokinase
Tissue plasminogen activator
Single-chain urinary plasminogen activator
Anistreplase

HEPARIN

(Heparin sodium injection 1000 units/mL)

Heparin is an anticoagulant that inhibits reactions that lead to clotting. It is indicated in prophylaxis and treatment of venous thrombosis and its extensions, pulmonary embolism (PE), peripheral arterial embolism, and atrial fibrillation with embolization; diagnosis and treatment of acute and chronic consumption coagulopathies (DIC); and prevention of postoperative deep venous thrombosis.

Commercial heparin is a sulfated mucopolysaccharide of repeating units of D-glucosamine, D-glucuronic acid, and L-iduronic acid. The comparative pharmacology of heparin and coumarin is shown in Tables 17 and 18.

The use of heparin and other anticoagulants is contraindicated in the presence of active hemorrhage, potential hemorrhage (acid pepsin disease), and hemorrhagic disorders (hemophilia).

Heparin and other anticoagulants should be used with extreme caution in patients with traumatic injuries to the central nervous system or the eyes because it is very difficult to control hemorrhage in these areas. The possible existence of an aneurysm must be considered in an untreated hypertensive patient.

Anticoagulant therapy during pregnancy is indicated for the treatment and prophylaxis of venous thromboembolic disease and systemic embolism associated with valvular heart disease or prosthetic heart valves. However, there are special problems that need to be considered when deciding on optimal anticoagulant therapy in pregnant women. Heparin does not cross the placenta and is probably safe for the fetus. However, long-term heparin therapy is occasionally associated with maternal hemorrhage and rarely with symptomatic osteoporosis. Coumarin derivatives cross the placenta and are potentially teratogenic, particularly in the first trimester. Neonatal hemorrhage is a risk if warfarin is administered to the pregnant mother near term.

Anticoagulant therapy should be monitored carefully in patients with severe hepatic or renal failure, vitamin K deficiency, or alcoholism, and those with arthritis who are taking acetylsalicylic acid in large quantities. Furthermore, anticoagulants are extensively metabolized and their metabolites excreted, which can have an important bearing in patients suffering from renal disorders.

HEPARIN CALCIUM

(Calciparine)

HEPARIN SODIUM

(Heparin Lock Flush, Hep-Lock, Heplock U/P, Liquaemin sodium)

Heparin (5000 to 7500 units IV push) is used in the treatment of pulmonary embolism, in prophylaxis of embolism, in open-heart surgery, in disseminated intravascular coagulation, and in an effort to maintain patency of IV indwelling catheters.

HEPATITIS A VACCINE, INACTIVATED

(Havrix suspension 720 EL.U/0.5 mL of viral antigen, Vaqta injectable 25 U/0.5 mL of HAV protein, injectable 50 U/1 mL of HAV protein.

Hepatitis A is an antiviral vaccine that provides active immunization. It is used as an active immunization of patients 2 years and older against disease caused by hepatitis A virus.

HEPATITIS B IMMUNE GLOBULIN, HUMAN (HBIG)

(H-BIG, Hep-B Gammagee, HyperHep)

Hepatitis B immune globulin, a hepatitis B prophylaxis product (0.6 ml/kg IM) is used within seven days of exposure to hepatitis B.

TABLE 17
Pharmacology of Heparin and Coumarin

Properties Studied	Heparin	Coumarin
Chemistry	High negative charge	
Occurrence	Naturally occurring in most tissues	Synthetic
Mechanism of action	Activates plasma antithrombin, blocks thromboplastin generation, neutralizes tissue thromboplastin	Inhibits the synthesis of factors II, VII, IX, and X by blocking the action of vitamin K
Pharmacokinetics		
Route of administration	Subcutaneously, intravenously	Orally
Onset	Minutes (10–20)	48 hrs
Duration	4 hr (subcutaneously)	2–10 days
Protein binding and metabolism	In liver by heparinase; inactive metabolite is excreted by the kidney	Bound to albumin (99%), side-chain reduction to alcohol (dextrowarfarin), oxidation to 7-hydroxywarfarin (levowarfarin)
Antagonists	Protamine sulfate, a strongly basic protein, forms a complex with heparin to an inactive compound; 1 mg protamine for 100 units of heparin	Vitamin K, whole blood, fresh plasma

TABLE 18
Comparison of Hirudin and Heparin as Anticoagulants

Heparin	Hirudin
Heteropolysaccharide with various chain lengths (5,000–25,000 Da)	Polypeptide (7,000 Da)
Needs antithrombin III as a cofactor	Direct interaction with thrombin
Heparin/antithrombin III complexes react also with various other factors of the coagulation/fibrinolysis cascades	Selective for thrombin
High affinity for numerous other compounds (e.g., platelets, endothelium)	Pharmacologically inert
May cause thrombocytopenia and bleeding	No side effect observed
Low-molecular-weight heparins (approx. 3,000–5,000 Da) with special properties available	Smaller synthetic hirudin derivatives (approx. 2,000 Da) inhibit thrombin effectively

HEPATITIS B VACCINE, RECOMBINANT (INACTIVATED)

(Engerix-B, Recombivax HB, Recombivax HB dialysis formulation)

Hepatitis B vaccine (20 mcg IM followed by a second dose of 20 mcg IM 30 days later) is used in immunization against infection from all known subtypes of hepatitis B; primary preexposure prophylaxis against hepatitis B; or postexposure prophylaxis (when given with hepatitis B immune globulin).

Immunization may be active or passive. Active immunization involves stimulation with an antigen to develop immunologic defenses against a future exposure. Passive immunization involves administration of preformed antibodies to an individual who is already exposed or is about to be exposed to an antigen.

Active immunization, vaccination, involves administration of an antigen as a whole, killed organism, an attenuated (live) organism, or a specific protein or peptide constituent of an organism. Booster doses often are required, especially when killed (inactivated) organisms are used as the immunogen. In the United States, vaccination has sharply curtailed or practically eliminated a variety of major infections, including diphtheria, measles, mumps, pertussis, rubella, tetanus, *Haemophilus influenzae* type b, and pneumococcus.

Although most vaccines have targeted infectious diseases, a new generation of vaccines may provide complete or limited protection from specific cancers or autoimmune diseases. Because T-cells optimally are activated by peptides and costimulatory ligands that are both present on antigen-presenting cells (APCs), one approach for vaccination has consisted of immunizing patients with APCs expressing a tumor antigen. The first generation of anticancer vaccines used whole cancer cells or tumor-cell lysates as a source of antigen in combination with various adjuvants, relying on host APCs to process and present tumor-specific antigens.

Passive immunization is indicated when an individual is deficient in antibodies because of a congenital or acquired immunodeficiency, when an individual with a high degree of risk is exposed to an agent and there is inadequate time for active immunization (e.g., measles, rabies, **hepatitis B**), or when a disease is already present but can be ameliorated by passive antibodies (e.g., botulism, diphtheria, tetanus). Passive immunization may be provided by several different products:

Immune globulin intravenous
Cytomegalovirus immune globulin
Respiratory syncytial virus immune globulin
Hepatitis B immune globulin
Rabies immune globulin
Rho(D) immune globulin
Tetanus immune globulin

for hepatitis B, rabies, tetanus, varicella-zoster, cytomegalovirus, and respiratory syncytial virus. Rho(D) immune globulin is a specific hyperimmune globulin for prophylaxis against hemolytic disease of the newborn due to Rh incompatibility between mother and fetus. All such plasma-derived products carry the theoretical risk of transmission of infectious disease.

HEPOXILINS

Hepoxilins are monohydroxy-epoxide derivatives of arachidonic acid that release intracellular calcium and open potassium channels. Hepoxilins appear to have proinflammatory actions in the skin, but inhibit the actions of inflammatory agents in the human neutrophil. Hepoxilin receptors have recently been identified that are coupled to G-proteins (see Figure 84).

HETASTARCH (HYDROXYETHYL STARCH; HES)

(Hespan injection 6 g per 100 mL in 0.9% sodium chloride)

Hetastarch is a plasma expander that produces expansion of plasma volume. It does not have oxygen-carrying capacity or contain plasma protein, so it is not a blood or plasma substitute. It is indicated as an adjunct therapy for plasma volume expansion in shock caused by hemorrhage, burns, surgery, sepsis, or other trauma; and as an adjunct in leukapheresis to improve harvesting and increase yield of granulocytes.

HETASTARCH

(HES, Hydroxyethyl Starch) (Hespan)

Hetastarch, an amylopectin derivative and plasma volume expander (500 to 1000 ml IV), is used in shock and cardiopulmonary bypass surgery.

HIRUDIN

The saliva of the medicinal leech contains a battery of substances that interfere with the hemostatic mechanisms of the host. One of these compounds is hirudin, a potent

HICCUP: Treatment of

Hiccup, or singultus, is a spasmodic, involuntary contraction of the inspiratory muscles, associated with delayed, abrupt glottic closure, causing a peculiar sound, expressed by different words around the world. They are:

Czkawka	Polish	Hoquet	French
Geehouk	Hebrew	Ikota	Russian
Hakka	Arabic	Lozingas	Greek
Hiccup, hiccough	English	Nac	Vietnamese
Hicka	Swedish	Schluckauf	German
Hiçkirik	Turkish	Sekseke	Parsi
Hik	Dutch	Singhiozzo	Italian
Hikke	Norwegian, Danish	Singultus	Latin
Hipo	Spanish	Sughitz	Romanian
Hirik	Kurd	Tale	Chinese

Hiccup is a forceful, involuntary inspiration commonly experienced by fetuses, children, and adults. Its purpose is unknown, and its pathophysiology still poorly understood. Short hiccup bouts are mostly associated with gastric distention or alcohol intake. They resolve spontaneously or with simple folk remedies and do not require medical attention. In contrast, prolonged hiccup is a rare but disabling condition that can induce depression, weight loss, and sleep deprivation. A wide variety of pathological conditions can cause chronic hiccup: myocardial infarction, brain tumor, renal failure, prostate cancer, and abdominal surgery are only a few of these conditions.

Drugs that have been shown to be effective in treating hiccup are:

Amitriptyline	Chlorpromazine	Mephenesin	Orphenadrine
Baclofen	Diphenylhydantoin	Metoclopramide	Valproic acid
Carbamazepine	Haloperidol	Nifedipine	

Baclofen, chlorpromazine, or metoclopramide are most effective.

HIRSUTISM: Treatment of

Hirsutism results from the change of fine, vellus hair to visible, thickened, terminal hair under the influence of dihydrotestosterone, a biologically active form of testosterone. This androgen-dependent hair growth develops in defined patterns. Terminal hair is a normal phenomenon and is often found on the upper lip, the chin, around the nipples and the midline of the lower abdomen.

Drugs causing hirsutism are:

Androgens
Anabolic steroids
Some progestogens
Danazol

Drugs causing hyperprolactinemia
High-dose phenothiazines
Metoclopramide

Patient distress is the prime indication for therapy. Drug treatment should be continued for 12 months before assessing response. Spironolactone is generally the drug tried first. Ovarian hormones, e.g., medroxyprogesterone acetate plus ethinyl estradiol, or cyproterone acetate plus ethinyl estradiol may be added if response is inadequate.

anticoagulant that maintains the fluidity of the ingested blood, and the most potent inhibitor of thrombin. Upon binding to thrombin, the cleavage of fibrinogen and subsequent clot formation are prevented. The potency and specificity of hirudin suggest it as a useful antithrombin III-independent alternative to heparin for the control of thrombosis (Table 18).

HISTAMINE

Histamine is synthesized in enterochromaffin-like cells, mucosal mast cells, and nerves, according to the following reaction:

$$\text{Histidine} \xrightarrow{\text{Histidine decarboxylase}} \text{Histamine}$$

Histamine is metabolized by histamine *N*-methyltransferase to *N*-methylhistamine, which is then deaminated by monoamine oxidase type B into methylimidazole acetic acid. Histamine is also found in platelets, leukocytes, and basophils in the skin, lungs, and gastric mucosa, as well as to a certain extent in blood, plasma, sputum, gastric juice, blister fluid, and pus. Histamine is stored mostly in mast cells.

Histamine may be used diagnostically to identify patients with pheochromocytoma (it increases the release of catecholamines) and to distinguish pernicious anemia (a lack of acid release indicates achlorhydria).

Histamine is involved in the immunoglobulin E-mediated immune responses that initiate and maintain a host of inflammatory and allergic reactions, including lysosomal enzyme release from neutrophils, lymphocyte proliferation in response to mitogens, lymphocyte-mediated cytolysis, and antibody production and secretion (see Figure 59).

Histamine, as a normal constituent of the gastric mucosa, controls both microcirculation and gastric secretion. The gastric secretagogues are acetylcholine, histamine, and gastrin (see Figure 34). The action of acetylcholine is blocked by atropine, and the action of histamine is blocked by

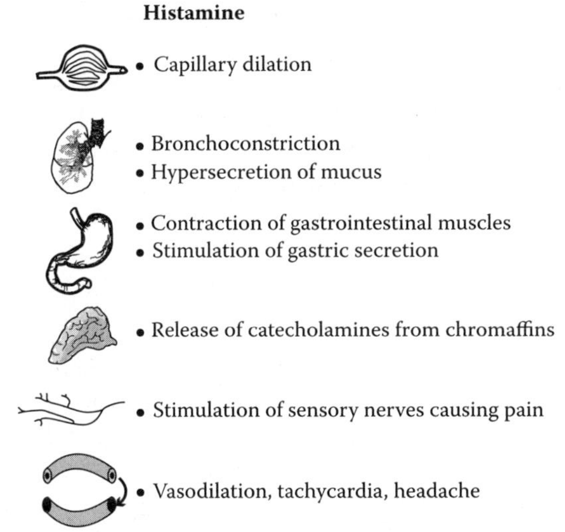

FIGURE 59 The release of histamine is stimulated by **numerous drugs** including **reserpine**, **codeine**, **meperidine**, **hydralazine**, **morphine**, ***d*-tubocurarine**, **dextrans**, and **papaverine**.

cimetidine, burimamide, and metiamide. No specific antagonist is available for gastrin.

The histamine release in the brain, and perhaps other sites, involves exocytosis, as this potassium-induced release is a calcium-dependent process. Histamine is released by many factors. For example, histamine is released by numerous drugs including reserpine, codeine, meperidine, hydralazine, morphine, *d*-tubocurarine, dextrans, papaverine, and compound 48/80. However, the different histamine storage sites show certain degrees of specificity. For example, the histamine in mast cells is not released following potassium-induced depolarization or by reserpine, factors that release histamine from neurons. Conversely, compound 48/80, which releases histamine from mast cells, is not able to release histamine from neurons.

In the peripheral system, histamine causes capillary dilation and increased permeability, bronchoconstriction and contraction of gastrointestinal muscles, stimulation of chromaffin cells releasing catecholamines, vasodilation, tachycardia, headache, stimulation of exocrine secretion causing hypersecretion of mucus in the lungs, and stimulation of gastric secretion (see Figure 34).

The diversified actions of histamine are brought forth through their interaction with different types of receptors, which are described in the following sections.

Histamine$_1$ (H_1) receptors mediate such actions as bronchoconstriction and the contraction of smooth muscles in the gastrointestinal tract. These effects are blocked by classic antihistaminics such as pyrilamine.

Stimulation of the H_2 receptors elicits a variety of responses, the most widely studied of which is gastric acid secretion from the parietal cells of the gastric glands. However, many other effects mediated by H_2 receptors are manifested in peripheral tissues. These include the positive chronotropic action in the auricular muscle, the inotropic action in the ventricular muscle, and the lipolytic effect in fat cells. In addition, the extensive use of cimetidine has led to the synthesis and marketing of more specific and efficacious analogs with pharmacologic properties (see Table 10).

H_3 receptors suppress gastric acid secretion, and this is evoked by cholinergic stimuli. H_3 receptors exist outside the parietal cells and seem to be located on cholinergic and nonadrenergic neurons of the myenteric plexus, where they inhibit the release of neurotransmitters. The agonist and antagonist for H_3 receptors are alpha-methylhistamine and thioperamide, respectively.

HISTOPLASMIN

(Histolyn-CYL, Histoplasmin diluted)

Histoplasmin, a histoplasma capsulatum antigen (0.1 mLof 1:100 dilution interdermally 5 to 10 cm apart into the volar surface of the forearm) is used to assess cell-mediated immunity and in suspected histoplasmosis.

HISTRELIN ACETATE

(Supprelin)

Histrelin, a gonadotropin-releasing hormone, is used in centrally mediated idiopathic or neurogenic precocious puberty (see also Table 15).

HOMATROPINE HYDROBROMIDE

(Lolab)

Homatropine is a moderately long-acting mydriatic and cycloplegic that is used for refraction (1 to 2 drops into each eye) in the treatment of inflammatory conditions of the uveal tract; for preoperative and postoperative states when mydriasis is required; and in axial lens opacities.

HUMAN IMMUNODEFICIENCY VIRUS (HIV) INFECTION: Treatment for

HIV is a single-stranded RNA virus that contains a virally encoded DNA polymerase enzyme, reverse transcriptase (RT). The HIV RT is the enzyme responsible for transcribing viral RNA into DNA, a cytoplasmic event. Following reverse transcription, the HIV DNA enters the cell nucleus and, through the action of another viral enzyme (integrase), is incorporated into the host cell genome. It is this event, the incorporation into host DNA that makes HIV infection a chronic, lifelong disease, because each time the lymphocyte is activated and the DNA transcribed and translated, new HIV virions are created and released.

The classification of antiretroviral agents for HIV infection is primarily based upon the stage of the life cycle that is interrupted by the therapeutic intervention. The primary steps in the life cycle include: (1) viral binding to cell surface receptors; (2) viral entry and uncoating; (3) transcription to DNA via the action of viral reverse transcriptase; (4) integration into the host DNA via the action of viral integrase; (5) transcription of the proviral DNA to mRNA and viral RNA and the translation of other viral proteins; (6) glycosylation of viral proteins; (7) viral assembly; and (8) budding of new viral particles through the host cell membrane (a time during which the action of HIV protease is evident). Each of these stages is currently under investigation in order to examine the potential value at each point of interference with HIV replication.

The medical aspects of HIV infection include:

AIDS-related complex (weight loss, chronic diarrhea, fever, thrush, herpes zoster, fatigue)
Opportunistic infections and cancer
End-stage renal disease
Blindness (cytomegalovirus)
HIV encephalopathy and dementia

The psychological aspects of HIV infection include:

Major depression, regression, and suicidal impulses
Delirium
Substance abuse
Antisocial personality
Bereavement

Patients with a clinical diagnosis of AIDS should undergo long-term therapy with reverse transcriptase inhibitors such as zidovudine (AZT, 1200 mg every 4 hours). Protease inhibitors or antiviral agents such as acyclovir may potentiate the beneficial effects of AZT. In addition, patients should be treated prophylactically for Pneumocystis carinii pneumonia; such regimens include sulfadoxine and pyrimethamine (Fansidar), dapsone, or aerolized pentamidine. Dextran sulfate is also useful because it blocks the binding of HIV to target cells (see Figure 107).

The currently approved reverse transcriptase inhibitors are:

- Didanosine
- Stavudine
- Zalcitabine
- Zidovudine

Protease inhibitors are:

- Indinavir sulfate (Crixivan)
- Ritonavir (Norvir)
- Saquinavir mesylate (Invirase)

HYALURONIC ACID DERIVATIVES

(Hyalgan solution 20 mg sodium hyaluronate per 2 mL)

Hyaluronic acid improves elasticity and viscosity of synovial fluid. It is indicated in the treatment of pain of osteoarthritis of the knee in patients who have failed to respond adequately to conservative nonpharmacologic therapy and to simple analgesics (e.g., acetaminophen); and mid to deep dermal implantation for correction of moderate to severe facial wrinkles and folds, such as nasolabial folds (Restylane).

HYALURONIDASE

(Amphadase solution for injection 150 units/mL (bovine source), Vitrase powder for injection, lyophilized 6200 units (ovine source), solution for injection 200 units/mL (ovine source))

It modifies the permeability of connective tissue through the hydrolysis of hyaluronic acid, which temporarily decreases the viscosity of the cellular cement and promotes diffusion of injected fluids or of localized transudates, thus facilitating their absorption.

Hyaluronidase, an enzyme, is used as an adjunct to increase absorption and dispersion of other injected drugs, as an adjunct to increase the absorption rate of fluids given by hypodermoclysis, and as an adjunct in excretion urography.

HYDRALAZINE HYDROCHLORIDE

(Apresoline tablets 25 mg)

Hydralazine is a peripheral vasodilator that directly relaxes vascular smooth muscle to cause peripheral vasodilation, decreasing arterial BP and peripheral vascular resistance. It is used in the treatment of both essential hypertension (oral form) and severe essential hypertension (parenteral form).

Hydralazine is the drug most often used in the treatment of moderate to severe hypertension. The decrease in total

---

HUNTINGTON'S DISEASE: The Search for Treatment Continues

Huntington's disease (HD) is a progressive degenerative disorder of the central nervous system inherited as an autosomal dominant trait. Clinically, the disorder is characterized by choreoathetosis (with age of onset typically in the late thirties or early forties) and neuropsychiatric disturbance. The striatum is particularly vulnerable to the degenerative disease process, with selective loss of medium spiny neurons and decreased levels of associated neurotransmitters, including substance P, GABA, met-enkephalin, and dynorphin. Although the underlying pathophysiology is unknown, recent theories concerning pathogenesis have involved mitochondrial abnormalities and excitotoxin-mediated damage. The gene for HD has recently been discovered and characterized as an unstable CAG trinucleotide repeat sequence on the short arm of chromosome 4 (now known as IT15). The direct test now available for the HD gene has facilitated disease diagnosis, particularly for those with unclear family history or chorea of uncertain origin; presymptomatic testing is also available.

There is no cure for HD, which, as a rule, terminates fatally 10 to 20 years after clinical onset. There is no treatment for the dementia, but the movement disorder may respond to drugs that interfere with dopaminergic inhibition of striatal output neurons. These include dopamine D_2-receptor-blocking drugs such as haloperidol, 0.5 to 4 mg orally four times daily, or chlorpromazine, 25 to 50 mg orally three times daily; and drugs that deplete dopamine from nerve terminals, such as reserpine, 0.5 to 5 mg orally daily, or tetrabenazine (unavailable in the United States), 12.5 to 50 mg orally three times daily. Drugs that potentiate GABAergic or cholinergic neurotransmission are generally ineffective.

---

peripheral resistance it brings about causes reflex elevation of the heart rate and enhanced cardiac output. This cardiac acceleration, which may precipitate an angina attack in susceptible individuals, can be blocked with beta-adrenergic-blocking agents (see Table 26). Propranolol also has a synergistic effect in reducing blood pressure. Hydralazine use can produce headache, palpitations, and gastrointestinal complications. The long-term administration of large doses causes a reversible lupus erythematosus-like syndrome. Hydralazine does not alter sympathetic functions.

Hydralazine was one of the first orally active antihypertensive drugs to be marketed in the United States; however, the drug initially was used infrequently because of tachycardia and tachyphylaxis. With a better understanding of the compensatory cardiovascular responses that accompany use of arteriolar vasodilators, hydralazine combined with sympatholytic agents and diuretics with greater therapeutic success. Nonetheless, its role in the treatment of hypertension has markedly diminished on account of the subsequent introduction of a new class of antihypertensive drugs.

Hydralazine causes direct relaxation of arteriolar smooth muscle. The molecular mechanisms mediating this action are not clear, but may ultimately involve a fall in intracellular calcium concentrations. Although a variety of changes in cellular signaling pathways are influenced by hydralazine, precise molecular targets that explain its capacity to dilate arteries remain uncertain. The drug does not dilate epicardial coronary arteries or relax venous smooth muscle. **Hydralazine**-induced vasodilation is associated with powerful stimulation of the sympathetic nervous system, likely due to baroreceptor-mediated reflexes, which results in increased heart rate and contractility, increased plasma renin activity, and fluid retention; all of these effects counteract the antihypertensive effect of hydralazine. Although most of the sympathetic activity is due to a baroreceptor-mediated reflex, **hydralazine** may stimulate the release of norepinephrine from sympathetic nerve terminals and augment myocardial contractility directly.

Most of the effects of hydralazine are confined to the cardiovascular system. The decrease in blood pressure after administration of hydralazine is associated with a selective decrease in vascular resistance in the coronary, cerebral, and renal circulations, with a smaller effect in skin and muscle. Because of preferential dilation of arterioles over veins, postural hypotension is not a common problem; hydralazine lowers blood pressure equally in the supine and upright positions.

Hydralazine is well absorbed through the gastrointestinal tract but the systemic bioavailability is low (16% in fast acetylators and 35% in slow acetylators). Hydralazine is *N*-acetylated in the bowel and/or the liver. The half-life of **hydralazine** is 1 hour, and systemic clearance of the drug is about 50 mL/kg per minute.

Two types of adverse effects occur after the use of **hydralazine**. The first, which are extensions of the pharmacological effects of the drug, include headache, nausea, flushing, hypotension, palpitations, tachycardia, dizziness, and angina pectoris. Myocardial ischemia occurs because of the increased O_2 demand induced by the baroreceptor-reflex-induced stimulation of the sympathetic nervous system and also because hydralazine does not dilate the epicardial coronary arteries; thus, the arteriolar dilation it produces may cause a "steal" of blood flow away from the ischemic region. Following parenteral administration to patients with coronary artery disease, the myocardial ischemia may be sufficiently severe and protracted to cause frank myocardial infarction. For this reason, parenteral administration of **hydralazine** is not advisable in hypertensive patients with coronary artery disease, hypertensive agents with multiple cardiovascular risk factors, or in older patients. In addition, if the drug is used alone, there may be salt retention with development of high-output congestive heart failure. When combined with a β-adrenergic-receptor blocker and a diuretic, **hydralazine** is better tolerated. The maximum recommended dose of **hydralazine** is 200 mg per day to minimize the risk of drug-induced lupus syndrome.

HYDROCHLOROTHIAZIDE
(Essidrix, Hydro-Diuril)

The thiazide diuretics, also called sulfonamide or benzothiadiazide diuretics, vary in their actions. For instance, the potency of hydrochlorothiazide is ten times greater than that of chlorothiazide (Diuril), but the two drugs have equal efficacy. The duration of action of hydrochlorothiazide, which is 6 to 12 hours, is equal to that of chlorothiazide. On the other hand, chlorthalidone (Hygroton) has a duration of action lasting 48 hours. Some thiazide derivatives inhibit carbonic anhydrase, which is unrelated to their diuretic activity. Those that are active in this respect may at sufficient dose have the same effect as acetazolamide on bicarbonate excretion. They cause a moderate loss of sodium (5 to 10% of the filtered load), chloride, and water, and the clearance of free water is impaired. They may cause metabolic alkalosis (resorption of bicarbonate and loss of hydrogen ions), hyperuricemia (enhanced resorption of uric acid), or hypokalemia (see also Figure 17).

Thiazide diuretics are used in the treatment of edema of cardiac and gastrointestinal origin and to bring about a state of intravascular volume depletion. Because this depleted intravascular volume is replenished from the interstitial (edematous) sites, the thiazide diuretics should not be administered too frequently. For example, hydrochlorothiazide is given q. other day and chlorthalidone is given once q. 2 to 3 days.

In small doses, thiazide diuretics are extremely effective in controlling essential hypertension. They exert their effects initially by bringing about volume depletion, then reduce the peripheral resistance and sensitivity of vascular receptor sites to catecholamine. Thiazide diuretics are also used in conjunction with antihypertensive medications.

The thiazides decrease the urinary calcium concentration by diminishing glomerular filtration and also enhance the urinary magnesium level.

The thiazide diuretics can reduce free water formation in patients with diabetes insipidus, in whom large amounts of free water are eliminated.

The loss of potassium can produce hypokalemia, which is particularly dangerous in patients receiving digitalis because it increases the risk of arrhythmias. Hypokalemia can be offset either by giving a potassium supplement (potassium chloride), or by the concurrent use of a potassium-sparing diuretic. However, the caregiver should not adopt both measures, because hyperkalemia will result. Hyperglycemia is a potential hazard for patients with diabetes mellitus. Hyperuricemia can precipitate an acute attack of gout, but usually only in those patients who either have already had gout or have a propensity toward it. As thiazides can cause a decrease in the GFR, they should not be used in patients whose renal function is less than one-third of normal. The risk of thiazide-induced hypercalcemia should be kept in mind in patients with conditions such as malignancies or hyperparathyroidism that are associated with hypercalcemia (see also Table 25).

HYDROCHLOROTHIAZIDE/TRIAMTERENE (HCTZ/TRIAMTERENE)

(Maxzide 25 mg tablets 37.5 mg triamterene/25 mg hydrochlorothiazide)

Hydrochlorothiazide/triamterene is a diuretic combination. **Hydrochlorothiazide** inhibits reabsorption of sodium and chloride in the ascending loop of Henle and early distal tubules. **Triamterene** interferes with sodium reabsorption at the distal tubule. The combination provides additive diuretic activity and antihypertensive effects and minimizes potassium depletion. They are indicated in the treatment of edema or hypertension in patients who have, or are at risk of developing, hypokalemia.

An early strategy for the management of hypertension was to alter Na^+ balance by restriction of salt in the diet. Pharmacological alteration of Na^+ balance became practical with the development of the orally active thiazide diuretics. These and related diuretic agents have antihypertensive effects when used alone, and they enhance the efficacy of virtually all other antihypertensive drugs. On account of these considerations, coupled with the very large favorable experience with **Triamterene** (Dyrenium, Maxzide) and **amiloride** (Midamor), these are the only two drugs of this class in clinical use. Both drugs cause small increases in NaCl excretion and usually are employed for their antikaliuretic actions to offset the effects of other diuretics that increase K^+ excretion. Consequently, triamterene and amiloride, along with **spironolactone**, often are classified as potassium (K^+)-sparing diuretics.

The exact mechanism for reduction of arterial blood pressure by diuretics is not certain. Initially, the drugs decrease extracellular volume by interacting with a thiazide-sensitive Na-Cl cotransporter in the kidney, leading to a fall in cardiac output. However, the hypotensive effect is maintained during long-term therapy because of reduced vascular resistance; cardiac output returns to pretreatment values and extracellular volume returns almost to normal because of compensatory responses such as activation of the renin-angiotensin system. How this occurs is unknown; however, thiazides promote vasodilation in isolated vessels from laboratory animals and humans.

Hydrochlorothiazide may open Ca^{2+}-activated K^+ channels, leading to hyperpolarization of vascular smooth muscle cells, which leads in turn to closing of L-type Ca^{2+} channels and a lower probability of opening, resulting in decreased Ca^{2+} entry and reduced vasoconstriction. **Hydrochlorothiazide** also inhibits vascular carbonic anhydrase, which hypothetically may alter smooth-cell systolic pH and thereby cause opening of Ca^{2+}-activated K^+ channels with the consequences noted earlier. The relevance of this intriguing finding to the observed antihypertensive effects of thiazides is speculative.

When a thiazide-class diuretic is utilized as the sole antihypertensive drug (monotherapy), its dose-response curve for lowering blood pressure in patients with hypertension should be kept in mind. Antihypertensive effects can be achieved in many patients with as little as 12.5 mg of **chlorthalidone** (Hygroton) or **hydrochlorothiazide** (Hydrodiuril) daily. Furthermore, when used as monotherapy, the maximal daily dose of thiazide-class diuretics usually should not exceed 25 mg of **hydrochlorothiazide** or chlorthalidone (or equivalent). Even though more diuresis can be achieved with higher doses of these diuretics, evidence indicates that doses higher than this are not generally more efficacious in patients with normal renal function. These doses of **hydrochlorothiazide** are not at the top of the dose-response curve for adverse effects such as K^+ wasting and inhibition of uric acid excretion, emphasizing the importance of knowledge about the dose-response relationships for both beneficial and adverse effects.

Urinary K^+ loss can be a problem with thiazides. Angiotensin-converting enzyme (ACE) inhibitors and angiotensin-receptor antagonists will attenuate diuretic-induced loss of potassium to some degree, and this is a consideration if a second drug is required to achieve further blood pressure reduction beyond that attained with the diuretic alone. Because the diuretic and hypotensive effects of these drugs are greatly enhanced when they are given in combination, care should be taken to initiate combination therapy with low doses of each of these drugs. Administration of ACE inhibitors or angiotensin-receptor antagonists together with other K^+-sparing agents or with K^+ supplements requires great caution; combining K^+-sparing agents with each other or with K^+ supplementation can cause potentially dangerous hyperkalemia in some patients.

In contrast to the limitation on the dose of thiazide-class diuretics used as monotherapy, the treatment of severe hypertension that is unresponsive to three or more drugs may require larger doses of the thiazide-class diuretics. Indeed, hypertensive patients may become refractory to drugs that block the sympathetic nervous system or to vasodilator drugs, because these drugs engender a state in which the blood pressure is very volume-dependent. Therefore, it is appropriate to consider the use of thiazide-class diuretics in doses of 50 mg of a daily **hydrochlorothiazide** equivalent when treatment with appropriate combinations and doses of three or more drugs fail to yield adequate control of the blood pressure. Alternatively, there may be a need to use higher-capacity diuretics such as furosemide, especially if renal function is not normal, in some of these patients. Dietary Na^+ restriction is a valuable adjunct to the management of such refractory patients and will minimize the dose of diuretic that is required. This can be achieved by a modest restriction of Na^+ intake to 2 g daily. More stringent Na^+ restriction is not feasible for most patients. Because the degree of K^+ loss relates to the amount of Na^+ delivered to the distal tubule, such restriction of Na^+ can minimize the development of hypokalemia and alkalosis. The effectiveness of thiazides as diuretics or antihypertensive agents is progressively diminished when the glomerular filtration rate falls below 30 ml/min. One exception is metolazone, which retains efficacy in patients with this degree of renal insufficiency.

Amiloride is a K^+-sparing diuretic that has some efficacy in lowering blood pressure in patients with hypertension. Spironolactone also lowers blood pressure but has some significant adverse effects, especially in men (e.g., impotence, gynecomastia, and benign prostatic hyperplasia). As a result of their capacity to inhibit loss of K^+ in the urine, these drugs are used in the medical treatment of patients with hyperaldosteronism, a syndrome that can lead to hypokalemia. **Triamterene** is a K^+-sparing diuretic that decreases the risk of hypokalemia in patients treated with a thiazide diuretic, but does not have efficacy in lowering blood pressure by itself. These agents should be used cautiously with frequent measurements of K_+ concentrations in plasma in patients predisposed to hyperkalemia. Patients taking spironolactone, amiloride, or **trlamterene** should be cautioned regarding the possibility that concurrent use of K^+-containing salt substitutes could produce hyperkalemia. Renal insufficiency is a relative contraindication to the use of K^+-sparing diuretics. Concomitant use of an ACE inhibitor or an angiotensin-receptor antagonist magnifies the risk of hyperkalemia with these agents.

HYDROCODONE

(Dicodid; Hycodan)

In this synthetic derivative of codeine, a ketone group replaces the –OH of codeine at position 6, and two H atoms are added at positions 7 and 8. It thus bears the same relation to codeine as dihydromorphinone (Dilaudid) does to morphine. It is marketed as the tartrate under the trade names Dicodid and Hycodan and is used chiefly for the relief of cough.

HYDROCODONE BITARTRATE/ACETAMINOPHEN

(Anexsia 5/500 tablets 5 mg hydrocodone bitartrate/500 mg acetaminophen)

Hydrocodone bitartrate is an opioid analgesic combination that inhibits synthesis of prostaglandins, binds to opiate receptors in CNS, and peripherally blocks pain impulse generation; produces antipyresis by direct action on the hypothalamic heat-regulating center; causes cough suppression by direct central action in the medulla; and may produce generalized CNS depression. They are indicated in the management of mild to moderate pain.

Aspirin, **acetaminophen**, the other nonnarcotic nonsteroidal antiinflammatory drugs (NSAIDs) used to treat pain and inflammation, and the drugs used for hyperuricemia and gout.

Most currently available traditional NSAIDs (tNSAIDs) act by inhibiting the prostaglandin G/H synthase enzymes, colloquially known as the **cyclooxygenases**. The inhibition of cyclooxygenase-2 (COX-2) is thought to mediate, in large part, the antipyretic, analgesic, and antiinflammatory actions of tNSAIDs, while the simultaneous inhibition of cyclooxygenase-1 (COX-1) largely but not exclusively accounts for unwanted adverse effects in the gastrointestinal tract.

Acetaminophen is a very weak antiinflammatory drug; it is effective as an antipyretic and analgesic agent at typical doses that partly inhibit COXs, but appears to have fewer gastrointestinal side effects than the tNSAIDs.

All NSAIDs, including selective COX-2 inhibitors, are antipyretic, analgesic, and antiinflammatory, with the exception of acetaminophen, which is antipyretic and analgesic but is largely devoid of antiinflammatory activity.

When employed as analgesics, these drugs usually are effective only against pain of low to moderate intensity, such as dental pain. Although their maximal efficacy is generally much less than the opioids, NSAIDs lack the unwanted adverse effects of opiates in the CNS, including respiratory depression and the development of physical dependence. NSAIDs do not change the perception of sensory modalities other than pain. Chronic postoperative pain or pain arising from inflammation is controlled particularly well by NSAIDs, whereas pain arising from the hollow viscera usually is not relieved. An exception to this is menstrual pain. The release of prostaglandins by the endometrium during menstruation may cause severe cramps and other symptoms of primary dysmenorrhea; treatment of this condition with NSAIDs has met with considerable success. Not surprisingly, the selective COX-2 inhibitors such as **rofecoxib** and **etoricoxib** are also efficacious in this condition.

HYDROCODONE BITARTRATE/CHLORPHENIRAMINE MALEATE

(S-T Forte 2 liquid 2.5 mg hydrocodone bitartrate and 2 mg chlorpheniramine maleate)

Hydrocodone bitartrate/chlorpheniramine maleate is an antitussive combination. **Hydrocodone** suppresses cough reflex; stimulates opiate receptors in the CNS and peripherally blocks pain impulse generation. **Chlorpheniramine** competitively antagonizes histamine at H_1-receptor sites. They provide relief of cough and rhinorrhea; and symptomatic relief of stubborn cough and runny nose caused by cold or allergy.

The following are the therapeutic and side effects of a number of H_1 antagonists based on their chemical structures.

Dibenzoxepin Tricyclics (Doxepin). **Doxepin**, the only drug in this class, is marketed as a tricyclic antidepressant. However, it is also a remarkably potent H_1 antagonist. It can cause drowsiness and is associated with anticholinergic effects. Doxepin is much better tolerated by patients who have depression than by those who do not. In nondepressed patients, sometimes even very small doses, e.g., 20 mg, may be poorly tolerated because of disorientation and confusion.

Ethanolamines (Prototype: Diphenhydramine). These drugs possess significant antimuscarinic activity and have a pronounced tendency to induce sedation. About half of those treated with conventional doses experience somnolence. The incidence of GI side effects, however, is low with this group.

Ethylenediamines (Prototype: Pyrilamine). These include some of the most specific H_1 antagonists. Although their central effects are relatively feeble, somnolence occurs in some patients. GI side effects are quite common.

Alkylamines (Prototype: Chlorpheniramine). These are among the most potent H_1 antagonists. The drugs are less prone than some H_1 antagonists to producing drowsiness and are more suitable agents for daytime use, but again, a significant proportion of patients do experience sedation. Side effects involving CNS stimulation are more common than with other groups.

First-Generation Piperazines. The oldest member of this group, chlorcyclizine, has a more prolonged action and produces a comparatively low incidence of drowsiness. Hydroxyzine is a long-acting compound that is used widely for skin allergies; its considerable CNS-depressant activity may contribute to its prominent antipruritic action. Cyclizine and meclizine have been used primarily to counter motion sickness, although promethazine and diphenhydramine (dimenhydrinate) are more effective.

Second-Generation Piperazines (Cetirizine). Cetirizine is the only drug in this class. It has minimal anticholinergic effects. It also has negligible penetration into the brain but is associated with a somewhat higher incidence of drowsiness than the other second-generation H_1 antagonists.

Phenothiazines (Prototype: Promethazine). Most drugs of this class are H_1 antagonists and also possess considerable anticholinergic activity. Promethazine, which has prominent sedative effects, and its many congeners are used primarily for their antiemetic effects.

First-Generation Piperidines (Cyproheptadine, Phenindamine). Cyproheptadine uniquely has both antihistamine and antiserotonin activity. Cyproheptadine and phenindamine cause drowsiness and also have significant anticholinergic effect.

Second-Generation Piperidines (Prototype: Terfenadine). Terfenadine and astemizole were withdrawn from the market. Current drugs in this class include loratadine, desloratadine, and fexofenadine. These agents are highly selective for H_1 receptors, lack significant anticholinergic actions, and penetrate poorly into the CNS. Taken together, these properties appear to account for the low incidence of side effects of piperidine antihistamines.

HYDROCODONE BITARTRATE/GUAIFENESIN

(Pneumotussin 2.5 cough syrup, 2.5 mg hydrocodone bitartrate and 200 mg guaifenesin)

Hydrocodone bitartrate/guaifenesin is an antitussive and expectorant combination. **Hydrocodone** suppresses cough reflex; stimulates opiate receptors in the CNS and peripherally blocks pain impulse generation. **Guaifenesin** may enhance output of respiratory tract fluid by reducing adhesiveness and surface tension, enhancing removal of viscous mucus, and making nonproductive coughs more productive and less frequent. They are indicated in the symptomatic relief of irritating nonproductive cough associated with upper and lower respiratory congestion.

HYDROCODONE BITARTRATE/IBUPROFEN

(Vicoprofen tablets 7.5 mg hydrocodone bitartrate and 200 mg ibuprofen)

Hydrocodone bitartrate/ibuprofen is an analgesic combination. **Hydrocodone** suppresses the cough reflex; stimulates opiate receptors in the CNS and peripherally blocks pain impulse generation. **Ibuprofen** decreases inflammation, pain, and fever, probably through inhibition of cyclooxygenase activity and prostaglandin synthesis. They are indicated for short-term (generally less than 10 days) management of acute pain; not indicated for treatment of osteoarthritis or rheumatoid arthritis.

HYDROCODONE BITARTRATE/HOMATROPINE METHYLBROMIDE

(Hycodan tablets, syrup 5 mg hydrocodone bitartrate and 1.5 mg homatropine MBr)

Hydrocodone bitartrate/homatropine methylbromide is an antitussive combination. **Hydrocodone** suppresses the cough reflex; stimulates opiate receptors in the CNS and peripherally blocks pain impulse generation. **Atropine** inhibits action of acetylcholine or other cholinergic stimuli at postganglionic cholinergic receptors. They are used for symptomatic relief of cough.

The class of drugs referred to here as muscarinic receptor antagonists includes (1) the naturally occurring alkaloids, atropine and scopolamine; (2) semisynthetic derivatives of these alkaloids, which primarily differ from the parent compounds in their disposition in the body or their duration of action; and (3) synthetic congeners, some of which show selectivity for particular subtypes of muscarinic receptors. Noteworthy agents among the synthetic derivatives are **homatropine** and **tropicamide**, which have a shorter duration of action than atropine, and **methylatropine**, **ipratropium**, and **tiotropium**, which are quaternized and do not cross the blood–brain barrier or readily cross membranes. The latter two agents are given by inhalation in the treatment of chronic obstructive pulmonary disease and are pending approval for use in bronchial asthma. **Ipratropium** also has an FDA-approved indication for perennial- and common cold-associated rhinorrhea. The synthetic derivatives possessing partial receptor selectivity include **pirenzepine**, used in the treatment of acid-peptic disease in some countries, and **tolterodine**, **oxybutynin**, and several others, used in the treatment of urinary incontinence.

Muscarinic receptor antagonists prevent the effects of ACh by blocking its binding to muscarinic cholinergic receptors at neuroeffector sites on smooth muscle, cardiac muscle, and gland cells; in peripheral ganglia; and in the CNS. In general, muscarinic receptor antagonists cause little blockade at nicotinic receptor sites. However, the quaternary ammonium antagonists generally exhibit a greater degree of nicotinic-blocking activity, and consequently are more likely to interfere with ganglionic or neuromuscular transmission.

HYDROCODONE BITARTRATE/PSEUDOEPHEDRINE HYDROCHLORIDE

(Detussin liquid 5 mg hydrocodone bitartrate and 60 mg pseudoephedrine hydrochloride)

Hydrocodone bitartrate/pseudoephedrine hydrochloride is an antitussive preparation. **Hydrocodone** suppresses cough reflex; stimulates opiate receptors in the CNS and peripherally blocks pain impulse generation. **Pseudoephedrine** causes vasoconstriction and subsequent shrinkage of nasal mucous membranes by alpha-adrenergic stimulation, which promotes nasal drainage. They are indicated for suppression of cough and relief of nasal congestion and other symptoms associated with the common cold, allergies, hay fever, sinusitis, and other respiratory illnesses.

HYDROCORTISONE

Hydrocortisone is an adrenocorticoid with both glucocorticoid and mineralocorticoid properties. It is a weak antiinflammatory agent but a potent mineralocorticoid, having potency similar to that of cortisone and twice that of prednisone. Hydrocortisone (or cortisone) is usually the drug of choice for replacement therapy in patients with adrenal insufficiency. It is usually not used for immunosuppressant activity because of the extremely large doses necessary and the unwanted mineralocorticoid effects.

Hydrocortisone and hydrocortisone cypionate (Cortef) may be administered orally. Hydrocortisone sodium phosphate may be administered by IM, SC, or IV injection, or by IV infusion, q. 12-hour interval. Hydrocortisone sodium succinate (A-hydroCort, Lifocort, Solu-Cortef) may be administered by IM or IV injection or IV infusion q. 2 to 10 hours, depending on the clinical situation. Hydrocortisone acetate is a suspension that may be administered by intra-articular, intrasynovial, intrabursal, intralesional, or soft tissue injection. It has a slow onset but a long duration of action. The injectable forms are usually used only when the oral dosage forms cannot be used (see also Table 11).

When administered in high doses or for prolonged therapy, hydrocortisone suppresses release of adrenocorticotropic hormone (ACTH) from the pituitary gland, and the adrenal cortex stops secreting endogenous corticosteroids. Because hydrocortisone suppresses immune response, patients should not be given live virus vaccines.

Hydrocortisone should be used with extreme caution in patients with GI ulceration, renal disease, hypertension, osteoporosis, diabetes mellitus, thromboembolic disorders, seizures, myasthenia gravis, congestive heart failure (CHF), tuberculosis, hypoalbuminemia, hypothyroidism, cirrhosis of the liver, emotional instability, psychotic tendencies, hyperlipidemias, glaucoma or cataracts, because the drug may exacerbate these conditions (see Tables 11 and 14).

HYDROCORTISONE (SYSTEMIC)

(Cortef, Cortenema, Hydrocortone)

HYDROCORTISONE (TOPICAL)

(Acticort, CaldeCORT, Cetacort, Cort-Dome, Cortizone, Dermacort, Dermi Cort, Dermolate, Dermtex HC, HC-JEL, HI-COR, H_2 Cort, Hydro-Tex, Hytone, Nutracort, Penecort, Racet-SE, Synacort)

HYDROCORTISONE ACETATE

(Biosone, Cortifoam)

HYDROCORTISONE ACETATE

(Cortaid, Cort-Dome, Corticaine, Lanacort, Orabase-HCA, Pharma-Cort, Rhulicort)

Hydrocortisone, a topical glucocorticoid with antiinflammatory properties, is indicated in inflammation of corticosteroid-responsive dermatoses, including those on the face, groin, armpits, and under the breasts; and in seborrheic dermatitis of the scalp.

HYDROCORTISONE ACETATE/PRAMOXINE HYDROCHLORIDE

(Analpram HC cream 1% hydrocortisone acetate/1% pramoxine hydrochloride)

Hydrocortisone acetate/pramoxine hydrochloride is a corticosteroid combination. **Hydrocortisone** depresses formation, release and activity of endogenous mediators of inflammation, as well as modifying the body's immune response. **Pramoxine** stabilizes the neuronal membrane of nerve endings with which it comes in contact. They are indicated in topical relief of the inflammatory and pruritic manifestations of corticosteroid-responsive dermatoses.

Keratolytic agents—including **lactic acid**, **glycolic acid**, **salicylic acid**, **urea**, and **sulfur**—are employed to treat various forms of hyperkeratosis ranging from calluses and verrucae to severe xerosis. Lactic and glycolic acid are α-hydroxy acids that are thought to disrupt ionic bonds and thus diminish corneocyte cohesion.

Salicylic acid is a β-hydroxy acid that is thought to function through solubilization of intercellular cement, again reducing corneocyte adhesion. It appears to eliminate the stratum corneum layer by layer from the outermost level downward. This contrasts with the α-hydroxy acids, which preferentially diminish cellular cohesion between the corneocytes at the lowest levels of the stratum corneum.

Urea is an antimicrobial agent that denatures and dissolves proteins and increases skin absorption and retention of water. Sulfur is antiseptic, antiparasitic, antiseborrheic, and keratolytic, accounting for its myriad uses in dermatology.

Keratolytics are available in a multitude of formulations for treating skin diseases. Prolonged use of salicylic acid preparations over large areas, especially in children and patients with renal and hepatic impairment, can result in salicylism. Irritation is a common side effect with higher concentrations. Lactic acid (Lac-hydrin, others) is an emollient that contains 12% lactic acid, which is an effective moisturizer indicated for the treatment of xerosis and ichthyosis vulgaris.

Glycolic acid is marketed in multiple cosmetic preparations (4 to 10%) and is used for the treatment of xerosis, ichthyosis, and photoaging.

HYDROCORTISONE ACETATE/UREA

(Carmol HC cream 1% hydrocortisone acetate and 10% urea)

Hydrocortisone acetate/urea is a corticosteroid combination. **Hydrocortisone** depresses formation, release, and activity of endogenous mediators of inflammation as well as modifying the body's immune response. **Urea** has hydrating and keratolytic properties. They are indicated in the relief of inflammatory and pruritic manifestations of corticosteroid-responsive dermatoses.

HYDROCORTISONE CYPIONATE

(Cortef)

HYDROCORTISONE SODIUM PHOSPHATE

(HydroCortone Phosphate)

HYDROCORTISONE SODIUM SUCCINATE

(A-hydroCort, Efcortelan, Lifocort, Solu-Cortef)

Hydrocortisone salts, possessing glucocorticoid-mineralocorticoid properties, are used in severe inflammation or adrenal insufficiency, in shock (other than adrenal crisis), and as an adjunctive treatment of ulcerative colitis and proctitis (see also Table 11).

HYDROFLUMETHIAZIDE

(Diucardin, Saluron)

Hydroflumethiazide, a thiazide diuretic with antihypertensive properties (25 to 200 mg p.o. daily), is used in edema or hypertension (see also Figure 17).

HYDROMORPHONE HYDROCHLORIDE

(Dilaudid tablets 1 mg, Dilaudid-HP)

Hydromorphone hydrochloride is an opioid analgesic that relieves pain by stimulating opiate receptors in CNS; it also causes respiratory depression, inhibition of cough reflex, peripheral vasodilation, inhibition of intestinal peristalsis, sphincter of Oddi spasm, stimulation of chemoreceptors that cause vomiting, and increased bladder tone. It is indicated for the relief of moderate to severe pain; and control of persistent nonproductive cough.

Hydromorphone, an opioid analgesic (1 to 6 mg p.o. q. 4 to 6 hours p.r.n.), is used in moderate to severe pain (see also Figure 68).

HYDROXYCHLOROQUINE SULFATE

(Plaquenil sulfate tablets 200 mg)

Hydroxychloroquine sulfate is a 4-aminoquinoline compound that interferes with parasitic nucleoprotein (DNA/RNA) synthesis and parasite growth or causes lysis of parasite or infected erythrocytes. In rheumatoid arthritis, it may suppress formation of antigens responsible for symptom-producing hypersensitivity reactions. It is indicated for prophylaxis and treatment of acute attacks of malaria caused by *Plasmodium vivax*, *Plasmodium malariae*, and *Plasmodium ovale*, and susceptible strains of *Plasmodium falciparum*. It is also used for treatment of chronic discoid and systemic lupus erythematosus (SLE) and acute or chronic rheumatoid arthritis in patients not responding to other therapies.

Hydroxychloroquine, a 4-amino-quinoline derivative with antimalarial and antiinflammatory properties (400 mg p.o. weekly), is used in suppressive prophylaxis of malarial attacks.

HYDROXYPROGESTERONE CAPROATE IN OIL

(Delalutin)

Hydroxyprogesterone is a long-acting progestin with a duration of action of 9 to 17 days. It is administered intramuscularly in a dose of 375 mg in primary and secondary amenorrhea, dysfunctional uterine bleeding, and metrorrhagia.

Hydroxyprogesterone suppresses ovulation, causes thickening of cervical mucus, and induces sloughing of the endometrium. It inhibits growth progression of progestin-sensitive uterine cancer tissue by an unknown mechanism.

The concomitant use of hydroxyprogesterone and bromocriptine may cause amenorrhea or galactorrhea, thus interfering with the action of bromocriptine. Concurrent use of these drugs is not recommended.

Hydroxyprogesterone is contraindicated in patients with a history of thromboembolic disorders because of its potential for causing these disorders; in patients with severe hepatic disease because impaired hepatic metabolism may cause the drug to accumulate in patients with breast or genital cancer because it may induce tumor growth; in patients with undiagnosed abnormal vaginal bleeding because the cause should be determined; and in pregnant or breast-feeding women.

Hydroxyprogesterone should be used cautiously in patients with existing conditions that might be aggravated by fluid and electrolyte retention, such as cardiac or renal disease, epilepsy, or migraine. Caution is also advised in administering this agent to diabetic patients (because decreased glucose tolerance may occur) or to patients with a history of mental depression.

HYDROXYUREA

(Hydrea)

Hydroxyurea, an antimetabolite with antineoplastic properties (60 to 80 mg/kg p.o. for a minimum of six weeks), is used in the treatment of melanoma; chronic myelocytic leukemia; recurrent, metastatic, or inoperable ovarian cancer; squamous cell carcinoma of the head and neck; polycythemia vera; and essential thrombocytosis (see also Figure 15).

HYDROXYZINE

(Atarax)

Oral hydroxyzine (50 to 100 mg q.i.d.) is indicated for symptomatic relief of anxiety and tension associated with psychoneurosis and as an adjunct in organic disease states in which anxiety is manifest. Hydroxyzine is used for the management of pruritus due to allergic conditions such as chronic urticaria, atopic and contact dermatoses, and in histamine-mediated pruritus. It is also used as a sedative, as a preanesthetic medication, and following general anesthesia.

Intramuscular hydroxyzine (100 mg q. 4 hours) is indicated for the acutely disturbed or hysterical patient; the acute or chronic alcoholic with anxiety withdrawal symptoms or delirium tremens; as pre- and postoperative and pre- and postpartum adjunctive medication to permit reduction in narcotic dosage, allay anxiety and control emesis; and as an adjunctive therapy in asthma.

Hydroxyzine is a piperazine antihistaminic agent that suppresses activity in the subcortical area of the CNS. It has skeletal muscular relaxant properties and exhibits antiemetic, analgesic, and bronchodilating actions.

Hydroxyzine may be teratogenic in experimental animals and should not be used in pregnancy. It causes drowsiness, and caution should be exercised while performing tasks requiring alertness. Hydroxyzine potentiates the CNS depressant effects of narcotics and barbiturates.

HYOSCYAMINE

(Cystospaz)

HYOSCYAMINE SULFATE

(Anaspaz, Bellaspaz, Cystospaz-M, Levsin, Levsin drops, Levsinex, Timecaps, Neoquess)

Hyoscyamine, a belladonna alkaloid with anticholinergic properties (0.125 to 0.25 mg p.o. t.i.d.), is used in GI tract disorders caused by spasm, and as an adjunctive therapy for peptic ulcers.

HYPERBARIC-OXYGEN THERAPY

Hyperbaric oxygen—100% oxygen at 2 to 3 times the atmospheric pressure at sea level—can result in arterial oxygen tension in excess of 2000 mmHg and oxygen tension in tissue of almost 400 mmHg. Such doses of oxygen have a number of beneficial biochemical, cellular, and physiological effects. Hyperbaric oxygen therapy has been used in carbon monoxide poisoning, compromised skin grafts, decompression sickness, anemia, arterial gas embolism, radiation-induced tissue injury, clostridial myonecrosis, necrotizing fascilitis, refractory osteomyelitis, acute traumatic ischemic injury, problem wounds, and thermal burns.

HYPERGLYCEMIA: Drug-Induced

β_2-adrenergic receptor agonists	Marijuana
Ca^{2+}-channel blockers	Morphine
Clonidine	Nalidixic acid
Diazoxide	Nicotine
Diuretics	Oral contraceptives
Epinephrine	Pentamidine
Glucocorticosteroids	Phenytoin
H_2-receptor blockers	Sulfinpyrazone
Heparin	

HYPERTENSION: Treatment of

Drugs	Adverse Effects
	Angiotensin-Converting Enzyme (ACE) Inhibitors
Captopril	Cough; hypotension, particularly with a diuretic or volume depletion; loss of taste with anorexia; skin rash; bronchospasm; acute renal failure with bilateral renal artery stenosis or stenosis of the artery to a solitary kidney; cholestatic jaundice; angioedema; hyperkalemia if also on potassium supplements or potassium-retaining diuretics; blood dyscrasias and renal damage are rare except in patients with renal dysfunction, and particularly in patients with collagen-vascular disease; may increase fetal mortality and should not be used during pregnancy

Drugs	Adverse Effects
Enalapril	Similar to captopril; pancreatitis
Lisinopril	Similar to captopril
Ramipril	Similar to captopril
	Calcium-Channel Blockers
Diltiazem	Similar to verapamil, but less likely to cause constipation
Isradipine	Similar to nifedipine
Nicardipine	Similar to nifedipine
Nifedipine	Similar to verapamil, but more likely to cause edema, and less likely to cause constipation or AV block; may cause tachycardia; arthralgias
Verapamil	Heart failure; hypotension; AV block; constipation; dizziness; edema; headache; bradycardia
	Diuretics
	Thiazide-Type
Bendroflumethiazide	
Benzthiazide	
Chlorthalidone	Hyperuricemia; hypokalemia; hypomagnesemia; hyperglycemia; hyponatremia; hypercalcemia; pancreatitis; rashes and other allergic reactions; increased serum low-density lipoprotein cholesterol and triglyceride concentrations, may be transient; depression; impotence
Chlorothiazide	
Cyclothiazide	
Hydrochlorothiazide	
Hydroflumethiazide	
Indapamide	
Methyclothiazide	
Metolazone	
Polythiazide	
Quinethazone	
Trichlormethiazide	
	Loop Diuretics
Bumetanide Furosemide	Dehydration; circulatory collapse; thromboembolism; hypokalemia; hypomagnesemia; hypocalcemia; hyperglycemia; metabolic alkalosis; hyperuricemia; blood dyscrasias; rashes; lipid changes as with thiazide-type diuretics
	Potassium-Retaining
Amiloride	Hyperkalemia; GI disturbances; rash; headache
Spironolactone	Hyperkalemia; hyponatremia; gynecomastia; agranulocytosis; menstrual abnormalities; GI disturbances; rash
Triamterene	Hyperkalemia; GI disturbances; increased blood urea nitrogen; metabolic acidosis; nephrolithiasis
	Drugs with Peripheral Sympatholytic Action
	Beta-Adrenergic-Blocking Drugs
Acebutolol	Similar to propranolol, but has intrinsic sympathomimetic activity and is relatively cardioselective, with less lipid changes and resting bradycardia and more antinuclear antibodies; occasional drug-induced lupus erythematosus
Atenolol	Similar to propranolol; relatively cardioselective
Betaxolol	Similar to propranolol; relatively cardioselective
Carteolol	Similar to propranolol, but has intrinsic sympathomimetic activity and less resting bradycardia and lipid changes; asthenia and muscle cramps
Labetalol	Similar to propranolol, but has intrinsic sympathomimetic activity and more orthostatic hypotension; fever; hepatotoxicity
Metoprolol	Similar to propranolol; is relatively cardioselective
Nadolol	Similar to propranolol
Penbutolol	Similar to propranolol, but has intrinsic sympathomimetic activity and fewer bradycardia and lipid changes
Pindolol	Similar to propranolol, but has intrinsic sympathomimetic activity and fewer resting bradycardia and lipid changes
Propranolol	Fatigue; depression; bradycardia; decreased exercise tolerance; congestive heart failure; aggravates peripheral vascular disease; GI disturbances; increased airway resistance; masks symptoms of hypoglycemia; Raynaud's phenomenon; vivid dreams or hallucinations; organic brain syndrome; rare blood dyscrasias and other allergic disorders; increased serum triglycerides, decreased HDL cholesterol; generalized pustular psoriasis; transient hearing loss; sudden withdrawal can lead to exacerbation of angina and myocardial infarction
Timolol	Similar to propranolol
	Peripheral Adrenergic Neuron Antagonists
Guanadrel	Similar to guanethidine, but less diarrhea
Guanethidine	Orthostatic hypotension; exercise hypotension; diarrhea; may aggravate bronchial asthma; bradycardia; sodium and water retention; retrograde ejaculation
Reserpine	Psychic depression; nightmares; nasal stuffiness; drowsiness; GI disturbances; bradycardia

Drugs	Adverse Effects
	Alpha-Adrenergic Blockers
Prazosin	Syncope with first dose; dizziness and vertigo; palpitations; fluid retention; headache; drowsiness; weakness; anticholinergic effects; priapism; urinary incontinence
Terazosin	Similar to prazosin
Doxazosin	Similar to prazosin, but with less hypotension after first dose
	Drugs with Central Sympatholytic Action
Clonidine	Severe insomnia and rebound hypertension; headache; cardiac arrhythmias after sudden withdrawal; CNS reactions similar to methyldopa, but more sedation and dry mouth; bradycardia; contact dermatitis from patches
Guanabenz	Similar to clonidine
Guanfacine	Similar to clonidine, but milder
Methyldopa	Sedation and other CNS symptoms; fever; orthostatic hypotension; bradycardia; GI disorders, including colitis; hepatitis; cirrhosis; hepatic necrosis; Coombs' positive hemolytic anemia; lupuslike syndrome; immune thrombocytopenia; red cell aplasia
	Direct Vasodilators
Hydralazine	GI disturbances; tachycardia; aggravation of angina; headache and dizziness; fluid retention; nasal congestion; rashes and other allergic reactions; lupuslike syndrome; hepatitis; glomerulonephritis
Minoxidil	Tachycardia; aggravation of angina; marked fluid retention; possible pericardial effusion; hair growth on face and body; coarsening of facial features; thrombocytopenia; leukopenia

HYPERTENSIVE EMERGENCIES: Treatment of

Drugs	Class	Comments
		Parenteral
Nitroprusside	Arteriolar and venous vasodilator	Thiocyanate toxicity with prolonged or too rapid infusion; should not be used in pregnancy
Nitroglycerin	Venous vasodilator, arteriolar vasodilator	Headache, tachycardia
Diazoxide	Arteriolar vasodilator	Not for patients with angina pectoris, myocardial infarction, dissecting aneurysm or pulmonary edema; can increase blood sugar; will arrest active labor
Trimethaphan	Ganglionic blocker	Preferred by many for emergency treatment of aortic dissection
Labetalol	Alpha- and beta-adrenergic blocker	80 to 90% response rate; can be followed by same drug taken orally
Hydralazine	Arteriolar vasodilator	May precipitate angina, myocardial infarction; not used for aortic dissection; main use is in pregnancy
Propranolol (Inderal; others)	Beta-adrenergic blocker	Useful as adjunct to potent vasodilators to prevent or treat excessive tachycardia; will not lower blood pressure
Enalaprilat	Angiotensin-converting enzyme inhibitor	Sometimes excessive response; not for use in pregnancy
		Oral
Nifedipine	Calcium-entry blocker	Sometimes excessive response
Clonidine	Central sympatholytic	Sedation prominent; rebound hypertension can occur
Captopril	Angiotensin-converting enzyme inhibitor	Excessive response with renal artery stenosis or after diuretics; not for use in pregnancy

HYPNOTICS

Benzodiazepines
Estazolam
Flurazepam
Quazepam
Temazepam
Triazolam

Barbiturates
Amobarbital
Pentobarbital
Secobarbital

Nonbarbiturate, nonbenzodiazepines
Chloral hydrate
Ethchlorvynol
Methyprylon

Antihistamines
Diphenhydramine
Doxylamine

HYPOGLYCEMIA: Drug-Induced

Angiotensin-converting enzyme inhibitors	Naproxen
β-adrenergic receptor antagonists	Pentamidine
Bromocriptine	
Calcium salts	Pyridoxine
Clofibrate	Salicylates
Ethanol	Sulbactam/ampicillin
Indomethacin	Sulfonamides
Lithium salts	Tetracycline
Mebendazole	Theophylline

HYPOTHALAMIC HORMONES

Agents	Actions
Thyrotropin-releasing hormone (TRH)	Stimulates both thyrotropin (TSH) and prolactin
Gonadotropin-releasing hormone (GnRH) also known as luteinizing hormone releasing hormone (LHRH)	Stimulates both luteinizing hormone (LH) and follicle-stimulating hormone (FSH)
Corticotropin-releasing hormone (CRH)	Stimulates adrenocorticotropin (ACTH)
Growth-hormone-releasing hormone (GHRH)	Stimulates growth hormone
Somatostatin	Inhibits growth hormone
Prolactin inhibitory factor (dopamine)	Inhibits prolactin

I

IBANDRONATE SODIUM

(Boniva tablets 2.5 mg)

Ibandronate is a bisphosphonate that inhibits osteoclast activity and reduces bone resorption and turnover. It is indicated in the treatment and prevention of osteoporosis in postmenopausal women.

IBOPAMINE

Activation of dopamine$_1$ (DA_1) and dopamine$_2$ (DA_2) receptors reduces blood pressure. DA is not useful as an antihypertensive agent because of its alpha-adrenoreceptor activity. However, extensive studies in patients with hypertension have demonstrated that, after administration of alpha-adrenoreceptor-blocking agents, arterial pressure is decreased with maintenance or improvement of renal blood flow.

Ibopamine is the diisobutryic ester of *N*-methyl dopamine (epinine). Epinine is released from ibopamine by plasma esterases after oral ingestion. Epinine is a DA_1-agonist that produces greater alpha-adrenoreceptor actions than DA; in addition, it is a potent beta$_2$-adrenoreceptor agonist. Ibopamine has been studied extensively for the treatment of congestive heart failure. A large number of invasive studies have shown that oral ingestion of 50 to 300 mg of ibopamine increases the cardiac index and decreases systemic vascular resistance. Diuretic and natriuretic effects also have been reported in several studies.

Unlike with levodopa, nausea and vomiting do not occur with ibopamine, apparently because ibopamine does not penetrate the chemoreceptor trigger zone in the area postrema. Ibopamine may cause heartburn. Large doses of ibopamine have been shown to produce transient elevations of pulmonary wedge pressure in some patients with severe congestive heart failure (CHF), but this effect does not appear to be a serious problem with smaller doses.

IBUPROFEN

(Advil tablets 200 mg)

Ibuprofen is a NSAID that decreases inflammation, pain, and fever, probably through inhibition of cyclooxygenase activity and prostaglandin synthesis. It is indicated in the relief of symptoms of rheumatoid arthritis, osteoarthritis, mild to moderate pain, primary dysmenorrhea, and reduction of fever.

Ibuprofen has analgesic, antipyretic, and antiinflammatory actions. It is indicated in the treatment of primary dysmenorrhea (400 mg q. 4 hours), in the management of fever (5 to 10 mg/kg), and for relief of the signs and symptoms of rheumatoid arthritis and osteoarthritis (300 to 800 mg q.i.d).

Ibuprofen should be administered cautiously to patients with a history of gastrointestinal (GI) disease, hepatic or renal disease, cardiac decompensation, systemic lupus erythematosus, or bleeding abnormalities, because the drug may worsen these conditions.

Patients with known "triad" symptoms (aspirin hypersensitivity, rhinitis/nasal polyps, and asthma) are at high risk of bronchospasm. Concomitant use of ibuprofen with anticoagulants and thrombolytic drugs (coumarin derivatives, heparin, streptokinase, or urokinase) may potentiate anticoagulant effects. Bleeding problems may occur if ibuprofen is used with other drugs that inhibit platelet aggregation, such as azlocillin, parenteral carbenicillin, dextran, dipyridamole, mezlocillin, piperacillin, sulfinpyrazone, ticarcillin, valproic acid, cefamandole, cefoperazone, moxalactam, plicamycin, salicylates, or other antiinflammatory agents. Ibuprofen may displace highly protein-bound drugs from binding sites. Toxicity may occur with coumarin derivatives, phenytoin, verapamil, or nifedipine. Increased nephrotoxicity may occur with gold compounds, other antiinflammatory agents, or acetaminophen. Ibuprofen may decrease the renal clearance of methotrexate and lithium. Antacids may decrease the absorption of ibuprofen. Ibuprofen may decrease effectiveness of diuretics and antihypertensive medications. Concomitant use with diuretics may increase nephrotoxicity. Concomitant use with furosemide and thiazides may decrease their effectiveness. Clinical manifestations of overdose include dizziness, drowsiness, paresthesia, vomiting, nausea, abdominal pain, headache, sweating, nystagmus, apnea, and cyanosis (see also Table 3).

IBUTILIDE FUMARATE

(Corvert solution 0.1 mg/mL)

Ibutilide is an antiarrhythmic agent that prolongs atrial and ventricular action potential duration and refractoriness by activation of a slow inward current (predominantly sodium). It is indicated for rapid conversion of recent onset atrial fibrillation or atrial flutter to sinus rhythm.

Ibutilide: Ibutilide (Corvert) is an I_{Kr} blocker that in some systems also activates an inward Na^+ current. The action-potential-prolonging effect of the drug may arise from either mechanism. **Ibutilide** is administered as a rapid infusion (1 mg over 10 minutes) for the immediate conversion of atrial fibrillation or flutter to sinus rhythm. The drug's efficacy rate is higher in patients with atrial flutter (50 to 70%) than in those with atrial fibrillation (30 to 50%). In atrial fibrillation, the conversion rate is lower in those in whom the arrhythmia has been present for weeks or months compared with those in whom it has been present for days. The major toxicity with ibutilide is **torsade de pointes**, which occurs in up to 6% of patients and requires immediate cardioversion in up to one-third of these. The drug undergoes extensive first-pass metabolism, and so is not used orally. It is eliminated by hepatic metabolism and has a half-life of 2 to 12 hours (average of 6 hours).

IDARUBICIN

(Idamycin PFS solution for injection 1 mg/mL)

Idarubicin is an anthracycline, which is a DNA-intercalating analog of daunorubicin, which has an inhibitory effect nucleic acid synthesis and interacts with the enzyme topoisomerase II.

Idarubicin, an antibiotic with antineoplastic activity (12 mg/m2 daily by slow IV injection), is indicated in the treatment of acute myelocytic leukemia in adults, including fragment, antigen-binding, classification M^1 through M^7, in combination with other approved antileukemic agents.

Daunorubicin, **doxorubicin**, **epirubicin**, **idarubicin**, and **mitoxantrone**, anthracycline antibiotics, are among the most important antitumor agents. They are derived from the fungus *Streptococcus peucetius* var. caesius. **Idarubicin** and epirubicin are analogs of the naturally produced anthracyclines, differing only slightly in chemical structure but having somewhat distinct patterns of clinical activity. Daunorubicin and **idarubicin** have been used primarily in the acute leukemias, whereas doxorubicin and epirubicin display broader activity against human solid tumors. These agents, which all possess potential for generating free radicals, cause an unusual and often irreversible cardiomyopathy, the occurrence of which is related to the total dose of the drug. The structurally similar agent mitoxantrone has useful activity against prostate cancer and AML, and is used in high-dose chemotherapy. **Mitoxantrone**, an anthracenedione, has significantly less cardiotoxicity than do the anthracyclines.

IDOXURIDINE

(IDU, Herplex, Stoxik)

Idoxuridine (1 drop into infected eye/hr during the day and q. 2 hours at night) is indicated in the treatment of herpes simplex keratitis. By altering normal DNA synthesis, idoxuridine inhibits the reproduction of herpes simplex virus. IDU replaces thymidine in the enzymatic step of viral replication, produces faulty DNA, and hence a structure that loses its ability to infect and destroy ocular tissue. Corticosteroids can accelerate the spread of a viral infection and are usually contraindicated in herpes simplex epithelial infections. Idoxuridine occasionally causes irritation, pain, pruritus, inflammation or edema of the eyes or lids; and allergic reactions, photophobia, corneal clouding, stippling, and punctate defects in the corneal epithelium. The punctate defects may be a manifestation of the infection, as healing usually takes place without interruption of therapy.

IFOSFAMIDE

(Ifex powder for injection)

Ifosfamide is a nitrogen mustard. Ifosfamide requires metabolic activation by microsomal liver enzymes to produce biologically active metabolites. Enzymatic oxidation of the chloroethyl side chains and subsequent dealkylation produces the major urinary metabolites, dichloroethyl ifosfamide and dichloroethyl cyclophosphamide. The alkylated metabolites of ifosfamide interact with DNA. It is indicated in germ cell testicular cancer.

Ifosfamide is an oxazaphosphorine, similar to cyclophosphamide. Cyclophosphamide has two chloroethyl groups on the exocyclic nitrogen atom, whereas one of the two-chloroethyl groups of ifosfamide is on the cyclic phosphoamide nitrogen of the oxazaphosphorine ring. Ifosfamide is activated in the liver by CYP3A4. The activation of **ifosfamide** proceeds more slowly, with greater production of dechlorinated metabolites and chloroacetaldehyde. These differences in metabolism likely account for the higher doses of **ifosfamide** required for equitoxic effects, the greater neurotoxicity of ifosfamide, and the possible differences in antitumor spectrum of the two agents.

Although initially considered an antimetabolite, the triazene derivative 5-(3,3-dimethyl-*l*-triazeno)-imidazole-4-carboxamide, usually referred to as **dacarbazine** or DTIC, functions through alkylation.

The alkylating agents differ in their patterns of antitumor activity and in the sites and severity of their side effects. Most cause dose-limiting toxicity to bone marrow elements, and to a lesser extent, intestinal mucosa. Most alkylating agents, including **nitrogen mustard**, **melphalan**, **chlorambucil**, **cyclophosphamide**, and **ifosfamide**, cause acute myelosuppression, with a nadir of the peripheral blood granulocyte count at 6 to 10 days and recovery in 14 to 21 days. Cyclophosphamide has lesser effects on peripheral blood platelet counts than do the other agents. Busulfan suppresses all blood elements, particularly stem cells, and may produce a prolonged and cumulative myelosuppression lasting months or even years. For this reason, it is used as a preparative regimen in allogenic bone marrow transplantation. **Carmustine** and other **chloroethylnitrosoureas** cause delayed and prolonged suppression of both platelets and granulocytes, reaching a nadir 4 to 6 weeks after drug administration and reversing slowly thereafter.

Both cellular and humoral immunity are suppressed by alkylating agents, which have been used to treat various autoimmune diseases. Immunosuppression is reversible at doses used in most anticancer protocols.

In addition to effects on the hematopoietic system, alkylating agents are highly toxic to dividing mucosal cells, leading to oral mucosal ulceration and intestinal denudation. The mucosal effects are particularly significant in high-dose chemotherapy protocols associated with bone marrow reconstitution, as they predispose to bacterial sepsis arising from the gastrointestinal tract. In these protocols, cyclophosphamide, melphalan, and thiotepa have the advantage of causing less mucosal damage than the other agents.

CNS toxicity is manifest in the form of nausea and vomiting, particularly after intravenous administration of nitrogen mustard or BCNU. Ifosfamide is the most neurotoxic of this class of agents, producing altered mental status, coma, generalized seizures, and cerebellar ataxia. These side effects have been linked to the release of chloroacetaldehyde from the phosphate-linked chloroethyl side chain of ifosfamide. High-dose busulfan may cause seizures; in addition, it accelerates the clearance of phenytoin, an antiseizure medication.

Ifosfamide in high doses for transplant causes a chronic, and often irreversible, renal toxicity. Proximal, and less commonly distal, tubules may be affected, with difficulties in Ca^{2+} and Mg^{2+} reabsorption, glycosuria, and renal tubular acidosis. Nephrotoxicity is correlated with the total dose of drug received and increases in frequency in children less than 5 years of age. The syndrome has been attributed to chloroacetaldehyde and/or acrolein excreted in the urine.

In summary, ifosfamide, an alkylating agent with antineoplastic properties (1.2 g/m^2/day IV for 5 days), is indicated in the treatment of testicular cancer. In addition, ifosfamide has been used in lung cancer, Hodgkin's and non-Hodgkin's lymphoma, breast cancer, acute and chronic lymphocytic leukemia, ovarian cancer, and sarcomas.

ILOPROST

(Ventavis inhalation solution 20 mcg)

Iloprost is a prostacyclin analog that dilates systemic and pulmonary arterial vascular beds. It is indicated in the treatment of pulmonary arterial hypertension.

IMATINIB

(Gleevec tablets 100 mg)

Imatinib is a protein-tyrosine-kinase inhibitor. Imatinib inhibits proliferation and induces apoptosis in BCR-ABL positive cell lines as well as fresh leukemic cells from Philadelphia chromosome-positive (Ph+) chronic myeloid leukemia (CML). Imatinib inhibits tumor growth of BCR-ABL transfected murine myeloid cells and BCR-ABL positive leukemia lines derived from CML patients in blast crisis. It also inhibits the receptor tyrosine kinases for platelet-derived growth factor (PDGF) and stem cell factor (SCF), c-Kit, and inhibits PDGF- and SCF-mediated cellular events. It is indicated in the treatment of newly diagnosed adult patients with Ph+ CML in chronic phase; patients with Ph+ CML in blast crisis, accelerated phase, or in chronic phase after failure of interferon-alpha treatment; children with Ph+ chronic phase CML whose disease has recurred after stem cell transplant or who are resistant to interferon-alpha therapy; and treatment of gastrointestinal stromal tumors (GIST).

Protein kinases are ubiquitous and critical components of signal transduction pathways that transmit information concerning extracellular or cytoplasmic conditions to the nucleus, thereby influencing gene transcription and/or DNA synthesis. The human genome contains approximately 550 protein kinases and an additional 130 protein phosphatases that regulate the activity of the various protein kinases. The protein kinases can be classified into three different categories: tyrosine kinases, with specific activity for tyrosine residues only, serine/threonine kinases, with activity for serine and threonine residues only, and kinases with activity for all three residues. Tyrosine kinases can be further subdivided into proteins that have an extracellular ligand binding domain (receptor tyrosine kinases) and enzymes that are confined to the cytoplasm and/or nuclear cellular compartment (nonreceptor tyrosine kinases). Abnormal activation of specific protein tyrosine kinases has been demonstrated in many human neoplasms, making them attractive molecular targets for cancer therapy. **Imatinib** and **Gefitinib** are two of these protein kinase inhibitors.

IMIPENEM-CILASTATIN

(Primaxin IV powder for injection 250 mg imipenem equivalent and 250 mg cilastatin equivalent)

Imipenem inhibits bacterial cell wall synthesis. Cilastatin prevents metabolism of imipenem, resulting in increased urinary recovery and decreased renal toxicity. They are indicated in the treatment of serious infections of the lower respiratory tract and urinary tract, intra-abdominal and gynecologic infections, bacterial septicemia, bone and joint infections, skin and skin structure infections, endocarditis, and polymicrobic infections due to susceptible microorganisms.

IMIPENEM-CILASTATIN SODIUM

(Primaxin I.M., Primaxin I.V.)

Imipenem, a carbapanem (thienamycin class), beta-lactam antibiotic (750 mg IM q. 12 hours), is indicated in mild to moderate lower respiratory tract, skin and skin-structure, or gynecologic infections; mild-to-moderate intra-abdominal infections; in serious respiratory and urinary tract infections; intra-abdominal, gynecologic, bone, joint, or skin infections; bacterial septicemia; or endocarditis.

IMIPRAMINE

(Tofranil)

The dibenzapine derivatives are called tricyclic antidepressants and include imipramine (Tofranil), desipramine (Norpramin), amitriptyline (Elavil), nortriptyline (Aventyl), protriptyline (Vivactil), and doxepin (Adapin).

Imipramine is demethylated to desipramine, and amitriptyline is demethylated to nortriptyline. Both metabolites are active antidepressants. Tricyclic antidepressants bind to plasma proteins to the extent of 90%, and, because of their extensive first-pass metabolism in the liver, they have very low and variable bioavailability. In circumstances when it is desirable to measure the plasma concentrations of these

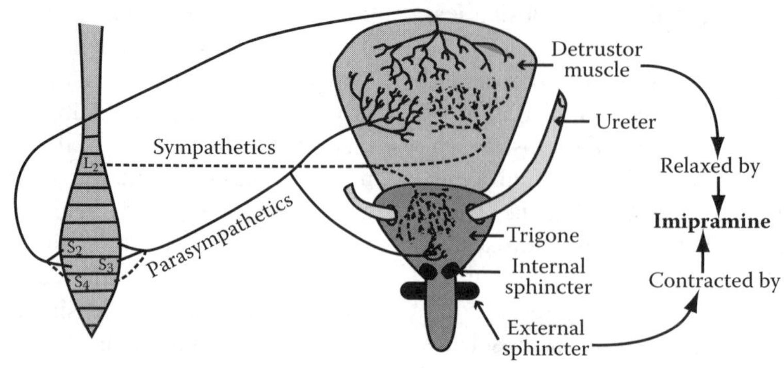

Figure 60 The anticholinergic effect of **imipramine** has been used successfully in managing **enuresis**.

drugs, the concentrations of their active metabolites should also be measured (Figure 60).

They resemble the phenothiazide derivatives such as chlorpromazine in structure and function. Like the phenothiazine derivatives (e.g., chlorpromazine), tricyclic antidepressants (e.g., imipramine) may reduce the seizure threshold and precipitate seizures in epileptic patients, and may cause cholestatic jaundice, movement disorders, and hematologic side effects.

Unlike the phenothiazine derivatives, the tricyclic antidepressants may increase motor activity, are antidepressant, have a very slow onset and long duration of action, and have a relatively narrow margin of safety and a strong anticholinergic effect. In fact, dry mouth is the most common side effect, and other anticholinergic effects, such as tachycardia, loss of accommodation, constipation, urinary retention, and paralytic ileus, have been reported (see Tables 5 and 7).

Tricyclic antidepressants, like some of the phenothiazine derivatives, are sedative in nature. Those compounds containing a tertiary amine (imipramine, amitriptyline, and doxepin) are the most sedative. Those compounds containing a secondary amine (nortriptyline and desipramine) are less so, and protriptyline has no sedative effect (see Tables 5 and 7).

Tricyclic antidepressants, like some of the phenothiazine derivatives (e.g., thoriodazine), have an anticholinergic property. Amitriptyline is the strongest in this regard, and desipramine is the weakest.

The tricyclic antidepressants also have cardiovascular actions. In particular, they cause orthostatic hypotension by obtunding the various reflex mechanisms involved in maintaining blood pressure.

Antidepressants may block the uptake of norepinephrine or serotonin (see Table 5).

In addition to possessing anticholinergic properties, antidepressants exhibit affinity for alpha$_1$- and alpha$_2$-adrenergic receptors, histaminergic (H_1) receptors, and dopaminergic (D_2) receptors (see Table 5).

The first-generation tricyclic antidepressants, the monoamine oxidase inhibitors, and the newer agents can cause sedation, insomnia, orthostatic hypotension, or nausea. Because of their anticholinergic properties, they may also produce cardiac toxicities. A primary indication for the use of tricyclic antidepressants is endogenous depression. Before treating an endogenous depression, however, it should first be differentiated from sadness. Disabling depression and its vegetative symptoms generally respond to tricyclic antidepressants but sadness does not, though it does respond to changes in environmental events. The effective dose of tricyclic antidepressants, which are equivalent drugs, is chosen empirically. The less sedative agents are chosen for apathetic and withdrawn patients. Because the margin of safety for these agents is narrow, they should not be prescribed in large quantities for a depressed patient who may use them to attempt suicide. The anticholinergic effect of imipramine has been used successfully in managing enuresis (see Figure 41).

The pain associated with diabetic peripheral neuropathy, trigeminal neuralgia, or cancer may predispose such patients to depression. Tricyclic antidepressants have been shown to be effective adjuncts in managing these and similar conditions. Some episodic phobias are regarded as "masked" depression and thus respond to treatment with tricyclic antidepressants. Fluoxetine, in addition to its antidepressant property, has been used as an appetite suppressant. Imipramine and desipramine have been used as antibulimic substances. Desipramine has been used as part of the treatment of alcoholism. Because depression has led to relapsed drinking in alcoholics striving to maintain sobriety, treatment with antidepressants may reverse or prevent these depressive symptoms. They may also correct the biochemical abnormalities hypothesized to underlie both depression and alcoholism, thus helping to ensure abstinence in recovering alcoholics.

Currently, overdoses of tricyclics are one of the most serious types of poisoning encountered in clinical practice because depressed patients who are treated with these drugs are also those who are the most prone to using them for suicidal purposes.

The diagnostic triad of coma, seizures, and cardiac arrhythmias should raise the suspicion of tricyclic overdose if there is otherwise no verified history of drug intake. Cardiac arrhythmias and conduction abnormalities are the major distinguishing features. A trial dose of intravenously administered physostigmine (1 to 4 mg) may suggest the diagnosis, because this will awaken the comatose patient or mitigate the arrhythmias. The effects of physostigmine are transient, and it is not a definitive treatment. Other problems encountered in such poisonings include neuromuscular irritability, delirium, hyperpyrexia, hypotension, and bladder or bowel paralysis. The cardiac arrhythmias are life threatening, so the patient must be closely monitored, with facilities available for possible resuscitation. Drugs such as quinidine and procainamide are contraindicated, but lidocaine, propranolol, or phenytoin have been used safely and effectively. The arterial blood gas levels, pH, and electrolyte concentrations should be monitored so that metabolic acidosis or hypokalemia can be identified that would further aggravate the arrhythmias. Electrical pacing may be required if the antiarrhythmic drugs fail. Hyperpyrexia is treated by cooling. Seizures may be managed by intravenous doses of diazepam.

IMIQUIMOD

(Aldara cream 5%)

Imiquimod is a topical immunomodulator. Imiquimod induces mRNA encoding cytokines, including interferon-alpha at the treatment site. It is indicated in the treatment of external genital and perianal warts/condyloma acuminata; treatment of clinically typical, nonhyperkeratotic, nonhypertrophic actinic keratosis on the face or scalp in immunocompetent adults; and treatment of biopsy-confirmed, primary superficial basal cell carcinoma in immunocompetent adults, with a maximum tumor diameter of 2 cm located on the trunk, neck, or extremities.

Imiquimod [1-(2-methylpropyl)-1*H*-imdazo[4,5-c]quino-lin-,4,amine] is a novel immunomodulatory agent that is effective for topical treatment of condylomata acuminata and certain other dermatologic conditions. It lacks direct antiviral or antiproliferative effects *in vitro* but rather induces cytokines and chemokines with antiviral and immunomodulating effects. **Imiquimod** shows antiviral activity in animal models after systemic or topical administration. When applied topically as a 5% cream to genital warts in humans, it induces local IFN-α, -β, and -γ TNF-α responses, and causes reductions in viral load and wart size. When applied topically (three times weekly for up to 16 weeks), **imiquimod** cream is associated with complete clearance of treated genital and perianal warts in about 50% of patients, with response rates being higher in women than in men. The median time to clearance is 8 to 10 weeks; relapses are not uncommon. Application is associated with local erythema in about 20% of patients, excoriation/flaking in 18 to 26%, itching in 10 to 20%, burning in 5 to 12%, and less often, erosions or ulcerations.

IMMUNE GLOBULIN

(Gamma Globulin; IG; Immune Serum Globulin; ISG)

IMMUNE GLOBULIN FOR IM USE

(IGIM) (Gamastan, Gammar)

IMMUNE GLOBULIN FOR IV USE

(IGIV) (Gamimune N, Gammagard, Gammar-IV, Iveegam, Sandoglobulin, Venoglobulin-1)

Immune globulin is indicated in patients with agammaglobulinemia or hypogammaglobulinemia.

IMMUNE GLOBULIN INTRAMUSCULAR (ISG)

(BayGam injection)

Immune globulin intramuscular is an immune globulin that replaces normal human IgG antibodies. It is indicated in passive immunization against or modification of hepatitis A; prevention or modification of measles in susceptible persons exposed less than 6 days previously; passive immunization against varicella in immunocompromised patients if varicella zoster immune globulin (VZIG) is not available and IGIM can be given promptly; and IgG replacement therapy in certain persons with hypoglobulinemia or agammaglobulinemia.

Intravenous Immunoglobulin (**IVIG**): In recent years, indications for the use of IVIG have expanded beyond replacement therapy for agammaglobulinemia and other immunodeficiencies include a variety of bacterial and viral infections, and an array of autoimmune and inflammatory diseases as diverse as thrombocytopenic purpura, Kawasaki's disease, and autoimmune skin, neuromuscular, and neurologic diseases. Although the mechanism of action of IVIG in immune modulation remains largely unknown, proposed mechanisms include modulation of expression and function of Fc receptors on leukocytes and endothelial cells, interference with complement activation and cytokine production, provision of antiidiotypic antibodies, and effects on the activation and effector function of T- and B-lymphocytes. Although IVIG is effective in many autoimmune diseases, its spectrum of efficacy and appropriate dosing (especially duration of therapy) are unknown. Additional controlled studies of IVIG are needed to identify proper dosing, cost–benefit, and quality-of-life parameters.

IMMUNE GLOBULIN IV (IGIV)

(Carimune NF powder for injection)

Immune globulin is an immune globulin that replaces normal human IgG antibodies; and promotes opsonization, fixes complement, and neutralizes bacteria, viruses, fungi, and parasites, and their toxins. It is indicated in the treatment of primary immunodeficiency states in patients unable to produce sufficient amounts of IgG antibodies.

IMMUNIZATION: Agents Used in

Passive Immunization

Antitoxins	
Botulism	
Diphtheria	
Tetanus	
Immunoglobulins	
Endotoxin (IgM)	Rubella
Hepatitis A or B	Tetanus
Pertussis	Vaccinia
Poliomyelitis	Varicella
Rabies	

Active Immunization

Bacterial	**Viral**
Cholera	Hepatitis B
Diphtheria	Influenza
Hemophilus	Measles
Meningococci	Mumps
Pertussis	Poliomyelitis
Pneumococci	Rabies
Tetanus	Rubella
Tuberculosis (BCG)	Smallpox
Typhoid	Yellow fever

IMMUNOSUPPRESSIVE MEDICATIONS

Agents	Actions	Side Effects
Glucocorticoids	Rheumatoid arthritis	Cushing's syndrome
	Systemic lupus erythematosus	Ulcers
	Autoimmunity	
	Transplantation	
Cyclophosphamide	Rheumatoid arthritis	Myelosuppression
	Systemic lupus erythematosus	Alopecia
		GI symptoms
		Cystitis
		Infertility
Azathioprine	Rheumatoid arthritis	Myelosuppression
	Systemic lupus erythematosus	GI symptoms
	Polymyositis	Hepatotoxicity
	Collagen diseases	
	Transplantation	
Methotrexate	Psoriasis	Myelosuppression
	Arthritis	Enteritis
	Dermatomyositis	Pulmonary fibrosis
Cyclosporine A	Systemic lupus erythematosus	Hepatotoxic
	Type I diabetes	Renotoxic
	Psoriasis	Neurotoxic
	Uveitis	Hypertension
	Transplantation	

IMMUNOTHERAPY OF CANCER

Tumor immunology is a scientific discipline that is driven by clinical translation. For many decades, scientists both at the bench and at the bedside have struggled with determining the role immunity may play in tumor eradication, if any. For many years, the major question driving the field was whether human tumors were immunogenic. Over the last decade, literally thousands of immunogenic proteins related to tumors have been identified, resulting in a host of new targets for immunomodulation.

Successful active immunization against cancer has long been a goal of tumor immunologists. Generating a native endogenous immune response against cancer offers many advantages as compared with more standard anticancer therapies. Stimulating a cellular immune response would allow cancer cells to potentially be eradicated at multiple metastatic sites as competent T-cells can "home" to antigen. Successful vaccination would generate immunological memory, allowing the eradication of tumors at times of disease relapse, which may take place years after primary therapy. The identification of specific tumor antigens has fueled the development of a variety of vaccine technologies aimed at increasing the magnitude of the tumor-specific immune response. Furthermore, technologies have been developed to quantitatively and reproducibly measure tumor immunity. Immunological monitoring techniques have evolved from novel laboratory tools to robust clinical assays capable of estimating the potency of immune-based therapies.

Vaccines for protection against infectious agents have been one of the most successful interventions in medicine. However, few vaccines are utilized to treat ongoing established infections. Similarly, cancer vaccines have had little success in eradicating growing cancers. The last several years have led to the development of a variety of clinical strategies that may prove more effective in established disease states. Adoptive T-cell therapy, donor lymphocyte infusion after transplant, or infusions of novel cytokines may all boost tumor-specific T-cell immunity above the level that can be achieved with vaccination alone. Indeed, stimulating the "graft-versus-leukemia effect" with donor lymphocyte infusion in subjects who have relapsed after allogeneic transplants for hematopoietic malignancy has become a standard of care and a lifesaving measure. Thus, immune-based strategies can be developed both to prevent relapse in minimal residual disease states, as well as to treat existing cancers.

The last decade of research in tumor immunology has seen the adoption of a multitude of immune-based therapies into the standard practice of oncology. Monoclonal antibodies targeting tumor antigens have revolutionized cancer treatment for patients with lymphoma, breast cancer, and other solid tumors. Antibody therapy has now been shown to have both biological, as well as immunological, effects. Antibodies targeting growth factor receptors will bind to inhibit cell signaling and limit unregulated growth. However, the binding of a monoclonal antibody may also activate immune system cells to respond to antigens expressed by tumors, thus stimulating endogenous immunity.

Finally, the role of the tumor microenvironment is critical in modulating and shaping the tumor-specific immune response. Advances in recent years have pointed to the most important mechanisms limiting the immune response in cancer patients, and these environmental influences can be modulated *in vivo* with novel reagents. Thus, treatments are directed both at initiating and expanding a cancer-specific immune response, as well as reigning in the environment from preventing the function of immune effectors. Clearly, combination immune-based approaches may be more potent than any strategy used in isolation.

Discovery of Target Molecules for Cancer Immunotherapy by Genetic and Bioinformatic Approaches

It has been a long-standing vision of scientists studying tumor immunology to use the immune system's effectors for the therapy of cancer by directing them against target molecules expressed selectively on tumor cells. Different genetic approaches for discovery of such target candidates have been developed over the last 15 years and are being pursued. The classical approaches apply expression cloning using either cancer-reactive T-lymphocytes or autoantibodies in crude patient sera as probes to identify target molecules of spontaneous immune responses. Recent concepts utilizing high-density microarray analysis, subtractive library approaches, or *in silico* cloning aim at the identification of genes with cancer cell-associated expression and subsequently address the immunogenicity of such molecules with reverse immunology.

Current Strategies for the Identification of Immunogenic Epitopes of Tumor Antigens

Peptide-based cancer immunotherapy relies on the identification of epitopes recognized by T-lymphocytes. Because of the high degree of polymorphism of human leukocyte antigens and issues of tumor escape from the immune response, the availability of a wide choice of diverse epitopes is essential for the therapist. There are a number of different approaches for identifying new class I- and class II-restricted target antigens appropriate for immunotherapy. The strategy of "reverse immunology" is applied for prediction of tumor-associated antigens by *in silico* screening sequences of selected proteins for peptides with high binding affinity to different human leukocyte antigen molecules. Subsequently, these peptides are synthesized and tested experimentally.

Natural-Killer Cells in Cancer Immunotherapy

Natural-killer (NK) cells are a class of lymphocytes distinct in their ability to identify and kill transformed self-cells without priming. Recognition is via receptors that bind unique but common surface molecules induced on these cells. These properties characterize NK cells as unique effectors for use in immunotherapy.

The Role of Immune Monitoring in Evaluating Cancer Immunotherapy

Just as cancer vaccines have evolved tremendously over the past decades, so too have the methods used to monitor the immune responses that they are intended to induce.

DNA Vaccines for Cancer Immunotherapy

The introduction of selected genes by direct injection of DNA represents a general strategy for short-term gene expression *in vivo*. DNA vaccines may be especially useful for cancer immunotherapy because DNA allows transient expression of tumor-associated antigens and immunostimulatory proteins by a relatively nonimmunogenic vector.

Dendritic Cells

Dendritic cells (DCs) have been called "nature's adjuvant" because of their remarkable ability to elicit adaptive, antigen-specific immunity. Immature DCs are highly specialized to capture antigens, but are poor at priming or activating T-cells. Following antigen capture or in a proinflammatory environment, DCs undergo a process of maturation in which antigen-carrying capacity is greatly reduced as T-cell priming and activating capacity are increased.

DCs are tightly regulated by expression of chemokine receptors whose expression varies according to the maturation state, microenvironmental milieu, and type of DC. Three principal subsets of human DCs are recognized: Langerhans' DCs, myeloid DCs, and plasmacytoid DCs. Much is now known regarding the lineage origins and specialized functions of these subsets, although much remains to be learned, and controversies abound.

Anti-Idiotype Antibody Vaccines for the Immunotherapy of Cancer

Certain anti-idiotypic (Id) antibodies that bind to the antigen-combining sites of antibodies can effectively mimic the three-dimensional structures and functions of the external antigens and can be used as surrogate antigens for active specific immunotherapy. Several monoclonal anti-Id antibodies that mimic distinct human tumor-associated antigens have been developed and characterized. CeaVac (anti-Id 3H1) is an internal image anti-Id antibody that mimics a distinct and specific epitope of carcinoembryonic antigen (CEA) and can be used as a surrogate for CEA. Extensive preclinical studies, as well as results obtained from clinical trials, suggest that vaccination with 3H1 has the potential to augment survival benefits. Anti-Id 3H1 easily breaks immune tolerance to CEA and induces anti-CEA antibody, as well as $CD4^+$ T-helper, responses in colorectal cancer patients and also in mice transgenic for CEA.

Autologous Tumor-Derived Heat Shock Protein Vaccine as a New Paradigm for Individualized Cancer Therapeutics

Heat shock proteins (HSPs) are a group of highly conserved and abundant molecules across all organisms. HSPs are molecular chaperones that are further induced in response to the accumulation of misfolded proteins in the cell. They are essential in chaperoning proteins and maintaining the correct conformation of protein substrates. Recently, these molecules have been implicated in bridging innate and adaptive immunity, owing to their ability to chaperone antigenic peptides and their surprising property of being able to modulate the functional status of professional antigen-presenting cells.

Tumor-Reactive T-Cells for Adoptive Immunotherapy

Adoptive T-cell therapy is based on specificity and efficacy, two essentials known to be necessary for successful cancer therapy. Tumor-reactive T-cells potentially display both characteristics in terms of antigen recognition and antitumor activity. In recent years, novel technologies have been established for the identification, isolation, activation, and expansion of human T-cells, which have greatly facilitated the further development of adoptive T-cell transfer regimens. Lessons learned from the first clinical trials revealed that the complexity of the *in vivo* environment interferes with the efficacy of transferred T-cells, such as tolerance induction and outgrowth of tumor escape variants. The results from these studies can be concluded by the following critical, but nevertheless encouraging, statement: "Tumor regressions observed after adoptive T-cell transfer are too frequent to be spontaneous." As these trials are not solely conducted for treating cancer patients, but also for research purposes, the resulting scientific observations have increased our understanding of T-cell activation, homing, and survival, as well as of the possibility of disrupting regulatory mechanisms. The knowledge drawn from the first generation of transfer studies can be implemented in the next generation of clinical trials. T-cell-based immunotherapy regimens are currently being combined with other immunological strategies in order to coordinate an effective attack against tumors. Further development of combinatorial therapies involving immunological and molecular technologies will offer the means to tailor adoptive transfer of T-cell immunity for each cancer patient.

T-Cell Adoptive Immunotherapy of Cancer

The T-cells of many cancer patients are naturally sensitized to tumor-associated antigens or can readily be sensitized with even simple vaccination maneuvers. Adoptive immunotherapy (AIT) constitutes a coordinated effort to harvest and activate such T-cells, propagate them in culture, and adoptively transfer them back into patients as therapy. Recent modifications in culture techniques, coupled with the administration of nonmyeloablative chemotherapy, have markedly improved the clinical impact of AIT in melanoma patients. Whereas such results clearly validate the capacity of AIT to cause regression of macroscopic tumors, not just micrometastases, it remains difficult to predict which patients receiving autologous T-cells will respond to AIT, and it remains poorly understood why tumor regressions tend to be partial and impermanent at best in the clinical setting. Continuing insights from preclinical mouse studies illuminate the complexities of AIT treatment failure and point to many underlying correctable elements, such as the inadvertent coadoptive transfer of passenger suppressor cells and both positive and negative impacts of culture on effector T-cell trafficking and apoptotic susceptibility. In addition, current investigations demonstrate distinctive and often synergistic roles for $CD4^+$ and $CD8^+$ subsets in AIT, which have so far not been superseded merely by giving higher doses of either subset alone. Despite the currently nonoverlapping contributions of $CD4^+$ and $CD8^+$ subsets to therapeutic outcome, it is anticipated that continuing strides in culture techniques may ultimately produce $CD4^+$ and $CD8^+$ subsets that each possess true stand-alone potency as adoptive monotherapy.

Retroviral-Mediated Gene Transfer for Engineering Tumor-Reactive T-Cells

Immunotherapy for cancer has taken several approaches including vaccinating patients to elicit T-cell responses to tumor antigens and adoptive transfer of tumor-reactive T- cells to patients. Vaccination has historically been ineffective in generating objective clinical responses. Whereas adoptive cell transfer therapy has shown some promise, the difficulties in obtaining the large number of requisite tumor-reactive T-cells warrant investigation into alternate models of immunotherapy. A novel approach is the retroviral-mediated transfer of genes encoding recognition of tumor antigens into peripheral blood T-cells. By cloning genes for T-cell receptors that mediate antitumor reactivity and introducing them into a patient's own T-cells, we can rapidly generate the large number of T cells necessary for adoptive transfer therapy for any patient, regardless of the patient's immune status.

Harnessing the Potential of Graft-versus-Tumor

The curative potential of allogeneic hematopoietic stem cell transplantation in treating cancer is derived in large part from the donor immune system reacting against host or tumor cell antigens to generate a graft-versus-tumor (GVT) effect. Whereas early animal models suggested this allogeneic immune response, evidence for its role in human transplantation was not realized until the late 1970s and early 1980s, when the association between graft-versus-host disease and tumor response became clear. In this section, the animal and human data that established the

GVT effect as the major therapeutic component of allogeneic hematopoietic stem cell transplantation are reviewed, and ongoing efforts to understand and build on GVT as a therapeutic modality for other tumor types are described. The current thinking on the biology of the effectors and modulators of GVT are discussed. The progress that has been made in clinical application of immunotherapy in the autologous setting and of solid tumor therapy in the allogeneic setting is reviewed. Finally, the potential for continued advances in the efficacy and safety of immunotherapy for cancer is explored, as reflected in recent and ongoing efforts to apply the growing understanding of alloreactivity toward fulfillment of the potential for targeted antitumor therapies.

Tumor-Induced Immune Suppression and Immune Escape

A large body of evidence supports the notion that both the adaptive and nonadaptive immune systems play an important role in the control of tumor progression in patients with malignant disease. These findings have provided the rationale for the development of active specific immunotherapy for the treatment of malignant disease. The enthusiastic application of active specific immunotherapy in a large number of patients has conclusively shown that:

- Several of the immunization strategies used elicit a **tumor antigen** (TA)-specific immune response.
- The results of immunomonitoring assays in patients treated with active specific immunotherapy have poor, if any, predictive value of clinical responses.
- Irrespective of the TA or immunization strategy used, clinical responses have only occasionally been observed.
- Disease frequently progresses and recurs in spite of induction and/or persistence of TA-specific immune responses.

These disappointing findings are likely to reflect, at least in part, the ability of tumor cells to manipulate the ongoing TA-specific immune response as well as evade immune recognition and destruction, utilizing multiple mechanisms. The latter include tumor cell-induced qualitative and/or quantitative defects in the generation and maintenance of TA-specific immune responses, tumor cell-induced immune suppression, and/or changes in the antigenic profile of tumor cells because of their genetic instability.

The Tumor Microenvironment

After more than 30 years of crusading against cancer, targeting mostly the tumor cell cycle, the need for novel therapeutic strategies has become increasingly clear. Survival and expansion of tumor cells cannot be achieved in the absence of a favorable microenvironment, the main components of which are leukocytes, vascular cells, and fibroblasts. This tumor microenvironment critically provides growth factors and survival signals for tumor cell proliferation, secretes angiogenic factors that control tumor vascularization, and directs invasion and metastasis through adhesion molecule interactions. In addition, a successful antitumor immune response is prevented by multiple mechanisms of evasion orchestrated by nontumor cells. Understanding how the tumor microenvironment modulates the immune response is vital to designing new potential ways of boosting anticancer immunity.

Manipulation of Lymphocyte Homeostasis for Enhancing Antitumor Immunity

Our appreciation of how the immune system recognizes and destroys cancer has led to the advancement of innovative approaches to be used for the treatment of cancer patients. The concept of immunotherapy is based on the body's immune system's ability to combat potentially dangerous assaults to the host such as those occurring from infection, but also those from transformed malignant cells. T-lymphocytes are capable of eliminating transformed cells after recognizing specific tumor antigens expressed on their cell surfaces. Thus, one immediate goal of tumor immunology is the development of effective approaches to harness the immune system's natural tendency to eliminate cancer. However, the processes that govern the total size and diversity of the T-cell pool represent a major barrier for the induction of effective antitumor immune responses. It is proposed that cancer vaccines intended to generate effective antitumor responses have been unsuccessful to control disease because of inadequate T-cell activation, the fleeting duration of antitumor T-cell responses, and an active suppressor system that downplay immune responses.

Manipulating Immunological Checkpoints to Maximize Antitumor Immunity

Initial clinical trials have demonstrated the safety and bioactivity of cancer vaccines, but vaccine-induced immune responses have seldom translated into clinically meaningful tumor regressions, particularly in advanced disease. It is increasingly clear that tumor-specific immune tolerance represents a layered system of controls that keep the immune system turned off. Immunoregulatory checkpoints map locoregionally to the tumor microenvironment and draining lymph nodes, and arise from the dynamic interactions between the tumor and the immune system. It is now apparent that cancer vaccines will have to be combined with other therapeutics that abrogate immune tolerance, further amplify vaccine-induced T-cell responses, or modify the tumor microenvironment to make it more conducive to the concerted action of innate and antigen-specific immune effector mechanisms.

Interleukin-2 as Cancer Therapy

Interleukin (IL)-2 is the only interleukin that has fully evolved from a partially purified product of activated T-cells to a commercially approved, bacterially produced recombinant human protein. Since 1992, IL-2 has been marketed for the treatment of advanced renal cancer, and its approval for advanced melanoma followed several years later. Whereas early efforts to characterize the mechanisms of action of IL-2 led to heightened understanding of cellular and cytokine interactions in malignancy and nonmalignant states, more recent efforts have focused on improving the therapeutic index of IL-2-based therapy. Optimal combinations of IL-2 with other agents such as antibodies, chemotherapeutics, and other cytokines for use in solid tumors, hematological malignancies, and nonmalignant diseases remain under active investigation. Other strategies that have emerged from the relative success of IL-2-based therapies include the development of immunocytokines and other structures containing an active IL-2 molecule covalently bound to a second molecule that redirects effector cells, prolongs the half-life, or alters the pharmacology of the IL-2 molecule. The use of IL-2 in immunization strategies is another area of active investigation, particularly for vaccine approaches that include *ex vivo* sensitization of T-cells to tumor antigens by antigen-presenting cells. Complementing the rapid advances in IL-2-based therapeutic manipulations of immune effector subsets is the recent discovery of IL-2-receptor-bearing regulatory T-cells and other counter-regulatory mechanisms of control or "escape" that will require careful study as more effective immunotherapy regimens are designed.

Biological and Clinical Properties of the type 1 Interferons

Interferons (IFNs) are class 2 cytokines that carry out important physiological functions in higher vertebrates, particularly in the regulation of host adaptive and innate immune responses. Virus and other innate immune stimuli induce expression of type 1 IFNs, which then act on responsive cells to establish an antiviral state. Type 1 IFN effects are mediated by the protein products of IFN-responsive genes, the identities and functions of which are only now starting to emerge fully. In a clinical setting, type 1 IFNs, IFN-α in particular, have shown effectiveness against a variety of malignancies. Current efforts aimed at improving pharmacokinetic and pharmacodynamic profiles of IFNs, identifying subtypes with novel biological activities and/or establishment of combined treatment modalities involving type 1 IFNs should lead to future improvements in therapeutic effectiveness.

Promising Γ-Chain Cytokines for Cancer Immunotherapy

The molecular identification of a plethora of T-cell tumor antigens that can serve as targets for many human cancers, and the clinical development of techniques to administer tumor vaccines, represent important advances toward the development of T-cell-specific immunotherapy for cancer. Despite this progress, current clinical results demonstrate that tumor vaccines, as single agents, are generally not potent enough to induce regression of existing tumors or long lasting enough to provide durable adjuvant benefit. Similarly, the full effectiveness of adoptive cellular therapies for cancer immunotherapy has not yet been realized because of difficulties in sustaining T-cells *in vivo* following adoptive transfer. Thus, the present challenge for the field of tumor immunology is to develop clinically applicable approaches for amplifying the T-cell-specific immunity induced by tumor vaccines and for augmenting survival of cells delivered in the context of adoptive therapies. The family of cytokines that signals through the common cytokine γ-chain (γ_c) demonstrates potent effects on T-cell development, expansion, and viability. IL-2, a prototypic member of this family, has already demonstrated antitumor effects in some settings. However, recent studies have demonstrated that other members of the γ_c cytokine family possess characteristics that render them more favorable than IL-2 for amplifying T-cell-specific immunity toward tumors. IL-7, IL-15, and IL-21 have all shown promise in preclinical models of tumor immunotherapy. IL-7 is notable for its capacity to serve as an immunorestorative agent, as well as its ability to augment both CD4 and CDS immune responses, with a particular capacity to amplify low-affinity, subdominant immune responses that are characteristically induced by tumor antigens. IL-15 provides potent survival and differentiation signals to both CDS memory cells and natural-killer cells, features that are likely to be translatable in the context of both tumor vaccines and adoptive immunotherapy. IL-21 is less well studied than IL-7 or IL-15, but appears able to amplify responses to other cytokines, especially IL-15, thus further augmenting effector and memory cell expansion. Thus, a large amount of preclinical data suggest that integration of one or several new γ_c cytokines into immunotherapy regimens for cancer will play an important role in moving this field closer to clinical efficacy.

Antibody Therapy for Solid Tumors

Over the last several years the use of **monoclonal antibody** (MAb) **therapy** for the treatment of human malignancy has advanced from experimental therapy to the standard of care for some malignancies. The success of MAb therapy stems not only from the ability to humanize the antibody, thus decreasing the inherent immunogenicity of the approach, but also from targeting appropriate proteins. Human cancers associated with the overexpression of particular growth factor receptors such as HER-2/neu, **epidermal growth factor receptor**, and vascular endothelial growth factor, have been impacted by commercially available antibodies.

Antibody Therapy for Non-Hodgkin's Lymphoma
Monoclonal antibodies have made a significant impact on the treatment of **non-Hodgkin's lymphoma** (NHL), and there has been a dramatic increase in clinical data regarding their use. The anti-CD20 antibody, **rituximab**, has shown substantial single-agent activity in both indolent and **aggressive B-cell lymphomas**. Rituximab is now standard therapy in relapsed indolent NHL, and it is the frontline treatment in combination with **cyclophosphamide/doxorubicin/vincristine/prednisone** chemotherapy for patients with large **B-cell lymphoma**. Combinations of rituximab with other cytotoxic agents or cytokines are currently being explored in a number of different studies, and some of these combinations show promise for the future. Other antibodies directed at different targets on lymphoma cells, such as **epratuzumab**, **apolizumab**, **alemtuzumab**, and **galiximab**, have also shown clinical activity in early trials. The radio-conjugated anti-CD20 antibodies ^{90}**yttrium ibritumomab tiuxetan** and ^{131}**iodine tositumomab** also have significant clinical activity in low-grade B-cell NHL, and the former has demonstrated superior complete response rates when compared with rituximab. The challenge for the future will be to determine the place of each antibody in the treatment of NHL.

INAMRINONE
(Inocor injection 5 mg/mL)

Inamrinone is an inotropic agent having positive inotropic effects with vasodilator activity. It is indicated in short-term management of CHF in patients whose condition can be closely monitored and who have not responded adequately to digitalis, diuretics, or vasodilators.

INDAPAMIDE
(Lozol tablets 1.25 mg)

Indapamide is a thiazide diuretic that enhances excretion of sodium, chloride, and water by interfering with transport of sodium ions across renal tubular epithelium. It is indicated in the treatment of edema associated with CHF, hepatic cirrhosis, renal dysfunction, and corticosteroid or estrogen therapy; and management of hypertension.

Indapamide is a sulfonamide diuretic that has been used for treatment of hypertension (2.5 to 5.0 mg/day). It has been proposed as an alternative antihypertensive agent with both diuretic and vasodilatory capability and a more favorable side-effect profile than the thiazides. Indapamide exerts its antihypertensive effect by two mechanisms. It appears to have a modest diuretic effect while also relaxing vascular smooth muscle. As a diuretic, indapamide increases the excretion of sodium, chloride, and water by interfering with the transport of sodium across the renal tubular epithelium. Its principal site of action remains controversial but is probably either at the diluting segment of the loop of Henle or the proximal segment of the distal tubule (see also Table 25 and Figure 17).

In studies with healthy volunteers, the bioavailability of indapamide after a single oral dose is about 90%. Coadministration with food or antacids does not significantly reduce the bioavailability. Peak plasma concentrations occur at 0.5 to 2 hours and remain fairly constant for up to 8 hours. Indapamide is widely distributed throughout the body with an apparent volume of distribution around 25 L. Indapamide has been shown to cause a significant reduction in total peripheral resistance and mean arterial pressure. Cardiac index and heart rate are essentially unchanged. Compared with the thiazide diuretics, indapamide causes little increase in the percentage of filtered sodium excreted. Indapamide administration causes a significant increase in plasma renin activity. Plasma aldosterone concentrations are increased by around 50%, and urinary aldosterone excretion is more than doubled with chronic indapamide therapy. Unlike the thiazide diuretics, 2.5 mg/day of indapamide has little effect on the glomerular filtration rate or effective renal plasma flow in hypertensive patients. Indapamide is indicated as a first-line treatment of the salt and fluid retention associated with congestive heart failure (CHF). Studies have shown that it can be as safe and effective in the treatment of pitting edema (both from CHF and other causes) as hydrochlorothiazide. It has also been shown to decrease urinary calcium excretion in patients with idiopathic hypercalciuria. Indapamide does cause a statistically significant reduction in mean serum potassium value.

IN VITRO FERTILIZATION: Drugs for

In vitro fertilization (IVF) has resulted in thousands of pregnancies for infertile couples. Clomifene (clomiphene citrate), human menopausal gonadotrophin (hMG; menotropins), and subsequent generations of products are commonly used as stimulation agents. In conjunction with the stimulation agents, gonadotrophin-releasing hormone (GnRH) agonists and human chorionic gonadotrophin (hCG) serve as adjuvants for successful control of all events in the induction process. Midazolam, nuperidine, or fentanyl may be used for oocyte recovery. If full anesthesia is required for gamete intrafallopian tube transfer or zygote intrafallopian tube transfer, balanced anesthesia with nitrous oxide and an opioid appears to be the most appealing option.

INDECAINIDE HYDROCHLORIDE

(Decabid)

Indecainide is a class 1C antiarrhythmic agent structurally similar to aprindine. Similar to encainide (Enkaid) and flecainide (Tambocor), indecainide suppresses premature ventricular complexes (PVCs) and depresses intramyocardial conduction. Indecainide prolongs the PR and QRS intervals, significantly increasing intraventricular conduction time without significantly affecting atrial or ventricular refractoriness. There appear to be no significant hemodynamic effects. Indecainide is absorbed well orally, is metabolized in the liver to desisopropyl indecainide, and is excreted in the urine. The side effects of indecainide are dizziness, headache, blurry vision, impotence, lightheadedness, confusion, and thought disorders.

INDENOLOL

Indenolol is a new antihypertensive agent with beta$_1$-adrenoceptor antagonist and beta$_2$-adrenoceptor agonist properties.

INDINAVIR SULFATE

(Crixivan capsules 100 mg)

Indinavir sulfate is a protease inhibitor that inhibits human immunodeficiency virus (HIV) protease, the enzyme that cleaves viral polyprotein precursors into functional proteins in HIV-infected cells. Inhibition of this enzyme by indinavir results in formation of immature noninfectious viral particles. It is indicated in the treatment of HIV infection in combination with other antiretroviral agents.

Indinavir (800 mg/t.i.d.) is an inhibitor of the HIV protease, which is an enzyme required for the proteolytic cleavage of the viral polyprotein precursors into the individual functional proteins found in infectious HIV. Indinavir binds to the protease active site and inhibits the activity of the enzyme. This inhibition prevents cleavage of the viral polyproteins resulting in the formation of immature noninfectious viral particles. Cross-resistance between indinavir and HIV reverse-transcriptase inhibitors is unlikely because the enzyme targets involved are different. Cross-resistance was noted between indinavir and the protease inhibitor ritonavir. Varying degrees of cross-resistance have been noted between indinavir and other HIV protease inhibitors. Indinavir is metabolized in the liver, and seven metabolites have been identified, and 20% of indinavir is excreted unchanged in the urine.

Nephrolithiasis, including flank pain with or without hematuria (including microscopic hematuria), has been reported in approximately 4% of patients receiving crixivan in clinical trials. In general, these events were not associated with renal dysfunction and resolved with hydration and temporary interruption of therapy (e.g., 1 to 3 days).

Indinavir should not be administered concurrently with terfenadine, astemizole, cisapride, triazolam, and midazolam because competition for cytochrome P450 3A4 by indinavir could result in inhibition of the metabolism of these drugs and create the potential for serious and/or life-threatening events (i.e., cardiac arrhythmias, prolonged sedation).

Indinavir is a peptidomimetic hydroxyethylene HIV protease inhibitor. It is formulated as the sulfate salt to yield better solubility and more consistent plasma concentrations as compared with the free base. The molecule was based on a renin inhibitor with some similarity to a phenylalanine-proline cleavage site in the HIV polyprotein, although **indinavir** is not itself a renin inhibitor. Indinavir is tenfold times more potent against the HIV-1 protease than that of HIV-2, and its 95% inhibitory concentration (IC_{95}) for wild-type HIV-1 ranges from 25 to 100 nM.

Indinavir is selectively toxic by potently inhibiting the HIV-encoded protease but not host-encoded aspartyl proteases. Indinavir reversibly binds to the active site of HIV protease, preventing polypeptide processing and subsequent virus maturation. Virus particles are produced in the presence of indinavir but are noninfectious.

Viral replication in the presence of **indinavir** selects for drug-resistant virus. The primary **indinavir** resistance mutations occur at HIV protease codons 46 (a methionine-to-isoleucine or leucine), 82, and 84. However, secondary resistance mutations can accumulate at codons 10, 20, 24, 46, 54, 63, 71, 82, 84, and 90, and these are associated with clinical **indinavir** resistance as well as cross-resistance to other HIV protease inhibitors.

Indinavir is absorbed rapidly after oral administration, with peak concentrations achieved in approximately 1 hour. Unlike other drugs in this class, food can adversely affect indinavir bioavailability; a high-calorie, high-fat meal reduces plasma concentrations by 75%. Absorption is unaffected by light low-fat meals. Therefore, indinavir must be taken while fasting or with a low-fat meal. **Indinavir** has the lowest protein binding of the HIV protease inhibitors, with only 60% of drug bound to plasma proteins. As a consequence, indinavir has higher fractional CSF penetration than other drugs in this class, although the clinical significance of this is unknown.

Indinavir undergoes extensive hepatic metabolism by CYP3A4. Indinavir and its metabolites are eliminated primarily in feces (81% of parent drug and metabolites). Plasma indinavir concentrations may increase with moderate liver disease, and dose reduction may be required. The short half-life of indinavir makes thrice-daily (every 8 hours) dosing necessary. However, **indinavir** clearance is greatly reduced by low doses of ritonavir, which also overcomes the deleterious effect of food on bioavailability. This allows indinavir to be dosed twice daily regardless of meals.

A unique and common adverse effect of indinavir is **crystalluria** and **nephrolithiasis**. This stems from the poor solubility of the drug, which is lower at pH 7.4 than at pH 3.5. Precipitation of indinavir and its metabolites in urine can cause renal colic, and nephrolithiasis occurs in approximately 3% of patients. Patients must drink sufficient fluids to maintain dilute urine and prevent renal complications. Risk of nephrolithiasis is related to higher plasma drug concentrations, which presumably produce higher urine concentrations, regardless of whether or not the drug is combined with ritonavir.

Indinavir frequently causes unconjugated **hyperbilirubinemia**, and 10% of patients develop an indirect serum bilirubin concentration of greater than 2.5 mg/dL. This is generally asymptomatic and is not associated with serious long-term sequelae. As with other HIV protease inhibitors, prolonged administration of indinavir is associated with the HIV **lipodystrophy** syndrome, especially fat accumulation. **Indinavir** has been associated with hyperglycemia and can induce a relative state of insulin resistance in healthy HIV-seronegative volunteers following a single 800-mg dose. Dermatologic complications have been reported, including hair loss, dry skin, dry and cracked lips, and ingrown toenails. Gastrointestinal side effects are less common with indinavir than with other HIV protease inhibitors.

Patients taking indinavir should drink at least 2 L of water daily to prevent renal complications. As indinavir solubility decreases at higher pH, antacids or other buffering agents should not be taken at the same time. Didanosine formulations containing an antacid buffer should not be taken within 2 hours before or 1 hour after **indinavir**. Like most other HIV protease inhibitors, **indinavir** is metabolized by CYP3A4 and is a moderately potent CYP3A4 inhibitor. Indinavir should not be coadministered with other CYP3A4 substrates that have a narrow therapeutic index.

Indinavir raises rifabutin concentrations and increases rifabutin toxicity; the rifabutin daily dose, therefore, should be reduced by 50%. Drugs that induce CYP3A4 may lower indinavir concentrations and should be avoided. **Rifampin** lowers the indinavir AUC by 90% and is contraindicated; efavirenz, nevirapine, and rifabutin lower **indinavir** levels less substantially (by 25% to 35%) and may necessitate an increased indinavir dose.

Large clinical trials have demonstrated both virologic and survival benefit of indinavir three times daily in combination with **zidovudine** and **lamivudine**. Twice-daily administration of the same total daily dose of indinavir (without ritonavir) was less efficacious, possibly reflecting inadequate trough concentrations with less frequent dosing. However, when combined with ritonavir and nucleoside analogs, twice-daily indinavir produces viral load reductions comparable with those of other HIV protease inhibitor regimens.

INDOMETHACIN

(Indocin)

Indomethacin, which has analgesic, antipyretic, and antiinflammatory actions, is indicated in moderate to severe rheumatoid arthritis (25 mg t.i.d.), in moderate to severe ankylosing spondylitis, in moderate to severe osteoarthritis, in bursitis or tendinitis (75 to 150 mg daily), and in acute gouty arthritis (50 mg t.i.d.) (see Figure 14 and Table 3).

The patency of the ductus arteriosus is maintained in part by prostaglandin. Indomethacin induces constriction of the ductus during the neonatal period, whereas infusion of prostaglandin E_1 maintains its patency (Figure 61).

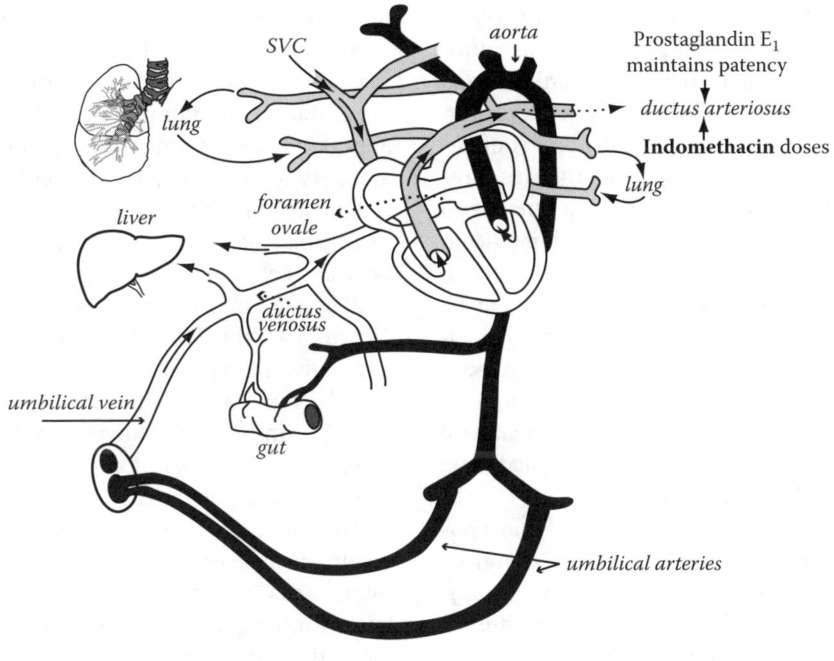

Figure 61 The patency of the ductus arteriosus is maintained in part by a prostaglandin. **Indomethacin** induces constriction of the ductus during the neonatal period, whereas infusion of prostaglandin E_1 maintains its patency.

Concomitant use of indomethacin with anticoagulants and thrombolytic drugs (coumarin derivatives, heparin, streptokinase, or urokinase) may potentiate anticoagulant effects. Bleeding problems may occur if indomethacin is used with other drugs that inhibit platelet aggregation, such as azlocillin, parenteral carbenicillin, dextran, dipyridamole, mezlocillin, piperacillin, sulfinpyrazone, ticarcillin, valproic acid, cefamandole, cefoperazone, moxalactam, plicamycin, salicylates, or steroids, which may cause increased GI adverse effects, including ulceration and hemorrhage. Aspirin may decrease the bioavailability of indomethacin. Because of the influence of prostaglandins on glucose metabolism, concomitant use with insulin or oral hypoglycemic agents may potentiate hypoglycemic effects. Indomethacin may displace highly protein-bound drugs from binding sites. Toxicity may occur with coumarin derivatives, phenytoin, verapamil, or nifedipine; increased nephrotoxicity may occur with gold compounds, other antiinflammatory agents, or acetaminophen. Indomethacin may decrease the renal clearance of methotrexate and lithium. Concurrent use with antihypertensive medications and diuretics may decrease their effectiveness. Concurrent use with triamterene is not recommended due to potential nephrotoxicity. Other diuretics may also predispose patients to nephrotoxicity. Clinical manifestations of overdose include dizziness, nausea, vomiting, intense headache, mental confusion, drowsiness, tinnitus, sweating, blurred vision, paresthesias, and convulsions. Patients over age 60 may be more susceptible to the toxic effects of indomethacin. The effects of indomethacin on renal prostaglandins may cause fluid retention and edema, a significant drawback for elderly patients and those with congestive heart failure.

Indomethacin was the product of a laboratory search for drugs with antiinflammatory properties. It was introduced in 1963 for the treatment of rheumatoid arthritis and related disorders. It is a nonselective COX inhibitor. Although indomethacin still is used clinically and is effective, toxicity and the availability of safer alternatives have limited its use. **Sulindac** was developed in an attempt to find a less toxic, but effective, congener of indomethacin and also is a nonselective COX inhibitor.

Indomethacin has prominent antiinflammatory and analgesic–antipyretic properties similar to those of the salicylates. **Indomethacin** is a more potent inhibitor of the cyclooxygenases than is aspirin, but patient intolerance generally limits its use to short-term dosing. Indomethacin has analgesic properties distinct from its antiinflammatory effects, and there is evidence for central and peripheral actions.

Indomethacin also inhibits the motility of polymorphonuclear leukocytes and depresses the biosynthesis of mucopolysaccharides. It also may have a direct, cyclooxygenase-independent vasoconstrictor effect. Observational studies have raised the possibility that indomethacin may increase the risk of myocardial infarction and stroke, but controlled clinical trials to address this hypothesis have not been performed.

Oral **indomethacin** has excellent bioavailability. Peak concentrations occur 1 to 2 hours after dosing. Indomethacin is 90% bound to plasma proteins and tissues. The concentration of the drug in the CSF is low, but its concentration in synovial fluid is equal to that in plasma within 5 hours of administration.

Between 10 and 20% of **indomethacin** is excreted unchanged in the urine, partly by tubular secretion. The majority is converted to inactive metabolites, including those formed by *O*-demethylation (about 50%), conjugation with glucuronic acid (about 10%), and *N*-deacylation. Free and conjugated metabolites are eliminated in the urine, bile, and feces. There is enterohepatic cycling of the conjugates and probably of **indomethacin** itself. The half-life in plasma is variable, perhaps because of enterohepatic cycling, but averages about 2.5 hours.

The total plasma concentration of **indomethacin** plus its inactive metabolites is increased by concurrent administration of **probenecid**, but it is not clear if concomitant use requires dose adjustment. Indomethacin does not interfere with the uricosuric effect of probenecid.

Indomethacin does not directly modify the effect of warfarin, but platelet inhibition and gastric irritation increase the risk of bleeding; concurrent administration is not recommended. Indomethacin antagonizes the natriuretic and antihypertensive effects of **furosemide** and thiazide diuretics and blunts the antihypertensive effect of β-receptor antagonists, AT_1-receptor antagonists, and ACE inhibitors.

A high rate of intolerance limits the long-term analgesic use of **indomethacin** (Indocin). Likewise, it is not used commonly as an analgesic or antipyretic unless the fever has been refractory to other agents (e.g., Hodgkin's disease).

Indomethacin is effective for relieving joint pain, swelling, and tenderness, increasing grip strength, and decreasing the duration of morning stiffness. It is estimated to be approximately 20 times more potent than aspirin. Overall, about two-thirds of patients benefit from treatment with indomethacin, which typically is initiated at 25 mg two or three times daily. In some patients, 100 mg taken at night provides better nighttime analgesia and relief from morning stiffness. Failure to obtain adequate symptom relief with 100 mg within 7 to 10 days is an indication to try an alternative therapy.

When tolerated, **indomethacin** often is more effective than aspirin in the treatment of ankylosing spondylitis and osteoarthritis. It also is very effective in the treatment of acute gout, although it is not uricosuric.

Indomethacin is FDA approved for closure of persistent patent ductus arteriosus. A typical regimen involves the intravenous administration of 0.1 to 0.2 mg/kg every 12 hours for three doses. Successful closure can be expected in more than 70% of neonates treated with the drug. Such therapy is indicated primarily in premature infants who weigh between 500 and 1750 g, who have a hemodynamically significant patent ductus arteriosus, and in whom other supportive maneuvers have been attempted. Unexpectedly, treatment with **indomethacin** also may decrease the incidence and severity of intraventricular hemorrhage in low-birth-weight neonates. The principal limitation of treating neonates is renal toxicity, and therapy is stopped if the output of urine falls to less than 0.6 ml/kg per hour. Renal failure, enterocolitis, thrombocytopenia, or hyperbilirubinemia are contraindications to the use of indomethacin.

INDORAMIN

Indoramin, a vasodilator, is an alpha-adrenergic antagonist and an effective antihypertensive medication. In addition, it has cardiac stabilizing properties. The doses used for the treatment of peripheral vascular disease are lower than those used for the treatment of hypertension. Both these effects are consistent with competitive postsynaptic alpha-adrenoreceptor antagonism. Absence of tachycardia can be attributed to a combination of postsynaptic alpha-receptor selectivity and myocardial membrane-stabilizing properties. Cardiac function remains essentially unchanged in humans. The unique mode of action of indoramin suggests that it may be especially beneficial in hypertensive patients with coexisting asthma, migraine, or vasospastic symptoms. Sedation is a side effect that may limit the dose in some patients, but mild sedation can be an advantage in those patients with anxiety, tension headaches, and insomnia among their pretreatment symptomatology. Coprescription with a diuretic reduces the required dose of indoramin and the incidence of sedation. Cerebrovascular accidents due to rebound hypertension after abrupt discontinuation of other antihypertensive agents are not observed with indoramin. No evidence of tolerance has been obtained, and the incidence of postural hypotension appears to be extremely low (see also Figure 49).

INFLIXIMAB

(Remicade powder for injection 100 mg)

Infliximab is an immunomodulator that neutralizes the biological activity of tumor necrosis factor alpha (TNF-α) by binding to its soluble and transmembrane forms and inhibits TNF-α receptor binding. It is indicated in reducing signs and symptoms and to induce and maintain clinical remission of moderate to severe Crohn's disease; in reducing the number of draining enterocutaneous and rectovaginal fistulas and maintaining fistula closure in Crohn's disease; in combination with methotrexate to reduce signs and symptoms, inhibit progression of structural damage, and improve physical function in patients with moderately to severely active rheumatoid arthritis who have had inadequate response to methotrexate; and for reducing signs and symptoms of active ankylosing spondylitis.

Infliximab (Remicade, cA2), a chimeric immunoglobulin (25% mouse, 75% human) that binds to and neutralizes TNF-α, represents a new class of therapeutic agents for treating **inflammatory bowel disease** (IBD). Although a great many of both pro- and antiinflammatory cytokines are generated in the inflamed gut in IBD, there is some rationale for targetingTNF-α because it is one of the principal cytokines mediating the T_H1 immune response characteristic of **Crohn's disease**.

Infliximab (5 mg/kg infused intravenously at intervals of several weeks to months) decreases the frequency of acute flares in approximately two thirds of patients with moderate to severe Crohn's disease and also facilitates the closing of enterocutaneous fistulas associated with Crohn's disease. Its longer-term role in Crohn's disease is evolving, but emerging evidence supports its efficacy in maintaining remission and in recurrence of fistulas.

Infliximab was designed specifically to target TNF-α. It also may have more complex actions. **Etaneracept**, another anti-TNF-α therapy that uses a circulating receptor to clear soluble TNF-α, blocks its biologic effects but is ineffective in Crohn's disease. **Infliximab** binds membrane-bound TNF-α and may cause lysis of these cells by antibody-dependent or cell-mediated cytotoxicity. Thus, **infliximab** may deplete specific populations of subepithelial inflammatory cells. These effects, together with its mean terminal plasma half-life of 8 to 10 days, may explain the prolonged clinical effects of infliximab.

The use of infliximab as a biologic response modifier raises several important considerations. Both acute (fever, chills, urticaria, or even anaphylaxis) and subacute (serum sickness-like) reactions may develop after infliximab infusion. Anti-double-stranded DNA antibodies develop in 9% of patients, but a frank lupus-like syndrome occurs only rarely. Antibodies to **infliximab** can decrease its clinical efficacy; strategies to minimize the development of these antibodies (e.g., treatment with glucocorticoids or other immunosuppressives) may be critical to preserving infliximab efficacy for either recurrent or chronic therapy. Other proposed strategies to overcome the problem of "antibody resistance" include increasing the dose of **infliximab** or decreasing the interval between infusions.

Infliximab therapy is associated with increased incidence of respiratory infections; of particular concern is potential reactivation of tuberculosis or other **granulomatous infections** with subsequent dissemination. The FDA recommends that candidates for infliximab therapy should be tested for latent tuberculosis with purified protein derivative, and patients who test positive should be treated prophylactically with **isoniazid**. However, anergy with a false-negative skin test has been noted in some patients with Crohn's disease, and some experts routinely perform chest radiographs to look for active or latent pulmonary disease. **Infliximab** also is contraindicated in patients with severe congestive heart failure and should be used cautiously in class I or II patients. As with the immunosupressives, there is concern about the possible increased incidence of **non-Hodgkin's lymphoma**, but a causal role has not been established. Finally, the significant cost of **infliximab** is an important consideration in some patients.

Additional anti-TNF therapies are being evaluated in treating Crohn's disease, including a more humanized monoclonal antibody (CDP571) that should be less antigenic, and **thalidomide** (Thalomid), a drug with significant anti-TNF-α effects.

Despite the fact that ulcerative colitis does not appear to have a T_H1-type immune response mediated through TNF-α, some studies have shown a beneficial effect of TNF-α modulation in this disorder as well. Clearly, this area of IBD therapy is evolving rapidly as new drugs emerge and clinical experience increases.

INFLUENZA VIRUS VACCINE, TRIVALENT TYPES A&B

(Purified surface antigen) (Fluvirin)

INFLUENZA VIRUS VACCINE, TRIVALENT TYPES A&B (SPLIT VIRUS)

(Fluogen, Flu-Shield, Fluzone (split virus)

INFLUENZA VIRUS VACCINE, TRIVALENT TYPES A&B (WHOLE VIRUS)

(Fluzone) (whole-virus)

Influenza viral vaccine is used in annual influenza prophylaxis in high-risk patients.

INHIBIN

The pituitary hormones responsible for regulating gonadal functions are luteinizing hormone (LH) and follicle-stimulating hormone (FSH). In males, LH stimulates the Leydig's cells to synthesize testosterone; FSH stimulates the Sertoli's cells to synthesize inhibin and androgen-binding protein, and, in conjunction with high intratesticular concentrations of testosterone, initiates and maintains spermatogenesis. In females, LH stimulates androgen synthesis, and FSH increases estrogen and inhibin synthesis in the granulosa cells. Both LH and FSH are released from the gonadotroph cells of the anterior pituitary in response to the hypothalamic hormone gonadotropin-releasing hormone (GnRH; also known as LH-releasing hormone). GnRH is a decapeptide with the following structure: pyro Glu-His-Trp-Ser-Tyr-Gly-Leu-Arg-Pro-Gly-NH_2 (also see Table 15).

INSOMNIA: Treatment with Benzodiazepines

Drugs	Duration of Action	Onset of Action
Clonazepam	Long	Intermediate
Diazepam	Long	Rapid
Estazolam	Intermediate	Rapid to intermediate
Flurazepam	Long	Rapid to intermediate
Lorazepam	Intermediate	Intermediate
Oxazepam	Short to intermediate	Intermediate to slow
Quazepam	Long	Rapid
Temazepam	Intermediate	Intermediate to slow
Triazolam	Short	Intermediate
Zolpidem	Short	Rapid

INSULIN

Diabetes mellitus results from disturbances in the metabolism of carbohydrates, lipids, and proteins. Normally, the blood glucose level is maintained within a range of 80 to 130 mg/mL. When the level rises above 180 mg/mL, the glucose spills into the urine, causing glucosuria. The utilization of glucose by most tissues, including muscle and adipose tissue, is insulin-dependent. The brain is an exception in that its utilization of glucose is insulin-independent. In the absence of insulin, the organs other than brain are able to make use of amino acids and fatty acids as alternate sources of energy.

The release of insulin is closely coupled with the glucose level. Hypoglycemia results in a low level of insulin and a high level of glucagon, and hence favors the processes of glycogenolysis and gluconeogenesis. Growth hormone is one of the glucose counterregulatory hormones. It is released in response to hypoglycemia and has intrinsic hyperglycemic actions as well as causing insulin resistance.

Following ingestion of a meal or the administration of glucose (e.g., in a glucose tolerance test), the glucose level rises, causing the release of insulin and inhibiting the release of hyperglycemic glucagon. Excess glucose is transformed into glycogen in the liver and the muscles. The high level of amino acids and free fatty acid fosters the respective formation of proteins in the muscles and triglycerides in the adipose tissues. In a nondiabetic fasting subject, the ensuing hypoglycemia not only discourages the release of insulin but also activates the homeostatic mechanisms that block the action of insulin and convert the storage of forms of fuel into utilizable glucose. Consequently, a number of hormones including glucagon, epinephrine, and glucocorticoid, are released, and these convert glycogen into glucose, triglyceride into free fatty acids, and proteins into amino acids (gluconeogenesis), respectively. Furthermore, the uptake and utilization of glucose in the peripheral tissues decrease. The muscles and other tissues utilize amino acids and free fatty acids, thus providing the brain with an adequate supply of glucose. In a diabetic individual who suffers from a deficiency of insulin, all of the aforementioned measures that apply to a fasting individual may also take place. However, the consumption of a meal or the administration of glucose will instead cause pronounced hyperglycemia because the insulin-dependent utilization of glucose by muscles and adipose tissues is lacking. The elevated glucose level thus surpasses the renal threshold, and glucose may appear continuously in the urine. The osmotic diuretic effects of glucose cause polyuria and polydipsia, and the chronic glucosuria may lead to urinary tract infection. Because the conversion to triglycerides does not take place, free fatty acids are metabolized to ketone bodies, causing ketonuria or ketoacidosis (acetone or fruity breath). The continuous destruction of muscular proteins may ultimately lead to muscle wasting and weight loss.

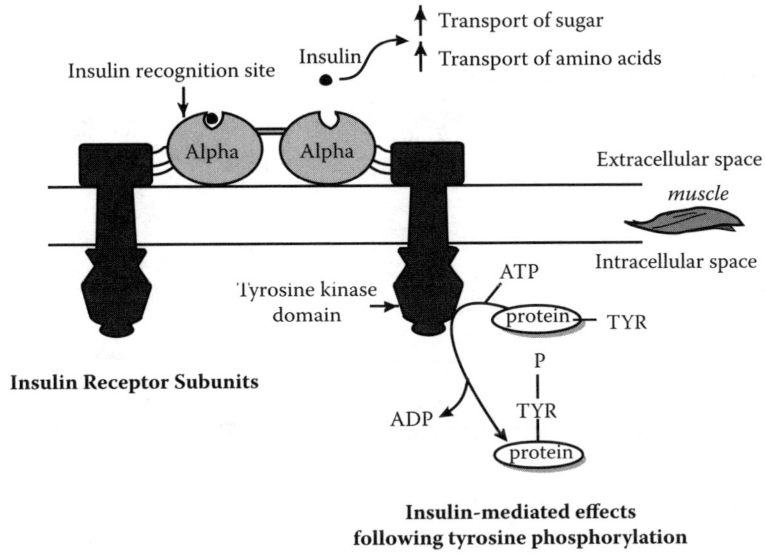

Figure 62 When insulin binds to specific membrane receptors on target cells, it enhances the transport of sugar and amino acids, stimulates anabolic pathways, and stimulates growth and development by triggering RNA and DNA synthesis.

There are two types of diabetes mellitus: type I, or insulin-dependent diabetes mellitus, and type II, or non-insulin-dependent diabetes mellitus. Type I diabetic patients may have islet-cell antibodies and human leukocyte antigens (HLA). They are dependent on insulin to prevent ketosis and have insulinopenia. Affected individuals consist mostly of children and young adults. Type II diabetic patients, who are non-insulin-dependent, are not prone to ketosis. This type of diabetes is not an autoimmune disorder nor associated with HLA. The patients are generally older (>40 years), may or may not be obese, and may or may not have been treated with insulin for the control of their hyperglycemia. The signs and symptoms of diabetes consist of thirst, anorexia, nausea, vomiting, abdominal pain, headache, drowsiness, weakness, coma, severe acidosis, air hunger (Kussmaul's breathing), sweetish odor of the breath, hyperglycemia, decreased blood bicarbonate level, decreased blood pH, and plasma that is strongly positive for ketone bodies. There are a number of complications that arise as the result of poorly treated or unstabilized diabetes. Vascular complications may be manifested by microangiopathy (thickening of the capillary basement membrane), intracapillary glomerulosclerosis (thickening of the glomerular capillary basement membrane, which leads to a nephrotic syndrome characterized by edema, albuminuria, and/or renal failure), and microangiopathy of the blood vessels supplying the retina (diabetic retinopathy). In fact, diabetes is still the leading cause of blindness in the world. In addition, there may be atherosclerosis of the peripheral arteries. Diabetic neuropathy may be associated with neuropathic ulcer, ptosis, diplopia, stabismus, loss of deep tendon reflexes, ankle drop, wrist drop, paresthesia, hyperalgesia, hyperesthesia, and orthostatic hypotension (because of autonomic dysfunction). When insulin binds to specific membrane receptors on target cells, this initiates a wide spectrum of biologic activities. It enhances the transport of sugar and amino acids, stimulates anabolic pathways, and stimulates growth and development by triggering RNA and DNA synthesis (see Figure 62).

The insulin receptor is a disulfide-linked oligomer consisting of two alpha and two beta chains, with molecular weights of 130,000 and 95,000, respectively. Cross-linking studies using ^{125}Iodine-labeled insulin have shown that the insulin-binding domain is situated primarily in the alpha subunit. In addition, it has been observed that proteolysis of the beta subunit does not appreciably influence insulin binding. Insulin binding to the alpha subunit was found to induce rapid phosphorylation of the intracellular domain of the beta subunit. The beta subunit contains a putative ATP-binding site and an intrinsic tyrosine-specific kinase as part of the receptor. The enzymatic activity of the receptor is activated by insulin binding, which results in increased tyrosine phosphorylation of the beta subunit as well as the production of a number of other cell proteins (Figure 54). The insulin receptor is internalized, and this action terminates the insulin signal at the surface of the cell. Once internalized, some of the receptors are degraded and others are recycled back to the membrane. In addition, phosphatases are able to dephosphorylate the phosphorylated insulin receptor. This dephosphorylation reduces kinase activity and decreases the responsiveness to insulin. A number of disorders are associated with the development of insulin resistance. Although some cases are due to autoimmune responses, such as the development of antiinsulin or

TABLE 19
Properties of Insulin Preparations

Types	Added Protein	Zinc Content (mg/100 U)	Action (hr) Onset	Peak	Duration
Rapid					
Regular (crystalline)	None	0.01–0.04	0.3–0.7	2–4	5–8
Semilente	None	0.2–0.25	0.5–1.0	2–8	12–16
Intermediate					
NPH (Isophane)	Protamine	0.016–0.40	1–2	6–12	18–24
Lente	None	0.2–0.25	1–2	6–12	18–24
Slow					
Ultralente	None	0.2–0.25	4–6	16–18	20–36
Protamine zinc	Protamine	0.2–0.25	4–6	14–20	24–36

antiinsulin receptor antibodies, insulin resistance often results from defects at the cellular level in the insulin receptor or in post-receptor function. The drug therapy of diabetes mellitus includes eliminating obesity (which causes resistance to both endogenous and exogenous forms of insulin), exercising (to promote glucose utilization and reduce insulin requirement), dieting (to restrict intake of excess amounts of carbohydrates), and taking insulin (primarily in polyuric, polydipsic, and ketonuric patients). Insulin preparations are fast-, intermediate-, or long-acting, as summarized in Table 19.

Crystalline (regular) insulin may be used as a supplemental injection or for instituting corrective measures in the management of infection and trauma, for postoperative stabilization, and for the rehabilitation of patients recovering from ketoacidosis and coma. In addition, NPH contains regular insulin.

Ultralente or semilente insulin is used to eliminate nocturnal and early morning hyperglycemia. Hypoglycemia is a primary complication of insulin therapy and may result from either an excess of insulin or a lack of glucose, or both. Severe hypoglycemia may cause headache, confusion, double vision, drowsiness, and convulsions. The treatment of this hypoglycemia may include the administration of glucose or glucagon. Lipodystrophy can also result from insulin therapy and is characterized by atrophy of subcutaneous fat. Insulin edema is manifested by a generalized retention of fluid. Insulin resistance arises when there is an excess insulin requirement that exceeds 200 units per day. The release of insulin is enhanced by certain physiologic substances (glucose, leucine, arginine, gastrin, secretin, and pancreozymin) and by certain pharmacologic agents (oral hypoglycemic agents). The release of insulin is also inhibited by some physiologic substances (epinephrine and norepinephrine) as well as by some pharmacologic substances (thiazide diuretics, diazoxide, and chlorpromazine).

INSULIN PREPARATIONS

Short-acting insulins

Standard insulin
- Regular Iletin I
- Regular insulin
- Semilente Iletin I
- Semilente insulin

Purified
- Beef regular Iletin II
- Pork regular Iletin II
- Regular purified pork insulin
- Velosulin
- Semilente purified pork

Human (purified)
- Humulin R
- Humulin BR
- Velosulin
- Novolin R
- Novolin R PenFill

Intermediate-acting insulins

NPH (standard)
- NPH Iletin I
- NPH insulin

NPH (purified)
- Beef NPH Iletin II
- Pork NPH Iletin II
- NPH purified pork
- Insulatard NPH

NPH (human)
- Humulin N
- Insulatard NPH
- Novolin N
- Novolin N PenFill

Lente (standard)
- Lente Iletin I
- Lente insulin

Lente (purified)
- Lente Iletin II
- Lente purified pork

Lente (human)
- Novolin L
- Humulin L

NPH-regular combination (70%/30%)

Purified
- Mixtard (70% NPH, 30% regular)

Human
- Novolin 70/30
- Novolin 70/30 PenFill
- Humulin 70/30
- Mixtard 70/30

Long-acting insulins

- Protamine zinc and Iletin I
- Ultralente Iletin I
- Ultralente insulin

Purified
- Protamine Zinc and Iletin II
- Ultralente purified beef

INSULIN (REGULAR)

(Humulin R, Novolin R, Novolin R PenFill, Pork regular Iletin II, Regular insulin, Regular Iletin 1, Regular [concentrated] Iletin II, Regular purified pork insulin, Velosulin human)

PROMPT INSULIN ZINC SUSPENSION

(Semilente)

INSULIN ZINC SUSPENSION (LENTE)

(Humulin l, Lente Iletin I, Lente Iletin II, Lente l, Novolin L)

PROTAMINE ZINC INSULIN SUSPENSION (ULTRALENTE)

(Humulin U Ultralente)

ISOPHANE INSULIN SUSPENSION (NPH)

(Humulin N, NPH Iletin I, NPH-N, Novolin N, Novolin N PenFill, Pork NPH Iletin II)

ISOPHANE INSULIN SUSPENSION AND INSULIN INJECTION (70% ISOPHANE INSULIN AND 30% INSULIN INJECTION)

(Humulin 70/30, Novolin 70/30, Novolin 70/30 PenFill)

ISOPHANE INSULIN SUSPENSION AND INSULIN INJECTION (50% ISOPHANE INSULIN AND 50% INSULIN INJECTION

(Humulin 50/50)

Insulin, a pancreatic hormone, is used in diabetic ketoacidosis and ketosis-prone and juvenile-onset diabetes mellitus, and in diabetes inadequately controlled by diet and oral hypoglycemics (see Table 19 and Figure 54).

INTERFERON ALFA-N3

(Alteron N)

Interferon, a biological response modifier with antineoplastic properties, is indicated in the treatment of condylomata acuminata (see also Figure 107).

INTERFERON ALFA-2A, RECOMBINANT

(Roferon-A)

INTERFERON ALFA-2B, RECOMBINANT

(Intron A)

Interferon, a biological response modifier with antineoplastic activity, is used in hairy cell leukemia, condylomata acuminata, Kaposi's sarcoma, chronic hepatitis C (non-A, non-B), and chronic hepatitis B (see also Figure 107).

INTERFERON BETA-1B

(Betaseron)

Interferon, a biological response modifier with antiviral and immunoregulating properties, is used to reduce the frequency of exacerbation in patients with relapsing–remitting multiple sclerosis (see also Figure 107).

INTERFERON ALFA-2A

(Roferon-A solution for injection 3 million IU/mL)

Interferon alfa-2a is an immunomodulator. Interferon alfa-2a has antiproliferative and immunomodulatory activities. Its elimination half-life is 3.7 to 8.5 hr after IV infusion. **Adult** use: for hairy cell leukemia, AIDS-related Kaposi's sarcoma, chronic myelogenous leukemia; **pediatric** use: for chronic myelogenous leukemia.

INTERFERON ALFA-2B

(Intron A powder for injection)

Interferon alfa-2b is an immunomodulator. It causes inhibition of virus replication in virus-infected cells, suppression of cell proliferation, and such immunomodulating activities as enhancement of the phagocytic activity of macrophages and augmentation of the specific cytotoxicity of lymphocytes for target cells. It is indicated in hairy cell leukemia; condylomata acuminata; AIDS-related Kaposi sarcoma; chronic hepatitis B; chronic non-A/non-B hepatitis (hepatitis C); and malignant melanoma; and follicular non-Hodgkin's lymphoma.

Although interferons (alpha, beta, and gamma) initially were identified by their antiviral activity, these agents also have important immunomodulatory activities. The interferons bind to specific cell-surface receptors that initiate a series of intracellular events: induction of certain enzymes, inhibition of cell proliferation, and enhancement of immune activities, including increased phagocytosis by macrophages and augmentation of specific cytotoxicity by T-lymphocytes. Recombinant **interferon alfa-2b** (IFN-alpha$_2$, intron A) is obtained from *Escherichia coli* by recombinant expression. It is a member of a family of naturally occurring small proteins with molecular weights of 15,000 to 27,600 daltons, produced and secreted by cells in response to viral infections and other inducers. Interferon alfa-2b is indicated in the treatment of a variety of tumors, including hairy cell leukemia, malignant melanoma, follicular lymphoma, and AIDS-related Kaposi's sarcoma. It also is indicated for infectious diseases, chronic hepatitis B, and condylomata acuminata. In addition, it is supplied in combination with **ribavirin** (Rebetron) for treatment of chronic hepatitis C in patients with compensated liver function not previously treated with interferon alfa-2b or who have relapsed after interferon alfa-2b therapy. Flu-like symptoms, including fever, chills, and headache are the most common adverse effects after **interferon alfa-2b** administration. Adverse experiences involving the cardiovascular system (hypotension, arrhythmias, and rarely cardiomyopathy and myocardial infarction) and CNS (depression, confusion) are less-frequent side effects.

Interferon gamma-lb (Actimmune) is a recombinant polypeptide that activates phagocytes and induces their generation of oxygen metabolites that are toxic to a number of microorganisms. It is indicated to reduce the frequency and severity of serious infections associated with chronic granulomatous disease. Adverse reactions include fever, headache, rash, fatigue, GI distress, anorexia, weight loss, myalgia, and depression.

Interferon beta-la (Avonex, Rebif), a 166-amino acid recombinant glycoprotein, and interferon beta-lb (Betaseron), a 165-amino acid recombinant protein, have antiviral and immunomodulatory properties. They are PDA approved for the treatment of relapsing and relapsing–remitting multiple sclerosis to reduce the frequency of clinical exacerbations. The mechanism of their action in multiple sclerosis is unclear.

INTERFERON ALFA-2B, RECOMBINANT/RIBAVIRIN

(Rebetron injection/capsules)

Interferon alfa-2b is an immunomodulator. Interferon alfa-2b inhibits virus replication in virus-infected cells and suppresses cell proliferation; although the exact mechanism of action of ribavirin is not know, it has antiviral inhibitory activity against respiratory syncytial virus, influenza virus, and herpes simplex virus. It is indicated in the treatment of chronic hepatitis C in patients with compensated liver disease previously untreated with alpha interferon or who have relapsed after alpha interferon therapy.

INTERFERON ALFA-N3

(Alferon N solution 5 million IU/mL)

Interferon alfa-n3 is an immunomodulator. These small proteins bind to specific cell membranes and initiate complex sequences, intracellular events, including induction of certain enzymes that produce antiproliferative action against tumor cells and inhibit viral replication in virus-infected cells. They are used in the treatment of condyloma acuminatum.

INTERFERON ALFACON-I

(Infergen injection 9 mcg)

Interferon alfacon-I is an immunomodulator. These small protein molecules bind to specific cell-surface receptors and initiate complex sequences of intracellular events, including production of enzymes and other products with antiviral, antiproliferative, and immunomodulatory effects. They are indicated in the treatment of chronic hepatitis C virus (HVC) infection in patients older than 18 years of age with compensated liver disease who have anti-HCV serum antibodies and/or the presence of HCV RNA.

Interferons (IFNs) are potent cytokines that possess antiviral, immunomodulating, and antiproliferative activities. These proteins are synthesized by host cells in response to various inducers and, in turn, cause biochemical changes leading to an antiviral state in cells. Three major classes of human interferons with significant antiviral activity currently are recognized: α (>18 individual species), β, and γ. Clinically used recombinant α IFNs are nonglycosylated proteins of approximately 19,500 daltons.

IFN-α and IFN-β may be produced by nearly all cells in response to viral infection and a variety of other stimuli, including double-stranded RNA and certain cytokines (e.g., interleukin-1, interleukin-2, and tumor necrosis factor). IFN-γ production is restricted to T-lymphocytes and natural killer cells responding to antigenic stimuli, mitogens, and specific cytokines. **IFN-α** and IFN-β exhibit antiviral and antiproliferative actions; stimulate the cytotoxic activity of lymphocytes, natural killer cells, and macrophages; and upregulate class I major histocompatibility (MHC) antigens and other surface markers. IFN-γ has less antiviral activity but more potent immunoregulatory effects, particularly macrophage activation, expression of class II MHC antigens, and mediation of local inflammatory responses.

Most animal viruses are inhibited by IFNs, although many DNA viruses are relatively insensitive. Considerable differences in sensitivity to the effects of IFNs exist among different viruses and assay systems. The biological activity of IFN usually is measured in terms of antiviral effects in cell culture and generally is expressed as international units (IU) relative to reference standards.

Following binding to specific cellular receptors, IFNs activate the JAK-STAT signal-transduction pathway and lead to the nuclear translocation of a cellular protein complex that binds to genes containing an IFN-specific response element. This, in turn, leads to synthesis of over two dozen proteins that contribute to viral resistance mediated at different stages of viral penetration. Inhibition of protein synthesis is the major inhibitory effect for many viruses. IFN-induced proteins include 2′5′-oligoadenylate [2-5(A)] synthetase and a protein kinase, either of which can inhibit protein synthesis in the presence of double-stranded RNA.

INTERFERON BETA-1A

(Avonex powder for injection)

Interferon beta-1a is an interferon beta, which has antiviral, antiproliferative, and immunoregulatory activities. It binds to specific cell membrane receptors that induce the expression of a number of gene products that mediate the biological actions of interferon beta-la. It is indicated for the treatment of relapsing forms of multiple sclerosis to slow accumulation of physical disability and decrease the frequency of clinical exacerbations.

Interferon beta-la (Avonex, Rebif), a 166-amino acid recombinant glycoprotein, and interferon beta-lb (Betaseron), a 165-amino acid recombinant protein, have antiviral and immunomodulatory properties. They are FDA approved in the treatment of relapsing and relapsing–remitting multiple sclerosis to reduce the frequency of clinical exacerbations. The mechanism of their action in multiple sclerosis is unclear. Flu-like symptoms (fever, chills, myalgia) and injection-site reactions have been common adverse effects.

Specific therapies are aimed at resolving acute attacks, reducing recurrences and exacerbations, and slowing the progression of disability. Nonspecific therapies focus on maintaining function and quality of life. For acute attacks, pulse glucocorticoids are often employed (typically, 1 g/day of methyl-**prednisolone** administered intravenously for 3 to 5 days). There is no evidence that tapered doses of oral prednisone are useful or even desirable.

For relapsing–remitting attacks, immunomodulatory therapies are approved: **beta-1 interferons** (interferon beta-la, interferon beta-lb, and glatiramer acetate [Copaxone]). The interferons suppress the proliferation of T-lymphocytes, inhibit their movement into the CNS from the periphery, and shift the cytokine profile from pro- to antiinflammatory types.

For relapsing–remitting attacks and for secondary progressive MS, the alkylating agent **cyclophosphamide** and the anthracenedionene-derivative **mitoxantrone** (Novatrone) are currently used in patients refractory to other immunomodulators. These agents, used primarily for cancer chemotherapy, have significant toxicities. Although cyclophosphamide in patients with MS may not be limited by an accumulated dose exposure, mitoxantrone can be tolerated only up to an accumulated dose of 100 to 140 mg/m^2. The utility of interferon therapy in patients with secondary progressive MS is unclear. In primary progressive MS, with no discrete attacks and less observed inflammation, suppression of inflammation seems to be less helpful. A minority of patients at this stage will respond to high doses of glucocorticoids.

Each of the agents mentioned above has side effects and contraindications that may be limiting: infections (for glucocorticoids); hypersensitivity and pregnancy (for immunomodulators); and prior anthracycline/anthracenedione use, mediastinal irradiation, or cardiac disease (mitoxantrone). With all of these agents, it is clear that the earlier they are used, the more effective they are in preventing disease relapses. What is not clear is whether any of these agents will prevent or diminish the later onset of secondary progressive disease, which causes the more severe form of disability. Given the fluctuating nature of this disease, only long-term studies lasting decades will answer this question.

A number of other new immunomodulatory therapies are completing phase III trials. One is a monoclonal antibody, natalizumab (Antegren), directed against the adhesion molecule α_4 integrin; natalizumab binds to α_4 integrin and antagonizes interactions with integrin heterodimers containing α_4 integrin, such as $\alpha_4\beta_1$ integrin that is expressed on the surface of activated lymphocytes and monocytes. Preclinical data suggest that an interaction of $\alpha_4\beta_1$ integrin with VCAM-1 (vascular cellular-adhesion molecule 1) is critical for T-cell trafficking from the periphery into the CNS; thus, blocking this interaction would hypothetically inhibit disease exacerbations. In fact, phase II clinical trials have demonstrated a significant decrease in the number of new lesions as determined by magnetic resonance imaging and clinical attacks in MS patients receiving natalizumab. Monoclonal antibodies directed against the IL-2 receptor are also entering phase II clinical trials.

INTERFERON GAMMA-1B

(Actimmune injection 100 mcg)

Interferon gamma-1b is an immunomodulator. It produces potent phagocyte activating effects, including generation of toxic oxygen metabolites within phagocytes, which mediate killing of microorganisms. Activities include enhancement of oxidative metabolism of tissue macrophages and enhancement of antibody-dependent cellular cytotoxicity and NK cell activity (see Figure 107). It is indicated in the reduction of frequency and severity of serious infections associated with chronic granulomatous disease.

Interferon-γ (IFN-γ) (Actimmune) activates macrophages to kill *M. tuberculosis*. Aerosol delivery of IFN-γ to the lungs of patients with multidrug-resistant tuberculosis results in wide pulmonary distribution and enhanced local immune stimulation.

IFNs are potent cytokines that possess antiviral, immunomodulating, and antiproliferative activities. These proteins are synthesized by host cells in response to various inducers and, in turn, cause biochemical changes leading to an antiviral state in cells. Three major classes of human interferons with significant antiviral activity currently are recognized: α (>18 individual species), β, and γ. Clinically used recombinant α IFNs are nonglycosylated proteins of approximately 19,500 daltons.

IFN-α and IFN-β may be produced by nearly all cells in response to viral infection and a variety of other stimuli, including double-stranded RNA and certain cytokines (e.g., interleukin-1, interleukin-2, and tumor necrosis factor). **IFN-γ** production is restricted to T-lymphocytes and natural killer cells responding to antigenic stimuli, mitogens, and specific cytokines. IFN-α and IFN-β exhibit antiviral and antiproliferative actions; stimulate the cytotoxic activity of lymphocytes, natural killer cells, and macrophages; and upregulate class I major histocompatibility (MHC) antigens and other surface markers. IFN-γ has less antiviral activity but more potent immunoregulatory effects, particularly macrophage activation, expression of class II MHC antigens, and mediation of local inflammatory responses.

INTERLEUKIN-2

(IL-2)

Interleukin-2 is a lymphokine with immunoregulatory properties that is indicated in metastatic renal cell carcinoma. In addition, interleukin-2 is used in cell transfer therapy in cancer patients. Cell transfer therapy is a new approach to strengthening the innate ability of the immune system to fight against cancer. In this therapy, lymphocytes are isolated and cultured with interleukin-2 for 3 days to yield lymphokine-activated

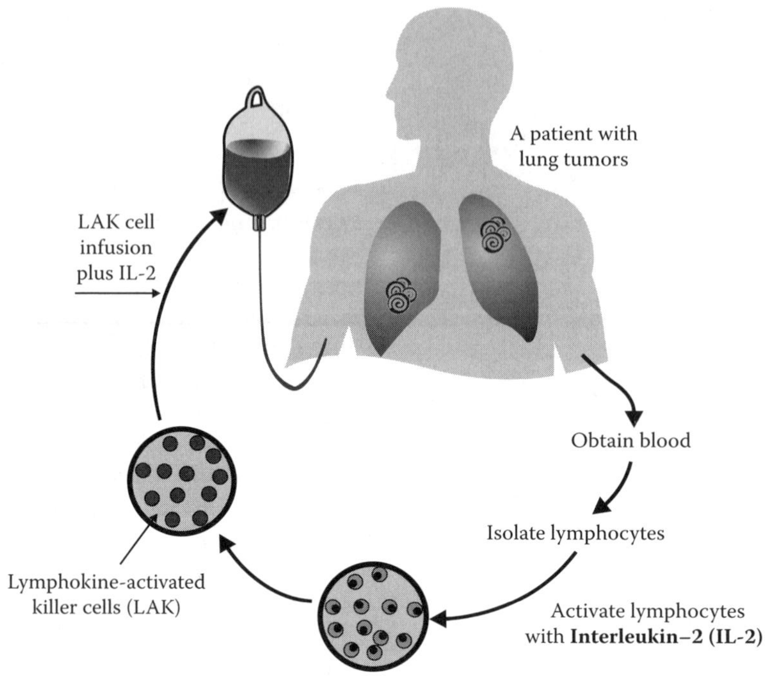

Figure 63 Cell transfer therapy is a new approach to strengthening the innate ability of the immune system to fight against cancer. In this therapy, lymphocytes are isolated and cultured with **interleukin-2** for three days to yield **lymphokine-activated killer cells**, which are then administered to patients along with interleukin-2.

killer cells, which are then administered to patients along with interleukin-2 (see Figure 63; and Cytokines).

INVERT SUGAR

(Travert)

Invert sugar, a carbohydrate (1000 ml of 5% solution by IV infusion), is indicated for nonelectrolyte fluid replacement and caloric supplementation solution.

IODINE

Iodides such as potassium iodide and Lugol's solution, which contains 5% iodine and 10% potassium iodide, exert their beneficial effects by inhibiting organification, inhibiting the release of thyroid hormones, and decreasing (inhibiting proteolysis) the size and vascularity of the thyroid gland. This makes them useful for preparing the patient for surgery. Iodine 131 is given orally in older patients for the treatment of thyrotoxicosis. It accumulates in the storage follicles and emits beta rays with a half-life of 5 days. Radioactive iodine, which crosses the placental barrier, is contraindicated in pregnant women (see Table 20). The treatment of thyrotoxicosis in younger patients may include the administration of an antithyroid drug such as propylthiouracil or methimazole. These agents are very slow in their onset of action, often taking years for remission to be apparent. The most serious side effect of these drugs is agranulocytosis. In the event of multinodular goiters, subtotal thyroidectomy may be indicated. Potassium iodide is next administered as a preoperative measure to diminish vascularity of the thyroid. In addition to surgery, radioactive iodine is being used increasingly in younger patients. The major complication following either surgery or treatment with radioactive iodine may be hypothyroidism, which then requires replacement therapy with levothyroxine.

TABLE 20
Comparison of Features of Antithyroid Drug and Iodine 131 Therapy for Hyperthyroidism

Features	Drug Therapy	Iodine 131 Therapy
Dosage	Daily	Single dose
Initial response	4–6 wk	8–12 wk
Side effects	Uncommon	Rare
Hypothyroidism	Uncommon	Common
Inadequate therapy	Uncommon	Rare
Need for continuous or repeated therapy	Common	Rare
Long-term outcome	Euthyroidism or hyperthyroidism	Hypothyroidism
Outcome dependent on contoured TSab production	Yes	No
Use during pregnancy	Acceptable	Never

IODINE-CONTAINING PRODUCTS

Oral Preparations
Amiodarone
Calcium iodide (e.g., calcidrine syrup)
Echothiophate iodide (ophthalmic solution)
Hydriodic acid syrup
Idoxuridine ophthalmic solution
Iodinated glycerol
Iodine-containing vitamins
Iodochlorhydroxyquin
Iodoquinol (diiodohydroxyquin)
Kelp
Lugol's solution
Niacinamide hydroiodide + potassium iodide (e.g., Iodo-Niacin)
Ponaris nasal emollient
Potassium iodide (e.g., Quadrinal)
Saturated solution of potassium iodide
Parenteral Preparations
Sodium iodide, 10% solution
Radiology Contrast Agents
Diatrizoate meglumine sodium
Iohexol
Iopanoic acid
Iothalamate
Ipodate
Metrizamide
Propyliodone
Topical Antiseptics
Iodine tincture
Iodochlorhydroxyquin cream
Iodoform gauze
Iodoquinol (diiodohydroxyquin) cream
Providone iodine

IODIXANOL

Iodixanol, a new isosmotic nonionic contrast agent similar to iohexol, is used in the cardiac catheterization laboratory. Iodixanol and iohexol are safe and effective in patients undergoing cardiac angiography.

IODOQUINOL

(Diiodohydroxyquin) (Amebaquin, Moebiquin, Yodoxin)

Iodoquinol, an 8-hydroxyquinoline iodinated compound possessing amebicidic properties (630 to 650 mg p.o. t.i.d. for 20 days), is indicated in the treatment of intestinal amebiasis.

IPECAC SYRUP

(Ipecac fluid extract is 14 times stronger than ipecac syrup.)

Ipecac, an emetic, contains emetine and cephaeline. It is used in a dose of 15 to 30 mL with 200 to 300 mL of water in drug overdosage and certain cases of poisoning. Ipecac may fail to exert its emetic effects on an empty stomach. Ipecac causes vomiting by irritating the stomach and by stimulating the chemotrigger zone for emesis (see also Figure 73). Ipecac exerts its emetic effects in 20 minutes. Activated charcoal will absorb ipecac syrup, and hence they should not be used together. Ipecac syrup is contraindicated in patients with poisoning caused by alkalis or corrosive agents because of hazard of further esophageal or mediastinal injury; in patients with poisoning from petroleum distillates; in patients who are semiconscious, unconscious, comatose, or in shock; and in patients with seizures, severe inebriation, depressed gag reflexes, or strychnine poisoning, because of hazards of aspiration, pneumonitis, bronchospasm, or pulmonary edema. When ipecac syrup does not cause emesis, absorption of the alkaloid emetine may occur and may cause heart conduction disturbances, atrial fibrillation, or fatal myocarditis. Ipecac syrup may be abused by bulimic and anorexic patients. It has been implicated as the causative factor of severe cardiomyopathies, and even death, in several persons with eating disorders who used it regularly to induce vomiting.

IPRATROPIUM BROMIDE

(Atrovent)

Ipratropium (2 inhalations, 36 mcg/q.i.d.) is a bronchodilator that is used in the treatment of bronchospasm associated with chronic obstructive pulmonary diseases including chronic bronchitis and emphysema. Ipratropium is a muscarinic cholinergic receptor blocking agent that inhibits its vagally mediated actions in bronchial smooth muscle. Ipratropium exerts its effect locally, is not absorbed in the lung, and is not found in a significant amount in the systemic circulation. The IV-administered ipratropium does not penetrate the blood–brain barrier. Ipratropium does not alter pulmonary gas exchange, pulse rate, or blood pressure. Ipratropium has been used concomitantly with other drugs, including sympathomimetic bronchodilators, methylxanthines, steroids, and cromolyn sodium, commonly used in the treatment of chronic obstructive pulmonary disease, without causing adverse drug reactions. Ipratropium causes dryness of the oropharynx. If sprayed into the eyes, it may cause blurring of vision, and hence could aggravate narrow-angle glaucoma (see also Figure 94).

IPRATROPIUM BROMIDE/ALBUTEROL SULFATE

(Combivent aerosol 18 mcg ipratropium bromide and 103 mcg albuterol sulfate per actuation)

Ipratropium bromide/albuterol sulfate is an anticholinergic preparation. **Albuterol** produces bronchodilation by relaxing bronchial smooth muscle through beta$_2$-receptor stimulation. **Ipratropium** antagonizes action of acetylcholine on bronchial smooth muscle in lungs, causing bronchodilation. They are indicated in the treatment of bronchospasm associated with COPD in patients requiring more than 1 bronchodilator.

IPSAPIRONE

The anxiolytic agents consist of benzodiazepine derivatives and azaspirodecanedione derivatives, which include buspirone, gepirone, and ipsapirone. The introduction of novel anxiolytic agents such as buspirone, which interacts with the serotonergic system, has suggested that serotoninergic fibers may be the final pathway through which anxiolytic effects are expressed. Buspirone has a chemical structure that is distinct from that of the benzodiazepines. Without this structural homology, it is not surprising that buspirone does not interact with the GABA receptors. Furthermore, the clinical profile of buspirone appears to be anxioselective, with a much reduced potential for abuse (see also Table 9). Although the benzodiazepines are now viewed as having a direct action at a binding site coupled to the gamma-aminobutyric acid (GABA) receptor (see Figure 50), this view was predated by the suggestion that serotoninergic systems interacted with the benzodiazepines. This view was spawned by the observation that benzodiazepines inhibit the firing of serotoninergic neurons in the dorsal raphe nucleus, decrease brain serotonin turnover (levels of 5-hydroxyindole acetic acid), and reverse the proconflict effects of direct serotoninergic stimulation of the dorsal raphe. As with buspirone, lesions of the serotoninergic system abolish diazepam's efficacy in a conflict test. A body of data supports the candidacy of serotonin as a mediator of the anxiolytic effects of benzodiazepines downstream from the GABA receptor. There is a convincing body of evidence that several types of serotonin (5-HT) receptors exist in the mammalian brain, two of which are well characterized: 5-HT_1 and 5-HT_2 sites. The 5-HT_1 sites can be further subdivided into at least three distinct subsets, which differ in their regional distribution and functions and are currently termed 5-HT_{1A}, 5-HT_{1B}, and 5-HT_{1C} sites. The 5-HT receptors in the hippocampus and other parts of the limbic system are primarily of the 5-HT_{1A} type. It is therefore tempting to speculate that drugs that display a high degree of selectivity for these receptor sites can selectively affect anxiety states. A breakthrough in that direction came with the discovery that buspirone, a drug with anxiolytic activity in humans, can help elucidate the role of 5-HT in anxiety. Buspirone, gepirone, and ipsapirone may therefore offer new therapeutic directions in the treatment of anxiety.

IRBESARTAN

(Avapro tablets 75 mg)

Irbesartan is an angiotensin-II-receptor antagonist that antagonizes the effect of angiotensin II (vasoconstriction and aldosterone secretion) by blocking the angiotensin II (AT_1 receptor) in vascular smooth muscle and the adrenal gland, producing decreased BP. It is indicated in the treatment of hypertension; and nephropathy in type 2 diabetes.

The importance of angiotensin II in regulating cardiovascular function has led to the development of nonpeptide antagonists of the AT_1, an angiotensin-II receptor for clinical use. **Losartan** (Cozaar), **candesartan** (Atacand), **irbesartan** (Avapro), **valsartan** (Diovan), **telmisartan** (Micardis), and **eprosartan** (Teveten) have been approved for the treatment of hypertension. By antagonizing the effects of angiotensin II, these agents relax smooth muscle and thereby promote vasodilation, increase renal salt and water excretion, reduce plasma volume, and decrease cellular hypertrophy. Angiotensin-II-receptor antagonists also theoretically overcome some of the disadvantages of ACE inhibitors, which not only prevent conversion of angiotensin I to angiotensin II but also prevent ACE-mediated degradation of bradykinin and substance P.

There are two distinct subtypes of angiotensin-II receptors, designated as type 1 (AT_1) and type 2 (AT_2). The AT_1 angiotensin-II-receptor subtype is located predominantly in vascular and myocardial tissue and also in brain, kidney, and adrenal glomerulosa cells, which secrete **aldosterone**. The AT_2 subtype of angiotensin II receptor is found in the adrenal medulla, kidney, and in the CNS, and may play a role in vascular development. Because the AT_1 receptor mediates feedback inhibition of renin release, renin and angiotensin-II concentrations are increased during AT_1-receptor antagonism. The clinical consequences of increased angiotensin-II effects on an uninhibited AT_2 receptor are unknown; however, emerging data suggest that the AT_2 receptor may elicit antigrowth and antiproliferative responses.

IRINOTECAN

(Camptosar injection 20 mg/mL)

Irinotecan is a DNA topoisomerase inhibitor. Irinotecan is a derivative of camptothecin. Camptothecins interact specifically with the enzyme topoisomerase I, which relieves torsional strain in DNA by inducing reversible single-strand breaks. It is indicated in the metastatic cancer of the colon or rectum after standard treatment with fluorouracil.

Irinotecan (CPT-11). **Irinotecan hydrochloride** (CPT-11) is a potent anticancer drug, but late-onset gastrointestinal toxic effects, such as severe diarrhea, make it difficult to use CPT-11 safely. After intravenous administration, CPT-11 is converted to SN-38, an active metabolite, by carboxy esterase. SN-38 is subsequently conjugated with glucuronic acid in the liver. SN-38 and SN-38 glucuronide are then excreted into the bile by MRP2. Some studies have shown that the inhibition of MRP2-mediated biliary excretion of SN-38 and its glucuronide by coadministration of probenecid reduces the drug-induced diarrhea.

Higher response rates are seen when 5-FU is used in combination with other agents, such as **cyclophosphamide** and **methotrexate** (breast cancer), **cisplatin** (head and neck cancer), and with **oxaliplatin** or **irinotecan** in colon cancer. The combination of 5-FU and oxaliplatin or irinotecan has become the standard first-line treatment for patients with metastatic colorectal cancer. The use of 5-FU in combination regimens has improved survival in the adjuvant treatment for breast cancer, and with **oxaliplatin** and **leucovorin**, for colorectal cancer. 5-FU also is a potent radiation sensitizer. Beneficial effects also have been reported when combined with irradiation for cancers of the esophagus, stomach, pancreas, cervix, anus, and head and neck. 5-FU is used widely with very favorable results for the topical treatment of premalignant keratoses of the skin and multiple superficial basal cell carcinomas.

IRON

The iron-deficiency anemias are caused by excessive loss of or an inadequate intake of iron. In women, menstruation and pregnancy may increase the iron requirement. Iron deficiency in men, as well as women, may be due to blood loss resulting from hemorrhage associated with gastric ulcer or neoplasm. In children, iron deficiency is due to a nutritionally inadequate diet. In the body, the total content of iron in men and women constitutes 50 and 35 mg per kilogram of body weight, respectively. Of this iron content, approximately 60% is associated with hemoglobin, 13% is associated with myoglobin and iron-containing enzymes, and the remaining 27% is located in the storage sites. Men and women differ with regard to their storage of iron, which is substantially lower in women due to menstruation. Menstrual losses are greater with the use of intrauterine devices and are decreased when estrogen-containing oral contraceptives are used.

Iron is primarily obtained from the diet, with an average daily intake of approximately 12 to 15 mg. Under normal circumstances, only 10% (1 mg) of the ingested iron is absorbed. However, in the event of iron-deficiency anemia, this increases to approximately 40%. Of course, the iron requirement is increased during growth and development, as the result of menstruation, pregnancy, and blood donation, and in an extensive number of pathologic conditions causing anemia. In addition, the long-term ingestion of certain drugs such as aspirin may alter the daily requirement. Iron is absorbed better in ferrous (Fe^{2+}) than in the ferric (Fe^{3-}) form. The extent of absorption of iron from the duodenum is thought to be regulated by mucosal proteins, and this process is referred to as mucosal block. The absorbed iron is either stored in mucosal ferritin, or is transported to plasma and bound to transferrin. Ordinarily, iron excretion and elimination are regulated to equal the amount of iron absorption. A major portion of iron (>60%) in the body is collected by bone marrow and incorporated into hemoglobin in the erythrocytes. In general, four atoms of iron are incorporated into one molecule of hemoglobin. When the erythrocytes are destroyed by the reticuloendothelium after 120 days in the circulation, the released iron is returned to transferrin and ferritin.

Extensive numbers of oral preparations are available for the treatment of iron deficiency. In general, the ferrous salts (ferrous sulfate, ferrous gluconate, and ferrous fumerate) are better absorbed than the ferric salts (ferric sulfate). Ferrous calcium citrate is most used in patients during pregnancy to provide iron as well as calcium. The parenteral iron medications available include iron-dextran (ferric hydroxide and high-molecular-weight dextran) for intramuscular use, dextriferron (a complex of ferric hydroxide and partially hydrolyzed dextran) for intravenous use, and saccharated iron oxide (a complex of ferric hydroxide and sucrose) for intravenous use. These preparations are reserved for those cases in which oral preparations are not tolerated, absorbed, or rapid enough in their onset of action, or are otherwise not suitable for noncompliant patients. A lethal dose of iron consists of 12 g of an iron preparation containing 1 or 2 g of elemental iron. Therefore, iron toxicity rarely occurs in adults but is frequently seen in children. The mortality rate among untreated children is high (45%). The initial signs and symptoms of iron poisoning are gastrointestinal and usually consist of nausea, vomiting, and diarrhea. If untreated, acidosis, cyanosis, and circulatory collapse may ensue. If the patient survives, there may be gastric scarring and pyloric stenosis resulting from the corrosive action of the iron preparation. Treatment should include induced vomiting and lavage if the poisoning is discovered early, catharsis to hasten evacuation, sodium bicarbonate therapy to combat the acidosis, and the administration of deferoxamine (Desferal), a specific iron-chelating agent. A dose of 100 mg of deferoxamine is able to bind 8.5 mg of iron. The chelating effects of deferoxamine are maximum at an acidic pH; therefore, when given orally, deferoxamine must be administered before the sodium bicarbonate. In the event of iron poisoning, deferoxamine may also be administered intramuscularly. Besides its usefulness in counteracting the effects of iron poisoning, deferoxamine has been used in disorders that involve iron overload such as ocular hemosiderosis or hemochromatosis.

IRON DEXTRAN

(DexFerrum injection 50 mg iron/mL)

Iron dextran is an iron product that replenishes hemoglobin and depleted iron stores. It is indicated in the treatment of iron deficiency anemia when oral administration of iron is unsatisfactory or impossible.

IRON SUCROSE

(Venofer injection 20 mg/mL)

Iron sucrose is an iron product that replenishes hemoglobin (Hgb) and depleted iron stores. It is indicated in the treatment of iron deficiency anemia in patients undergoing chronic hemodialysis who are receiving erythropoietin therapy.

When oral iron therapy fails, parenteral iron administration may be an effective alternative. The rate of response to parenteral therapy is similar to that which follows usual oral doses. Common indications are iron malabsorption (e.g., **sprue**, **short bowel syndrome**), severe oral iron intolerance, as a routine supplement to total parenteral nutrition, and in patients who are receiving erythropoietin.

Parenteral iron also has been given to iron-deficient patients and pregnant women to create iron stores, something that would take months to achieve by the oral route. Parenteral iron therapy should be used only when clearly indicated, as acute hypersensitivity, including anaphylactic and anaphylactoid reactions, can occur in 0.2 to 3% of patients. The belief that the response to parenteral iron, especially **iron dextran**, is faster than oral iron is open to debate. In otherwise healthy individuals, the rate of hemoglobin response is determined by the balance between the severity of the anemia (the level of erythropoietin stimulus) and the delivery of iron to the marrow from iron absorption and iron stores. When a large intravenous dose of **iron dextran** is given to a severely anemic patient, the hematologic response can exceed that seen with oral iron for 1 to 3 weeks. Subsequently, however, the response is no better than that seen with oral iron.

ISOCARBOXAZID

(Marplan tablets 10 mg)

Isocarboxazid is an MAO inhibitor, which blocks activity of enzyme MAO, thereby increasing monoamine (e.g., epinephrine, norepinephrine, serotonin) concentrations in CNS. It is indicated in the treatment of depression. Isocarboxazid (30 mg/kg) is a monoamine oxidase inhibitor (MAO) indicated for the treatment of depressed patients who have become refractory to tricyclic antidepressants or electroconvulsive therapy and depressed patients in whom tricyclic antidepressants are contraindicated. Isocarboxazid is absorbed rapidly and completely from the GI tract and is excreted primarily in the urine within 24 hours. Isocarboxazid is contraindicated in patients with uncontrolled hypertension and seizure disorders because the drug may precipitate hypertensive reactions and lower the seizure threshold. Isocarboxazid should be used cautiously in patients with a history of severe headaches, angina pectoris, or other cardiovascular diseases, type I and type II diabetes, Parkinson's disease and other motor disorders, hyperthyroidism, pheochromocytoma, renal or hepatic insufficiency, and bipolar disease (reduce dosage during manic phase). Foods containing high concentrations of tyramine or other pressor amines may precipitate hypertensive crisis. Isocarboxazid enhances the pressor effects of amphetamines, ephedrine, phenylephrine, phenylpropanolamine, and related drugs, and may result in serious cardiovascular toxicity. Concomitant use of isocarboxazid with disulfiram may cause tachycardia, flushing, or palpitations. Concomitant use with general anesthetics, which are normally metabolized by MAO, may cause severe hypotension and excessive CNS depression; isocarboxazid should be discontinued for at least one week before using these agents. Isocarboxazid decreases the effectiveness of local anesthetics (for example, procaine and lidocaine), resulting in poor nerve block.

ISCHEMIC STROKE: Treatment of

Vascular disorders of the nervous system may be an abnormality of the vessel wall (atheromatous thrombosis), occlusion by embolus, rupture of a vessel, progressive obliteration of the lumen (with or without diminished cardiac output), altered viscosity, or vascular permeability. Whatever the process, the result is one of the ischemic or hemorrhagic stroke syndromes. Here, stroke refers to any sudden focal neurologic deficit, e.g., hemiparesis, loss of consciousness, hemianopia.

In establishing which pathologic process is responsible for a specific stroke syndrome, recognition of the mode of onset of the neurologic deficit is important. The suddenness of onset, rapidity of evolution, and pattern of deficits determined from examination will usually allow an accurate diagnosis.

Thrombotic stroke may be sudden or may have a stuttering onset over hours or several days, often in a stepwise fashion with sudden accumulating increments.

Embolic stroke is almost always abrupt in onset and complete within minutes.

Hemorrhagic stroke may have a sudden onset with evolution to maximal deficit occurring in a smooth fashion over several hours.

Therapy for stroke is undergoing major changes. Many of the changes parallel the advances made in the therapy for myocardial infarction. Acute intervention with cytoprotective and thrombolytic agents is undergoing active investigation. Cytoprotective therapy includes drugs that act to prevent cell death during ischemia and reperfusion. These agents include calpain inhibitors, voltage-sensitive calcium- and sodium-channel antagonists, receptor-mediated calcium-channel antagonists [including *N*-methyl-*d*-aspartate (NMDA) and α-amino-3-hydroxy-5-methyl-4-isoxazole propionic acid (AMPA) antagonists], glutamate-synthesis inhibitors, glutamate-release antagonists, γ-aminobenzoic acid (GABA) antagonists, 5-HT (serotonin)-receptor agonists, gangliosides, antioxidants, growth factors, antiapoptotic agents, and antiadhesion molecules. Thrombolysis is effective in myocardial infarction. Thrombolysis is undergoing evaluation in stroke with streptokinase, anisoylated plasminogen streptokinase activator complex (APSAC), tissue plasminogen activator (t-PA: including recombinant t-PA), urokinase, and single-chain urokinase (scu-PA). Both systemic and selective administration are being evaluated. Preventive therapy with both antiplatelet and anticoagulant drugs sheds new light on how best to stratify patients in terms of a risk–benefit ratio.

Use it cautiously and in reduced dosage with alcohol, barbiturates, and other sedatives, narcotics, dextromethorphan, and tricyclic antidepressants. Cocaine and vasoconstrictors in local anesthetics may precipitate a hypertensive response (see also Figure 80).

ISOETHARINE HYDROCHLORIDE

(Arm-a-Med, Beta-2, Bisorine, Bronkosol, Dey-Dose, Dey-Lute, Dispos-a-Med)

ISOETHARINE MESYLATE

(Bronkometer)

Isoetharine, a sympathomimetic agent with bronchodilating properties (aerosol inhaler 340 mcg/metered spray), is indicated in the treatment of bronchial asthma and reversible bronchospasm that may occur with bronchitis and emphysema (see also Figure 94).

ISOFLURANE

(Forane)

Isoflurane is a 1-chloro-2,2,2-trifluoroethyl difluoromethyl ether. The chemical and physical properties of isoflurane are similar to those of its isomer enflurane. It is not flammable in air or oxygen. Isoflurane allows a smooth and rapid induction (10 minutes) of, and emergence from, general anesthesia. The clinical signs by which depth of anesthesia is judged include progressive decreases in blood pressure and in respiratory volume and rate, as well as an increase in heart rate. Systemic arterial blood pressure decreases progressively with increasing depth during anesthesia with isoflurane, as it does with halothane and enflurane. However, in contrast to the latter agents, cardiac output is well maintained with isoflurane. Depression of renal blood flow, the rate of glomerular filtration, and urinary flow accompanies anesthesia with isoflurane, as with all the volatile anesthetic agents. However, all changes in renal function observed during anesthesia are rapidly reversed during recovery. Only 0.02% of the isoflurane that enters the body is metabolized; this fraction is markedly less than the extent of metabolism of halothane or enflurane. The small quantities of fluoride and trifluoracetic acid that are generated as degradation products of isoflurane are insufficient to cause cell damage, which accounts for the lack of renal or hepatic toxicity. Isoflurane does not appear to be a mutagen, teratogen, or carcinogen (see also Table 16).

ISOMETHEPTENE MUCATE/ DICHLORALPHENAZONE/ ACETAMINOPHEN

(Midrin capsules 65 mg isometheptene mucate, 100 mg dichloralphenazone, 325 mg APAP)

Isometheptene mucate is an antituberculosis agent that interferes with lipid and nucleic acid biosynthesis in actively growing tubercle bacilli. It is indicated in the treatment of all forms of tuberculosis. Isometheptene mucate is a migraine combination. **Isometheptene** mucate acts as sympathomimetic to constrict dilated cranial and cerebral arterioles. **Dichloralphenazone** is a mild sedative that reduces emotional reaction to pain of vascular and tension headaches. **Acetaminophen** is a mild analgesic. They are indicated in relief of tension and vascular headaches. The FDA has classified the drug as possibly effective in treatment of migraine headaches.

ISONIAZID

(INH)

Isoniazid (300 mg/day in a single dose), which acts against actively growing tubercle bacilli, is indicated for the treatment and chemoprophylaxis of tuberculosis. Isoniazid is bactericidal in nature and interferes with lipid and nucleic acid biosynthesis in the growing organism. It is absorbed completely from the GI tract and diffuses readily into cell body fluids, including cerebrospinal fluid. It is metabolized in the liver by acetylation and is excreted (50%) unchanged in the urine. Isoniazid may cause severe and fatal hepatitis, and the incidence is much higher in elderly subjects. The regular consumption of ethanol enhances the incidence of isoniazid-induced hepatitis. Isoniazid may cause pyridoxine deficiency and peripheral neuropathy, which necessitates a daily dose (10 to 50 mg) of pyridoxine. Isoniazid causes optic neuritis, and periodic ophthalmologic examinations during isoniazid therapy are recommended even when visual symptoms do not occur. Isoniazid does interact with other medications. Isoniazid inhibits the activity of monoamine oxidase, and adverse interactions may occur with tyramine-containing foods such as aged cheeses. It also inhibits diamine oxidase causing exaggerated responses (e.g., headache, palpitations, sweating, hypotension, flushing, diarrhea, itching) to foods containing histamine (e.g., tuna, sauerkraut juice, yeast extract). Overdosage with isoniazid causes nausea, vomiting, dizziness, slurring of speech, blurring of vision, and visual hallucinations (including bright colors and strange designs). With marked overdosage, respiratory distress and CNS depression, progressing rapidly from stupor to profound coma, are to be expected along with severe, intractable seizures. Ingestion of 80 to 150 mg/kg usually results in severe seizures and a high likelihood of fatality. Severe metabolic acidosis, acetonuria, and hyperglycemia are typical laboratory findings.

ISOPROPAMIDE IODIDE

(Darbid)

Isopropamide (5 mg q. 12 hours) is indicated as an adjunctive therapy in the treatment of peptic ulcer. It is a muscarinic cholinergic-receptor antagonist that decreases the motility of the gastrointestinal tract and inhibits gastric acid secretion. Isopropamide is poorly absorbed from the GI tract, does not cross the blood–brain barrier, is excreted in the urine as metabolites, and in the feces as unchanged drug (see also Table 4 and Figure 34).

Isopropamide is contraindicated in patients with narrow-angle glaucoma because drug-induced cycloplegia and mydriasis may increase intraocular pressure; and in patients with obstructive uropathy, obstructive GI tract disease, severe ulcerative colitis, myasthenia gravis, paralytic ileus, intestinal atony, or toxic megacolon, because the drug may exacerbate these conditions.

Isopropamide should be administered cautiously to patients with autonomic neuropathy, hyperthyroidism, coronary artery disease, cardiac arrhythmias, CHF, or ulcerative colitis because the drug may exacerbate the symptoms of these disorders; to patients with hepatic or renal disease because toxic accumulation may occur; to patients over age 40 because the drug increases the glaucoma risk; to patients with hiatal hernia associated with reflux esophagitis because the drug may decrease lower esophageal sphincter tone; and in hot or humid environments because the drug may predispose the patient to heatstroke. Clinical effects of overdose include curare-like symptoms and such peripheral effects as headache, dilated, nonreactive pupils, blurred vision, flushed, hot, dry skin, dryness of mucous membranes, dysphagia, decreased or absent bowel sounds, urinary retention, hyperthermia, tachycardia, hypertension, and increased respiration.

ISOPROTERENOL

(Aerolone, Isuprel, Vapo-Iso)

ISOPROTERENOL HYDROCHLORIDE

(Isuprel, Isuprel Mistometer, Norisodrine)

ISOPROTERENOL SULFATE

(Medihaler-Iso)

Isoproterenol, a sympathomimetic amine with bronchodilating and cardiac stimulant properties, is indicated in the treatment of complete heart block, after closure of ventricular septal defect, to prevent heart block, as maintenance therapy in AV block, as treatment of bronchospasm during mild acute asthma attacks, bronchospasm in chronic obstructive pulmonary disease, bronchospasm during mild acute asthma attacks or in chronic obstructive pulmonary disease, acute asthma attacks unresponsive to inhalation therapy or control of bronchospasm during anesthesia, for bronchodilation, emergency treatment of cardiac arrhythmias, immediate temporary control of atropine-resistant hemodynamically significant bradycardia, and as adjunct therapy in the treatment of shock.

Isoproterenol (aerosol: delivers 131 mcg/dose in fine mist) is indicated in the treatment of bronchospasm associated with acute and bronchial asthma, pulmonary emphysema, bronchitis, and bronchiectasis. Parenteral isoproterenol is indicated as an adjunct to fluid and electrolyte replacement therapy in the treatment of hypovolemic and septic shock, low cardiac output states, CHF, and cardiogenic shock. Sublingual or rectal isoproterenol is indicated in Adams–Stokes syndrome and atrioventricular heart block. Isoproterenol relaxes bronchial smooth muscle by direct action on beta$_2$-adrenergic receptors, relieving bronchospasm, increasing vital capacity, decreasing residual volume in the lungs, and facilitating passage of pulmonary secretions. It also produces relaxation of GI and uterine smooth muscle via stimulation of beta$_2$ receptors. Peripheral vasodilation, cardiac stimulation, and relaxation of bronchial smooth muscle are the main therapeutic effects. Isoproterenol acts on beta$_1$-adrenergic receptors in the heart, producing a positive chronotropic and inotropic effect. It usually increases cardiac output. In patients with AV block, isoproterenol shortens conduction time and increases the rate and strength of ventricular contraction. Isoproterenol is contraindicated in patients with preexisting cardiac arrhythmias, especially tachycardia (including tachycardia caused by digitalis toxicity) because of the drug's cardiac stimulant effects. Clinical manifestations of overdose include exaggeration of common adverse reactions, particularly cardiac arrhythmias, extreme tremors, nausea and vomiting, and profound hypotension.

ISOSORBIDE

(Ismotic)

Isosorbide, an osmotic diuretic (1 to 5 mg/kg p.o.), is used for short-term reduction of intraocular pressure from glaucoma.

ISOSORBIDE

(Isordil)

Isosorbide dinitrate (sublingual, chewable, and oral medications) is indicated in the treatment and prevention of angina pectoris. Isosorbide dinitrate reduces myocardial oxygen demand through peripheral vasodilation, resulting in decreased venous filling pressure and, to a lesser extent, decreased arterial impedance. These combined effects result in decreased cardiac work and, consequently, reduced myocardial oxygen demands. The drug also redistributes coronary blood flow from epicardial to subendocardial regions. Isosorbide dilates peripheral vessels, helping to manage pulmonary edema and congestive heart failure caused by decreased venous return to the heart. Arterial vasodilatory effects also decrease arterial impedance and thus left-ventricular workload, benefiting the failing heart. These combined effects may help some patients with acute myocardial infarction. Clinical effects of overdose result primarily from vasodilation and methemoglobinemia and include hypotension, persistent throbbing headache, palpitations, visual disturbance, flushing of the skin and sweating (with skin later becoming cold and cyanotic), nausea and vomiting, colic and bloody diarrhea, orthostasis, initial hyperpnea, dyspnea, slow respiratory rate, bradycardia, heart block, increased intracranial pressure with confusion, fever, paralysis, and tissue hypoxia from methemoglobinemia, which can lead to cyanosis, metabolic acidosis, coma, clonic convulsions, and circulatory collapse.

Death may result from circulatory collapse or asphyxia (see also Figures 69 and 70).

ISOSORBIDE DINITRATE

(Dilatrate-SR, Iso-Bid, Isochron, Isonate, Isonate TR, Isordil, Isotrate, Onset-5, Sorate, Sorbide TD, Sorbitrate, Sorbitrate SA)

Isosorbide, an antianginal nitrate with vasodilating properties (2.5 to 10 mg sublingually), is indicated in the treatment or prophylaxis of acute anginal attacks and treatment of chronic ischemic heart disease (see also Figures 69 and 70).

ISOSORBIDE MONONITRATE

(Imdur, Ismo, Monoket)

Isosorbide, an antianginal nitrate (20 mg p.o. b.i.d.), is indicated in prevention of angina pectoris due to coronary artery disease (see also Figures 60 and 61).

ISOSORBIDE MONONITRATE

(ISMO tablets 20 mg)

Isosorbide mononitrate is a nitrate. It causes relaxation of smooth muscle of venous and arterial vasculature. It is indicated in prevention of angina pectoris.

Organic nitrates are available in a number of formulations that include rapid-acting nitroglycerin tablets or spray for sublingual administration, short-acting oral agents such as isosorbide dinitrate (Isordil, Sorbitrate, others), long-acting oral agents such as isosorbide mononitrate (Imdur), topical preparations such as nitroglycerin ointment and transdermal patches, and intravenous nitroglycerin. The nitrate preparations are relatively safe and effective agents whose principal action in the treatment of CHF is reduction of left-ventricular filling pressures. This preload reduction is due to an increase in peripheral venous capacitance. Nitrates will cause a decline in pulmonary and systemic vascular resistance, particularly at higher doses, although this response is less marked and less predictable than with nitroprusside. These drugs do have a selective vasodilator effect on the epicardial coronary vasculature and may enhance both systolic and diastolic ventricular function by increasing coronary flow; the clinical relevance of this coronary vasodilator effect in patients with epicardial coronary obstruction remains controversial.

ISOTRETINOIN

(Accutane)

Isotretinoin, a retinoic acid derivative with antiacne properties, is indicated in the treatment of severe cystic acne unresponsive to conventional therapy. In addition, it has been used in keratinization disorders resistant to conventional therapy.

ISOTRETINOIN (13-CIS-RETINOIC ACID)

(Accutane capsules 10 mg)

Isotretinoin is a first-generation retinoid that reduces sebum secretion and sebaceous gland size, inhibits sebaceous gland differentiation, and alters sebum lipid composition. It is indicated in the treatment of severe acne.

Retinoids include natural compounds and synthetic derivatives of retinol that exhibit vitamin A activity. Retinoids have many important functions throughout the body, including roles in vision, regulation of cell proliferation and differentiation and bone growth, immune defense, and tumor suppression. Because vitamin A affects normal epithelial differentiation, it was investigated as a treatment for cutaneous disorders but was abandoned initially because of unfavorable side effects. Molecular modifications yielded compounds with vastly improved margins of safety. First-generation retinoids include **retinol**, **tretinoin** (all-*trans*-retinoic acid), **isotretinoin** (13-*cis*-retinoic acid), and **alitretinoin** (9-*cis*-retinoic acid). Second-generation retinoids, also known as aromatic retinoids, were created by alteration of the cyclic end group and include **acitretin**. Third-generation retinoids contain further modifications and are called arotinoids. Members of this generation include **tazarotene** and **bexarotene**. **Adapalene**, a derivative of naphthoic acid with retinoid-like properties, does not fit precisely into any of the three generations.

Retinoic acid (RA) exerts its effects on gene expression by activating two families of receptors—**retinoic acid receptors** (RARs) and the **retinoid X receptors** (RXRs)—that are members of the **thyroid/steroid hormone receptor superfamily**. Retinoids (ligands) bind transcription factors (nuclear receptors), and the ligand-receptor complex then binds to the promoter regions of target genes to regulate their expression. The gene products formed contribute to the desirable pharmacological effects of these drugs and their unwanted side effects. Additional complexity arises because each receptor has three isoforms (α, β, and γ) that form homo- and heterodimers. Retinoid-responsive tissues express one or more RAR and RXR subtypes in various combinations that determine activity locally. Human skin contains mainly RARα and RARβ.

Oral **isotretinoin** (accutane) is approved for the treatment of severe nodulocystic **acne vulgaris**. The drug has remarkable efficacy in severe acne and may induce prolonged remissions after a single course of therapy. It normalizes keratinization in the sebaceous follicle, reduces sebocyte number with decreased sebum synthesis, and reduces **Propionibacterium acnes**, the organism that proves inflammation in acne.

Isotretinoin is administered orally. The recommended dose is 0.5 to 2 mg/kg per day for 15 to 20 weeks. Lower doses are effective but are associated with shorter remissions. The cumulative dose also is important, so smaller doses for longer periods can be used to achieve a total dose in the range of 120 mg/kg. Approximately 40% of patients will relapse, usually within 3 years of therapy, and may require retreatment. Preteens and patients with acne conglobata or androgen excess are at increased risk of relapse. However, mild relapses may respond to conventional management with topical and systemic antiacne agents.

Isotretinoin is prescribed for severe, **recalcitrant nodular acne**, moderate acne unresponsive to oral antibiotics, and acne that produces scarring. It also is used commonly for other related disorders, such as **Gram-negative folliculitis**, **acne rosacea**, and **hidradenitis suppurativa**.

Dose-dependent adverse effects on the skin and mucous membranes are observed most commonly, including cheilitis, mucous membrane dryness, epistaxis, dry eyes, blepharoconjunctivitis, erythematous eruptions, and xerosis. Alteration of epidermal surfaces may facilitate *Staphylococcus aureus* colonization and, rarely, subsequent infection. Hair loss, exuberant granulation tissue formation, photosensitivity, and dark adaptation dysfunction are rarer occurrences.

Systemic side effects generally are less significant with short-term therapy. Transitory elevations in serum transaminases occur rarely. Hyperlipidemia is frequent, with 25% of patients developing increased triglyceride levels and, less frequently, increased cholesterol and low-density lipoproteins (LDL) and decreased high-density lipoproteins (HDL). Myalgia and arthralgia are common complaints. Headaches occur and rarely are a symptom of pseudotumor cerebri. Use of isotretinoin concomitantly with tetracycline antibiotics may increase the risk of pseudotumor cerebri. Controversy exists regarding the potential linking of isotretinoin to depression, suicidal thoughts, and suicide. Epidemiological studies to date have not shown an association between **isotretinoin** and depression or suicide, perhaps because acne itself may be a risk factor for depression. Some physicians have proposed a causal relationship with mood changes and depression in a limited number of patients. These uncontrolled clinical observations have not been examined in a rigorous, prospective manner. In addition, there is a paucity of data on the effect of retinoids on adult brain function. Long-term therapy may produce skeletal side effects, including diffuse idiopathic skeletal hyperosteoses, and extraskeletal ossification.

High doses of isotretinoin produce partial regression of multiple **basal cell carcinomas** but are more effective in suppressing the formation of new tumors, as demonstrated in patients with **xeroderma pigmentosum**. **Isotretinoin** also prevents second primary tumors in patients who have had a previous squamous cell carcinoma of the head and neck. **Isotretinoin** also is effective for oral leukoplakia. Topical tazarotene has shown efficacy in some basal cell carcinomas. Cutaneous T-cell lymphoma has been shown to respond to several types of topical and systemic retinoids, including bexarotene. The benefits of long-term retinoid use in malignant lymphomas such as cutaneous T-cell lymphoma must be balanced by appreciation of retinoid toxicity and the chronicity of the disease.

ISOXSUPRINE HYDROCHLORIDE

(Vasodilan tablets 10 mg)

Isoxsuprine is a peripheral vasodilator, which stimulates skeletal beta receptors to produce vasodilation; stimulates cardiac function (increased contractility, heart rate, and cardiac output) and relaxes the uterus. At higher doses, it inhibits platelet aggregation and decreases blood viscosity. It is indicated for treatment of cerebral vascular insufficiency, peripheral vascular disease caused by arteriosclerosis obliterans, thromboangitis obliterans, and Raynaud's disease.

ISRADIPINE

(DynaCirc capsules 2.5 mg)

Isradipine is a calcium-channel-blocking agent with antihypertensive properties that reduces systemic vascular resistance and blood pressure by inhibiting movement of calcium ions across cell membrane in systemic and coronary vascular smooth muscle and myocardium. It is indicated in the treatment of hypertension (see also Table 13).

Voltage-sensitive Ca^{2+} channels (L-type or slow channels) mediate the entry of extracellular Ca^{2+} into smooth muscle and cardiac myocytes and sinoatrial (SA) and atrioventricular (AV) nodal cells in response to electrical depolarization. In both smooth muscle and cardiac myocytes, Ca^{2+} is a trigger for contraction, albeit by different mechanisms. Ca^{2+}-channel antagonists, also called **Ca^{2+}-entry blockers**, inhibit Ca^{2+} channel function. In vascular smooth muscle, this leads to relaxation, especially in arterial beds. These drugs also may produce negative inotropic and chronotropic effects in the heart.

An increased concentration of cytosolic Ca^{2+} causes increased contraction in cardiac vascular smooth muscle cells. The entry of extracellular Ca^{2+}-is more important in initiating the contraction of cardiac myocytes (Ca^{2+}-induced Ca^{2+} release). The release of Ca^{2+} from intracellular storage sites also contributes to contraction of vascular smooth muscle, particularly in some vascular beds. Cytosolic Ca^{2+} concentrations may be increased by various contractile stimuli. Thus, many hormones and neurohormones increase Ca^{2+} influx through so-called receptor-operated channels, whereas high external concentrations of K^+ and depolarizing electrical stimuli increase Ca^{2+} influx through voltage-sensitive, or "potential operated," channels. The Ca^{2+}-channel antagonists produce their effects by binding to the α_1 subunit of the L-type Ca^{2+} channels and reducing Ca^{2+} flux through the channel.

Nifedipine given intravenously increases forearm blood flow with little effect on venous pooling; this indicates a selective dilation of arterial resistance vessels. The decrease in arterial blood pressure elicits sympathetic reflexes, with resulting tachycardia and positive inotropy. Nifedipine also has direct negative inotropic effects *in vitro*. However, nifedipine relaxes vascular smooth muscle at significantly lower concentrations than those required for prominent direct effects on the heart. Thus, arteriolar resistance and blood pressure are lowered, contractility and segmental ventricular function are improved, and heart rate and cardiac output are increased modestly. After oral administration of nifedipine, arterial dilation increases peripheral blood flow; venous tone does not change.

The other dihydropyridines—**amlodipine**, **felodipine**, **isradipine**, **nicardipine**, **nisoldipine**, and **nimodipine**—share many of the cardiovascular effects of nifedipine. Amlodipine is a dihydropyridine that has a slow absorption and a prolonged effect. With a plasma half-life of 35 to 50 hours, plasma levels and effect increase over 7 to 10 days of daily administration of a constant dose. **Amlodipine** produces both peripheral arterial vasodilation and coronary dilation, with a hemodynamic profile similar to that of nifedipine. However, there is less reflex tachycardia with amlodipine, possibly because the long half-life produces minimal peaks and troughs in plasma concentrations. **Felodipine** may have even greater vascular specificity than does nifedipine or amlodipine. At concentrations producing vasodilation, there is no negative inotropic effect. Like nifedipine, felodipine indirectly activates the sympathetic nervous system, leading to an increase in heart rate. Nicardipine has antianginal properties similar to those of nifedipine and may have selectivity for coronary vessels. **Isradipine** also produces the typical peripheral vasodilation seen with other dihydropyridines, but because of its inhibitory effect on the SA node, little or no rise in heart rate is seen. This inhibitory effect does not extend to the cardiac myocytes, however, because no cardiodepressant effect is seen. Despite the negative chronotropic effect, isradipine appears to have little effect on the AV node, so it may be used in patients with AV block or combined with a β-adrenergic-receptor antagonist.

In general, because of their lack of myocardial depression and, to a greater or lesser extent, lack of negative chronotropic effect, dihydropyridines are less effective as monotherapy in stable angina than are verapamil, diltiazem, or a β-adrenergic-receptor antagonist. Nisoldipine is more than 1000 times more potent in preventing contraction of human vascular smooth muscle than in preventing contraction of human cardiac muscle *in vitro*, suggesting a high degree of vascular selectivity. Although **nisoldipine** has a short elimination half-life, a sustained-release preparation has been developed that is efficacious as an antianginal agent. Nimodipine has high lipid solubility and was developed as an agent to relax the cerebral vasculature. It is effective in inhibiting cerebral vasospasm and has been used primarily to treat patients with neurological defects associated with cerebral vasospasm after subarachnoid hemorrhage.

ITRACONAZOLE

(Sporanox capsules 100 mg)

Itraconazole is a triazole antifungal agent that inhibits the C-demethylation step in the synthesis of ergosterol, which is a vital component of fungal cell membranes. **Injection**: used in treatment of aspergillosis, blastomycosis, histoplasmosis, and the empiric treatment of febrile neutropenic patients with suspected fungal infections. **Capsules**: used in treatment of asper-gillosis, blastomycosis, histoplasmosis, and onychomycosis (nonimmunocompromised patients only). **Oral solution**: used in treatment of oropharyngeal or esophageal candidiasis and empiric treatment of febrile neutropenic patients with suspected fungal infections.

Itraconazole (Sporonox) is available as a capsule and two solution formulations, one for oral and one for intravenous administration. The capsule form of the drug is best absorbed in the fed state, but the oral solution is better absorbed in the fasting state, providing peak plasma concentrations that are more than 150% of those obtained with the capsule. Both the oral solution and intravenous formulation are solubilized in a 40:1 weight ratio of **itraconazole** hydroxypropyl-β-cyclodextrin, so that administration of 200 mg of **itraconazole** provides 8 g of this excipient. **Itraconazole** is metabolized in the liver. It is both a substrate for and a potent inhibitor of CYP3A4. Itraconazole is present in plasma with an approximately equal concentration of a biologically active metabolite, hydroxy-**itraconazole**. Bioassays may report up to 3.3 times as much itraconazole in plasma as do physical methods such as high-performance liquid chromatography, depending on the susceptibility of the bioassay organism to hydroxy-itraconazole. The native drug and metabolite are >99% bound to plasma proteins. Neither appears in urine or CSF. The half-life of itraconazole at steady state is approximately 30 to 40 hours. Steady-state levels of **itraconazole** are not reached for 4 days and those of hydroxy-itraconazole for 7 days; thus, loading doses are recommended when treating deep mycoses. Severe liver disease will increase itraconazole plasma concentrations, but azotemia and hemodialysis have no effect. Some 80 to 90% of intravenously administered hydroxypropyl-β-cyclodextrin is excreted in the urine, and the compound accumulates in the presence of azotemia. Intravenous administration of **itraconazole** is contraindicated in patients with a creatinine clearance below 30 ml/min because of concern about potential hydroxypropyl-β-cyclodextrin toxicity. It is not carcinogenic but is teratogenic in rats, and is contraindicated in the treatment of onychomycosis during pregnancy or for women contemplating pregnancy.

Itraconazole given as a capsule is the drug of choice for patients with indolent, nonmeningeal infections due to ***B. dermatitidis***, ***H. capsulatum***, ***P. brasiliensis***, and ***C. immitis***. This dosage form also is useful in therapy of indolent invasive aspergillosis outside the CNS, particularly after the infection has been stabilized with **amphotericin B**. The intravenous formulation is approved for the initial 2 weeks of therapy with **blastomycosis**, histoplasmosis, and indolent aspergillosis, and for empirical therapy of febrile neutropenic patients not responding to antibacterial antibiotics and at high risk of fungal infections. The intravenous route would be most appropriate for patients unable to tolerate the oral formulation or unable to absorb **itraconazole** because of decreased gastric acid production. Approximately half the patients with distal subungual onychomycosis respond to

itraconazole. Although not an approved use, **itraconazole** is a reasonable choice for treatment of **pseudallescheriasis**, an infection not responding to amphotericin B therapy, as well as cutaneous and extracutaneous sporotrichosis, tinea corporis, and extensive tinea versicolor. HTV-infected patients with disseminated histoplasmosis or *Penicillium marneffei* infections have a decreased incidence of relapse if given prolonged **itraconazole** "maintenance" therapy. It is as yet unclear whether patients responding to highly active antiretroviral therapy (HAART) will require less than lifelong therapy for *P. marneffei* and disseminated histoplasmosis. **Itraconazole** is not recommended for maintenance therapy of cryptococcal meningitis in HIV-infected patients because of a high incidence of relapse. Long-term therapy has been used in non-HIV-infected patients with allergic bronchopulmonary aspergillosis to decrease the dose of glucocorticoids and reduce attacks of acute bronchospasm.

Itraconazole, a synthetic triazole with antifungal properties, is indicated in the treatment of blastomycosis (pulmonary and extra-pulmonary), histoplasmosis (including chronic cavitary pulmonary disease and disseminated nonmeningeal histoplasmosis) and aspergillosis (pulmonary and extra-pulmonary) in patients who are intolerant of or refractory to amphotericin B therapy. In addition, itraconazole has been used in the treatment of superficial mycoses (dermatophytoses, pityriasis versicolor, sebopsoriasis, candidiasis [vaginal, oral or chronic mucocutaneous], and onychomycosis), systemic mycoses (candidiasis, cryptococcal infections [meningitis, disseminated], dimorphic infections [paracoccidioidomycosis, coccidioidomycosis]), subcutaneous mycoses (sporotrichosis, chromomycosis), cutaneous leishmaniasis, fungal keratitis, alteranariosis, and zygomycosis. Itraconazole is an orally active, broad-spectrum, triazole antifungal agent that has a higher affinity for fungal cytochrome P450 than ketoconazole but a low affinity for mammalian cytochrome P450. Itraconazole has a broader spectrum of activity than other azole antifungals and shows interesting pharmacokinetic features in terms of its tissue distribution. These properties have resulted in reduced treatment times for a number of diseases such as vaginal candidiasis, as well as effective oral treatment of several deep mycoses, including aspergillosis and candidiasis (see also Figure 21).

IVERMECTIN

Ivermectin is a potent macrocyclic lactone causing paralysis in many nematodes and arthropods through an influx of chloride ions across the cell membrane. It is currently the drug of choice for human onchocerciasis and shows potent microfilaricidal activity against the other major filarial parasites of humans (*Wuchereria bancrofti*, *Brugia malayi*, *Loa loa*, and *Mansonella ozzardi*) but not against *M. perstans*. Ivermectin also has excellent efficacy in both human strongyloidiasis and cutaneous larva migrans for which good alternative treatments have not been available, and it is as effective as currently available drugs against the intestinal nematodes *Ascaris lumbriocoides*, *Trichuris trichiura*, and *Enterobius vermicularis*; against the human hookworms, it shows only partial efficacy. Preliminary studies indicate that ivermectin has the potential to become the drug of choice for ectoparasitic infections (mites, lice) of humans as well.

J

JAPANESE ENCEPHALITIS VIRUS VACCINE, INACTIVATED

(Je-Vax)

Japanese encephalitis virus vaccine is indicated for primary immunization (1 mL/SC on days 0, 7, and 30) and booster immunization (1 mL/SC after 2 years) against Japanese encephalitis.

JIMSON WEED

The atropine series contains a number of very closely allied alkaloids of which the chief are atropine, hyoscyamine, and hyoscine or scopolamine. They are found in the roots and leaves of many plants of the *Solanaceae* order, notably belladonna (*Atropa belladonna*), henbane (*Hyoscyamus niger*), the thorn apple or jimson weed (*Datura stramonium*), and some members of the *Duboisia* and *Scopolia* species. These plants were used during the Middle Ages to form the "sorcerer's drugs" and have been smoked, chewed, or imbibed in the form of decoctions by primitive people for the hallucinations and frenzy that they produce.

Atropine and its allied drugs (hyoscyamine, scopolamine, homatropine, etc.) are autonomic blocking agents that inhibit the action of the postganglionic cholinergic nerves and were, therefore, formerly designated as depressants of the parasympathetic system, or as antiparasympathomimetic agents. These drugs differ from nicotine and curare, which are also depressants of the parasympathetic system but which act as blocking agents on preganglionic cholinergic nerves. Atropine in therapeutic doses has no effect on the nicotinic actions of acetylcholine but specifically blocks all muscarinic responses of injected acetylcholine, whether excitatory as in the intestine, or inhibitory as in the heart. It fails, however, to block all cholinergic nerve stimulations and also exerts effects that are not explicable on the basis of its antagonism to acetylcholine. In addition to their action in blocking the muscarinic effects of acetylcholine, atropine and its allies exert important effects on the central nervous system (see also Figures 12 and 26).

K

KALLIDIN

As autocoids, bradykinin and kallidin increase vascular permeability, produce vasodilation, increase the synthesis of prostaglandins, and cause edema and pain. Extensive evidence exists that bradykinin and other kallidin substances contribute to the pathogenesis of the inflammatory response that occurs in acute and chronic diseases, including allergic reactions, arthritis, asthma, sepsis, viral rhinitis, and inflammatory bowel diseases. Bradykinin (Arg-Pro-Pro-Gly-Phe-Ser-Pro-Phe-Arg), a nonapeptide, and kallidin, a decapeptide, are derived from kininogens. Both tissue and plasma kallikreins are involved in the synthesis of bradykinin and kallidin (Figure 30), and both have a short plasma half-life of only 15 seconds. The kinins are catabolized by kininase II, which is also known as angiotensin-converting enzyme (see Figure 24). Kinin receptors are classified as either kinin B_1 or kinin B_2. Kinin-B_1 receptors, which are located in the aorta and mesenteric veins, respond to kinin agonists in the following order of potency:

des Arg^{10}-kallidin > des Arg^{10}-bradykinin > kallidin > [try(Mc^8)] bradykinin.

Kinin-B_2 receptors, which are located in the jugular vein and carotid artery, respond to kinin agonists in the following order of potency:

kallidin > [try(Mc^8)]bradykinin > bradykinin > des Arg^{10}-kallidin > des Arg^9-bradykinin.

Analogs of des Arg^9-bradykinin or des Arg^{10}-kallidin are selective antagonists for kinin-B_1 receptors. Analogs of [$Dphen^7$] bradykinin are antagonists for kinin-B_2 receptors. Activation of the B_2-kinin receptors, in virtually all the tissues so far described, leads to stimulation of phosphatidylinositol (PI)-specific phospholipase C, resulting in the formation of inositol phosphates and diacylglycerol, and subsequent elevations in the intracellular calcium concentration. In addition, bradykinin-induced increases in the intracellular calcium concentrations of human airway smooth muscle appear to be mediated both by activation of PLC-PI turnover and by calcium influx via receptor-operated calcium channels.

KANAMYCIN SULFATE

(Kantrex capsules 500 mg)

Kanamycin sulfate is an aminoglycoside antibiotic that inhibits its production of bacterial protein, causing cell death. **Parenteral**: used in short-term treatment of serious infections caused by susceptible strains of microorganisms, especially Gram-negative bacteria. **Oral**: used in short-term adjunctive therapy for suppression of intestinal bacteria and treatment of hepatic coma.

The antibacterial activity of gentamicin, tobramycin, kanamycin, netilmicin, and amikacin is primarily directed against aerobic, Gram-negative bacilli. Kanamycin, like streptomycin, has a more limited spectrum compared with other aminoglycosides and, in particular, it should not be used to treat infections caused by *Serratia* or *P. aeruginosa*. Kanamycin may be used as an initial therapy for one or more of the following organisms: *Escherichia coli*, *Proteus* sp. (both indole-positive and indole-negative), *Enterobacter aerogenes*, *Klebsiella pneumoniae*, *Serratia marcescens*, and *Acinetobacter* sp. It may be used as initial therapy with a penicillin or cephalosporin before obtaining results of susceptibility testing (see also Figure 88). Aminoglycosides are bactericidal and inhibit protein synthesis in susceptible microorganisms. They exert this effect by (1) interfering with the initiation complex of peptide formation, (2) misreading the code on the messenger RNA template, which causes the incorporation of inappropriate amino acid into peptide, and (3) rupturing the polysomes into monosomes, which become nonfunctional. Resistance to aminoglycosides may be due to one or a combination of the following mechanisms: interference with the transport of aminoglycoside into bacterial cells, deletion of receptors on the 30S ribosomal subunit, thus preventing the functioning of aminoglycosides, and the bacterial biotransformation of aminoglycosides to inactive forms.

In addition, because the initial transport of aminoglycosides into bacterial cells is an oxygen-dependent process, microorganisms that are able to grow under anaerobic conditions show or develop resistance. The aminoglycosides are poorly absorbed from the gastrointestinal tract and, for this reason, are administered intramuscularly. Furthermore, because they do not penetrate into the central nervous system, they may have to be given intrathecally or intraventricularly in the treatment of meningitis. Aminoglycosides are excreted by glomerular filtration, which is greatly reduced in the presence of renal impairment, thus leading to toxic blood levels. The most serious toxic reactions following aminoglycoside therapy are cochlear damage and vestibular impairment, which lead to vertigo and disturb the ability to maintain postural equilibrium. Aminoglycosides given during pregnancy can cause deafness in the newborn. Nephrotoxicity and reversible neuromuscular blockade causing respiratory paralysis have also been seen following the use of high doses (see also Table 23).

The aminoglycoside group includes **gentamicin**, **tobramycin**, **amikacin**, **netilmicin**, **kanamycin**, **streptomycin**, and **neomycin**. These drugs are used primarily to treat infections caused by aerobic Gram-negative bacteria;

streptomycin is an important agent for the treatment of tuberculosis. In contrast to most inhibitors of microbial protein synthesis, which are bacteriostatic, the aminoglycosides are bactericidal inhibitors of protein synthesis. Mutations affecting proteins in the bacterial ribosome, the target for these drugs, can confer marked resistance to their action. However, most commonly, resistance is due to acquisition of plasmids or transposon-encoding genes for aminoglycoside-metabolizing enzymes, or from impaired transport of the drug into the cell. Thus, there can be cross-resistance between members of the class.

These agents contain amino sugars linked to an aminocyclitol ring by glycosidic bonds. They are polycations, and their polarity is responsible in part for pharmacokinetic properties shared by all members of the group. For example, none is absorbed adequately after oral administration, inadequate concentrations are found in cerebrospinal fluid (CSF), and all are excreted relatively rapidly by the normal kidney. Although aminoglycosides are widely used and are important agents, serious toxicity limits their usefulness. All members of the group share the same spectrum of toxicity, most notably nephrotoxicity and ototoxicity, which can involve the auditory and vestibular functions of the eighth cranial nerve.

The use of **kanamycin** has declined markedly because its spectrum of activity is limited compared with other aminoglycosides, and it is among the most toxic.

Kanamycin sulfate (Kantrex) is available for injection and oral use. The parenteral dose for adults is 15 mg/kg per day (two to four equally divided and spaced doses), with a maximum of 1.5 g/day. Children may be given up to 15 mg/kg per day.

Kanamycin is all but obsolete, and there are few indications for its use. It has been employed to treat tuberculosis in combination with other effective drugs. It has no therapeutic advantage over streptomycin or amikacin and probably is more toxic; either should be used instead, depending on susceptibility of the isolate.

Kanamycin can be administered orally as adjunctive therapy in cases of hepatic encephalopathy. The dose is 4 to 6 g/day for 36 to 72 hours; quantities as large as 12 g/day (in divided doses) have been given. It is ototoxic and nephrotoxic. Like neomycin, its oral administration can cause malabsorption and superinfection.

KAOLIN/PECTIN

(Kao-Spen suspension 5.2 g)

Kaolin/pectin is an antidiarrheal combination that absorbs fluid, and binds and removes digestive tract irritants. They are used for symptomatic treatment of diarrhea. Kaopectate (190 mg kaolin/mL and 4.34 mg pectin/mL) is an antidiarrheal agent. By being absorbent, it recovers excess fluid in bowel dysfunction. It is contraindicated in obstructive bowel dysfunction. When used concomitantly, kaolin/pectin may impair absorption of the following drugs: antidyskinetics, antimuscarinics (especially atropine), chloroquine, dicyclomine, digoxin or digitalis glycosides, lincomycin, phenothiazines, tetracycline antibiotics, and xanthines (especially caffeine, theophylline, aminophylline, dyphylline, and oxtriphylline).

Hydrophilic and poorly fermentable colloids or polymers such as **carboxymethylcellulose** and **calcium polycarbophil** absorb water and increase stool bulk (calcium polycarbophil absorbs 60 times its weight in water). They usually are used for constipation but are sometimes useful in mild chronic diarrheas in patients suffering from irritable bowel syndrome. The mechanism of this effect is not clear, but they may work as gels to modify stool texture and viscosity and to produce a perception of decreased stool fluidity. Some of these agents also may bind bacterial toxins and bile salts. Clays such as **kaolin** (a **hydrated aluminum silicate**) and other silicates such as **attapulgite** (magnesium aluminum disilicate, Diasorb) bind water avidly (attapulgite absorbs eight times its weight in water) and may also bind enterotoxins. However, this effect is not selective and may involve other drugs and nutrients; hence these agents are best avoided within 2 to 3 hours of taking other medications. A mixture of **kaolin and pectin** (a plant polysaccharide) is a popular over-the-counter remedy (**Kaopectolin**) and may provide useful symptomatic relief of mild diarrhea.

KETAMINE HYDROCHLORIDE

(Ketalar)

Ketamine hydrochloride is a general anesthetic that produces a rapid-acting anesthetic state with profound analgesia, normal pharyngeal–laryngeal reflexes, normal or slightly enhanced skeletal muscle tone, cardiovascular and respiratory stimulation and, occasionally, transient and minimal respiratory depression. It is indicated in diagnostic and surgical procedures that do not require skeletal muscle relaxation, induction of anesthesia, and supplementation of low-potency agents, such as nitrous oxide.

Ketamine is used as a sole anesthetic agent for diagnostic and surgical procedures that do not require skeletal muscle relaxation. It is best suited for short procedures, but it can be used with additional doses for longer procedures. It is also used for the induction of anesthesia prior to the administration of other general anesthetics and to supplement low-potency agents, such as nitrous oxide.

Ketamine is a rapid-acting general anesthetic producing an anesthetic state characterized by profound analgesia, normal pharyngeal-laryngeal reflexes, normal or slightly enhanced skeletal muscle tone, cardiovascular and respiratory stimulation and, occasionally, a transient and minimal respiratory depression.

Emergence from ketamine's anesthesia may be associated with psychological manifestations such as pleasant dream-like states, vivid imagery, hallucinations and emergence delirium, sometimes accompanied by confusion, excitement, and irrational behavior. The duration is ordinarily a few hours; however, recurrences have been seen up to 24 hours postoperatively. No residual psychological effects are known. Ketamine should be used cautiously in patients with hypertension and cardiac decompensation. Halothane blocks the cardiovascular stimulatory effects of ketamine. Barbiturates and narcotics prolong the recovery time following ketamine. Ketamine may prolong the action of tubocurarine and cause prolonged respiratory depression (see also Figure 82).

Ketamine is an arylcyclohexylamine, a congener of phencyclidine. It is supplied as a racemic mixture even though the S-isomer is more potent with fewer side effects. Although more lipophilic than thiopental, **ketamine** is water soluble and available as 10-, 50-, and 100-mg/mL solutions in sodium chloride plus the preservative benzethonium chloride.

Ketamine (Ketalar, others) has unique properties that make it useful for anesthetizing patients at risk for hypotension and bronchospasm and for certain pediatric procedures. However, significant side effects limit its routine use. **Ketamine** rapidly produces a hypnotic state quite distinct from that of other anesthetics. Patients have profound analgesia, unresponsiveness to commands, and amnesia but may have their eyes open, move their limbs involuntarily, and breathe spontaneously. This cataleptic state has been termed **dissociative anesthesia**.

Ketamine typically is administered intravenously but also is effective by intramuscular, oral, and rectal routes. The induction doses are 0.5 to 1.5 mg/kg IV, 4 to 6 mg/kg IM, and 8 to 10 mg/ml. Onset of action after an intravenous dose is similar to that of the other parenteral anesthetics, but the duration of anesthesia of a single dose is longer. For anesthetic maintenance, ketamine occasionally is continued as an infusion (25 to 100 μg/kg per minute). Ketamine does not elicit pain on injection or true excitatory behavior as described for **methohexital**, although involuntary movements produced by ketamine can be mistaken for anesthetic excitement.

The onset and duration of an induction dose of **ketamine** are determined by the same distribution/redistribution mechanism operant for all the other parenteral anesthetics.

Ketamine is hepatically metabolized to norketamine, which has reduced CNS activity; norketamine is further metabolized and excreted in urine and bile. **Ketamine** has a large volume of distribution and rapid clearance that make it suitable for continuous infusion without the drastic lengthening in duration of action seen with thiopental. Protein binding is much lower with **ketamine** than with the other parenteral anesthetics.

Ketamine has indirect sympathomimetic activity. Ketamine's behavioral effects are distinct from those of other anesthetics. The **ketamine**-induced cataleptic state is accompanied by nystagmus with pupillary dilation, salivation, lacrimation, and spontaneous limb movements with increased overall muscle tone. Although ketamine does not produce the classic anesthetic state, patients are amnestic and unresponsive to painful stimuli. **Ketamine** produces profound analgesia, a distinct advantage over other parenteral anesthetics.

Unlike other parenteral anesthetics, ketamine increases cerebral blood flow and intracranial pressure (ICP) with minimal alteration of cerebral metabolism. These effects can be attenuated by concurrent administration of thiopental and/or benzodiazepines along with hyperventilation. However, given that other anesthetics actually reduce ICP and cerebral metabolism, ketamine is relatively contraindicated for patients with increased intracranial pressure or those at risk for cerebral ischemia. In some studies, **ketamine** increased intraocular pressure (IOP), and its use for induction of patients with open eye injuries is controversial. The effects of ketamine on seizure activity appear mixed, without either strong pro- or anticonvulsant activity. Emergence delirium characterized by hallucinations, vivid dreams, and illusions is a frequent complication of ketamine that can result in serious patient dissatisfaction and can complicate postoperative management. Delirium symptoms are most frequent in the first hour after emergence and appear to occur less frequently in children. Benzodiazepines reduce the incidence of emergence delirium.

Unlike other anesthetics, induction doses of ketamine typically increase blood pressure, heart rate, and cardiac output. The cardiovascular effects are indirect and are most likely mediated by inhibition of both central and peripheral catecholamine reuptake. Ketamine has direct negative inotropic and vasodilating activity, but these effects usually are overwhelmed by the indirect sympathomimetic action. Thus, ketamine is a useful drug, along with **etomidate**, for patients at risk of hypotension during anesthesia. Although not arrhythmogenic, **ketamine** increases myocardial oxygen consumption and is not an ideal drug for patients at risk for myocardial ischemia.

The respiratory effects of **ketamine** are perhaps the best indication for its use. Induction doses of ketamine produce small and transient decreases in minute ventilation, but respiratory depression is less severe than with other general anesthetics. Ketamine is a potent bronchodilator due to its indirect sympathomimetic activity and perhaps some direct bronchodilating activity. Thus, **ketamine** is particularly well suited for anesthetizing patients at high risk for bronchospasm.

KETANSERINE

Several of the newer antihypertensive medications have multiple sites of action. For example, labetalol, dilevalol, carvedilol, and celiprolol are beta-adrenergic receptors that also have vasodilating properties. Because serotonin may play a role in the pathogenesis, maintenance, and progression of hypertensive disease, ketanserine has been developed as a new antihypertensive medication that exhibits selective antagonism for the serotonin$_2$ receptor and has a somewhat weaker alpha$_1$-adrenergic-receptor antagonist activity. Urapidil is a vasodilator that elicits central hypotensive activity by stimulating serotonin$_{1A}$ receptors. Indenolol, another new antihypertensive agent, is a beta$_1$-receptor antagonist and a beta$_2$-vascular-adrenergic-receptor agonist.

KETOCONAZOLE

(Nizoral tablets 200 mg)

Ketoconazole is an antifungal agent that impairs synthesis of ergosterol, allowing increased permeability in fungal cell membrane and leakage of cellular components. It is indicated in the treatment of susceptible systemic and cutaneous fungal infections (see Figure 64). Topical: used for seborrheic dermatitis, tinea corporis, tinea cruris, tinea pedis, and tinea versicolor.

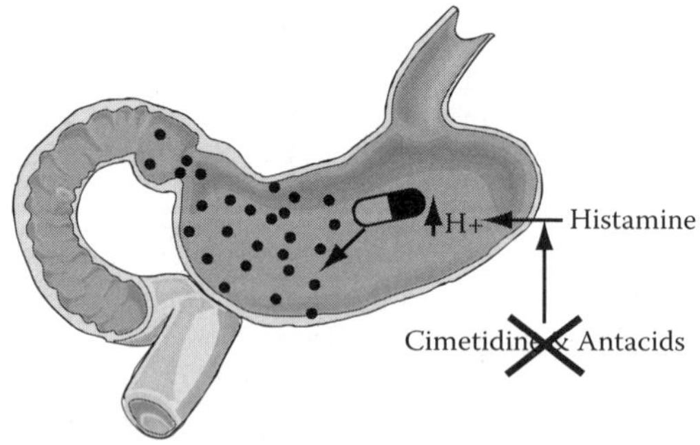

FIGURE 64 Ketoconazole has a broad therapeutic potential for a number of superficial and systemic fungal infections.

Ketoconazole (200 mg daily) is indicated in the treatment of the following systemic fungal infections: candidiasis, chronic mucocutaneous candidiasis, oral thrush, candiduria, blastomycosis, coccidiomycosis, histoplasmosis, chromomycosis, and paracoccidioidomycosis. Moreover, it is effective in the treatment of severe recalcitrant cutaneous dermatophyte infections not responding to topical therapy or oral griseofulvin or in patients unable to take griseofulvin. Ketoconazole, a broad-spectrum antifungal agent, impairs the synthesis of ergosterol, the main sterol of fungal cell membranes, allowing increased permeability and leakage of cellular components. Ketoconazole dissolves in an acidic solution. Therefore, antacids, histamine$_2$-receptor-blocking agents, or anticholinergic agents reduce its oral absorption and bioavailability (Figure 21). Peak plasma concentration of ketoconazole is achieved within 2 hours and is bound to albumin to the extent of 95 to 99%. Ketoconazole is metabolized in the liver to inactive metabolites and is excreted mainly (90%) in the bile and feces. Renal failure does not alter the dosing regimen. As ketoconazole penetrates poorly into CSF, it is not used in fungal meningitis.

Ketoconazole has been associated with hepatic toxicity, hence necessitating liver function tests before, during, and after termination of the therapy. Ketoconazole reduces the serum level of testosterone, which returns to normal levels after discontinuation of therapy. It increases the plasma levels, bioavailability, or actions of oral anticoagulants, astemizole, terfenidine, corticosteroids, and cyclosporine, but decreases that of theophylline.

KETOPROFEN

(Orudis)

Ketoprofen (50 to 75 mg p.o. t.i.d.), an analgesic, antipyretic, and antiinflammatory agent, is indicated in the treatment of rheumatoid arthritis and osteoarthritis. Ketoprofen is absorbed completely from the gastrointestinal tract and is highly protein bound. It is metabolized in the liver, and the metabolites are excreted in the urine. Like other nonsteroidal antiinflammatory agents, ketoprofen should be administered cautiously to patients with a history of peptic ulcer disease, renal dysfunction, or hepatic dysfunction, and to those predisposed to fluid retention, such as those with congestive heart failure and hypertension, because ketoprofen may increase the risk of fluid retention and edema. Patients with aspirin hypersensitivity, rhinitis/nasal polyps, and asthma are at high risk of bronchospasm. Concomitant use of ketoprofen with anticoagulants and thrombolytic drugs (coumarin derivatives, heparin, streptokinase, or urokinase) may potentiate anticoagulant effects. Bleeding problems may occur if ketoprofen is used with other drugs that inhibit platelet aggregation, such as azlocillin, parenteral carbenicillin, dextran, dipyridamole, mezlocillin, piperacillin, sulfinpyrazone, ticarcillin, valproic acid, cefamandole, cefoperazone, moxalactam, and plicamycin. Because of the influence of prostaglandins on glucose metabolism, concomitant use with insulin or oral hypoglycemic agents may potentiate hypoglycemic effects. Ketoprofen may displace highly protein-bound drugs from binding sites. Toxicity may occur with coumarin derivatives, phenytoin, verapamil, or nifedipine. Increased nephrotoxicity may occur with gold compounds, other antiinflammatory agents, or acetaminophen. Ketoprofen may decrease the renal clearance of methotrexate and lithium. It may decrease the effectiveness of antihypertensive agents and diuretics. Concomitant use with diuretics may increase nephrotoxic potential. Concomitant use with diuretics or antihypertensives may decrease their effectiveness (see also Table 3).

Ketoprofen (Orudis, Oruvail) shares the pharmacological properties of other propionic acid derivatives and is available for sale without a prescription in the United States. A more potent S-enantiomer is available in Europe. In addition to COX inhibition, **ketoprofen** may stabilize lysosomal membranes and antagonize the actions of bradykinin. It is unknown if these actions are relevant to its efficacy in humans. Ketoprofen demonstrates a pharmacokinetic profile similar to **fenoprofen**. It has a half-life in plasma of about 2 hours except in the elderly, in whom it is slightly prolonged. **Ketoprofen** is conjugated with glucuronic acid in the liver, and the conjugate is excreted in the urine. Patients with impaired renal function eliminate the drug more slowly.

Approximately 30% of patients experience mild gastrointestinal side effects with ketoprofen, which are decreased if the drug is taken with food or antacids. **Ketoprofen** can cause fluid retention and increased plasma concentrations of creatinine. These effects generally are transient and asymptomatic and are more common in patients who are receiving diuretics or in those older than 60. Thus, renal function should be monitored in such patients.

KETOROLAC TROMETHAMINE

(Toradol)

Ketorolac, a nonsteroidal antiinflammatory agent (30 to 60 mg IM), is used in short-term management of pain (see also Table 3).

KETOROLAC TROMETHAMINE (OPHTHALMIC)

(Acular solution 0.5%)

Ketorolac, a nonsteroidal antiinflammatory agent (one drop of 0.5% solution instilled in the conjunctival sac), is used for relief of ocular itching caused by seasonal allergic conjunctivitis (see also Table 3).

Ketorolac tromethamine is an analgesic, which decreases inflammation, pain, and fever through inhibition of prostaglandin synthesis. **Oral**, **IM**, **IV** use: in adults—short-term management of moderately severe, acute pain; **IM**, **IV** use: in children 2 years of age and older—moderately severe, acute pain. **Ophthalmic forms**: use in adults and children 3 years of age and older. Ocular use: for temporary relief of ocular itching caused by seasonal allergic conjunctivitis and treatment of postoperative inflammation in patients who have undergone cataract extraction. Ocular LS use: for reduction of ocular pain and burning/stinging following corneal refractive surgery. Ocular PF use: for reduction of ocular pain and photophobia following incisional refractive surgery.

Ketorolac is a potent analgesic but only a moderately effective antiinflammatory drug. It is one of the few NSAIDs approved for parenteral administration. It has greater systemic analgesic than antiinflammatory activity. Like other tNSAIDs, it inhibits platelet aggregation and promotes gastric ulceration. Ketorolac also has antiinflammatory activity when topically administered in the eye.

Ketorolac has a rapid onset of action, extensive protein binding, and a short duration of action. Oral bioavailability is about 80%. Urinary excretion accounts for about 90% of eliminated drug, with about 10% excreted unchanged and the remainder as a glucuronidated conjugate. The rate of elimination is reduced in the elderly and in patients with renal failure.

Ketorolac (administered as the tromethamine salt Toradol, Ultram) has been used as a short-term alternative (less than 5 days) to opioids for the treatment of moderate to severe pain and is administered intramuscularly, intravenously, or orally. Unlike opioids, tolerance, withdrawal, and respiratory depression do not occur. Like other NSAIDs, aspirin sensitivity is a contraindication to the use of ketorolac. Typical doses are 30 to 60 mg (intramuscular), 15 to 30 mg (intravenous), and 5 to 30 mg (oral). **Ketorolac** is used widely in postoperative patients, but it should not be used for routine obstetric analgesia. Topical (ophthalmic) **ketorolac** is FDA approved for the treatment of seasonal allergic conjunctivitis and postoperative ocular inflammation after cataract extraction.

Side effects at usual oral doses include somnolence, dizziness, headache, gastrointestinal pain, dyspepsia, nausea, and pain at the site of injection.

KETOTIFEN FUMARATE

(Zaditor solution 0.025%)

Ketotifen is an ophthalmic antihistamine that inhibits release of mediators from cells involved in hypersensitivity reactions. It is indicated in temporary prevention of itching of eyes caused by allergic conjunctivitis.

Topical antihistamines include **emedastine difumarate** (Emadine) and **levocabastine hydrochloride** (Livostin). **Cromolyn sodium** (Crolom), which prevents the release of histamine and other autacoids from mast cells, has found limited use in treating conjunctivitis that is thought to be allergen-mediated, such as vernal conjunctivitis. **Lodoxamide tromethamine** (Alomide) and **pemirolast** (Alamast) mast-cell stabilizers also are available for ophthalmic use. **Nedocromil** (Alocril) also is primarily a mast-cell stabilizer with some antihistamine properties. **Olopatadine hydrochloride** (Patanol), **ketotifen fumarate** (Zaditor), and **azelastine** (Optivar) are H_1 antagonists with mast-cell-stabilizing properties. **Epinastine** (Elestat) antagonizes H_1 and H_2 receptors and exhibits mast-cell-stabilizing activity.

L

LABETALOL HYDROCHLORIDE

(Normodyne tablets 100 mg)

Labetalol hydrochloride is an alpha-adrenergic blocker/beta-adrenergic blocker that selectively blocks alpha-1 receptors and nonselectively blocks beta receptors to decrease BP, heart rate, and myocardial oxygen demand. It is indicated in the management of hypertension.

Labetalol (100 mg b.i.d.), either by itself or with a thiazide diuretic, may be used in the treatment of hypertension. Labetalol, an alpha$_1$- and beta-adrenergic-blocking agent, causes a dose-dependent fall of blood pressure without causing reflex tachycardia or impairing renal function. Labetalol is absorbed completely, reaching peak plasma levels in 1 to 2 hours. It undergoes extensive first-pass effects, is conjugated with glucuronic acid, and the metabolite is excreted in the urine and via bile in the feces. Labetalol is contraindicated in bronchial asthma, overt cardiac failure, third-degree heart block, cardiogenic shock, and severe bradycardia. Labetatol may prevent the premonitory signs and symptoms, such as tachycardia or hypoglycemia, seen in patients with diabetes mellitus. Like other beta-adrenergic-blocking agents, labetalol may also reduce the release of insulin in response to hyperglycemia. Therefore, in patients taking labetalol, the dosage of insulin may need to be readjusted. Beta-adrenergic-blocking agents may attenuate the effectiveness of adrenergic-receptor agonists used in the management of bronchial asthma. Cimetidine increases the bioavailability of labetalol, and halothane augments the myocardial depressant property of labetalol. Labetalol augments the hypertensive effects of nitroglycerine but blocks the nitroglycerine-induced tachycardia.

Labetalol (Normodyne, Trandate, others) is representative of a class of drugs that act as competitive antagonists at both α_1 and β receptors. **Labetalol** has two optical centers.

The pharmacological effects of **labetalol** have become clearer since the four isomers were separated and tested individually. The R,R isomer is about four times more potent as a β-receptor antagonist than is racemic **labetalol,** and it accounts for much of the β-blockade produced by the mixture of isomers, although it no longer is in development as a separate drug (dilevalol). As an α_1 antagonist, this isomer is less than 20% as potent as the racemic mixture. The R,S isomer is almost devoid of both α- and β-blocking effects. The S,R isomer has almost no β-blocking activity, yet is about five times more potent as an α_1-blocker than is racemic labetalol. The S,S isomer is devoid of β-blocking activity and has a potency similar to that of racemic labetalol as an α_1-receptor antagonist. The R,R isomer has some intrinsic sympathomimetic activity at β_2-adrenergic receptors; this may contribute to vasodilation. Labetalol also may have some direct vasodilating capacity.

The actions of **labetalol** on both α_1 and β receptors contribute to the fall in blood pressure observed in patients with hypertension. α_1-Receptor blockade leads to relaxation of arterial smooth muscle and vasodilation, particularly in the upright position. The β_1-blockade also contributes to a fall in blood pressure, in part by blocking reflex sympathetic stimulation of the heart. In addition, the intrinsic sympathomimetic activity of labetalol at β_2 receptors may contribute to vasodilation.

Labetalol is available in oral form for therapy of chronic hypertension and as an intravenous formulation for use in hypertensive emergencies. **Labetalol** has been associated with hepatic injury in a limited number of patients.

Although **labetalol** is completely absorbed from the gut, there is extensive first-pass clearance; bioavailability is only about 20 to 40% and is highly variable. Bioavailability may be increased by food intake. The drug is rapidly and extensively metabolized in the liver by oxidative biotransformation and glucuronidation; very little unchanged drug is found in the urine. The rate of metabolism of labetalol is sensitive to changes in hepatic blood flow. The elimination half-life of the drug is about 8 hours. The half-life of the R,R isomer of labetalol (dilevalol) is about 15 hours. **Labetalol** provides an interesting and challenging example of pharmacokinetic–pharmacodynamic modeling applied to a drug that is a racemic mixture of isomers with different kinetics and pharmacological actions.

LACTOFERRIN

Lactoferrin is a 703-amino-acid glycoprotein originally isolated from milk. Plasma lactoferrin is predominantly neutrophil-derived, but indications are that it may also be produced by other cells. Lactoferrin in body fluids is found in the iron-free form, the monoferric form, and in the diferric form. Three isoforms of lactoferrin have been isolated, i.e., two with RNAse activity (lactoferrin-beta and lactoferrin-gamma) and one without RNAse activity (lactoferrin-alpha). Receptors for lactoferrin can be found on intestinal tissue, monocytes/macrophages, neutrophils, lymphocytes, platelets, and on certain bacteria. A wide spectrum of functions is ascribed to lactoferrin. These range from a role in the control of iron availability to immune modulation.

LACTOGEN

Early in pregnancy, glucose homeostasis is altered by the increasing levels of estrogen and progesterone, which lead to beta-cell hyperplasia and an increased insulin response to a glucose load. During the second half of pregnancy, rising levels of human placental lactogen and other contrainsulin hormones synthesized by the placenta modify maternal utilization of glucose and amino acids. The actions of lactogen are responsible, in part, for the diabetogenic state associated with pregnancy.

LACTULOSE

(Cephulac, Cholac, Chronulac, Constilac, Constulose, Duphalac, Enulose, Generiac, Lactulose PSE)

Lactulose, a disaccharide with laxative properties (20 to 30 g p.o. t.i.d.), is used to prevent and treat portal-systemic encephalopathy, including hepatic precoma and coma in patients with severe hepatic disease.

LACTULOSE

(Cephulac solution 10 g lactulose/15 mL)

Lactulose is a hyperosmotic agent, which produces increased osmotic pressure within colon and acidifies its contents, resulting in increased stool water content and stool softening. It causes migration of ammonia from blood into colon, where it is converted to ammonium ion and expelled through laxative action. It is indicated in the treatment of constipation; and prevention and treatment of portal-systemic encephalopathy, including stages of hepatic precoma and coma.

Lactulose (Cephulac, Chronulac, and others) is a synthetic disaccharide of galactose and fructose that resists intestinal disaccharidase activity.

This and other nonabsorbable sugars such as **sorbitol** and **mannitol** are hydrolyzed in the colon to short-chain fatty acids, which stimulate colonic propulsive motility by osmotically drawing water into the lumen. Sorbitol and **lactulose** are equally efficacious in the treatment of constipation caused by **opioids** and **vincristine**, of constipation in the elderly, and of idiopathic chronic constipation. They are available as 70% solutions, which are given in doses of 15 to 30 mL at night, with increases as needed up to 60 mL per day in divided doses. Effects may not be seen for 24 to 48 hours rafter dosing is begun. Abdominal discomfort or distention and flatulence are relatively common in the first few days of treatment but usually subside with continued administration. A few patients dislike the sweet taste of the preparations; dilution with water or administering the preparation with fruit juice can mask the taste.

Lactulose also is used to treat **hepatic encephalopathy**. Patients with severe liver disease have an impaired capacity to detoxify ammonia coming from the colon, where it is produced by bacterial metabolism of fecal urea. The drop in luminal pH that accompanies hydrolysis to short-chain fatty acids in the colon results in "trapping" of the ammonia by its conversion to the polar ammonium ion. Combined with the increases in colonic transit, this therapy lowers circulating ammonia levels. The therapeutic goal in this condition is to give sufficient amounts of lactulose (usually 20 to 30 g, 3 to 4 times per day) to produce two to three soft stools a day with a pH of 5 to 5.5.

LAMIVUDINE (3TC)

(Epivir tablets 150 mg)

Lamivudine is a nucleoside reverse transcriptase inhibitor, which inhibits replication of HIV and hepatitis B virus (HBV). HIV infection: **Epivir** is used in combination with other antiretroviral agents for the treatment of HIV infection. Chronic hepatitis B: **Epivir-HBV** is used in the treatment of chronic hepatitis B associated with evidence of hepatitis B viral replication and active liver inflammation.

Lamivudine, the (-)-enantiomer of 2′,3′-dideoxy-3′-thiacytidine, is a nucleoside analog that inhibits HIV reverse transcriptase and HBV DNA polymerase. It inhibits HBV replication *in vitro* by 50% at concentrations of 4 to 7 ng/mL with negligible cellular cytotoxicity. Cellular enzymes convert lamivudine to the triphosphate, which competitively inhibits HBV DNA polymerase and causes chain termination. The intracellular $t_{1/2}$ of the triphosphate averages 17 to 19 hours in HBV-infected cells, so infrequent dosing is possible.

Lamivudine triphosphate is a potent inhibitor of the DNA polymerase; reverse transcriptase of HBV, and oral lamivudine is active in animal models of hepadnavirus infection. **Lamivudine** shows enhanced antiviral activity in combination with **adefovir** or **penciclovir** against hepadnaviruses. Point mutation in the YMDD motif of HBV DNA polymerase results in a 40 to 10^4 times reduction in *in vitro* susceptibility. **Lamivudine** resistance confers cross-resistance to related agents such as **emtricitabine** and clevudine and is often associated with an additional non-YMDD mutation that confers cross-resistance to famciclovir. **Lamivudine**-resistant HBV retains susceptibility to adefovir and partially to entecavir. Viruses bearing YMDD mutations are less replication competent *in vitro* than wild-type HBV. However, lamivudine resistance is associated with elevated HBV DNA levels, decreased likelihood of HbeAg loss or seroconversion hepatitis exacerbations, and progressive fibrosis and graft loss in transplant recipients.

Following oral administration, lamivudine is absorbed rapidly with a bioavailability of about 80% in adults. Peak plasma levels average approximately 1000 ng/mL after 100-mg doses. **Lamivudine** is distributed widely in a volume comparable with total-body water. The plasma $t_{1/2}$ of elimination averages about 9 hours, and approximately 70% of the dose is excreted unchanged in the urine. About 1% is metabolized to an inactive *trans*-sulfoxide metabolite. In HBV-infected children, doses of 3 mg/kg per day provide plasma exposure and trough plasma levels comparable with those in adults receiving 100 mg daily. Dose reductions are indicated for moderate renal insufficiency (creatinine clearance <50 ml/min). Trimethoprim decreases the renal clearance of lamivudine.

At the doses used for chronic HBV infection, lamivudine generally has been well tolerated. Aminotransferase increases after therapy occur more often in lamivudine recipients, and flares in posttreatment aminotransferase elevations (>500 IU/mL) occur in about 15% of patients after cessation.

Lamivudine is approved for the treatment of chronic HBV hepatitis in adults and children. In adults, doses of 100 mg/day for 1 year cause suppression of HBV DNA levels, normalization of aminotransferase levels in 41% or more of patients, and reductions in hepatic inflammation in over 50% of patients. Seroconversion with antibody to HbeAg occurs in fewer than 20% of recipients at 1 year. In children aged 2 to 17 years, lamivudine (3 mg/kg per day to a maximum of 100mg for 1 year) is associated with normalization of aminotransferase levels in about one-half and seroconversion to anti-Hbe in about one-fifth of cases. In those without emergence of resistant variants, prolonged therapy is associated with sustained suppression of HBV DNA, continued histological improvement, and an increased proportion of patients experiencing a virological response (loss of HbeAg and undetectable HBV DNA). Prolonged therapy is associated with an approximate halving of the risk of clinical progression and development of hepatocellular carcinoma in those with advanced fibrosis or cirrhosis. However, the frequency of lamivudine-resistant variants increases progressively with continued drug administration, and frequencies of 38%, 53%, and 67% have been found after 2, 3, and 4 years of treatment, respectively. The risk of resistance development is higher after transplantation and in HIV/HBV-coinfected patients.

Combined use of IFN or pegIFN alfa-2a with **lamivudine** has not improved responses in HBeAg-positive patients consistently. The addition of lamivudine to pegINF alfa-2a for 1 year of therapy does not improve post-treatment response rates in HBeAg-negative patients. In HIV and HBV coinfections, higher lamivudine doses are associated with antiviral effects and, uncommonly, anti-HBe seroconversion. Administration of lamivudine before and after liver transplantation may suppress recurrent HBV infection.

LAMIVUDINE/ZIDOVUDINE

(Combivir tablets 150 mg lamivudine/300 mg zidovudine)

Lamivudine/zidovudine is a nucleoside analog reverse-transcriptase inhibitor combination that inhibits replication of HIV by incorporation into HIV DNA and producing an incomplete, nonfunctional DNA. They are indicated in the treatment of HIV infection.

LAMOTRIGINE

(Lamictal tablets 25 mg)

Lamotrigine is an anticonvulsant that is chemically unrelated to existing antiepileptic drugs (AEDs). One proposed mechanism suggests inhibition of voltage-sensitive sodium channels, thereby stabilizing neuronal membranes, that modulates presynaptic transmitter release of excitatory amino acids (e.g., glutamate, aspartate). **Bipolar disorder**: use in maintenance treatment of bipolar I disorder to delay the time to occurrence of mood episodes in patients treated for acute mood episodes with standard therapy. **Epilepsy**: use as adjunctive therapy in the treatment of partial seizures in adults and as adjunctive therapy in the generated seizures of Lennox–Gastaut syndrome in pediatric and adult patients; conversion to monotherapy in adults with partial seizures who are receiving treatment with a single enzyme-inducing antiepileptic agent. **Lamotrigine** (Lamictal) is a phenyltriazine derivative initially developed as an antifolate agent based on the incorrect idea that reducing folatc would effectively combat seizures. Structure–activity studies indicate that its effectiveness as an antiseizure drug is unrelated to its antifolate properties.

Lamotrigine suppresses tonic hind-limb extension in the maximal electroshock model and partial and secondarily generalized seizures in the kindling model, but does not inhibit clonic motor seizures induced by pentylenetetrazol. **Lamotrigine** blocks sustained repetitive firing of mouse spinal cord neurons and delays the recovery from inactivation of recombinant Na^+ channels, mechanisms similar to those of **phenytoin** and **carbamazepine**. This may well explain lamotrigine's actions on partial and secondarily generalized seizures. However, as mentioned below, **lamotrigine** is effective against a broader spectrum of seizures than phenytoin and carbamazepine, suggesting that **lamotrigine** may have actions in addition to regulating recovery from inactivation of Na^+ channels. The mechanisms underlying its broad spectrum of actions are incompletely understood. One possibility involves **lamotrigine's** inhibition of glutamate release in rat cortical slices treated with veratridine, a Na^+-channel activator, raising the possibility that lamotrigine inhibits synaptic release of glutamate by acting at Na^+ channels themselves.

Lamotrigine is completely absorbed from the gastrointestinal tract and is metabolized primarily by glucuronidation. The plasma half-life of a single dose is 15 to 30 hours. Administration of phenytoin, carbamazepine, or phenobarbital reduces the half-life and plasma concentrations of **lamotrigine**. Conversely, addition of valproate markedly increases plasma concentrations of lamotrigine, likely by inhibiting glucuronidation. Addition of lamotrigine to valproic acid produces a reduction of valproate concentrations by approximately 25% over a few weeks. Concurrent use of lamotrigine and carbamazepine is associated with increases of the 10,11-epoxide of carbamazepine and clinical toxicity in some patients.

Lamotrigine is useful for monotherapy and add-on therapy of partial and secondarily generalized tonic-clonic seizures in adults and Lennox–Gastaut syndrome in both children and adults. **Lennox–Gastaut syndrome** is a disorder of childhood characterized by multiple seizure types, mental retardation, and refractoriness to antiseizure medication.

The most common adverse effects are dizziness, ataxia, blurred or double vision, nausea, vomiting, and rash when

lamotrigine was added to another antiseizure drug. A few cases of **Stevens–Johnson syndrome** and disseminated intravascular coagulation have been reported. The incidence of serious rash in pediatric patients (approximately 0.8%) is higher than in the adult population (0.3%).

LANATOSIDE C

The most important and often-used drugs in the treatment of congestive heart failure are the cardiac glycosides, which may exist and occur naturally in the body. Unfortunately, the margin of safety for these drugs is very narrow (therapeutic index 3.0). Toxicity can develop readily, and careful attention to the pharmacokinetic principles is absolutely crucial. The cardiac glycosides are obtained from numerous natural sources, including *Digitalis lanata* and *Digitalis purpurea* (white and purple foxglove), squill (Mediterranean sea onion), oleander, lily of the valley, and other plants. Among the useful available cardiac glycosides are the following:

Digitalis purpurea	*Digitalis lanata*	*Strophanthus gratus*
Digitoxin	Digoxin	Ouabain
Digoxin	Lanatoside C	
Digitalis leaf	Deslanoside	

Of these, only digoxin and digitoxin and, to a certain extent, ouabain are used extensively. The molecular structures of the cardiac glycosides, including digoxin, have three common components: a steroid nucleus (aglycones or genins), a series of sugar residues in the C3 position, and a five- or six-membered lactone ring in the C17 position.

The sugar residue in digoxin and digitoxin is –*O*-digitoxose-digitoxose-digitoxose. Digoxin varies from digitoxin in having a hydroxy group at C12. Glycosides possess both lipophilic residues (a steroid nucleus) and hydrophilic residues (a lactone ring and OH group). These residues and other factors strongly influence the pharmacokinetic profiles of these cardiac glycosides. Digitoxin is excreted extensively unchanged by the kidney. Renal insufficiency alters its half-life and safety. An elevated blood urea nitrogen (BUN) level signals the diminished capacity to eliminate digoxin. A direct relationship exists between the clearance of digoxin and that of creatine, which, in addition to BUN, may be used to assess a patient's ability to excrete digoxin (see also Table 12).

LANSOPRAZOLE

(Prevacid tablets)

Lansoprazole is an *H. pylori* agent/proton-pump inhibitor, which suppresses gastric acid secretion by blocking "acid (proton) pump" within gastric parietal cells. Lansoprazole, structurally related to omeprazole, is a benzimidazole derivative with antisecretory and antiulcer activities. It inhibits the acid pump activity at the final stage of the enzyme process and therefore reduces the acid secretion of parietal cells. Lansoprazole is converted to active metabolites in the acid environment of the cells (see also Figure 72).

It is used for oral short-term treatment of active duodenal ulcer; to maintain healing of duodenal ulcers; short-term treatment of all grades of erosive esophagitis; maintenance of healing of erosive esophagitis; long-term treatment of pathological hypersecretory conditions, including **Zollinger–Ellison syndrome**; in combination with amoxicillin plus **clarithromycin** or **amoxicillin** alone (in patients intolerant or resistant to clarithromycin) for the eradication of *H. pylori* in patients with active or recurrent duodenal ulcers; short-term treatment and symptomatic relief of active benign gastric ulcer (including nonsteroidal antiinflammatory drug [NSAID]-associated gastric ulcer in patients who continue NSAID use and for reducing risk of NSAID-associated gastric ulcer in patients with a history of NSAID-associated gastric ulcer); treatment of heartburn and other symptoms of gastroesophageal reflux disease (GERD); and IV short-term treatment (up to 7 days) of all grades of erosive esophagitis.

The most potent suppressors of gastric acid secretion are inhibitors of the gastric H^+, K^+-ATPase (**proton pump**). In typical doses, these drugs diminish the daily production of acid (basal and stimulated) by 80% to 95%. Five proton-pump inhibitors are available for clinical use: **omeprazole** (Prilosec, Rapinex, Zegerid) and its S-isomer, **esomeprazole** (Nexium), **lansoprazole** (Prevacid), **rabeprazole** (Aciphex), and **pantoprazole** (Protonix). These drugs have different substitutions on their pyridine and/or benzimidazole groups but are remarkably similar in their pharmacological properties. Omeprazole is a racemic mixture of R- and S-isomers; the S-isomer, esomeprazole (S-omeprazole), is eliminated less rapidly than R-omeprazole, which theoretically provides a therapeutic advantage because of the increased half-life. Despite claims to the contrary, all proton-pump inhibitors have equivalent efficacy at comparable doses.

Proton-pump inhibitors are prodrugs that require activation in an acid environment. After absorption into the systemic circulation, the prodrug diffuses into the parietal cells of the stomach and accumulates in the acidic secretory canaliculi. Here, it is activated by proton-catalyzed formation of a tetracyclic sulfenamide trapping the drug so that it cannot diffuse back across the canalicular membrane. The activated form then binds covalently with sulfhydryl groups of cysteines in the H^+, K^+-ATPase, irreversibly inactivating the pump molecule. Acid secretion resumes only after new pump molecules are synthesized and inserted into the luminal membrane, providing a prolonged (up to 24- to 48-hour) suppression of acid secretion, despite the much shorter plasma half-lives (0.5 to 2 hours) of the parent compounds. Because they block the final step in acid production, the proton-pump inhibitors are effective in acid suppression regardless of other stimulating factors.

To prevent degradation of proton-pump inhibitors by acid in the gastric lumen, oral dosage forms are supplied in different formulations: (1) enteric-coated drugs contained inside gelatin capsules (omeprazole, esomeprazole, and **lansoprazole**); (2) enteric-coated granules supplied as a powder for suspension (**lansoprazole**); (3) enteric-coated tablets (pantoprazole, rabeprazole, and omeprazole); and (4) powdered drug combined with sodium bicarbonate (omeprazole). The delayed-release and enteric-coated tablets dissolve only at alkaline pH, while admixture of omeprazole with sodium bicarbonate simply neutralizes stomach acid; both strategies substantially improve the oral bioavailability of these acid-labile drugs. Until recently, the requirement for enteric coating posed a challenge to the administration of proton-pump inhibitors in patients for whom the oral route of administration is not available. These patients and those requiring immediate acid suppression now can be treated parenterally with pantoprazole or **lansoprazole**, both of which are approved for intravenous administration in the United States. A single intravenous bolus of 80 mg of pantoprazole inhibits acid production by 80% to 90% within an hour, and this inhibition persists for up to 21 hours, permitting once-daily dosing to achieve the desired degree, of hypochlorhydria. The FDA-approved dose of intravenous pantoprazole for gastroesophageal reflux disease is 40 mg daily for up to 10 days. Higher doses (e.g., 160 to 240 mg in divided doses) are used to manage hypersecretory conditions such as the **Zollinger–Ellison syndrome**.

LANTHANUM CARBONATE

(Fosrenol tablets)

Lanthanum carbonate is a phosphate binder that inhibits gastrointestinal (GI) absorption of phosphate by forming highly insoluble lanthanum phosphate complex with dietary phosphate released from food during digestion. It is indicated for reducing serum phosphate in patients with end-stage renal disease.

LARONIDASE

(Aldurazyme injection 2.9 mg laronidase/5 mL)

Laronidase is an endocrine and metabolic agent, which provides exogenous enzyme for uptake into lysosomes and increases the catabolism of glycosaminoglycans. It is indicated in the treatment of patients with **Hurler and Hurler–Scheie forms of mucopolysaccharidosis I** (MPS I); and patients with the Scheie form who have moderate to severe symptoms.

LATANOPROST

(Xalatan ophthalmic solution 0.005%)

Latanoprost is an ophthalmic/prostaglandin agonist, which is a prostaglandin $F_{2\alpha}$ analog that reduces intraocular pressure (IOP) by increasing the output of aqueous humor. It is indicated in reduction of elevated IOP in patients with open-angle glaucoma or ocular hypertension.

Latanoprost is as effective as other medications in the treatment of glaucoma, which is the second cause of irreversible blindness in the world. Topical beta-adrenergic-receptor-blocking agents, timolol maleate, betaxolol, levobunolol, and metipranolol, are the most widely used medications. Apraclonidine, a new alpha$_2$-adrenergic agonist decreases aqueous humor formation without effect on outflow. Epinephrine and dipivefrin are effective. Systemic carbonic anhydrase inhibitors acetazolamide, dichlorphenamide, and methazolamide are used in chronic glaucoma when topical therapy is insufficient and in acute glaucoma when very high intraocular pressure needs to be controlled quickly. Latanoprost, a phenyl-substituted prostaglandin F_2 alpha, (one drop of 0.006% once or twice daily) has been shown to be effective in the treatment of ocular hypertension, primary open-angle glaucoma, and capsular glaucoma. Latanoprost has been effectively combined with twice daily ophthalmic timolol (0.5%) in patients who are not adequately controlled on timolol alone. Latanoprost reduces IOP by increasing uveoscleral outflow without effects on aqueous flow. The only apparent side effect is darkening of the pigment of eyes, such as hazel, that are made up of multiple colors. It will not change the eye color of someone whose eyes are uniformly blue or uniformly brown. Hazel or green eyes may change, and it may cause brown or blue eyes to darken if they have faded with aging.

The goal in glaucoma is to prevent progressive glaucomatous optic-nerve damage with minimum risk and side effects from either topical or systemic therapy. With these general principles in mind, a stepped medical approach may begin with a topical prostaglandin analog. Due to their once-daily dosing, low incidence of systemic side effects, and potent IOP lowering effect, prostaglandin analogs have largely replaced β-adrenergic-receptor antagonists as first-line medical therapy for glaucoma. The prostaglandin analogs consist of **latanoprost** (Xalatan), **travoprost** (Travatan), **bimatoprost** (Lumigan), and **unoprostone** (Rescula).

Prostaglandin $PGF_{2\alpha}$ was found to reduce IOP but has intolerable local side effects. Modifications to the chemical structure of $PGF_{2\alpha}$ have produced a number of analogs with a more acceptable side-effect profile. In primates and humans, $PGF_{2\alpha}$ analogs appear to lower IOP by facilitating aqueous outflow through the accessory uveoscleral outflow pathway. The mechanism by which this occurs is unclear. $PGF_{2\alpha}$ and its analogs (prodrugs that are hydrolyzed to $PGF_{2\alpha}$) bind to FP receptors that link to G_{q11} and thence to the PLC-IP3-Ca^{2+} pathway.

LAXATIVES

Rapid-acting laxatives (2 hours)	Intermediate-acting laxatives (6 hours)
Osmotive laxatives	**Stimulant laxatives**
Sodium phosphates	Diphenylmethane derivatives
Magnesium sulfate	Phenolphthalein
Milk of magnesia	Bixacodyl
Magnesium citrate	Anthraquinone derivatives
Castor oil	Senna
	Cascara sagrada
Slow-acting laxatives (24 hrs)	
Bulk-forming laxatives	**Surfactant laxatives**
Bran	Docusates
Psyllium preparations	Poloxamers
Methylcellulose	**Lactulose**
Calcium polycarbophil	

LAXATIVES AND CATHARTICS

Although often used interchangeably, the terms *laxative* and *cathartic* do have slightly different meanings. A laxative effect refers to the excretion of a soft, formed stool; catharsis implies a more fluid and complete evacuation.

Irritant agents used in the treatment of constipation include cascara sagrada, castor oil, senna, rhubarb, phenolphthalein, and acetphenolisatin. Phenolphthalein is a constituent of many over-the-counter preparations, including Ex-Lax and Feen-A-Mint. Most of these agents, with the exception of castor oil, are slow in their onset of action (24 hours). Phenolphthalein is thought to exert its effect by inhibiting the movement of water and sodium from the colon into the blood and by stimulating mucus secretion. If misused on a prolonged basis, a consequential loss of mucus may lower the plasma protein level. Castor oil is hydrolyzed to ricinoleic acid, the active cathartic. It has an onset of action of 2 to 6 hours. The misuse of any of these agents has been shown to cause hypokalemia, dehydration, and a cathartic colon (resembling ulcerative colitis). Phenolphthalein-containing products may color alkaline urine red.

Bulk saline laxatives fall into two categories: inorganic salts (magnesium sulfate, magnesium citrate, milk of magnesia, sodium sulfate, and sodium phosphate), and organic hydrophilic colloids (methylcellulose, carboxymethylcellulose [Metamucil], plantago seed, agar, psyllium, bran, and fruits). They exert their effects by absorbing and retaining water, increasing bulk, stimulating colonic peristaltic movements, and lubricating and hydrating the desiccated fecal materials.

These agents are more effective when administered with water. The onset of action of organic salts is relatively fast (2 to 6 hours) and that of colloids is relatively slow (1 to 3 days). These agents, which are very effective and safe, should not be used when the intestinal lumen has been narrowed. The prolonged use of saline cathartics may create problems for certain individuals. For example, magnesium salts have been known to cause hypermagnesemia, coma, and death in patients with renal insufficiency. Sodium salts may also be responsible for causing congestive heart failure (CHF). The lubricants consist of mineral oil and dioctyl sodium sulfonsuccinate (Colace). Colace is used in the pharmaceutical industry as an emulsifying and dispersing substance. Both agents are taken orally. These agents, which do not influence peristalsis, soften desiccated stools or delay the desiccation of fecal materials. They are especially useful in patients with painful bowel movements resulting from inspissated stools or inflammation of the anal sphincter such as occurs with hemorrhoids or anal fissures. Colace is also useful for patients in whom the consequences of "straining at stool" may be harmful. When used for a long time, mineral oil may come to interfere with the absorption of fat-soluble vitamins and other essential nutrients. Lipid pneumonitis may evolve if mineral oil is used as a vehicle for drugs that are taken nasally.

Laxatives are used to hasten the elimination and reduce the absorption of a poison that has been taken. Laxatives are used before and after treatment with antihelmintic drugs. Laxatives are used to clean the gastrointestinal tract before radiographic techniques are performed.

LAZAROIDS

The 21-aminosteroids (lazaroids) are inhibitors of lipid membrane peroxidation and appear to function as oxygen free radical scavengers. The therapeutic potential of the lazaroid, tirilazad mesylate, has been extensively studied in several CNS disorders. Tirilazad and related compounds have been found to be highly beneficial in spinal cord trauma. Clinical studies using tirilazad in subarachnoid hemorrhage have been more promising. It has been shown to be beneficial in terms of reducing vasospasm and cerebral infarction associated with subarachnoid hemorrhage.

LEFLUNOMIDE

(Arava tablets, 10 mg)

Leflunomide is an antirheumatic agent. It is an isoxazole immunomodulatory agent that inhibits dihydro-orotate dehydrogenase and has antiproliferative and antiinflammatory activity. It is indicated in the treatment of active rheumatoid arthritis (RA) to reduce signs and symptoms and to retard structural damage.

Leflunomide (Arava) is a pyrimidine-synthesis inhibitor indicated for the treatment of adults with rheumatoid arthritis. This drug has found utility in the treatment of polyomavirus nephropathy seen in immunosuppressed renal transplant recipients and is increasingly being used for that purpose. There are no studies showing efficacy, however, compared with control patients treated with withdrawal or reduction of immune-suppression alone in BK virus nephropathy. The drug inhibits dihydro-orotate dehydrogenase in the *de novo* pathway of pyrimidine synthesis. It is hepatotoxic and can cause fetal injury when administered to pregnant women.

LEGIONNAIRES' DISEASE: Treatment of

Legionnaires' disease is characterized by a nonproductive cough, pulse–temperature dissociation, abnormalities in results of liver function tests, diarrhea, hyponatremia, hypophosphatemia, myalgia, confusion, and multiple rigors.

The treatment of Legionnaires' disease is summarized below:

Antimicrobial Agent(s)	Dosage
First choice	
Erythromycin (± rifampin)	Intravenous: 500 mg to 1 g every 6 hours
	Oral: 500 mg (base) every 6 hours
Second choices	
Azithromycin	Oral: 500 mg on day 1, then 250 mg daily for another 4 days
or Clarithromycin	Oral: 250 mg every 12 hours
	Intravenous: 400 mg every 12 hours
or Ciprofloxacin	Oral: 500 mg every 12 hours
or Ofloxacin	Oral or intravenous: 400 mg every 12 hours
or Doxycycline (± rifampin)	Intravenous: 200 mg every 12 hours for two doses, then 200 mg every 24 hours
	Oral: 200 mg once, then either 100 mg every 12 hours or 200 mg every 24 hours
Trimethoprim-sulfamethoxazole (TMP-SMZ)	Intravenous or oral: 5 mg of TMP component per kg every 8 hours

LENOGRASTIM

Lenograstim (recombinant glycosylated human granulocyte colony-stimulating factor; rHuG-CSF, is a hematopoietic growth factor (HGF) that acts primarily to stimulate proliferation and differentiation of committed progenitor cells of the granulocyte-neutrophil lineage into functionally mature neutrophils. Lenograstim is a useful adjunct to chemotherapy for the treatment of nonmyelogenous malignancies, including myeloblastive chemotherapy followed by bone marrow transplantation (see also Cytokines).

LEPIRUDIN

(Refludan powder for injection 50 mg)

Lepirudin is a thrombin inhibitor. One molecule of lepirudin (rDNA) binds to 1 molecule of thrombin and blocks the thrombogenic activity of thrombin. It is indicated in anticoagulation in patients with heparin-induced thrombocytopenia and associated thromboembolic disease to prevent further thromboembolic complications.

Heparin-induced thrombocytopenia (platelet count <150,000/ml or a 50% decrease from the pretreatment value) occurs in about 0.5% of medical patients 5 to 10 days after initiation of therapy with standard heparin. The incidence of thrombocytopenia is lower with low-molecular-weight heparin. Thrombotic complications that can be life threatening or lead to amputation occur in about one-half of the affected heparin-treated patients and may precede the onset of thrombocytopenia. The incidence of heparin-induced thrombocytopenia and thrombosis is higher in surgical patients. Venous thromboembolism occurs most commonly, but arterial thromboses causing limb ischemia, myocardial infarction, and stroke also occur. Bilateral adrenal hemorrhage, skin lesions at the site of subcutaneous heparin injection, and a variety of systemic reactions may accompany heparin-induced thrombocytopenia. The development of IgG antibodies against complexes of heparin with platelet factor 4, (or, rarely, other chemokines) appears to cause all of these reactions. These complexes activate platelets by binding to FcγIIa receptors, which results in platelet aggregation, release of more platelet factor 4, and thrombin generation. The antibodies also may trigger vascular injury by binding to platelet factor 4 attached to heparin sulfate on the endothelium.

Heparin should be discontinued immediately if unexplained thrombocytopenia or any of the clinical manifestations mentioned above occur 5 or more days after beginning heparin therapy, regardless of the dose or route of administration. The onset of heparin-induced thrombocytopenia may occur earlier in patients who have received heparin within the previous 3 to 4 months and have residual circulating antibodies. The diagnosis of heparin-induced thrombocytopenia can be confirmed by a heparin-dependent platelet activation assay or an assay for antibodies that react with heparin/platelet factor 4 complexes. As thrombotic complications may occur after cessation of therapy, an alternative anticoagulant such as **lepirudin**, **argatroban**, or **danaparoid** should be administered to patients with heparin-induced thrombocytopenia. Low-molecular-weight heparins should be avoided, because these drugs often cross-react with standard heparin in heparin-dependent antibody assays. Warfarin may precipitate venous limb gangrene or multicentric skin necrosis in patients with heparin-induced thrombocytopenia and should not be used until the thrombocytopenia has resolved and the patient is adequately anticoagulated with another agent.

Lepirudin (Refludan) is a recombinant derivative (Leu^1-Thr^2-63-desulfohirudin) of hirudin, a direct thrombin inhibitor present in the salivary glands of the medicinal leech. It is a 65-amino-acid polypeptide that binds tightly to both the catalytic site and the extended substrate recognition site (exosite I) of thrombin. **Lepirudin** is approved in the United States for treatment of patients with heparin-induced thrombocytopenia. It is administered intravenously at a dose adjusted to maintain the aPTT at 1.5 to 2.5 times the median of the laboratory's normal range for aPTT. The drug is excreted by the kidneys and has a half-life of about 1.3 hours. Lepirudin should be used cautiously in patients with renal failure, as it can accumulate and cause bleeding in these clients. Patients may develop antihirudin antibodies that occasionally cause a paradoxical increase in the aPTT; therefore, daily monitoring of the aPTT is recommended. There is no antidote for **lepirudin**.

LETROZOLE

(Femara tablets 2.5 mg)

Letrozole is an aromatase inhibitor. A nonsteroidal competitive inhibitor of the aromatase enzyme system, it inhibits the conversion of androgens to estrogens. It is indicated as an extended adjuvant treatment of early breast cancer in postmenopausal women who have received 5 years of adjuvant **tamoxifen** therapy; first-line treatment of postmenopausal women with hormone receptor positive or hormone receptor unknown locally advanced or metastatic cancer; and in advanced breast cancer in postmenopausal women with disease progression following. Third-generation aromatase inhibitors developed in the 1990s, include the type 1 steroidal agent exemestane and the type 2 nonsteroidal imidazoles **anastrozole** and **letrozole**. Currently, third-generation AIs are most commonly used for the treatment of early-stage and advanced breast cancer.

In postmenopausal women with primary breast cancer, **letrozole** inhibits whole body aromatization and reduces local aromatization within the tumors. The drug has no significant effect on the synthesis of adrenal steroids or thyroid hormone and does not alter levels of a range of other hormones. **Letrozole** also reduces cellular markers of proliferation to a significantly greater extent than tamoxifen in human estrogen-dependent tumors that overexpress **human epidermal growth factor receptors** (HER)1 and/or HER2/neu.

Letrozole increases the levels of bone resorption markers in healthy postmenopausal women and in those with a history of breast disease but without current active disease. **Letrozole** has not demonstrated a consistent effect on serum lipid levels in healthy women or postmenopausal women with breast cancer.

Letrozole is rapidly absorbed after oral administration and maximum plasma levels are reached about 1 hour after ingestion. **Letrozole** has a bioavailability of 99.9%. Steady-state plasma concentrations of letrozole are reached after 2 to 6 weeks of treatment. Following metabolism by CYP2A6 and CYP3A4, letrozole is eliminated as an inactive carbinol metabolite mainly *via* the kidneys. Due to the low total body clearance (2.21 L/h), the elimination half-life is about 40 to 42 hours.

Letrozole (Femara), 2.5 mg administered orally once daily, has shown efficacy in the treatment of postmenopausal women with early-stage or advanced, hormone-receptor-positive breast cancer.

In early-stage disease, extending adjuvant endocrine therapy with letrozole (beyond the standard 5-year period of tamoxifen) improved disease-free survival compared with placebo and improved overall survival in the subset of patients with positive axillary nodes.

In advanced breast cancer, **letrozole** is superior to tamoxifen as first-line treatment; time to disease progression is significantly longer and objective response rate is significantly greater with letrozole, but median overall survival is similar between groups. As second-line therapy of advanced breast cancer that has progressed on antiestrogen therapy, **letrozole** shows efficacy equivalent to that of anastrozole and similar to or better than that of megestrol.

Similarly to tamoxifen, **letrozole** generally is well tolerated; the most common treatment-related adverse events are hot flushes, nausea, and hair thinning. In patients with tumors that progressed on antiestrogen therapy, letrozole was tolerated at least as well as, or better than, **megestrol**. In the trial of extended adjuvant therapy, adverse events reported more frequently with letrozole than placebo were hot flashes, arthralgia, myalgia, and arthritis, but cessation of **letrozole** was no more frequent than placebo in this double-blind trial. A greater number of new diagnoses of osteoporosis occurred among women receiving letrozole, but the long-term effects on bone mineral density or lipid metabolism have yet to be determined.

LEUCOVORIN CALCIUM (FOLINIC ACID)

(Wellcovorin tablets 5 mg)

Leucovorin calcium is a folic acid derivative, which acts as an antidote to drugs that antagonize folic acid, such as **methotrexate**. Oral and parenteral: used in treatment to diminish toxicity and counteract effect of overdosage of folic acid antagonists. Parenteral: used in treatment of megaloblastic anemia caused by folic acid deficiency when oral therapy is not feasible.

Tumor cells acquire resistance to methotrexate as the result of several factors, which include the deletion of a high-affinity, carrier-mediated transport system for reduced folates, an increase in the concentration of dihydrofolate reductase, and the formation of a biochemically altered reductase with reduced affinity for methotrexate. To overcome this resistance, higher doses of methotrexate need to be administered. The effects of methotrexate may be reversed by the administration of leucovorin, the reduced folate. This leucovorin "rescue" prevents or reduces the toxicity of methotrexate, which is expressed as mouth lesions (stomatitis), injury to the gastrointestinal epithelium (diarrhea), leukopenia, and thrombocytopenia.

Antifolate chemotherapy occupies a special place in the history of cancer treatment, as this class of drugs produced the first striking, although temporary, remissions in **leukemia**, and the first cure of a solid tumor, **choriocarcinoma**. These advances provided great impetus to the development of chemotherapy for cancer. Interest in folate antagonists further increased with the development of curative combination therapy for **childhood acute lymphocytic leukemia**; in this therapy, methotrexate played a critical role in both systemic treatment and intrathecal therapy. Introduction of high-dose regimens with "rescue" of host toxicity by the reduced folate, **leucovorin** (folinic acid, citrovorum factor, 5-formyl tetrahydrofolate, N^5-formyl FH_4), further extended the effectiveness of this drug to both systemic and CNS lymphomas, osteogenic sarcoma, and leukemias. Most recently, **pemetrexed**, an analog that differs from methotrexate in its transport properties and sites of action, has proven useful in treating **mesothelioma** and lung cancer.

LEUPROLIDE ACETATE

(Lupron depot microspheres for injection, lyophilized 3.75 mg, microspheres for injection)

Leuprolide acetate is a gonadotropin-releasing hormone (GnRH) analog and a synthetic luteinizing hormone-releasing hormone (LHRH) agonist of greater potency than naturally occurring GnRH. It occupies pituitary GnRH receptors and thus desensitizes them, inhibiting gonadotropin secretion required for gonadal production of testosterone and estrogen. It is indicated for palliative treatment of advanced prostatic cancer (alone or in combination with **flutamide**); management of endometriosis in women over 18 years (depot preparation); treatment of children with central precocious puberty (CPP [pediatric injection or depot pediatric]); and uterine leiomyomata (depot preparation).

The most common form of androgen deprivation therapy (ADT) involves chemical suppression of the pituitary with GnRH agonists. GnRH agonists cause an initial surge in levels of luteinizing hormone (LH) and follicle-stimulating hormone (FSH), followed by inhibition of gonadotropin release. This results in reduction of testicular production of testosterone to castrate levels. GnRH agonists in common use include **leuprolide** (Lupron, others), **goserelin** (Zoladex), **triptorelin** (Trelstar), and **buserelin** (Suprefact).

Long-acting GnRH agonists are used for palliative therapy of hormonally responsive tumors (e.g., prostate or breast cancer), generally in conjunction with agents that block steroid biosynthesis or action to avoid transient increases in hormone levels. Because it does not transiently increase sex steroid production, an extended-release form of the GnRH antagonist abarelix (Plenaxis) also is marketed for use in prostate cancer patients in whom serious adverse consequences might accompany any stimulus to tumor growth (e.g., in patients with spinal cord metastases where increased tumor growth could lead to paralysis) The GnRH agonists also are used to suppress steroid-responsive conditions such as endometriosis, uterine leiomyomas, and acute intermittent porphyria. Depot preparations of **goserelin** (Zoladex), **leuprolide** (Lupron depot, Elegard) or **triptorelin** (Trelstar LA), which can be administered subcutaneously or intramuscularly monthly or every 3 months can be used in these settings and may be particularly useful for pharmacological castration in disorders such as paraphilia, for which strict patient compliance is problematic.

The long-acting agonists generally are well tolerated, and side effects are those that would be predicted to occur when gonadal steroidogenesis is inhibited (e.g., hot flashes, vaginal dryness and atrophy, decreased bone density). Because of these effects, therapy in non-life-threatening diseases such as **endometriosis** or **uterine leiomyomas** generally is limited to 6 months unless add-back therapy with estrogens and/or progestins is incorporated into the regimen. In addition to these predicted effects, abarelix has been associated with a significant incidence of hypersensitivity reactions, and its therapeutic role remains to be defined.

LEVALBUTEROL HYDROCHLORIDE

(Xopenex solution of inhalation 0.31 mg levalbuterol per 3 mL, solution for inhalation 0.63 mg levalbuterol per 3 mL)

Levalbuterol hydrochloride is a sympathomimetic agent that produces bronchodilation by relaxing bronchial smooth muscles via beta$_2$-adrenergic receptor stimulation. It is indicated in the treatment or prevention of bronchospasm in patients with reversible obstructive airway disease. **Short-acting β_2-adrenergic-receptor agonists** include **albuterol** (Proventil, Ventolin), **levalbuterol**, the (R)-enantiomer of **albuterol** (Xopenex), **metaproterenol** (Alupent), **terbutaline** (Brethaire), and **pirbuterol** (Maxair). These drugs are used for acute inhalation treatment of bronchospasm. Terbutaline (Brethine, Bricanyl), albuterol, and metaproterenol also are available in oral dosage forms. Each of the inhaled drugs has an onset of action within 1 to 5 minutes and produces bronchodilation that lasts for about 2 to 6 hours. When given in oral dosage forms, the duration of action is somewhat longer (oral terbutaline, for example, has a duration of action of 4 to 8 hours). Although there are slight differences in the relative β_2/β_1-receptor potency ratios among the drugs, all of them are selective for the β_2 subtype.

The most effective drugs in relaxing airway smooth muscle and reversing bronchoconstriction are short-acting β_2-adrenergic-receptor agonists. They are the preferred treatment for rapid symptomatic relief of dyspnea associated with asthmatic bronchoconstriction. Although these drugs are prescribed on an as-needed basis, it is imperative that guidelines be given to the patient so that reliance on relief of symptoms during times of deteriorating asthma does not occur. When the asthma symptoms become persistent, the patient should be reevaluated so that drugs aimed at controlling, in addition to reversing, the disease can be described.

Salmeterol xinafoate (Serevent) and **formoterol** (Foradil) are long-lasting adrenergic agents with very high selectivity for the β_2-receptor subtype. Inhalation of salmeterol provides persistent bronchodilation lasting over 12 hours. The mechanism underlying the extended duration of action of salmeterol is not yet fully understood. The extended side chain on salmeterol renders it 10,000 times more lipophilic than albuterol. The lipophilicity regulates the diffusion rate away from the receptor determining the degree of partitioning in the lipid bilayer of the membrane. Subsequent to binding the receptor the less lipophilic, short-acting agonists are removed rapidly from the receptor environment by diffusion in the aqueous phase. Unbound salmeterol, by contrast, persists in the membrane and only slowly dissociates from the receptor environment.

LEVAMISOLE

In addition to its antiviral actions, interferon has an antiproliferative effect and modifies the functions of macrophages and natural killer cells. Thymosin, a protein synthesized by the epitheloid component of the thymus, may be potentially valuable in patients with DiGeorge's syndrome or other T-cell deficiency states. Levamisole augments T-cell-mediated immunity and may be of value in the immunodeficiency associated with Hodgkin's disease.

LEVETIRACETAM

(Keppra tablets 250 mg)

Levetiracetam is an anticonvulsant that selectively prevents hypersynchronization of epileptiform burst firing and propagation of seizure activity. It is indicated as an adjunctive therapy in partial onset seizures in adults with epilepsy.

The ideal antiseizure drug would suppress all seizures without causing any unwanted effects. Unfortunately, the drugs used currently not only fail to control seizure activity in some patients, but frequently cause unwanted effects that range in severity from minimal impairment of the CNS to death from aplastic anemia or hepatic failure. The clinician who treats patients with epilepsy is thus faced with the task of selecting the appropriate drug or combination of drugs that best controls seizures in an individual patient at an acceptable level of untoward effects. As a general rule, complete control of seizures can be achieved in up to 50% of patients, whereas another 25% can be improved significantly. The degree of success varies as a function of seizure type, cause, and other factors.

To minimize toxicity, treatment with a single drug is preferred. If seizures are not controlled with the initial agent at adequate plasma concentrations, substitution of a second drug is preferred to the concurrent administration of another agent. However, multiple-drug therapy may be required, especially when two or more types of seizure occur in the same patient.

Levetiracetam (Keppra) is a pyrrolidine, the racemically pure S-enantiomer of α-ethyl-2-oxo-l-pyrrolidineacetamide. **Levetiracetam** exhibits a novel pharmacological profile insofar as it inhibits partial and secondarily generalized tonic–clonic seizures in the kindling model, yet is ineffective against maximum electroshock- and pentylenetetrazol-induced seizures, findings consistent with clinical effectiveness against partial and secondarily generalized tonic–clonic seizures. The mechanism by which levetiracetam exerts these antiseizure effects is unknown. No evidence for an action on voltage-gated Na^+ channels or either GABA- or glutamate-mediated synaptic transmission has emerged. A stereoselective binding site has been identified in rat brain membranes and the synaptic vesicle protein SVZA has been shown to be a brain-binding target of **levetiracetam**.

Levetiracetam is rapidly and almost completely absorbed after oral administration and is not bound to plasma proteins. Ninety-five percent (95%) of the drug and its inactive metabolite are excreted in the urine, 65% of which is unchanged drug; 24% of the drug is metabolized by hydrolysis of the acetamide group. It neither induces nor is a high-affinity substrate for CYP isoforms or glucuronidation enzymes and thus is devoid of known interactions with other antiseizure drugs, oral contraceptives, or anticoagulants.

A double-blind, placebo-controlled trial of adults with refractory partial seizures demonstrated that addition of **levetiracetam** to other antiseizure medications was superior to placebo. Insufficient evidence is available with respect to use of **levetiracetam** as monotherapy for partial or generalized epilepsy.

The drug is well tolerated. The most frequently reported adverse effects are somnolence, asthenia, and dizziness.

LEVOBUNOLOL

(AK-Beta solution 0.25%)

Levobunolol a beta-adrenergic-blocking ophthalmic agent, which reduces IOP by reducing aqueous humor production, is indicated in the treatment of IOP in chronic open-angle glaucoma or ocular hypertension. β-Receptor antagonists are very useful in the treatment of chronic open-angle glaucoma. Six drugs currently are available: **carteolol** (Ocupress, others), **betaxolol** (Betaoptic, others), **levobunolol** (Betagan, others), **metipranolol** (Optipranolol, others), **timolol** (Timoptic, others), and **levobetaxolol** (Betaxon). Timolol, levobunolol, carteolol, and metipranolol are nonselective, whereas betaxolol and levobetaxolol are β_1 selective. None of the agents has significant membrane-stabilizing or intrinsic sympathomimetic activities. Topically administered blockers have little or no effect on pupil size or accommodation and are devoid of blurred vision and night blindness often seen with miotics. These agents decrease the production of aqueous humor, which appears to be the mechanism for their clinical effectiveness.

The drugs generally are administered as eye drops and have onset in approximately 30 minutes with a duration of 12 to 24 hours. While topically administered β-blockers usually are well tolerated, systemic absorption can lead to adverse cardiovascular and pulmonary effects in susceptible patients. They therefore should be used with great caution in glaucoma patients at risk of adverse systemic effects of β-receptor antagonists (e.g., patients with bronchial asthma, severe chronic obstructive pulmonary disease [COPD], or those with bradyarrhythmias). Recently three β-blockers (betaxolol, metipranolol, and timolol) also have been observed to confer protection to retinal neurons, apparently related to their ability to attenuate neuronal Ca^{2+} and Na^+ influx. Betaxolol is the most effective antiglaucoma drug at reducing Na^+/Ca^{2+} influx. It is thought that β-blockers may be able to blunt ganglion cell death in glaucoma and that levobetaxolol may be a more important neuroprotectant than timolol because of its greater capacity to block Na^+ and Ca^{2+} influx.

LEVOBUNOLOL HYDROCHLORIDE

(Betagan)

Levobunolol, a beta-adrenergic-receptor-blocking agent (instill 1 to 2 drops of 0.25% solution b.i.d. in each eye), is used in the treatment of chronic open-angle glaucoma and ocular hypertension.

LEVOCABASTINE

Levocabastine is a highly specific and potent histamine H_1-receptor antagonist that has been specifically developed for the topical treatment of allergic rhinoconjunctivitis. Levocabastine is some 15,000 times more potent than chlorpheniramine, expressing antihistaminic activity at doses below 0.002 mg/kg. In addition, it has a highly specific binding affinity for H_1-receptors with no evidence of anticholinergic, antiserotonergic, or antidopaminergic activity at doses considerably in excess of therapeutically effective concentrations. Terfenadine, astemizole, loratadine, and cetirizine are second-generation antihistaminic agents that are relatively nonsedating.

LEVODOPA

In the management of Parkinson's disease, two major precursors of dopamine, namely L-tyrosine and levodopa, have been investigated. L-Tyrosine has proved ineffective for two reasons: (1) tyrosine hydroxylase is the rate-limiting enzyme, and it must be bypassed in order to raise the concentration of dopamine, and (2) there is some evidence that the action of tyrosine hydroxylase is defective in parkinsonism. Levodopa is an inert chemical, but its metabolite dopamine is pharmacologically active. The amount of levodopa prescribed depends on the severity of the parkinsonism. It is the current practice to give L-dopa in combination with carbidopa, a peripheral dopa-decarboxylase inhibitor. In this combination (Sinemet), doses of only several hundred milligrams of levodopa daily, instead of several thousand milligrams if given alone, are necessary for achieving the desired control (see also Figure 33).

The first signs of improvement are usually a subjective feeling of well-being accompanied by increased vigor. The symptoms yield in the following sequence: first the akinesia, then the rigidity, and finally the tremor, which disappears slowly and incompletely. If the drug is stopped, the symptoms reappear in the reverse order: tremor, rigidity, and then akinesia. The postural abnormality responds less effectively to medications. Among the adverse reactions encountered during the first months of levodopa therapy is nausea, usually without vomiting. This emetic action of levodopa is often troublesome and seems to be aggravated by the consumption of coffee. Eliminating coffee, or drinking decaffeinated coffee instead, usually overcomes this problem. Enhancing the dose of carbidopa attenuates the emetic actions of levodopa. The use of a phenothiazine antiemetic (such as clorpromazine, which blocks the dopamine receptor sites in the brain and therefore counteracts the beneficial effects of levodopa) is discouraged. The development of involuntary movements may limit the usefulness of levodopa. This peak dose dyskinesia is usually manifested in the form of choreic movements that involve the hands, arms, legs, and face. Oromandibular dystonia develops in 10% of the patients. In addition, increased oral activity with constant chewing, biting, opening and closing of the mouth, and intermittent protrusions of the tongue are the most frequent side effects. The abnormal involuntary movements usually occur during the period of maximum benefit from levodopa, which is usually 1 to 2 hours after each dose, and may last from several minutes up to 1 to 2 hours. To avoid these involuntary movements, the frequency of drug administration must usually be increased and the individual dose of levodopa decreased.

The beneficial and side effects of levodopa may be mediated via different receptor sites. For example, the beneficial effects of levodopa may be brought about by the dopamine$_1$ (D_1) receptor, whereas the dyskinesia may be brought about by the dopamine$_2$ (D_2) receptor. D_2-receptor-blocking agents such as oxiperomide and tiapride are able to reduce levodopa-induced dyskinesia without exacerbating the parkinsonian symptomatology. The conventional phenothiazines (such as chlorpromazine) and butyrophenones (such as haloperidol) block both D_1 and D_2 receptors. Therefore, these drugs are not suitable for the management of levodopa-induced dyskinesia.

Levodopa should be used with caution in patients with various cardiovascular disorders. The peripheral decarboxylation of levodopa markedly increases the concentration of dopamine in the blood. Dopamine is a pharmacologically active catecholamine that influences alpha- and beta-adrenergic receptors.

Therapeutic doses of levodopa produce cardiac stimulation by activating the beta$_1$-receptor site in the heart. In some elderly patients, it may produce cardiac arrhythmias. The cardiac stimulation is blocked by propranolol, the beta-adrenergic-receptor-blocking agent (see Figure 83). Propranolol has also been shown to be effective in suppressing tremor. Particular cardiac conditions that warrant careful attention when the use of levodopa is considered are angina pectoris and a history of cardiac arrhythmias. Psychiatric syndromes, peptic ulcer, and glaucoma are also contraindications to its use.

The on–off phenomenon is a sudden loss of effectiveness with the abrupt onset of akinesia ("off" effects) that may last for minutes or hours. This is followed by an equally sudden return of effectiveness ("on" effects) that may even be accompanied by hyperkinesia. The effect is so sudden that it has been compared to the action of a light switch being turned on and off. The use of levodopa is associated with a 10 to 20% frequency of the on–off phenomenon, whereas a 50% frequency is seen with levodopa use alone. The mechanism underlying this on–off phenomenon is not known. Most probably it is due to the sudden unavailability of dopamine to its receptor sites. For example, it has been shown that the on–off phenomenon is greatly relieved in patients who are on low protein diets. Dietary amino acids compete with levodopa for absorption from the gut and for transport across the blood–brain barrier. During the "off" period, the plasma level of levodopa is low. Dopamine receptor agonists are able to alleviate the symptoms, indicating that the receptor site is active.

The on–off effect should be differentiated from the wearing-off or end-of-dose response. Wearing off is clearly related to the dosage and blood level of levodopa. As the disease progresses and the number of nigral striatal neurons decreases, less dopamine can be stored in the striatum. This necessitates the constant replenishment of levodopa from the blood, so that the bioavailability of plasma levodopa becomes an important factor.

The true on–off phenomenon, which is rarely seen before the second year of treatment, probably is related more to the pharmacodynamic properties of the receptors themselves. The receptor mechanisms are turned off as suddenly as they are also turned on.

LEVODOPA-CARBIDOPA

(Sinemet)

Levodopa, a precursor of dopamine (100 mg), and carbidopa, an inhibitor of peripheral dopa decarboxylase (10 mg), in combination are used in the treatment of Parkinson's disease (see also Figure 33).

LEVOFLOXACIN

(Levaquin tablets 250 mg)

Levofloxacin is a fluoroquinolone/ophthalmic/antibiotic that interferes with microbial DNA synthesis. It is indicated in the treatment of acute maxillary sinusitis, acute bacterial exacerbation of chronic bronchitis, nosocomial pneumonia, community-acquired pneumonia, skin and skin structure infections, chronic bacterial prostatitis, urinary tract infection (UTI), inhalational anthrax (postexposure), and acute pyelonephritis caused by susceptible strains of specific microorganisms. Ophthalmic use is for the treatment of conjunctivitis caused by susceptible strains of aerobic Gram-positive and aerobic Gram-negative microorganisms.

The first quinolone, **nalidixic acid**, was isolated as a by-product of the synthesis of chloroquine. It has been available for the treatment of urinary tract infections for many years. The introduction of fluorinated 4-quinolones, such as **ciprofloxacin** (Cipro), **moxifloxacin** (Avelox), and **gatifloxacin** (Tequin), represents a particularly important therapeutic advance because these agents have broad antimicrobial activity and are effective after oral administration for the treatment of a wide variety of infectious diseases. Relatively few side effects appear to accompany the use of these fluoroquinolones, and microbial resistance to their action does not develop rapidly. Rare and potentially fatal side effects, however, have resulted in the withdrawal from the market of temafloxacin (immune hemolytic anemia), trovafloxacin (hepatotoxicity), grepafloxacin (cardiotoxicity), and clinafloxacin (phototoxicity). In all these cases, the side effects were so infrequent as to be missed by prerelease clinical trials and detected only by postmarketing surveillance.

LEVOMETHADYL ACETATE HYDROCHLORIDE

(Orlaam)

Levomethadyl acetate hydrochloride, a synthetic diphenylheptane derivative and an opioid receptor agonist (20 to 40 mg p.o.), is used in the management of opiate dependence.

LEVONORGESTREL

(Norplant system)

Levonorgestrel, a progestin with contraceptive properties, is used in long-term (up to 5 years), reversible prevention of pregnancy (see also Figure 55). High doses of diethylstilbestrol and other estrogens once were used for postcoital contraception (the "**morning-after pill**") but never received FDA approval for this indication. The FDA has now approved two preparations for postcoital contraception. PLAN-B is two doses of the "minipill" (0.75 mg of levonorgestrel per pill) separated by 12 hours. Preven is two 2-pill doses of a high-dose oral contraceptive (0.25 mg of **levonorgestrel** and 0.05 mg of ethinyl estradiol per pill) separated by 12 hours. This is sometimes referred to as the "**Yuzpe**" **method** after the Canadian physician who pioneered its use. The FDA also has declared other products with the same or very similar composition safe and effective for use as emergency contraceptive pills.

The first dose of such preparations should be taken anytime within 72 hours after intercourse, and this should be followed 12 hours later by a second dose. This treatment reduces the risk of pregnancy following unprotected intercourse by approximately 60% for the Yuzpe method and 80% for **levonorgestrel** alone. With either preparation, effectiveness appears to increase the sooner after intercourse the pills are taken.

LEVOPROPOXYPHENE NAPSYLATE

(Novrad)

Unlike dextropropoxyphene (Darvon), levopropoxyphene has no analgesic or respiratory depressant properties.

LEVORPHANOL TARTRATE

(Levo-Dromoran)

Levorphanol (2 to 3 mg p.o.) is a synthetic morphinan derivative which is recommended for moderate to severe pain, often as an adjunct with anesthetics. It exerts its analgesic action in 20 minutes and has a duration of action of 4 hours. Levorphanol is conjugated with glucuronic acid in the liver and is excreted in the urine. Levorphanol should be administered cautiously during labor and delivery, as it crosses the placental barrier and may cause severe respiratory depression in premature infants. Like morphine, levorphanol is contraindicated in severe head injury where the intracranial pressure may be high. Levorphanol should be administered cautiously to patients with renal or hepatic dysfunction because drug accumulation or prolonged duration of action may occur; to patients with pulmonary disease (asthma, chronic obstructive pulmonary disease) because the drug depresses respiration and suppresses the cough reflex; to patients undergoing biliary tract surgery because the drug may cause biliary spasm; to patients with convulsive disorders because the drug may precipitate seizures; to elderly or debilitated patients, who are more sensitive to both therapeutic and adverse drug effects; and to patients prone to physical or psychic addiction because of the high risk of addiction to this drug (see also Figure 68).

Numerous CNS drugs including narcotics, analgesics, general anesthetics, antihistamines, phenothiazines, barbiturates, benzodiazepines, sedative–hypnotics, tricyclic antidepressants, alcohol, and muscle relaxants, potentiate the respiratory and CNS depression, sedation, and hypotensive effects of levorphanol.

Levorphanol, when combined with anticholinergic medications, may cause paralytic ileus. The most common signs and symptoms of levorphanol overdose are CNS depression, respiratory depression, and miosis. Naloxone will reverse levorphanol-induced respiratory depression. (Because the duration of action of levorphanol is longer than that of naloxone, repeated antagonist dosing is necessary.)

LEVOSULPIRIDE

Levosulpiride is the (–) enantiomer of sulpiride, an antiemetic, antidyspeptic, and antipsychotic drug. However, levosulpiride is a more potent antiemetic compound than sulpiride. Levosulpiride (50 to 300 mg/day) is effective in depressive and somatoform disorders, as well as in the treatment of negative symptoms in schizophrenic patients.

LEVOTHYROXINE SODIUM

(Synthroid)

Levothyroxine is indicated in the treatment of hypothyroidism (0.05 mg initially); of myxedema coma (0.4 mg IV initially); of thyroid-stimulating hormone (TSH) suppression in thyroid cancer; of euthyroid and nodules goiter; and of thyroid suppression therapy (2.6 mcg/kg/day for 7 to 10 days). Levothyroxine increases the metabolic rate of tissue. It affects protein and carbohydrate metabolism, promotes gluconeogenesis, increases the utilization and mobilization of glycogen stores, stimulates protein synthesis, and regulates cell growth and differentiation. The orally administered levothyroxine exerts its full effects within one week. It is distributed widely, and the highest levels are found in the liver and the kidneys. Levothyroxine, which is extensively protein bound, becomes metabolized by deiodination. The half-life of levothyroxine is 6 to 7 days. Levothyroxine is contraindicated in patients with thyrotoxicosis, acute myocardial infarction, and uncorrected adrenal insufficiency because the drug increases tissue metabolic demands. Levothyroxine also is contraindicated for treating obesity because it is ineffective and can cause life-threatening adverse reactions. Levothyroxine should be used cautiously in patients with angina or other cardiovascular disease because of the risk of increased metabolic demands, and in patients with diabetes mellitus because of reduced glucose tolerance. Concomitant use of levothyroxine with tricyclic antidepressants or sympathomimetics may increase the effects of any or all of these drugs and may lead to coronary insufficiency or cardiac arrhythmias. Clinical manifestations of overdose include the signs and symptoms of hyperthyroidism, including weight loss, increased appetite, palpitations, nervousness, diarrhea, abdominal cramps, sweating, tachycardia, increased blood pressure, widened pulse pressure, angina, cardiac arrhythmias, tremor, headache, insomnia, heat intolerance, fever, and menstrual irregularities (see also Figures 66, 97, and 98).

LIDOCAINE HYDROCHLORIDE/EPINEPHRINE

(Xylocaine with epinephrine injection 0.5%)

Lidocaine hydrochloride is a local anesthetic/vasopressor preparation. **Lidocaine** stabilizes neuronal membranes by inhibiting the ionic fluxes required for the initiation and conduction of impulses, thereby effecting local anesthetic action. **Epinephrine** stimulates both alpha and beta receptors within sympathetic nervous system; relaxes smooth muscle of bronchi and iris and is an antagonist of histamine. They are indicated for production of local or regional anesthesia by infiltration techniques such as percutaneous injection, by peripheral nerve block techniques such as brachial plexus and intercostals, and by central neural techniques such as lumbar and caudal epidural blocks.

Lidocaine (Xylocaine, others), an aminoethylamide is the prototypical amide local anesthetic. **Lidocaine** produces faster, more intense longer lasting, and more extensive anesthesia than does an equal concentration of procaine. **Lidocaine** is an alternative choice for individuals sensitive to ester-type local anesthetics.

Lidocaine is absorbed rapidly after parenteral administration and from the gastrointestinal and respiratory tracts. Although it is effective when used without any vasoconstrictor, epinephrine decreases the rate of absorption, such that the toxicity is decreased and the duration of action usually is prolonged. In addition to preparations for injection, an iontophoretic, needle-free drug-delivery system for a solution of **lidocaine** and epinephrine (**Iontocaine**) is available. This system generally is used for dermal procedures and provides anesthesia to a depth of up to 10 mm.

A **lidocaine** transdermal patch (**Lidoderm**) is used in relief of pain associated with postherpetic neuralgia. The combination of lidocaine (2.59%) and prilocaine (2.5%) in an occlusive dressing (**Emla anesthetic disc**) is used as an anesthetic prior to venipuncture, skin graft harvesting, and infiltration of anesthetics into genitalia.

Lidocaine is dealkylated in the liver by CYPs to monoethylglycine xylidide and glycine xylidide, which can be metabolized further to monoethylglycine and xylidide. Both monoethylglycine xylidide and glycine xylidide retain local anesthetic activity. In humans, about 75% of the xylidide is excreted in the urine as the further metabolite 4-hydroxy-2, 6-dimethylaniline.

The side effects of **lidocaine** seen with increasing dose include drowsiness, tinnitus, dysgeusia, dizziness, and twitching. As the dose increases, seizures, coma, and respiratory depression and arrest will occur. Clinically significant cardiovascular depression usually occurs at serum **lidocaine** levels that produce marked CNS effects. The metabolites monoethylglycine xylidide and glycine xylidide may contribute to some of these side effects.

Lidocaine has a wide range of clinical uses as a local anesthetic; it has utility in almost any application where a local anesthetic of intermediate duration is needed. Lidocaine also is used as an antiarrhythmic agent.

Lidocaine is indicated for production of local or regional anesthesia by the infiltration technique, and by central neural techniques such as lumbar and caudal epidural blocks.

Lidocaine produces faster, more intense, longer-lasting, and more extensive anesthesia than does an equal concentration of procaine. Unlike procaine, it is an aminoethylamide and is the prototypical member of this class of local anesthetics. It is a good choice for individuals sensitive to ester-type local anesthetics. Although it is effective when used without any vasoconstrictor, in the presence of epinephrine, the rate of absorption and the toxicity are decreased, and the duration of action usually is prolonged (see also Figure 80).

Lidocaine, given intravenously, is indicated in the acute management of ventricular arrhythmias. Lidocaine blocks both open and inactivated cardiac Na^+ channels. Recovery from block is very rapid, so lidocaine exerts greater effects in depolarized (e.g., ischemic) and/or rapidly driven tissues. Lidocaine is not useful in atrial arrhythmias, probably because atrial action potentials are so short that the Na^+ channel is in the inactivated state only briefly and diastolic (recovery) times are relatively long.

Lidocaine decreases automaticity by reducing the slope of phase 4 and altering the threshold for excitability. Action potential duration usually is unaffected or is shortened; such shortening may be due to the block on the few Na^+ channels that inactivate late during the cardiac action potential. Lidocaine usually exerts no significant effect on PR or QRS duration; QT is unaltered or slightly shortened.

Lidocaine is dealkylated in the liver by mixed-function oxidases to monoethylglycine xylidide and glycine xylidide, which can be metabolized further to monoethylglycine and xylidide. Both monoethylglycine and glycine xylidide retain local anesthetic activity. In human beings, about 75% of xylidide is excreted in the urine as the further metabolite, 4-hydroxy-2,6-dimethylaniline. Clinical effects of overdose include signs and symptoms of CNS toxicity, such as convulsions and/or respiratory depression and cardiovascular toxicity.

LIDOCAINE HYDROCHLORIDE/PRILOCAINE

(EMLA cream, 2.5% lidocaine and 2.5% prilocaine)

Lidocaine hydrochloride is a topical/local anesthetic preparation. It stabilizes neuronal membranes by inhibiting the ionic fluxes required for the initiation and conduction of impulses, thereby affecting local anesthetic action. It is indicated as a topical anesthetic for use on normal intact skin for local analgesia or genital mucous membranes for superficial minor surgery and as pretreatment for infiltration anesthesia

LINCOMYCIN

(Lincocin)

Lincomycin, which resembles erythromycin, in a dose of 500 mg t.i.d., is indicated in the treatment of serious infections due to susceptible strains of streptococci, pneumococci, and staphylococci resistant to other antibiotics. Lincomycin inhibits protein synthesis by interfering with the formation of initiation complexes and with aminoacyl translocation reactions. The receptor for lincomycins on the 50S subunit of the bacterial ribosome is a 23S rRNA, perhaps identical to the receptor for erythromycins (see also Figure 88). Thus, these two drug classes may block each other's attachment and may interfere with each other. Resistance to lincomycin appears slowly, perhaps as a result of chromosomal mutation. Plasmid-mediated resistance has not been established with certainty. Resistance to lincomycin is not rare among streptococci, pneumococci, and staphylococci. *C. difficile* strains are regularly resistant.

Lincomycin is widely distributed in the body but does not appear in the CNS in significant concentrations. It is about 90% protein bound. Excretion is mainly through the liver, bile, and urine. Lincomycin's common adverse effects are diarrhea, nausea, and skin rashes. Impaired liver function (with or without jaundice) and neutropenia sometimes occur. Severe diarrhea and enterocolitis have followed clindamycin administration and place a serious restraint on its use.

LINDANE

(Gamma benzene hexachloride) (G-Well, Kwell, Kwildane, Scabene)

Lindane, a chlorinated hydrocarbon insecticide with scabicidal and pediculicidal properties (1% cream, lotion, shampoo), is used in scabies and pediculosis.

LINDANE

(Lindane lotion 1%, shampoo 1%)

Lindane exerts its action by being directly absorbed into the parasite and ova. **Lotion**: used in treatment of *Sarcoptes scabiei* (scabies) in patients who have failed to respond to adequate doses or are intolerant of other approved therapies. **Shampoo**: used in treatment of *Pediculus capitis* (head lice) and *Pediculus pubis* (crab lice) and their ova in patients who have failed to respond to adequate doses or are intolerant of other approved therapies.

Infestations with ectoparasites such as body lice and scabies are common throughout the world. These conditions have a significant impact on public health in the form of disabling pruritus, secondary infection, and in the case of the body louse, transmission of life-threatening illnesses such as **typhus**. Topical and oral medications are available to treat these infestations.

Perhaps the best known antiectoparasitic medication is 1% **γ-benzene hexachloride lotion**, also known as **lindane**.

Lindane has been used as a commercial insecticide as well as a topical medication. It is highly effective in the treatment of **ectoparasites**. Neurotoxicity, although a concern with the use of lindane, is a rare side effect when the medication is used correctly. However, the FDA has defined lindane as a second-line drug in treating **pediculosis** and **scabies** and has highlighted the potential for neurotoxicity in children and adults weighing less than 110 pounds. The lotion is applied in a thin layer from the neck down, left in place for 8 to 12 hours or overnight, and removed by thorough washing at the end of the 8- to 12-hour period. The treatment may be repeated in 1 week. To avoid problems with neurotoxicity, the lotion should be applied only in a thin coat to dry skin, should not be applied immediately after bathing, and should be kept away from the eyes, mouth, and open cuts or sores. A 1% lindane shampoo also is available for head and body lice.

A second topical agent that is very useful in the treatment of ectoparasites is **permethrin**.

Permethrin is a synthetic derivative of the insecticide **pyrethrum**, which was obtained originally from ***Chrysanthemum cinerariaefolium***. Neurotoxicity associated with this compound is extremely rare. A 5% cream (Acticin, Elimite, others) is available in the treatment of scabies. This is used as an 8- to 12-hour or overnight application. A 1% permethrin cream rinse (NIX) also is available for the treatment of lice.

Ivermectin (Stromectol), an anthelmintic drug used traditionally to treat onchocerciasis, also is effective in the off-label treatment of scabies.

LINEZOLID

(Zyvox tablets 400 mg)

Linezolid is an **oxazolidinone** that prevents the formation of a functional 70S initiation complex, which is essential to the bacterial translation process. It is indicated in the treatment of vancomycin-resistant *Enterococcus faecium* infections; treatment of nosocomial pneumonia, complicated and uncomplicated skin and skin structure infections, and community-acquired pneumonia caused by susceptible strains of specific organisms.

Linezolid (Zyvox) is a synthetic antimicrobial agent of the oxazolidinone class.

Linezolid is active against Gram-positive organisms including staphylococci, streptococci, enterococci, Gram-positive anaerobic cocci, and Gram-positive rods such as *Corynebacterium* spp. and *Listeria* monocytogenes. It has poor activity against most Gram-negative aerobic or anaerobic bacteria. It is bacteriostatic against enterococci and staphylococci and bactericidal against streptococci. MICs are ≤ 2 μg/mL against strains of *E. faecium, E. faecalis, S. pyogenes, S. pneumoniae*, and *viridans* strains of streptococci. MICs are ≤ 4 μg/mL for strains of *S. aureus* and coagulase-negative staphylococci. *Mycobacterium tuberculosis* is moderately susceptible, with MICs of 2 μg/mL. Because of its unique mechanism of action, linezolid is active against strains that are resistant to multiple other agents, including penicillin-resistant strains of *S. pneumoniae*; methicillin-resistant, vancomycin-intermediate, and vancomycin-resistant strains of staphylococci; and vancomycin-resistant strains of enterococci.

Linezolid inhibits protein synthesis by binding to the P site of the 50S ribosomal subunit and preventing formation of the larger ribosomal-fMet-tRNA complex that initiates protein synthesis. As mentioned above, there is no cross-resistance with other drug classes. Resistance in enterococci and staphylococci is due to point mutations of the 23S rRNA. As multiple copies of 23S rRNA genes are present in bacteria, resistance generally requires mutations in two or more copies.

Linezolid is well absorbed after oral administration and may be administered without regard to food. With oral bioavailability approaching 100%, dosing for oral and intravenous preparations is the same. Peak serum concentrations average 12 to 14 μg/mL 1 to 2 hours after a single 600-mg dose in adults and approximately 20 μg/mL at steady state with dosing every 12 hours. The half-life is approximately 4 to 6 hours. Linezolid is 30% protein-bound and distributes widely to well-perfused tissues, with a 0.6 to 0.7 L/kg volume of distribution.

Linezolid is broken down by nonenzymatic oxidation to aminoethoxyacetic acid and hydroxyethyl glycine derivatives. Approximately 80% of the dose of linezolid appears in the urine, 30% as active compound, and 50% as the two primary oxidation products. Ten percent of the administered dose appears as oxidation products in feces. Although serum concentrations and half-life of the parent compound are not appreciably altered by renal insufficiency, oxidation products accumulate in renal insufficiency, with half-lives increasing by approximately 50 to 100%. The clinical significance of this is unknown, and no dose adjustment in renal insufficiency is currently recommended. **Linezolid** and its breakdown products are eliminated by dialysis; therefore, the drug should be administered after hemodialysis. One case report noted sustained therapeutic concentrations of linezolid in peritoneal dialysis fluid with oral administration of 600 mg of linezolid twice daily.

Linezolid is FDA approved for treatment of infections caused by vancomycin-resistant *E. faecium*; nosocomial pneumonia caused by methicillin-susceptible and methicillin-resistant strains of *S. aureus*; community-acquired pneumonia caused by penicillin-susceptible strains of *S. pneumoniae*; complicated skin and skin-structure infections caused by streptococci and methicillin-susceptible and -resistant strains of *S. aureus*; and uncomplicated skin and skin-structure infections. In noncomparative studies, **linezolid** (600 mg twice daily) has had clinical and microbiological cure rates in the range of 85 to 90% in treatment of a variety of infections (soft tissue, urinary tract, and bacteremia) caused by vancomycin-resistant *E. faecium*. A 200-mg, twice-daily dose was less effective, with clinical and microbiological cure rates of approximately 75 and 59%, respectively. The 600-mg, twice-daily dose, therefore, should be used for treatment of infections caused by enterococci. A 400-mg, twice-daily dosage regimen is recommended only for treatment of uncomplicated skin and skin-structure infections.

The drug seems to be well tolerated, with generally minor side effects (e.g., gastrointestinal complaints, headache, rash). Myelosuppression, including anemia leukopenia, pancytopenia, and thrombocytopenia, has been reported in patients receiving linezolid. Thrombocytopenia or a significant reduction in platelet count has been associated with **linezolid** in 2.4% of treated patients, and its occurrence is related to duration of therapy. Platelet counts should be monitored in patients with risk of bleeding preexisting thrombocytopenia, or intrinsic or acquired disorders of platelet function (including those potentially caused by concomitant medication) and in patients receiving courses of therapy lasting beyond 2 weeks. **Linezolid** is a weak, nonspecific inhibitor of monoamine oxidase. Patients receiving concomitant therapy with an adrenergic or serotonergic agent or consuming more than 100 mg of tyramine a day may experience palpitations, headache, or hypertensive crisis. Peripheral and optic neuropathy, which seem to be reversible upon drug discontinuation, have been reported with prolonged use. Linezolid is neither a substrate nor an inhibitor of CYPs.

LINOLEIC ACID

All naturally occurring prostaglandins are derived through the cyclization of 20-carbon unsaturated fatty acids such as arachidonic acid, which in turn is synthesized from the essential fatty acid, linoleic acid.

Besides serving as a precursor for the synthesis of prostaglandins, arachidonic acid is also a precursor for the synthesis of prostacyclin, thromboxanes, and leukotrienes.

LIOTHYRONINE

(Cytomel, Cytomine)

Liothyronine, a thyroid preparation, has a short half-life and hence is used diagnostically in the T_3-suppression test.

LIOTHYRONINE SODIUM (TRIIODOTHYRONINE)

(Cytomel tablets 5 mcg)

Liothyronine sodium is a thyroid hormone that increases metabolic rate of body tissues and is needed for normal growth and maturation. It is indicated for the replacement or supplemental therapy in hypothyroidism; in TSH suppression for treatment or prevention of euthyroid goiters (e.g., thyroid nodules, multinodular goiters, enlargement in chronic thyroiditis); and as a diagnostic agent in suppression tests to differentiate suspected hyperthyroidism from euthyroidism; and in treatment of myxedema coma/precoma (IV).

LIOTRIX

(Euthyroid; Thyrolar)

Liotrix, a thyroid preparation, is a combination of T_4 and T_3, and is standardized to yield a T_4 to T_3 ratio of 4 to 1 (see also Figure 66).

LIOTRIX

(Thyrolar 1/4 tablets 3.1 mcg)

Liotrix is a thyroid hormone that increases the metabolic rate of body tissues and is needed for normal growth and maturation. It is indicated for replacement or supplemental therapy in hypothyroidism; pituitary TSH suppression in treatment or prevention of various types of euthyroid goiters, including thyroid nodules, subacute or chronic lymphocytic thyroiditis (Hashimoto's), multinodular goiter, and management of thyroid cancer; and as a diagnostic agent in suppression tests to differentiate suspected and hyperthyroidism or thyroid gland autonomy.

LIPID-LOWERING DRUGS

Drugs	Actions
HMG-CoA Reductase Inhibitors	
Fluvastatin Lovastatin Pravastatin Simvastatin	Inhibit HMG-CoA (3-hydroxy-3-methyl-glutaryl-coenzyme A) reductase, the enzyme that catalyzes the rate-limiting step in cholesterol synthesis
Bile-Acid-Binding Resins	
Cholestyramine Colestipol	Lower concentration of LDL cholesterol
Fibric Acid Derivatives	
Gemfibrozil Clofibrate Bezafibrate	Lowers VLDL and can increase HDL cholesterol concentrations
Nicotinic Acid	
Niacin	Decreases triglyceride

HMG-CoA reductase inhibitors are the drugs of first choice for treatment of most patients with hypercholesterolemia. They are more effective and better tolerated than other lipid-lowering drugs, and have been shown to decrease mortality from coronary artery disease.

LISINOPRIL

(Prinivil tablets 2.5 mg, Zestril)

Lisinopril is an angiotensin I-converting enzyme (ACE) inhibitor. It competitively inhibits ACE, prevents angiotensin I conversion to angiotensin II, and is a potent vasoconstrictor that also stimulates aldosterone secretion. Results are a decrease in sodium and fluid retention, a decrease in BP, and increase in diuresis. It is indicated in the treatment of hypertension; treatment of heart failure not responding to diuretics and digitalis; and treatment of acute MI within 24 hours in hemodynamically stable patients.

Lisinopril (Prinivil, Zestril), the third ACE inhibitor approved for use in the United States, is the lysine analog of enalaprilat; unlike **enalapril**, lisinopril itself is active. *In vitro*, lisinopril is a slightly more potent ACE inhibitor than is enalaprilat. **Lisinopril** is absorbed slowly, variably, and incompletely (about 30%) after oral administration (not reduced by food); peak concentrations in plasma are achieved in about 7 hours. It is cleared as the intact compound by the kidney, and its half-life in plasma is about 12 hours. **Lisinopril** does not accumulate in tissues. The oral dosage of **lisinopril** ranges from 5 to 40 mg daily (single or divided dosage), with 5 and 10 mg daily being appropriate for the initiation of therapy for heart failure and hypertension, respectively. A daily dose of 2.5 mg is recommended for patients with heart failure who are hyponatremic or have renal impairment.

Agents with positive inotropic actions that may be used in the management of CHF include the cardiac glycosides (e.g., digoxin and digitoxin), dopaminergic analogs (e.g., dobutamine), phosphodiesterase inhibitors (e.g., amrinone and milrinone), angiotensin antagonists (e.g., captopril, enalapril, and lisinopril), and vasodilators (nitrates and hydralazine). Lisinopril, an ACE inhibitor, increases the left-ventricular ejection fraction in patients with CHF, and the drug's effectiveness is not diminished in the presence of impaired renal function. Lisinopril (10 mg once a day) may be used in patients with uncomplicated essential hypertension not on diuretic therapy. Lisinopril (5 mg once a day) may be used with diuretics and digitalis in congestive heart failure (see Figure 23).

LISINOPRIL/HYDROCHLOROTHIAZIDE

(Prinzide 10/12.5 mg tablets)

Lisinopril/hydrochlorothiazide is antihypertensive combination. **Lisinopril** competitively inhibits angiotensin I-converting enzyme and prevents angiotensin I conversion to angiotensin II, reversing the potassium loss associated with the diuretic. **Hydrochlorothiazide** increases chloride, sodium, and water excretion by interfering with transport of sodium ions across renal tubular epithelium. They are indicated in the treatment of hypertension.

LITHIUM CARBONATE

(Eskalith)

Lithium is given orally as a salt, and the particular salt does not affect the therapeutic action. Lithium's anionic partner—carbonate, chloride acetate, citrate, or sulfate—serves only as an inert vehicle. Carbonate is by far the most widely used lithium salt. In addition, lithium carbonate contains more lithium, weight for weight, than do the other lithium salts. Because lithium is not bound to any plasma or tissue proteins, it is widely distributed throughout the body. Lithium ions are eliminated mainly by the kidneys. There is a direct relationship between the amount of sodium chloride ingested and the fraction of filtered lithium resorbed, in that the lower the sodium intake, the greater is the lithium retention. The contraindications are significant cardiovascular (CV) or renal diseases that would compromise its excretion. Lithium is unique among the psychopharmacologic compounds in that it rarely has any undesirable effects on emotional or intellectual functioning. A few unwanted effects are seen in the somatic sphere, and these fall into three overlapping categories.

1. Initially, when the maintenance dose of lithium is being established, the patient may experience gastrointestinal discomfort such as nausea, vomiting, diarrhea, stomach pain, muscular weakness, unusual thirst, frequent urination, and a slight feeling of being dazed, tired, and sleepy. These early side effects disappear once the patient is stabilized.
2. From the beginning of treatment, patients exhibit slight and barely noticeable hand tremors, which do not respond to antiparkinsonian agents.
3. After several months of continuous therapy with lithium, diabetes insipidus and goiter may develop. The kidney tubules then become insensitive to the action of antidiuretic hormone, and its administration is ineffective. Either a dose reduction or discontinuation of the lithium corrects this side effect without leaving any residual pathology. In the presence of goiter, the patient remains euthyroid. It has been reported that the administration of small amounts of thyroxine may counteract this side effect. Lithium is thought to exert its effect by interfering with the calcium-mediated release of norepinephrine increasing the uptake of norepinephrine, and decreasing the sensitivity of postsynaptic receptor sites to norepinephrine. In addition, there is increasing evidence that lithium exerts its therapeutic action by interfering with the polyphosphoinositide metabolism in the brain and by preventing inositol recycling through the uncompetitive inhibition of inositol monophosphatase.

The uses of lithium fall into two categories: established and innovative. Among its established uses, lithium salts are used to treat acute mania and as a prophylactic measure to prevent the recurrence of bipolar manic-depressive illness. As innovative agents, lithium salts have been used with certain success in the management of the following illnesses or conditions. In combination with tricyclic antidepressants, lithium is used in treating recurrent endogenous depression. In combination with neuroleptics, it is used in the management of schizoaffective disorders. In combination with neuroleptics, it is used to control schizophrenia. Lithium is also used in the case of patients with alcoholism associated with depression and has been used to correct the neutropenia that occurs during cancer chemotherapy. Lithium has been investigated for use in subduing aggressive behaviors in nonpsychotic but possibly brain-damaged patients. Its use has also been investigated in the management of inappropriate secretion of antidiuretic hormone.

LITOXETINE

Litoxetine is a new selective and potent inhibitor of serotonin receptors that has antiemetic effects against cisplatin-induced emesis. The clinical use of the majority of serotoninergic antidepressants such as fluoxetin and fluvoxamine is associated with gastrointestinal discomfort which appears to be due to stimulation of 5-HT_3 receptors. Litoxetine, by antagonizing 5-HT_3 receptors, may limit nausea and vomiting associated with fluoxetin or fluvoxamine (see also Figure 73).

LOCAL ANESTHETICS

Ester Compounds	Amide Compounds
Chloroprocaine	Bupivacaine
Procaine	Etidocaine
Tetracaine	Lidocaine
	Mepivacaine
	Prilocaine

Epinephrine is used in combination with a local anesthetic to reduce its uptake, prolong its duration of action, produce a bloodless field of operation, and protect against systemic effects. Local anesthetic solutions containing epinephrine should not be used in areas supplied by end arteries such as in the digits, ear, nose, and penis, because of the threat of ischemia and subsequential gangrene. Furthermore, under no circumstances should anesthetic solutions containing epinephrine be used intravenously in patients with cardiac arrhythmias. In general, solutions designed for multiple doses should not be used for spinal or epidural anesthesia (see also Figure 73).

LODOXAMIDE TROMETHAMINE

(Alomide)

Lodoxamide, a substance that stabilizes mast cells and has antiallergic properties (1 to 2 drops of 0.1% solution into each affected eye), is used in the treatment of vernal keratoconjunctivitis, vernal conjunctivitis, and vernal keratitis.

LOMEFLOXACIN HYDROCHLORIDE

(Maxaquin tablets 400 mg)

Lomefloxacin hydrochloride is a fluoroquinolone that interferes with microbial DNA synthesis. It is indicated in the treatment of infections of the lower respiratory tract and urinary tract caused by susceptible organisms; and in the prevention of UTIs in patients undergoing transurethral or transrectal procedures.

Lomefloxacin, a fluoroquinolone broad-spectrum antibiotic (400 mg p.o. daily for 10 to 14 days), is used in acute bacterial exacerbations of chronic bronchitis caused by *Haemophilis influenzae* or *Moraxella* (*Branhamella*) *catarrhalis*; in uncomplicated urinary tract infections (cystitis) caused by *Escherichia coli*, *Klebsiella pneumoniae*, *Proteus mirabilis*, or *Staphylococcus saprophyticus*; in complicated urinary tract infections caused by *E. coli*, *K. pneumoniae*, *P. mirabilis*, and *Pseudomonas aeruginosa*; and it is possibly effective against infections caused by *Citrobacter diversus* or *Enterobacter cloacae*; and for the prophylaxis of infections after transurethral surgical procedures (see also Figure 85).

LOMUSTINE

(CeeNU capsules 10 mg)

Lomustine is a nitrosourea. Its mechanism of action involves the inhibition of both DNA and RNA synthesis through DNA alkylation. Lomustine has been shown to affect a number of cellular processes including RNA, protein synthesis, and the processing of ribosomal and nucleoplasmic messenger RNA; DNA base component structure; and the rate of DNA synthesis and DNA polymerase activity. It is cell-cycle nonspecific. It is indicated in the treatment of brain tumors and Hodgkin's disease in adults and children.

Carmustine (BNCU), lomustine (CCNU), and semustine (methyl-CCNU) generate alkyl carbonium ions and isocyanate molecules and hence are able to interact with DNA and other macromolecules. These agents, which are lipid soluble, cross the blood–brain barrier and are therefore effective in treating brain tumors. They are bone marrow depressants.

The nitrosoureas, which include compounds such as 1,3-*bis*-(2-chloroethyl)-*l*-nitrosourea (carmustine; BCNU), 1-(2-chloroethyl)-3-cyclohexyl-1-nitrosourea (**lomustine**; CCNU), and its methyl derivative (semustine; methyl-CCNU), as well as the antibiotic streptozocin (streptozotocin), exert their cytotoxicity through the spontaneous breakdown to an alkylating intermediate, the 2-chloroethyl diazonium ion.

Cytotoxic actions: The most important pharmacological actions of the alkylating agents are those that disturb DNA synthesis and cell division. The capacity of these drugs to interfere with DNA integrity and function and to induce cell death in rapidly proliferating tissues provides the basis for their therapeutic and toxic properties. Whereas certain alkylating agents may have damaging effects on tissues with normally low mitotic indices—for example, liver, kidney, and mature lymphocytes—these tissues usually are affected in a delayed time frame. Acute effects are manifest primarily against rapidly proliferating tissues, Lethality of DNA alkylation depends on the recognition of the adduct, the creation of DNA strand breaks by repair enzymes, and an intact apoptotic response. The actual mechanism(s) of cell death related to DNA alkylation are not yet well characterized.

LOOP DIURETICS

The major loop diuretics are furosemide (Lasix) and ethacrynic acid (Edecrin). Furosemide is chemically related to the thiazide diuretics, but ethacrynic acid is not. These agents inhibit the active resorption of chloride (and sodium) in the thick, ascending medullary portion of the loop of Henle and also in the cortical portion of the loop or the distal tubule. The diuresis they produce, which is similar to that seen with the thiazides, predominantly causes a loss of chloride, sodium, and potassium, but HCO_3 excretion is not increased. Although large volumes of fluid can be excreted with the use of these agents, the ability of the kidney to produce either a dilute or concentrated urine is greatly diminished. These agents are the most efficacious of all the diuretics now on the market, usually producing about a 20% loss in the filtered load of sodium (furosemide, 15 to 30%; ethacrynic acid, 17 to 23%). Loop diuretics are ordinarily taken orally, but can be given intravenously if a very rapid onset of action is sought, as when used in combination with antihypertensive medications in the management of a hypertensive crisis. Furosemide and ethacrynic acid undergo some active renal tubular secretion as well as glomerular filtration. A minor portion is excreted by the liver. Loop diuretics are used for treating the following conditions:

- Edema of cardiac, hepatic, or renal origin, including acute pulmonary edema and hypertensive crisis
- Acute renal failure, to maintain urine flow, though an excessive loss of extracellular fluid volume can cause a decrease in the GFR
- Hypercalemia

Excessive volume depletion, hyponatremia, and hypotension are major risks associated with the use of loop diuretics, and the side effects of hypokalemia, hyperuricemia, and hyperglycemia are always present. Loop diuretics should not be used concurrently with ototoxic aminoglycoside antibiotics (i.e., streptomycin, gentamicin, kanamycin, tobramycin) (see also Table 25 and Figure 17).

LOPERAMIDE HYDROCHLORIDE

(Diar-aid tablets 2 mg, Imodium capsules 2 mg)

Loperamide hydrochloride is an antidiarrheal agent that slows intestinal motility, affects water and electrolyte movement through intestine, inhibits peristalsis, reduces daily fecal volume, increases viscosity and bulk density of stool, and diminishes loss of fluid and electrolytes. It is indicated in the control and symptomatic relief of acute nonspecific or chronic diarrhea; and in the reduction in volume of ileostomy output.

Loperamide (Imodium, others), like **diphenoxylate**, is a piperidine derivative. It slows gastrointestinal motility by effects on the circular and longitudinal muscles of the intestine presumably as a result of its interactions with opioid receptors in the intestine. Some part of its antidiarrheal effect may be due to a reduction of gastrointestinal secretion. In controlling chronic diarrhea, loperamide is as effective as diphenoxylate. In clinical studies, the most common side effect is abdominal cramps. Little tolerance develops to 1 s constipating effect.

In human volunteers taking large doses of **loperamide**, concentrations of drug in plasma peak about 4 hours after ingestion; this long latency may be due to inhibition of GI motility and to enterohepatic circulation of the drug. The apparent elimination half-life is 7 to 14 hours. **Loperamide** is poorly absorbed after oral administration and, in addition, apparently does not penetrate well into the brain because of *P*-glycoprotein transporter widely expressed in the brain endothelium. Mice with deletions of one of the genes encoding the *P*-glycoprotein transporter have much higher brain levels and significant central effects after administration of loperamide. Inhibition of *P*-glycoprotein by many clinically used drugs, such as quinidine and verapamil, possibly could lead to enhanced central effects of loperamide.

In general, **loperamide** is unlikely to be abused parenterally because of its low solubility; large doses of loperamide given to human volunteers do not elicit pleasurable effects typical of opioids. The usual dosage is 4 to 8 mg/day; the daily dose should not exceed 16 mg.

Loperamide has been shown to be effective against traveler's diarrhea, used either alone or in combination with antimicrobial agents (trimethoprim, trimethoprim-sulfamethoxazole, or a fluoroquinolone). **Loperamide** also has been used as adjunct treatment in almost all forms of chronic diarrheal disease, with few adverse effects. Loperamide lacks significant abuse potential and is more effective in treating diarrhea than diphenoxylate. Overdosage, however, can result in CNS depression (especially in children) and paralytic ileus. In patients with active inflammatory bowel disease involving the colon, **loperamide** should be used with great caution, if at all, to prevent development of toxic megacolon.

Loperamide N-oxide, an investigational agent, is a site-specific prodrug; it is chemically designed for controlled release of loperamide in the intestinal lumen, thereby reducing systemic absorption.

Loperamide (4 mg initially and not exceeding 16 mg/day) is indicated in the control and symptomatic relief of acute nonspecific diarrhea and chronic diarrhea associated with inflammatory bowel diseases. In addition, it may be used to control traveler's diarrhea or to reduce the volume of discharge from ileostomies. The antidiarrheal agents are codeine, diphenoxylate, and atropine (Lomotil), and loperamide. Because it causes less addiction than codeine, loperamide is now the most commonly used antidiarrheal agent. These agents achieve their effects by reducing the propulsive activity of the gut, enhancing the contact time between the intestinal mucosal and the luminal contents, and enhancing active chloride absorption, hence opposing the secretory effects of toxin. Loperamide should not be used in acute diarrhea associated with organisms that penetrate the intestinal mucosa (enteroinvasive *Escherichia coli*, *Salmonella*, and *Shigella*) or in pseudomembranous colitis associated with broad-spectrum antibiotics. Opioid antidiarrheal agents should not be used in cases of severe ulcerative colitis threatened by impending toxic megacolon or in patients with shigellosis, because they prolong duration of the disease.

LOPINAVIR/RITONAVIR

(Kaletra capsules, soft gelatin 133.3 mg lopinavir/ 33.3 mg ritonavir, solution, oral 80 mg lopinavir/ 20 mg ritonavir per mL)

Lopinavir is a protease inhibitor combination. **Lopinavir** inhibits HIV protease, the enzyme required to form functional proteins in HIV-infected patients. **Ritonavir** inhibits the cytochrome P450 (CYP) 3A-mediated metabolism of lopinavir, increasing lopinavir plasma concentrations. They are indicated in the treatment of HIV infections in combination with other antiviral agents.

Lopinavir is a peptidomimetic HIV protease inhibitor that is structurally similar to ritonavir but is three- to tenfold more potent against HIV-1 *in vitro*. **Lopinavir** is active against both HIV-1 and HIV-2; its IC_{50} for wild-type HIV variants in the presence of 50% human serum ranges from 65 to 290 nM. **Lopinavir** is available only in coformulation with low doses of **ritonavir**, which is used to inhibit CYP3A4 metabolism and increase concentrations of lopinavir.

Lopinavir is selectively toxic by potently inhibiting the HIV-encoded protease but not host-encoding aspartyl proteases. Protease-specific resistance mutations are identified with less frequency in patients taking lopinavir than with other HIV protease inhibitors. Treatment-naive patients who fail a first regimen containing lopinavir generally do not have HIV protease mutations but may have genetic resistance to the other drugs in the regimen. For treatment-experienced patients, accumulation of four or more HIV protease inhibitor resistance mutations is associated with a reduced likelihood of virus suppression after starting lopinavir. Mutation associated with lopinavir failure in treatment-experienced patients include those at HIV protease codons 10, 20, 24, 32, 33, 36, 46, 47, 50, 53, 54, 63, 71, 73, 82, 84, and 90. There is no evidence that exposure to the low doses of ritonavir in the lopinavir-ritonavir coformulation selects for ritonavir-specific resistance mutations.

Lopinavir is only available as a coformulation with low doses of ritonavir. When administered orally without ritonavir, lopinavir plasma concentrations were exceedingly low mainly owing to first-pass metabolism. Both the first-pass metabolism and systemic clearance of lopinavir are very sensitive to inhibition by **ritonavir**. A single 50-mg dose of ritonavir increased the lopinavir AUC by 77 times compared with that produced with 400 mg lopinavir alone; 100 mg ritonavir increased the lopinavir AUC by 155-fold. Lopinavir trough concentrations were increased 50- to 100-fold by coadministration of low doses of ritonavir. Multiple-dose pharmacokinetic studies have not been conducted with lopinavir in the absence of ritonavir. Adding 100 mg **ritonavir** twice daily to the lopinavir–ritonavir coformulation (a total of 200 mg twice daily of ritonavir) has only a modest further effect on lopinavir concentrations, increasing the mean steady-state AUC by 46%.

Lopinavir is absorbed rapidly after oral administration. A moderate- to high-fat meal increases oral bioavailability by up to 50%, and it is therefore recommended that the drug be taken with food. Although the capsules contain lopinavir–ritonavir in a fixed 4:1 ratio, the observed plasma concentration ratio for these two drugs following oral administration is nearly 20:1, reflecting the sensitivity of lopinavir to the inhibitory effect of ritonavir on CYP3A4. Lopinavir undergoes extensive hepatic oxidative metabolism by CYP3A4. Approximately 90% of total drug in plasma is the parent compound, and less than 3% of a dose is eliminated unchanged in the urine. Both **lopinavir** and **ritonavir** are highly bound to plasma proteins, mainly to α_1-acid glycoprotein, and therefore have a low fractional penetration into CSF and semen. Unlike ritonavir, the *in vitro* IC_{50} of lopinavir is not affected by physiological concentrations of albumin.

The most common adverse events reported with the lopinavir–ritonavir coformulation have been gastrointestinal including loose stools, diarrhea, nausea, and vomiting. These are less frequent and less severe than those reported with the 600-mg twice-daily standard dose of **ritonavir**. The most common abnormalities include elevated total cholesterol and triglycerides. Because the same adverse effects occur with **ritonavir**, it is unclear whether the side effects are due to ritonavir, lopinavir, or both.

In comparative clinical trials, lopinavir has antiretroviral activity at least comparable with that of other potent HIV protease inhibitors and better than that of nelfinavir. A lopinavir-based regimen was one of the two preferred regimens for treatment-naive HIV-infected adults in 2004. **Lopinavir** also has considerable and sustained antiretroviral activity in patients who failed previous HIV protease inhibitor-containing regimens. In one study, 70 subjects who had failed therapy with one previous HIV protease inhibitor were treated for 2 weeks with lopinavir, followed by the addition of nevirapine. At 48 weeks, 60% of subjects had plasma HIV-1 RNA levels of less than 50 copies/mL despite substantial phenotypic resistance to other HIV protease inhibitors. Because plasma concentrations of lopinavir generally are much higher than those required to suppress HIV replication *in vitro*, the drug may be capable of suppressing HIV isolates with low-level protease inhibitor resistance.

LORACARBEF

(Lorabid pulvules (capsules) 200 mg)

Loracarbef is a cephalosporin/antibiotic that binds to proteins in the bacterial cell wall, which inhibits cell wall synthesis. It is indicated in the treatment of otitis media, acute maxillary sinusitis, pharyngitis, tonsillitis, infection of lower respiratory tract, skin and skin structures, and urinary tract caused by susceptible strains of specific microorganisms.

Loracarbef, a synthetic beta lactam antibiotic of the carbacephem class (200 to 400 mg p.o. q. 12 hours), is used in the treatment of secondary bacterial infections of acute bronchitis, acute bacterial exacerbations or chronic bronchitis, of pneumonia, pharyngitis, tonsillitis, sinusitis, acute otitis media, uncomplicated skin and skin-structure infections, impetigo, uncomplicated cystitis, and in uncomplicated pyelonephritis.

LORATIDINE

(Alavert tablets, orally)

It is a peripherally selective piperidine histamine receptor blocker, which competitively antagonizes histamine at the H_1-receptor site. It is indicated in the temporary relief of symptoms caused by hay fever or other upper respiratory allergies (runny nose, sneezing, itchy/watery eyes, itching of the nose or throat); and in the treatment of chronic idiopathic urticaria.

Second-generation H_1-receptor antagonists lack anticholinergic side effects and are described as nonsedating largely because they do not cross the blood–brain barrier. They include **cetirizine** (Zyrtec), **loratadine** (Claritin), **desloratidine** (Clarinex), and **fexofenadine hydrochloride** (Allegra). Although second-generation nonsedating H_1-receptor blockers are as effective as the first-generation H_1 blockers, they are metabolized by CYP3A4 and, to a lesser extent, by CYP2D6 and should not be coadministered with medications that inhibit these enzymes (e.g., imidazole antifungals and macrolide antibiotics).

H_2-receptor blockers include **cimetidine** (Tagamet), **ranitidine** (Zantac), **famotidine** (Pepcid), and **nizatidine** (Axid). Besides their use in combination with H_1-receptor blockers for pruritus, the H_2-receptor blockers have immunomodulating effects, and this property has been exploited in children to treat warts.

Terfenadine, astemizole, loratadine, and cetirizine are second-generation antihistaminic agents that are relatively nonsedating. Other H_1-receptor antagonists currently undergoing clinical trials are azelastine, ebastine, and levocabastine. Loratadine is readily absorbed, with its onset of action beginning within 1 to 3 hours, reaching a maximum at 8 to 12 hours, and lasting in excess of 24 hours. Because peak plasma concentration may be delayed by 1 hour with a meal, the drug should be administered on an empty stomach.

Loratidine is about 98% bound to plasma protein. The drug does not readily cross the blood–brain barrier. Loratidine is extensively metabolized to an active metabolite called descarboethoxyloratadine. Approximately 80% of the total dose administered can be found equally distributed between urine and feces. The mean elimination half-life is 8.4 hours for loratadine. Loratidine overdosage (40 mg) causes somnolence, tachycardia, and headache.

LORATADINE/PSEUDOEPHEDRINE SULFATE

(Claritin-D 12 hour tablets 120 mg pseudoephedrine sulfate and 5 mg loratadine)

Loratadine/pseudoephedrine sulfate is an antihistamine/decongestant. **Loratadine** competitively antagonizes histamine at the H_1 receptor. **Pseudoephedrine** causes vasoconstriction and subsequent shrinkage of nasal mucous membranes by alpha-adrenergic stimulation, promoting nasal drainage. They are indicated in the relief of seasonal allergic rhinitis.

LORAZEPAM

(Ativan)

Lorazepam (2 to 3 mg/day) is indicated for the management of anxiety disorders or for the short-term relief of the symptoms of anxiety or anxiety associated with depressive symptoms. In addition, it may be used as a preanesthetic medication producing sedation, relief of anxiety, and a decreased ability to recall events related to surgery.

The pharmacology of benzodiazepine derivatives differs significantly from that of the neuroleptics, in that the benzodiazepines have no psychoplegic (antipsychotic) activity and cause no extrapyramidal, autonomic, or endocrine side effects. In addition, unlike the neuroleptics, which lower the seizure threshold, these substances are anticonvulsants. In addition, they are anxiolytics, muscle relaxants, and mild sedatives. Although the benzodiazepine derivatives do not produce pronounced autonomic or CV side effects, they can reduce or block the emotionally induced changes in cardiovascular functions, probably through actions on the limbic system.

Compounds such as oxazepam and lorazepam, which possess inactive metabolites, are relatively short acting, whereas compounds such as prazepam, with several active metabolites, have longer disposition half-lives. Consequently, it may be necessary to reduce the doses of those benzodiazepines with active metabolites.

Lorazepam is absorbed from the gastrointestinal tract at a slightly more rapid rate than oxazepam, with peak plasma concentrations occurring about 2 hours after the administration of a single oral dose. Steady-state plasma levels may vary considerably between individuals during repeated dosing, as is the case with other benzodiazepines. Age has no effect on steady-state concentrations, but clearance is slightly reduced in elderly subjects. Unlike diazepam or chlordiazepoxide, the absorption of lorazepam from intramuscular injection sites is predictable, producing a pattern of absorption similar to that observed with oral doses. Like other benzodiazepines, lorazepam has a relatively large volume of distribution of 0.9 L/kg. More than 90% of circulating lorazepam is bound to plasma proteins. As with oxazepam, glucuronidation to an inactive metabolite is the primary metabolic pathway of lorazepam, although very small amounts of other metabolites (hydroxylorazepam and quinazolinone derivatives) have been identified in humans. As with oxazepam, liver disease does not appreciably alter either the elimination half-life or the plasma clearance of lorazepam. Similarly, in the context of severe renal impairment the elimination half-life of unchanged lorazepam is not altered (see also Table 9).

LOSARTAN

Losartan, a nonpeptide, biphenylimidazole potassium salt, is the first agent in a new class of effective antihypertensive drugs called angiotensin-II (Ang II)-receptor blockers used for treatment of hypertension. Losartan works by blocking the binding of Ang II selectively at the type 1 Ang II receptor (AT1), thereby inhibiting all known actions of Ang II that are associated with hypertension (see also Figure 24).

LOSARTAN POTASSIUM

(Cozaar tablets 25 mg)

Losartan is an angiotensin II antagonist. It antagonizes the effect of angiotension II (vasoconstriction and aldosterone secretion) by blocking the angiotensin II receptor (AT receptor) in vascular smooth muscle and the adrenal gland, producing decreased blood pressure (BP). It is indicated in the treatment of hypertension; nephropathy in type 2 diabetic patients; and reduces risk of stroke in patients with hypertension and left-ventricular hypertrophy.

LOSARTAN POTASSIUM/HYDROCHLOROTHIAZIDE

(Hyzaar tablets 12.5 mg hydrochlorothiazide/50 mg losartan potassium)

Losartan is an antihypertensive combination. **Losartan** antagonizes the effect of angiotensin II (vasoconstriction and aldosterone secretion) by blocking the angiotensin II receptor (ATI receptor) in vascular smooth muscle and the adrenal gland, producing decreased BP; **hydrochlorothiazide** inhibits reabsorption of sodium and chloride in the ascending loop of Henle and early distal tubules. They are indicated in hypertension.

The angiotensin II-receptor blockers (ARBs) available for clinical use bind to the AT receptor with high affinity and generally are more than 10,000-fold selective for the AT_2 receptor versus the AT_1 receptor. There are two distinct subtypes of angiotensin II receptors, designated as type 1 (AT_1) and type 2 (AT_2). The AT_1 angiotensin II-receptor subtype is located predominantly in vascular and myocardial tissue and also in brain, kidney, and adrenal glomerulosa cells, which secrete aldosterone. The AT_2 subtype of angiotensin II receptor is found in the adrenal medulla, kidney, and in the CNS, and may play a role in vascular development. The rank-order affinity of the AT_2 receptor for ARBs is **candesartan** = **omesartan** > **irbesartan** = **eprosartan** > **telmisartan** = **valsartan** = EXP 3174 (the active metabolite of losartan) > **losartan**. Although binding of ARBs to the AT_1 receptor is competitive, the inhibition by ARBs of biological responses to angiotensin II often is insurmountable; i.e., the maximal response to angiotensin II cannot be restored in the presence of the ARB regardless of the concentration of angiotensin II added to the experimental preparation. Of the currently available ARBs, candesartan suppresses the maximal response to angiotensin II the most, whereas insurmountable blockade by irbesartan, eprosartan, telmisartan, and valsartan is less. Although **losartan** antagonism is surmountable, its active metabolite, EXP 3174, causes some degree of insurmountable blockade. The mechanism of insurmountable antagonism by ARBs may be due to slow dissociation kinetics of the compounds from the AT_1 receptor; however, a number of other factors may contribute, such as ARB-induced receptor internalization and alternative binding sites for ARBs on the AT_1 receptor. Regardless of the mechanism, insurmountable antagonism has the theoretical advantage of sustained receptor blockade even with increased levels of endogenous ligand and with missed doses of drug. Whether this theoretical advantage translates into an enhanced clinical performance remains to be determined.

The importance of angiotensin II in regulating CV function has led to the development of nonpeptide antagonists of the AT_1 angiotensin II receptor for clinical use. **Losartan** (Cozaar), candesartan (Atacand), irbesartan (Avapro), valsartan (Diovan), telmisartan (Micardis), and eprosartan (Teveten) have been approved for the treatment of hypertension. By antagonizing the effects of angiotensin II, these agents relax smooth muscle and thereby promote vasodilation, increase renal salt and water excretion, reduce plasma volume, and decrease cellular hypertrophy. Angiotensin-II-receptor antagonists also theoretically overcome some of the disadvantages of ACE inhibitors, which not only prevent conversion of angiotensin I to angiotensin II but also prevent ACE-mediated degradation of bradykinin and substance P.

LOVASTATIN

(Mevacor)

Lovastatin (20 mg daily) is indicated for reduction of LDL and total cholesterol levels in patients with primary hypercholesterolemia (types IIa, IIb).

Lovastatin, an inactive lactone, is hydrolyzed to the beta-hydroxy acid, which specifically inhibits 3-hydroxy-3-methylglutaryl-coenzyme A reductase (HMG-CoA reductase). This enzyme is an early (and rate-limiting) step in the synthetic pathway of cholesterol. At therapeutic doses, the enzyme is not blocked, and biologically necessary amounts of cholesterol can still be synthesized. These reductase inhibitors are structural analogs of 3-hydroxy-3-methylglutaryl-coenzyme A (HMG-CoA). The first drug in this class was compactin. A close congener, lovastatin, is widely used. Simvastatin, pravastatin, and fluvastatin are similar drugs.

Lovastatin is absorbed to the extent of 30% and undergoes an extensive first-pass hepatic extraction. Lovastatin is converted to the active B hydroxy acid form in the liver. Other metabolites include the 6, hydroxy derivative and two unidentified compounds. About 80% of lovastatin is excreted primarily in feces, about 10% in urine. Concomitant administration with cholestyramine or colestipol may enhance lipid-reducing effects but may decrease bioavailability

LOWER RESPIRATORY TRACT INFECTIONS: Treatment of

Lower respiratory tract infections (LRTI) may be grouped according to their clinical picture and differing etiology: bronchitis (acute bronchitis, exacerbation of chronic bronchitis) and pneumonia [primary (community acquired), secondary (nosocomial), atypical]. Additionally, severe cases of LRTIs (mostly pneumonia) should be treated according to the degree of severity.

Acute bronchitis is usually a viral infection which, unless there is a special disposition, does not require antibiotic therapy. For the initial oral chemotherapy of bacterial infections of the lower respiratory tract (chronic bronchitis, pneumonia) the effective and well tolerated cephalosporins, macrolides, and amoxicillin plus β-lactamase inhibitor are recommended. In complicated cases with severe underlying disease, longer history or frequent exacerbations, quinolones should be given if Gram-negative infections are suspected or if initial therapy with other substances has failed. If *Legionella*, *Mycoplasma*, or *Chlamydia* spp., so-called atypical pathogens, are involved, macrolide antibiotics are the therapy of first choice. Special attention should be given to the increase in resistance against co-trimoxazole (trimethoprim-sulfamethoxazole) and tetracyclines. In hospitals where primary pneumonias are treated preferentially by intravenous medication, therapy should be switched to oral antibiotics as soon as feasible (follow-up therapy).

For severely ill patients with secondary pneumonia and underlying disease, second-generation cephalosporins with aminoglycosides, or monotherapy with third-generation cephalosporins are recommended. In very severe, high-risk cases, third-generation cephalosporins, combinations with high-dosage quinolones or ureidopenicillins plus β-lactamase inhibitors are suitable.

of lovastatin. Concomitant administration of cyclosporine, erythromycin, gemfibrozil, or niacin may increase risk of severe myopathy or rhabdomyolysis. Lovastatin may increase the anticoagulant effects of warfarin.

LOXAPINE HYDROCHLORIDE
(Loxitane C, Loxitane I.M.)

LOXAPINE SUCCINATE
(Loxitane)

Loxapine, a dibenzoxazepine compound, represents a new subclass of tricyclic antipsychotic agents, chemically distinct from the thioxanthenes, butyrophenones, and phenothiazines. Chemically, it is a 2-chloro-11-(4-methyl-1-piperazinyl)-dibenz[b,f](1,4)-oxazepine. It is present in capsules as the succinate salt, and in the concentrate and parenteral forms primarily as the hydrochloride salt.

Loxapine (10 mg b.i.d.) is indicated for the treatment of psychotic disorders. It exerts its antipsychotic effects in part by blocking postsynaptic dopamine receptors. It causes moderate sedation, possesses anticholinergic properties, and produces extensive movement disorders such as akathisia, dystonia, parkinsonism, tardive dyskinesia, and neuroleptic malignant syndrome.

Loxapine is absorbed rapidly and completely from the GI tract. Sedation occurs in 30 minutes. Loxapine is distributed widely into the body, including breast milk. Peak effect occurs at 1 1/2 to 3 hours; steady-state serum level is achieved within 3 to 4 days. The drug is 91 to 99% protein bound.

The drug is metabolized extensively by the liver, forming a few active metabolites; duration of action is 12 hours. Most of the drug is excreted as metabolites in urine, some is excreted in feces via the biliary tract. About 50% of the drug is excreted in urine and feces within 24 hours. Similar to phenothiazine derivatives such as chlorpromazine, loxapine should be used cautiously in patients with cardiac disease (arrhythmias, congestive heart failure, angina pectoris, valvular disease, or heart block), encephalitis, Reye's syndrome, head injury, respiratory disease, epilepsy and other seizure disorders, glaucoma, prostatic hypertrophy, urinary retention, hepatic or renal dysfunction, Parkinson's disease, or pheochromocytoma. Overdosage with loxapine causes CNS depression characterized by deep, unarousable sleep and possible coma, hypotension or hypertension, extrapyramidal symptoms, abnormal involuntary muscle movements, agitation, seizures, arrhythmias, ECG changes, hypothermia or hyperthermia, and autonomic nervous system dysfunction (see also Tables 5 through 7).

LUGOL'S SOLUTION

Iodides such as potassium iodide and Lugol's solution, which contain 5% iodine and 10% potassium iodide, exert their beneficial effects by inhibiting organification, inhibiting the release of thyroid hormones, and decreasing (inhibiting proteolysis) the size and vascularity of the gland. This makes them useful for preparing the patient for surgery (see also Figure 66).

LUTEINIZING HORMONE

The pituitary hormones responsible for regulating gonadal function are LH and FSH. In males, LH stimulates the Leydig's cells to synthesize testosterone; FSH stimulates the Sertoli's cells to synthesize inhibin and androgen-binding protein and, in conjunction with high intratesticular concentrations of testosterone, initiates and maintains spermatogenesis. In females, LH stimulates androgen synthesis, and FSH increases estrogen and inhibin synthesis in the granulosa cells. Both LH and FSH are released from the gonadotroph cells of the anterior pituitary in response to the hypothalamic hormone GnRH (also known as LH-releasing hormone). GnRH is a decapeptide with the following structure: pyro Glu-His-Trp-Ser-Tyr-Gly-Leu-Arg-Pro-Gly-NH_2 (see also Table 15).

LUTROPIN ALFA

(Luveris powder for injection)

Lutropin alfa is a gonadotropin that increases estradiol secretion, thereby supporting FSH-induced follicular development. Lutropin alfa is coadministered with follitropin alfa for stimulation of follicular development in infertile, hypogonadotropic, hypogonadal women with profound LH deficiency.

LYMPHOCYTE IMMUNE GLOBULIN

(Antithymocyte globulin [equine]) (Atgam)

Lymphocyte immune globulin, an immunoglobulin with immunosuppressive properties (15 mg/kg/day IV for 14 days), is used in the prevention or treatment of acute renal allograft rejection, in aplastic anemia, skin allotransplantation, and in bone marrow allotransplantation (see also Figure 28).

LYMPHOCYTE IMMUNE GLOBULIN

(Atgam solution for injection 50 mg/mL)

Lymphocyte immune globulin is an immune globulin. Antilymphocytic effect is believed to reflect an alteration of the function of the T-lymphocytes. It is indicated for moderate to severe aplastic anemia; and treatment of acute allograft rejection in renal transplantation.

LYMPHOKINES

Because tumor growth is associated with the progressive impairment of immunologic competence, a therapeutic goal is the enhancement of cell-mediated immunity. Cell-mediated immunity may be augmented by nonspecific stimulants such as levamisole, lymphokines, and interferon, which stimulate the antitumor activity of NK cells. Cell-mediated immunity may also be stimulated by specific stimulants such as vaccines, which are composed of killed or inactivated tumor cells or tumor cell fragments. The full range of immunotherapy's usefulness remains to be realized.

LYPRESSIN

(Diapid)

Vasopressin (Pitressin) may be administered either subcutaneously or intramuscularly. It has a duration of action of 2 to 8 hours. Vasopressin tannate (pitressin tannate) is a suspension and should be injected intramuscularly only. It has a duration of action of 2 to 3 days. Desmopressin acetate (DDAVP) is used topically. Lypressin is administered as an intranasal spray. All these agents may be used in the treatment of central diabetes insipidus (vasopressin sensitive) (see also Figure 102).

M

MACROLIDE ANTIBIOTICS

Azithromycin
Clarithromycin
Erythromycin

MAFENIDE

(Sulfamylon)

Mafenide, a topical antibacterial agent (8.5% cream) is indicated as an adjunctive treatment of second- and third-degree burns.

MAGALDRATE

(Aluminum-magnesium complex) (Lowsium, Riopan, Riopan Plus)

Magaldrate, an antacid (540 mg between meals), by neutralizing gastric acid and inactivating pepsin, is used in the management of acid-pepsin disease.

MAGALDRATE (HYDROXYMAGNESIUM ALUMINATE)

(Iosopan liquid 540 mg/5 mL)

Magaldrate is an antacid that neutralizes gastric acid, thereby increasing pH of the stomach and duodenal bulb. It increases lower esophageal sphincter tone and inhibits smooth muscle contraction and gastric emptying. It is indicated in symptomatic relief of upset stomach associated with hyperacidity, including heartburn, gastroesophageal reflux, acid indigestion, and sour stomach; and relief of hyperacidity, associated with peptic ulcer, gastritis, peptic esophagitis, gastric hyperacidity, and hiatal hernia.

MAGNESIUM CITRATE

(Citrate of Magnesia)

Magnesium citrate is a mineral/laxative. It attracts and retains water in intestinal lumen, thereby increasing intraluminal pressure and inducing the urge to defecate. It is indicated for short-term treatment of constipation and evacuation of the colon for rectal and bowel evaluation.

MAGNESIUM HYDROXIDE

(Milk of Magnesia, Magnesia Magma)

Magnesium hydroxide, an antacid with laxative properties (6 to 20 ml/p.o.), is used as an antacid, as a laxative in constipation, and in bowel evacuation before surgery.

MAGNESIUM OXIDE

(Mag-Ox 400 tablets 400 mg)

Magnesium oxide is an antacid that neutralizes gastric acid and thereby increases pH of the stomach and duodenal bulb; it also increases lower esophageal sphincter tone. It is indicated in the symptomatic relief of upset stomach associated with hyperacidity, including heartburn, gastroesophageal reflux, acid indigestion and sour stomach; relief of hyperacidity associated with peptic ulcer, gastritis, peptic esophagitis, gastric hyperacidity and hiatal hernia. It is also used for treatment of hypomagnesemia, or magnesium depletion resulting from malnutrition, restricted diet, alcoholism, or magnesium-depleting drugs.

MAGNESIUM SALICYLATE

(Analate, Arthrin, Doan's pills, Efficin, Magan, Mobidin)

Magnesium salicylate (500 mg) is indicated in the relief of the signs and symptoms of rheumatoid arthritis, osteoarthritis, bursitis, and other musculoskeletal disorders. Magnesium salicylate is a nonsteroidal antiinflammatory agent with antipyretic and analgesic properties. Salicylic acid is the active moiety released into the plasma by magnesium salicylate. It is enzymatically biotransformed through two pathways to salicyluric acid and salicylphenolic glucuronide and eliminated in the urine. Oral salicylates are absorbed rapidly, partly from the stomach but mostly from the upper intestine. Salicylic acid is rapidly distributed throughout all body tissues and most transcellular fluids, mainly by pH-dependent passive processes. It can be detected in synovial, spinal, and peritoneal fluid, in saliva, and in milk. It readily crosses the placental barrier. From 50 to 90% of salicylic acid is bound to plasma proteins, especially albumin. Magnesium salicylate is contraindicated in patients with advanced chronic renal insufficiency.

MAGNESIUM SULFATE

(Epsom salt)

Magnesium sulfate is an anticonvulsant. Magnesium has a CNS-depressant effect; prevents/controls seizures by blocking neuromuscular transmission and decreasing the amount of acetylcholine liberated at the end plate by motor nerve impulse. Orally, it attracts/retains water in the intestinal lumen, thereby increasing intraluminal pressure and inducing the urge to defecate.

Parenteral: used for seizure prevention and control in severe preeclampsia or eclampsia without deleterious CNS depression in the mother, fetus, or newborn; as replacement therapy in magnesium deficiency, especially in acute hypomagnesemia accompanied by signs of tetany similar to those observed in hypocalcemia; to correct or prevent hypomagnesemia by addition to total parenteral nutrition admixture hypertension, encephalopathy, and convulsions in children with acute nephritis; inhibition of premature labor; as treatment of life-threatening ventricular arrhythmias; for prevention and treatment of nutritional magnesium deficiency; and as a laxative.

Purgation: The rationale for using an osmotic cathartic is to minimize absorption by hastening the passage of the toxicant through the gastrointestinal tract. Few, if any, controlled clinical data are available on the effectiveness of cathartics in the treatment of poisoning. Cathartics generally are considered harmless unless the poison has injured the gastrointestinal tract. Cathartics are indicated after the ingestion of enteric-coated tablets, when the time after ingestion is greater than 1 hour, and for poisoning by volatile hydrocarbons. Sorbitol is the most effective, but sodium sulfate and **magnesium sulfate** also are used; all act promptly and usually have minimal toxicity. However, magnesium sulfate should be used cautiously in patients with renal failure or in those likely to develop renal dysfunction, and Na^+-containing cathartics should be avoided in patients with congestive heart failure (CHF).

Whole-bowel irrigation (WBI) is a technique that not only promotes defecation but also eliminates the entire contents of the intestines. This technique uses a high-molecular-weight **polyethylene glycol** and **isosmolar electrolyte solution** (PEG–ES) that does not alter serum electrolytes. It is available commercially as **Golytely** and **Colyte**. A position statement on WBI, issued by the American. Academy of Clinical Toxicology and the European Association of Poisons Centres and Clinical Toxicologists, indicates that WBI should not be used routinely in the management of the poisoned patient. Even though volunteer studies have shown substantial decreases in the bioavailability of certain ingested drugs, evidence from controlled clinical trials is lacking. WBI may be considered in cases of acute poisoning by sustained-release or enteric-coated drugs and possibly toxic ingestions of iron, lead, zinc, or packets of illicit drugs.

MALATHION

(Ovide lotion 0.5%)

Malathion is a pediculicide that inhibits cholinesterase activity. It is used in the treatment of head lice (*Pediculus humanus capitis*) and their ova of the scalp hair.

MANIC SYMPTOMS: Drugs that Induce

Alcohol	Disulfiram
Amantadine	Ephedrine
Amphetamines	Hallucinogens
Anabolic steroids	Indomethacin
Anticholinergics	Isoniazid
Anticonvulsants	Levodopa
Antidepressants	Monoamine oxidase inhibitors
Baclofen	Methylphenidate
Benzodiazepines	Metoclopramide
Bromides	Niridazole
Bronchodilators	Phenylpropanolamine
Caffeine	Procainamide
Calcium	Procarbazine
Captopril	Quinacrine
Cimetidine	Sympathomimetics
Cocaine	Theophylline
Corticosteroids (ACTH)	Thyroid supplements
Decongestants	Tolmetin
Diltiazem	Yohimbine

In addition, withdrawal from certain medications, such as baclofen, clonidine, corticosteroids, or tricyclic antidepressants, may cause manic symptoms.

MANNITOL

(Osmitrol)

The osmotic diuretics and related agents consist of mannitol, urea (Ureaphil), glycerin (Glycerol, Osmoglyn), and isosorbide (Hydronol). Mannitol and urea are nonelectrolytes that are freely filterable and undergo very little or no metabolism or renal tubular resorption. When given in sufficient quantities, these drugs increase the osmolarity of plasma and the amount of both the glomerular filtrate and the renal tubular fluid. The presence of such a drug in the lumen prevents the resorption of much of the water, hence the urine volume is increased. They do not prevent the active resorption of sodium from the tubular fluid, but some additional sodium is excreted as a normal constituent of the increased volume of urine. Osmotic diuretics are not effective in removing the edematous fluid caused by sodium retention, but can maintain the flow of urine even when the glomerular filtration rate (GFR) is decreased. Osmotic diuretics are given by intravenous infusion in a hypertonic solution, and they are excreted by glomerular filtration (see also Figure 17 and Table 25).

MAPROTILINE HYDROCHLORIDE

(Ludiomil tablets 25 mg)

Maprotiline hydrochloride is a tricyclic antidepressant that inhibits norepinephrine (but not serotonin) reuptake. It is indicated in depression and anxiety associated with depression.

Maprotiline (75 mg/day), a tricyclic antidepressant, is indicated for the treatment of depressive illness in patients with depressive neurosis (dysthymic disorder) and manic-depressive illness, depressed type (major depressive disorder). Also, it is effective for the relief of anxiety associated with depression. Its properties are compared with that of imipramine and are listed in Tables 5 through 7.

MASOPROCOL

(Actinex)

Masoprocol, a dicatechol compound with antipsoriatic and antineoplastic properties (10% cream), is used in actinic (solar) keratoses.

MAZINDOL

(Mazanor, Sanorex)

Mazindol, an imidazoisoindol, is used as a short-term adjunct regimen in exogenous obesity. In addition, mazindol has been used in the treatment of cocaine misuse and narcolepsy.

MEASLES, MUMPS, AND RUBELLA VIRUS VACCINE, LIVE

(M-M-R-II powder for injection mixture of 3 viruses: at least 1,000 measles $TCID_{50}$ [tissue culture infectious doses], at least 20,000 mumps $TCID_{50}$ and at least 1,000 rubella $TCID_{50}$ per 0.5 mL dose)

Measles, mumps, and rubella vaccine live is a viral vaccine that induces protective antibodies against measles, mumps, and rubella viruses. It is indicated for vaccination of individuals known to be susceptible to measles, mumps, or rubella; and for prevention of occurrence of congenital rubella syndrome (CRS) among offspring of women who contract rubella during pregnancy. It is the preferred immunizing agent for most children and many adults.

MEASLES AND RUBELLA VIRUS VACCINE, LIVE, ATTENUATED

(M-R-Vax II)

This vaccine is used in measles and rubella immunization.

MEASLES VIRUS VACCINE, LIVE, ATTENUATED

(Attenuvax)

This viral vaccine is used for immunization.

MEBENDAZOLE

(Vermox tablets)

Mebendazole is a benzimidazole that kills parasitic worms by blocking glucose uptake, thus depleting stored glycogen. Without glycogen, parasites cannot reproduce or survive. It is indicated in the treatment of *Trichuris trichuria* (whipworm), *Enterobius vermicularis* (pinworm), *Ascaris lumbricoides* (roundworm), *Ancylostoma duodenale* (common hookworm), or *Necator americanus* (American hookworm), in single infection or mixed infections.

Mebendazole inhibits the formation of the worms' microtubules and irreversibly blocks glucose uptake by the susceptible helminths, thereby depleting endogenous glycogen stored within the parasite, which is required for its survival and reproduction. Mebendazole does not affect blood glucose concentrations in the host.

Mebendazole is absorbed poorly after oral administration, and most of it is excreted unchanged in the feces.

Mebendazole exerts its effects slowly (3 days), and effectiveness of treatment depends on the degree of infection or resistance of the parasites to treatment. Phenytoin or carbamazepine reduce the plasma level of mebendazole. The major nematode parasites of humans include **soil-transmitted helminths** (STHs; sometimes referred to as "**geohelminths**") and the filarial nematodes.

The major STH infections, which include ascariasis, trichuriasis, and hookworm infection, are among the most prevalent infections in developing countries. Because STH worm burdens are higher in school-aged children than in any other single group, the WHO and the Partnership for Child Development (PCD) advocate using schools and schoolteachers to administer broad-spectrum anthelmintics on a periodic and frequent basis. The most widely used agents employed for reducing morbidity are the benzimidazole anthelmintics (BZAs), either **albendazole** (Albenza and Zentel) or mebendazole (Vermox). A single dose of a BZA reduces worm burdens and subsequently improves host iron and hemoglobin status, physical growth, cognition, educational achievement, and school absenteeism, as well as having a positive influence on the entire community, namely through a reduction in the spread of ascariasis and trichuriasis. In 2001, the World Health Assembly adopted a resolution urging that by 2010 member states should regularly administer anthelmintics to 75% of all school-age children at risk for morbidity. Concerns with this recommendation include: (1) the sheer scope of the undertaking; (2) the high rates of posttreatment STH reinfection that occur in areas of high transmission; (3) the possibility that widespread treatment will lead to the emergence of BZA drug resistance; and (4) the observation that focusing exclusively on school-aged children would miss populations that are vulnerable to hookworm infection, such as preschool children and women of reproductive age.

In addition to targeting STH infections among school-aged children, there is an ongoing attempt to employ anthelmintics that eliminate lymphatic filariasis (LF) and onchocerciasis (river blindness) over the next 10 to 20 years. The term elimination refers to the reduction of disease incidence to zero or close to zero, with a requirement for ongoing control efforts. The major goal for LF and onchocerciasis elimination is to interrupt arthropod-borne transmission by administering combination therapy with either diethylcarbamazine and albendazole (in LF-endemic regions such as India and Egypt), or **ivermectin** and **albendazole** (in LF regions where onchocerciasis and/or loiasis are coendemic). These drugs target the microfilarial stages of the parasite, which circulate in blood and are taken up by arthropod vectors where further parasite development takes place. Both control programs rely heavily on the generosity of major drug companies that donate ivermectin and albendazole.

Ascaris lumbricoides, known as the "roundworm," parasitizes an estimated 1.2 billion people worldwide. Ascariasis may affect from 70 to 90% of persons in some tropical regions, but it also is seen in temperate climates. People become infected by ingesting food or soil contaminated with embryonated *A. lumbricoides* eggs. The highest ascaris worm burdens occur in school-aged children in whom the parasite can cause intestinal obstruction or hepatobiliary ascariasis.

More effective, less toxic compounds largely have replaced older ascaricides. **Mebendazole**, **pyrantel pamoate** (Antiminth, others), and **albendazole** are preferred agents. **Piperazine** also is effective but is used less often because of occasional neurotoxicity hypersensitivity reactions. Cure with any of these drugs is achieved in nearly 100% of cases, and all infected persons should be treated. **Mebendazole** and albendazole are preferred for therapy of asymptomatic to moderate ascariasis. Both of these benzimidazoles are ascaricidal and have a broad spectrum of activity against mixed infections with other gastrointestinal nematodes. Albendazole is useful against infections with some systemic nematodes and some cestodes as well. Both compounds should be used with caution to treat heavy *Ascaris* infections, alone or with hookworms. In rare instances, hyperactive ascarids may migrate to unusual loci and cause serious complications such as appendicitis, occlusion of the common bile duct, intestinal obstruction, and intestinal perforation with peritonitis. Therapy with nonascaricidal agents such as **pyrantel** is preferred by some clinicians for heavy *Ascaris* infections because this agent paralyzes the worms prior to their expulsion. Surgery still may be required despite the use of these agents. Pyrantel is considered safe for use during pregnancy, whereas the BZAs should be avoided during the first trimester. Pyrantel and albendazole are considered "investigational" drugs for treatment of ascariasis in the United States, even though they are approved for other indications.

Toxocariasis, a zoonotic infection caused by the canine ascarid *Toxocara canis*, is a common helminthiasis in North America and Europe. Possibly, it has displaced pinworm as the most common helminthic infection in the United States. The three major syndromes caused by *T. canis* infection are visceral larva migrans (VLM), ocular larva migrans (OLM), and covert toxocariasis (CT). CT has been postulated to represent an underappreciated cause of asthma and seizures. The specific treatment of VLM is reserved for patients with severe, persistent, or progressive symptoms. Albendazole is the drug of choice. In contrast, the role of anthelmintic drugs in the treatment of OLM and CT is controversial. In the case of the former, surgical management often is indicated, sometimes accompanied by systemic or topical steroids.

Unlike thiabendazole, **mebendazole** does not cause significant systemic toxicity in routine clinical use, even in the presence of anemia and malnutrition. This probably reflects its low systemic bioavailability. Transient symptoms of abdominal pain, distention, and diarrhea have occurred in cases of massive infestation and expulsion of gastrointestinal worms. Rare side effects in patients treated with high doses of mebendazole include allergic reactions, alopecia, reversible neutropenia, agranulocytosis, and hypospermia. Reversible elevation of serum transaminases is not uncommon in this population. **Mebendazole** treatment may be associated with occipital seizures. **Mebendazole** is a potent embryotoxin and teratogen in laboratory animals; effects may occur in pregnant rats at single oral doses as low as 10 mg/kg. Thus, despite a lack of evidence for teratogenicity in humans, it generally is advised that mebendazole not be given to pregnant women or to children less than 2 years of age. It also should not be used in patients who have experienced allergic reactions to the agent.

MECAMYLAMINE HYDROCHLORIDE

(Inversine tablets 2.5 mg)

Mecamylamine hydrochloride is an antiadrenergic agent that has a potent ganglionic blocking property. It is indicated in the treatment of moderately severe to essential hypertension; and uncomplicated malignant hypertension. Blockade of sympathetic ganglia interrupts adrenergic control of arterioles and results in vasodilation, improved peripheral blood flow in some vascular beds, and a fall in blood pressure.

Generalized ganglionic blockade also may result in atony of the bladder and gastrointestinal tract, cycloplegia, xerostomia, diminished perspiration and, by abolishing circulatory reflex pathways, postural hypotension. These changes represent the generally undesirable features of ganglionic blockade, which severely limit the therapeutic efficacy of ganglionic-blocking agents.

MECHLORETHAMINE HYDROCHLORIDE

(Mustargen)

Mechlorethamine (0.4 mg/kg for each course) is indicated in the palliative treatment of Hodgkin's disease (stages III and IV), lymphosarcoma, chronic myelocytic or chronic lymphocytic leukemia, polycythemia vera, mycosis fungoides, and bronchogenic carcinoma. Mechlorethamine is an alkylating agent with cytotoxic, mutagenic, and radiomimetic actions that inhibit rapidly proliferating cells. Mechlorethamine is highly toxic and is a potent vesicant. Extravasation of mechlorethamine into subcutaneous tissues results in painful inflammation and induration.

The adverse reactions of mechlorethamine are thrombosis and thrombophlebitis (local toxicity). Bone marrow depression and gastrointestinal problems such as nausea and severe vomiting begin 1 to 3 hours after use and may persist for 24 hours. A maculopapular skin eruption and erythema multiforme have occurred. Alopecia occurs infrequently. Delayed menses, oligomenorrhea, temporary or permanent amenorrhea, and, in male patients, impaired spermatogenesis, azoospermia, and total germinal aplasia have occurred, especially in those receiving combination therapy, such as in MOPP therapy (mechlorethamine, Oncovin [vincristine], procarbazine, and prednisone). Spermatogenesis may return in patients in remission, but this may occur several years after chemotherapy has been discontinued.

Mechlorethamine was the first clinically used nitrogen mustard and is the most reactive of the drugs in this class.

Severe local reactions of exposed tissues necessitate rapid intravenous injection of mechlorethamine for most clinical uses. In either water or body fluids, at rates affected markedly by pH, mechlorethamine rapidly undergoes chemical degradation as it combines with either water or cellular nucleophiles, and the parent compound disappears within minutes from the bloodstream.

Mechlorethamine HCl (Mustargen) was formerly used primarily in the combination chemotherapy regimen MOPP (**mechlorethamine**, **vincristine** [**Oncovin**], **procarbazine**, and **prednisone**) in patients with Hodgkin's disease. It is given by intravenous bolus administration in doses of 6 mg/m^2 on days 1 and 8 of the 28-day cycles of each course of treatment. It has been largely replaced by cyclophosphamide, melphalan, and other more stable alkylating agents. It also is used topically for treatment of cutaneous T-cell lymphoma as a solution that is rapidly mixed and applied to affected areas of skin.

The major acute toxic manifestations of **mechlorethamine** are nausea and vomiting, lacrimation, and myelosuppression. Leukopenia and thrombocytopenia limit the amount of drug that can be given in a single course.

Like other alkylating agents, nitrogen mustard blocks reproductive infection and may produce menstrual irregularities or premature ovarian failure in women, and oligospermia in men. Because fetal abnormalities can be induced, this drug as well as other alkylating agents should not be used in the first trimester of pregnancy, and should only be used with caution in later stages of pregnancy. Breast-feeding must be terminated before therapy with mechlorethamine is initiated.

Local reactions to extravasation of **mechlorethamine** into the subcutaneous tissue result in a severe, brawny, tender induration that may persist for a long time. If the local reaction is unusually severe, a slough may result. If it is obvious that extravasation has occurred, the involved area should be promptly infiltrated with a sterile isotonic solution of sodium thiosulfate (167 mM); an ice compress then should be applied intermittently for 6 to 12 hours. Thiosulfate reacts avidly with nitrogen mustard and thereby protects tissue constituents.

Mechlorethamine hydrochloride (Mustargen) and **carmustine** (bischloronitrosourea, BCNU, BICNU) are used topically to treat cutaneous T-cell lymphoma. Both can be applied as a solution or in ointment form. It is important to monitor complete blood counts and liver function tests because systemic absorption can cause bone marrow suppression and hepatitis. Other side effects include allergic contact dermatitis, irritant dermatitis, secondary cutaneous malignancies, and pigmentary changes. Carmustine also can cause erythema and posttreatment telangiectasias.

MECLIZINE HYDROCHLORIDE

(Antivert tablets 12.5 mg)

Meclizine is an anticholinergic drug that acts on the CNS to decrease vestibular stimulation and depress labyrinthine activity. It is indicated in the prevention and treatment of nausea, vomiting, and dizziness of motion sickness; possibly as effective treatment for vertigo of vestibular dysfunction origin.

Meclizine (25 to 50 mg 1 hour prior to travel) is indicated in prevention and treatment of nausea, vomiting, and dizziness of motion sickness. Meclizine has antiemetic, anticholinergic, and antihistaminic properties. It reduces the sensitivity of the labyrinthine apparatus. The action may be mediated through neuronal pathways to the vomiting center (VC), from the chemoreceptor trigger zone (CTZ), peripheral nerve pathways, or other CNS centers (see also Figure 73).

Meclizine may produce drowsiness and hence should be used cautiously while completing tasks that require alertness. Because of its anticholinergic properties, it should be used cautiously in patients with glaucoma, obstructive disease of the GI or GU tract, and in elderly male subjects with possible prostatic hypertrophy. This drug may have a hypotensive action, which becomes confusing or dangerous in postoperative patients.

Meclizine may potentiate the CNS depressant effects of alcohol, barbiturates, and anxiolytic agents. Its overdosage will cause drowsiness, restlessness, excitation, nervousness, insomnia, euphoria, blurred vision, diplopia, vertigo, tinnitus, and auditory and visual hallucinations.

Available H_1 antagonists: Summarized in the following text are the therapeutic and side effects of a number of H_1 antagonists based on their chemical structures.

Dibenzoxepin Tricyclics (**Doxepin**): Doxepin, the only drug in this class, is marketed as a tricyclic antidepressant. However, it also is a remarkably potent H_1 antagonist. It can cause drowsiness and is associated with anticholinergic effects. Doxepin is much better tolerated by patients who have depression than by those who do not. In nondepressed patients, sometimes even very small doses, e.g., 20 mg, may be poorly tolerated because of disorientation and confusion.

Ethanolamines (**Prototype**: **Diphenhydramine**): These drugs possess significant antimuscarinic activity and have a pronounced tendency to induce sedation. About half of those treated with conventional doses experience somnolence. The incidence of GI side effects, however, is low with this group.

Ethylenediamines (**Prototype**: **Pyrilamine**): These include some of the most specific H_1 antagonists. Although their central effects are relatively feeble, somnolence occurs in a fair proportion of patients. GI side effects are quite common.

Alkylamines (**Prototype**: **Chlorpheniramine**): These are among the most potent H_1 antagonists. The drugs are less prone to produce drowsiness than some H_1 antagonists and are more suitable agents for daytime use, but again, a significant proportion of patients do experience sedation. Side effects involving CNS stimulation are more common than with other groups.

First-Generation Piperazines: The oldest member of this group, **chlorcyclizine**, has a more prolonged action and produces a comparatively low incidence of drowsiness.

Hydroxyzine is a long-acting compound that is used widely for skin allergies; its considerable CNS-depressant activity may contribute to its prominent antipruritic action. **Cyclizine** and **meclizine** have been used primarily to counter motion sickness, although promethazine and diphenhydramine (dimenhydrinate) are more effective.

Second-Generation Piperazines (Cetirizine): Cetirizine is the only drug in this class. It has minimal anticholinergic effects. It also has negligible penetration into the brain but is associated with a somewhat higher incidence of drowsiness than the other second-generation H_1 antagonists.

Phenothiazines (Prototype: Promethazine): Most drugs of this class are H_1 antagonists and also possess considerable anticholinergic activity. Promethazine, which has prominent sedative effects, and its many congeners are used primarily for their antiemetic effects.

First-Generation Piperidines (Cyproheptadine, Phenindamine): Cyproheptadine uniquely has both antihistamine and antiserotonin activity. Cyproheptadine and phenindamine cause drowsiness and also have significant anticholinergic effects.

Second-Generation Piperidines (Prototype: Terfenadine): Terfenadine and astemizole were withdrawn from the market. Current drugs in this class include loratadine, desloratadine, and fexofenadine. These agents are highly selective for H_1 receptors, lack significant anticholinergic actions, and penetrate poorly into the CNS. Taken together, these properties appear to account for the low incidence of side effects of piperidine antihistamines.

MECLOFENAMATE SODIUM

(Meclofenamate sodium capsules 50 mg)

Meclofenamate is indicated in the relief of mild to moderate pain (50 mg/6 hours); in the treatment of primary dysmenorrhea (100 mg t.i.d.); and in acute and chronic rheumatoid arthritis and osteoarthritis (200 to 400 mg/day in 3 to 4 equal doses). Meclofenamate is a nonsteroidal antiinflammatory agent that has analgesic and antipyretic properties. The menstrual cycle is associated with two potentially incapacitating events: dysmenorrhea and the premenstrual syndrome. Substantial evidence indicates that the excessive production of prostaglandin F_{2a} is the major source of painful menstruation. The nonsteroidal antiinflammatory drugs such as aspirin, ibuprofen, meclofenamate, mefenamic acid, and naproxen are used to treat dysmenorrhea.

Meclofenamate is rapidly absorbed, with peak plasma concentration occurring in 1 hour. It is extensively metabolized to an active metabolite (3-hydroxymethyl metabolite of meclofenamic acid) and at least six other less well-characterized minor metabolites. Only this active metabolite has been shown to inhibit cyclooxygenase activity *in vitro* with approximately one-fifth the activity of meclofenamate sodium. The 3-hydroxymethyl metabolite of meclofenamic acid with a mean half-life of approximately 15 hours does accumulate following multiple dosing. Approximately 70% of the administered dose is excreted by the kidneys, with 8 to 35% excreted as conjugated species of meclofenamic acid and its active metabolite.

Concomitant use of meclofenamate with anticoagulants and thrombolytic drugs (coumarin derivatives, heparin, streptokinase, or urokinase) may potentiate anticoagulant effects. Bleeding problems may occur if used with other drugs that inhibit platelet aggregation, such as azlocillin, parenteral carbenicillin, dextran, dipyridamole, mazlocillin, piperacillin, sulfinpyrazone, ticarcillin, valproic acid, cefamandole, cefoperazone, moxalactam, plicamycin, salicylates, or other antiinflammatory agents. Alcohol, corticotropin, or steroids may increase adverse GI effects caused by meclofenamate, which may include ulceration and hemorrhage. Aspirin may decrease the bioavailability of meclofenamate.

Because of the influence of prostaglandins on glucose metabolism, concomitant use with insulin or oral hypoglycemic agents may potentiate hypoglycemic effects. Meclofenamate may displace highly protein-bound drugs from binding sites. Toxicity may occur with coumarin derivatives, phenytoin, verapamil, or nifedipine. Meclofenamate may decrease the renal clearance of methotrexate and lithium. It may decrease the clinical effectiveness of diuretics and antihypertensives. Concomitant use with diuretics may increase nephrotoxicity. Clinical manifestations of meclofenamate overdose include CNS stimulation, irrational behavior, marked agitation, and generalized seizures. Renal toxicity may follow this phase of CNS stimulation.

MEDIUM CHAIN TRIGLYCERIDES

(M.C.T. oil)

Medium chain triglycerides (15 ml p.o. t.i.d.) are used in conditions of inadequate digestion or absorption of food fats, chylous ascites, or chylous thorax.

MEDROXYPROGESTERONE ACETATE

(Amen tablets 10 mg)

Medroxyprogesterone acetate (MPA) inhibits secretion of pituitary gonadotropins, thereby preventing follicular maturation and ovulation (contraceptive effect); inhibits spontaneous uterine contraction; transforms proliferative endometrium into secretory endometrium; produces anti-neoplastic effect in advanced endometrial or renal carcinoma. **PO**: used in treatment of secondary amenorrhea and abnormal uterine bleeding caused by hormonal imbalance; reduction of incidence of endometrial hyperplasia in nonhysterectomized postmenopausal women receiving 0.625 mg conjugated estrogen. **Parenteral**: used for prevention of pregnancy; and adjunctive and palliative treatment of inoperable, recurrent, and metastatic endometrial or renal carcinoma.

The established benefits of estrogen therapy in postmenopausal women include amelioration of vasomotor symptoms and the prevention of bone fractures and urogenital atrophy.

Vasomotor symptoms: The decline in ovarian function at menopause is associated with vasomotor symptoms in most women. The characteristic hot flashes may alternate with chilly sensations, inappropriate sweating, and (less commonly) paresthesias. Treatment with estrogen is specific and is the most efficacious pharmacotherapy for these symptoms. If estrogen is contraindicated or otherwise undesirable, other options may be considered.

MPA may provide some relief of vasomotor symptoms for certain patients, and the α_2-adrenergic agonist **clonidine** diminishes vasomotor symptoms in some women, presumably by blocking the CNS outflow that regulates blood flow to cutaneous vessels. In many women, hot flashes diminish within several years; when prescribed for this purpose, the dose and duration of estrogen use should thus be the minimum necessary to provide relief.

Osteoporosis is a disorder of the skeleton associated with the loss of bone mass. The result is thinning and weakening of the bones and an increased incidence of fractures, particularly compression fractures of the vertebrae and minimal-trauma fractures of the hip and wrist. The frequency and severity of these fractures and their associated complications (e.g., death and permanent disability) are a major public health problem, especially as the population continues to age. Osteoporosis is an indication for estrogen therapy, which clearly is efficacious in decreasing the incidence of fractures. However, because of the risks associated with estrogen use, first-line use of other drugs should be carefully considered. Nevertheless, it is important to note that the majority of fractures in the postmenopausal period occur in women without a prior history of osteoporosis, and estrogens are the most efficacious agents available for prevention of fractures at all sites in such women.

The primary mechanism by which estrogens act is to decrease bone resorption; consequently, estrogens are more effective in preventing, rather than restoring, bone loss. Estrogens are most effective if treatment is initiated before significant bone loss occurs, and their maximal beneficial effects require continuous use; bone loss resumes when treatment is discontinued. An appropriate diet with adequate intake of Ca^{2+} and vitamin D and weight-bearing exercise enhance the effects of estrogen treatment. Public health efforts to improve diet and exercise patterns in girls and young women also are rational approaches to increase bone mass.

Loss of tissue lining the vagina or bladder leads to a variety of symptoms in many postmenopausal women. These include dryness and itching of the vagina, dyspareunia, swelling of tissues in the genital region, pain during urination, a need to urinate urgently or often, and sudden or unexpected urinary incontinence. When estrogens are being used solely for relief of vulvar and vaginal atrophy, local administration as a vaginal cream, ring device, or tablets may be considered.

The incidence of cardiovascular disease is low in premenopausal women, rising rapidly after menopause, and epidemiological studies consistently showed an association between estrogen use and reduced cardiovascular disease in postmenopausal women. Furthermore, estrogens produce a favorable lipoprotein profile, promote vasodilation, inhibit the response to vascular injury, and reduce atherosclerosis. Studies such as these led to the widespread use of estrogen for prevention of cardiovascular disease in postmenopausal women. As discussed previously, several randomized, prospective studies unexpectedly indicated that the incidence of heart disease and stroke in older postmenopausal women treated with conjugated estrogens and a progestin was initially increased, although the trend reversed with time. Although it is not clear if similar results would occur with different drugs/doses or in different patient populations, estrogens (alone or in combination with a progestin) should not be used for the treatment or prevention of cardiovascular disease.

Compounds with biological activities similar to those of **progesterone** have been variously referred to in the literature as **progestins**, **progestational agents**, **progestagens**, **progestogens**, **gestagens**, or **gestogens**.

The progestins include the naturally occurring hormone progesterone, 17α-acetoxyprogesterone derivatives in the pregnane series, 19-nortestosterone derivatives (estranes), and norgestrel and related compounds in the gonane series. **MPA** and **megestrol acetate** are C21 steroids with selective activity very similar to that of progesterone itself. MPA and oral micronized progesterone are widely used with estrogens for menopausal hormone therapy and other situations in which a selective progestational effect is desired, and a depot form of MPA is used as a long-acting injectable contraceptive. The 19-nortestosterone derivatives were developed for use as progestins in oral contraceptives, and although their predominant activity is progestational, they exhibit androgenic and other activities. The gonanes are a more recently developed series of "19-nor" compounds, containing an ethyl rather than a methyl substituent in the 13-position, and they have diminished androgenic activity. These two classes of 19-nortestosterone derivatives are the progestational components of all oral and some long-acting injectable contraceptives.

Aside from bleeding irregularities, headache is the most commonly reported untoward effect of depot **MPA**. Mood changes and weight gain also have been reported, but controlled clinical studies of these effects are not available. It is of more concern that many studies have found decreases in HDL levels and increases in LDL levels, and that there have been several reports of decreased bone density. These effects may be due to reduced endogenous estrogens because depot **MPA** is particularly effective in lowering gonadotropin levels. Numerous human studies have not found any increases in breast, endometrial, cervical, or ovarian cancer in women receiving **MPA**. Because of the time required to completely eliminate the drug, the contraceptive effect of this agent may remain for 6 to 12 months after the last injection.

MEDROXYPROGESTERONE ACETATE

(Amen, Curretab, Depo-Provera, Provera)

Medroxyprogesterone, a progestin, is used in abnormal uterine bleeding from hormonal imbalance, in secondary amenorrhea, and for female contraception. In addition, it has been used in paraphilia in male subjects.

MEFENAMIC ACID

(Ponstel capsules 250 mg)

Mefenamic acid is a NSAID, which decreases inflammation, pain, and fever, probably through inhibition of cyclooxygenase activity and prostaglandin synthesis. It is indicated in the relief of moderate pain lasting less than 1 week; and in treatment of primary dysmenorrhea.

Mefenamic acid (500 mg p.o. initially, then 250 mg every 4 hours), which inhibits prostaglandin synthesis, is indicated in the treatment of moderate pain and in the management of primary dysmenorrhea. The duration of therapy should not exceed 1 week. It is a nonsteroidal antiinflammatory agent with analgesic and antipyretic properties. Mefenamic acid is absorbed rapidly and completely from the GI tract. It is highly protein-bound and is metabolized in the liver. Mefenamic acid is excreted mainly in urine with some biliary excretion. The plasma half-life is around two hours.

Concomitant use of mefenamic acid with anticoagulants and thrombolytic drugs (coumarin derivatives, heparin, streptokinase, or urokinase) may potentiate anticoagulant effects. Bleeding problems may occur if mefenamic acid is used with other drugs that inhibit platelet aggregation, such as azlocillin, parenteral carbenicillin, dextran, dipyridamole, mezlocillin, piperacillin, sulfinpyrazone, ticarcillin, valproic acid, cefamandole, cefoperazone, moxalactam, plicamycin, aspirin, or other antiinflammatory agents. Alcohol, corticotropin, or steroids may cause increased GI adverse reactions, including ulceration and hemorrhage. Aspirin may decrease the bioavailability of mefenamic acid.

Because of the influence of prostaglandins on glucose metabolism, concomitant use with insulin or oral hypoglycemic agents may potentiate hypoglycemic effects. Mefenamic acid may displace highly protein-bound drugs from binding sites. Toxicity may occur with coumarin derivatives, phenytoin, verapamil, or nifedipine. Increased nephrotoxicity may occur with gold compounds, other antiinflammatory agents, or acetaminophen. It may decrease the renal clearance of methotrexate and lithium. Mefenamic acid may decrease the clinical effectiveness of diuretics and antihypertensives. Concomitant use with diuretics may increase nephrotoxicity. Clinical manifestations of overdose include CNS stimulation, irrational behavior, marked agitation, and generalized seizures. Renal toxicity may follow this phase of CNS stimulation.

The fenamates are a family of NSAIDs first discovered in the 1950s that are derivatives of *N*-phenylanthranilic acid. They include **mefenamic**, **meclofenamic**, and **flufenamic acids**. They have no clear advantages over several other NSAIDs, and frequently cause GI side effects.

Mefenamic acid (Ponstel, Ponstan [United Kingdom], Dysman [United Kingdom]) and meclofenamate sodium [Meclomen] have been used mostly in the short-term treatment of pain in soft-tissue injuries, dysmenorrhea, and in rheumatoid and osteoarthritis. These drugs are not recommended for use in children or pregnant women.

Mefenamic acid and meclofenamate, but not flufenamic acid, are available in the United States. All three are available in Europe. They are used rarely for chronic therapy of the arthritides.

Mefenamic acid and meclofenamate are *N*-substituted phenylanthranilic acids.

The fenamates are typical NSAIDs. **Mefenamic acid** has central and peripheral actions, and it (and perhaps other fenamates) may antagonize directly certain effects of prostaglandins, although it is not clear that receptor blockade is attained at therapeutic concentrations.

These drugs are absorbed rapidly and have short durations of action. In humans, approximately 50% of a dose of mefenamic acid is excreted in the urine, primarily as the 3-hydroxymethyl and 3-carboxyl metabolites and their conjugates. Twenty percent (20%) of the drug is recovered in the feces, mainly as the unconjugated 3-carboxyl metabolite.

Approximately 25% of users develop gastrointestinal side effects at therapeutic doses. Roughly 5% of patients develop a reversible elevation of hepatic transaminases. Diarrhea, which may be severe and associated with steatorrhea and inflammation of the bowel, also is relatively common. Autoimmune hemolytic anemia is a potentially serious but rare side effect.

The fenamates are contraindicated in patients with a history of gastrointestinal disease. If diarrhea or rash occur, these drugs should be stopped at once. Vigilance is required for signs or symptoms of hemolytic anemia.

MEFLOQUINE HYDROCHLORIDE

(Mefloquine hydrochloride tablets 250 mg)

Mefloquine is an antimalarial preparation that acts as a blood schizonticide. It is indicated in the treatment of mild to moderate malaria caused by mefloquine-susceptible strains of *Plasmodium falciparum* or *P. vivax*; and prevention of malaria caused by *P. falciparum* or *P. vivax*. Patients with acute *P. vivax* need subsequent treatment with 9-aminoquinolone to prevent relapse.

MEGESTROL ACETATE

(Megace suspension 40 mg/mL)

Megestrol acetate is a progestin that inhibits secretion of pituitary gonadotropins, thereby preventing follicular maturation and ovulation (contraceptive effect); inhibits spontaneous uterine contraction; and transforms proliferative endometrium into secretory endometrium. It is indicated as a palliative treatment of advanced inoperable, recurrent, or metastatic carcinoma of breast or endometrium.

Compounds with biological activities similar to those of **progesterone** have been variously referred to in the literature as **progestins**, **progestational agents**, **progestagens**, **progestogens**, **gestagens**, or **gestogens**. The progestins include the naturally occurring hormone progesterone, 17α-acetoxyprogesterone derivatives in the pregnane series, 19-nortestosterone derivatives (estranes), and norgestrel and related compounds in the gonane series. **MPA** and **megestrol acetate** are C21 steroids with selective activity very similar to that of progesterone itself. MPA and oral micronized progesterone are widely used with estrogens for menopausal hormone therapy and other situations in which a selective progestational effect is desired, and a depot form of MPA is used as a long-acting injectable contraceptive. The 19-nortestosterone derivatives were developed for use as progestins in oral contraceptives, and although their predominant activity is progestational, they exhibit androgenic and other activities. The gonanes are a more recently developed series of "19-nor" compounds, containing an ethyl rather than a methyl substituent in the 13-position, and they have diminished androgenic activity. These two classes of 19-nortestosterone derivatives are the progestational components of all oral and some long-acting injectable contraceptives.

Megestrol is indicated in the treatment of anorexia, cachexia, or an unexplained significant weight loss in patients with a diagnosis of AIDS. In addition, it has been recommended as a palliative treatment of advanced carcinoma of the breast or endometrium (i.e., recurrent, inoperable, or metastatic disease). Megestrol, a progestin, inhibits growth and causes regression of progestin-sensitive breast and endometrial cancer tissue by an unknown mechanism. An antiluteinizing effect mediated via the pituitary has been postulated. Evidence also suggests a local effect as a result of the marked changes from direct instillation of progestational agents into the endometrial cavity. The precise mechanism by which megestrol produces effects in anorexia and cachexia is unknown.

Megestrol is absorbed from the GI tract, is highly bound to plasma proteins, and is stored in adipose tissue. It is metabolized in the liver, and the metabolites are eliminated by the kidneys. Megestrol is contraindicated in patients with a history of thromboembolic disorder because the drug may be associated with thromboembolic disease; in patients with severe hepatic disease because drug accumulation may occur; in patients with undiagnosed abnormal vaginal bleeding because the drug may stimulate growth of some tumors; and in pregnant or breast-feeding women because of the potential for adverse effects on the fetus or neonate.

Megestrol should be used cautiously in patients with conditions that might be aggravated by fluid and electrolyte retention such as cardiac or renal disease, epilepsy, or migraine. Caution is also advised in administering this agent to diabetic patients because decreased glucose tolerance may occur, or to patients with a history of mental depression because the drug may exacerbate these effects. Weight gain is a frequent side effect of megestrol acetate. This effect has been associated with increased appetite, not necessarily with fluid retention.

Thromboembolic phenomena, including thrombophlebitis and pulmonary embolism, have occurred on rare occasions. Nausea, vomiting, edema, breakthrough bleeding, dyspnea, tumor flare (with or without hypercalcemia), hyperglycemia, alopecia, carpal tunnel syndrome, and rash have been reported.

MELARSOPROL

(Arsobal)

Trypanosomiasis is produced by protozoa of the genus *Trypanosoma* and leads to Gambian or mid-African sleeping sickness (*T. gambiense*), Rhodesian or East African sleeping sickness (*T. rhodesiense*), and Chagas' disease, which is seen in the populations of Central and South America (*T. cruzi*). Agents effective in the treatment of trypanosomiasis are the aromatic diamidines (pentamidine, stilbamidine, and propamidine). Pentamidine is the preferred drug for the prevention and early treatment of *T. gambiense* infections; however, it cannot penetrate the CNS. Melarsoprol is the drug recommended for *T. gambiense* infections that do not respond to pentamidine or for managing the late meningoencephalitic stages of infection. It does reach the CNS. Nifurtimox (Lampit) is the drug of choice for treating the acute form of Chagas' disease. Suramin (Naphuride) is effective only in the therapy of African sleeping sickness.

MELATONIN

Melatonin is the major hormone produced in the pineal gland. The concentration of the hormone in blood is increased during the hours of darkness, whereas a low concentration occurs during daylight. Its secretion is controlled by an endogenous rhythm-generating system that is entrained by light. Melatonin has a role in cuing circadian rhythms (notably the sleep–wake rhythm) and promoting sleep, and it contributes significantly to the circadian rhythm in body temperature.

Administration of melatonin or bright-light treatment has established therapeutic actions in circadian rhythm sleep disorders, including disorders associated with jet lag, shift work, delayed-phase sleep disorder, periodic sleep disorder in blindness, and sleep and behavioral disorders in children with multiple brain damage. The effects of bright light or melatonin treatment follow a phase-response curve. Evening bright-light treatment causes a phase delay in the sleep–wake cycle, and morning light causes a phase advance. Melatonin treatment produces effects that are nearly the mirror image of those caused by bright light.

Few clinical trials have been done in insomnias that are not associated with circadian rhythm disorders. Large doses of melatonin may have a therapeutic effect in chronic insomnia. Insomnia that coincides with diminished melatonin secretion occurs in aging and following treatment with beta-adrenoceptor blockers. Trials of melatonin treatment for these sleep disorders have yet to be published. A decrease in melatonin concentration has been reported in most studies of depressed patients. Treatment with drugs that enhance noradrenergic transmission or with tryptophan or 5-methoxypsoralen cause both a therapeutic response and an increase in melatonin secretion; however, no treatment trials of melatonin have been reported in depressed patients.

MELOXICAM

(Mobic tablets 7.5 mg)

Meloxicam is a NSAID, which decreases inflammation, pain, and fever, probably through inhibition of cyclooxygenase activity and prostaglandin synthesis. It is indicated in relief of signs and symptoms of osteoarthritis and rheumatoid arthritis. Most NSAIDs inhibit both COX-1 and COX-2 with little selectivity, although some, conventionally thought of as tNSAIDs—diclofenac, **meloxicam**, and **nimesulide**—exhibit selectivity for COX-2 that is close to that of **celecoxib** *in vitro*. Indeed, meloxicam achieved approval in some countries as a selective inhibitor of COX-2. The hypothesis that the antiinflammatory effects of NSAIDs would be accompanied by a lower ulcerogenic potential propelled efforts to design drugs with greater selectivity for COX-2 versus Cox-1. These efforts led to approval and marketing of **rofecoxib**, **celecoxib**, and **valdecoxib** as selective COX-2 inhibitors, known as the coxibs, and the development of others (e.g., **etoricoxib** and **lumiracoxib**). Based on whole blood assays, several previously marketed NSAIDs also have selectivity ratios comparable to those of the least-selective of the novel COX-2 inhibitors, celecoxib. These include **meloxicam**, **nimesulide**, and **diclofenac**. **Meloxicam** (Mobic) was approved recently by the FDA for use in osteoarthritis.

The recommended dose for **meloxicam** is 7.5 to 15 mg once daily for osteoarthritis, and 15 mg once daily for rheumatoid arthritis.

Meloxicam demonstrates roughly tenfold COX-2 selectivity on average in *ex vivo* assays. However, this is quite variable, and a clinical advantage or hazard has yet to be established. Indeed, even with surrogate markers, the relationship to dose is nonlinear. There is significantly less gastric injury compared to piroxicam (20 mg/day) in subjects treated with 7.5 mg/day of meloxicam, but the advantage is lost with 15 mg/day. As in the case of diclofenac, **meloxicam** would not seem like a desirable alternative to prescribing celecoxib to patients at increased risk of myocardial infarction or stroke.

MELPHALAN

(Alkeran tablets 2 mg)

Melphalan is a nitrogen mustard. It is a bifunctional, alkylating agent of the bischloroethylamine type. Its cytotoxicity appears to be related to the extent of its interstrand cross-linking with DNA. Like other bifunctional alkylating agents, it is active against resting and rapidly dividing tumor cells. Melphalan (phenylalanine mustard) properties (150 mcg/kg/day p.o. for 7 days) is indicated in the treatment of multiple myeloma, testicular seminoma, non-Hodgkin's lymphoma, osteogenic sarcoma, breast cancer, and nonresectable advanced ovarian cancer. The general pharmacological and cytotoxic actions of **melphalan**, the phenylalanine derivative of nitrogen mustard, are similar to those of other **mechlorethamines**. The drug is not a vesicant.

When given orally, melphalan is absorbed in an incomplete and variable manner, and 20 to 50% of the drug is recovered in the stool. The drug has a half-life in plasma of approximately 45 to 90 minutes, and 10 to 15% of an administered dose is excreted unchanged in the urine. Patients with decreased renal failure may develop unexpectedly severe myelosuppression.

Melphalan (Alkeran) for multiple myeloma is used in doses of 6 to 8 mg daily for a period of 4 days, in combination with other agents. A rest period of up to 4 weeks should then intervene. The usual intravenous dose is 15 mg/m^2 infused over 15 to 20 minutes. Doses are repeated at 2-week intervals for four doses and then at 4-week intervals based on response and tolerance. Dosage adjustments should be considered based on blood cell counts and in patients with renal impairment.

Melphalan also may be used in myeloablative regimens followed by bone marrow or peripheral blood stem cell reconstitution. For this use, the dose is 180 to 200 mg/m^2.

The clinical toxicity of melphalan is mostly hematological and is similar to that of other alkylating agents. Nausea and vomiting are less frequent. Alopecia does not occur at standard doses, and changes in renal or hepatic function have not been observed.

MEMANTINE HYDROCHLORIDE

(Namenda tablets 5 mg)

Memantine hydrochloride is an *N*-methyl-D-aspartate (NMDA) receptor antagonist. It is postulated that memantine exerts its therapeutic effect as a low to moderate affinity, noncompetitive nervous system NMDA receptor antagonist by binding preferentially to the NMDA receptor-operated cation channels.

Memantine, a NMDA receptor blocker that neutralizes the effect of glutamate at striatal and subthalamic levels, has shown beneficial effects in the treatment of some parkinsonian patients chronically treated with levodopa, who demonstrated increased motor deterioration. In addition, it is indicated for treatment of moderate to severe dementia of Alzheimer's disease (AD).

A major approach to the treatment of AD has involved attempts to augment the cholinergic function of the brain. An early approach was the use of precursors of acetylcholine synthesis, such as **choline chloride** and **phosphatidyl choline** (lecithin). Although these supplements generally are well tolerated, randomized trials have failed to demonstrate any clinically significant efficacy.

A somewhat more successful strategy has been the use of inhibitors of acetylcholinesterase (AChE), the catabolic enzyme for acetylcholine. **Physostigmine**, a rapidly acting, reversible AChE inhibitor, produces improved responses in animal models of learning, and some studies have demonstrated mild transitory improvement in memory following physostigmine treatment in patients with AD. The use of physostigmine has been limited because of its short half-life and tendency to produce symptoms of systemic cholinergic excess at therapeutic doses.

Four inhibitors of AChE currently are approved by the FDA for treatment of Alzheimer's disease: **tacrine** (1,2,3,4-tetrahydro-9-aminoacridine; Cognex), **donepezil** (Aricept), **rivastigmine** (Excelon), and **galantamine** (Razadyne). Tacrine is a potent centrally acting inhibitor of AChE. Studies of oral tacrine in combination with lecithin have confirmed that there is indeed an effect of tacrine on some measures of memory performance, but the magnitude of improvement observed with the combination of lecithin and tacrine is modest at best. The side effects of tacrine often are significant and dose-limiting; abdominal cramping, anorexia, nausea, vomiting, and diarrhea are observed in up to one-third of patients receiving therapeutic doses, and elevations of serum transaminases are observed in up to 50% of those treated. Because of significant side effects, tacrine is not used widely clinically. Donepezil is a selective inhibitor of AChE in the CNS with little effect on AChE in peripheral tissues. It produces modest improvements in cognitive scores in Alzheimer's disease patients and has a long half-life, allowing once-daily dosing. Rivastigmine and galantamine are dosed twice daily and produce a similar degree of cognitive improvement. Adverse effects associated with donepezil, rivastigmine, and galantamine are similar in character but generally less frequent and less severe than those observed with tacrine; they include nausea, diarrhea, vomiting, and insomnia. Donepezil, rivastigmine, and galantamine are not associated with the hepatotoxicity that limits the use of tacrine.

An alternative strategy for the treatment of AD is the use of the NMDA glutamate-receptor antagonist **memantine** (Namenda). **Memantine** produces a use-dependent blockade of NMDA receptors. In patients with moderate to severe AD, use of **memantine** is associated with a reduced rate of clinical deterioration. Whether this is due to a true disease-modifying effect, possibly reduced excitotoxicity, or is a symptomatic effect of the drug is unclear. Adverse effects of **memantine** usually are mild and reversible, and may include headache or dizziness.

MENINGOCOCCAL VACCINE

(Menomune-A/C/Y/W-135 injection 50 mcg)

Meningococcal vaccine is a bacterial vaccine that induces production of bactericidal antibodies specific to capsular polysaccharides of serogroups A, C, Y, and W-135.

Menomune is an active immunization against invasive meningococcal disease caused by serogroups A, C, Y, and W-135; it may be used to prevent and control outbreaks of serogroup C meningococcal disease. **Menactra** is used for active immunization of adolescents and adults, 11 to 55 years of age, against invasive meningococcal disease caused by *Neisseria meningitidis* serogroups A, C, Y, and W-135.

MENOTROPINS

(Pergonal powder or pellet for injection)

Menotropins are gonadotropins that stimulate ovarian follicular growth in women who do not have primary ovarian failure. **Women**: it is used in conjunction with human chorionic gonadotropin (hCG), for multiple follicular development and ovulation induction in patients who have previously received pituitary suppression. **Men**: it is used in conjunction with hCG for stimulation of spermatogenesis in primary or secondary hypogonadotropic hypogonadism caused by a congenital factor or prepubertal hypophysectomy, and in secondary hypogonadotropic hypogonadism caused by hypophysectomy, craniopharyngioma, cerebral aneurysm, or chromophobe adenoma.

Gonadotropins are purified from human urine or prepared using recombinant DNA technology. Several preparations of urinary gonadotropins have been developed. **Chorionic gonadotropin** (Pregnyl, Novarel, Profasi, others), which mimics the action of luteinizing hormone (LH), is obtained from the urine of pregnant women. Urine from postmenopausal women is the source of **menotropins** (Pergonal, Repronex), which contain roughly equal amounts of follicle-stimulating hormone (FSH) and LH, as well as a number of other urinary proteins. Because of their relatively low purity, menotropins are administered intramuscularly to decrease the incidence of hypersensitivity reactions. **Urofollitropin** (uFSH; Bravelle) is a highly purified FSH prepared by immunoconcentration with monoclonal antibodies and is pure enough to be administered subcutaneously.

MEPENZOLATE BROMIDE

(Cantil tablets 25 mg)

Mepenzolate bromide is a quaternary anticholinergic agent that diminishes gastric acid and pepsin secretion; it suppresses spontaneous contractions of the colon. It is a postganglionic parasympathetic inhibitor. Mepenzolate, an anticholinergic agent with gastrointestinal antispasmodic properties (25 to 50 mg p.o. q.i.d.), is used as an adjunctive therapy in peptic ulcer, irritable bowel syndrome, and neurologic bowel disturbances.

MEPERIDINE HYDROCHLORIDE

(Demerol tablets 50 mg)

Meperidine hydrochloride is an opioid analgesic that relieves pain by stimulating opiate receptors in the CNS; it also causes respiratory depression, peripheral vasodilation, inhibition of intestinal peristalsis, sphincter of Oddi spasm, stimulation of chemoreceptors that cause vomiting and increased bladder tone.

Oral and parenteral: used for relief of moderate to severe pain; **parenteral**: used for preoperative sedation; support of anesthesia; obstetrical analgesia.

The pharmacology of meperidine resembles that of morphine, with the following exceptions: the antitussive and antidiarrheal effects of meperidine are minimal; meperidine does not produce miosis; and it may even cause mydriasis. Meperidine's duration of action is extremely short, and hence it is used as an analgesic during diagnostic procedures such as cystoscopy, gastroscopy, pneumoencephalography, and retrograde pyelography. It is also used as a preanesthetic medication and an obstetric analgesic. Because meperidine has atropine-like actions, toxic doses produce a mixed picture of morphine and atropine poisoning. In a narcotic addict who has developed tolerance to the depressant effects of morphine, meperidine poisoning resembles that of atropine and is characterized by mydriasis, tachycardia, dry mouth, excitement, and convulsions. The atropine-like effects of morphine are not reversed by naloxone, a narcotic antagonist (see also Figure 68).

The structural formulas of meperidine, a phenylpiperidine: **Meperidine** is predominantly a μ-receptor agonist, and it exerts its chief pharmacological action on the CNS and the neural elements in the bowel. It is no longer recommended for the treatment of chronic pain because of concerns over metabolite toxicity. It should not be used for longer than 48 hours or in doses greater than 600 mg/day.

Meperidine produces a pattern of effects similar but not identical to that described for morphine. Its analgesic effects are detectable about 15 minutes after oral administration, peak in about 1 to 2 hours, and subside gradually. The onset of analgesic effect is faster (within 10 minutes) after subcutaneous or intramuscular administration, and the effect reaches a peak in about 1 hour that corresponds closely to peak in concentrations in plasma. In clinical use, the duration of effective analgesia is approximately 1.5 to 3 hours. In general, 75 to 100 mg **meperidine** hydrochloride pethidine (Demerol) given parenterally, is approximately equivalent to 10 mg morphine, and in equianalgesic doses, meperidine produces as much sedation, respiratory depression, and euphoria as does morphine. In terms of total analgesic effect, **meperidine** is about one-third as effective when given orally as when administered parenterally. A few patients may experience dysphoria.

Peak respiratory depression is observed within 1 hour of intramuscular administration, and there is a return toward normal starting in about 2 hours. Like other opioids, **meperidine** causes pupillary constriction, increases the sensitivity of the labyrinthine apparatus, and has effects on the secretion of pituitary hormones similar to those of morphine. Meperidine sometimes causes CNS excitation, characterized by tremors, muscle twitches, and seizures; these effects are due largely to accumulation of a metabolite, **normeperidine**. As with morphine, respiratory depression is responsible for an accumulation of CO_2 which, in turn, leads to cerebrovascular dilation, increased cerebral blood flow, and elevation of cerebrospinal fluid pressure.

The effects of **meperidine** on the cardiovascular system generally resemble those of morphine, including the ability to release histamine on parenteral administration. Intramuscular administration of **meperidine** does not affect heart rate significantly, but intravenous administration frequently produces a marked increase in heart rate.

Meperidine has effects on certain smooth muscles qualitatively similar to those observed with other opioids. It does not cause as much constipation as does morphine even when given over prolonged periods of time; this may be related to its greater ability to enter the CNS, thereby producing analgesia at lower systemic concentrations. As with other opioids, clinical doses of **meperidine** slow gastric emptying sufficiently to delay absorption of other drugs significantly.

The uterus of a nonpregnant woman usually is mildly stimulated by meperidine. Administered before an oxytocic, **meperidine** does not exert any antagonistic effect. Therapeutic doses given during active labor do not delay the birth process; in fact, the frequency, duration, and amplitude of uterine contraction sometimes may be increased. The drug does not interfere with normal postpartum contraction or involuntary contraction of the uterus, and it does not increase the incidence of postpartum hemorrhage.

Meperidine is absorbed by all routes of administration, but the rate of absorption may be erratic after intramuscular injection. The peak plasma concentration usually occurs at about 45 minutes, but the range is wide. After oral administration, only about 50% of the drug escapes first-pass metabolism to enter the circulation, and peak concentrations in plasma usually are observed in 1 to 2 hours.

In humans, meperidine is hydrolyzed to **meperidinic** acid, which, in turn, is partially conjugated. Meperidine also is N-demethylated to normeperidine, which then may be hydrolyzed to normeperidinic acid and subsequently conjugated. **Meperidine** is metabolized chiefly in the liver, with a half-life of about 3 hours. In patients with cirrhosis, the bioavailability of meperidine is increased to as much as 80%, and the half-lives of both meperidine and normeperidine are prolonged. Approximately 60% of **meperidine** in plasma is protein bound. Only a small amount is excreted unchanged.

The pattern and overall incidence of untoward effects that follow the use of **meperidine** are similar to those observed after equianalgesic doses of morphine, except that constipation and urinary retention may be less common. Patients who experience nausea and vomiting with morphine may not do so with **meperidine**; the converse also may be true. As with other opioids, tolerance develops to some of these effects. The contraindications generally are the same as for other opioids. In patients or addicts who are tolerant to the depressant effects of meperidine, large doses repeated at short intervals may produce an excitatory syndrome including hallucinations, tremors, muscle twitches, dilated pupils, hyperactive reflexes, and convulsions. These excitatory symptoms are due to the accumulation of normeperidine, which has a half-life of 15 to 20 hours compared with 3 hours for meperidine. Opioid antagonists can block the convulsant effect of normeperidine in the mouse. Because normeperidine is eliminated by the kidney and the liver, decreased renal or hepatic function increases the likelihood of such toxicity.

Severe reactions may follow the administration of **meperidine** to patients being treated with monoamine oxidase (MAO) inhibitors. Two basic types of interactions can be observed. The most prominent is an excitatory reaction (**serotonin syndrome**) with delirium, hyperthermia, headache, hyper- or hypotension, rigidity, convulsions, coma, and death. This reaction may be due to the ability of meperidine to block neuronal reuptake of serotonin and the resulting serotonergic overactivity. Therefore, meperidine and its congeners should not be used in patients taking MAO inhibitors. **Dextromethorphan** also inhibits neuronal serotonin uptake and should be avoided in these patients. **Tramadol** inhibits uptake of norepinephrine and serotonin, and should not be used concomitantly with MAO inhibitors. Similar interactions with other opioids have not been observed clinically. Another type of interaction, a potentiation of opioid effect owing to inhibition of hepatic CYPs, also can be observed in patients taking MAO inhibitors, necessitating a reduction in the doses of opioids.

Chlorpromazine increases the respiratory-depressant effects of meperidine, as do tricyclic antidepressants; this is not true of diazepam. Concurrent administration of drugs such as **promethazine** or chlorpromazine also may greatly enhance meperidine-induced sedation without slowing clearance of the drug. Treatment with phenobarbital or phenytoin increases systemic clearance and decreases oral bioavailability of meperidine; this is associated with an elevation of the concentration of normeperidine in plasma. As with morphine, concomitant administration of an **amphetamine** has been reported to enhance the analgesic effects of meperidine and its congeners while counteracting sedation.

The major use of meperidine is for analgesia. Unlike morphine and its congeners, meperidine is not used for the treatment of cough or diarrhea. Single doses of meperidine also appear to be effective in the treatment of postanesthetic shivering. **Meperidine**, 25 to 50 mg, is used frequently with antihistamines, corticosteroids, acetaminophen, or NSAIDs to prevent or ameliorate infusion-related rigors and shaking chills that accompany the intravenous administration of **amphotericin B**, **aldesleukin** (interleukin-2), **trastuzumab**, and **alemtuzumab**.

Meperidine crosses the placental barrier and, even in reasonable analgesic doses, causes a significant increase in the percentage of babies who show delayed respiration, decreased respiratory minute volume, or decreased oxygen saturation, or who require resuscitation. Fetal and maternal respiratory depression induced by meperidine can be treated with naloxone. The fraction of drug that is bound to protein is lower in the fetus; concentrations of free drug thus may be considerably higher than in the mother. Nevertheless, **meperidine** produces less respiratory depression in the newborn than an equianalgesic dose of morphine or methadone.

MEPHENTERAMINE SULFATE

(Wyamine)

Mephenteramine is indicated in the treatment of hypotension secondary to ganglionic blockage and that occurring following spinal anesthesia. Although not recommended as corrective therapy for shock of hypotension secondary to hemorrhage, mephenteramine may be used as an emergency measure to maintain blood pressure until blood or blood substitutes become available. Mephenteramine sulfate is a mixed-acting sympathomimetic amine that acts both directly and indirectly by releasing norepinephrine. The increase in blood pressure produced by mephenteramine is due to an increase in cardiac output resulting from enhanced cardiac contraction and, to a lesser extent, due to increased peripheral resistance.

Mephenteramine-induced pressor response occurs almost immediately and persists 15 to 30 minutes after IV injection; after IM injection, onset is within 5 to 15 minutes, persisting 1 to 4 hours. Mephenteramine is metabolized in the liver by N-demethylation and p-hydroxylation. Mephenteramine is excreted in urine within 24 hours as unchanged drug and metabolites.

The antihypertensive effects of guanethidine may be partially or totally reversed by the mixed-acting sympathomimetics. Halogenated hydrocarbon anesthetics may sensitize the myocardium to the effects of catecholamines. Use of vasopressors may lead to serious arrhythmias. MAO inhibitors, such as tranylcypromine, increase the pressor response to mixed-acting vasopressors. Possible hypertensive crisis and intracranial hemorrhage may occur. This interaction may also occur with furazolidone, an antimicrobial with MAO inhibitor activity. In obstetrics, if vasopressor drugs are used either to correct hypotension or are added to the local anesthetic solution, some oxytocics may cause severe persistent hypertension in the presence of mephenteramine. The pressor response of mephenteramine may be attenuated by tricyclic antidepressants, which block the uptake of norepinephrine.

MEPHENYTOIN

(Mesantoin)

Mephenytoin is demethylated to 5-ethyl-5-phenylhydantoin (Nirvanol), which is an active anticonvulsant. Mephenytoin binds to plasma protein to the extent of 40%, with an elimination half-life of 7 hours. Mephenytoin causes sedation, whereas phenytoin does not. The incidence of dose- and time-dependent side effects of mephenytoin is lower than that seen with phenytoin. On the other hand, the incidence of severe and fatal hypersensitivity reactions is far higher than that reported for phenytoin. Therefore, mephenytoin is not the first drug of choice. It is used for the treatment of tonic–clonic, simple partial, and complex partial seizures in patients who have become refractory to phenytoin or other drugs.

MEPHOBARBITAL

(Mebaral tablets 32 mg)

Mephobarbital is a barbiturate sedative and hypnotic agent. It depresses sensory cortex, decreases motor activity, alters cerebellar function, and produces drowsiness, sedation, and hypnosis. It is indicated as a sedative for relief of anxiety, tension, and apprehension; and as an anticonvulsant for the treatment of grand mal epilepsy.

Mephobarbital (Mebaral) is *N*-methylphenobarbital. It is N-demethylated in the hepatic endoplasmic reticulum, and most of its activity during long-term therapy can be attributed to the accumulation of phenobarbital. Consequently, the pharmacological properties, toxicity, and clinical uses of **mephobarbital** are the same as those for phenobarbital.

The barbiturates can produce all degrees of depression of the CNS, ranging from mild sedation to general anesthesia. Certain barbiturates, particularly those containing a 5-phenyl substituent (e.g., phenobarbital and mephobarbital), have selective anticonvulsant activity. The antianxiety properties of the barbiturates are inferior to those exerted by the benzodiazepines.

Except for the anticonvulsant activities of phenobarbital and its congeners, the barbiturates possess a low degree of selectivity and therapeutic index. Thus, it is not possible to achieve a desired effect without evidence of general depression of the CNS. Pain perception and reaction are relatively unimpaired until the moment of unconsciousness, and in small doses, the barbiturates increase the reaction to painful stimuli. Hence they cannot be relied on to produce sedation or sleep in the presence of even moderate pain.

Hypnotic doses of barbiturates increase the total sleep time and alter the stages of sleep in a dose-dependent manner. Like the benzodiazepines, these drugs decrease sleep latency, the number of awakenings, and the durations of rapid-eye-movement (REM) and slow-wave sleep. During repetitive nightly administration, some tolerance to the effects on sleep occurs within a few days, and the effect on total sleep time may be reduced by as much as 50% after 2 weeks of use. Discontinuation leads to rebound increases in all the parameters reported to be decreased by barbiturates.

Mephobarbital is indicated for use as a sedative for the relief of anxiety, tension, and apprehension, and as an anticonvulsant for the treatment of grand mal (400 to 600 mg/day) and petit mal epilepsies (6 to 12 mg/kg p.o./day). Mephobarbital, which is more lipid soluble than phenobarbital, becomes metabolized to phenobarbital. The pharmacologic characteristics of mephobarbital are similar to those of phenobarbital, and it is therefore used as an alternate drug. It has been reported that mephobarbital causes less sedation and hypersensitivity reactions than phenobarbital. Similar to phenobarbital, mephobarbital inhibits posttetanic potentiation and especially raises the seizure threshold. The precise mechanism of action of mephobarbital is not known, though two dissimilar mechanisms have been advanced. In the first, phenobarbital and mephobarbital, by inhibiting aldehyde reductase, are thought to interfere with the metabolism of aldehyde generated by biogenic amines such as dopamine, norepinephrine, and serotonin. The accumulation of these aldehydes in the CNS has depressing properties, and this reduces the neuronal sensitivity to excitation. In the second theory, phenobarbital and mephobarbital are thought to enhance the presynaptic release of gamma aminobutyric acid (GABA) and, at the same time, reduce the postsynaptic uptake of GABA. About 50% of an oral dose of mephobarbital is absorbed from the GI tract; action begins within 30 to 60 minutes and lasts 10 to 16 hours. Mephobarbital is distributed widely throughout the body. It is metabolized by the liver to phenobarbital; about 75% of a given dose is converted in 24 hours. Therapeutic blood levels of phenobarbital are 15 to 40 mcg/mL.

Mephobarbital is excreted primarily in urine; small amounts are excreted in breast milk. Mephobarbital is contraindicated in near-term pregnancy because of the hazard of respiratory depression and neonatal coagulation defects; in patients with severe respiratory disease or status asthmaticus because it may cause respiratory depression; or in patients with a history of porphyria or marked hepatic impairment because it may exacerbate porphyria. The drug should be used with caution in patients taking alcohol, CNS depressants, MAO inhibitors, narcotic analgesics, or anticoagulants. Symptoms of acute overdose include CNS and respiratory depression, areflexia, oliguria, tachycardia, hypotension, hypothermia, and coma. Shock may occur.

MEPIVACAINE HYDROCHLORIDE

(Carbocaine)

Mepivacaine is indicated in production of local or regional analgesia and anesthesia by local infiltration, peripheral nerve block techniques, and central neural techniques including epidural and caudal blocks (see also Figure 31).

Local anesthetics block the generation and the conduction of nerve impulses, presumably by increasing the threshold for electrical excitation in the nerve, by slowing the propagation of the nerve impulse, and by reducing the rate of rise of the action potential. In general, the progression of anesthesia is related to the diameter, myelination, and conduction velocity of affected nerve fibers. Clinically, the order of loss of nerve function is as follows: pain, temperature, touch, proprioception, and skeletal muscle tone. Systemic absorption of local anesthesia produces effects on the cardiovascular and central nervous systems. At blood concentrations achieved with normal therapeutic doses, changes in cardiac conduction, excitability, refractoriness, contractility, and peripheral vascular resistance are minimal. However, toxic concentrations depress cardiac conduction and excitability, which may lead to atrioventricular block and ultimately to cardiac arrest. In addition, myocardial contractility is depressed and peripheral vasodilation occurs, leading to decreased cardiac output and arterial blood pressure. Mepivacaine's potency and speed of action are similar to those of lidocaine, with an onset of action of 5 minutes and a duration of action of 15 to 30 minutes. Local anesthetics rapidly cross the placenta, and when used for epidural, paracervical, caudal, or pudendal block anesthesia, can cause varying degrees of maternal, fetal, and neonatal toxicity.

MEPROBAMATE

(Equanil, tablets 200 mg)

Meprobamate is an antianxiety agent. It produces CNS depressant action at multiple sites, including thalamic and limbic systems. It is indicated in the management of anxiety (see Table 9). Many drugs with diverse structures have been used for their sedative–hypnotic properties, including **paraldehyde** (introduced before the barbiturates), **chloral hydrate**, **ethchlorvynol**, **glutethimide**, **methyprylon**, **ethinamate**, and **meprobamate** (introduced just before the benzodiazepines).

Meprobamate is a bis-carbamate ester; it was introduced as an antianxiety agent in 1955, and this remains its only approved use in the United States. However, it also became popular as a sedative–hypnotic drug, and it is discussed here mainly because of its continued use for such purposes. The question of whether the sedative and antianxiety actions of **meprobamate** differ is unanswered, and clinical proof of the efficacy of meprobamate as a selective antianxiety agent in human beings is lacking.

The pharmacological properties of **meprobamate** resemble those of the benzodiazepines in a number of ways. **Meprobamate** can release suppressed behaviors in experimental animals at doses that cause little impairment of locomotor activity, and although it can cause widespread depression of the CNS, it cannot produce anesthesia. However, ingestion of large doses of **meprobamate** alone can cause severe or even fatal respiratory depression, hypotension, shock, and heart failure. Meprobamate appears to have a mild analgesic effect in patients with musculoskeletal pain, and it enhances the analgesic effects of other drugs.

Meprobamate is well absorbed when administered orally. Nevertheless, an important aspect of intoxication with meprobamate is the formation of **gastric bezoars** consisting of undissolved **meprobamate** tablets; hence, treatment may require endoscopy, with mechanical removal of the bezoar. Most of the drug is metabolized in the liver, mainly to a side-chain hydroxy derivative and a glucuronide; the kinetics of elimination may depend on the dose. The half-life of meprobamate may be prolonged during its chronic administration, even though the drug can induce some hepatic CYPs.

The major unwanted effects of the usual sedative doses of meprobamate are drowsiness and ataxia; larger doses produce considerable impairment of learning and motor coordination and prolongation of reaction time. Like the benzodiazepines, **meprobamate** enhances the CNS depression produced by other drugs.

The abuse of meprobamate has continued despite a substantial decrease in the clinical use of the drug. Carisoprodol (Soma), a skeletal muscle relaxant whose active metabolite is **meprobamate**, also has abuse potential, and has become a popular "street drug." **Meprobamate** is preferred to the benzodiazepines by subjects with a history of drug abuse. After long-term medication, abrupt discontinuation evokes a withdrawal syndrome usually characterized by anxiety, insomnia, tremors, and, frequently, hallucinations; generalized seizures occur in about 10% of cases. The intensity of the symptoms depends on the dosage ingested.

6-MERCAPTOPURINE

(6-MP)

6-Mercaptopurine (2.5 mg/kg/day) is indicated for remission induction and maintenance therapy of acute lymphatic (lymphocytic, lymphoblastic) leukemia, and for acute myelogenous leukemia. Mercaptopurine competes with hypoxanthine and guanine for the enzyme hypoxanthine–guanine phosphoribosyltransferase and is converted to thioinosinic acid (TIMP). This intracellular nucleotide inhibits several reactions involving inosinic acid (IMP). In addition, 6-methylthioinosinate (MTIMP) is formed by the methylation of TIMP. Both TIMP and MTIMP inhibit *de novo* purine ribonucleotide synthesis. Radiolabeled 6-MP may be recovered from deoxyribonucleic acid (DNA) in the form of deoxythioguanosine. Some mercaptopurine is converted to nucleotide derivatives of 6-thioguanine. The absorption of 6-mercaptopurine is incomplete, averaging 50%, and its entry into cerebrospinal fluid is negligible. Mercaptopurine becomes catabolized by methylation of the sulfhydryl group and oxidation by the enzyme xanthine oxidase. Allopurinol inhibits xanthine oxidase and retards the catabolism of mercaptopurine and its active metabolites. Plasma half-life averages 21 and 47 minutes in children and in adults, respectively. Metabolites of mercaptopurine appear in urine within 2 hours after administration. After 24 hours, >50% of a dose can be recovered in the urine as intact drug and metabolites. There is complete cross-resistance between mercaptopurine and thioguanine. The most consistent dose-related toxicity is bone marrow suppression, which may be manifested by anemia, leukopenia, or thrombocytopenia (see also Figure 15).

The induction of complete remission of acute lymphatic leukemia is frequently associated with marrow hypoplasia. Maintenance of remission generally involves multiple drug regimens whose component agents cause myelosuppression. Anemia, leukopenia, and thrombocytopenia are frequently observed. Dosages and schedules are adjusted to prevent life-threatening cytopenias. Hepatotoxicity occurs with doses of greater than 2.5 mg/kg/day.

MEROPENEM

(Merrem powder for injection 500 mg)

Meropenem is a carbapenem that inhibits cell wall synthesis. It is indicated in the treatment of intra-abdominal infections in adults and children at least 3 months old, and in meningitis in children of at least 3 months when caused by susceptible microorganisms.

Meropenem (Merrem IV) is a dimethylcarbamoyl pyrolidinyl derivative of **thienamycin**. It does not require coadministration with cilastatin because it is not sensitive to renal dipeptidase. Its toxicity is similar to that of imipenem except that it may be less likely to cause seizures (0.5% of **meropenem**- and 1.5% of imipenem-treated patients seized). Its *in vitro* activity is similar to that of imipenem, with activity against some imipenem-resistant *P. aeruginosa* but less activity against Gram-positive cocci. Clinical experience with meropenem demonstrates therapeutic equivalence with imipenem.

Imipenem-cilastatin is effective for a wide variety of infections, including urinary tract and lower respiratory infections; intra-abdominal and gynecological infections; and skin, soft tissue, bone, and joint infections. The drug combination appears to be especially useful for the treatment of infections caused by cephalosporin-resistant nosocomial bacteria, such as *Citrobacter freundii* and *Enterobacter* spp. It would be prudent to use imipenem for empirical treatment of serious infections in hospitalized patients who have recently received other β-lactam antibiotics because of the increased risk of infection with cephalosporin- and/or penicillin-resistant bacteria. Imipenem should not be used as monotherapy for infections owing to *P. aeruginosa* because of the risk of resistance developing during therapy.

MESALAMINE (5-ASA)

(Asacol tablets, delayed release 400 mg)

Mesalamine is a GI agent that reduces inflammation of colon topically by preventing production of substances involved in the inflammatory process such as arachidonic acid.

It is indicated in the treatment of active, mild to moderate distal ulcerative colitis, proctosigmoiditis, or proctitis.

Mesalamine (5-aminosalicylic acid; Asacol, others) is a salicylate that is used for its local effects in the treatment of inflammatory bowel disease. The drug is not effective orally because it is poorly absorbed and is inactivated before reaching the lower intestine. It currently is available as a suppository and rectal suspension enema (Rowasa) for treatment of mild to moderate proctosigmoiditis; and as a rectal suppository (Canasa, others) for the treatment of distal ulcerative colitis, proctosigmoiditis, or proctitis. Two oral formulations that deliver drug to the lower intestine, olsalazine (sodium azodisalicylate, a dimer of 5-aminosalicylate linked by an azo bond; Dipentum) and **mesalamine** formulated in a pH-sensitive polymer-coated oral preparation (Asacol) and controlled-release capsule (Pentasa), are efficacious in treatment of inflammatory bowel disease, in particular ulcerative colitis. Sulfasalazine (salicylazosulfapyridine; Azulfidine) contains **mesalamine** linked covalently to sulfapyridine; it is absorbed poorly after oral administration, but it is cleaved to its active components by bacteria in the colon. The drug is of benefit in the treatment of inflammatory bowel disease, principally because of the local actions of **mesalamine**. Sulfasalazine and olsalazine also have been used in the treatment of rheumatoid arthritis and ankylosing spondylitis.

First-line therapy for mild to moderate ulcerative colitis generally involves **mesalamine (5-aminosalicylic acid**, or **5-ASA)**. The archetype for this class of medications is **sulfasalazine** (Azulfidine), which consists of 5-ASA linked to sulfapyridine by an azo bond. Although this drug was developed originally as therapy for rheumatoid arthritis, clinical trials serendipitously demonstrated a beneficial effect on the gastrointestinal symptoms of subjects with concomitant ulcerative colitis. Sulfasalazine represents one of the first examples of an oral drug that is delivered effectively to the distal gastrointestinal tract. Given individually, either 5-ASA or sulfapyridine is absorbed in the upper gastrointestinal tract; the azo linkage in sulfasalazine prevents absorption in the stomach and small intestine, and the individual components are not liberated for absorption until colonic bacteria cleave the bond. 5-ASA is now regarded as the therapeutic moiety, with little, if any, contribution by sulfapyridine.

Although mesalamine is a salicylate, its therapeutic effect does not appear to be related to cyclooxygenase inhibition; indeed, traditional nonsteroidal antiinflammatory drugs actually may exacerbate IBD. Many potential sites of action have been demonstrated *in vitro* for either sulfasalazine or **mesalamine**: inhibition of the production of IL-1 and TNF-α, inhibition of the lipoxygenase pathway, scavenging of free radicals and oxidants, and inhibition of NF-κβ, a transcription factor pivotal to production of inflammatory mediators. Specific mechanisms of action of these drugs have not been identified.

Although not active therapeutically, sulfapyridine causes many of the side effects observed in patients taking sulfasalazine. To preserve the therapeutic effect of 5-ASA without the side effects of sulfapyridine, several second-generation 5-ASA compounds have been developed. They are divided into two groups: prodrugs and coated drugs. Prodrugs contain the same azo bond as sulfasalazine but replace the linked sulfapyridine with either another 5-ASA (olsalazine, Dipentum) or an inert compound (balsalazide, Colazide). Thus, these compounds act at similar sites along the gastrointestinal tract as does sulfasalazine. The alternative approaches employ either a delayed-release formulation (**Pentasa**) or a pH-sensitive coating (**Asacol**). Delayed-release **mesalamine** is released throughout the small intestine and colon, whereas pH-sensitive **mesalamine** is released in the terminal ileum and colon. These different distributions of drug delivery have potential therapeutic implications.

Inflammatory bowel disease (IBD) is a chronic disease that affects women in their reproductive years; thus the issue of pregnancy often has a significant impact on medical management. In general, decreased disease activity increases fertility and improves pregnancy outcomes. At the same time, limiting medication during pregnancy is always desired but sometimes conflicts with the goal of controlling the disease.

Mesalamine and glucocorticoids are FDA category B drugs that are used frequently in pregnancy and generally are considered safe, whereas **methotrexate** is clearly contraindicated in pregnant patients. The use of thiopurine immunosuppressives is more controversial. Because these medications are given long term, both their initiation and discontinuation are major management decisions. Although there are no controlled trials of these medications in pregnancy, considerable experience has emerged over the last several years. There does not appear to be an increase in adverse outcomes in pregnant patients maintained on thiopurine-based immunosuppressives. Nonetheless, decisions regarding the use of these medications in patients contemplating pregnancy are complex, and necessarily must involve consideration of risks and benefits involved.

MESNA

(Mesnex tablets 400 mg)

Mesna is a cytoprotective agent. It is used to reduce the incidence of ifosfamide-induced hemorrhagic cystitis. Mesna disulfide is reduced to the free thiol compound, mesna, which reacts chemically with the urotoxic ifosfamide metabolites, resulting in their detoxification. It is indicated in prevention of ifosfamide-induced hemorrhagic cystitis.

If one restricts the definition of receptors to macromolecules, then several drugs may be said not to act on receptors as such. Some drugs specifically bind small molecules or ions that are found normally or abnormally in the body. One example is the therapeutic neutralization of gastric acid by a base (antacid). Another example is the use of **2-mercaptoethane sulphonate** (**mesna**), a free-radical scavenger eliminated rapidly by the kidneys, to bind to reactive metabolites associated with some cancer chemotherapeutic agents and thus to minimize their untoward effects on the urinary tract. Other agents act according to nonpharmacological colligative properties without a requirement for highly specific chemical structure. For example, certain relatively benign compounds, such as mannitol, can be administered in quantities sufficient to increase the osmolarity of various body fluids and thereby cause appropriate changes in the distribution of water. Depending on the agent and route of administration, this effect can be exploited to promote diuresis, catharsis, expansion of circulating volume in the vascular compartment, or reduction of cerebral edema. In a similar fashion, the introduction of cholesterol-binding agents orally (e.g., **cholestyramine resin**) can be used in the management of hypercholesterolemia to decrease the amount of cholesterol absorbed from the diet.

Certain drugs that are structural analogs of normal biological chemicals may be incorporated into cellular components and may thereby alter their function. This property has been termed a counterfeit incorporation mechanism and has been particularly useful with analogs of pyrimidines and purines that can be incorporated into nucleic acids; such drugs have clinical utility in antiviral and cancer chemotherapy.

Although mucosal and bone marrow toxicities occur predictably and acutely with conventional doses of these drugs, other organ toxicities may occur after prolonged or high-dose use; these effects can appear after months or years, and may be irreversible and even lethal. All alkylating agents have caused pulmonary fibrosis, usually several months after treatment. In high-dose regimens, particularly those employing busulfan or BCNU, vascular endothelial damage may precipitate veno-occlusive disease (VOD) of the liver, an often fatal side effect that is successfully reversed by the investigational drug defibrotide. The nitrosoureas and ifosfamide, after multiple cycles of therapy, may lead to renal failure. **Cyclophosphamide** and **ifosfamide** release a nephrotoxic and urotoxic metabolite, **acrolein**, which causes a severe hemorrhagic cystitis, a side effect that in high-dose regimens can be prevented by coadministration of 2-mercaptoethanesulfonate (**mesna** or Mesnex), which conjugates acrolein in urine. Ifosfamide in high doses for transplant causes a chronic, and often irreversible, renal toxicity. Proximal, and less commonly distal, tubules may be affected, with difficulties in Ca^{2+} and Mg^{2+} reabsorption, glycosuria, and renal tubular acidosis. Nephrotoxicity is correlated with the total dose of drug received, and increases in frequency in children less than 5 years of age. The syndrome has been attributed to chloroacetaldehyde and/or acrolein excreted in the urine.

MESORIDAZINE BESYLATE

(Serentil)

Mesoridazine has been used effectively in schizophrenia, behavioral problems in mental deficiency and chronic brain syndrome, alcoholism, and psychoneurotic manifestations associated with neurotic components of personality disorders.

Mesoridazine, a metabolite of thioridazine, is thought to exert its antipsychotic effects by postsynaptic blockade of CNS dopamine receptors, thereby inhibiting dopamine-mediated effects. Mesoridazine has many other central and peripheral affects; it produces both alpha and ganglionic blockade and counteracts histamine- and serotonin-mediated activities. Mesoridazine and thioridazine cause fewer movement disorders (see Phenotheazine Derivatives). Mesoridazine is metabolized to inactive metabolites, which are excreted by the kidneys. Overdosage of mesoridazine causes CNS depression characterized by deep, unarousable sleep, convulsive seizures, and cardiac arrhythmias (see also Table 2).

METAPROTERENOL SULFATE

(Alupent aerosol 75 mg as micronized powder in inert propellant (100 inhalations))

Metaproterenol sulfate is a sympathomimetic agent that relaxes bronchial smooth muscle through beta-2-receptor stimulation. It is indicated in the treatment of bronchial asthma and reversible bronchospasm associated with bronchitis and emphysema; and control of acute asthma attacks in children of at least 6 years (inhalation solution only).

The methylxanthines consist of aminophylline, dyphylline, enprofylline, and pentoxifylline. Aminophylline (theophylline ethylenediamine) is the most widely used of the soluble theophyllines. Its main therapeutic effect is bronchodilation. In addition, it causes CNS stimulation, cardiac acceleration, diuresis, and gastric secretion. Aminophylline is available in an oral, rectal (pediatric), or intravenous solution, which is used in the treatment of status asthmaticus. Although it is a less effective bronchodilator than beta-adrenergic agonists, it is particularly useful in preventing nocturnal asthma (see also Figure 94).

Metaproterenol (called **orciprenaline** in Europe), along with **terbutaline** and **fenoterol**, belongs to the structural class of **resorcinol bronchodilators** that have hydroxyl groups at positions 3 and 5 of the phenyl ring (rather than at positions 3 and 4 as in catechols). Consequently, **metaproterenol** is resistant to methylation by catechol-O-methyl transferase (COMT), and a substantial fraction (40%) is absorbed in active form after oral administration. It is excreted primarily as glucuronic acid conjugates. Metaproterenol is considered to be β_2 selective, although it probably is less selective than albuterol or terbutaline, and hence is more prone to cause cardiac stimulation.

Effects occur within minutes of inhalation and persist for several hours. After oral administration, onset of action is slower, but effects last 3 to 4 hours. **Metaproterenol** (Alupent, others) is used for the long-term treatment of **obstructive airway diseases**, asthma, and for treatment of **acute bronchospam**. Side effects are similar to the short- and intermediate-acting sympathomimetic bronchodilators.

Short-acting β_2-adrenergic-receptor agonists include **albuterol** (Proventil, Ventolin), **levalbuterol**, the (R)-enantiomer of albuterol (Xopenex), **metaproterenol** (Alupent), **terbutaline** (Brethaire), and **pirbuterol** (Maxair). These drugs are used for acute inhalation treatment of bronchospasm. Terbutaline (Brethine, bricanyl), albuterol, and **metaproterenol** also are available in oral dosage form. Each of the inhaled drugs has an onset of action within 1 to 5 minutes and produces bronchodilation that lasts for about 2 to 6 hours. When given in oral dosage forms, the duration of action is somewhat longer (oral terbutaline, for example, has a duration of action of 4 to 8 hours). Although there are slight differences in the relative β_2/β_1-receptor potency ratios among the drugs, all of them are selective for the β_2 subtype.

The most effective drugs in relaxing airway smooth muscle and reversing bronchoconstriction are short-acting β_2-adrenergic-receptor agonists. They are the preferred treatment for rapid symptomatic relief of dyspnea associated with asthmatic bronchoconstriction. Although these drugs are prescribed on an as-needed basis, it is imperative that guidelines be given to the patient so that reliance on relief of symptoms during times of deteriorating asthma does not occur. When the asthma symptoms become persistent, the patient should be reevaluated so that drugs aimed at controlling, in addition to reversing, the disease can be prescribed.

Long-acting β-adrenergic-receptor agonists—Salmeterol xinafoate (Serevent) and **formoterol** (Foradil) are long-lasting adrenergic agents with very high selectivity for the β_2-receptor subtype. Inhalation of salmeterol provides persistent bronchodilation lasting over 12 hours. The mechanism underlying the extended duration of action of salmeterol is not yet fully understood. The extended side chain on salmeterol renders it 10,000 times more lipophilic than albuterol. The lipophilicity regulates the diffusion rate away from the receptor by determining the degree of partitioning in the lipid bilayer of the membrane. Subsequent to binding the receptor, the less-lipophilic, short-acting agonists are removed rapidly from the receptor environment by diffusion in the aqueous phase. Unbound salmeterol, by contrast, persists in the membrane and only slowly dissociates from the receptor environment.

METARAMINOL

(Aramine)

Metaraminol is indicated in prevention and treatment of the acute hypotensive state occurring with spinal anesthesia, adjunctive treatment of hypotension due to hemorrhage, reactions to medications, surgical complications, and shock associated with brain damage due to trauma or tumor. The pressor effects of metaraminol begin 1 to 2 minutes after IV infusion, 10 minutes after IM injection, and 5 to 20 minutes after SC injection. The effects last from about 20 minutes to 1 hour. Metaraminol is a sympathomimetic amine that increases both systolic and diastolic blood pressure by vasoconstriction, and this effect is accompanied by a marked reflex bradycardia. It has a direct effect on alpha-adrenergic receptors, and its prolonged infusions can deplete norepinephrine from sympathetic nerve endings. Metaraminol increases venous tone, causes pulmonary vasoconstriction, and elevates pulmonary pressure even when cardiac output is reduced. Pressor effect is decreased, but not reversed, by alpha-adrenergic-blocking agents. The antihypertensive effects of guanethidine may be partially or totally reversed by the mixed-acting sympathomimetics. Halogenated hydrocarbon anesthetics may sensitize the myocardium to the effects of catecholamines. Use of vasopressors may lead to serious arrhythmias. MAO A inhibitors, such as tranylcypromine, increase the pressor response to mixed-acting vasopressors. Possible hypertensive crisis and intracranial hemorrhage may occur. This interaction may also occur with furazolidone, an antimicrobial agent with MAO inhibitory properties. The pressor response of metaraminol is reduced by tricyclic antidepressants such as desipramine.

METAXALONE

(Skelaxin)

Metaxalone (800 mg t.i.d.), a centrally acting muscle relaxant, is indicated as an adjunct to rest, physical therapy, and other measures for the relief of discomfort associated with acute painful musculoskeletal conditions. It has no direct action on the contractile mechanism, or myoneural function. It should be administered cautiously to individuals with hepatic impairment. Metaxalone is a CNS-depressant and potentiates the CNS depressant effects of ethanol.

METFORMIN HYDROCHLORIDE

(Glucophage tablets 500 mg)

Metformin hydrochloride is a biguanide that decreases blood glucose by decreasing hepatic glucose production. It may also decrease intestinal absorption of glucose and increase response to insulin. Metformin is indicated as an adjunct to diet and exercise to lower blood glucose in patients with type 2 diabetes mellitus. Metformin IR tablets and oral solution are indicated in patients 10 years of age and older. The ER tablets are indicated in patients 17 years of age and older. In combination with a sulfonylurea or insulin to improve glycemic control, metformin is indicated in patients 17 years of age and older.

Metformin (Glucophage, others) and **phenformin** were introduced in 1957, and **buformin** was introduced in 1958. The latter was of limited use, but metformin and phenformin were used widely. Phenformin was withdrawn in many countries during the 1970s because of an association with lactic acidosis. **Metformin** has been associated only rarely with that complication, and has been used widely in Europe and Canada; it became available in the United States in 1995. **Metformin** given alone or in combination with a sulfonylurea improves glycemic control and lipid concentrations in patients who respond poorly to diet or to a sulfonylurea alone.

Metformin is antihyperglycemic, not hypoglycemic. It does not cause insulin release from the pancreas, and generally does not cause hypoglycemia even in large doses. It has no significant effects on the secretion of glucagon, cortisol, growth hormone, or somatostatin. **Metformin** reduces glucose levels primarily by decreasing hepatic glucose production and by increasing insulin action in muscle and fat. At a molecular level, these actions are mediated at least in part by activation of the cellular kinase AMP-activated protein kinase (AMP kinase). The mechanism by which metformin reduces hepatic glucose production is controversial, but most data indicate an effect on reducing **gluconeogenesis**. **Metformin** also may decrease plasma glucose by reducing the absorption of glucose from the intestine, but this action has not been shown to have clinical relevance.

Metformin is absorbed mainly from the small intestine. The drug is stable, does not bind to plasma proteins, and is excreted unchanged in the urine. It has a half-life of about 2 hours. The maximum recommended daily dose of metformin in the United States is 2.5 g given in three doses with meals.

Patients with renal impairment should not receive **metformin**. Other contraindications include hepatic disease, a past history of lactic acidosis (of any cause), cardiac failure requiring pharmacological therapy, or chronic hypoxic lung disease. The drug also should be discontinued temporarily prior to the administration of intravenous **contrast media** and prior to any surgical procedure. The drug should not be readministered any sooner than 48 hours after such procedures, and should be withheld until renal function is determined to be normal. These conditions all predispose to increased lactate production and hence to the potentially fatal complication of lactic acidosis. The reported incidence of lactic acidosis during metformin treatment is less than 0.1 cases per 1000 patient-years, and the mortality risk is even lower.

Acute side effects of **metformin**, which occur in up to 20% of patients, include diarrhea, abdominal discomfort, nausea, metallic taste, and anorexia. These usually can be minimized by increasing the dosage of the drug slowly and taking it with meals. Intestinal absorption of vitamin B_{12} and folate often is decreased during chronic metformin therapy, and calcium supplements reverse the effect of metformin on vitamin B_{12} absorption.

Consideration should be given to stopping treatment with metformin if the plasma lactate level exceeds 3 mM, or in the setting of decreased renal or hepatic function. It also is prudent to stop metformin if a patient is undergoing a prolonged fast or is treated with a very-low-calorie diet. Myocardial infarction or septicemia mandates immediate drug discontinuation. **Metformin** usually is administered in divided doses two or three times daily. The maximum effective dose is 2.5 g/day. It lowers hemoglobin A_{1c} values by about 2%, an effect comparable with that of the sulfonylureas. **Metformin** does not promote weight gain, and can reduce plasma triglycerides by 15 to 20%. There is a strong consensus that reduction in hemoglobin A_{1c} by any therapy (insulin or oral agents) diminishes microvascular complications. **Metformin**, however, is the only therapeutic agent that has been demonstrated to reduce macrovascular events in type 2 diabetes mellitus. It can be administered in combination with sulfonylureas, thiazolizinediones, and/or insulin. Fixed-dose combinations containing metformin and glyburide (**Glucovance**, others), glipizide (**Metaglip**), and rosiglitazone (**Avandamet**) are available.

METHACYCLINE HYDROCHLORIDE

(Rondomycin)

Methacycline is a broad-spectrum tetracycline antibiotic that is synthetically derived from oxytetracycline. Methacycline (600 mg/day) is indicated in infections caused by Gram-positive bacteria, *Rickettsia*, *Mycoplasma*, *Amoeba*, and *Chlamydia*. It binds to the 30S subunit of the bacterial ribosome in such a way that the binding of the aminoacyl-transfer RNA to the acceptor site on the messenger RNA ribosome complex is blocked (see also Figure 96). Tetracyclines are effective in the treatment of Rocky Mountain spotted fever, murine typhus, recrudescent epidemic typhus, scrub typhus, Q fever, lymphogranuloma venereum, psittacosis, tularemia, brucellosis, gonorrhea, certain urinary tract infections, granuloma inguinale, chancroid, syphilis, and disease due to *Bacteroides* and *Clostridium.*

Tetracyclines in general cause toxic and hypersensitivity reactions. These consist commonly of gastrointestinal irritations that are disabling, and may necessitate discontinuation of the medications. With continuous usage, tetracyclines may alter the normal flora, allowing the growth of *Pseudomonas*, *Proteus*, staphylococci-resistant coliforms, *Clostridium*, and *Candida* organisms. These superinfections should be recognized and treated appropriately with vancomycin and other drugs (see also Figure 100). Tetracyclines have been known to cause hepatic necrosis, especially when given in large intravenous doses or when taken by pregnant women or patients with preexisting liver impairment. Tetracycline preparations whose potency has expired can cause renal tubular acidosis. With the exception of doxycycline, tetracyclines accumulate in patients with renal impairment. They also produce nitrogen retention, especially when given with diuretics. Tetracyclines bind to calcium and then become deposited in bone, causing damage to developing bone and teeth.

METHADONE HYDROCHLORIDE

(Dolophine hydrochloride tablets 5 mg)

Methadone hydrochloride is an opioid analgesic that relieves pain by stimulating opiate receptors in the CNS; it also causes respiratory depression, peripheral vasodilation, inhibition of intestinal peristalsis, sphincter of Oddi spasm, stimulation of chemoreceptors that cause vomiting and increased bladder tone.

The primary use of methadone is in the management of severe pain; and detoxification and temporary maintenance treatment of narcotic addiction. Pharmacologically, methadone is very similar to morphine, with the following exceptions: methadone is effective orally; its onset and duration of action are longer than morphine's; tolerance to methadone develops very slowly, and, if abruptly withdrawn, the abstinence syndrome develops more slowly, is less intense, and is more prolonged than the abstinence syndrome of morphine; and the abuse potential of methadone is lower than morphine's. Like morphine, methadone is used in the management of pain. It is also used in the detoxification and treatment of narcotic addiction (see also Figure 68). Methadone is a long-acting μ-receptor agonist with pharmacological properties qualitatively similar to those of morphine.

The analgesic activity of the racemate is almost entirely the result of its content of L-methadone, which is 8 to 50 times more potent than the D isomer; D-methadone also lacks significant respiratory depressant action and addiction liability, but it does possess antitussive activity.

The outstanding properties of methadone are its analgesic activity, its efficacy by the oral route, its extended duration of action in suppressing withdrawal symptoms in physically dependent individuals, and its tendency to show persistent effects with repeated administration. Miotic and respiratory-depressant effects can be detected for more than 24 hours after a single dose, and on repeated administration, marked sedation is seen in some patients. Effects on cough, bowel motility, biliary tone, and the secretion of pituitary hormones are qualitatively similar to those of morphine.

Methadone is absorbed well from the gastrointestinal tract and can be detected in plasma within 30 minutes of oral ingestion; it reaches peak concentrations at about 4 hours. After therapeutic doses, about 90% of methadone is bound to plasma proteins. Peak concentrations occur in the brain within 1 or 2 hours of SC or IM administration, and this correlates well with the intensity and duration of analgesia. **Methadone** also can be absorbed from the buccal mucosa.

Methadone undergoes extensive biotransformation in the liver. The major metabolites, the results of N-demethylation and cyclization to form pyrrolidines and pyrroline, are excreted in urine and bile along with small amounts of unchanged drug. The amount of **methadone** excreted in urine is increased when urine is acidified. The half-life of methadone is approximately 15 to 40 hours.

Methadone appears to be firmly bound to protein in various tissues, including brain. After repeated administration, there is gradual accumulation in tissues. When administration is discontinued, low concentrations are maintained in plasma by slow release from extravascular binding sites; this process probably accounts for the relatively mild but protracted withdrawal syndrome.

Side effects, toxicity, and conditions that alter sensitivity, as well as the treatment of acute intoxication, are similar to those described for morphine. During long-term administration, there may be excessive sweating, lymphocytosis, and increased concentrations of prolactin, albumin, and globulins in the plasma. **Rifampin** and **phenytoin** accelerate the metabolism of methadone and can precipitate withdrawal symptoms.

Volunteer postaddicts who receive subcutaneous or oral **methadone** daily develop partial tolerance to the nauseant, anorectic, miotic, sedative, respiratory-depressant, and cardiovascular effects of **methadone**. Tolerance develops more slowly to **methadone** than to morphine in some patients, especially with respect to the depressant effects; this may be related in part to cumulative effects of the drug or its metabolites. Tolerance to the constipating effect of methadone does not develop as fully as tolerance to other effects. The behavior of addicts who use methadone parenterally is strikingly similar to that of morphine edicts, but many former heroin users treated with oral methadone show virtually no overt behavioral effects.

Development of physical dependence during the long-term administration of methadone can be demonstrated by drug withdrawal or by administration of an opioid antagonist. Subcutaneous administration of 10 to 20 mg methadone to former opioid addicts produces definite euphoria equal in duration to that caused by morphine, and its overall abuse potential is comparable with that of morphine.

The primary uses of **methadone hydrochloride** (Dolophine, others) are relief of chronic pain, treatment of opioid abstinence syndromes, and treatment of heroin users. It is not used widely as an antiperistaltic agent. It should not be used in labor.

METHAMPHETAMINE HYDROCHLORIDE (DESOXYEPHEDRINE HYDROCHLORIDE)

(Desoxyn tablets 5 mg)

Methamphetamine hydrochloride is an amphetamine that activates noradrenergic neurons causing CNS and respiratory stimulation; and stimulates the satiety center in the brain, causing appetite suppression. It is indicated for treatment of attention deficit disorder in children; it is a short-term exogenous obesity adjunct.

Methamphetamine (2.5 to 5 mg p.o. daily) has been used in the management of obesity, narcolepsy, and attention deficit hyperactivity impulse disorder. Methamphetamine, which releases norepinephrine and dopamine, stimulates the CNS. It is absorbed from the GI tract after oral administration, is distributed throughout the body, crosses the placenta, and is found in breast milk. It is metabolized in the liver and is excreted in the urine. Methamphetamine is contraindicated in patients with hyperthyroidism, glaucoma, angina pectoris, or any degree of hypertension or other severe cardiovascular disease because it may cause hazardous arrhythmias and changes in blood pressure. The simultaneous use of methamphetamine and a monoamine oxidase inhibitor such as tranylcypromine should be discouraged. Methamphetamine should be used with caution in patients with diabetes mellitus; in patients who are elderly, debilitated, asthenic, or psychopathic; in patients who have a history of suicidal or homicidal tendencies; and in children with Gilles de la Tourette's syndrome. Amphetamine-induced CNS stimulation, superimposed on CNS depression, can cause seizures. Concomitant use with MAO inhibitors (or drugs with MAO-inhibiting activity, such as furazolidone), or within 14 days of such therapy, may cause hypertensive crisis; use with antihypertensives may antagonize their effects. Concomitant use with antacids, sodium bicarbonate, or acetazolamide enhances reabsorption of methamphetamine and prolongs duration of action, whereas use with ascorbic acid enhances methamphetamine excretion and shortens duration of action. Use with phenothiazines or haloperidol decreases methamphetamine effects. Barbiturates antagonize methamphetamine by CNS depression, whereas caffeine or other CNS stimulants produce additive effects. Patients using methamphetamine have an increased risk of arrhythmias during general anesthesia. Methamphetamine may alter insulin requirements. Symptoms of overdose include increasing restlessness, tremor, hyperreflexia, tachypnea, confusion, aggressiveness, hallucinations, and panic; fatigue and depression usually follow the excitement stage. Other symptoms may include arrhythmias, shock, alterations in blood pressure, nausea, vomiting, diarrhea, and abdominal cramps; death is usually preceded by convulsions and coma.

Methamphetamine (Desoxyn) is closely related chemically to amphetamine and ephedrine. In the brain, methamphetamine releases dopamine and other biogenic amines, and inhibits neuronal and vesicular monoamine transporters as well as MAO.

Small doses have prominent central stimulant effects without significant peripheral actions; somewhat larger doses produce a sustained rise in systolic and diastolic blood pressures, due mainly to cardiac stimulation. Cardiac output is increased, although the heart rate may be slowed. Venous constriction causes peripheral venous pressure to increase. These factors tend to increase the venous return and thus cardiac output. Pulmonary arterial pressure is raised, probably owing to increased cardiac output. Methamphetamine is a schedule II drug under federal regulations and has high potential for abuse. It is widely used as a cheap, accessible recreational drug, and methamphetamine abuse is a widespread phenomenon. Its illegal production in clandestine laboratories throughout the United States is common. Methamphetamine is used principally for its central effects, which are more pronounced than those of amphetamine and are accompanied by less prominent peripheral actions.

Subjective effects similar to those of **cocaine** are produced by **amphetamine**, **dextroamphetamine**, **methamphetamine**, **phenmetrazine**, **methylphenidate**, and **diethylpropion**. Amphetamines increase synaptic dopamine primarily by stimulating presynaptic release rather than by blockade of reuptake, as is the case with cocaine. Intravenous or smoked methamphetamine produces an abuse/dependence syndrome similar to that of cocaine, although clinical deterioration may progress more rapidly. In animal studies, **methamphetamine** in doses comparable with those used by human abusers produces neurotoxic effects in dopamine and serotonin neurons. **Methamphetamine** can be produced in small, clandestine laboratories starting with ephedrine, a widely available non-prescription stimulant. Oral stimulants, such as those prescribed in a weight-reduction program, have short-term efficacy because of tolerance development. Only a small proportion of patients introduced to these appetite suppressants subsequently exhibits dose escalation or drug seeking from various physicians; such patients may meet diagnostic criteria for abuse or addiction. **Fenfluramine** (no longer marketed in the United States) and **phenylpropanolamine** (no longer marketed in the United States) reduce appetite with no evidence of significant abuse potential. **Mazindol** (no longer marketed in the United States) also reduces appetite, with less stimulant properties than amphetamine.

Khat is a plant material widely chewed in East Africa and Yemen for its stimulant properties; these are due to the alkaloidal **cathinone**, a compound similar to amphetamine. **Methcathinone**, a congener with similar effects, has been synthesized in clandestine laboratories, but widespread use in North America has not been reported.

METHANDROSTENOLONE

(Dianabol)

Methandrostenolone is an androgenic steroid with anabolic actions (see also Table 8).

Because androgens have significant effects on muscle mass and on body weight when administered to hypogonadal men, it was assumed, but never proven, that androgens in pharmacological doses could promote growth of muscle above the levels produced by the normal testicular secretion. This assumption was based on the belief that anabolic and androgenic actions are different, and a concerted effort was made to devise pure "anabolic" steroids that have no androgenic effects. In fact, androgenic and anabolic effects do not result from different actions of the same hormone but represent the same action in different tissues; androgen-responsive muscle contains the same receptor that mediates the action of the hormones in other target tissues. All anabolic hormones tested to date are also androgenic. In appropriate doses, most anabolic agents can be used for replacement of androgen. For example, methandrostenolone, which has a greater effect on nitrogen balance per unit weight than methyltestosterone, is a potent androgen and has been used for replacement therapy in hypogonadal men. Nevertheless, androgens have been tried in a variety of clinical situations other than hypogonadism with the hope that improvement in nitrogen balance and muscle development would outweigh any deleterious side effects.

METHANTHELINE BROMIDE

(Banthine)

Methantheline (50 to 100 mg p.o. q. 6 hours), an anticholinergic agent, is used as an adjunctive therapy in peptic ulcer. It blocks the action of acetylcholine at neuroaffector sites, inhibiting gastric acid secretion and pancreatic secretions. Methantheline is contraindicated in patients with narrow-angle glaucoma because drug-induced cycloplegia and mydriasis may increase intraocular pressure (IOP); and in patients with obstructive uropathy, obstructive GI tract disease, severe ulcerative colitis, myasthenia gravis, paralytic ileus, intestinal atony, or toxic megacolon. Methantheline should be administered cautiously to patients with autonomic neuropathy, hyperthyroidism, coronary artery disease, cardiac arrhythmias, congestive heart failure, or ulcerative colitis because toxic accumulation may occur; in patients over age 40, because the drug increases the glaucoma risk; in patients with hiatal hernia associated with reflux esophagitis because the drug may decrease lower esophageal sphincter tone; and in hot or humid environments because the drug may predispose the patient to heatstroke. The concurrent administration of antacids decreases the oral absorption of methantheline, which should be administered at least one hour before antacids. Clinical signs of overdosage with methantheline include curare-like symptoms and such peripheral effects as headache; dilated, nonreactive pupils; blurred vision; flushed, hot, dry skin; dryness of mucous membranes; dysphagia; decreased or absent bowel sounds; urinary retention; hyperthermia; tachycardia; hypertension; and increased respiration.

METHAQUALONE

(Quaalude)

Methaqualone has been used for daytime sedation and in patients with simple insomnia. It is useful for patients who cannot tolerate barbiturates.

METHARBITAL

(Gemonil)

Metharbital, 5,5-diethyl-*l*-methylbarbituric acid, an N-substituted derivative of barbital, shares the anticonvulsant properties of phenobarbital. It is claimed to be particularly effective in young children for the control of massive spasms resulting from underlying brain damage, and in myoclonic seizures. In equivalent doses, it is less depressing than phenobarbital. Metharbital is administered initially in doses of 50 mg (infants and children) and 100 mg (adults) one to three times daily, orally. This dosage may be increased gradually depending on tolerance, up to 600 to 800 mg if needed to control seizures.

METHAZOLAMIDE

(Methazolamide tablets 25 mg)

Methazolamide is a carbonic anhydrase inhibitor that inhibits carbonic anhydrase enzyme, reducing the rate of aqueous humor secretion and, thus, lowering IOP. It is indicated in the treatment of ocular conditions where lowering IOP is likely to be of therapeutic benefit (e.g., chronic open-angle glaucoma, secondary glaucoma, and preoperatively in acute angle-closure glaucoma).

Acetazolamide (Diamox) is the prototype of a class of agents that have limited usefulness as diuretics but have played a major role in the development of fundamental concepts of renal physiology and pharmacology.

When sulfanilamide was introduced as a chemotherapeutic agent, **metabolic acidosis** was recognized as a side effect. This observation led to the demonstration that sulfanilamide is an inhibitor of carbonic anhydrase. Subsequently, an enormous number of sulfonamides were synthesized and tested for the ability to inhibit carbonic anhydrase; of these compounds, acetazolamide has been studied most extensively. Three carbonic anhydrase inhibitors currently are available in the United States—**acetazolamide**, **dichlorphenamide** (Daranide), and **methazolamide** (GlaucTabs). The common molecular motif of available carbonic anhydrase inhibitors is an unsubstituted sulfonamide moiety.

Proximal tubular epithelial cells are richly endowed with the zinc metalloenzyme carbonic anhydrase, which is found in the luminal and basolateral membranes (type IV carbonic anhydrase, an enzyme tethered to the membrane by a glycosylphosphatidylinositol linkage), as well as in the cytoplasm (type II carbonic anhydrase). Carbonic anhydrase plays a key role in $NaHCO_3$ reabsorption and acid secretion.

In the proximal tubule, the free energy in the Na^+ gradient established by the basolateral Na^+ pump is used by a Na^+–H^+ antiporter (also referred to as a Na^+–H^+ exchanger [NHE]) in the luminal membrane to transport H^+ into the tubular lumen in exchange for Na^+. In the lumen, H^+ reacts with filtered HCO_3^- to form $H_2CO_3^-$, which decomposes rapidly to CO_2 and water in the presence of carbonic anhydrase in the brush border. Normally, the reaction between CO_2 and water occurs slowly, but carbonic anhydrase reversibly accelerates this reaction several thousand times. CO_2 is lipophilic and rapidly diffuses across the luminal membrane into the epithelial cell, where it reacts with water to form $H_2CO_3^-$, a reaction catalyzed by cytoplasmic carbonic anhydrase. (The actual reaction catalyzed by carbonic anhydrase is $OH^- + CO_2 \rightarrow HCO_3^-$; however, $H_2O \rightarrow OH^- + H^+$, and $HCO_3 + H^+ \rightarrow H_2CO_3$, so the net reaction is $H_2O + CO_2 \rightarrow H_2CO_3$). Continued operation of the Na^+–H^+ antiporter maintains a low proton concentration in the cell, so $H_2CO_3^-$ ionizes spontaneously to form H^+ and HCO_3^-, creating an electrochemical gradient for HCO_3^- across the basolateral membrane. The electrochemical gradient for HCO_3^- is used by a Na^+– HCO_3^- symporter (also referred to as the Na^+– HCO_3^- cotransporter [NBC]) in the basolateral membrane to transport Na HCO_3^- into the interstitial space. The net effect of this process is transport of Na HCO_3^- from the tubular lumen to the interstitial space, followed by movement of water (isotonic reabsorption). Removal of water concentrates Cl^- in the tubular lumen, and consequently, Cl^- diffuses down its concentration gradient into the interstitium via the paracellular pathway.

METHAZOLAMIDE

(Neptazane)

Methazolamide (50 to 100 mg p.o. b.i.d. or t.i.d.), a carbonic anhydrase inhibitor, decreases the formation of aqueous humor, lowering IOP, and hence is indicated as an adjunctive treatment for the treatment of open-angle glaucoma. Methazolamide is absorbed orally, and distributes into plasma, erythrocytes, extracellular fluid, bile, aqueous humor, and granulocyte colony-stimulating factor (CSF). It is metabolized partially in the liver and is partially (20 to 30%) excreted in the urine.

Methazolamide is contraindicated in patients with hepatic insufficiency, low potassium or sodium levels, hyperchloremic acidosis, or severe renal impairment because of the potential for enhanced electrolyte imbalances. It should be used cautiously in patients with respiratory acidosis or other severe respiratory problems because the drug may produce acidosis; in patients with diabetes because it may cause hyperglycemia and glycosuria; in patients taking cardiac glycosides because they are more susceptible to digitalis toxicity from methazolamide-induced hypokalemia; and in patients taking other diuretics. Methazolamide alkalizes urine, thus decreasing excretion of amphetamines, procainamide, quinidine, and flecainide. Methazolamide increases excretion of salicylates, phenobarbital, and lithium, lowering plasma levels of these drugs and necessitating dosage adjustments.

METHDILAZINE

METHDILAZINE HYDROCHLORIDE

(Tacacryl)

Methdilazine, a phenothiazine derivative with antihistaminic properties (8 mg p.o. b.i.d.), is used in pruritis.

METHENAMINE AND METHENAMINE SALTS

(Methenamine hippurate)

Methenamine is an antiinfective agent. In acidic urine, methenamine is hydrolyzed to ammonia and formaldehyde, which is bactericidal to certain bacteria in urine. Acid salts (methenamine mandelate and hippurate) have some nonspecific bacteriostatic activity and help to maintain low urine pH. It is indicated in suppression or elimination of bacteriuria associated with pyelonephritis, cystitis, and other chronic UTIs; in treatment of infected residual urine, sometimes accompanying neurologic disease or diabetes.

METHENAMINE HIPPURATE

(Hiprex, Urex)

METHENAMINE MANDELATE

(Mandameth, Mandelamine, Mandelamine Forte Suspension)

Methenamine, a urinary tract antiinfective agent, is used in long-term prophylaxis or suppression of chronic urinary tract infections (methenamine hippurate), and in the treatment of urinary tract infections associated with neurogenic bladder.

Methenamine mandelate decomposes in solution to generate formaldehyde which, in a concentration of 20 μg/ml, inhibits all bacteria causing urinary tract infections (see Figure 65). Therefore, methenamine mandelate is indicated in suppression or elimination of bacteriuria associated with pyelonephritis, cystitis, and other chronic urinary tract infections. The nonspecific antibacterial action of formaldehyde is effective against Gram-positive and Gram-negative organisms, and fungi. *E. coli*, enterococci, and staphylococci are usually susceptible. *Enterobacter aerogenes* and *Proteus vulgaris* are generally resistant. Urea-splitting organisms (e.g., *Proteus*, *Pseudomonas*) may be resistant because they raise the pH of the urine, inhibiting the release of formaldehyde. An effective urine concentration of formaldehyde must persist for a minimum of two

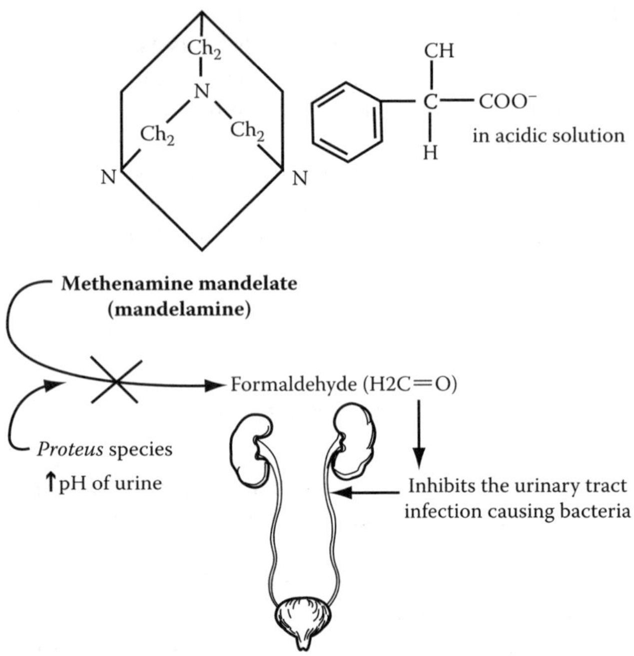

FIGURE 65 **Methenamine mandelate** decomposes in solution to generate **formaldehyde**, which inhibits all bacteria that cause urinary tract infections. Urea-splitting microorganisms raise the pH of the urine and hence inhibit the release of formaldehyde and the action of methenamine.

hours. Methenamine is effective clinically against most common urinary tract pathogens. It has demonstrable antibacterial activity *in vitro* against *E. coli, Micrococcus pyogenes, E. aerogenes, P. aeruginosa*, and *P. vulgaris* at pH 5 to 6.8. The minimal inhibitory concentrations are significantly lower in more acidic media; therefore, efficacy can be increased by urine acidification. Methenamine is particularly suited for therapy of chronic infections because bacteria and fungi do not develop resistance to formaldehyde. Sodium bicarbonate and acetazolamide can decrease the effectiveness of methenamine by alkalinizing the urine and inhibiting the conversion of methenamine to formaldehyde. Methenamine is absorbed orally. However, because of the ammonia produced, it is contraindicated in patients suffering from hepatic insufficiency (see Figure 65).

The urinary tract antiseptics inhibit the growth of many species of bacteria. They cannot be used to treat systemic infections because effective concentrations are not achieved in plasma with safe doses. However, because they are concentrated in the renal tubules, they can be administered orally to treat infections of the urinary tract. Furthermore, effective antibacterial concentrations reach the renal pelvis and the bladder. Treatment with such drugs can be thought of as local therapy—only in the kidney and bladder.

Methenamine is a urinary tract antiseptic and prodrug that owes its activity to its capacity to generate formaldehyde. **Methenamine** is hexamethylenetetramine (hexamethylenamine).

The compound decomposes in water to generate formaldehyde, according to the following reaction:

$$NH_4(CH_2)_6 + 6H_2O + 4H^+ \rightarrow 4NH^+_4 + 6HCHO$$

At pH 7.4, almost no decomposition occurs; however, the yield of formaldehyde is 6% of the theoretical amount at pH 6 and 20% at pH 5. Thus, acidification of the urine promotes the formaldehyde-dependent antibacterial action. The reaction is fairly slow, and 3 hours are required to reach 90% completion.

Nearly all bacteria are sensitive to free aldehyde at concentrations of about 20 μg/mL. Urea-splitting microorganisms (e.g., *Proteus* spp.) tend to raise the pH of the urine and thus inhibit the release of formaldehyde. Microorganisms do not develop resistance to formaldehyde.

Methenamine is absorbed orally, but 10 to 30% decomposes in the gastric juice unless the drug is protected by an enteric coating. Because of the ammonia produced, **methenamine** is contraindicated in hepatic insufficiency. Excretion in the urine is nearly quantitative. When the urine pH is 6 and the daily urine volume is 1000 to 1500 mL, a daily dose of 2 g will yield a concentration of 18 to 60 μg/mL of formaldehyde; this is more than the MIC for most urinary tract pathogens. Various poorly metabolized acids can be used to acidify the urine. Low pH alone is bacteriostatic, so acidification serves a double function. The acids commonly used are **mandelic acid** and **hippuric acid** (Uerx, Hiprex).

Gastrointestinal distress frequently is caused by doses greater than 500 mg four times a day, even with enteric-coated tablets. Painful and frequent micturition, albuminuria, hematuria, and rashes may result from doses of 4 to 8 g/day given for longer than 3 to 4 weeks. Once the urine is sterile, a high dose should be reduced. Because systemic **methenamine** has low toxicity at the typically used doses, renal insufficiency does not constitute a contraindication to the use of methenamine alone, but the acids given concurrently may be detrimental. **Methenamine** mandelate is contraindicated in renal insufficiency. Crystalluria from the mandelate moiety can occur. Methenamine combines with sulfamethizole and perhaps other sulfonamides in the urine, which results in mutual antagonism.

Methenamine is not a primary drug for the treatment of acute urinary tract infections, but it is of value for chronic suppressive treatment. The agent is most useful when the causative organism is *E. coli*, but it usually can suppress the common Gram-negative offenders, and often *S. aureus* and *S. epidermidis* as well. *E. aerogenes* and *P. vulgaris* are usually resistant. Urea-splitting bacteria (mostly *Proteus*) make it difficult to control the urine pH. The physician should strive to keep the pH below 5.5.

METHICILLIN SODIUM

(Staphcillin)

Methicillin, a penicillinase-resistant penicillin (4 to 12 g IM or IV daily), is used in systemic infections caused by susceptible organisms (see also Table 23).

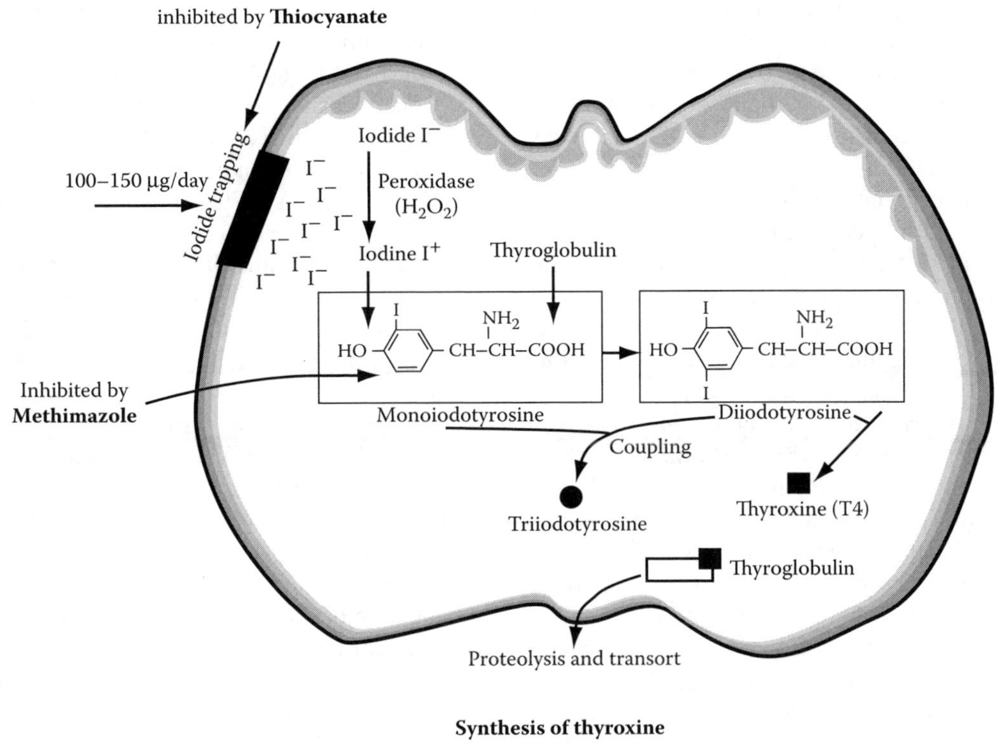

FIGURE 66 Methimazole inhibits the synthesis of thyroid hormone by interfering with the incorporation of iodine into tyrosine and the formation of iodothyronine.

METHIMAZOLE

(Tapazole tablets 5 mg)

Methimazole is an antithyroid agent that inhibits synthesis of thyroid hormones. It is indicated in long-term therapy of hyperthyroidism; and amelioration of hyperthyroidism in preparation for subtotal thyroidectomy or radioactive iodine therapy.

Methimazole (15 to 60 mg p.o. daily until patients are euthyroid) is indicated in the treatment of hyperthyroidism. Propylthiouracil, carbimazole, and methimazole, thyroid hormone antagonists, exert their effects by inhibiting iodide organification, and by inhibiting the formation of diiodothyronine (DIT) (see Figure 66).

These agents possess a thiocarbamide moiety

$$\overset{\displaystyle S}{\overset{\|}{\text{(-N-C-R)}}}$$

which is essential for their antithyroid actions. The onset of their beneficial effects is slow and takes 3 to 4 weeks. In preparation for thyroidectomy, methimazole inhibits the synthesis of the thyroid hormone and causes a euthyroid state, reducing surgical problems during thyroidectomy; as a result, the mortality for a single-stage thyroidectomy is low. Iodide reduces the vascularity of the gland, making it less friable. For treating thyrotoxic crisis (thyrotoxicosis), propylthiouracil (PTU), theoretically, is preferred over methamazole because it inhibits peripheral deiodination of thyroxine to triiodothyronine. Methimazole is absorbed orally, crosses the placental barrier, and is concentrated in the thyroid gland. It is metabolized in the liver and partially (7%) excreted unchanged. Clinical manifestations of overdose include nausea, vomiting, epigastric distress, fever, headache, arthralgia, pruritus, edema, and pancytopenia.

The **antithyroid drugs** that have clinical utility are the **thioureylenes**, which belong to the family of thionamides. **Propylthiouracil** may be considered as the prototype.

The antithyroid compounds currently used in the United States are **propylthiouracil** (6-*n*-propylthiouracil) and **methimazole** (*l*-methyl-2-mercaptoimidazole; Tapazole). In Great Britain and Europe, carbimazole (Neo-mercazole), a carbethoxy derivative of **methimazole**, is available, and its antithyroid action is due to its conversion to methimazole after absorption. Measurements of the course of organification of radioactive iodine by the thyroid show that absorption of effective amounts of propylthiouracil follows within 20 to 30 minutes of an oral dose, and that the duration of action of the compounds used clinically is brief. The effect of a dose of 100 mg of propylthiouracil begins to wane in 2 to 3 hours, and even a 500-mg dose is completely inhibitory for only 6 to 8 hours. As little as 0.5 mg of **methimazole** similarly decreases the organification of radioactive iodine in the thyroid gland, but a single dose of 10 to 25 mg is needed to extend the inhibition to 24 hours.

The half-life of propylthiouracil in plasma is about 75 minutes, whereas that of **methimazole** is 4 to 6 hours. The drugs are concentrated in the thyroid, and methimazole, derived from the metabolism of carbimazole, accumulates after carbimazole is administered. Drugs and metabolites appear largely in urine.

Propylthiouracil and **methimazole** cross the placenta and also can be found in breast milk.

The incidence of side effects from propylthiouracil and **methimazole** as currently used is relatively low. The overall incidence as compiled from published cases by early investigators was 3% for propylthiouracil and 7% for **methimazole**, with 0.44% and 0.12% of cases, respectively, developing the most serious reaction, **agranulocytosis**. The development of agranulocytosis with **methimazole** is probably dose related, but no such relationship exists with propylthiouracil. Further observations have found little, if any, difference in side effects between these two agents, and suggest that an incidence of agranulocytosis of approximately 1 in 500 is a maximal figure. Agranulocytosis usually occurs during the first few weeks or months of therapy but may occur later. Because it can develop rapidly, periodic white cell counts usually are of little help. Patients should immediately report the development of sore throat or fever, which usually heralds the onset of this reaction. Agranulocytosis is reversible upon discontinuation of the offending drug, and the administration of recombinant human **CSF** may hasten recovery. Mild granulocytopenia, if noted, may be due to thyrotoxicosis or may be the first sign of this dangerous drug reaction. Caution and frequent leukocyte counts are then required.

The most common reaction is a mild, occasionally purpuric, urticarial papular rash. It often subsides spontaneously without interrupting treatment, but it sometimes calls for the administration of an antihistamine, corticosteroids, or changing to another drug (cross-sensitivity to propylthiouracil and **methimazole** is uncommon). Other less frequent complications are pain and stiffness in the joints, paresthesias, headache, nausea, skin pigmentation, and loss of hair. Drug fever, hepatitis, and nephritis are rare, although abnormal liver function tests are not infrequent with higher doses of propylthiouracil. Although vasculitis was previously thought to be a rare complication, **antineutrophilic cytoplasmic antibodies** (ANCAs) have been reported to occur in about 50% of patients receiving propylthiouracil, and rarely with **methimazole**.

The antithyroid drugs are used in the treatment of hyperthyroidism in the following three ways: (1) as definitive treatment, to control the disorder in anticipation of a spontaneous remission in **Graves' disease**; (2) in conjunction with radioactive iodine to hasten recovery while awaiting the effects of radiation; and (3) to control the disorder in preparation for surgical treatment.

The usual starting dose for propylthiouracil is 100 mg every 8 hours or 150 mg every 12 hours. When doses larger than 300 mg daily are needed, further subdivision of the time of administration to every 4 to 6 hours is occasionally helpful. **Methimazole** is effective when given as a single daily dose because of its relatively long plasma and intrathyroidal half-life, as well as its long duration of action. Failures of response to daily treatment with 300 to 400 mg of propylthiouracil or 30 to 40 mg of **methimazole** are most commonly due to noncompliance. Delayed responses also are noted in patients with very large **goiters,** or those in whom iodine in any form has been given beforehand. Once euthyroidism is achieved, usually within 12 weeks, the dose of antithyroid drug can be reduced, but not stopped, lest an enhanced recurrence of Graves' disease occurs.

The thyrotoxic state usually improves within 3 to 6 weeks after the initiation of antithyroid drugs. The clinical response is related to the dose of antithyroid drug, the size of the goiter, and pretreatment serum T_3 concentrations. The rate of response is determined by the quantity of stored hormone, the rate of turnover of hormone in the thyroid, the half-life of the hormone in the periphery, and the completeness of the block in synthesis imposed by the dosage given. When large doses are continued, and sometimes with the usual dose, hypothyroidism may develop as a result of overtreatment. The earliest signs of hypothyroidism call for a reduction in dose; if they have advanced to the point of discomfort, thyroid hormone in full replacement doses can be given to hasten recovery; then the lower maintenance dose of antithyroid drug is instituted for continued therapy. Despite initial suggestions to the contrary, there is no benefit of combination levothyroxine and **methimazole** therapy on either remission rates or on changes in serum concentrations of thyroid-stimulating immunoglobulins.

After treatment is initiated, patients should be examined and thyroid function tests (serum-free thyroxine index and total triiodothyronine concentrations) measured every 2 to 4 months. Once euthyroidism is established, follow-up every 4 to 6 months is reasonable.

Control of hyperthyroidism usually is associated with a decrease in goiter size, but if the thyroid enlarges, hypothyroidism probably has been induced. When this occurs, the dose of the antithyroid drug should be significantly decreased and/or levothyroxine can be added once hypothyroidism is confirmed by laboratory testing.

Antithyroid drugs have been used in many patients to control the hyperthyroidism of Graves' disease until a remission occurs. Early investigators reported that 50% of patients so treated for 1 year remained well without further therapy for long periods, perhaps indefinitely. More recent reports have indicated that a much smaller percentage of patients sustain remissions after such treatment. Increased dietary iodine has been implicated in the latter, less favorable rates.

Unfortunately, there is no way of predicting before treatment is begun which patients will eventually achieve a lasting remission and who will relapse. It is clear that a favorable outcome is unlikely when the disorder is of long standing, the thyroid is quite large, or various forms of treatment have failed. To complicate the issue further, remission and eventual hypothyroidism may represent the natural history of Graves' disease.

During treatment, a positive sign that a remission may have taken place is reduced size of the goiter. The persistence of goiter often indicates failure, unless the patient becomes hypothyroid. Another favorable indication is continued freedom from all signs of hyperthyroidism when the maintenance dose is small. Finally, a decrease in thyroid-stimulating immunoglobulins, suppression of ^{123}I thyroid uptake when thyroxine or triiodothyronine is given, and a normal serum thyroid-stimulating hormone (TSH) response to thyrotropin-releasing hormone (TRH) may be helpful in predicting a remission in some patients, although these tests are not routinely performed.

Because antithyroid drug therapy, radioactive iodine, and subtotal thyroidectomy all are effective treatments for Graves' disease, there is no worldwide consensus among endocrinologists as to the best approach to therapy. Prolonged drug therapy of Graves' disease in anticipation of a remission is most successful in patients with small goiters or mild hyperthyroidism. Those with large goiters or severe disease usually require definitive therapy with either surgery or radioactive iodine (^{131}I). Radioactive iodine remains the treatment of choice of many endocrinologists in the United States. Many investigators consider coexisting ophthalmopathy to be a relative contraindication for radioactive iodine therapy because worsening of ophthalmopathy has been reported after radioactive iodine, although this remains controversial. Others suggest that development of hypothyroidism, regardless of the treatment, is the strongest risk factor for progression of ophthalmopathy. Smoking may also be a risk factor for worsening ophthalmopathy. In older patients, depleting the thyroid gland of preformed hormone by treatment with antithyroid drugs is advisable prior to therapy with radioactive iodine, thus preventing a severe exacerbation of the hyperthyroid state during the subsequent development of radiation thyroiditis. Subtotal thyroidectomy is advocated for Graves' disease in young patients with large goiters, children who are allergic to antithyroid drugs, pregnant women (usually in the second trimester) who are allergic to antithyroid drugs, and patients who prefer surgery over antithyroid drugs of radioactive iodine. Radioactive iodine or surgery is indicated for definitive therapy in toxic nodular goiter because remissions following antithyroid drug therapy do not occur.

Thyrotoxicosis occurs in about 0.2% of pregnancies and is caused most frequently by Graves' disease. Antithyroid drugs are the treatment of choice; radioactive iodine is clearly contraindicated. Historically, propylthiouracil has been preferred over **methimazole** because transplacental passage was thought to be lower; however, both propylthiouracil and **methimazole** cross the placenta equally. Current data suggest that either may be used safely in the pregnant patient. Recent reports from Scandinavia, where carbimazole is used more frequently than propylthiouracil, have suggested that carbimazole administration is rarely associated with congenital gut abnormalities. The antithyroid drug dosage should be minimized in order to keep the serum-free thyroxine index in the upper half of the normal range or slightly elevated. As pregnancy progresses, Graves' disease often improves, and it is not uncommon for patients either to be on a very low dose or off antithyroid drugs completely by the end of pregnancy. Therefore, the antithyroid drug dose should be reduced, and maternal thyroid function should be frequently monitored in order to decrease chances of fetal hypothyroidism. Relapse or worsening of Graves' disease is common after delivery, and patients should be monitored closely. Propylthiouracil is the drug of choice in nursing women because very small amounts of the drug appear in breast milk and do not appear to affect thyroid function in the suckling baby. However, doses of **methimazole** up to 20 mg daily in nursing mothers have been shown to have no effect on thyroid function in the baby.

Several drugs that have no intrinsic antithyroid activity are useful in the symptomatic treatment of thyrotoxicosis. Adrenergic-receptor antagonists are effective in antagonizing the sympathetic/adrenergic effects of thyrotoxicosis, thereby reducing tachycardia, tremor, and stare, and relieving palpitations, anxiety, and tension. Either **propranolol**, 20 to 40 mg four times daily, or **atenolol**, 50 to 100 mg daily, is usually given initially. Propranolol or esmolol can be given intravenously if needed. Propranolol, in addition to its adrenergic-receptor-antagonist action, has weak inhibitory effects on peripheral $T_4 \rightarrow T_3$ conversion. Calcium-channel blockers (**diltiazem**, 60 to 120 mg four times daily) can be used to control tachycardia and decrease the incidence of supraventricular tachyarrhythmias. These drugs should be discontinued once the patient is euthyroid.

Other drugs that are useful in the rapid treatment of the severely thyrotoxic patient are agents that inhibit the peripheral conversion of thyroxine to triiodothyronine. **Dexamethasone** (0.5 to 1 mg two to four times daily), and the iodinated radiological contrast agents **iopanoic acid** (Telepaque, 500 to 1000 mg once daily), and **sodium ipodate** (Oragrafin, 500 to 1000 mg once daily) are effective in preoperative preparation. Neither iopanoic acid nor sodium ipodate is available in the United States. **Cholestyramine** has been used in severely toxic patients to bind thyroid hormones in the gut and thus block the enterohepatic circulation of the iodothyronines.

METHOCARBAMOL

(Robaxin tablets 500 mg)

Methocarbamol is a centrally acting skeletal muscle relaxant. A carbamate derivative of guaifenesin (1.5 g p.o. q.i.d.), methocarbamol is used as an adjunct in acute, painful musculoskeletal conditions and in supportive therapy in tetanus management.

METHOCARBAMOL/ASPIRIN

(Methocarbamol w/ASA tablets 400 mg methocarbamol and 325 mg aspirin)

This compound may cause relaxation of skeletal muscle via general CNS depression. Aspirin inhibits prostaglandin synthesis, resulting in analgesia, antiinflammatory activity, and inhibition of platelet aggregation. It is indicated as an adjunct to rest, physical therapy, and other measures for the relief of discomfort associated with acute, painful, musculoskeletal conditions.

METHOHEXITAL SODIUM

(Brevital)

Methohexital (1 mg/kg in 1% solution given at a rate of 1 mL/5 seconds) is used for induction of anesthesia lasting 5 to 7 minutes. Maintenance of anesthesia may be accomplished by intermittent injections of 1% solution or by continuous IV drip of a 0.2% solution. Intermittent injections of about 20 to 40 mg (2 to 4 ml of a 1% solution) may be given as required, usually every 4 to 7 minutes. For continuous drip, the average rate of administration is about 3 mL of a 0.2% solution/min (1 drop/second). Methohexital should not be mixed in the same syringe or administered simultaneously during IV infusion through the same needle with acid solutions, such as atropine sulfate, metocurine iodide, and succinylcholine chloride.

METHOTREXATE

(Amethopterin)

Methotrexate is a folic acid antagonist that binds to dihydrofolate reductase, thus interfering with the synthesis of the active cofactor tetrahydrofolic acid, which is necessary for the synthesis of thymidylate, purine nucleotides, and the amino acids serine and methionine. Methotrexate is used for the following types of cancer:

Acute lymphoid leukemia: During the initial phase, vincristine and prednisone are used; methotrexate and mercaptopurine are used for maintenance therapy; in addition, methotrexate is given intrathecally, with or without radiotherapy, to prevent meningeal leukemia

Diffuse histiocytic lymphoma: Cyclophosphamide, vincristine, methotrexate, and cytarbine (COMA)

Mycosis fungoides: Methotrexate

Squamous cell, large-cell anaplastic, and adenocarcinoma: Doxorubicin and cyclophosphamide, or methotrexate

Head and neck squamous cell: *Cis*-platinum and bleomycin, or methotrexate

Choriocarcinoma: Methotrexate

Tumor cells acquire resistance to methotrexate as a result of several factors, which include deletion of a high-affinity, carrier-mediated transport system for reduced folates, an increase in the concentration of dihydrofolate reductase, and the formation of a biochemically altered reductase with reduced affinity for methotrexate. To overcome this resistance, higher doses of methotrexate need to be administered. The effects of methotrexate may be reversed by the administration of leucovorin, the reduced folate. This leucovorin "rescue" prevents or reduces the toxicity of methotrexate, which is expressed as mouth lesions (stomatitis), injury to the gastrointestinal epithelium (diarrhea), leukopenia, and thrombocytopenia.

METHOTRIMEPRAZINE HYDROCHLORIDE

(Levoprome)

Methotrimeprazine, a propylamino phenothiazine, with sedative, analgesic, and antipyretic properties, is used to induce preanesthetic sedation and analgesia, and postoperative analgesia.

METHOXAMINE HYDROCHLORIDE

(Vasoxyl)

Methoxamine, a sympathomimetic agent with alpha-adrenergic-stimulating effects (3 to 5 mg IV injected slowly), is indicated in supporting, restoring, or maintaining blood pressure during anesthesia. It produces potent and prolonged pressor action without causing cardiac acceleration. Methoxamine occasionally causes bradycardia, which is abolished by atropine. It should be used cautiously in patients with hyperthyroidism, bradycardia, partial heart block, myocardial diseases, or severe arteriosclerosis. Bretylium may potentiate the action of methoxamine on adrenergic receptors, possibly resulting in arrhythmias; guanethidine may increase the pressor response of methoxamine, possibly resulting in severe hypertension; halogenated hydrocarbon anesthetics do sensitize the myocardium to the effects of catecholamines. Methoxamine and halothane may lead to serious arrhythmias. Methoxamine is used in obstetrics to correct hypotension or is added to the local anesthetic solution. Some oxytocics may cause severe and persistent hypertension; and tricyclic antidepressants, such as imipramine, potentiate the pressor effects of methoxamine.

METHOXSALEN

(8-MOP capsules 10 mg)

Methoxsalen is a psoralen that acts as a photosensitizer. A psoralen derivative with pigmenting properties (12 to 20 mg p.o.), methoxsalen is used to induce repigmentation in vitiligo.

Photochemotherapy with psoralen-containing plant extracts was employed for the treatment of vitiligo in Egypt and India as early as 1500 B.C. Orally administered **8-methoxypsoralen** followed by UVA (PUVA) is FDA approved for the treatment of vitiligo, psoriasis, and cutaneous T-cell lymphoma.

Psoralens belong to the **furocoumarin** class of compounds, which are derived from the fusion of a **furan** with a **coumarin**. They occur naturally in many plants, including limes, lemons, figs, and parsnips. Two psoralens,

8-methoxypsoralen (**methoxsalen**) and **4, 5, 8-trimethylpsoralen** (trioxsalen, Trisoralen) are available in the United States. **Methoxsalen** is used primarily because of its superior gastrointestinal absorption.

The psoralens are absorbed rapidly after oral administration. Photosensitivity typically is maximal 1 to 2 hours after ingestion of **methoxsalen**. There is significant but saturable first-pass elimination in the liver, which may account for variations in plasma levels among individuals after a standard dose. **Methoxsalen** has a serum half-life of approximately 1 hour, but the skin remains sensitive to light for 8 to 12 hours. Despite widespread drug distribution throughout the body, it is photoactivated only in the skin where the UVA penetrates.

The mechanism by which PUVA induces photosensitivity is not known. The action spectrum for oral PUVA is between 320 and 400 nm. Two distinct photoreactions take place. Type I reactions involve the oxygen-independent formation of mono- and bifunctional adducts in DNA. Type II reactions are oxygen-dependent and involve sensitized transfer of energy to molecular oxygen. The therapeutic effects of PUVA in psoriasis may result from a decrease in DNA-dependent proliferation after adduct formation. Perhaps more importantly, PUVA can alter cytokine profiles and cause immunocyte apoptosis, thereby interrupting immunopathologic processes.

PUVA promotes melanogenesis in normal skin. Increased pigmentation results from augmented transfer of melanosomes from melanocytes to keratinocytes; however, there is no change in the size of melanosomes or in their distribution pattern.

Methoxsalen is supplied in soft gelatin capsules (Oxsoralen-Ultra) and hard gelatin capsules (8-MOP). The dose is 0.4 mg/kg for the soft capsule and 0.6 mg/kg for the hard capsule taken 1.5 to 2 hours before UVA exposure. A lotion containing 1% **methoxsalen** (Oxsoralen) also is available for topical application. It can be diluted for use in bath water to minimize systemic absorption. The risk of phototoxicity is increased with topical PUVA therapy. In U.S. and European multicenter cooperative studies of PUVA for the treatment of psoriasis, initial clearance rates approaching 90% were achieved. Relapse occurs within 6 months of cessation of treatment in many patients, which has prompted efforts to design maintenance protocols.

PUVA also is used to repigment the leukoderma of vitiligo. Success rates are highest in young individuals with recent onset of disease involving nonacral areas. Localized vitiligo can be treated with topical PUVA and more extensive disease with systemic administration. PUVA also is employed in the treatment of cutaneous T-cell lymphoma, atopic dermatitis, alopecia areata, lichen planus, urticaria pigmentosa, and as a preventive modality in some forms of photosensitivity.

The major acute side effects of PUVA include nausea, blistering, and painful erythema. PUVA-induced redness and blistering generally peak within 48 to 72 hours.

Chronic PUVA therapy accelerates photoaging and the development of actinic keratoses, nonmelanoma skin cancer, and melanoma. Squamous cell carcinomas occur at 10 times the expected frequency. In patients receiving 250 or more treatments, there is an increased risk of melanoma. Careful monitoring of patients for cutaneous carcinoma therefore is essential.

Extracorporeal photopheresis (ECP) is a form of pheresis therapy that has proven effective in the treatment of cutaneous T-cell lymphoma. After oral administration of **methoxsalen**, leukocytes are separated from whole blood using an ECP device and then exposed to UVA radiation. The irradiated cells then are returned to the patient. Multiple mechanisms probably contribute to the effectiveness of this procedure. ECP simultaneously and efficiently induces apoptosis of disease-causing T-cells and conversion of monocytes to functional dendritic cells by processing and presenting the unique antigenic determinants of pathogenic T-cell clones, the dendritic cells either initiate a clinically relevant anticutaneous T-cell lymphoma cytotoxic response or suppress the activity of autoreactive T-cell clones.

Photodynamic therapy (PDT) combines the use of photosensitizing drugs and visible light for the treatment of various dermatological disorders, particularly nonmelanoma skin cancer and precancerous actinic keratoses. The concept is predicated on the insight that tumor tissue selectively absorbs greater amounts of porphyrins than surrounding nontumor tissue. The agents most widely employed in PDT are porphyrins, their precursors, or derivatives thereof. The photosensitized chemical reaction is oxygen-dependent. Light delivered to the skin is absorbed by porphyrin molecules. These molecules transfer their energy to oxygen, forming reactive oxygen species that result in injury or destruction of lipid-rich membranes and subsequent tissue damage.

Methotrexate: The antimetabolite **methotrexate** is a folic acid analog that competitively inhibits dihydrofolate reductase. Methotrexate has been used for moderate to severe psoriasis since 1951. It suppresses immunocompetent cells in the skin, and it also decreases the expression of cutaneous lymphocyte-associated antigen (CLA)-positive T-cells and endothelial cell E-selectin, which may account for its efficacy in psoriasis. It is useful in treating a number of other dermatological conditions, including **pityriasis lichenoides et varioliformis**, **lymphomatoid papulosis**, **sarcoidosis**, **pemphigus vulgaris**, **pityriasis rubra pilaris**, **lupus erythematosus**, **dermatomyositis**, and **cutaneous T-cell lymphoma**.

METHOXYFLURANE

(Penthrane)

Methoxyflurane is the most potent of the inhalational anesthetics. It is metabolized extensively to fluoride and other nephrotoxic products. Because methoxyflurane does not alter uterine contraction during labor, it is valuable for obstetric anesthesia. Its toxic effects on the respiration and cardiovascular systems are similar to those produced by halothane. Methoxyflurane reduces renal blood flow and the glomerular filtration rate (see also Table 16).

METHSCOPOLAMINE BROMIDE

(Pamine tablets 2.5 mg)

Methscopolamine is a quaternary anticholinergic agent that competitively inhibits action of acetylcholine at muscarinic receptors. Methscopolamine, an anticholinergic agent with gastrointestinal antispasmodic properties (2.5 to 5 mg p.o. one-half hour before meals), is used as an adjunctive therapy in peptic ulcer and irritable bowel syndrome (IBS).

Anticholinergic agents ("spasmolytics" or "antispasmodics") often are used in patients with IBS. The most common agents of this class available in the United States are nonspecific antagonists of the muscarinic receptor and include the tertiary amines **dicyclomine** (Bentyl) and **hyoscyamine** (Levsin, others), and the quaternary ammonium compounds **glycopyrrolate** (Robinul) and **methscopolamine** (Pamine). The advantage of the latter two compounds is that they have a limited propensity to cross the blood–brain barrier and hence a lower risk for neurological side effects such as light-headedness, drowsiness, or nervousness. These agents typically are given either on an as-needed basis (with the onset of pain) or before meals to prevent the pain and fecal urgency that predictably occur in some patients with IBS (with presumed exaggerated gastrocolic reflex).

Dicyclomine is given in doses of 10 to 20 mg orally every 4 to 6 hours as necessary. Hyoscyamine is available in many forms, including oral capsules, tablets, elixir, drops, a nonaerosol spray (0.125 to 0.25 mg every 4 hours as needed), and an extended-release form for oral use (0.375 mg every 12 hours as needed). Glycopyrrolate also comes in extended-release tablets (2 mg once or twice a day), in addition to a standard-release form (1 mg up to three times a day). **Methscopolamine** is provided as 2.5-mg tablets, and the dose is 1 or 2 tablets, three to four times a day.

METHSUXIMIDE

(Celantin)

Methsuximide belongs to the succinimide family (ethosuximide and phensuximide), which share a common heterocyclic (succinimide) ring. Methsuximide is a nonpolar chemical compound that is water soluble and slightly lipophilic. Its exact effects on excitable membranes are not known. An antagonistic against absence and partial seizures, methsuximide may have more than one mechanism of action, including effects on transmitter release; calcium uptake into presynaptic endings; and conductance of sodium, potassium, and chloride. Methsuximide is quickly absorbed through the gastrointestinal tract, and peak plasma levels are achieved in 2 to 4 hours. The drug is distributed evenly throughout the body, and penetrates brain and fat tissue better than ethosuximide. Because its protein binding and solubility are poor, methsuximide equilibrates with cerebrospinal fluid. It is rapidly metabolized to *N*-desmethylmethsuximide or 2-methyl-2-phenyl succinimide in hours, and has a mean half-life of 1.4 hours. Methsuximide has a wide spectrum of antiepileptic activity and is effective in complex partial seizures, generalized tonic–clonic seizures, and absence seizures. Furthermore, methsuximide is an effective adjunctive agent in the management of refractory complex partial seizures.

Common adverse experiences such as gastrointestinal disturbance, lethargy, somnolence, fatigue, and headache may be seen with methsuximide, but these usually are transient and dose related. Other adverse experiences include hiccups, irritability, ataxia, blurred vision or diplopia, inattention, dysarthria, and psychic changes. In some patients, headache, photophobia, and hiccups require withdrawal of methsuximide. Transient leukopenia has been reported. Delayed profound coma after methsuximide overdose has been described.

Methsuximide increases the serum concentrations of phenobarbital and phenytoin, and reduces that of carbamezepine.

METHYCLOTHIAZIDE

(Aquatensen, Enduron, Ethon)

Methyclothiazide, a thiazide diuretic with antihypertensive properties (0.05 to 0.2 mg/kg p.o. daily), is used in edema or hypertension (see also Figure 17 and Table 25).

METHYL ALCOHOL

Methyl alcohol is used as an industrial solvent and as an adulterant that is added to ethyl alcohol to prevent its consumption. Methyl alcohol is metabolized to formaldehyde and formic acid, according to the following reactions:

$$\text{Methanol} \xrightarrow[\text{dehydrogenase}]{\text{Alcohol}} \text{formaldehyde} \xrightarrow[\text{dehydrogenase}]{\text{Alcohol}} \text{formic acid}$$

Besides producing all of the CNS effects discussed for ethyl alcohol, methyl alcohol consumption leads to acidosis and blindness. The treatment of methyl alcohol poisoning may include water and electrolyte replacement along with the administration of sodium bicarbonate to combat the acidosis. Ethyl alcohol may also be administered intravenously because it is a preferred substrate by liver alcohol dehydrogenase, thus allowing methyl alcohol to be excreted unmetabolized in the urine.

METHYLCELLULOSE

(Cellothyl, Citrucel, Cologel)

Methylcellulose, an absorbent and bulk-forming substance with laxative properties (one tablespoon powder in 240 mL water daily), is indicated in the treatment of chronic constipation.

METHYLDOPA AND METHYLDOPATE HYDROCHLORIDE

(Methyldopa tablets 250 mg methyldopa, tablets 500 mg methyldopa, methyldopate hydrochloride injection 50 mg/mL)

Methyldopa is a centrally acting antiadrenergic agent that causes central alpha-adrenergic stimulation, which inhibits sympathetic cardioaccelerator and vasoconstrictor centers; reduces plasma renin activity; and reduces standing and supine BP. It is indicated in the treatment of hypertension.

Alpha-methyldopa is used for the control of mild to severe hypertension. It is converted to alpha-methylnorepinephrine, whose main hypotensive effect is due to stimulation of presynaptic alpha$_2$-adrenergic receptors that leads to a reduction in the release of norepinephrine. In addition, it reduces the peripheral vascular resistance without altering the heart rate or cardiac output. Postural hypotension is mild and infrequent. Alpha-methyldopa can cause sedation, and tolerance to it can develop. Coomb's test will be positive (25%) in patients who are taking the drug. Alpha-methyldopa has a long onset and a short duration of action. It is especially useful in the management of hypertension complicated by renal dysfunction because it does not alter either renal blood flow or the glomerular filtration rate. It is contraindicated in patients with liver disease and may produce hepatitis-like symptoms (see also Figure 33).

Attention-deficit/hyperactivity disorder (ADHD), first evident in childhood, is characterized by excessive motor activity, difficulty in sustaining attention, and impulsiveness. Children with this disorder frequently are troubled by difficulties in school, impaired interpersonal relationships, and excitability. Academic underachievement is an important characteristic. A substantial number of children with this syndrome have characteristics that persist into adulthood, although in modified form. Behavioral therapy may be helpful in some patients. Catecholamines may be involved in the control of attention at the level of the cerebral cortex. A variety of stimulant drugs have been utilized in the treatment of ADHD, and they are particularly indicated in moderate to severe cases. **Dextroamphetamine** has been demonstrated to be more effective than placebo. **Methylphenidate** is effective in children with ADHD and is the most common intervention. Treatment may start with a dose of 5 mg of methylphenidate in the morning and at lunch; the dose is increased gradually over a period of weeks depending on the response as judged by parents, teachers, and the clinician. The total daily dose generally should not exceed 60 mg; because of its short duration of action, most children require two or three doses of methylphenidate each day. The timing of doses is adjusted individually in accordance with rapidity of onset of effect and duration of action.

Methylphenidate, dextroamphetamine, and amphetamine probably have similar efficacy in ADHD and are the preferred drugs in this disorder. Pemoline appears to be less effective, although like sustained-release preparations of methylphenidate (Ritalin SR, Concerta, Meta-Date), and amphetamine (Adderal XR), it may be used once daily in children and adults. Potential adverse effects of these medications include insomnia, abdominal pain, anorexia, and weight loss that may be associated with suppression of growth in children. Minor symptoms may be transient or may respond to adjustment of dosage or administration of the drug with meals. Other drugs that have been utilized include tricyclic antidepressants, antipsychotic agents, and clonidine.

Methyldopa (Aldomet) is a centrally acting antihypertensive agent. It is a prodrug that exerts its antihypertensive action via an active metabolite. Although used frequently as an antihypertensive agent in the past, methyldopa's significant adverse effects limit its current use in the United States to treatment of hypertension in pregnancy, where it has a record for safety.

Methyldopa (α-methyl-3,4-dihydroxy-L-phenylalanine), an analog of 3,4-dihydroxyphenylalanine (DOPA), is metabolized by the L-aromatic amino acid decarboxylase in adrenergic neurons to α-methyldopamine, which then is converted to α-methylnorepinephrine. α-Methylnorepinephrine is stored in the secretory vesicles of adrenergic neurons, substituting for norepinephrine (NE) itself. Thus, when the adrenergic neuron discharges its neurotransmitter, α-methylnorepinephrine is released instead of norepinephrine.

Because α-methylnorepinephrine is not as potent as norepinephrine as a vasoconstrictor, its substitution for norepinephrine in peripheral adrenergic neurosecretory vesicles does not alter the vasoconstrictor response to peripheral adrenergic neurotransmission. Rather, α-methylnorepinephrine acts in the CNS to inhibit adrenergic neuronal outflow from the brain stem. Methylnorepinephrine probably acts as an agonist at presynaptic α_2-adrenergic receptors in the brain stem, attenuating NE release and thereby reducing the output of vasoconstrictor adrenergic signals to the peripheral sympathetic nervous system.

Methyldopa reduces vascular resistance without causing much change in cardiac output or heart rate in younger patients with uncomplicated essential hypertension. In older patients, however, cardiac output may be decreased as a result of decreased heart rate and stroke volume; this is secondary to relaxation of veins and a reduction in preload. The fall in arterial pressure is maximal 6 to 8 hours after an oral or intravenous dose. Although the decrease in supine blood pressure is less than that in the upright position, symptomatic orthostatic hypotension is less common with **methyldopa** than with drugs that act exclusively on peripheral adrenergic neurons or autonomic ganglia; this is because methyldopa attenuates, but does not completely block, baroreceptor-mediated vasoconstriction. For this reason, it is well tolerated during surgical anesthesia. Any severe hypotension is reversible with volume expansion. Renal blood flow is maintained, and renal function is unchanged during treatment with **methyldopa**.

Plasma concentrations of norepinephrine fall in association with the reduction in arterial pressure, and this reflects the decrease in sympathetic tone. Renin secretion also is reduced by methyldopa, but this is not a major effect of the drug and is not necessary for its hypotensive effects. Salt and water often are gradually retained with prolonged use of methyldopa, and this tends to blunt the antihypertensive effect. This has been termed "pseudo-tolerance," and can be overcome with concurrent use of a diuretic.

Because methyldopa is a prodrug that is metabolized in the brain to the active form, its concentration in plasma has less relevance for its effects than that for many other drugs. When administered orally, methyldopa is absorbed by an active amino acid transporter. Peak concentrations in plasma occur after 2 to 3 hours. The drug is distributed in a relatively small apparent volume (0.4 L/kg) and is eliminated with a half-life of about 2 hours. The transport of methyldopa into the CNS is apparently also an active process. **Methyldopa** is excreted in the urine primarily as the sulfate conjugate (50 to 70%) and as the parent drug (25%). The remaining fraction is excreted as other metabolites, including methyldopamine, methylnorepinephrine, and *O*-methylated products of these catecholamines. The half-life of methyldopa is prolonged to 4 to 6 hours in patients with renal failure.

In spite of its rapid absorption and short half-life, the peak effect of methyldopa is delayed for 6 to 8 hours even after intravenous administration, and the duration of action of a single dose is usually about 24 hours; this permits once- or twice-daily dosing. The discrepancy between the effects of **methyldopa** and the measured concentrations of the drug in plasma is most likely related to the time required for transport into the CNS, conversion to the active metabolite storage of α-methyl norepinephrine, and its subsequent release in the vicinity of relevant α_2 receptors in the CNS. This is a good example of the potential for a complex relationship between a drug's pharmacokinetics and its pharmacodynamics. Patients with renal failure are more sensitive to the antihypertensive effect of methyldopa, but it is not known if this is due to alteration in excretion of the drug or to an increase in transport into the CNS.

In addition to lowering blood pressure, the active metabolite of methyldopa acts on α_2-adrenergic receptors in the brain stem to inhibit the centers that are responsible for wakefulness and alertness. Thus, methyldopa produces sedation that is largely transient. A diminution in psychic energy may persist in some patients, and depression occurs occasionally. Medullary centers that control salivation also are inhibited by α-adrenergic receptors, and methyldopa may produce dryness of the mouth. Other side effects that are related to the pharmacological effects in the CNS include a reduction in libido, parkinsonian signs, and hyperprolactinemia that may become sufficiently pronounced to cause **gynecomastia** and **galactorrhea**. It seems possible that accumulation of α-methyldopamine in dopaminergic neurons could account for some central effects. In individuals who have sinoatrial node dysfunction, methyldopa may precipitate severe bradycardia and sinus arrest, including that which occurs with carotid sinus hypersensitivity.

Methyldopa also produces some adverse effects that are not related to its pharmacological action. Hepatotoxicity, sometimes associated with fever, is an uncommon but potentially serious toxic effect of methyldopa. Prompt diagnosis of hepatotoxicity requires a low threshold for considering the drug as a cause for hepatitis-like symptoms (e.g., nausea, anorexia) and screening for hepatotoxicity (e.g., with determination of hepatic transaminases) after 3 weeks and again 3 months after initiation of treatment. The incidence of **methyldopa**-induced hepatitis is unknown, but about 5% of patients will have transient increases in hepatic transaminases in plasma. Hepatic dysfunction usually is reversible with prompt discontinuation of the drug, but will recur if methyldopa is given again; a few cases of fatal hepatic necrosis have been reported. It is advisable to avoid the use of methyldopa in patients with hepatic disease.

Methyldopa can cause hemolytic anemia. At least 20% of patients who receive methyldopa for a year develop a positive Coombs test (antiglobulin test) that is due to autoantibodies directed against the Rh antigen on erythrocytes. The development of a positive Coombs test is not necessarily an indication to stop treatment with methyldopa; 1 to 5% of these patients will develop a hemolytic anemia that requires prompt discontinuation of the drug. The Coombs test may remain positive for as long as a year after discontinuation of methyldopa, but the hemolytic anemia usually resolves within a matter of weeks. Severe hemolysis may be attenuated by treatment with glucocorticoids. Adverse effects that are even more rare include leukopenia, thrombocytopenia, red cell aplasia, lupus erythematosus-like syndrome, lichenoid and granulomatous skin eruptions, myocarditis, retroperitoneal fibrosis, pancreatitis, diarrhea, and malabsorption.

Methyldopa is an effective antihypertensive agent that has been replaced by other drugs in many parts of the world. It is a preferred drug for treatment of hypertension during pregnancy based on its effectiveness and safety for both mother and fetus.

The usual initial dose of **methyldopa** is 250 mg twice daily, and there is little additional effect with doses above 2 g per day. Administration of a single daily dose of methyldopa at bedtime minimizes sedative effects, but administration twice daily is required for some patients.

METHYLENE BLUE

(Urolene blue)

Methylene blue, a thiazide dye with urinary tract antiseptic properties (55 mg p.o. t.i.d.), is used in cystitis, urethritis, and chronic urolithiasis; in methemoglobinemia and cyanide poisoning; and in chronic methemoglobinemia.

METHYLERGONOVINE MALEATE

(Methergine tablets 0.2 mg)

Methylergonovine is a uterine stimulant that acts directly on smooth muscle of the uterus and increases tone, rate, and amplitude of rhythmic contractions, thereby inducing a rapid and sustained tetanic uterotonic effect that shortens the third stage of labor and reduces blood loss. It is indicated for management after delivery of placenta; postpartum atony and hemorrhage; subinvolution; and under full obstetric supervision, may be given in the second stage of labor following delivery of the anterior shoulder.

Methylergonovine (0.2 mg IM after delivery of placenta) increases the strength, duration, and frequency of uterine contractions and decreases uterine bleeding following placental delivery. It induces a rapid and sustained tetanic uterotonic effect that shortens the third stage of labor and reduces blood loss. The onset of action of methylergonovine when given intramuscularly is 2 to 5 minutes, and a maximum concentration is reached in 30 minutes. The excretion of methylergonovine appears to be both renal and hepatic in nature. Methylergonovine should be given intravenously slowly (within 60 seconds) and cautiously because sudden hypertension may ensue. It may be given orally (0.2 mg t.i.d.) for a maximum of one week to control uterine bleeding. The adverse reactions of methylergonovine include nausea, vomiting, hypertension, dizziness, headache, tinnitus, diaphoresis, palpitations, temporary chest pain, and dyspnea.

METHYLPHENIDATE HYDROCHLORIDE

(Ritalin)

Methylphenidate is indicated for the treatment of children with ADHD (5 to 10 mg p.o. daily) and for adults with narcolepsy (10 mg p.o. t.i.d.). Methylphenidate, a CNS stimulant and an analeptic, releases norepinephrine and hence stimulates the reticular activating system and the cerebral cortex. Its actions resemble those produced by amphetamine. Similar to other sympathomimetic agents, methylphenidate should be used with caution in patients with symptomatic cardiovascular disease, hyperthyroidism, angina pectoris, moderate to severe hypertension, or advanced arteriosclerosis because it may cause dangerous arrhythmias and blood pressure changes.

Methylphenidate should not be used with monoamine oxidase inhibitors such as tranylcypromine. Symptoms of overdose may include euphoria, confusion, delirium, coma, toxic psychosis, agitation, headache, vomiting, dry mouth, mydriasis, self-injury, fever, diaphoresis, tremors, hyperreflexia, muscle twitching, seizures, flushing, hypertension, tachycardia, palpitations, and arrhythmias.

Methylphenidate is a piperidine derivative that is structurally related to amphetamine. **Methylphenidate** (Ritalin, others) is a mild CNS stimulant with more prominent effects on mental than on motor activities. However, large doses produce signs of generalized CNS stimulation that may lead to convulsions. Its pharmacological properties are essentially the same as those of the amphetamines. **Methylphenidate** also shares the abuse potential of the amphetamines and is listed as a schedule II controlled substance in the United States. Methylphenidate is effective in the treatment of narcolepsy and ADHD.

Methylphenidate is readily absorbed after oral administration and reaches peak concentrations in plasma in about 2 hours. The drug is a racemate; its more potent (+) enantiomer has a half-life of about 6 hours, and the less potent (−) enantiomer has a half-life of about 4 hours. Concentrations in the brain exceed those in plasma. The main urinary metabolite is a deesterified product, ritalinic acid, which accounts for 80% of the dose. The use of **methylphenidate** is contraindicated in patients with glaucoma.

Dexmethylphenidate (Focalin) is the *d*-threo enantiomer of racemic methylphenidate. It is FDA approved for the treatment of ADHD and is listed as a schedule II controlled substance in the United States.

METHYLPREDNISOLONE

(Medrol)

Methylprednisolone is an intermediate-acting glucocorticoid with no mineralocorticoid properties (see also Tables 11 and 14). Glucocorticoids are used in:

- **Endocrine disorders** (e.g., primary or secondary adrenal cortical insufficiency)
- **Rheumatic disorders** (e.g., ankylosing spondylitis, acute or subacute bursitis, or tenosynovitis)
- **Collagen disease** (e.g., lupus erythematosus, acute rheumatic carditis)
- **Dermatologic diseases** (e.g., severe erythema multiforme, bullous dermatitis herpetiformis)
- **Ophthalmic disorders** (e.g., allergic conjunctivitis, keratitis)
- **Respiratory disorders** (e.g., bronchial asthma, seasonal allergic rhinitis)
- **Hematologic disorders** (e.g., idiopathic thrombocytopenic purpura, acquired hemolytic anemia)
- **Neoplastic diseases** (e.g., leukemias and lymphomas)
- **Edematous states** (e.g., nephrotic syndrome)
- **Gastrointestinal diseases** (e.g., ulcerative colitis, Crohn's disease)
- **Diseases of CNS** (e.g., multiple sclerosis)

In addition, glucocorticoids are used in spinal conditions. For example, methylprednisolone (32 mg/day) is used to reduce mortality in severe alcoholism and hepatitis; and methylprednisolone (IV within 8 hours of injury) is used to improve neurogenic function in acute spinal cord injury (see also Table 14).

There are two categories of toxic effects from therapeutic use of glucocorticoids: acute adrenal insufficiency due to too rapid withdrawal of corticosteroids after long-term use, resulting in fever, myalgia, arthralgia, malaise, anorexia, nausea, desquamation of skin, orthostatic hypotension, dizziness, fainting, dyspnea, and hypoglycemia; and cushingoid changes from continued use of large doses, resulting in moonface, central obesity, striae, hirsutism, acne, ecchymoses, hypertension, osteoporosis, myopathy, sexual dysfunction, diabetes, hyperlipidemia, peptic ulcer, increased susceptibility to infection, and electrolyte and fluid imbalance.

METHYLPREDNISOLONE
(Systemic) (MedroL)

METHYLPREDNISOLONE ACETATE
(dep-Medalone, Depoject, Depo-Medrol, Depopred, Depo-Predate, Duralone, Durameth, Medralone, Medrone, M-Prednisol, Rep-Ped)

METHYLPREDNISOLONE SODIUM SUCCINATE
(A-MethaPred, Solu-Medrol)

Methylprednisolone, a glucocorticoid with antiinflammatory and immunosuppressant properties, is used in the treatment of severe inflammation or immunosuppression. In addition, methylprednisolone has been used in the treatment or minimization of motor/sensory defects caused by acute spinal cord injury (see also Tables 11 and 14).

METHYLSALICYLATE
(Oil of wintergreen)

Paraamino salicylic acid has bacteriostatic activity against *Mycobacterium tuberculosis*. Methyl salicylate (oil of wintergreen) has been used in the past as a counterirritant. Salicylic acid (20% solution) has keratolytic properties and is used to remove cornified epidermis (corn). Because salicylic acid itself is too toxic for systemic use, the various salts of salicylate, including acetylsalicylic acid (aspirin), are used instead (see also Table 3).

METHYLTESTOSTERONE
(Android capsules 10 mg)

Methyltestosterone is an androgen that promotes growth and development of male reproductive organs, maintains secondary sex characteristics, increases protein anabolism, and decreases protein catabolism. It is indicated for replacement therapy in the following conditions associated with a deficiency or absence of endogenous testosterone: **primary hypogonadism** (congenital or acquired); **hypogonadotropic hypogonadism** (congenital or acquired); delayed puberty (males); and is used secondarily in advancing inoperable metastatic (skeletal) mammary cancer (females).

Methyltestosterone is used in male and female subjects with the following indications: hypogonadism, male climacteric, and impotence: 10 to 40 mg/day orally; androgen deficiency: 10 to 50 mg/day orally (5 to 25 mg buccal); postpubertal cryptorchidism: 30 mg/day orally; postpartum breast pain and engorgement: 80 mg/day orally for 3 to 5 days; and breast cancer: 50 to 200 mg/day orally (25 to 100 mg buccal). Methyltestosterone may cause edema. Retention of water in association with sodium chloride appears to be a consistent effect of the administration of androgen and accounts for much of the gain in weight, at least in short-term treatment. In the doses used to treat hypogonadism, retention of fluid usually does not lead to detectable edema, but edema may become troublesome when large doses are given in the treatment of neoplastic diseases. Edema also is common in patients with CHF or renal insufficiency, and in patients prone to edema from some other cause, such as cirrhosis of the liver or hypoproteinemia. Salt and water retention from androgens usually responds to the administration of natriuretics (see Table 8).

Methyltestosterone was the first androgen discovered to cause cholestatic hepatitis, but all androgens with 17 alpha-alkyl substitutions can cause this complication. Jaundice is the prominent clinical feature, and the underlying disturbance is stasis and accumulation of bile in the biliary capillaries of the central portion of the hepatic lobules without obstruction in the larger ducts. The hepatic cells usually exhibit only minor histological changes and remain viable. If jaundice occurs, it generally develops after 2 to 5 months of therapy. Alterations in various tests of hepatic function occur more commonly than jaundice and include increases in the concentration of bilirubin and the levels of aspartate aminotransferase and alkaline phosphatase in the plasma. The severity of the response is dependent on the dose of 17 alpha-alkyl-substituted testosterone analogs administered, and is particularly prominent when large amounts are given, as for palliation in neoplastic diseases. Disturbance of hepatic function has not been described with the parenteral use of testosterone esters. Consequently, testosterone esters should be administered instead of 17 alpha-substituted steroids in virtually all clinical situations (except hereditary angioneurotic edema). In particular, the use of 17 alpha-substituted esters should be avoided in patients with liver disease. Patients who have received 17 alpha-alkyl-substituted androgens for prolonged periods may develop hepatic adenocarcinoma. Most of the patients described received the derivatives for 1 to 7 years, and the complication may be more common in subjects with Fanconi's anemia. Androgens can decrease the concentration of thyroid-binding globulin in plasma and thereby influence thyroid function tests, increase the excretion of 17-ketosteroids, raise plasma LDL-cholesterol and lower plasma HDL-cholesterol concentrations, and increase the hematocrit. 17 alpha-alkyl-substituted steroids cause an increase in the hepatic synthesis and plasma concentrations of a variety of glycoproteins.

METHYLXANTHINES

Caffeine, theobromine, and theophylline are purine derivatives closely related to the xanthine bodies found in the urine and tissues of animals. Xanthine is 2:6 dioxypurine; caffeine is 1:3:7 trimethylxanthine; theobromine is 3:7 dimethylxanthine; and theophylline is 1:3 dimethylxanthine. They all resemble each other in most points of their pharmacological action, but they differ markedly in the relative intensity of their action on various functions. Thus, caffeine is the most potent CNS stimulant of the group; theobromine exerts the greatest action on the muscles; and theophylline is the most effective diuretic and coronary dilator. Theobromine has comparatively little effect on the CNS, whereas theophylline has no action on the muscles. Caffeine stimulates the CNS, in particular that part associated with psychical functions. Ideas become clearer; thought flows more easily and rapidly; and fatigue and drowsiness disappear.

METHYSERGIDE MALEATE

(Sansert)

Methysergide (4 to 8 mg daily) is indicated for prophylaxis of vascular headache. In addition, it is used for prevention or reduction of intensity and frequency in patients suffering from one or more severe vascular headaches per week or from vascular headaches that are so severe that preventive therapy is indicated, regardless of the frequency of attack. Methysergide is a semisynthetic ergot derivative that inhibits or blocks the effects of serotonin and ameliorates the attack in 1 to 2 days. Plasma serotonin levels are elevated during the preheadache phase of classical migraine and decreased during an attack. Without serotonin, the extracranial arteries are dilated and distended, resulting in headache. Methysergide may displace serotonin on receptor pressor sites of the walls of cranial arteries during a migraine attack and thereby preserve the vasoconstriction afforded by serotonin. Methysergide is a peripheral antagonist of serotonin, competitively blocking the serotonin receptor in the blood vessel. It also inhibits histamine release from mast cells and stabilizes platelets against spontaneous or induced release of serotonin. Centrally, methysergide may act as a serotonin agonist, especially in the midbrain. It has very weak uterotonic and emetic actions. Retroperitoneal fibrosis, pleuropulmonary fibrosis, and fibrotic thickening of cardiac valves may occur in patients receiving long-term methysergide therapy.

The use of methysergide is contraindicated in peripheral vascular disease, severe arteriosclerosis, severe hypertension, coronary artery disease, phlebitis or cellulitis of the lower limbs, pulmonary disease, collagen disease or fibrotic processes, impaired liver or renal function, and valvular heart disease (see also Figure 93).

The concurrent use of beta-adrenergic-receptor-blocking agents and methysergide may result in peripheral ischemia manifested by cold extremities with possible peripheral gangrene.

METIAMIDE

Metiamide, which was developed from burimamide by replacing a methylene group with an isoteric thio ether, is a histamine$_2$-(H_2) receptor antagonist with high specific activity, low toxicity, and good oral bioavailability in the treatment of acid-pepsin disease (see also Table 4).

Histamine, as a normal constituent of the gastric mucosa, controls both microcirculation and gastric secretion. The gastric secretagogs are acetylcholine, histamine, and gastrin. The action of acetylcholine is blocked by atropine, and the action of histamine is blocked by cimetidine, burimamide, and metiamide. No specific antagonist is available for gastrin. The histamine release in the brain and perhaps other sites involves exocytosis because this potassium-induced release is a calcium-dependent process. Histamine is released by many factors. For example, histamine is released by numerous drugs including reserpine, codeine, meperidine, hydralazine, morphine, *d*-tubocurarine, dextrans, and papaverine (see also Figure 59).

METIPRANOLOL

(OptiPranolol ophthalmic solution 0.3%)

Metipranolol is a beta-adrenergic-blocking agent, which reduces IOP, probably by reducing aqueous humor production and, to a minor extent, by slightly increasing outflow. It is indicated for treatment of elevated IOP in patients with ocular hypertension or glaucoma.

The β-receptor antagonists now are the next most common topical medical treatment. There are two classes of topical β-blockers. The nonselective ones bind to both β_1 and β_2 receptors and include **timolol maleate** and **hemihydrate**, **levobunolol**, **metipranolol**, and **carteolol**. There is one β_1-selective antagonist, **betaxolol**, available for ophthalmic use, but it is less efficacious than the nonselective β-blockers because the β receptors of the eye are largely of the β_2 subtype. However, because the β_1 receptors are found preferentially in the heart whereas the β_2 receptors are found in the lung, betaxolol is less likely to cause breathing difficulty. In the eye, the targeted tissues are the ciliary body epithelium and blood vessels, where β_2 receptors account for 75 to 90% of the total population. How β-blockade leads to decreased aqueous production and reduced IOP is uncertain. Production of aqueous humor seems to be activated by a β-receptor-mediated cyclic AMP-PKA pathway; β-blockade blunts adrenergic activation of this pathway by preventing catecholamine stimulation of the β receptor, thereby decreasing intracellular cAMP. Another hypothesis is that β-blockers decrease ocular blood flow, which decreases the ultrafiltration responsible for aqueous production.

When there are medical contraindications to the use of prostaglandin analogs or β-receptor antagonists, other agents, such as an α_2-adrenergic-receptor agonist or topical carbonic anhydrase inhibitor may be used as first-line therapy. The α_2-adrenergic agonists improve the pharmacologic profile of the nonselective sympathomimetic agent epinephrine and its derivative, **dipivefrin** (Propine). Epinephrine stimulates both α and β adrenergic receptors. The drug appears to decrease IOP by enhancing both conventional (via a β_2-receptor mechanism) and uveoscleral outflow (perhaps via prostaglandin production) from the eye. Although effective, epinephrine is poorly tolerated, principally due to localized irritation and hyperemia. Dipivefrin is an epinephrine prodrug that is converted into epinephrine by esterases in the cornea. It is much better tolerated but still is prone to cause epinephrine-like side effects. The α_2-adrenergic agonist **clonidine** is effective at reducing IOP, but also readily crosses the blood–brain barrier and causes systemic hypotension; as a result it no longer is used for glaucoma. In contrast, **apraclonidine** (Iopidine) is a relatively selective α_2-adrenergic agonist that is highly ionized at physiologic pH and therefore does not cross the blood–brain barrier. **Brimonidine** (Alphagan, others) is also a selective α_2-adrenergic agonist, but is lipophilic, enabling easy corneal penetration. Both apraclonidine and brimonidine reduce aqueous production and may enhance some uveoscleral outflow. Both appear to bind to pre- and postsynaptic α_2 receptors. By binding to the presynaptic receptors, the drugs reduce the amount of neurotransmitter release from sympathetic nerve stimulation and thereby lower IOP. By binding to postsynaptic α_2 receptors, these drugs stimulate the G_i pathway, reducing cellular cyclic AMP production, thereby reducing aqueous humor production.

The development of a topical carbonic anhydrase inhibitor took many years but was an important event because of the poor side-effect profile of oral carbonic anhydrase inhibitors (CAIs). **Dorzolamide** (Trusopt) and **brinzolamide** (Azopt) both work by inhibiting carbonic anhydrase (isoenzyme II), which is found in the ciliary body epithelium. This reduces the formation of bicarbonate ions, which reduces fluid transport and thus IOP.

Metoprolol (Lopressor, others) is a β_1-selective-receptor antagonist that is devoid of intrinsic sympathomimetic activity and membrane-stabilizing activity. The reflex sympathetic responses to heart failure may stress the failing heart and exacerbate the progress of the disease, and blocking those responses could be beneficial. A number of well-designed randomized clinical trials involving numerous patients have demonstrated that certain β-receptor antagonists are highly effective treatment for patients with all grades of heart failure secondary to left ventricular systolic dysfunction. The drugs have been shown to improve myocardial function, improve life quality, and to prolong life. From the point of view of the history of therapeutic advances in the treatment of CHF, it is interesting to note how this drug class has moved from being completely contraindicated to being the standard of care in many settings (see Figure 67).

Large trials have been conducted with **carvedilol**, **bisoprolol**, **metoprolol**, **xamoterol**, **bucindolol**, **betaxol**, **nebivolol**, and **talinolol**. Carvedilol, **metoprolol**, and bisoprolol all have been shown to reduce the mortality rate in large cohorts of patients with stable chronic heart failure regardless of severity. In the initial use of β-blockers for treating heart failure, the beginning effects often are neutral or even adverse. Benefits accumulate gradually over a period of weeks to months, although benefits from the third-generation vasodilator β-blocker carvedilol may be seen within days in patients with severe heart failure. There also is a reduction in the hospitalization of patients along with a reduction in mortality with fewer sudden deaths and deaths caused by progressive heart failure. These benefits

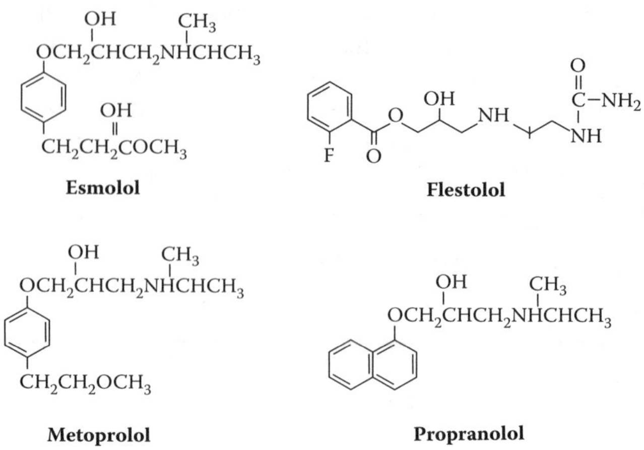

FIGURE 67 Metoprolol, a cardioselective beta_1-adrenergic receptor antagonist, is an antihypertensive agent used in the treatment of acute myocardial infarction.

extend to patients with asthma and with diabetes mellitus. Patients in atrial fibrillation and heart failure can also benefit from β-blockade. On the other hand, patients with heart failure and atrial fibrillation are associated with a higher mortality, and the benefit derived from β-blockers may not be comparable to those in sinus rhythm. Long-term β-blockade reduces cardiac volume, myocardial hypertrophy, and filling pressure, and increases ejection fraction (e.g., ventricular remodeling). β-Receptor antagonists impact mortality even before beneficial effects on ventricular function are observed, possibly due to prevention of arrhythmias or a reduction in acute vascular events.

Some patients are unable to tolerate β-blockers. Hopefully, ongoing trials will identify the common characteristics that define this population so that β-blockers can be avoided in these patients. Because of the real possibility of acutely worsening cardiac function, β-receptor antagonists should be initiated only by clinicians experienced in patients with CHF. As might be anticipated, starting with very low doses of drug and advancing doses slowly over time, depending on each patient's response, are critical for the safe use of these drugs in patients with CHF.

METIPRANOLOL HYDROCHLORIDE (OptiPranolol)

Metipranolol, a beta-adrenergic-blocking agent (instill 1 drop in each affected eye b.i.d.), is used in the treatment of ocular conditions in which lowering of IOP would be beneficial (ocular hypertension, chronic open-angle glaucoma).

METOCLOPRAMIDE (Maxolon tablets 10 mg)

Metoclopramide is an antidopaminergic/GI stimulant that stimulates upper GI tract motility, resulting in accelerated gastric emptying and intestinal transit and increased resting tone of lower esophageal sphincter. It exerts antiemetic properties through antagonism of central and peripheral dopamine receptors. **PO**: used in relief of symptoms associated with acute and recurrent diabetic gastroparesis; and short-term therapy of symptomatic, documented gastroesophageal reflux disease in adults who fail to respond to conventional therapy. **Parenteral**: used in prevention of nausea and vomiting associated with emetogenic cancer chemotherapy; prophylaxis of postoperative nausea and vomiting when nasogastric suction is undesirable; and facilitation of small-bowel intubation when tube does not pass pylorus with conventional maneuvers.

Oral metoclopramide is indicated in the treatment of diabetic gastroparesis (10 mg 30 minutes before each meal and at bedtime for 2 to 8 weeks) and symptomatic gastroesophageal reflux (10 to 15 mg orally up to 4 times daily 30 minutes before each meal and at bedtime for 4 to 12 weeks). Furthermore, parenteral metoclopramide is indicated in prevention of nausea and vomiting associated with emetogenic cancer chemotherapy, for prophylaxis of postoperative nausea and vomiting when nasogastric suction is undesirable, and as a single dose to facilitate small-bowel intubation when the tube does not pass the pylorus with conventional maneuvers.

Metoclopramide stimulates motility of the upper GI tract without stimulating gastric, biliary, or pancreatic secretions. It sensitizes the gastrointestinal tissues to the action of acetylcholine.

The antiemetic properties of metoclopramide appear to be a result of its antagonism of central and peripheral dopamine receptors. Dopamine produces nausea and vomiting by stimulation of the medullary chemoreceptor trigger zone (CTZ), and metoclopramide blocks stimulation of the CTZ by agents like levodopa or apomorphine that are known to increase dopamine levels or to possess dopamine-like effects. Metoclopramide also inhibits the central and peripheral effects of apomorphine and abolishes the slowing of gastric emptying caused by apomorphine.

Metoclopramide is contraindicated in the presence of GI hemorrhage, mechanical obstruction, or perforation. Because it is a dopamine-receptor-blocking agent, it causes extrapyramidal reactions such as dystonia and parkinsonism.

Metoclopramide increases gastric transit time, enhancing the absorption of substances absorbed in the small intestine (e.g., ethanol, cyclosporin) and decreasing the absorption of substances absorbed in the stomach (e.g., cimetidine, digoxin). Anticholinergic drugs and dopamine-function-enhancing substances such as levodopa reduce the effectiveness of metoclopramide. Because metoclopramide releases catecholamine, it should be used cautiously with monoamine oxidase inhibitors such as tranylcypromine. Because metoclopramide inhibits plasma cholinesterase, it increases the effectiveness of succinylcholine, a skeletal muscle relaxant.

Overdosage with metoclopramide causes drowsiness, disorientation, extrapyramidal reactions, muscle hypertonia, irritability, and agitation. Diphenhydramine, possessing anticholinergic and antihistaminic properties, may be used to treat the extrapyramidal reactions.

Metoclopramide (Reglan) and other substituted benzamides are derivatives of **paraaminobenzoic** acid and are structurally related to **procainamide**.

The mechanisms of action of **metoclopramide** are complex and involve 5-HT_4-receptor agonism, vagal and central 5-HT_3-antagonism, and possible sensitization of muscarinic receptors on smooth muscle, in addition to dopamine-receptor antagonism. **Metoclopramide** is one of the oldest true **prokinetic agents**; its administration results in coordinated contractions that enhance transit. Its effects are confined largely to the upper digestive tract, where it increases lower esophageal sphincter tone and stimulates antral and small-intestinal contractions. Despite having *in vitro* effects on the contractility of colonic smooth muscle, metoclopramide has no clinically significant effects on large-bowel motility.

Metoclopramide is absorbed rapidly after oral ingestion, undergoes sulfation and glucuronide conjugation by the liver, and is excreted principally in the urine, with a half-life of 4 to 6 hours. Peak concentrations occur within 1 hour after a single oral dose; the duration of action is 1 to 2 hours.

Metoclopramide has been used in patients with **gastroesophageal reflux disease** to produce symptomatic relief of, but not healing of, associated esophagitis. It clearly is less effective than modern acid-suppressive medications, such as **proton-pump inhibitors** or **histamine H_2-receptor antagonists**, and now rarely is used in this setting. Metoclopramide is indicated more often in symptomatic patients with **gastroparesis**, in whom it may cause mild to modest improvements of gastric emptying. **Metoclopramide** injection is used as an adjunctive measure in medical or diagnostic procedures such as intestinal intubation or contrast radiography of the GI tract. Although it has been used in patients with postoperative ileus, its ability to improve transit in disorders of small-bowel motility appears to be limited. In general, its greatest utility lies in its ability to ameliorate the nausea and vomiting that often accompany GI dysmotility syndromes. **Metoclopramide** has also been used in the treatment of persistent hiccups, but its efficacy in this condition is equivocal at best.

Metoclopramide is available in oral dosage forms (tablets and solution) and as a parenteral preparation for intravenous or intramuscular use. The usual initial oral dose range is 10 mg, 30 minutes before each meal and at bedtime. The onset of action is within 30 to 60 minutes after an oral dose. In patients with severe nausea, an initial dose of 10 mg can be given intramuscularly (onset of action 10 to 15 minutes) or intravenously (onset of action 1 to 3 minutes). For prevention of chemotherapy-induced emesis, metoclopramide can be given as an infusion of 1 to 2 mg per kg of body weight, administered over at least 15 minutes, beginning 30 minutes before the chemotherapy is begun and repeated as needed every 2 or 3 hours. Alternatively, a continuous intravenous infusion may be given (3 mg/kg of body weight before chemotherapy, followed by 0.5 mg/kg of body weight per hour for 8 hours). The usual pediatric dose for gastroparesis is 0.1 to 0.2 mg/kg of body weight per dose, given 30 minutes before meals and at bedtime.

The major side effects of metoclopramide include extrapyramidal effects, such as those seen with the phenothiazines. **Dystonias**, usually occurring acutely after intravenous administration, and **parkinsonian-like symptoms** that may occur several weeks after initiation of therapy generally respond to treatment with anticholinergic or antihistaminic drugs and are reversible upon discontinuation of metoclopramide. **Tardive dyskinesia** also can occur with chronic treatment (months to years) and may be irreversible. Extrapyramidal effects appear to occur more commonly in children and young adults and at higher doses. Like other dopamine antagonists, **metoclopramide** also can cause **galactorrhea** by blocking the inhibitory effect of dopamine on prolactin release, but this adverse effect is relatively infrequent in clinical practice. Methemoglobinemia has been reported occasionally in premature and full-term neonates receiving metoclopramide.

In contrast to **metoclopramide**, domperidone predominantly antagonizes the dopamine D_2 receptor with major involvement of other receptors. It is not available for use in the United States but has been used elsewhere (Motilium, others), and has modest prokinetic activity in doses of 10 to 20 mg three times a day. Although it does not readily cross the blood–brain barrier to cause extrapyramidal side effects, domperidone exerts effects in the parts of the CNS that lack this barrier, such as those regulating emesis, temperature, and prolactin release. As is the case with metoclopramide, domperidone does not appear to have any significant effects on lower gastrointestinal motility. Other D_2-receptor antagonists being explored as prokinetic agents include **levosulpiride**, the levoenantiomer of sulpiride.

METOCURINE IODIDE

(Metubine)

Metocurine, a skeletal muscle relaxant, is indicated as an adjunct to anesthesia, to facilitate endotracheal intubation (0.2 to 0.4 mg/kg), and to reduce the intensity of muscle contraction in pharmacologically or electrically induced convulsions. Metocurine is a methyl analog of tubocurarine, which produces nondepolarizing (competitive) neuromuscular blockade.

Histamine release with Metubine iodide occurs less frequently than with *d*-tubocurarine and is related to dosage and rapidity of administration. Effects on the cardiovascular system (e.g., changes in pulse rate, hypotension) are less than those reported with equivalent doses of *d*-tubocurarine and gallamine.

Because the main excretory pathway for Metubine iodide is through the kidneys, severe renal disease or conditions associated with poor renal perfusion (shock states) may result in prolonged neuromuscular blockade.

Following intravenous injection in the mother, placental transfer of Metubine iodide occurs rapidly, and, after 6 minutes, the fetal plasma concentration is approximately one-tenth the maternal level. Metocurine does not inhibit vagal transmission or sympathetic ganglionic blockade, and therefore produces minimal hemodynamic changes in humans. The relatively stable heart rate and blood pressure associated with its use make it a useful agent for patients with coronary artery disease and hypertension.

Parenteral administration of high doses of certain antibiotics may intensify or resemble the neuroblocking action of metocurine. These include neomycin, streptomycin, bacitracin, kanamycin, gentamicin, dihydrostreptomycin, polymyxin B, colistin, sodium colistimethate, and tetracyclines. If muscle relaxants and antibiotics must be administered simultaneously, the patient should be observed closely for any unexpected prolongation of respiratory depression. Certain general anesthetics have a synergistic action with neuromuscular blocking agents. Halothane and isoflurane potentiate the neuromuscular blocking action of other nondepolarizing agents and may be presumed to do so with Metubine iodide.

Administration of quinidine shortly after recovery may produce recurrent paranalysis. The use of magnesium sulfate in preeclamptic patients potentiates the effects of both depolarizing and nondepolarizing muscle relaxants (see also Figure 99).

The most frequently noted adverse reaction is prolongation of the drug's pharmacologic action. Neuromuscular effects may range from skeletal-muscle weakness to a profound relaxation that produces respiration insufficiency or apnea. Possible adverse reactions include allergic or hypersensitivity reactions to the drug or to its iodide content, and histamine release when large doses are administered rapidly. Signs of histamine release include erythema, edema, flushing, tachycardia, arterial hypotension, bronchospasm, and circulatory collapse. An overdose of Metubine iodide may result in prolonged apnea, cardiovascular collapse, and sudden release of histamine. Massive doses of metocurine are not reversible by the antagonists edrophonium or neostigmine and atropine. Overdosage may be avoided by the careful monitoring of response by means of a peripheral nerve stimulator. The primary treatment for residual neuromuscular blockade with respiratory paralysis or inadequate ventilation is maintenance of the patient's airway and manual or mechanical ventilation. Accompanying derangements of blood pressure, electrolyte imbalance, or circulating blood volume should be determined and corrected by appropriate fluid and electrolyte therapy. Residual neuromuscular blockade following surgery may be reversed by the use of anticholinesterase inhibitors such as neostigmine or pyridostigmine bromide and atropine.

METOLAZONE

(Zaroxolyn tablets 2.5 mg)

Metolazone is a thiazide diuretic that increases urinary excretion of sodium and chloride by inhibiting reabsorption in the ascending limb of the loop of Henle and early distal tubules. It is indicated in the treatment of edema and hypertension.

Metolazone is a quinazoline derivative with thiazide-like diuretic properties that is indicated in the treatment of edema associated with heart failure and hypertension (2.5 to 5 mg p.o./day). Metolazone increases urinary excretion of sodium and water by inhibiting sodium reabsorption in the cortical diluting tubule of the nephron, thus relieving edema. It may be more effective in edema associated with impaired renal function than thiazide or thiazide-like diuretics. Metolazone is thought to be a direct vasodilator, and by decreasing the body's sodium, reduces the total peripheral resistance. About 70 to 95% of metolazone is excreted unchanged in urine. Its half-life is about 14 hours in healthy subjects; it may be prolonged in patients with decreased creatinine clearance. Metolazone should be used cautiously in patients with severe renal disease because it may decrease glomerular filtration rate and precipitate azotemia; in patients with impaired hepatic function or liver disease because electrolyte changes may precipitate coma; and in patients taking digoxin because hypokalemia may predispose them to digitalis toxicity. Metolazone potentiates the hypotensive effects of most other antihypertensive drugs; this may be used to therapeutic advantage. Metolazone may potentiate the hyperglycemic, hypotensive, and hyperuricemic effects of diazoxide, and its hyperglycemic effect may increase insulin or sulfonylurea requirements in diabetic patients (see also Figure 17).

Metolazone may reduce renal clearance of lithium, elevating serum lithium levels, and may necessitate a 50% reduction in lithium dosage. It turns urine slightly more alkaline and may decrease urinary excretion of some amines, such as amphetamine and quinidine; alkaline urine may also decrease therapeutic efficacy of methenamine compounds such as methamine mandelate. Cholestyramine and colestipol may bind metolazone, preventing its absorption; give drugs 1 hour apart. Clinical signs of overdose include GI irritation and hypermotility, diuresis, and lethargy, which may progress to coma.

METOPROLOL TARTRATE

(Lopressor)

In the treatment of hypertension, a major use of beta-blockers is in combination with hydralazine. The direct vasodilators bring about reflex cardiac stimulation, and beta-blockers prevent these adverse effects (see also Figure 67). Beta-blockers also reduce blood pressure by exerting a central effect or a peripheral action, or both, which decreases renin activity. Metoprolol and atenolol are $beta_1$ selective, and they are safer agents in patients with asthma, diabetes mellitus, or low-renin hypertension. Some beta-blocking agents such as pindolol have intrinsic sympathomimetic activity and may be used in the treatment of pronounced bradycardia (sick sinus syndrome). Unlike propranolol, metoprolol is not a very lipid-soluble substance, does not enter the brain, and does not cause CNS toxicity (see Figure 70).

In the treatment of hypertension, metoprolol is used in an initial dose of 100 mg/day in single or divided doses, used alone or added to a diuretic. The dosage may be increased at weekly intervals until optimum blood pressure reduction is achieved. In the treatment of angina pectoris, metoprolol is used in an initial dose of 100 mg/day in two divided doses. Dosage may be gradually increased at weekly intervals until optimum clinical response is obtained or a pronounced slowing of heart rate occurs. The effective dosage range is 100 to 400 mg/day. In the treatment of myocardial infarction, treatment with metoprolol should be initiated as soon as possible after the patient's arrival in a coronary care or similar unit immediately after the patient is hemodynamically stable. The patient should receive three intravenous bolus doses of 5 mg each at 2-minute intervals. Then 50 mg of metoprolol is given orally every 6 hours for 48 hours, followed by a maintenance dose of 100 mg b.i.d.

METRIFONATE

(Bilarcil)

Metrifonate is an organophosphorous-inhibiting cholinesterase in *Schistosoma haematobium*. Because the plasma cholinesterase in the host is similarly inhibited, depolarizing neuromuscular blocking agents, other cholinesterase inhibitors, and agents metabolized by plasma cholinesterase should not be administered with metrifonate (see also Figure 79).

METRONIDAZOLE HYDROCHLORIDE

(Protostat)

Metronidazole is indicated in the treatment of symptomatic trichomoniasis in females and males when the presence of the trichomonad has been confirmed by appropriate laboratory procedures; and in the treatment of asymptomatic females when the organism is associated with endocervitis, cervicitis, or cervical erosion. Metronidazole is also indicated in the treatment of acute intestinal amebiasis (amebic dysentery and amebic liver abscess). It is indicated in the treatment of serious infections caused by susceptible anaerobic bacteria. Indicated surgical procedures should be performed in conjunction with metronidazole therapy. In a mixed aerobic and anaerobic infection, antibiotics appropriate for the treatment of the aerobic infection should be used in addition to metronidazole.

In the treatment of most serious anaerobic infections, metronidazole IV 15 mg/kg infused over one hour is usually administered initially. This may be followed by oral therapy with metronidazole at the discretion of the physician.

The nitro group of metronidazole is reduced inside the infecting organism; this reduction product disrupts DNA and inhibits nucleic acid synthesis. The drug is active in intestinal and extraintestinal sites. It is active against most anaerobic bacteria and protozoa, including *Bacteroides fragilis, B. metaninogenicus, Fusobacterium, Vellonella,*

Clostridium, Peptococcus, Peptostreptococcus, Entamoeba histolytica, Trichomonas vaginalis, Giardia lambia, and *Balantidum coli*. Metronidazole is absorbed orally, and its peak serum concentration occurs in 1 hour. It is distributed into most body tissues and fluids, including CSF, bone, bile, saliva, pleural and peritoneal fluids, vaginal secretions, seminal fluids, middle-ear fluid, and hepatic and cerebral abscesses. CSF levels approach serum levels in patients with inflamed meninges; they reach about 50% of serum levels in patients with uninflamed meninges. Less than 20% of metronidazole is bound to plasma proteins. It readily crosses the placenta. Metronidazole is metabolized to an active 2-hydroxymethyl metabolite and also to other metabolites. About 60 to 80% of the dose is excreted as the parent compound or its metabolites. About 20% of a metronidazole dose is excreted unchanged in urine; about 6 to 15% is excreted in feces. Metronidazole's half-life is 6 to 8 hours in adults with normal renal function; the half-life may be prolonged in patients with impaired hepatic function.

Concomitant use of metronidazole with oral anticoagulants prolongs prothrombin time. Concomitant use with alcohol inhibits alcohol dehydrogenase activity, causing a disulfiram-like reaction (nausea, vomiting, headache, abdominal cramps, and flushing) in some patients. Concomitant use with disulfiram may precipitate psychosis and confusion, and should be avoided. Concomitant use with barbiturates and phenytoin may diminish the antimicrobial effectiveness of metronidazole by increasing its metabolism, and may require higher doses of metronidazole. Concomitant use with cimetidine may decrease the clearance of metronidazole, thereby increasing its potential for causing adverse effects. Clinical signs of overdose include nausea, vomiting, ataxia, seizures, and peripheral neuropathy.

METYRAPONE TEST

The level of cortisol is thought to directly control the secretion of ACTH through a negative feedback mechanism that may be directed at both the hypothalamus and the anterior pituitary gland. Conversely, a reduced concentration of cortisol or cortisol-like substances eliminates the negative effect and enhances the release of ACTH (see also Figure 38).

The metyrapone test may be used diagnostically to evaluate the proper functioning of the anterior pituitary gland. When administered orally, metyrapone inhibits the activity of 11-beta-hydroxylase, which is necessary for the synthesis of cortisol, corticosterone, and aldosterone, promotes the release of corticotropin, which in turn increases production of the precursors (11-deoxycortisol and 11-deoxycorticosterone), and enhances the appearance of 17-hydroxycorticosteroids and 17-ketogenic steroids. In the event that the pituitary gland is nonfunctional, and therefore cannot stimulate ACTH secretion, the levels of these urinary metabolites will not increase.

MEXILETINE

(Mexitil)

Mexiletine (initially 200 mg/every 8 hours) is indicated in the treatment of documented, life-threatening ventricular arrhythmias, such as sustained ventricular tachycardia. Because of the proarrhythmic effects of mexiletine, its use with lesser arrhythmias is not recommended. The actions of mexiletine resemble those of lidocaine, which inhibits the inward sodium current, thus reducing the rate of rise of the action potential, phase O. Mexiletine decreases the effective refractory period (ERP) in Purkinje fibers. The decrease in ERP is of lesser magnitude than the decrease in action potential duration (APD), with a resulting increase in ERP/APD ratio. Mexiletine is a local anesthetic and a class IB antiarrhythmic compound with electrophysiologic properties similar to lidocaine. It is contraindicated in cardiogenic shock, and preexisting second- or third-degree AV block. Mexiletine is well absorbed (approximately 90%) from the GI tract. The absorption rate is reduced in situations in which gastric emptying time is increased. Narcotics, atropine, and magnesium-aluminum hydroxide may slow its absorption, whereas metoclopramide may accelerate its absorption.

Mexiletine is metabolized in the liver. The most active minor metabolite is *N*-methylmexiletine, which is <20% as potent as mexiletine. The urinary excretion of *N*-methylmexiletine is <0.5%.

Overdosage with mexiletine causes dizziness, drowsiness, nausea, hypotension, sinus bradycardia, paresthesia, seizures, intermittent left-bundle branch block, and temporary asystole. With massive overdoses, coma and respiratory arrest may occur (see also Figure 84).

MEZLOCILLIN SODIUM

(Mezlin)

Carbenicillin cures serious infections caused by *Pseudomonas* species and *Proteus* strains resistant to ampicillin. It is not absorbed from the GI tract, and therefore must be administered intraperitoneally. Carbenicillin indanyl is acid stable and hence can be given orally. Ticarcillin is four times more potent than carbenicillin in treating a *Pseudomonas aeruginosa* infection, and azlocillin is ten times more potent than carbenicillin against *Pseudomonas*. Mezlocillin and piperacillin are more active against *Klebsiella* infection than carbenicillin.

Mezlocillin is indicated for:

- **Lower respiratory tract infections**, including pneumonia and lung abscess caused by *Haemophilus influenzae, Klebsiella* sp. including *K. pneumoniae, Proteus mirabilis, Pseudomonas* sp. including *P. aeruginosa, E. coli*, and *Bacteroides* sp. including *B. fragilis*
- **Intra-abdominal infections**, including acute cholecystitis, cholangitis, peritonitis, hepatic abscess, and intra-abdominal abscess caused by susceptible *E. coli, P. mirabilis, Klebsiella* sp.,

Pseudomonas sp., *Streptococcus faecalis* (enterococcus), *Bacteroides* sp., *Peptococcus* sp., and *Peptostreptococcus* sp.

Urinary tract infections caused by susceptible *E. coli, P. mirabilis*, the indole-positive *Proteus* sp., *Morganella morganii, Klebsiella* sp., *Enterobacter* sp., *Serratia* sp., *Pseudomonas* sp., *S. faecalis* (enterococcus)

Uncomplicated gonorrhea due to susceptible *Neisseria gonorrhoeae*

Gynecological infections, including endometritis, pelvic cellulitis, and pelvic inflammatory disease associated with susceptible *N. gonorrhoeae, Peptococcus* sp., *Peptostreptococcus* sp., *Bacteroides* sp., *E. coli, P. mirabilis, Klebsiella* sp., and *Enterobacter* sp.

Skin and skin structure infections caused by susceptible *S. faecalis* (enterococcus), *E. coli, P. mirabilis*, the indole-positive *Proteus* sp., *P. vulgaris*, and *Providencia rettgeri, Klebsiella* sp., *Enterobacter* sp., *Pseudomonas* sp., *Peptococcus* sp., and *Bacteroides* sp.

Septicemia, including bacteremia caused by susceptible *E. coli, Klebsiella* sp., *Enterobacter* sp., *Pseudomonas* sp., *Bacteroides* sp., and *Peptococcus* sp.

Streptococcal infections caused by *Streptococcus* sp. including group A beta-hemolytic *Streptococcus* and *S. pneumoniae*; however, such infections are ordinarily treated with more narrow-spectrum penicillins

Mezlocillin's broad spectrum of activity makes it useful for treating mixed infections caused by susceptible strains of both Gram-negative and Gram-positive aerobic and anaerobic bacteria. It is not effective, however, against infections caused by penicillinase-producing *Staphylococcus aureus*.

Mezlocillin is effective in combination with an aminoglycoside in the treatment of life-threatening infections caused by *P. aeruginosa*. In the treatment of febrile episodes in immunosuppressed patients with granulocytopenia, it may be combined with an aminoglycoside or a cephalosporin. The rate of elimination of mezlocillin is dose-dependent and related to the degree of renal function impairment. Dosage adjustments are not required in patients with mild impairment of renal function.

MIANSERIN

Serotonergic antagonists such as methysergide represent the first class of drugs shown to be effective in migraine prophylaxis. Methysergide is an ergot derivative that has complex effects on serotonergic and other neurotransmitter systems. It has been shown to be effective in 60 to 80% of migraine patients and should be given for at least a 6-week trial. This agent is used most frequently for patients who complain of cluster headaches. Common side effects include nausea, vomiting, and diarrhea. A few patients have developed retroperitoneal fibrosis following prolonged use of methysergide. Therefore, it is recommended that this drug be administered for no more than 6 consecutive months. The patient should then discontinue the medication for at least 4 to 8 weeks, after which the drug can be reintroduced safely. Ergonovine (Ergotrate) is another ergot alkaloid that has been used prophylactically. Other 5-HT receptor antagonists (i.e., pizotifen, mianserin) have also been reported effective in migraine prophylaxis. Mianserin also has shown efficacy as an antidepressant. It does not alter the uptake of norepinephrine, serotonin, or dopamine. Mianserin blocks alpha-1- and alpha-2-adrenergic receptors and H_1-histamine receptors without having any anticholinergic effects. Mianserine is sedative in nature (see also Figure 94).

MICAFUNGIN SODIUM

(Mycamine powder for injection 50 mg)

Micafungin sodium is an antifungal agent that inhibits synthesis of 1,3-B-D-glucan, an essential component of fungal cell walls, but not present in mammalian cells. It is indicated in the treatment of esophageal candidiasis; and prophylaxis of *Candida* infections in patients undergoing hematopoietic stem-cell transplantation.

Screening natural products of fungal fermentation in the 1970s led to the discovery that echinocandins had activity against *Candida* and that the biologic activity was directed against formation of β(1,3) D-glucans in the cell wall. Selection of different echinocandins and their chemical modifications led first to the discovery of **cilofungin**. Clinical trials were stopped because of toxicity from the solubilizing agent. Further research has led to one drug approved for clinical use, **caspofungin**, and two compounds that are in development: **anidulafungin** and **micafungin**. All have the same mechanism of action but differing pharmacologic properties. Susceptible fungi include *Candida* species and *Aspergillus* species. ***In vitro*** resistance can be conferred in *C. albicans* by mutation in one of the genes that encodes β(1,3) D-glucan synthase. Azole-resistant isolates of *C. albicans* remain susceptible to echinocandins.

MICONAZOLE

(Monistat)

Miconazole is indicated in the treatment of the following severe systemic fungal infections: coccidioidomycosis, candidiasis, cryptococcosis, pseudoallescheriosis (petriellidosis, allescheriosis), paracoccidioidomycosis, and in the treatment of chronic mucocutaneous candidiasis.

In the treatment of fungal meningitis or *Candida* urinary bladder infections, IV infusion alone is inadequate. It must be supplemented with intrathecal administration or bladder irrigation.

Miconazole, an imidazole derivative, exerts a fungicidal effect by altering the permeability of the fungal cell membrane. Its mechanism of action may also involve an alteration of RNA and DNA metabolism or an intracellular accumulation of peroxides toxic to the fungal cell.

Miconazole is rapidly metabolized in the liver. About 14 to 22% of the administered dose is excreted in the urine, mainly as inactive metabolites. The terminal elimination half-life is 20 to 25 hours.

Rapid injection of undiluted miconazole may produce transient tachycardia or arrhythmia. Miconazole and amphotericin B are antagonistic both *in vitro* and *in vivo*. The antifungal activity of the two drugs, when used in combination, is less than that of either drug used alone. Miconazole enhances the effectiveness of anticoagulants and increases the serum level of phenytoin. It has caused rash, pruritis, and phlebitis at the site of infusion. A transient decrease in hematocrit has been noted.

MIDAZOLAM

(Versed)

Midazolam (IM) is indicated for causing preoperative sedation and impairment of preoperative events. When given intravenously, it is used for producing conscious sedation prior to short diagnostic or endoscopic procedures, either alone or with a narcotic. It is used for induction of general anesthesia, before administration of other anesthetic agents, and to supplement nitrous oxide and oxygen (balanced anesthesia) for short surgical procedures. Intravenously administered midazolam has been associated with respiratory depression and respiratory arrest, especially when used for conscious sedation. In some cases, where this was not recognized promptly and treated effectively, death or hypoxic encephalopathy resulted. Midazolam, like other members of benzodiazepine derivatives, exerts its CNS depressant effects by enhancing and facilitating GABAergic transmission (see Figure 50). It decreases cerebrospinal fluid pressure and IOP. Barbiturates, alcohol, or other CNS depressants may increase the risk of underventilation or apnea and contribute to prolonged effect when used with midazolam. Narcotic premedication also depresses ventilatory response to carbon dioxide stimulation.

Narcotics (e.g., morphine, meperidine, and fentanyl), secobarbital, or fentanyl and droperidol (Innovar) used as premedications accentuate the hypnotic effect of midazolam (see also Table 9). A moderate (15%) reduction in induction dosage of thiopental is required following IM use of midazolam for premedication. The dosage of inhalational anesthetics may need to be reduced when midazolam is used as an induction agent. The IV administration decreases the minimum alveolar concentration (MAC) of halothane required for general anesthesia. Symptoms of overdosage include sedation, somnolence, confusion, impaired coordination and reflexes, coma, and untoward effects on vital signs. Flumazenil (Romazicon) may be used to antidote the effects of midazolam (see Figure 50).

MIDODRINE HYDROCHLORIDE

(ProAmatine tablets 2.5 mg)

Midodrine hydrochloride is a vasopressor that activates arteriolar and venous α-adrenergic receptors, resulting in an increase in vascular tone and elevation of BP. It is indicated in the treatment of symptomatic orthostatic hypotension in patients whose lives are considerably impaired despite standard clinical care, including support stockings, fluid expansion, and lifestyle changes.

Midodrine (proamatine) is an orally effective α_1-receptor agonist. It is a prodrug; its activity is due to its conversion to an active metabolite, **desglymidodrine**, which achieves peak concentrations about 1 hour after a dose of midodrine. The half-life of desglymidodrine is about 3 hours. Consequently, the duration of action is about 4 to 6 hours. **Midodrine**-induced rises in blood pressure are associated with both arterial and venous smooth muscle contraction. This is advantageous in the treatment of patients with **autonomic insufficiency** and **postural hypotension**. A frequent complication in these patients is supine hypertension. This can be minimized by avoiding dosing prior to bedtime and elevating the head of the bed. Very cautious use of a short-acting antihypertensive drug at bedtime may be useful in some patients. Typical dosing, achieved by careful titration of blood pressure responses, varies between 2.5 and 10 mg three times daily.

In some patients in shock, hypotension is so severe that vasoconstricting drugs are required to maintain a blood pressure that is adequate for CNS perfusion. Alpha agonists such as norepinephrine, phenylephrine, metaraminol, mephentermine, **midodrine**, **ephedrine**, **epinephrine**, **dopamine**, and **methoxamine** all have been used for this purpose. This approach may be advantageous in patients with hypotension due to failure of the sympathetic nervous system (e.g., after spinal anesthesia or injury). However, in patients with other forms of shock, such as cardiogenic shock, reflex vasoconstriction generally is intense, and a receptor agonist may further compromise blood flow to organs such as the kidneys and gut and adversely increase the work of the heart. Indeed, vasodilating drugs such as **nitroprusside** are more likely to improve blood flow and decrease cardiac work in such patients by decreasing afterload if a minimally adequate blood pressure can be maintained.

Patients with orthostatic hypotension (excessive fall in blood pressure with standing) often represent a pharmacological challenge. There are diverse causes for this disorder, including the **Shy–Drager syndrome** and idiopathic autonomic failure. Therapeutic approaches include physical maneuvers and a variety of drugs (**fludrocortisone**, **prostaglandin synthesis inhibitors**, **somatostatin analogs**, **caffeine**, **vasopressin analogs**, and **dopamine antagonists**). A number of sympathomimetic drugs also have been used in treating this disorder. The ideal agent would enhance venous constriction prominently and produce relatively little arterial constriction so as to avoid supine hypertension. No such agent currently is available. Drugs used in this disorder to activate α_1 receptors include both direct- and indirect-acting agents. **Midodrine** shows promise in treating this challenging disorder.

MIFEPRISTONE

(Mifeprex tablets 200 mg)

Mifepristone is an abortifacient that competes with progesterone at progesterone-receptor sites. It is indicated in the termination of intrauterine pregnancy through day 49 of pregnancy. The first report of an antiprogestin, RU 38486 (often referred to as RU-486) or **mifepristone**, appeared in 1981; this drug is available for the termination of pregnancy. Antiprogestins also have several other potential applications, including uses as contraceptives, to induce labor, and to treat uterine leiomyomas, endometriosis, meningiomas, and breast cancer.

Mifepristone is a derivative of the 19-norprogestin norethindrone containing a dimethyl-aminophenol substituent at the 11β-position. It effectively competes with both progesterone and glucocorticoids for binding to their respective receptors. **Mifepristone** was initially thought to be a pure antiprogestin; this is its predominant activity in most situations, but it also has some agonist activity. Thus, it is now considered a **progesterone-receptor modulator** (**PRM**) due to its context-dependent activity.

Other PRMs and pure progesterone antagonists now have been synthesized, and most contain an 11β-aromatic group. Another widely studied antiprogestin is **onapristone** (or ZK 98299), which is similar in structure to **mifepristone** but contains a methyl substituent in the 13α rather than 13β orientation. More selective PRMs, such as **asoprisnil**, are being studied experimentally.

In the presence of progestins, mifepristone acts as a competitive receptor antagonist for both progesterone receptors. While **mifepristone** acts primarily as an antagonist *in vivo*, it exhibits some agonist activity in certain *in vivo* and *in vitro* contexts. In contrast, onapristone appears to be a pure progesterone antagonist both *in vivo* and *in vitro*. PR complexes of both compounds antagonize the actions of progesterone–PR complexes and also appear to preferentially recruit corepressors.

When administered in the early stages of pregnancy, **mifepristone** causes decidual breakdown by blockade of uterine progesterone receptors. This leads to detachment blastocyst, which decreases hCG production. This in turn causes a decrease in progesterone secretion from the corpus luteum, which further accentuates decidual breakdown. Decreased endogenous progesterone coupled with blockade of progesterone receptors in the uterus increases uterine prostaglandin levels and sensitizes the myometrium to their contractile actions. **Mifepristone** also causes cervical softening, which facilitates expulsion of the detached blastocyst.

Mifepristone can delay or prevent ovulation depending upon the timing and manner of administration. These effects are due largely to actions on the hypothalamus and pituitary rather than the ovary, although the mechanisms are unclear.

If administered for one or several days in the mid- to late-luteal phase, mifepristone impairs the development of a secretory endometrium and produces menses. PR blockade at this time is the pharmacological equivalent of progesterone withdrawal, and bleeding normally ensues within several days and lasts for 1 to 2 weeks after antiprogestin treatment.

Mifepristone also binds to glucocorticoid and androgen receptors and exerts antiglucocorticoid and antiandrogenic actions. A predominant effect in humans is blockade of the feedback inhibition by cortisol of ACTH secretion from the pituitary, thus increasing both corticotropin and adrenal steroid levels in the plasma. Onapristone also binds to both glucocorticoid and androgen receptors, but has less antiglucocorticoid activity than mifepristone.

Mifepristone is orally active with good bioavailability. Peak plasma levels occur within several hours, and the drug is slowly cleared with a plasma half-life of 20 to 40 hours. In plasma, it is bound by α_1-acid glycoprotein, which contributes to its long half-life. Metabolites are primarily the mono- and di-demethylated products (which are thought to have pharmacological activity) formed via CYP3A4-catalyzed reactions, and to a lesser extent, hydroxylated compounds. The drug undergoes hepatic metabolism and enterohepatic circulation, and metabolic products are found predominantly in the feces.

Mifepristone (Mifeprex), in combination with **misoprostol** or other prostaglandins, is available for the termination of early pregnancy. When **mifepristone** is used to produce a medical abortion, a prostaglandin is given 48 hours after the antiprogestin to further increase myometrial contractions and ensure expulsion of the detached blastocyst. Intramuscular **sulprostone**, intravaginal **gemeprost**, and oral misoprostol have been used. The success rate with such regimens is >90% among women with pregnancies of 49 days' duration or less. The most severe untoward effect is vaginal bleeding, which most often lasts from 8 to 17 days but is only rarely (0.1% of patients) severe enough to require blood transfusions. High percentages of women also have experienced abdominal pain and uterine cramps, nausea, vomiting, and diarrhea due to the prostaglandin. Women receiving chronic glucocorticoid therapy should not be given **mifepristone** because of its antiglucocorticoid activity, and the drug should be used very cautiously in women who are anemic or receiving anticoagulants. Women over 35 years old with cardiovascular risk factors should not be given **sulprostone** because of possible heart failure.

Other investigational or potential uses for **mifepristone** that are under development include the induction of labor after fetal death; the induction of labor at the end of the third trimester; treatment of endometriosis, leiomyomas, breast cancer, and meningiomas; and as a postcoital or luteal-phase contraceptive. A major concern about long-term use is the possibility of unopposed estrogenic effects, but this concern could be allayed by further development of selective PR modulators.

MIGLITOL

(Glyset tablets 25 mg, tablets 50 mg)

Miglitol is an alpha-glucosidase inhibitor that inhibits intestinal enzymes that digest carbohydrates, thereby reducing carbohydrate digestion after meals, which lowers postprandial glucose elevation in diabetics. It is used in patients with non-insulin-dependent diabetes mellitus (NIDDM) who have failed dietary therapy. It may be used alone or in combination with sulfonylureas.

α-Glucosidase inhibitors reduce intestinal absorption of starch, dextrin, and disaccharides by inhibiting the action of α-glucosidase in the intestinal brush border. Inhibition of this enzyme slows the absorption of carbohydrates; the postprandial rise in plasma glucose is blunted in both normal and diabetic subjects.

α-Glucosidase inhibitors do not stimulate insulin release and therefore do not result in hypoglycemia. These agents may be considered as monotherapy in elderly patients or in patients with predominantly postprandial hyperglycemia. α-Glucosidase inhibitors typically are used in combination with other oral antidiabetic agents and/or insulin. The drugs should be administered at the start of a meal. They are poorly absorbed.

Acarbose (precose), an oligosaccharide of microbial origin, and **miglitol** (Glyset), a **desoxynojirimycin derivative**, also competitively inhibit **glucoamylase** and **sucrase** but have weak effects on pancreatic α-amylase. They reduce postprandial plasma glucose levels in type 1 and type 2 diabetes mellitus subjects. α-Glucosidase inhibitors can significantly improve hemoglobin A_{1c} levels in severely hyperglycemic type 2 diabetes mellitus patients. However, in patients with mild to moderate hyperglycemia, the glucose-lowering potential of α-glucosidase inhibitors (assessed by hemoglobin A_1 levels) is about 30% to 50% of that of other oral antidiabetic agents.

α-Glucosidase inhibitors cause dose-related malabsorption, flatulence, diarrhea, and abdominal bloating. Titrating the dose of drug slowly (25 mg at the start of a meal for 4 to 8 weeks, followed by increases at 4- to 8-week intervals to a maximum of 75 mg before each meal) reduces gastrointestinal side effects. Smaller doses are given with snacks. Acarbose is most effective when given with a starchy, high-fiber diet with restricted amounts of glucose and sucrose. If hypoglycemia occurs when α-glucosidase inhibitors are used with insulin or an insulin secretagogue, glucose rather than sucrose, starch, or maltose should be administered.

MIGLUSTAT

(Zavesca capsules 100 mg)

Miglustat is an endocrine and metabolic agent that causes a competitive and reversible inhibitor of the enzyme glucosylceramide synthase. It is indicated in the treatment of adult patients with mild to moderate type 1 **Gaucher disease** for whom enzyme replacement therapy is not an option (e.g., hypersensitivity).

MIGRAINE HEADACHES: Treatment of

Drugs and Dosages

Aspirin, 650 mg every 4 hours
Aspirin, 650 mg with butalbital, 50 mg
Aspirin, 300 mg, with caffeine, 50 mg, and butalbital, 50 mg
Acetaminophen, 650 mg every 4 hours
Acetaminophen, 325 mg, with butalbital, 50 mg
Dihydroergotamine, 1 mg IM or IV at onset and every hour
Ergotamine, 1 mg
Ergotamine, 1 mg, plus caffeine, 100 mg
Ergotamine, 2 mg, plus caffeine, 100 mg (suppository)
Ibuprofen, 400–800 mg three times a day
Indomethacin, 50 mg three times a day
Naproxen sodium, 550 mg, then 275 mg every 6 to 8 hours
Sumatriptan, 6 mg subcutaneously

The medication to be chosen depends on the severity and/or frequency of attacks and the response of the patients.

MILRINONE LACTATE

(Primacor)

Agents with positive inotropic actions that may be used in the management of CHF include the cardiac glycosides (e.g., digoxin and digitoxin), dopaminergic analogs (e.g., dobutamine), phosphodiesterase inhibitors (e.g., amrinone and milrinone), angiotensin antagonists (e.g., captopril, enalapril, and lisinopril), and vasodilators (nitrates and hydralazine).

Milrinone is a member of a new class of bipyridine inotropic/vasodilator agents with phosphodiesterase inhibitor activity. It is a positive inotrope and vasodilator, with little chronotropic activity, different in structure and mode of action from either the digitalis glycosides or catecholamines (see also Figures 23 and 42).

At relevant inotropic and vasorelaxant concentrations, milrinone is a selective inhibitor of peak III cAMP phosphodiesterase isozyme in cardiac and vascular muscle. This inhibitory action is consistent with cAMP-mediated increases in intracellular ionized calcium and contractile protein phosphorylation and relaxation in vascular muscle. Additional experimental evidence also indicates that milrinone is not a beta-adrenergic agonist nor does it inhibit sodium–potassium adenosine triphosphatase activity as do the digitalis glycosides.

In patients with CHF, milrinone produces dose-related increases in the maximum rate of increase of left ventricular pressure. Milrinone has a direct inotropic effect and a direct arterial vasodilator activity. Both the inotropic and vasodilatory effects occur over the therapeutic range of plasma concentrations of 100 to 300 ng/mL. In addition to increasing myocardial contractility, milrinone improves diastolic function as evidenced by improvements in left ventricular diastolic relaxation.

In patients with depressed myocardial function, milrinone produces a prompt increase in cardiac output and decreases in pulmonary capillary wedge pressure and vascular resistance without a significant increase in heart rate or myocardial oxygen consumption. Overdosage of milrinone, which is a vasodilator, produces hypotension.

MINERALOCORTICOIDS

The mineralocorticoids influence salt and water metabolism and, in general, conserve sodium levels. They promote the resorption of sodium and the secretion of potassium in the cortical collecting tubules and possibly the connecting segment. They also elicit hydrogen secretion in the medullary collecting tubules. The main mineralocorticoid is aldosterone, with a daily secretion of 100 μg. Aldosterone is synthesized from 18-hydroxycorticosterone by a dehydrogenase. The consequence of 18-hydroxycorticosterone dehydrogenase deficiency is diminished secretion of aldosterone, and the clinical manifestations consist of sodium depletion, dehydration, hypotension, potassium retention, and enhanced plasma renin levels (see also Figure 17).

MINERAL OIL

(Agoral, Kondremul Plain, Milkinol, Neo-cultol, Nujol, Petrogalar Plain, Zymenol)

Mineral oil, a lubricant, is indicated in constipation or preparation for bowel studies or surgery.

MINOCYCLINE HYDROCHLORIDE

(Minocin)

Minocycline, a tetracycline, is indicated in syphilis or gonorrhea in patients sensitive to penicillin. In addition, it may be used in uncomplicated urethral, endocervical, or rectal infection, and in uncomplicated gonococcal urethritis in men (see also Figure 96). Tetracyclines enter bacterial cells by both passive diffusion and active transport, and then accumulate intracellularly. This does not occur in mammalian cells. The tetracyclines bind to the 30S subunit of the bacterial ribosome in such a way that the binding of the aminoacyl-transfer RNA to the acceptor site on the messenger RNA ribosome complex is blocked (see Figure 96).

Minocycline is active against many Gram-negative and Gram-positive organisms—*Mycoplasma, Rickettsia, Chlamydia,* and spirochetes; it may be more active against staphylococci than other tetracyclines. The potential vestibular toxicity and cost of minocycline limits its usefulness. It may be more active than other tetracyclines against *Nocardia asteroides*; it is also effective against *Mycobacterium marinum* infections. Minocycline has been used for meningococcal meningitis prophylaxis because of its activity against *Neisseria meningitidis*. The absorption of tetracyclines from the GI tract is nonuniform. Up to 30% of chlortetracycline is absorbed. The absorption rate for tetracycline, oxytetracycline, and demeclocycline ranges between 60 and 80%, whereas as much as 90 to 100% of doxycycline and minocycline is absorbed. The unabsorbed tetracycline may modify the intestinal flora. The absorption of tetracyclines is impaired by divalent cations (calcium, magnesium, and ferrous iron), by aluminum, and by extremely alkaline pHs. Tetracyclines are distributed widely throughout the body fluid, cross the placental barrier, and can accumulate in growing bones. The concentrations of chlortetracycline in spinal fluid are only one-fourth of those in plasma. Minocycline, a more lipid-soluble tetracycline, reaches a high concentration in tears and saliva and can eradicate the meningococcal carrier state.

The tetracyclines are metabolized in the liver and excreted mainly by the bile and urine. The concentrations of tetracyclines in the bile are 10 times higher than those in serum. Tetracyclines in general cause toxic and hypersensitivity reactions. These consist commonly of GI irritations that are disabling and may necessitate discontinuation of the medications. With continuous usage, tetracyclines may alter the normal flora, allowing the growth of *Pseudomonas*, *Proteus*, staphylococci-resistant coliforms, *Clostridium*, and *Candida* organisms. These superinfections should be recognized and treated appropriately with vancomycin and other drugs. Tetracyclines have been known to cause hepatic necrosis, especially when given in large intravenous doses or when taken by pregnant women or patients with preexisting liver impairment. Tetracycline preparations whose potency has expired can cause renal tubular acidosis (Fanconi's syndrome). With the exception of doxycycline, tetracyclines accumulate in patients with renal impairment. Tetracyclines also produce nitrogen retention, especially when given with diuretics. Tetracyclines bind to calcium and then become deposited in bone, causing damage to developing bone and teeth. The intravenous administration of tetracyclines has been observed to cause venous thrombosis.

MINOXIDIL

(Topical) (Rogaine)

Minoxidil (2% 1 mL of solution b.i.d.) is used in the treatment of male pattern baldness (alopecia androgenetica).

MINOXIDIL

(Loniten)

Minoxidil (10 to 40 mg/day) is indicated for severe hypertension that is symptomatic or associated with target organ damage and is not manageable with maximum therapeutic doses of a diuretic plus two other antihypertensives. Topical minoxidil (Rogaine) in 0.3 to 4.5% solution is used to stimulate vertex hair growth in individuals with alopecia androgenetica, expressed in males as baldness of the vertex of the scalp and in females as diffuse hair loss or thinning of the frontoparietal areas. There is no effect in patients with predominantly frontal hair loss. The mechanism is not known, but like minoxidil, some other arterial dilating drugs also stimulate hair growth when given systemically.

Minoxidil is a direct-acting peripheral vasodilator. The exact mechanism of action on the vascular smooth muscle is unknown. It does not interfere with vasomotor reflexes; therefore, it does not produce orthostatic hypotension. The drug does not affect CNS function. It appears to block calcium uptake through the cell membrane. Minoxidil reduces elevated systolic and diastolic blood pressure by decreasing peripheral vascular resistance. The blood pressure response to minoxidil is dose-related and proportional to the extent of hypertension. In humans, forearm and renal vascular resistance decline; forearm blood flow increases, whereas renal blood flow and GFR are preserved.

When used in severely hypertensive patients resistant to other therapy, frequently with an accompanying diuretic and beta-adrenergic blocker, minoxidil decreases the blood pressure and reverses encephalopathy and retinopathy. Minoxidil causes peripheral vasodilation and elicits a reduction of peripheral arteriolar resistance. This action, with the associated fall in blood pressure, triggers sympathetic, vagal inhibitory, and renal homeostasis mechanisms, including an increase in renin secretion that leads to increased cardiac rate and output, and salt and water retention. These adverse effects can usually be minimized by coadministration of a diuretic and a beta-adrenergic-blocking agent or other sympathetic nervous system suppressant. Although minoxidil does not cause orthostatic hypotension, its use in patients on guanethidine can result in profound orthostatic effects (see also Table 26).

MIRTAZAPINE

(Remeron tablets 15 mg)

Mirtazapine is a tetracyclic compound that enhances central nonadrenergic and serotonergic activity. It is indicated in the treatment of depression.

Tricyclic antidepressants are oxidized by hepatic microsomal enzymes, followed by conjugation with glucuronic acid, The major metabolite of **imipramine** is **desipramine**; biotransformation of imiprimine or desipramine occurs largely by oxidation to 2-hydroxy metabolites, which retain some ability to block the transport of amines and have particularly prominent cardiac depressant actions. In contrast, **amitriptyline** and its major demethylated by-product, **nortriptyline**, undergo preferential oxidation at the 10 position. The 10-hydroxy metabolites may have some biological activity, and may be less cardiotoxic than the 2-hydroxy metabolites of imipramine or desipramine. Conjugation of ring-hydroxylated metabolites with glucuronic acid extinguishes any remaining biological activity. The N-demethylated metabolites of several tricyclic antidepressants are pharmacologically active and may accumulate in concentrations approaching or exceeding those of the parent drug, to contribute variably to overall pharmacodynamic activity.

Amoxapine is oxidized predominantly to the 8-hydroxy metabolite and less to the 7-hydroxy metabolite. The 8-hydroxy metabolite is pharmacologically active, including antagonistic interactions with D_2-dopamine receptors. Amoxapine has some risk of extrapyramidal side effects, including tardive dyskinesia, reminiscent of those of the N-methylated congener loxapine, a typical neuroleptic.

Mirtazapine is also N-demethylated and undergoes aromatic hydroxylation. **Trazodone** and **nefazodone** both are N-dealkylated to yield **metachlorophenylpiperazine** (mCPP), an active metabolite with serotonergic activity. Bupropion yields active metabolites that include amphetamine-like compounds. **Clomipramine**, **fluoxetine**, **sertraline**, and **venlafaxine** are N-demethylated to **norclomipramine**, **norfluoxetine**, **norsertraline**, and **desmethylvenlafaxine**, respectively. As occurs with the tertiary-amine tricyclic antidepressants, the N-demethylated metabolites of serotonin reuptake inhibitors also are eliminated more slowly, and some are pharmacologically active. **Norclomipramine** contributes noradrenergic activity. Norfluoxetine is a very long-acting inhibitor of serotonin transport (elimination half-life approximately 10 days) that requires several weeks for elimination. Norfluoxetine also competes for hepatic CYPs and thereby elevates blood levels of other agents, including tricyclic antidepressants. These effects can persist for days after administration of the parent drug has been stopped. Norsertraline, though also eliminated relatively slowly (half-life of 60 to 70 hours), appears to contribute limited pharmacological activity or risk of drug interactions. **Nornefazodone** contributes little to the biological activity or duration of action of **nefazodone**.

With some notable exceptions, inactivation and elimination of most antidepressants occurs over a period of several days. Generally, secondary-amine tricyclic antidepressants and the N-demethylated derivatives of serotonin reuptake inhibitors have elimination half-lives about twice those of the parent drugs. Nevertheless, most tricyclics are almost completely eliminated within 7 to 10 days. An exceptionally long-acting tricyclic antidepressant is protriptyline (half-life of about 80 hours). Most MAO inhibitors are long acting because recovery from their effects requires the synthesis of new enzyme over a period of 1 to 2 weeks.

At the other extreme, **trazodone**, **nefazodone**, and venlafaxine have short half-lives (about 3 to 6 hours), as does the active 4-hydroxy metabolite of venlafaxine (half-life of about 11 hours). The half-life of bupropion is about 14 hours. Owing to rapid aromatic hydroxylation, the half-life of nefazodone is very short (about 3 hours). The shorter duration of action of these agents usually implies the need for multiple daily doses. Some short-acting antidepressants have been prepared in slow-release preparations (notably bupropion and venlafaxine), to allow less frequent dosing and potentially to temper side effect related to agitation and GI disturbance.

Antidepressants are metabolized more rapidly by children and more slowly by patients over 60 years of age as compared with young adults. Dosages are adjusted accordingly, sometimes to daily doses in children that far exceed those typically given to adults.

Weakness and fatigue are attributable to central effects of tricyclic antidepressants, particularly tertiary amines and **mirtazapine**, all of which have potent central antihistaminic effects. Trazodone and nefazodone also are relatively sedating. Other CNS effects include variable risk of confusion or delirium, in large part owing to atropine-like effects of tricyclic antidepressants. Epileptic seizures can occur; this is especially likely with daily doses of bupropion above 450 mg, maprotiline above 250 mg, or acute overdoses of amoxapine or tricyclics. The risk of cerebral or cardiac intoxication can increase if such agents are given in relatively high doses, particularly when combined with SSRIs that inhibit their metabolism. MAO inhibitors can induce sedation or behavioral excitation and have a high risk of inducing postural hypotension, sometimes with sustained mild elevations of diastolic blood pressure.

Another risk of antidepressants in vulnerable patients (particularly those with unrecognized bipolar depression) is switching, sometimes suddenly, from depression to hypomanic or manic excitement, or mixed, dysphoric-agitated, manic-depressive states. To some extent this effect is dose-related and is somewhat more likely in adults treated with tricyclic antidepressants than with serotonin reuptake inhibitors, bupropion, and perhaps with MAO inhibitors. Risk of mania with newer sedating antidepressants, including nefazodone and **mirtazapine**, also may be relatively low, but some risk of inducing mania can be expected with any treatment that elevates mood, including in children with unsuspected bipolar disorder.

MISOPROSTOL

(Cytotec tablets 100 mcg)

Misoprostol is a prostaglandin (PG) that represents a synthetic prostaglandin E_1 analog that inhibits gastric acid secretion and exerts mucosal-protective properties. It is indicated in prevention of gastric ulcers in high-risk patients who are taking NSAIDs.

There has been intense interest in the effects of the PGs on the female reproductive system. When given early in pregnancy, their action as **abortifacients** may be variable and often incomplete, and accompanied by adverse effects. PGs appear, however, to be of value in missed abortion and molar gestation, and they have been used widely for the induction of mid-trimester abortion. Several studies have shown that systemic or intravaginal administration of the PGE_1 analog **misoprostol** in combination with **mifepristone** (RU-486) or **methotrexate** is highly effective in the termination of early pregnancy.

PGE_2 or $PGE_{2\alpha}$ can induce labor at term. However, they may have more value when used to facilitate labor by promoting ripening and dilation of the cervix.

The capacity of several PG analogs to suppress gastric ulceration is a property of therapeutic importance. Of these, misoprostol (Cytotec), a PGE_1 analog, is approved by the Food and Drug Administration (FDA). **Misoprostol** appears to heal gastric ulcers about as effectively as the H_2-receptor antagonists; however, relief of ulcerogenic pain and healing of duodenal ulcers have not been achieved consistently with misoprostol. This drug currently is used primarily for the prevention of ulcers that often occur during long-term treatment with NSAIDs. In this setting, **misoprostol** appears to be as effective as the **proton-pump inhibitor omeprazole**.

PGE_1 (alprostadil) may be used in the treatment of impotence. Intracavernous injection of PGE_1 causes complete or partial erection in impotent patients who do not have disorders of the vascular system or cavernous body damage. The erection lasts for 1 to 3 hours and is sufficient for sexual intercourse. PGE_1 is more effective than **papaverine**. The agent is available as a sterile powder that is reconstituted with water for infections (**Caverject**).

Misoprostol, a prostaglandin E_1 analog with gastric mucosal protectant properties, is used in prevention of gastric ulcer induced by nonsteroidal antiinflammatory agents. In addition, it has been used in the treatment of duodenal or gastric ulcer.

MITHRAMYCIN

(Mithracin)

The mechanism of action of mithramycin is similar to dactinomycin's. It is used in patients with advanced disseminated tumors of the testes and for the treatment of hypercalcemia associated with cancer. Mithramycin may cause GI injury, bone marrow depression, hepatic and renal damage, and hemorrhagic tendency.

MITOMYCIN

(Mutamycin)

Mitomycin (20 mg/m^2 IV as a single dose at 6 to 8 week intervals) is indicated in therapy of disseminated adenocarcinoma of stomach or pancreas combined with other chemotherapeutic agents, and as a palliative treatment when other modalities fail. Mitomycin has been given by the intravesical route for the management of superficial bladder cancer. As an ophthalmic solution, mitomycin appears to be beneficial as an adjunct to surgical excision in the treatment of primary or recurrent pterygia. Mitomycin is an antibiotic with antitumor activity isolated from *Streptomyces caespitosus*. It selectively inhibits the synthesis of deoxyribonucleic acid (DNA). The guanine and cytosine content correlates with the degree of mitomycin-induced cross-linking. At high concentrations, cellular ribonucleic acid (RNA) and protein synthesis are also suppressed. Bone marrow suppression, notably thrombocytopenia and leukopenia, which may contribute to overwhelming infection in an already compromised patient, is the most serious syndrome of microangiopathic hemolytic anemia. Thrombocytopenia and irreversible renal failure have occurred. Acute shortness of breath and severe bronchospasm have occurred following the use of vinca alkaloids in patients who had previously or simultaneously received mitomycin. Onset of this acute respiratory distress occurs within minutes to hours after the vinca alkaloid injection. Bronchodilators, steroids, or oxygen produce symptomatic relief.

MITOTANE

(Lysodren tablets 500 mg)

Mitotane is an antineoplastic agent. The primary action is on the adrenal cortex. The production of adrenal steroids is reduced. The biochemical mechanism of action is unknown. Data suggest that the drug modifies the peripheral metabolism of steroids and directly suppresses the adrenal cortex. Use of mitotane alters the peripheral metabolism of cortisol, even though plasma levels of corticosteroids do not fall. The drug causes increased formation of 6-beta-hydroxycortisol. Mitotane, a chlorophenothane (DDT) analog with antineoplastic properties (1 to 6 g p.o. daily in divided doses), is used in the treatment of inoperable adrenocortical cancer.

The principal application of **mitotane** (*o,p'*-DDD), a compound chemically similar to the insecticides DDT and DDD, is in the treatment of neoplasms derived from the adrenal cortex. In studies of the toxicology of related insecticides, it was noted that the adrenal cortex was severely damaged, an effect caused by the presence of the *o,p'* isomer of DDD.

The mechanism of action of **mitotane** has not been elucidated, but its relatively selective attack on adrenocortical cells, normal or neoplastic, is well established. Thus, administration of the drug causes a rapid reduction in the levels of adrenocorticosteroids and their metabolites in blood and urine, a response that is useful both in guiding dosage and in following the course of **hyperadrenocorticism (Cushing's syndrome)** resulting from an adrenal tumor or adrenal hyperplasia. Damage to the liver, kidneys, or bone marrow has not been encountered.

Approximately 40% of **mitotane** is absorbed after oral administration. After daily doses of 5 to 15 g, concentrations of 10 to 90 μg/mL of unchanged drug and 30 to 50 μg/mL of a metabolite are present in the blood. After discontinuation of therapy, plasma concentrations of **mitotane** are still measurable for 6 to 9 weeks. Although the drug is found in all tissues, fat is the primary site of storage. A water-soluble metabolite of **mitotane** is found in the urine; approximately 25% of an oral or parenteral dose is recovered in this form. About 60% of an oral dose is excreted unchanged in the stool.

Mitotane (Lysodren) is administered in initial daily oral doses of 2 to 6 g, usually given in three or four divided portions, but the maximal tolerated dose may vary from 2 to 16 g per day. Treatment should be continued for at least 3 months; if beneficial effects are observed, therapy should be maintained indefinitely. **Spironolactone** should not be administered concomitantly because it interferes with the adrenal suppression produced by mitotane.

Treatment with mitotane is indicated for the palliation of inoperable adrenocortical carcinoma, producing symptomatic benefit in 30 to 50% of such patients.

Although the administration of mitotane produces anorexia and nausea in approximately 80% of patients, somnolence and lethargy in about 34%, and dermatitis in 15 to 20%, these effects do not contraindicate the use of the drug at lower doses. Because this drug damages the adrenal cortex, administration of adrenocorticosteroids is indicated, particularly in patients with evidence of adrenal insufficiency, shock, or severe trauma.

MITOXANTRONE

(Novantrone sterile solution for injection 2 mg/mL)

Mitoxantrone is an anthracenedione/immunomodulator. It has a cytocidal effect on proliferating and nonproliferating cultured human cells, suggesting lack of cell-cycle phase specificity. It is used in adult acute nonlymphocytic leukemia (ANLL) as adjunctive therapy; advanced hormone-refractory prostate cancer (in combination with corticosteroids); and secondary (chronic) progressive, progressive–relapsing, or worsening relapsing–remitting MS.

Mitoxantrone (12 mg/m^2 daily by IV infusion on days 1 to 3) is used as an initial treatment in combination with other approved drugs for **acute nonlymphocytic leukemia** (AML).

Valrubicin (Valstar) was approved in 1998 for intravesical therapy of **bacille Calmette–Guerin–refractory urinary bladder carcinoma** *in situ* in patients for whom immediate cystectomy would be associated with unacceptable morbidity or mortality. **Epirubicin** (4′-epidoxorubicm, Ellence) was approved by the FDA in 1999 as a component of adjuvant therapy following resection of early lymph-node-positive breast cancer.

A related anthracenedione, **mitoxantrone**, has been approved for use in AML. **Mitoxantrone** has limited ability to produce quinone-type free radicals and causes less cardiac toxicity than doxorubicin. It produces acute myelosuppression, cardiac toxicity, and mucositis as its major toxicities; the drug causes less nausea and vomiting and alopecia than doxorubicin. It also is used as a component of experimental high-dose chemotherapy regimens, with uncertain efficacy.

Mitoxantrone (Novantrone) is supplied for intravenous infusion. To induce remission in acute nonlymphocytic leukemia in adults, the drug is given in a daily dose of 12 mg/m^2 for 3 days as a component of a regimen that also includes cytosine arabinoside. **Mitoxantrone** also is used in **advanced hormone-resistant prostate cancer** in a dose of 12 to 14 mg/m^2 every 21 days. Mitoxantrone has been approved by the FDA for the treatment of late-stage, secondary progressive multiple sclerosis.

For relapsing–remitting attacks and for secondary progressive MS, the alkylating agent **cyclophosphamide** and the anthracenedionene-derivative **mitoxantrone** (Novatrone) are currently used in patients refractory to other immunomodulators. These agents, used primarily for cancer chemotherapy, have significant toxicities. Although cyclophosphamide in patients with MS may not be limited by an accumulated dose exposure, **mitoxantrone** can be tolerated only up to an accumulated dose of 100 to 140 mg/m^2. The utility of interferon therapy in patients with secondary progressive MS is unclear. In primary progressive MS, with no discrete attacks and less observed inflammation, suppression of inflammation seems to be less helpful. A minority of patients at this stage will respond to high doses of glucocorticoids.

Each of the agents mentioned previously has side effects and contraindications that may be limiting: infections (for glucocorticoids); hypersensitivity and pregnancy (for immunomodulators); and prior anthracycline/anthracenedione use, mediastinal irradiation, or cardiac disease (**mitoxantrone**). With all of these agents, it is clear that the earlier they are used, the more effective they are in preventing disease relapses. What is not clear is whether any of these agents will prevent or diminish the later onset of secondary progressive disease, which causes the more severe form of disability. Given the fluctuating nature of this disease, only long-term studies lasting decades will answer this question.

A number of other new immunomodulatory therapies are completing phase III trials. One is a monoclonal antibody, natalizumab (Antegren), directed against the adhesion molecule α_4 integrin; natalizumab binds to α_4 integrin and antagonizes interactions with integrin heterodimers containing α_4 integrin, such as $\alpha_4\beta_1$ integrin that is expressed on the surface of activated lymphocytes and monocytes. Preclinical data suggest that an interaction of $\alpha_4\beta_1$ integrin with VCAM-1 (**vascular cellular-adhesion molecule 1**) is critical for T-cell trafficking from the periphery into the CNS; thus, blocking this interaction would hypothetically inhibit disease exacerbations. In fact, phase II clinical trials have demonstrated a significant decrease in the number of new lesions as determined by magnetic resonance imaging and clinical attacks in MS patients receiving natalizumab. Monoclonal antibodies directed against the IL-2 receptor are also entering phase III clinical trials.

MIVACURIUM CHLORIDE

(Mivacron injection 0.5 mg/mL)

Mivacurium is a nondepolarizing neuromuscular blocker that binds competitively to cholinergic transmission. It is indicated as an adjunct to general anesthesia—facilitation of tracheal intubation. At present, only a single depolarizing agent, succinylcholine, is in general clinical use, whereas multiple competitive or nondepolarizing agents are available. Therapeutic selection should be based on achieving a pharmacokinetic profile consistent with the duration of the interventional procedure and minimizing cardiovascular compromise or other side effects. Two general classifications are useful because they are helpful in distinguishing side effects and pharmacokinetic behavior. The first relates to the duration of drug action, and these agents are categorized as long-, intermediate-, and short-acting. The persistent blockade and difficulty in complete reversal after surgery with **D-tubocurarine**, **metocurine**, **pancuronium**, and **doxacurium** led to the development of **vecuronium** and **atracurium**, agents of intermediate duration. This was followed by the development of a short-acting agent, **mivacurium**. Often, the long-acting agents are the more potent, requiring the use of low concentrations. The necessity of administering potent agents in low concentrations delays their onset. **Rocuronium** is an agent of intermediate duration but of rapid onset and lower potency. Its rapid onset allows it to be used as an alternative to succinylcholine in rapid-induction anesthesia and in relaxing the laryngeal and jaw muscles to facilitate tracheal intubation.

Mivacurium, a nondepolarizing neuromuscular-blocking agent (0.15 mg/kg IV push in 5 to 15 seconds), is used as an adjunct to general anesthesia to facilitate endotracheal intubation and to provide skeletal muscle relaxation during surgery or mechanical ventilation (see also Figure 99).

MOCLOBEMIDE

Moclobemide is a novel benzamide reversible inhibitor of monoamine oxidase A and has clinical efficacy in a wide spectrum of depressive illness including endogenous and nonendogenous depression in younger adults and in the elderly. Comparisons have shown similar efficacy to all main classes of antidepressants and much greater tolerability and safety in overdose than tricyclic antidepressants. Clinically, it is neither sedative nor alerting. There is no need for dietary restrictions for patients on moclobemide on a normal diet, and drug interactions are few and usually mild. Moclobemide should be used cautiously in patients who may be taking meperidine or serotonin reuptake inhibitors (see Figure 37).

MODAFINIL

(Provigil tablets 100 mg)

Modafinil is an analeptic. It is used to improve wakefulness in patients with excessive daytime spleepiness associated with narcolepsy, obstructive sleep apnea/hypopnea syndrome (OSAHS), and shift work sleep disorder (SWSD).

Numerous medications have been tried in placebo-controlled clinical trials with cocaine addicts, but finding a medication that consistently improves the results of behavior therapy alone has been elusive. Animal models suggest that enhancing GABAergic inhibition can reduce reinstatement of cocaine self-administration. This finding prompted a controlled clinical trial of topiramate (Topam-AX) that showed a significant improvement for this medication approved for use in epilepsy. Topiramate also was found to reduce the relapse rate in alcoholics, prompting current studies in patients dually dependent on cocaine and alcohol. Baclofen (Lioresal, others), a $GABA_B$ agonist, was found in a single-site trial to reduce relapse in cocaine addicts, and currently is being studied in a multiclinic trial. A different approach was taken using **modafinil** (Provigil), a medication that increases alertness and is approved for the treatment of **narcolepsy**. This medication was found to reduce the euphoria produced by cocaine and to relieve cocaine withdrawal symptoms. After a single-site, double-blind study found it effective in reducing relapse, **modafinil** is being studied in a multisite trial among cocaine-dependent patients.

MOEXIPRIL HYDROCHLORIDE

(Univasc tablets 7.5 mg)

Moexipril is an ACE inhibitor that competitively inhibits angiotensin-I-converting enzyme, preventing conversion of angiotensin I to angiotensin II, which is a potent vasoconstrictor and also stimulates aldosterone secretion from the adrenal cortex. This results in a decrease in sodium and fluid retention, a decrease in BP, and an increase in diuresis. It is indicated in the treatment of hypertension.

Angiotensin II is an important regulator of cardiovascular function. The ability to reduce levels of angiotensin II with orally effective inhibitors of ACE represents an important advance in the treatment of hypertension. **Captopril** (Capoten) was the first such agent to be developed for the treatment of hypertension. Since then, **enalapril** (Vasotec), **lisinopril** (Prinivil), **quinapril** (Accupril), **ramipril** (Altace), **benazepril** (Lotensin), **moexipril** (Univasc), **fosinopril** (Monopril), **trandolapril** (Mavik) and **perindopril** (Aceon) also have become available. These drugs have proven to be very useful for the treatment of hypertension because of their efficacy and their very favorable profile of adverse effects, which enhances patient adherence.

The ACE inhibitors appear to confer a special advantage in the treatment of patients with diabetes, slowing the development and progression of diabetic glomerulopathy. They also are effective in slowing the progression of other forms of chronic renal disease, such as **glomerulosclerosis**, and many of these patients also have hypertension. An ACE inhibitor is the preferred initial agent in these patients. Patients with hypertension and ischemic heart disease are candidates for treatment with ACE inhibitors; administration of ACE inhibitors in the immediate postmyocardial infarction period has been shown to improve ventricular function and reduce morbidity and mortality.

The endocrine consequences of inhibiting the biosynthesis of angiotensin II are of importance in a number of facets of hypertension treatment. Because ACE inhibitors blunt the rise in **aldosterone** concentrations in response to Na^+ loss, the normal role of aldosterone to oppose diuretic-induced natriuresis is diminished. Consequently, ACE inhibitors tend to enhance the efficacy of diuretic drugs. This means that even very small doses of diuretics may substantially improve the antihypertensive efficacy of ACE inhibitors; conversely, the use of high doses of diuretics together with ACE inhibitors may lead to excessive reduction in blood pressure and to Na^+ loss in some patients.

Moexipril (Univasc): **Moexipril** is another prodrug whose antihypertensive activity is almost entirely due to its deesterified metabolite, **moexiprilat**. **Moexipril** is absorbed incompletely, with bioavailability as moexiprilat of about 13%. Bioavailability is markedly decreased by food; therefore, the drug should be taken 1 hour before meals. The time to peak plasma concentration of moexiprilat is almost 1.5 hours, and the elimination half-life varies between 2 and 12 hours. The recommended dosage range is 7.5 to 30 mg daily in one or two divided doses. The dosage range is halved in patients who are taking diuretics or who have renal impairment.

MOLECULAR MEDICINE

Dramatic discoveries in **molecular medicine** along with concomitant rapid technological advances have revolutionized the diagnosis and treatment of a broad range of human diseases. Given the pace of new discovery, **genetic- and cell-based therapies** may well become a common part of the physician's armamentarium in the near future. Direct links between genetic mutations and diseases are being mapped almost routinely. Genomic approaches to diseases such as breast cancer have led to identification of previously unrecognized malignancies and the ability to prognosticate outcomes to therapy. The delicate interplay between adipocytes and regulation of insulin sensitivity, the roles of bone morphogenetic proteins in pulmonary hypertension, and the discovery of mutations involved in an array of cardiomyopathies are but a few of the important recent advances that have direct implications for patient care.

The basic patterns of genetic transmission in humans have been known for about a century, but are now coming to be understood at the molecular level. In addition to classical dominant, recessive, and **sex-linked inheritance**, more complex patterns have also been identified. These include maternal transmission of traits encoded in the mitochondrial genome, digenic traits determined by two distinct genes, and genomic imprinting. It is becoming clear that both rare and common genetic traits are determined by a complex interaction of multiple genetic and nongenetic factors.

The "rules" of segregation of alleles originally defined by **Gregor Mendel** explained much of the phenomena associated with inheritance and have been dogmatically applied in the field of genetics. However, there are situations in which the rules of Mendelian inheritance cannot explain observed phenomena. A variety of molecular mechanisms have been identified that explain certain phenomena that are not easily explained by traditional **Mendelian patterns of inheritance**. These non-Mendelian mechanisms differ on a molecular basis, but can be described as a group by the term "nontraditional mechanisms of inheritance" or "nontraditional inheritance." Stated simply, nontraditional inheritance refers to the pattern of inheritance of a trait or phenotype that occurs predictably, recurrently, and in some cases familially, but does not follow the rules of typical Mendelian autosomal or sex chromosome inheritance.

Cancer is a genetic disease, but there are many different types of genetic changes found within a cancer cell.

The study of relatively rare **cancer predisposition disorders** has provided crucial insights into basic mechanisms of cellular physiology and tumorigenesis.

The clinical implications of **pharmacogenetics** are vast, and many more are becoming apparent as research continues. Health care providers will increasingly need to take pharmacogenetics into consideration when prescribing medications. Each patient's history, physical condition, gender, and ethnicity must be considered when prescribing drugs. Specific genotypic testing of patients for polymorphisms that influence drug metabolism and action will become a clinical reality. **Silicone chip technology** utilizing **single-nucleotide polymorphisms** will be able to provide a practitioner with reliable and timely information in an office setting to guide practice. Genetics and pharmacology are no longer separate sciences.

Gene therapy offers the potential for cure of **hemophilia**, a sex-linked genetic bleeding disorder caused by deficiency of either **coagulation factor VIII** or **coagulation factor DC**. The features of hemophilia that make it a leading candidate for **gene therapy** include the fact that the factor VTC and factor IX genes have been identified and cloned, therapeutic benefit would result from achieving expression at plasma levels as low as 1% of normal, and a wide variety of gene transfer vectors and cell target types could be useful. The challenge is to obtain long-term gene expression at levels sufficient to prevent spontaneous bleeding, while avoiding unwanted toxicity or immune responses to the expressed clotting factor.

Cardiogenesis is a complex process involving different cell types, such as muscle, endothelial, neural crest, and matrix cells. These cells follow a "protocol" that emerges through changes in gene expression induced by developmental and mechanical cues. Data from human genetics and animal mutants suggest that most **congenital heart malformations** arise from gene alterations The next challenge will be to unravel the sequence of molecular decisions that result in the formation of heart and blood vessel from the first embryonic tissue layers. This knowledge is expected to result in novel strategies for diagnosis, treatment, or prevention of heart diseases.

Genetics is an emerging field in cardiovascular medicine. Remarkably, less than 50 years ago, genetics was a nascent field of basic research with little apparent relevance to cardiovascular science or any other medical subspecialty. Yet today, **cardiovascular genetics** is a discipline that fully integrates high-technology laboratory investigation and clinical medicine. From this unusual hybrid have emerged discoveries that precisely identify cause in heretofore "idiopathic" disorders that provide fundamental insights into disease processes, and that delineate subtypes in well-defined pathologies. Insights from these discoveries uproot traditional anatomic classifications of disease and integrate cell physiology and molecular biochemistry into the study of pathology. For researchers, practitioners, and patients alike, cardiovascular genetics has a growing impact on the definition and diagnosis of disease, on explaining prognosis, and expanding treatments.

The understanding of **cardiac excitation contraction coupling** and **β-adrenoreceptor signaling** continues to evolve. Defects in the steps of excitation contraction coupling and β-adrenergic signaling have been identified in human and experimental models of **heart failure**. Abnormalities in ionic channels, transporters, kinases, and various signaling pathways collectively contribute to the "failing phenotype." β-Adrenoceptors are widely expressed in human tissues and activated by neuronally released and circulating catecholamine. They are important mediators of the sympathoadrenal axis regulating numerous physiological events, including relaxation of vascular smooth muscle, cardiac inotropy, chronotropy, and lusitropy. The traditional view of signal transduction is changing because of the emergence of concepts in the complexity of **guanine nucleotide protein-coupled receptor** (GPCR)-**effector coupling**, an intracellular coupling.

The major complication of **coronary artery disease** (CAD) is myocardial injury and dysfunction from inadequate delivery of essential nutrients. Coronary obstruction can be severe before it limits blood flow, particularly under resting conditions, and thus this process can develop over years while remaining clinically silent. Inadequate blood flow that does not produce permanent myocardial cell damage is termed **myocardial ischemia**. Reduction or obstruction in flow sufficient in severity and duration to cause irreversible, clinically detectable **myocardial damage** is termed **myocardial infarction** (MI). Improved biochemical markers of myocyte injury with greater sensitivity and specificity (such as cardiac **troponin isoforms**) have made the detection of small amounts of myocardial injury feasible in a clinical setting. Detection of these markers identifies a subset of patients at higher risk for subsequent complications and increases the number of patients with **diagnosable infarction** who would previously have been considered to have suffered "only" an episode of ischemia. The clinical and biological spectrum from mild ischemia to substantial infarction appears to be a continuum rather than distinct categories.

The relationship between alterations in serum lipoprotein levels and heart disease risk was recognized more than 50 years ago. Since then, remarkable expansion has occurred in the knowledge of the genetics, molecular and cellular biology, and physiology of the lipoprotein metabolism system, leading to large-scale clinical trials of **lipid-lowering drugs** to test their efficacy in preventing acute coronary syndromes. The value of this approach has been repeatedly affirmed. As a result, the treatment of patients with lipid disorders constitutes one of the most common interventions in adult medical practice and remains the centerpiece of strategies aimed at reducing the incidence of **coronary heart disease** (CHD).

Hypertension is a complex, multifactorial condition defined by a consistently elevated arterial blood pressure.

If untreated, hypertension leads to morbidity and mortality primarily, secondary to heart disease (CHF, coronary artery disease, and left-ventricular hypertrophy), renal failure, or stroke. As with many disease states, the molecular etiology of hypertension could originate with one gene (monogenic) or several genes (polygenic). Few cases of hypertension in humans have been shown to be monogenic. Because essential hypertension (i.e., hypertension not caused by a secondary etiology such as renal artery stenosis) is likely a complex, polygenic disease, a major task of hypertension research has been to elucidate its genetic basis. Owing to the complexity of the task, investigators have used multiple genetic strategies in the basic science and clinical research settings. In addition, essential hypertension is a multifactorial state involving interactions between genetic, environmental, and demographic factors. Essential hypertension is likely to result from an elaborate interaction between a network of major and minor genes that mediate the pathophysiological process of elevating blood pressure. In addition, susceptibility genes that modify an individual's response to environment, age, sex, body mass index, and probably other unknown factors compound these genetic interactions. Multiple epistatic effects within and between the causative and susceptibility genes complicate this process. Thus, **essential hypertension** is a truly complex disease whose treatment and therapy depend not only on identifying candidate genes involved but also on dissecting their interactions with other factors.

Advances in genomics and proteomics have provided powerful tools to study the genetics of multifactorial diseases like hypertension. However, with the exception of monogenic forms of hypertension such as **familial hyperaldosteronism**, **Liddle's syndrome**, and mutations in **epithelial sodium channels** (ENaC), little progress has been made in identifying the underlying genetics of essential hypertension. Thus, there is great difficulty in studying a pathophysiologically heterogeneous disease like hypertension that varies by renin status and sodium dependency, among other factors.

Pathological cardiac hypertrophy develops in response to stresses, and can be concentric, eccentric, or both. An excess pressure load placed on the heart, for example, resulting from uncorrected hypertension or valvular disease, results in concentric hypertrophy. This hypertrophy is initially believed to be adaptive, normalizing systolic wall stress, though it is not clear that hypertrophy is necessary to maintain systolic function in the face of moderately elevated pressure loads. Eccentric hypertrophy results most often from volume loads such as those in valvular insufficiency. Finally, the hypertrophy that occurs in the remote noninfarcted myocardium, as part of the remodeling process following a myocardial infarction, may be both concentric and eccentric.

Cells that are terminally differentiated, by definition, cannot undergo hyperplastic growth. Rather, normal growth of these cells, which include cardiomyocytes, is hypertrophic. This form of hypertrophy, termed physiological hypertrophy, is both concentric (characterized by addition of sarcomeres in parallel, leading to increased width of the myocyte) and eccentric (characterized by the addition of sarcomeres in series, leading to increased length of the myocyte). Pathological cardiac hypertrophy develops in response to stresses, and can be concentric, eccentric, or both. An excess pressure load placed on the heart, for example, resulting from uncorrected hypertension or valvular disease, results in concentric hypertrophy. This hypertrophy is initially believed to be adaptive, normalizing systolic wall stress, though it is not clear that hypertrophy is necessary to maintain systolic function in the face of moderately elevated pressure loads. Eccentric hypertrophy results most often from volume loads such as those in valvular insufficiency. Finally, the hypertrophy that occurs in the remote noninfarcted myocardium, as part of the remodeling process following a **myocardial infarction** (MI), may be both concentric and eccentric.

If the load placed on the heart is not normalized (such as via effective antihypertensive therapy), the heart may continue to hypertrophy, eventually leading to elevated filling pressures and the so-called diastolic heart failure. The hypertrophied heart may also begin to decompensate, leading to progressive dilatation, systolic dysfunction, and heart failure on that basis. Not surprisingly, left-ventricular hypertrophy is a significant risk factor for the development of heart failure, increasing the risk of this end point by 6- to 17-fold. Furthermore, within 5 years of the first detection of left-ventricular hypertrophy, one-third of men and one-fourth of women are dead, usually from cardiac disease.

Given the importance of hypertrophy as a cardiac risk factor, investigators have begun to identify the molecular pathways that regulate the cardiac hypertrophic response in an attempt to identify novel pharmacological targets of potential clinical relevance. The focus of these investigations has been on the cell-surface receptors for agonists that are believed to trigger the hypertrophic response, such as **receptors for angiotensin** (Ang)-II, endothelin (ET)-l, and α- and β-adrenergic agents, and therapies directed at the Ang-II receptor have been effective in regressing hypertrophy and in reducing cardiovascular end points even in patients with diabetes. However, given the vast number of agents that have been reported to induce hypertrophy (see the following text), and the increasing evidence that hypertrophy is multifactorial in origin, focus has shifted to intracellular signaling pathways that may function as final common pathways necessary for the hypertrophic response, irrespective of the inciting stimuli. With the rapid advances in the development of small-molecule inhibitors of components of these pathways that can be used *in vivo*, it is essential to understand the signaling networks that regulate hypertrophic growth.

Ion channel mutations cause long QT syndrome, **Brugada syndrome**, **conduction disorders**, **catecholinergic ventricular tachycardia**, and some forms of familial atrial fibrillation and pre-excitation. Transgenic and gene-targeted mouse models of these disorders have further increased the understanding of links between ion channel mutations and these rare arrhythmia syndromes. It is important to realize, however, that the genetic basis of other inherited arrhythmic syndromes remains unclear, as does the role of genes that are not ion channels. In addition, the relationship of common genetic variants (polymorphisms) to arrhythmic risk is only beginning to be studied.

Elucidation of the genetic mechanisms that contribute to **cardiovascular pathology** has stimulated the development of gene therapy for cardiovascular disease. Gene therapy involves the introduction and expression of recombinant DNA with a goal of ameliorating or curing a disease condition. Gene therapy approaches have been developed to treat a variety of cardiovascular diseases, and many of these approaches have shown promise in animal models of human diseases. Nevertheless, clinical trials of cardiovascular gene therapy are at an early stage, and the place of gene therapy as a treatment for cardiovascular disease remains uncertain.

In the past decade, concepts in classification, pathogenesis, and histopathology of the **idiopathic interstitial pneumonias** have undergone considerable change. This evolution has had a substantial impact on the approach to the diagnosis and clinical management of these patients. Some of the changes have led to considerable confusion, especially with entities such as nonspecific interstitial pneumonia. A firm grasp of the basis for separating these disorders is essential for any physician involved with the care of these patients. The consensus statement from the American Thoracic Society (ATS) and the European Respiratory Society (ERS) defined the idiopathic interstitial pneumonias (IIPs) as a heterogeneous group of nonneoplastic disorders resulting from damage to the lung parenchyma by the varying patterns of inflammation and fibrosis, which are sufficiently different from one another to be designated as separate disease entities. The ATS/ERS IIPs classification includes seven clinico-radiological–pathological entities in order of relative frequency: **idiopathic pulmonary fibrosis** (IPF), **nonspecific interstitial pneumonia** (NSIP), **cryptogenic organizing pneumonia**, **respiratory bronchiolitis-associated interstitial lung disease** (RB-ILD), **desquamative interstitial pneumonitis** (DIP), **acute interstitial pneumonia**, and **lymphoid interstitial pneumonia**. As a group, they can be distinguished from other forms of diffuse parenchymal lung disease by clinical methods including history, physical examination, chest radiology and laboratory studies, and pathology. Achieving a correct diagnosis is a dynamic process. The final diagnosis is rendered only after the pulmonologist, radiologist, and pathologist have reviewed the clinical, radiological, and pathological data.

Understanding of the molecular basis of asthma has progressed significantly in the last decade. The roles of immune recognition and effector cells in orchestrating airway inflammation have been developed, and a picture of how these cells—as well as structural cells within the airways—control long-term tissue remodeling is emerging, which provides a comprehensive view of the pathophysiological processes involved in the disease. Phenotypic changes in the asthmatic bronchial epithelium and its interaction with other cells have been identified, which explain many features of asthma. Moreover, major steps have been taken in characterizing the genetic basis of the disease.

Chronic obstructive pulmonary disease (COPD) is a disease state characterized by airflow limitation that is not fully reversible, caused by a noxious agent. COPD is the fourth leading cause of mortality and affects more than 16 million people in the United States, a number that has increased about 40% since 1982. As COPD and other cigarette-related diseases become epidemic worldwide, the biology of emphysema is clearly complex and poorly understood, with limited translation into effective pharmacotherapy.

Pulmonary arterial hypertension results from the pathological elevation in pulmonary vascular resistance owing to a combination of increased vascular tone and vessel-wall remodeling. It is a heterogeneous disorder with the vascular phenotype dependent on the mechanism and severity of injury. What is clear is that with increasing duration and severity, pulmonary hypertension is associated with progressive vessel-wall remodeling, ultimately resulting in fixed, irreversible lesions. All three cell types within the vessel wall contribute to these vascular lesions through the combined effect of cell proliferation, cell migration, and matrix deposition. Current therapies are aimed at restoring vasodilator function although limiting mitogen-induced proliferation. New therapies need to reverse these vascular lesions by breaking down the extracellular matrix and inducing controlled regression (apoptosis) within the vessel wall. This provides the best chance to restore the pulmonary circulation to its natural low resistive state and reduce the morbidity and mortality associated with this disease.

Cystic fibrosis is a genetic disease that affects multiple organ systems yet leads to respiratory failure and premature death in most afflicted patients. Rapid advancements in our understanding of disease pathogenesis have occurred because of the cloning of the **cystic fibrosis transmembrane conductance regulator gene**. Recent work has shown that volume depletion of the periciliary fluid layer and mucus dehydration reduces mucus clearance and promotes the initiation and progression of CF lung disease. Therapies that correct dysregulated salt and water transport in the lung, either by correcting or bypassing the basic cystic fibrosis transmembrane conductance regulator defect, are now being developed, and hold great promise.

Gene therapy is under development for a variety of lung diseases, both those caused by single-gene defects, such as cystic fibrosis and α_1-antitrypsin deficiency; and multifactorial disease, such as cancer, asthma, lung fibrosis, and acute respiratory distress syndrome (ARDS). Both viral and nonviral approaches have been explored, the major limitation of the former being the inability to repeatedly administer, which renders this approach perhaps more applicable to conditions requiring single administration, such as cancer.

A pulmonary surfactant is required for adaptation to air breathing after birth and reducing surface tension at the air–liquid interface in the alveolus to maintain lung volumes during the respiratory cycle. Pulmonary surfactants are a complex mixture of proteins and lipids whose synthesis, packaging, secretion, and catabolism are tightly controlled at transcriptional and posttranscriptional levels. It is well established that the lack of a pulmonary surfactant causes **respiratory distress syndrome** (RDS) in preterm infants. Abnormalities in surfactant content, composition, and function are also associated with acute RDSs in older patients in a variety of clinical conditions associated with lung injury. As the genetic and cellular systems regulating surfactant homeostasis are increasingly understood, gene mutations and abnormalities in the pathways mediating surfactant homeostasis are being implicated in the pathogenesis of both acute and chronic pulmonary diseases.

Hormones provide a form of communication between different cells and from one organ to another. The dramatic effects of hormones on physiological functions such as growth and metabolism have promoted studies to elucidate their sources of production, sites of action, and how they are controlled. Because hormones exert their effects by binding to specific receptors, studies defining their mechanisms of action have also provided important paradigms for how receptors activate intracellular signaling cascades that lead to altered cellular responses.

Endocrine disorders ultimately involve abnormalities of hormone production or action. Etiologies of a relatively large number of these diseases with well-defined genetic bases have been identified.

Hormones can be divided generally into three major classes:

1. Derivatives of amino acids (e.g., dopamine and catecholamines)
2. Peptides and proteins (e.g., TRH or insulin)
3. Derivatives of steroids (e.g., estrogen or cortisol)

The completion of the human genome sequence has permitted the identification of additional signaling molecules of many different classes. The impact of this new information on the understanding of the pathophysiology of disease is already evidenced in terms of the ability to predict specific receptors or pathways that might harbor mutations in different disorders. Numerous examples exist of mutations in genes that encode hormones, their receptors, second messenger signaling pathways, and of the factors that transduce hormone signals

Diabetes mellitus affects approximately 5% of the general population with its prevalence varying among ethnic groups and geographic regions. Two types of diabetes, type 1 and type 2, account for approximately 10% and 90% of diabetes cases, respectively. Although these two disorders share a common phenotype, fasting and postprandial hyperglycemia, their etiology is distinct. Type 1 diabetes is characterized by **pancreatic β-cell deficiency** with a resulting absolute deficiency of **insulin**. The β-cell deficiency is most commonly secondary to autoimmune-mediated destruction. Type 2 diabetes, in contrast, is characterized by a deficiency of insulin action resulting from a combination of **insulin resistance** and relative **β-cell dysfunction** that is manifested as inadequate insulin secretion in the face of insulin resistance and hyperglycemia.

The familial clustering of both type 1 and type 2 diabetes has long suggested a genetic contribution to the etiology of the diseases. In the case of type 1 diabetes, the concordance rate among monozygotic twins is 30 to 40% compared with a concordance rate of 5 to10% among dizygotic twins. The risk of type 1 diabetes for siblings of an affected individual is approximately 6%, whereas the risk in the general population is approximately 0.4%. Although these data are consistent with a genetic contribution to the etiology of the disease, the lack of 100% concordance in monozygotic twins suggests that environmental factors make a significant contribution to the disease pathogenesis. These environmental factors are not clearly defined, but some studies suggest that certain viral infections or early childhood diet may affect the risk of type 1 diabetes. Prenatal exposure to rubella is a clear risk factor, as 20% of children with the **congenital rubella syndrome** develop type 1 diabetes. Other potential risk factors for which there are conflicting or unconfirmed data include enterovirus infections and early introduction of either cow's milk protein, cereal, or gluten into the diet. Familial clustering of disease is much more apparent in type 2 diabetes. The concordance rate among monozygotic twins is 50 to 90%, whereas approximately 40% of siblings and 30% of offspring of affected individuals develop either type 2 diabetes or impaired glucose tolerance. Again, these data are consistent with a significant genetic contribution to the development of type 2 diabetes but suggest that environmental influences are also important.

With the advent of molecular genetics, significant progress has been made in defining the genetics of rare, monogenic forms of diabetes as well as more typical type 1 and 2 diabetes. Progress is reflected in the classification of diabetes, which includes diagnostic categories of genetic defects in β-cell function and insulin action.

The cell types of the mature adenohypophysis are derived embryologically from somatic ectoderm associated with Rathke's pouch. Highly specific trophic factors determine a precise temporal and spatial development of cells expressing unique gene products. The six hormones of the anterior pituitary gland are expressed by at least five distinct hormone-producing cell populations, including **corticotrophs** (pro-opiomelanocortin, POMC), **somatotrophs** (growth hormone, GH), **lactotrophs** (prolactin, PRL), **thyrotrophs** (TSH), and **gonadotrophs** (FSH and LH). Each of these cells is identified by specific assays of polypeptide gene expression, including single-cell mRNA, immunoelectron microscopy, and immunocytochemical assays. The temporal ontogeny of these gene products is initially adrenocorticotropic hormone (ACTH) and α-subunit. Distinct GH- and PRL-expressing cells follow, and TSH, LH, and FSH are the final cell types to mature at 12 weeks.

Each of the anterior pituitary trophic hormones is induced by a respective hypothalamic-releasing hormone, and their transcription is regulated by negative feedback inhibition of their respective target hormones. Once the cell has been transformed, its ultimate growth characteristics and neoplastic behavior appear to be determined by several genes acting relatively distally, including ras and nm23.

Growth hormone (GH) is a multifunctional hormone produced in the pituitary that promotes postnatal growth of skeletal and soft tissues through a variety of effects. In addition to promoting growth of tissues, GH also exerts a variety of other biological effects, including lactogenic, diabetogenic, lipolytic, and protein anabolic effects, as well as sodium and water retention. The frequency of GH deficiency has been estimated at 1/4000 to 1/10,000 in various studies. Estimates of the proportion of GH-deficient cases having an affected parent, sibling, or child range from 3 to 30% in different studies. This occurrence of familial clustering suggests that a significant proportion of cases might have a genetic basis.

Insights into the molecular basis of numerous **thyroid disorders** have grown impressively. Careful clinical and biochemical phenotyping continues to be the essential first step in all attempts to unravel the underlying pathogenic mechanisms. Elucidation of the molecular basis has been enormously facilitated by the increasingly complete information on the human genome, growing knowledge about developmental processes, the complexity of signaling pathways, and mechanisms of hormone action. Aside from deepening the understanding of the mechanisms governing physiology and **pathology of the hypothalamic–pituitary–thyroid axis**, this increasingly dense knowledge has growing impact on diagnostic and therapeutic modalities.

The **parathyroid glands** play a crucial role in maintaining normal calcium homeostasis, primarily through their regulated secretion of parathyroid hormone. A variety of congenital and acquired causes of diminished parathyroid function exist, including developmental abnormalities and defective parathyroid hormone synthesis or release, and the genetic basis for many of these is known. Primary disorders of parathyroid hyperfunction, mostly owing to parathyroid gland tumors, can be familial or sporadic. Molecular pathogenetic insights into these disorders are substantial and have been exploited for clinical management.

Congenital adrenal hyperplasia (CAH) is a family of autosomal recessive disorders caused by mutations that encode for enzyme involved in one of the various steps of adrenal steroid synthesis. These defects result in the absence or the decreased synthesis of cortisol from its cholesterol precursor. The anterior pituitary secretes excess **ACTH** via feedback regulation by cortisol, which results in overstimulation of the adrenals and causes hyperplasia.

Symptoms owing to CAH can vary from mild to severe depending on the degree of the enzymatic defect. In the classical forms of CAH, defects in the **cytochrome P450s 21-hydroxylase (21-OH)** or **11β-hydroxylase (11β-OH)** cause varying degrees of genital ambiguity in females owing to shunting of excess cortisol precursors to the androgen synthesis pathway. Prenatal adrenal androgen excess causes virilization of female genitalia and postnatally results in advanced bone age and puberty in both females and males. Defects in androgen synthesis owing to defects in **β-hydroxysteroid dehydrogenase** (3β-HSD)$\Delta^{5,4}$-isomerase, in **17α-hydroxylase (17α-OH)/17,20-lyase**, and in the steroidogenic acute regulatory protein (StAR) result in inadequate prenatal virilization of males and depressed puberty in both sexes. Less severe, nonclassical forms of CAH present postnatally as signs of androgen excess.

The adrenal cortex plays a key role in regulating intermediary metabolism, fluid and electrolyte balance, and the response to stress. Molecular analyses of specific disorders resulting from either the diminished or enhanced production/action of **corticosteroids** have led to the identification of a number of genes that play key roles in adrenal function and corticosteroid action. These genes provide potential targets for novel therapies that may revolutionize our approaches to these rare adrenal diseases. In addition, understanding the molecular causes of these diseases has provided important insights into basic adrenal functions that may translate into improved therapy of more common disorders such as hypertension and obesity.

Multiple endocrine neoplasia type 1 (MEN1) is characterized by the combined occurrence of tumors of the parathyroid, pancreatic islets, and anterior pituitary. In addition, some patients may also develop adrenal cortical, carcinoid, **facial angiofibromas**, **collagenomas**, and **lipomatons tumors**. MEN1 is inherited as an autosomal-dominant disorder, and the gene causing MEN1 is located on chromosome 11q13. The MEN1 gene consists of 10 exons that encode a 610 amino acid protein, menin, which has a role in transcriptional regulation and genome stability. The mutations causing MEN1 are of diverse types and are scattered throughout the coding region. Mice deleted for a MEN1 allele develop endocrine tumors similar to those found in MEN1 patients. The availability of these mouse models for MEN1 will help to further elucidate the role of menin in regulating cell proliferation.

Multiple endocrine neoplasia is a genetic endocrine tumor syndrome characterized by the presence of medullary thyroid carcinoma (MTC), pheochromocytoma, and hyperparathyroidism. There are two major variants. Multiple endocrine neoplasia type 2A (MEN2A) or Sipple's syndrome has three clinical features: MTC, **pheochromocytoma**, and **hyperparathyroidism**; MEN2B has a different phenotype: MTC, pheochromocytoma, mucosal neuromas distributed throughout the mouth and gastrointestinal tract, and Marfanoid features including long thin arms and legs, an altered upper/lower body ratio, and pectus abnormalities. These clinical syndromes are caused by specific activating mutations of the **RET tyrosine kinase receptor**, important in neurological development of the gastrointestinal tract. MEN2 is one of a handful of genetic syndromes where the identification of a mutation leads to a specific action. Children with germ-line-activating mutations of RET are treated in early childhood with a total thyroidectomy to prevent the development of metastatic MTC.

The development of the male phenotype is a complex process that involves the active participation of genes involved at many levels, from those specifying gonadal differentiation to the **androgen receptor** (AR) itself. **Defective virilization** can be caused by defects anywhere along the pathway. Considering the clinical syndromes caused by known defects of genes such as steroid **5α-reductase II** and the AR, the pathogenesis of a large proportion of defects in virilization remains unexplained. It is conceivable that some might represent defects in genes required for normal AR function or at steps beyond the site of action of the AR itself (e.g., coactivators, or defects in genes activated by the AR).

The primary function of the human ovary is the production of **fertilizable gametes**, a role essential for the survival of the human species. Ovarian gametes are surrounded by somatic cells in a structure known as a **follicle**. The follicle is the essential unit of the ovary, providing both **oocytes** (eggs) and the steroid hormones necessary for female physical development and reproduction. The process of **folliculogenesis** involves the growth and maturation of the egg and division and differentiation of the somatic cells to the point of ovulation or release of a mature oocyte. Folliculogenesis takes many months—not just the 4 weeks of a menstrual cycle. Failure of ovarian follicular function results in infertility. Failure of follicle formation or early follicle loss can result in failure of pubertal progression and severe early osteoporosis. Less severe disruption or later follicle loss can result in **premature ovarian failure** (POF) or early menopause. Disruption of the normal balance of hormone production can alter the ovarian cycle and adversely affect other organ systems such as the central nervous or cardiovascular systems.

Ovarian gametogenesis has been described as intricate and delicately balanced. Although complicated, this process is also characterized by multiple redundancies providing robustness to the process that allows for compensation for isolated gene defects. Many processes that occur in embryonic development are also necessary for follicle development and normal ovarian function. Genes that regulate other developmental processes might also have a role in follicle development.

Lipolysis is the pathway by which adipocyte triglycerides are hydrolyzed and mobilized as free fatty acids, during periods when energy expenditure exceeds caloric intake. **Hormone-sensitive lipase** is the major enzyme involved in regulation of lipolysis. Numerous hormones acutely regulate lipolysis, but the most physiologically important are insulin (inhibitory) and catecholamines (stimulatory). Hormone-sensitive lipase is activated by phosphorylation in response to stimulatory hormones through a cAMP-mediated cascade. Conversely, insulin and other hormones that inhibit lipolysis decrease phosphorylation of hormone-sensitive lipase. Lipolysis can also be regulated over the longer term by changes in gene expression in response to growth hormone, cytokines, insulin, and glucose.

Sarcopenia is defined as an involuntary loss of skeletal muscle mass and function that occurs with advancing age. It has been associated with muscle weakness resulting in an increased prevalence of falls, loss of function and independence, and higher morbidity. As the elderly population increases, sarcopenia and its resulting disability will become increasingly important. There are 39 million Americans over the age of 65, with an expected increase of 6 million in the next 10 years.

The pathogenesis of sarcopenia is multifactorial. Disuse atrophy from physical inactivity can reduce mitochondrial function, enzyme activity, energy reserves, and increased susceptibility to **reactive oxygen species (ROS)-induced damage**. Dysregulation of muscle amino acid metabolism and protein turnover can result from inactivity, inadequate nutrition, and/or altered transcriptional or translational control of muscle protein synthesis. Traumatic injury may induce alterations in CNS function and neural stimulation and lead to muscular changes. Illness and medications frequently taken with advancing age can cause hormonal changes and reduced muscle blood flow. Other alterations such as disrupted expression of essential regulatory genes and inflammatory cytokine dysregulation might also contribute to sarcopenia in the older population.

Iron is a major component of the Earth's crust, but its own chemistry greatly limits utilization and also sets the basis for its toxicity. The capacity of readily exchanging electrons in aerobic conditions makes iron essential for fundamental cell functions, such as DNA synthesis, transport of oxygen and electrons, and cell respiration. However, because humans have no means to control iron excretion, excess iron, regardless of the route of entry, accumulates in parenchymal organs and threatens cell viability.

A number of disease states are caused by excessive accumulation of iron in the body. The term "primary" identifies diseases owing to a recognizable hereditary defect in proteins directly involved in iron homeostasis, as opposed to conditions in which iron overload is secondary to known factors or diseases.

Hereditary hemochromatosis (HH) is the most common cause of iron overload in humans. **Ferroportin-associated iron overload**, erroneously classified as type-4 hemochromatosis in genetic taxonomy, is likely the most common cause of hereditary hyperferritinemia beyond classic HH. The disorder, clinically recognized in 1999, has distinctive genetic, pathological, and clinical features.

The application of molecular biological and genetic techniques to the study of the luminal gastrointestinal tract epithelium has led to exciting advances in several broad areas. The study of **inflammatory bowel diseases** (IBD) has advanced greatly, with the identification of the first disease susceptibility gene for **Crohn's disease**, the tentative identification of other susceptibility loci for IBD, the creation of new animal models of IBD using gene knockout and transgenic technology, and the application of cellular and molecular techniques to develop novel therapies for IBD. The molecular mechanisms underlying intestinal digestion and absorption of nutrients have been further clarified by the cloning and characterization of **enterocytic genes** that play critical roles in the digestion and absorption of luminal nutrients. Their chromosomal localization, structure, and regulation of expression have been at least partially characterized. These studies have provided the groundwork for understanding the pathophysiology of several rare but well-described genetic disorders of small-intestinal transport, and have begun to clarify the mechanisms underlying more common gastrointestinal problems such as lactase deficiency.

Three **isoforms of nitric oxide synthase** (NOS) and two of **cyclooxygenase** (COX) are expressed in the normal kidney. Neuronal (type I) NOS is expressed heavily in the macula densa where it blunts the tubuloglomerular feedback response that increases afferent arteriolar tone in proportion to distal Nad delivery, and in the cortical and inner medullary collecting ducts where it impairs tubular Na^+ entry. Endothelial (type III) NOS is expressed in endothelial cells where it mediates the endothelium-derived relaxing factor response, and in the thick ascending limb where it inhibits tubular NaCl reabsorption. Inducible (type II) NOS is widely expressed after cytokine challenge. It participates in cell death following sepsis or ischemia of the kidney. COX-1 is expressed in endothelial and smooth-muscle cells of renal vasculature and in the medullary collecting ducts where it antagonizes arginine vasopressin and inhibits Na^+ reabsorption. COX-2 is expressed in the macula densa cells and adjacent thick ascending limb where it enhances renin secretion and inhibits tubular NaCl reabsorption. NOS and COX isoforms interact extensively to fulfill their major roles of adapting renal function to changes in salt and water intake or blood pressure.

Hypertension is an increase of blood pressure to levels greater than normal that arises because of a mismatch between the volume of the vascular tree and the volume of blood. Blood volume depends on total body sodium content, which is a balance between sodium intake and output. Total body sodium is controlled by variable excretion of sodium by the kidneys. To regulate sodium balance, the primary variable that the kidney monitors is not total body sodium but rather systemic blood pressure. Renal regulation of blood pressure is via the release of the peptide hormone **renin** from specialized renal cells. Release of renin ultimately leads to the production of **angiotensin II**. Angiotensin II increases total peripheral resistance and blood pressure and also leads to an increase in aldosterone. Aldosterone is a steroid hormone that increases sodium reabsorption in the distal nephron by activating **epithelial Na channels** (ENaCs). Thus, hypertension is a defect in one of these elements that control total body sodium balance.

Nephrogenic diabetes insipidus (NDI) is a rare disorder in which the kidney is unresponsive to the water-retaining action of **vasopressin** (**antidiuretic hormone**). Congenital NDI results from a genetic mutation in the V_2-receptor, AQP2, or other transport proteins such as the UT-B urea transporter, involved in generating a hypertonic renal medulla. Acquired NDI most commonly results from **lithium therapy**, but can also result from prolonged hypercalcemia protein malnutrition, hypokalemia, and following the release of unilateral or **bilateral ureteral obstruction**. The current therapeutic options for congenital NDI are limited and only partially beneficial in reducing the excessive urine output.

The **muscular dystrophies** are a group of inherited primary diseases of muscle that are characterized clinically by progressive, chronic weakness, and pathologically by degeneration of muscle fibers with necrosis and connective-tissue infiltration. This definition distinguishes muscular dystrophies from other primary diseases of muscle, including the **congenital myopathies** and **inflammatory myopathies**, although there are some areas of overlap.

The clinical course of muscular dystrophy varies widely between specific diseases from the rapidly fatal **Walker–Warburg disease** to the milder **Becker's muscular dystrophy**. There are four major categories of muscular dystrophy: **dystrophinopathies**, **limb-girdle muscular dystrophies** (LGMD), **congenital muscular dystrophies**, and the **syndromic muscular dystrophies**. These categories are largely based on the clinical characteristics of the diseases and do not reflect the differences in molecular and biochemical origins. An international collaborative effort in the mid-1980s led to positional cloning of **dystrophin**, the gene on the X-chromosome responsible for **Duchenne's muscular dystrophy**. Since then, the genes that cause more than a dozen other types of muscular dystrophy have been described (summarized at http://www.dmd.nl/). These proteins, with other associated muscle proteins that have not been shown to play a primary role in human disease, have been extensively studied. The majority of the proteins produced by these genes appear primarily to be structural in function and are linked to each other in the vicinity of the sarcolemma. Some of these proteins may also play a role in cellular signaling and repair. Very few are enzymes.

Rhabdomyosarcomas are the most common soft-tissue sarcomas in childhood, yet they are still a relatively rare tumor, with an incidence in the United States of 1.3-4.5/million children/year. The histological classification of rhabdomyosarcoma has historically relied on the expression of genes associated with skeletal muscle in some of the tumor cells, giving a subset of cells the appearance of skeletal muscle cells or myoblasts. Several histological subcategories of rhabdomyosarcomas have also been recognized. **Embryonal rhabdomyosarcomas** occur most frequently during the first 3 years after birth and account for about 50–60% of rhabdomyosarcomas. Additional distinctions can be made within the group of embryonal rhabdomyosarcomas; for example, there are the botyroid and spindle cell variants. **Alveolar rhabdomyosarcomas** are distinguished from embryonal rhabdomyosarcomas histologically by characteristic open spaces in pathology sections, reminiscent of alveoli in the lungs. Alveolar rhabdomyosarcomas account for approximately 20% of rhabdomyosarcomas and have a bimodal incidence distribution with peaks at approximately ages 3 and 15 years. A third group of pleomorphic or primitive rhabdomyosarcomas is not easily distinguished from other small round cell tumors of childhood, such as neuroblastoma, **Ewing's sarcoma**, **primitive neuroectodermal tumors**, and **non-Hodgkin's lymphoma** based on standard histology. For these primitive tumors, classification as rhabdomyosarcomas can be confirmed using antibodies or other molecular probes to genes characteristically expressed in skeletal muscle, such as desmin, or muscle creatine kinase.

Colorectal cancer is the third most common death-causing disease in the developed countries. It arises after a series of mutations in various tumor suppressor and protooncogenes, each of which are accompanied by specific alterations and pathological conditions. Recent advances have contributed a great deal of understanding of the molecular basis of events that lead to **colorectal tumorigenesis**. Mutation in the **adenomatous polyposis coli** (APC) gene is considered to be one of the earliest events in the development of colon cancer. The **familial adenomatous polyposis** and **hereditary nonpolyposis colorectal cancer** (HNPCC) are the most commonly inherited colorectal cancers. Familial adenomatous polyposis and HNPCC develop owing to mutations in APC and DNA mismatch repair (MMR) genes, respectively. The main functions of APC are known to regulate **β-catenin protein** levels through the **Wnt-signaling pathway**, involved in cell migration and cell–cell adhesion, and chromosomal stability. Mutations in the APC gene disrupt the normal functioning of these pathways and thus are involved in the development of colon cancer. Colorectal cancer also develops owing to alterations in the **transforming growth factor-β-signaling pathway**. Mutations in the pro-apoptotic gene Bax is found in many colon tumors from HNPCC patients.

Breast cancer is the most common malignancy and a leading cause of mortality in women in the Western world. More than 200,000 American women were diagnosed with breast cancer in 2004. The incidence of breast cancer varies with multiple factors including gender, age, ethnicity, family history, reproductive factors, socioeconomic class, exogenous and endogenous hormones, radiation exposure, genetic susceptibility, and so on. Like other human cancers, breast cancer is recognized as a genetic disease in that it is thought to result from a progressive accumulation of genetic changes. Initiation of breast cancer results from uncontrolled cell proliferation and/or aberrant programmed cell death as a consequence of cumulative alterations of tumor suppressor gene and/or protooncogene expression. Epigenetic changes such as DNA methylation or chromatin modeling can also contribute to modified gene expression. These changes can modulate expression of a variety of critical genes with diverse functions. Previously, the only biological factor of clinical import in breast cancer was steroid receptor expression because it has been an important predictive factor of response to endocrine therapy. However, over the last two decades, enormous advances have been made in the understanding of breast cancer at the molecular level. This understanding has revealed a large number of new targets that may play a role as risk, prognostic, or predictive factors and/or aid in the development of new effective therapies of breast cancer.

Lung cancer is the leading cause of cancer-related deaths worldwide today, with an estimated 169,500 new cases and 157,400 deaths predicted for 2001 in the United States. Human lung cancer is a disease of heterogeneous histology that can be divided into two major categories: **small-cell lung cancer** (SCLC) and **non-small-cell lung cancer** (NSCLC). SCLC represents approximately 25% of all lung cancer worldwide. The remaining 75% of lung cancers fall into one of three major subtypes of NSCLC **carcinomas**: **squamous cell carcinoma** (SCC), **adenocarcinoma**, and **large-cell carcinoma**. Tobacco smoking is the most important cause of lung cancer, with 80 to 90% of the disease arising in cigarette smokers. Early epidemiological studies of smoking-caused lung cancer indicated that SCC was the most frequently diagnosed type of lung cancer, followed by small-cell carcinoma. Adenocarcinoma of the lung is the most common histological type of lung cancer in the world, and is the most frequent type of lung cancer in women, nonsmokers, and in young people.

With the application of molecular biology and biotechnologies to human prostate cancer research, new targets in the lethal phenotypes of prostate cancer have been rapidly ascertained. How many are pharmacologically amenable and can be blocked with clinical relevance remains to be discovered. For all the emergent genetic and protein target insights, perhaps the greatest challenges will be the participation of more men with prostate cancer in translational research clinical trials that evaluate the new science of therapeutics designed specifically for prostate cancer

The incidence of cutaneous melanoma is increasing significantly and responds poorly to current therapies. At the root of this problem is the transformation of melanocytes, which normally synthesize **melanin** to protect the skin against **ultraviolet (UV) damage**, into highly invasive cells that can colonize many different regions of the body, reminiscent of their neural crest origin. Paradoxically, UV radiation increases the incidence of melanoma and the penetrance of melanoma susceptibility genes such as CDKNA2A. Abnormal expression of **cadherins**, **integrins**, and other cell-adhesion and matrix proteins are key in melanoma cell transformation and in transendothelial migration, a key step in metastasis.

Malignant CNS tumors that originate from brain tissue or from the brain's coverings (i.e., primary tumors) cause significant morbidity and mortality. Each year, seven to ten new cases of primary intracranial tumors are diagnosed per 100,000 population. Tumors of the glioma group are the most common primary brain tumors in adults, and the most important group of diffusely infiltrating gliomas are the astrocytomas and oligoden-drogliomas. The biological behavior of such tumors varies from slowly growing indolent lesions that may produce symptoms over many years to aggressive, rapidly growing neoplasms that can cause death within a year of diagnosis. Most gliomas are incurable because they infiltrate brain tissue, making it difficult to completely remove the tumor without damaging normal structures. Because of this, recurrences of such tumors are common, despite standard therapeutic efforts (usually radiation and/or chemotherapy).

The **acute myeloid leukemias** (AML) are a heterogeneous group of malignant diseases of **hematopoietic progenitor cells** with a spectrum of molecular genetic abnormalities, clinical characteristics, and variable outcomes with available treatments. For several decades, the cornerstone for treatment of AML has been empirically derived cytotoxic chemotherapy. Although this remains the foundation of treatment, advances have been made in the development of molecularly targeted therapies of AML based on an improved understanding of the genetic basis of the disease. Furthermore, emerging data indicate that AML can be viewed as a hierarchy, similar to that observed in the normal hematopoietic development, in which there is a critical population of leukemic stem cells that are necessary for continued growth and propagation of AML. These leukemic stem cells are likely to be the basis for relapsed disease after remission induction, and may perhaps be the best target for developing novel therapeutic approaches to the disease.

Acute lymphoblastic leukemia (ALL) is the most common malignancy among children and represents 80% and 10 to 20%, respectively, of childhood and adult acute leukemias. Advances in the understanding of childhood ALL have transformed the disease from a rapidly progressive and usually lethal disorder to a disease with an 80% cure rate. These improved outcomes are resulting from the development of multiagent, dose-intensive chemotherapy regimens, CNS prophylaxis, and improved supportive care. Parallel to the improved understanding of therapeutic approaches to ALL, knowledge of the pathogenesis of ALL has increased dramatically. However, uncovering the molecular mechanisms behind this disease has not yet produced targeted therapies that specifically act on these elements, as has been the case, for example, with tyrosine kinase inhibition for chronic myelogenous leukemia (CML). Such novel treatment approaches are needed in particular in adult ALL which, although morphologically indistinguishable from pediatric disease, has a considerably poorer response to chemotherapy and remains incurable in >50% of the cases. These differences in part result from differing molecular pathogenesis, which results in a higher proportion of tumors with *de novo* pan-drug resistance.

Chronic myelogenous leukemia is a clonal hematopoietic stem disorder characterized by excess numbers of myeloid cells that, over time, lose the capacity for terminal differentiation. A series of discoveries led to the identification of the **BCR-ABL tyrosine kinase** as the cause of the disease, and this provided the impetus for the development of specific agents that target this abnormality. This has also led to improved methods for diagnosis and molecular monitoring of patients with the disease.

Non-Hodgkin's lymphoma (NHL) is a complex and heterogeneous group of disorders characterized by clonal proliferation of lymphocytes at different stages of maturation. There are approximately 30 types of NHL with varying clinical, pathological, and genetic features. Understanding some of its biological features has provided insights into the clinical behavior of NHL. For example, lymphomas with high proliferative indices (like **Burkitt's and lymphoblastic lymphomas**) present with rapidly growing tumor masses, referred to clinically as **high-grade lymphomas**, and are rapidly fatal if not successfully treated. Histologically, these lymphomas have diffuse architecture, and intermediate- or large-cell morphology with large numbers of visible mitotic figures. In contrast, lymphomas with low proliferative indices (**follicular and small lymphocytic lymphomas** [SLLs]) have indolent clinical courses measured in years, affect older patients, and have small, mature-looking cell morphology. Ironically, the "aggressive," rapidly growing lymphomas are curable, whereas the indolent ones remain incurable with available therapeutic strategies.

Multiple myeloma (MM) is a hematopoietic malignancy characterized by the clonal expansion of mature B cells, a low proliferative index, clonal secretion of Ig, osteolytic bone destruction, and ultimate development of drug resistance. MM cells are thought to arise from post-germinal center (GC) plasma cells that have undergone immunoglobulin class switching and somatic hypermutation. Importantly, it is through these normal DNA recombinatorial processes of B-cell differentiation (Ig class switching and somatic hypermutation) that the initial transforming events in MM have been proposed to originate. Evidence for this hypothesis has been demonstrated through the identification of numerous immunoglobulin heavy chain (IgH) and light chain (IgL) translocations in MM and the premalignant monoclonal gammopathy of unknown significance (MGUS). Like their normal plasma-cell counterparts, MM cells home to the bone marrow (BM), remaining closely associated with their physical extracellular environment. MM cells become BM independent only in the most terminal phases and only after the acquisition of secondary or tertiary transforming mutations. These later DNA alterations are frequently somatic mutations and secondary Ig-translocations, leading to the constitutive activity of **oncogenes**.

Paroxysmal nocturnal hemoglobinuria (PNH) is a complex hematological disorder probably first described three centuries ago and regarded as a mystery until the 1980s when most of its pathophysiology was elucidated, followed by the 1990s, when the underlying molecular defect was finally unraveled. The original denomination, PNH, stresses only one component of the disease (i.e., a hyperhemolytic state). A more complete updated definition could read as follows: it is an acquired blood disorder characterized by the expansion of one or a few hematopoietic cell clones carrying a mutation in the X-linked **phosphatidylinositol glycan class A (PIG-A) gene**, which renders the cells unable to produce the **glycosyl-phosphatidylinositol (GPI) anchor**, against a background of a reduced bone marrow activity. Because of its complex pathophysiology, the disease has been variously classified among **hemolytic anemias**, **myelodysplasia**, **myeloproliferative disorders**, or **bone marrow failure syndromes**; indeed, PNH has some features of each of these.

Bone marrow failure is an encompassing term that describes the pancytopenia arising from a variety of clinical disease entities and etiologies. More specifically, the definition includes peripheral blood cytopenias that are caused by inadequate marrow production of either single or multiple cell lines. This can be because of either defective or insufficient marrow production.

Venous thrombosis is mostly caused by disturbances in the plasma coagulation system with platelet participation playing a minor role, whereas in arterial thrombosis, platelets play the predominant role, with some participation of the plasma coagulation system. This paradigm helps explain why **coagulation factor abnormalities**, such as **factor V Leiden**, or **deficiencies of protein C**, **protein S**, and **antithrombin** predominantly lead to **venous thromboembolism**. An understanding of the role of abnormalities predisposing to arterial thromboembolism, such as platelet receptor polymorphisms, is just emerging. At present, inconsistent findings of studies regarding the association of these polymorphisms with arterial thromboembolism limits their clinical usefulness.

Psoriasis is a chronic, inflammatory and hyperproliferative disease of the skin, scalp, nails, and joints, affecting 1 to 2% of the U.S. population. It is found worldwide; its frequency varies from 0 to 3% among different ethnic groups. Most of its variable clinical presentations eventuate into erythematous, scaly plaques with or without nail disease and arthritis. Susceptibility to psoriasis is unmistakably heritable, but the phenotype is controlled by multiple genes as well as environmental factors. Trauma, stress, and infections are important determinants of disease onset and severity. At the cellular level, psoriasis is characterized by markedly increased epidermal proliferation and incomplete differentiation; elongation, dilatation, and "leakiness" of the superficial plexus of dermal capillaries; and a mixed inflammatory and immune cell infiltrate of the epidermis and papillary dermis. A multitude of plausible pathomechanisms have been envisaged for psoriasis, with early concepts focusing on the now epidermal hyperplasia characteristic of this disease. There is wide agreement that psoriasis is driven by interactions between the innate and acquired immune systems in the skin and joints. However, the root cause of psoriasis remains unclear. This section reviews psoriasis' protean clinical manifestations, diagnosis, differential diagnosis, and management, and what has been accomplished to solve its long-standing riddle, particularly in the areas of immunology and genetics.

Atopic dermatitis, also known as **atopic eczema**, is a chronic inflammatory skin disease frequently seen in patients with a personal or family history of asthma and allergic rhinitis. There have been extraordinary strides made in the understanding of the immunopathogenesis of allergic diseases. In particular, this constellation of inherited illnesses is associated with activation of a specific group of **cytokine genes encompassing IL-3**, **IL-4**, **IL-5**, **IL-13**, and **granulocyte-macrophage colony-stimulating factor**. The molecular basis for selective activation of this cytokine gene cluster and its immunological consequences are being investigated. However, it is clear that allergic diseases result from a polygenic inheritance pattern that involves cytokine-gene activation and other less-well-defined gene products as well. In addition, the clinical expression of allergic diseases is highly dependent on a complex interaction between the host and its environment, for example, allergen exposure.

Systemic lupus erythematosus (SLE) is multisystem autoimmune disease characterized by the production of autoantibodies against a host of nuclear antigens. Lupus, the Latin word for wolf, has been used for at least seven centuries to describe the malar rash that some think resembles an animal bite. The disease was recognized initially as a skin disease. Hebra and Kaposi were the first to report systemic involvement of the disease. Their work published in 1874 described the association of lupus with anemia, lung involvement, mental status changes, and death. In three papers published between 1895 and 1903, **Sir William Osier** described the systematic involvement of lupus, the first detailed description recognizing the multiple systems affected by the disease.

Lupus affects multiple organ systems including the skin, joints, mucous and serosal membranes, kidneys, blood, lungs, and nervous system. The disease is more common in females and in African Americans. Despite advances, the pathogenesis of SLE is still incompletely understood.

Systemic sclerosis is an **autoimmune disease** of unknown origin characterized by excessive deposition of collagen and other connective tissue macromolecules in skin and multiple internal organs, severe alterations in the microvasculature, and humoral and cellular immunological abnormalities. Although the most apparent and almost universal clinical features of systemic sclerosis are related to the progressive thickening and fibrosis of the skin, some degree of involvement of multiple internal organs is uniformly present even when not clinically apparent.

Tuberous sclerosis, **neurofibromatosis 1 and 2**, **hereditary hemorrhage telangiectasia**, **anhidrotic ectodermal dysplasia**, and **icontinentia pigmenti** are pathological processes that affect signal transduction and transcriptional regulation. Elucidation of the molecular defects underlying these disorders has led to a better understanding of the mechanisms by which the skin and other organ systems develop and regulate cell growth and differentiation.

The extracellular matrix of connective tissue consists of a meshwork critical for organogenesis and homeostatic maintenance of tissues through complex protein supramolecular assembly and cell-matrix interactions. There are four principal groups of extracellular matrix components, viz., **collagen**, the **elastic fibers**, **noncollagenous glycoproteins**, and **glycosaminoglycan/proteoglycan macromolecules**. Understanding of the supramolecular organization of these fiber structures and their interactions with glycosaminoglycan/proteoglycan macromolecules as well as cellular components of the connective tissue, has allowed identification of critical metabolic and structural features that are prerequisites for normal physiological function of these proteins.

Atrichia with papular lesions (APL) is a rare autosomal-recessive form of total **alopecia**. Affected individuals are both without eyebrows and eyelashes, and never develop axillary and pubic hair. The scalp hair usually appears normal at birth, but falls out soon after. Defects in the human homolog of the **mouse hairless gene** (Hr) have been implicated as the molecular basis of this rare form of congenital hair loss.

Specific skin lesions associated with internal disorders result from metabolic defects. Excesses in specific aromatic amino acids owing to autosomal-recessive diseases cause distinctive skin lesions. **Excess phenylalanine** is associated with decreased hair and skin pigment, **tyrosine excess** with skin blisters and hyperkeratosis of the palms and soles, and homogentisic acid excess with deposition of colored polymers in the skin and cartilage. **Excessive iron** stimulates **melanin synthesis** in hemochromatosis. Storage of complete carbohydrates is responsible for vascular lesions in **Fabry's disease** and **fucosidosis**. Genetic defects of **porphyrin** synthesis cause increased sensitivity to visible light, leading to blisters. A defect in a **urea cycle enzyme** causes fragile hair in argininosuccinic aciduria.

The oral cavity is made up of complex and diverse tissues that provide a variety of highly specialized functions ranging from **neurosensory** (e.g., taste) to nutritional/digestive functions (e.g., salivary digestion and mastication). Not surprisingly, there is a substantial portion of the human genome used in making these unique diverse structures and allowing them to function appropriately. Consequently, there are hundreds of conditions affecting the soft and hard tissues of the oral cavity. Some of these conditions affect primarily or only the oral cavity, although others are associated with significant somatic manifestations.

Malformations of cortical development occur when the normal process of brain development is disrupted. With the widespread use of high-resolution neuroimaging, brain malformations are increasingly being recognized as a relatively common cause of refractory epilepsy, mental retardation, and other neurological disorders. The molecular and genetic bases of many cortical malformations have been elucidated in recent years, both expanding our understanding of the underlying biological processes in brain development and informing our approach to these disorders in clinical practice.

Muscular dystrophies are generally genetic changes resulting in degeneration (and regeneration) of muscle. Mutations of 29 different genes can cause specific types of muscular dystrophy. The most common form of muscular dystrophy is **Duchenne's muscular dystrophy**, caused by mutations in the **dystrophin gene** on the X-chromosome, resulting in an absence of the protein dystrophin. Mutations in the same gene cause the less common and less severe **Becker's muscular dystrophy**, characterized by a partial deficiency of the dystrophin protein.

Ion channels are integral membrane proteins that form water-filled pores and allow the rapid passage of ions across cell membranes. The importance of ion-channel function in health and disease states has long been recognized, particularly in medical therapeutics. Many drugs act directly on ion channels, including **local anesthetic agents**, **antiarrhythmics**, **antihypertensives**, **most antiepileptic drugs**, and **many psychoactive medications**. Mutations of ion-channel genes have been established as the cause of several human diseases, including more than 30 disorders affecting excitability in nerve, muscle, or special sensory organs and disorders of epithelial transport affecting kidney, lung, or gut.

Molecular genetic analysis of the **demyelinating neuropathies Charcot–Marie–Tooth disease,** and hereditary neuropathy with liability to pressure palsies, has uncovered a novel mutational mechanism whereby a reciprocal recombination involving a misaligned flanking repeat sequence results in both the Charcot–Marie–Tooth disease type-lA duplication and hereditary neuropathy with liability to pressure palsies deletion. These studies have illuminated the role that gene dosage may play in causing a disease phenotype, which has important implications for therapeutic strategies, and which may underlie the basis of the extreme clinical variability. The identification of these rearrangement mutations (duplication and deletion) has resulted in the availability of molecular procedures for establishing or excluding a secure diagnosis, enabling presymptomatic and prenatal diagnosis, and providing prognostic information.

Amyotrophic lateral sclerosis is a lethal, paralyzing disorder of motor neurons in the brain, brain stem, and spinal cord. Its onset, typically in the 6th decade of life, is age-dependent; mean onset is 55 years, and mean survival is 3 to 5 years. About 5 to 10% of cases are transmitted as an autosomal dominant trait familial amyotrophic lateral sclerosis.

Expansion of **trinucleotide repeat sequences** is the mutational mechanism in at least 16 neurological disorders, including **fragile X type A syndrome**, **myotonic dystrophy**, **spinobulbar muscular atrophy**, **Huntington's disease**, and several others. The discovery of trinucleotide repeat expansions provides a biological explanation for "anticipation," the increase in disease severity and decrease in age of onset from one generation to the next, observed in all of these disorders.

Parkinson's disease (PD), which is the most common neurodegenerative movement disorder, is clinically characterized by resting tremor, rigidity, bradykinesia, and postural instability. The pathological hallmarks of PD include **loss of dopaminergic neurons** in the substantia nigra pars compacta as well as the presence of abnormal protein deposits known as **Lewy bodies** in some of the surviving nigral neurons. The loss of dopaminergic neurons in the substantia nigra pars compacta results in striatal dopamine deficiency, which accounts for the motor impairments of patients with PD. Although the precise etiology remains unclear, several environmental and genetic factors have been implicated in the molecular pathogenesis of PD. This chapter will systematically discuss each of these factors and their putative pathogenic mechanisms.

Alzheimer's disease (AD), **Lewy body variant** (LEV) of AD, (which is now referred to as **dementia with Lewy bodies** [DLB]) and the **frontotemporal dementias** (FTD) are the three commonest causes of adult-onset dementia. These diseases present in mid to late adult life with progressive defects in memory and higher cognitive functions such as the performance of complex, learned motor tasks (apraxias), reasoning, and so on. The clinical features of AD and DLB (deficits in recent and immediate memory deficits, praxis, reasoning and judgment, and so on) stem from involvement of the temporal lobe, hippocampus, and the parietal association cortices, with lesser involvement of frontal lobes until late in the disease. DLB overlaps with AD, sharing most of the clinical and neuropathological features of AD, but differentiated by prominent visual hallucinations, sensitivity to phenothiazine tranquilizers, and the presence of Lewy bodies (α-synuclein-containing intraneuronal inclusions) in neocortical neurons. In contrast, in FTD, the clinical syndrome is overshadowed by behavioral disturbances (disinhibition, aggressivity, and so on) and speech disturbances (aphasia), which arise from involvement of the frontal neocortex. The FTD symptom complex frequently also includes additional features such as muscle rigidity, tremor, bradykinesia (parkinsonism), and muscle weakness (amyotrophy).

Prion diseases, or **transmissible spongiform encephalopathies** (TSEs), are CNS-degenerative disorders of a sporadic, familial, or acquired nature. They include **Creutzfeldt–Jakob disease** (CJD), **Gerstmann–Sträussler–Scheinker** (GSS) **syndrome**, **Kuru**, and **fatal familial insomnia** (FFI) in humans, and a number of encephalopathies of animals. The latter comprise scrapie of sheep, bovine spongiform encephalopathy (BSE) or "mad cow disease," chronic wasting diseases of deer and elk, and similar diseases of exotic ungulates. A large body of circumstantial evidence has accumulated indicating that BSE prions can provoke a variant form of CJD in humans.

Narcolepsy and other neurological sleep disorders are among the most common clinical ailments, and molecular research is beginning to shed light on the neurobiology of sleep and the mechanisms underlying specific disorders of sleep. **Neurofibromatosis (NF) 1 and 2** are genetically and phenotypically distinct genetic disorders characterized by the development of benign and malignant tumors. Advances in molecular genetics have resulted in the identification of the NF1 and NF2 genes and their encoded proteins, **neurofibromin** and **merlin/schwannomin**. Identification of these causative genes has led to an improved understanding of the molecular pathogenesis of NF1 and NF2, and has recently resulted in the development of targeted, biologically based therapies for tumors in NF1.

Damage to the adult brain or spinal cord commonly produces persistent dysfunction without recovery. To replace lost neuron stem cells, trophic factors, and transplantation of neural-competent cells might be relevant. Treatment of dysfunction based on the disconnection of surviving neurons requires the axonal regeneration from remaining neurons and a degree of plasticity in neuronal connectivity.

Unlike many single-gene neurological disorders such as **Huntington's disease**, **neurofibromatosis**, and **Rett's syndrome**, most psychiatric illnesses are etiologically complex. It is this complexity that stands as the major obstacle hindering risk-gene identification in psychiatry, and all of the diagnostic, therapeutic, and preventive advances that such discoveries might engender. Linkage and association analyses will probably be able to resolve some of the genetic complexity of many psychiatric conditions; but it is also likely that emerging disciplines, such as systems biology and functional genomics, will inform traditional genomic methods to hasten the compilation of a full catalog of susceptibility genes for psychiatric illness.

Different hypotheses explain the **etiology of depression**. Each focuses on different biological processes that contribute to explaining the clinical manifestation of depression and connect the regulation of mood to other biological processes such as the stress response and feeding behavior. Most likely, these different signaling pathways converge at a certain point to specifically control mood. This convergence point may control neurotransmission, in particular, long-term potentiation in the hippocampus. This opens the possibility that, by dissecting pathways activated by antidepressants, it would be possible to find new targets for novel drugs with a direct and specific mechanism of action, likely producing novel antidepressants with a higher potency, a faster action, and fewer side effects.

Despite a broad knowledge base about the **pathology of schizophrenia**, albeit fragmented and often inconsistent, no theme has emerged to link the illness with its molecular pathophysiology. There is insufficient certainty and consistency of findings to identify the critical molecular target on which to base therapeutic discovery. The most limiting aspect of schizophrenia therapeutics is this lack of critical knowledge with respect to its target pathophysiology, on which therapeutic strategies could be developed.

Autism is associated with abnormalities in key aspects of human behavior from the earliest stages of development throughout the life span. It is among the psychiatric disorders most strongly influenced by genetic factors. Although the understanding of the genes and molecular mechanisms involved in the pathogenesis of autism remains limited, several chromosomal regions have been identified that likely harbor autism susceptibility genes. Neuropathological studies have identified subtle differences in the number, morphology, and organization of neurons in specific brain regions. Modest changes exist in the level of expression of multiple molecules involved in neural development and neurotransmission. Structural neuroimaging studies have identified abnormalities in brain growth trajectories and have suggested that these trajectories may differ across substructures and tissues. Functional imaging studies have identified activation patterns in response to specific stimuli that reflect abnormalities in several key neural systems. Integration of findings across **gene–brain–behavior studies** is likely to provide important insights into the pathogenesis and neural mechanisms underlying this complex neurodevelopmental syndrome.

Drug addiction continues to exact enormous human and financial costs on society at a time when available treatments remain inadequately effective for most people. Given that advances in treating other medical disorders have resulted directly from research of the molecular and cellular pathophysiology of the disease process, an improved understanding of the basic neurobiology of addiction should likewise translate into more efficacious treatments.

MOLECULAR ONCOLOGY

Thomas Hodgkin's (1796–1866) criteria for determining a cancer's malignancy would still stand today: appearance of the tumor, tendency to spread, enlargement of neighboring lymph nodes, and general symptoms of wasting. Until the late-18th century, medicine was symptom oriented. Toward the early-19th century, the French clinicopathological school stressed symptoms of diagnostic significance and the primacy of physical signs. Louis Pasteur (1822–1895) did much to solve the problem of correlating microbes and disease, and Robert Koch formulated the now-famous postulates to prove the pathogenicity of microorganisms. In spite of extremely important therapeutic advances (such as antimicrobials, endocrine agents, and drugs based on receptor–ligand interactions or inhibition of enzyme catalytic sites), our diagnostic skills today appear to be more potent than our ability to cure. X-rays, CT scans, NMR, ultrasounds, radioisotopes, PET scans, endoscopies, and other high-tech procedures have gradually increased our diagnostic abilities and have decreased our strict dependence on the skilled elucidation of clinical physical signs. After the important discoveries of molecular biology and genetics in the second half of the 20th century, molecular medicine is seen as the main promise for medical progress in the coming century, but it will probably come at the inevitable price of increasing complexity.

For some time, many oncologists in large cancer centers have believed that better combinations of drugs would be found for treating cancer and cancer mortality would decrease, but they would not need to understand much about the mechanisms underlying the origin and spread of the disease. This rather empirical and optimistic approach led to a number of successful, albeit toxic, treatments for some uncommon cancers, such as tumors in children, several types of leukemias and lymphomas, and germ-cell cancers in young men.

Most clinicians believe that it will be through science and hard work, rather than magic or mere luck, that cancer will be defeated. To understand the prospects of cancer research, practicing clinicians and the public need some idea of the present state of knowledge on the subject. The problem is that, in the past 2.5 decades, an explosion of information, rather than knowledge, has occurred concerning the molecular aspects of cancer: >300 genes and their respective protein products have been described as directly or indirectly linked to cancer. The forest may be missed because of the trees. Cancer clinicians (including medical oncologists, radiotherapists, hematologists, general surgeons, gynecologists, and urologists) find it increasingly difficult to stay abreast of knowledge in the molecular aspects of these complex diseases. Some believe that relevant information eventually will pass from the molecular pathology laboratory to the cancer clinical units with the help of clever computer programmers. Before clinicians can decide on the curability or incurability of any given cancer and on which sequence and combination of drugs to use, they will need to consult a computer programmer and the molecular pathology laboratory.

The term **prognostic factor**, when used regarding patients with malignancies, has taken on several meanings. In general, a prognostic factor is considered to be useful because its results serve to separate a large heterogeneous population into smaller populations with more precisely predictable outcomes. In theory, if this separation is both reliable and disparate, one can apply therapy more efficiently to the population by exposing those most likely to need and benefit from the therapy while ensuring that the other group avoids needless toxicities.

In essence, the term **tumor marker** has come to describe a variety of molecules or processes that differ from the norm in malignant cells, tissues, or fluids in patients with malignancies. Assessment of these alterations from normal can be used to place patients into categories that are distinguished by different outcomes, either in the absence of specific therapy or after various treatments are applied.

Tumor markers can include changes at the genetic level (e.g., mutations, deletions, or amplifications), the transcriptional level (e.g., over- or underexpression), the translational or posttranslational level (e.g., increased or decreased quantities of protein, or abnormal glycosylation of proteins), and/or the functional level (e.g., histologic description of cellular grade or presence of neovascularization). Each of these can be assessed by one or more assays that use one or more methods with different reagents. This enormous heterogeneity of approaches is the root of considerable confusion regarding the value, in clinical terms, of a given tumor marker.

Over the past two decades, we have come to an understanding of cancer as a genetic disorder caused by the progressive accumulation of multiple genetic changes, which include point mutations, chromosomal rearrangements, viral insertions, and genomic amplifications and deletions. Gene amplifications, point mutations, viral insertions, and chromosomal rearrangements are dominant genetic damages that primarily target oncogenes whose gain of function (overexpression) leads to dysregulation of cell growth and transformation. Recessive point mutations and deletions mainly cause loss of function in **tumor suppressor genes** (TSGs) that control cell-cycle progression and DNA repair mechanisms.

Over several decades, we have experienced remarkable advances in the understanding of basic cellular and molecular biology. The cornerstones of this development were the discovery of **oncogenes** in human cancer and the identification of **TSGs**. The detailed characterization of different **cyclins** and **cyclin-dependent kinases** (CDK), responsible for the immediate regulation of various phases of the cell cycle, are other major achievements. The factors involved in cell-cycle regulation may have a role as diagnostic markers and possible targets for antiproliferative drugs.

Histopathologic analysis of tumors has been the linchpin of tissue diagnosis and hence classification. The information provided by histopathologists regarding tumor types and subtypes, tumor grade and stage forms the core body of information required for clinical management. With increasing use of sophisticated radiology (ultrasound, magnetic resonance imaging [MRI]) and the implementation of screening programs for various diseases (cervical and breast cancer), pathologists are faced with problems of classifying early and borderline lesions and trying to predict their natural history. It is hoped that the new molecular techniques will help provide a molecular classification that is more robust and clinically useful.

The concept of a **circulating tumor marker** applies to a secreted chemical product of a tumor cell such that the concentration of the chemical in the blood may in some way represent a quantifiable assessment of the tumor burden at that time. The earliest example is the protein produced from myeloma cells discovered by Bence Jones in the mid-19th century. Subsequently, a number of oncofetal and other proteins have proved useful and are widely available from antibody-based assays. This science is set to expand dramatically with an increase in our knowledge of the molecular pathology of cancer subtypes and the application of **genomic and proteomic analysis techniques**. One example is the measurement of serum DNA concentration. The DNA probably derives from necrosis and apoptosis. The specificity can be increased by analyzing tumor DNA, such as that with allelic imbalance of sequences subject in that tumor type to frequent allelic losses. Alternatively, mass spectroscopy of serum proteins may provide patterns diagnostic of particular cancers. For ovarian tumors, it has been suggested that a cluster pattern can distinguish patients with cancer; this approach seems less successful in diagnosing early prostate cancer.

Understanding the molecular, cellular, and tissue changes that occur during tumorigenesis is central to the cancer research effort. The translational aspects of this field—the development of clinical applications from the laboratory findings—are aimed at improving diagnosis, monitoring, and treatment of disease, targets that are facilitated by an appreciation of the mechanism underlying pathogenesis. Approaches used to achieve these goals can be divided into two broad classes. The first of these encompasses strategies designed to identify disease markers that can be used to develop screening tools with sufficient sensitivity and specificity to detect cancer in the general population, aid in clinical cancer diagnosis, predict prognosis, and identify patients with recurrent or metastatic disease. Second are studies aimed at improving therapy, by identifying either molecules and pathways that can be exploited as targets for disease intervention, or molecules that predict response or resistance to therapy, with the aim of patient stratification and individualization of treatment.

Components of **growth factor-signaling pathways** were among the earliest gene products implicated in cancer induction in animals and then inferred to be instrumental in human cancers. This discovery led to the general idea that inactivation of **TSGs** or activation of **protooncogenes** by mutation in cancer cells substituted in some way for the normal environmental cues that regulate cell proliferation and function.

Breast cancer is the most common cancer affecting women worldwide. In the United States alone, an estimated 211,000 new cases of breast cancer will be diagnosed each year. It is estimated that one in every eight American women will be diagnosed with breast cancer within the course of her lifetime. With more sensitive and accurate means of early detection and an ever-increasing number of drugs available to treat breast cancer, it is likely that women diagnosed today will live longer and may need more than one type of cancer therapy. Many cellular factors mediate breast transformation and tumor growth, including growth factors, members of **phosphorylation signaling cascades**, **oncogenes**, and **nuclear hormone receptors**. Although each of these factors has a role in the development of breast cancer, the **steroid hormone estrogen** is the primary promotional factor. Epidemiologic evidence has shown that a woman's overall lifetime exposure to endogenous estrogen, increased by early menarche, late menopause, and nulliparity, is the primary **risk factor for developing breast cancer**.

A number of complex changes take place between the time a cell is formed and the time it divides into two daughter cells. This process is known as the cell cycle. The morphologic changes associated with particular stages of the cell cycle are well known; however, a detailed understanding of the regulatory mechanisms controlling cell-cycle progression has only recently been elucidated. Understanding the biochemical and genetic mechanisms that control these cellular changes is fundamental to cell biology because it influences processes such as cell transformation, cell differentiation, and cell growth. A greater knowledge of the molecular mechanisms underlying the transformation of mammalian cells may allow the design of inhibitors of the specific biochemical processes responsible for abnormal cell proliferation or cancer.

These regulatory proteins belong to a unique family of kinases named "**cyclin-dependent kinases**" (CDKs). The identification of CDKs has led to a number of other related and important discoveries of the molecular mechanisms involved in the regulation of cell-cycle progression. A number of **protooncogenes** (cyclin Dl, CDC25, CDK4) and tumor suppressor genes (TSGs) (pRb, p53, p16) have been identified in the context of **cell-cycle regulation**. Together, these discoveries have enhanced our overall understanding of cell transformation and tumor biology.

Few of the basic research fields within oncology have experienced such an explosive growth as the area of **angiogenesis**. Intense effort in the laboratories of both academia and pharmaceutical companies has led to its own translation to the clinical research. The plethora of new and old compounds shown to be either angiogenic or antiangiogenic in several laboratories in *in vitro*, *ex vivo*, and *in vivo* models has led to a parallel increase in the number of new **antiangiogenic drugs** entering clinical oncology trials. Some advanced potential drugs have stumbled in mid- or late-clinical phases, however. In addition to these issues, much scientific debate has occurred, which has led to the repositioning of many antiangiogenic targets, clearly illustrating the vast activity in this field.

As basic research advances in the understanding of angiogenesis pathways, scientists learn more about the mechanism of action of both the **inducers and the blockers of the tumor-induced angiogenesis**. In this sense, the emerging area of translational research is leading to a better and more focused interaction between basic and clinical researchers, which will eventually lead to a better knowledge of how antiangiogenesis drugs work *in vivo*, and the definition of clinical trials that best use the potential of these new weapons in the fight against cancer.

Metastasis is the most life-threatening aspect of malignant neoplasm. When a tumor remains localized, its surgical removal generally results in the survival of the patient and, thus, the lesion is called benign. By contrast, when a tumor invades adjacent tissues and spreads to other anatomic sites, the possibility of cure becomes poor and the lesion is called malignant. Cancer can disseminate by **hematogenous spread** (e.g., sarcomas), by **lymphatic spread** (e.g., carcinomas), or by **seeding within natural body cavities** (e.g., ovarian carcinoma within the peritoneal cavity). The lymphatic and venous systems are highly interconnected, allowing disseminating cancer to pass from one system to the other. Clinical and pathologic observations point to the local/regional lymph node spread as an early-occurring event. Use of the **sentinel lymph node** is a promising staging method in the diagnoses of breast carcinoma and melanoma. Anatomy by itself does not fully explain the distribution of metastasis in different organs. The dissemination of cancer is a complex process, and the outcome depends on numerous interactions between the cancer cell and the host environment. During malignant progression, tumor cells must elude the **immunosurveillance mechanisms** and lose their responsiveness to the normal growth controls. To successfully develop metastatic foci, cancer cells detach from the primary tumor mass; penetrate the basement membrane and invade the surrounding host stroma; gain access to blood or lymphatic vessels by crossing subendothelial basement membrane and survive in the circulation; arrest and extravasate through the vessel walls; infiltrate the surrounding host tissue compartments; and finally grow in the newly colonized organ. The process is dynamic, and the diverse steps can take place at different times. The clinical patterns are different as well. When the primary tumor is first diagnosed, metastases may be detectable or may be present but not detected (occult). In the latter scenario, after removal of the primary lesion, metastases may appear shortly afterward. Alternatively, they may take a very long time to become detectable.

Despite significant advances in the treatment of solid tumors and hematologic malignancies, clinical drug resistance to anticancer therapy is still a frequent problem that often leads to treatment failure in cancer patients. Resistance to chemotherapy can be divided into intrinsic (or *de novo*) and acquired resistance. The former refers to tumors that are insensitive to cytotoxic drugs at diagnosis, such as pancreatic cancer, renal cancer, and malignant melanoma. Acquired drug resistance is common in tumors such as breast cancer, **SCLC**, and ovarian cancer that initially are highly responsive to anticancer therapy, but become resistant during the course of the disease. These tumors often develop resistance not only to previously used drugs but also to other compounds with different structures and mechanisms of action to which they have never been exposed.

Multiple cellular mechanisms have been identified that can contribute to the drug-resistance phenotype, including alterations in drug-transport systems, resulting in decreased intracellular drug concentration; changes in the activation or inactivation of drugs (metabolic resistance); alterations in drug targets; increased repair of drug-induced damage;

alterations in drug-induced apoptosis; and changes in signaling pathways. In addition, pharmacologic factors, such as inadequate dosing or route of delivery, may play a role in clinical resistance of tumors. These mechanisms can develop simultaneously, and multiple factors can contribute to the drug-resistance phenotype of tumor cells

Genetic information, in the form of DNA, must be protected for expression within the cell and transfer between generations. Although a number of mechanisms have been developed to allow for genetic diversity, multiple and redundant mechanisms work to avoid errors during DNA synthesis before cell duplication and/or to avoid the impact of mutagens from endogenous or exogenous sources. The DNA sequence can be changed as the result of copying errors introduced by **DNA polymerases** during replication and by environmental agents such as mutagenic chemicals and certain types of radiation. If DNA sequence changes, whatever their cause, are left uncorrected, both growing and nongrowing somatic cells could accumulate so many mutations that they could no longer function. Thus, the correction of DNA sequence errors in all types of cells is important for survival.

The human immune system can mount a specific response to cancer. Intense research is aimed at dissecting the intricacies of the interactions between the immune system and tumor cells. A driving force behind this research is the idea that cancer-directed immunity can be enhanced to improve the outcome for patients with the disease. The specificity of the immune response makes **cancer immunotherapy** extremely attractive because it offers the promise of reducing damage to bystander normal tissues and lessening the severe side effects associated with current cancer therapies. A variety of modalities can be incorporated into an immunotherapeutic approach, including vaccines, recombinant-antibodies (Abs), cytokines, and cellular and gene therapies. Moreover, techniques are now available to measure **antigen (Ag)-specific immunity** with great sensitivity and allow the biology of tumor-specific T-cells obtained from patients to be studied. These techniques provide the best evidence to date of the strengths and weaknesses of the human immune response to cancer. Formidable barriers remain, however, to the successful manipulation of tumor-specific immunity in cancer patients.

The development of innovative cancer drugs has generated much excitement. We stand poised to take advantage of our newfound understanding of the molecular basis of cancer to develop **innovative treatments** that are both more effective and less toxic than "traditional" **cytotoxic chemotherapy**.

The prospect of more-selective, target-based therapies is made possible through a detailed understanding of the molecular differences in structure and function between cancer and normal cells. This understanding has been achieved primarily in the last quarter of the 20th century by painstaking, hypothesis-driven molecular biology and genetic research, but has progressed rapidly with the sequencing of the human genome. The sequencing should be finalized shortly, 50 years after Watson and Crick elucidated the structure of DNA and the molecular mechanism of DNA replication and heredity.

The impact of the new wealth of genomic information will be enormous, and includes an emphasis on integrating traditional hypothesis-driven research with genomics, proteomics, and other "-omic" technologies. Discovering critical nodes in tumor cell rewiring is clearly one of the roles for "omics" research—the study of biologic systems on a global, massively parallel basis.

During the past several decades, cancer research has primarily focused on development of cytotoxic agents for treatments. These efforts have significantly improved the prognosis of some types of malignancies, including some leukemias, lymphomas, and testicular carcinoma. However, other tumors, including metastatic colorectal, breast, and lung carcinomas, are still associated with poor prognosis. Innovative approaches to understanding the cellular and molecular mechanisms of the process of carcinogenesis have provided new insights into the paradigm of cancer treatment by exploring the possibilities of early detection, chemoprevention, and treatment of premalignant disease.

Intraepithelial neoplasia (IEN) is characterized as moderate to severe dysplasia that occurs on the causal pathway from normal tissue to malignancy. Accumulation of genetic mutations manifests in the phenotypic changes associated with cancer, including loss of cell-cycle control and apoptosis. Because the process of carcinogenesis often requires many years, identification of IEN at early stages affords numerous opportunities for intervention of the malignant progression.

Prevention of cancer through development of **chemopreventive agents** for high-risk populations and interventions for early stage carcinogenesis are key strategies of current oncology research. Research in the fields of chemoprevention and treatment of carcinogenesis has led to identification of diagnostic methodologies and potential agents that reduce cancer risk. Techniques that show promise for early diagnosis of cancer and potential agents for chemoprevention in high-risk populations, and treatment of the early stages of carcinogenesis are being investigated in clinical studies to determine their ability to reduce cancer risk, morbidity, and mortality in selected populations

The most outstanding progress in molecular biology during the 20th century led from the understanding of the genetic code to the development of DNA technology, which led ultimately to **gene therapy**. These advances raised hopes that cancer could be cured using such an approach. The area of cancer gene therapy is vast and targets both malignant and nonmalignant cells for therapeutic gain. Gene therapy that targets malignant cells embraces a large spectrum of methods including the insertion of **tumor suppressor genes** (TSGs), **cytokine genes**, **toxin genes**, and **prodrug-activating genes**.

MOLINDONE HYDROCHLORIDE

(Moban)

Molindone (50 to 75 mg/day) is indicated in the management of the manifestations of psychotic disorders. Molindone is structurally unrelated to the phenothiazines, butyrophenones, or thioxanthenes, but it resembles the piperazine phenothiazines in its clinical action. It causes sedation, possesses anticholinergic properties and, similar to fluphenazine, produces movement disorders. Molindone is metabolized, and the metabolites are excreted in the urine. It lowers the seizure threshold and may cause seizures in patients with epilepsy and other seizure disorders. Concomitant use with sympathomimetics, including epinephrine, phenylephrine, phenylpropanolamine, and ephedrine (often found in nasal sprays), or appetite suppressants may decrease their stimulatory and pressor effects. Because of its alpha-blocking potential, molindone may cause epinephrine reversal—a hypotensive response to epinephrine.

Molindone may inhibit blood pressure response to centrally acting antihypertensive drugs, such as guanethidine, guanabenz, guanadrel, clonidine, methyldopa, and reserpine. Additive effects are likely after concomitant use of molindone with CNS depressants, including alcohol, analgesics, barbiturates, narcotics, tranquilizers, and general, spinal, or epidural anesthetics, or parenteral magnesium sulfate (oversedation, respiratory depression, and hypotension); antiarrhythmic agents, quinidine, disopyramide, or procainamide (increased incidence of cardiac arrhythmias and conduction defects); atropine or other anticholinergic drugs, including antidepressants, monoamine oxidase inhibitors, phenothiazines, antihistamines, meperidine, and antiparkinsonian agents (oversedation, paralytic ileus, visual changes, and severe constipation); nitrates (hypotension); and metrizamide (increased risk of convulsions). Beta-blocking agents may inhibit molindone metabolism, increasing plasma levels and toxicity. Concomitant use with propylthiouracil increases risk of agranulocytosis; concomitant use with lithium may result in severe neurologic toxicity, with an encephalitis-like syndrome and a decreased therapeutic response to molindone. Decreased therapeutic response to molindone may follow concomitant use with calcium-containing drugs such as phenytoin and tetracyclines, aluminum- and magnesium-containing antacids or antidiarrheals (decreased absorption), or caffeine (increased metabolism). Molindone may antagonize the therapeutic effect of bromocriptine on prolactin secretion; it may also decrease the vasoconstricting effects of high-dose dopamine and may decrease effectiveness and increase toxicity of levodopa (by dopamine blockade). Calcium sulfate in molindone tablets may inhibit the absorption of phenytoin or tetracyclines (see Table 2).

MOLSIDOMINE

Molsidomine is a prodrug for the formation of nitric oxide (NO). Its pharmacokinetics are characterized by rapid absorption and hydrolysis, taking a short time to achieve maximal systemic concentration of both the parent compound and its active metabolite. It has been used in the management of angina pectoris (see also Figure 30).

MOMETASONE FUROATE

(Asmanex Twisthaler powder for inhalation 220 mcg/actuation, Elocon ointment 0.1%, cream 0.1%, lotion 0.1%, Nasonex spray 50 mcg/spray (as monohydrate))

Mometasone furoate is a medium-potency topical corticosteroid that depresses formation, release, and activity of endogenous mediators of inflammation including prostaglandins, kinins, histamine, liposomal enzymes, and the complement system; and modifies the body's immune response. **Topical**: used for relief of inflammatory and pruritic manifestations of corticosteroid-responsive dermatoses. **Intranasal**: used for treatment of nasal symptoms of seasonal allergic and perennial allergic rhinitis; prophylaxis of nasal symptoms of seasonal allergic rhinitis; and treatment of nasal polyps. **Oral inhalation**: used for maintenance treatment of asthma as prophylactic therapy; in asthma patients requiring oral corticosteroid therapy, adding Asmanex Twisthaler may reduce or eliminate the need for oral corticosteroids.

MONOAMINE OXIDASE INHIBITORS

The monoamine oxidase inhibitors are used occasionally to treat depression. The hydrazine derivatives consist of isocarboxazid (Marplan) and phenelzine sulfate (Nardil). The nonhydrazine derivatives include tranylcypromine (Parnate).

Monoamine oxidase can metabolize monoamines by oxidative deamination and convert them to inactive acidic derivatives. Monoamine oxidase inhibitors seem to compete with physiologically active monoamine for the active site of the enzyme. In general, not only do these agents inhibit the oxidase that metabolizes amines but they also inhibit the oxidase that metabolizes drugs and essential nutrients. Hence, the incidence of drug–drug and drug–food interactions is extremely high with these agents. Monoamine oxidases have various applications. They may be used as a local anesthetic (cocaine), an antihistaminic (diphenylhydramine), or an antidepressant (tranylcypromine). Monoamine oxidase inhibitors have been used in the treatment of hypertension (direct blockade of sympathetic ganglion), angina pectoris (coronary dilation), narcolepsy (stimulating the reticular activating system), and depression (increasing the brain's norepinephrine pool). Needless to say, these agents should be used with extreme caution in conjunction with sympathomimetic amines, ganglionic-blocking agents, procaine, and anesthetic agents. They are contraindicated in patients with hyperthyroidism and in combination with tricyclic antidepressants. In the event of poisoning, adrenergic-blocking agents such as phentolamine may be effective for combating the hypertensive crisis.

The high incidence of drug–food and drug–drug interactions rules out monoamine oxidase inhibitors as antidepressants of first choice. However, there are circumstances

MONOAMINE OXIDASE INHIBITORS: Contemporary Treatment of Depression

Monoamine oxidase inhibitor (MAOI) antidepressants have been in use for nearly 40 years. At the present time, they are viewed as second- or third-line antidepressant medications for reasons of both efficacy and safety. The available MAOIs are phenelzine sulfate (Nardil), isocarboxazid (Marplan), and tranylcypromine sulfate (Parnate). Two additional MAOI antidepressants, moclobemide and brofaromine, are approved for use in Europe and/or Canada.

It was initially believed that the antidepressant effectiveness of MAOIs was the direct result of MAO inhibition. This acute effect decreases degradation of monoamines (e.g., norepinephrine, serotonin, or dopamine) stored in presynaptic neurons, thereby resulting in an increased amount of these neurotransmitters available at the synapse. More recent research indicates that this model does not fully explain the mechanism of MAOIs' efficacy. For example, the positive (+) stereoisomer of tranylcypromine is a poor antidepressant despite inhibiting MAO. The main pharmacologic difference between the negative (–) and + isomers of tranylcypromine is that the former has much weaker effects as a norepinephrine reuptake inhibitor in relation to its potency as an MAOI. The other MAOIs may also block the reuptake of selected neurotransmitters. However, like the non-MAOI uptake inhibitors, these acute effects often precede clinical antidepressant effects by weeks. More consistent with the 2- to 4-week lag in therapeutic effect, chronic treatment with a diverse number of MAOIs has been shown to reduce the number of α_2- and β-adrenergic and serotonin (5-HT_2) postsynaptic binding sites in the brain.

The high incidence of drug–food and drug–drug interactions rule out MAOIs as antidepressants of first choice. However, there are circumstances in which these agents may be used effectively and successfully. These are:

When a patient has not responded to a tricyclic antidepressant for an adequate trial period and with an appropriate dosage.

When a patient has developed allergic reactions to tricyclics.

When a patient has had previous depressive episodes that responded well to MAOIs.

in which these agents may be used effectively and successfully. These are: when a patient has not responded to a tricyclic antidepressant for an adequate trial period and with an appropriate dosage; when a patient has developed allergic reactions to tricyclics; and when a patient has had previous depressive episodes that responded well to monoamine oxidase inhibitors (see also Figure 37).

MONOCTANOIN

(Moctanin)

Monoctanoin, an esterified glycerol, is used to solubilize cholesterol gallstones that are retained in the biliary tract after cholecystectomy.

MONOIODOTYROSINE

(MIT)

The steps involved in the synthesis of thyroid hormones are depicted in Figure 66. First, the ingested iodide (100 to 150 mg/day) is actively transported (iodide trapping) and then accumulated in the thyroid gland. Following this, the trapped iodide is oxidized by a peroxidase system to active iodine, which iodinates the tyrosine residue of glycoprotein to yield monoiodotyrosine (MIT) and diiodotyrosine (DIT). This process is called iodide organification. The MIT and DIT combine to form T_4. T_3 and T_4 are released from thyroglobulin through the actions of pinocytosis and the proteolysis of thyroglobulin by lysosomal enzymes. In the circulation, 75% of T_4 is bound to thyroxine-binding globulin (TBG), and the remainder is mostly bound to thyroxine-binding prealbumin (TBPA). Approximately 0.05% of T_4 remains free. T_3 is similarly bound to TBG, allowing only 0.5% of it to remain in the free form.

MONTELUKAST SODIUM

(Singulair tablets 10 mg)

Montelukast sodium is a leukotriene receptor antagonist that blocks the effects of specific leukotrienes in the respiratory airways, thereby reducing bronchoconstriction, edema, and inflammation. It is indicated in the prophylaxis and chronic treatment of asthma in patients 12 months and older; and in relief of symptoms of seasonal allergic rhinitis in patients 2 years and older.

Seasonal allergic rhinitis (hay fever) is caused by deposition of allergens on the nasal mucosa, resulting in an immediate hypersensitivity reaction. This reaction usually is not accompanied by asthma because the allergenic particles are too large to be inhaled into the lower airways (e.g., pollens). Treatment for allergic rhinitis is similar to that for asthma. Topical glucocorticoids, including **beclomethasone** (Beconase), **mometasone** (Nasonex), **budesonide** (Rhinocort), **flunisolide** (Nasarel), **fluticasone** (Flonase), and **triamcinolone** (Nasacort), can be highly effective with minimal side effects, particularly if treatment is instituted immediately prior to the allergy season. Topical glucocorticoids can be administered twice daily (beclomethasone and flunisolide) or even once daily (budesonide, **mometasone**, fluticasone, and triamcinolone). **Cromolyn** usually requires dosing three to six times daily for full effects. Rare instances of local candidiasis have been reported with glucocorticoids and probably can be avoided by rinsing the mouth after use.

Unlike in asthma, antihistamines afford considerable, though incomplete, symptom relief in allergic rhinitis. Nasal decongestants rely on β-adrenergic agonists (e.g., pseudoephedrine and phenylephrine) as vasoconstrictors. Anticholinergic agents such as **ipratropium bromide** (Atrovent) are effective in inhibiting parasympathetic reflex-evoked secretions from serous glands lining the nasal mucosa.

MOPP THERAPY

The alkylating agents exert their antineoplastic actions by generating highly reactive carbonium ion intermediates that form a covalent linkage with various nucleophilic components on both proteins and DNA. The 7 position of the purine base guanine is particularly susceptible to alkylation, resulting in miscoding, depurination, or ring cleavage. Bifunctional alkylating agents are able to cross-link either two nucleic acid molecules or one protein and one nucleic acid molecule. Although these agents are very active from a therapeutic perspective, they are also notorious for their tendency to cause carcinogenesis and mutagenesis. Alkylating agents that have a nonspecific effect on the cell-cycle phase are the most cytotoxic to rapidly proliferating tissues.

The activity of nitrogen mustards depends on the presence of a bis-(2-chloroethyl) grouping:

$$N\begin{cases} CH_2\text{-}CH_2Cl \\ CH_2\text{-}CH_2Cl \end{cases}$$

This is present in mechlorethamine (Mustargen), which is used in patients with Hodgkin's disease and other lymphomas, usually in combination with other drugs, such as in MOPP therapy (**mechlorethamine**, **Oncovin** [vincristine], **procarbazine**, and **prednisone**). It may cause bone marrow depression.

MORICIZINE HYDROCHLORIDE

(Ethmozine)

Moricizine (600 to 900 mg/day given every 8 hours in three equally divided doses) is indicated in the treatment of documented ventricular arrhythmias, such as sustained ventricular tachycardia, that are life threatening. Because of the proarrhythmic effects of moricizine, its use should be reserved for patients in whom the benefits of treatment outweigh the risks. Moricizine is a class 1C antiarrhythmic agent with potent local anesthetic activity and myocardial-membrane-stabilizing effects. It shares some of the characteristics of the class 1A (disopyramide, procainamide, or quinidine), of class 1B (lidocaine, mexiletene, phenytoin, or tocainide), or class 1C agents (encainide, flecainide, or propafenone) in that it reduces the fast inward current carried by sodium ions. Moricizine shortens phase 2 and 3 repolarization, resulting in a decreased action potential duration and effective refractory period. A dose-related decrease in the maximum rate of phase 0 depolarization (V_{max}) occurs without effect on maximum diastolic potential or action potential amplitude. The sinus node and atrial tissue are not affected. Following oral administration, moricizine undergoes significant first-pass metabolism resulting in an absolute bioavailability of ~38%. Moricizine undergoes extensive biotransformation: <1% is excreted unchanged in the urine. There are at least 26 metabolites (see also Figure 84).

Cimetidine increases the plasma level of moricizine, and digoxin and moricizine cause an additive prolongation of the PR interval. Moricizine increases the clearance of theophylline. The most serious adverse reaction of moricizine is its tendency to cause arrhythmias. Palpitation, sustained ventricular tachycardia, cardiac chest pain, CHF, MI, hypotension, hypertension, syncope, supraventricular arrhythmias (including atrial fibrillations/flutter), cardiac arrest, bradycardia, pulmonary embolism, vasodilation, cerebrovascular events, and thrombophlebitis have occurred. CNS problems such as dizziness, headache, fatigue, hypesthesias, asthenia, nervousness, parasthesias, sleep disorders, tremor, anxiety, depression, euphoria, confusion, somnolence, agitation, seizure, coma, abnormal gait, hallucinations, nystagmus, diplopia, speech disorder, akathisia, memory loss, ataxia, abnormal coordination, dyskinesia, vertigo, and tinnitus have been reported. Urinary retention or frequency, dysuria, urinary incontinence, kidney pain, impotence, and decreased libido take place. Abdominal pain, dyspepsia, vomiting, diarrhea, anorexia, bitter taste, dysphagia, flatulence, and ileus are other side effects of moricizine.

MORPHINE SULFATE

The opium alkaloids, which are obtained from *Papaver somniferum*, contain two groups of compounds: those with phenanthrene derivatives, consisting of morphine (1 to 10%), codeine (0.7 to 2.5%), and thebaine (0.5 to 1.5%); and those with isoquinolone derivatives, consisting of papaverine (1%) and noscapine (5 to 10%). Morphine depresses the cerebral cortex, hypothalamus, and medullary centers. These effects are responsible for suppressing pain perception, including narcosis, depressing the cough center, depressing the vomiting center, and depressing respiration. In horses, morphine stimulates the spinal cord in a predictable fashion. This effect is short-lived in humans and is seldom seen when given in therapeutic doses. Initially, morphine stimulates the vomiting center, and emesis occurs early in cases of intoxication. Depression of the vomiting center then ensues late in intoxication. Morphine stimulates the vagus nerve, causing bradycardia, and stimulates the nucleus of the third cranial nerve (oculomotor), causing miosis.

The relief of pain brought about by morphine is selective, and other sensory modalities such as touch, vibration, vision, hearing, and the like are not obtunded. Morphine does not reduce the responsiveness of nerve endings to

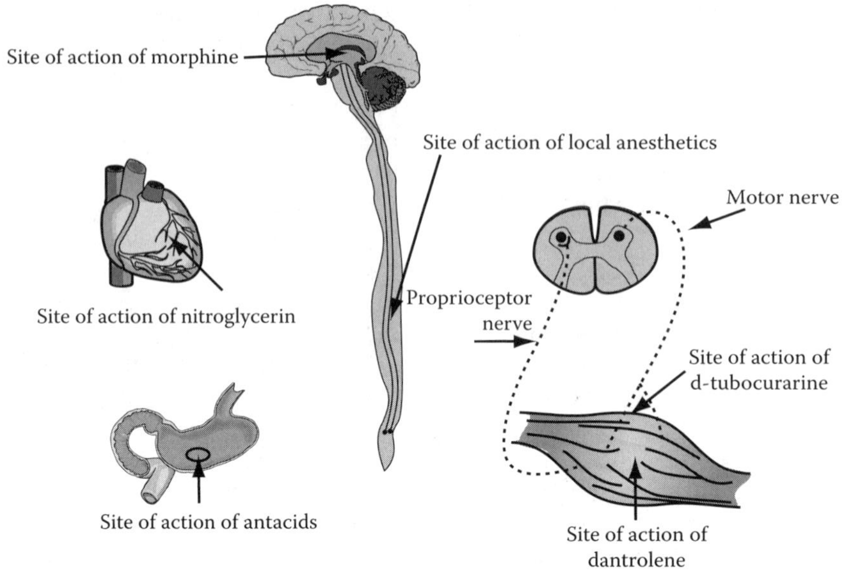

FIGURE 68 Morphine exerts its analgesic effects by **elevating the pain threshold** and especially by altering the patient's reactions to pain. Morphine induces analgesia by activating the **opioid**, **adrenergic**, and **serotonergic systems**.

noxious stimuli, nor does it impair the conduction of nerve impulses along the peripheral nerves, as seen following the administration of local anesthetics.

Morphine exerts its analgesic effects by elevating the pain threshold and especially by altering the patient's reactions to pain. It induces analgesia by activating the opioid, adrenergic, and serotoninergic (see Figure 68) systems. Analgesia results from the activation of those systems within the dorsal horn of the spinal cord that depress the transmission of pain sensation to the brain. This is accomplished by decreasing the release of pain transmitters such as substance P or by hyperpolarizing the interneurons within the dorsal horn, or both. Morphine activates these mechanisms by interacting with the μ receptors located on neurons in the dorsal cord. There is considerable evidence suggesting that this action depends on the activation of the adrenergic system within the dorsal horn. This in turn suggests that morphine analgesia could be potentiated by the addition of drugs such as clonidine that activate the adrenergic system. In addition, morphine appears to activate the endogenous supraspinal system that is normally activated by pain to protect the body from excessive nonessential pain stimulation. It appears that the translocation of calcium is the essential factor and that the basic mechanism of morphine results from alterations in the intracellular calcium concentration. This activity results from the interaction of morphine with μ receptors that, in turn, affect the G protein level, which then activates secondary transmitter systems. Certain antihistaminic substances have analgesic properties.

Morphine also alters a patient's reaction to pain. Patients report that the sensation of pain often exists, but, under the influence of morphine, they feel more at ease and comfortable. This euphoria is present in 90 to 95% of patients. Morphine may cause dysphoria in the remaining 5 to 10%. In a relatively small dose of 5 to 10 mg, it relieves the constant but dull pain originating from the viscera, such as that of coronary, pulmonary, and biliary origin. In somewhat larger doses (10 to 20 mg), morphine relieves the sharp, lancinating, and intermittent pain resulting from bone fractures and other physical injuries. Inoperable and terminal causes of neoplastic diseases usually require the administration of morphine or other narcotics in increasing doses that eventually lead to both tolerance and addiction. In the management of myocardial infarction, morphine, meperidine, pentazocine, methadone, and heroin have all been used as analgesics. In addition, streptokinase (a thrombolytic agent), atenolol or metoprolol (beta-adrenergic-receptor-blocking agents), and nitroglycerin (a vasodilator) have been advocated.

Chronic idiopathic pain syndrome is a common, disabling, and costly condition. It is believed to be of psychological origin but may involve both cerebral and peripheral physiologic mechanisms. Because it is often associated with depression, psychotropic drugs, notably the tricyclic antidepressants, may be required.

The spinal administration of morphine, with or without a local anesthetic, has been advocated for producing a sustained period of postoperative analgesia. However, adverse side effects from such analgesia include ventilatory depression, itching, and urinary retention. Morphine depresses all phases of respiration (respiratory rate, tidal volume, and minute volume) when given in subhypnotic and subanalgesic doses. In humans, a morphine overdose causes respiratory arrest and death. Therefore, morphine and other narcotic analgesics should be used with extreme caution in patients with asthma, emphysema, or cor pulmonale, and in disorders that may involve hypoxia, such as chest wound, pneumothorax, or bulbar poliomyelitis.

Morphine releases histamine and may cause peripheral vasodilation and orthostatic hypotension. The cutaneous blood vessels dilate around the "blush areas" such as the face, neck, and upper thorax. Morphine causes cerebral vasodilation (due to increased carbon dioxide retention secondary to respiratory depression), and hence it increases the cerebrospinal fluid pressure. Therefore, morphine should be used cautiously in patients with either meningitis or recent head injury. When given subcutaneously, morphine is absorbed poorly whenever there is either traumatic or hemorrhagic shock.

Very large doses of morphine can be used to produce anesthesia; however, the consequentially decreased peripheral resistance and blood pressure are troublesome. Fentanyl and sufentanil, which are potent and selective μ agonists, are less likely to cause hemodynamic instability during surgery, in part because they do not trigger the release of histamine.

Morphine reduces the activity of the entire gastrointestinal tract in that it reduces the secretion of hydrochloric acid, diminishes the motility of the stomach, and increases the tone of the upper part of the duodenum. These actions may delay passage of the stomach contents into the duodenum. Both pancreatic and biliary secretions are diminished, and this may also hinder digestion. In the large intestine, the propulsive peristaltic wave in the colon is reduced, the muscle tone including that of the anal sphincter is increased, and the gastrocolic reflex (defecation reflex) is reduced. These actions, in combination, cause constipation, which seems to be a chronic problem among addicts.

Opiate preparations, usually given as paregorics, are effective and fast-acting antidiarrheal agents. These agents are also useful postoperatively to produce solid stool following an ileostomy or colostomy. A meperidine derivative, diphenoxylate, is usually dispensed with atropine and sold as Lomotil. The atropine is added to discourage the abuse of diphenoxylate by narcotic addicts who are tolerant to massive doses of narcotic but not to the CNS-stimulant effects of atropine.

Morphine causes oliguria, and this results from (1) pronounced diaphoresis; (2) the relative hypotension and decreased glomerular filtration rate; and (3) the release of antidiuretic hormone from the neurohypophysis. In an elderly patient with prostatic hypertrophy, morphine may cause acute urinary retention. Morphine may reduce the effectiveness of a diuretic when both drugs are used in combination in the treatment of CHF.

Tolerance develops to the narcotic and analgesic actions of morphine, so that increasingly larger doses are needed to render patients pain free. Tolerance develops to many of morphine's effects such as analgesia, euphoria, narcosis, respiratory depression, hypotension, and antidiuresis. Morphine-induced bradycardia may be experienced. However, no tolerance develops to morphine-induced miosis or constipation. If the administration of morphine is discontinued, the tolerance is lost, and the preaddiction analgesic doses of morphine become effective once more.

In subjects who are addicted to morphine, the initial symptoms of the abstinence or withdrawal syndrome usually appear 6 to 12 hours after the last dose and consist of CNS irritability and feelings of fatigue, autonomic hyperactivity such as tachycardia and hypertension, gastrointestinal hyperactivity such as diarrhea, and autonomic supersensitivity such as insomnia and restlessness.

MORRHUATE SODIUM

(Scleomate injection 5%)

Morrhuate sodium is a sclerosing agent that causes venous intima inflammation and thrombus formation, which occludes the injected vein and subsequently forms fibrous tissue that results in partial or complete vein obliteration. It is indicated for obliteration of primary varicosed veins consisting of simple dilation with competent valves.

MOXIFLOXACIN HYDROCHLORIDE

(Avelox tablets 400 mg)

Moxifloxacin hydrochloride is a fluoroquinolone/antibiotic. It interferes with microbial DNA synthesis. Moxifloxacin is indicated in the treatment of acute bacterial sinusitis, acute bacterial exacerbation of chronic bronchitis, community-acquired pneumonia, uncomplicated skin and skin structure infections, and conjunctivitis caused by susceptible organisms.

MULTIMERIN

Multimerin is a large adhesive protein synthesized by megakaryocytes and stored within platelet alpha-granules. This novel protein was first discovered in platelets, using a monoclonal antibody raised against human platelets. Multimerin is extremely large and is comprised of variably sized, disulfide-linked multimers. The building blocks of the multimers are the p-155 and p-170 subunits. These subunits are derived by proteolysis of a common precursor protein.

Multimerin shares many similarities with von Willebrand factor, but, unlike the latter, it is not found in plasma. Within alpha-granules, multimerin is found in an eccentric location, colocalizing with von Willebrand factor. Platelet activation leads to multimerin release with expression of this protein on the activated platelet surface. Increased platelet surface expression of multimerin is a mark of platelet activation, both *in vitro* and *in vivo*. The function of multimerin remains to be discovered.

MULTIPLE SCLEROSIS: Treatment of

Multiple sclerosis (MS) is an inflammatory, demyelinating disease of the white matter of the CNS that commonly affects young adults. Two-thirds of patients have onset between the ages of 20 and 40 years; the peak period for onset is 25 to 30 years of age.

The disease is characterized by episodes of neurologic symptoms occurring over a period of days to weeks, followed by complete or incomplete remissions of various durations. Early signs and symptoms of MS commonly include fatigue, gait and limb ataxia, spasticity, dizziness, double vision, acute optic neuritis, and numbness and weakness in one or more limbs.

The classical lesions in MS, the plaques, are microscopically characterized by circumscribed demyelination in the presence of intact axons. Macrophages are the main cells involved in myelin destruction; attachment of superficial myelin lamellae to the macrophage surface, immunoglobulin deposition between macrophages and myelin lamellae, and production of complement and proteolytic enzymes all contribute to this process. Furthermore, T-lymphocytes, both the CD4 (helper) and CD8 (suppressor) phenotypes, are present in the perivascular lesions.

The initial successes in MS therapy involved the use of corticosteroid treatments to induce short-term improvements in neurological function, and symptomatic therapies for some of the complications of MS. More recently, with improved understanding of the immunological events occurring during progression of the disease, therapies that modify the natural history of the disease have become available. Interferon beta-1b (Betaseron) is the first new treatment for MS to be licensed by the U.S. FDA in the last 30 years.

Global immunosuppression with azathioprine and cyclophosphamide has been utilized with varying benefits for several decades. In addition, there have been recent reports of beneficial effects of immunosuppressive agents such as methotrexate and cladribine in patients with chronic progressive MS.

Several lines of evidence point to the involvement of immune mechanisms in MS. This suggests that immunotherapy may hold an answer for these patients. The goals of immunotherapy at present are to improve recovery from exacerbations, decrease the number and severity of relapses, and limit progression of the disease. Nonspecific immunosuppressive agents like corticotropin and corticosteroids are beneficial for acute exacerbations, but disease progression still occurs. Attempts to slow progression with azathioprine, cyclophosphamide, intravenous immune globulin, and cyclosporin have been only modestly successful and can cause serious adverse effects. Interferon-β_{1b} can reduce the number and severity of relapses in patients with relapsing–remitting MS; copolymer 1 and cladribine may hold promise as well. Better understanding of the immunologic basis of MS may lead to more specific immunotherapies with more lasting benefits.

MUMPS SKIN TEST ANTIGEN (MSTA)

Mumps antigen is used to assess cell-mediated immunity.

MUMPS VIRUS VACCINE, LIVE (Mumpsvax)

Mumps vaccine is used for immunization.

MUPIROCIN (PSEUDOMONIC ACID A) (Bactroban ointment 2%, cream 2%, Bactroban nasal ointment 2%)

Mupirocin is an antibiotic agent that inhibits bacterial protein synthesis. It is indicated in treatment of impetigo caused by *Staphylococcus aureus* and *Streptococcus pyogenes* (topical ointment); and treatment of secondarily infected traumatic skin lesions (up to 10 cm in length or 100 cm^2 in area).

Mupirocin (Bactroban) is derived from a fermentation product of *Pseudomonas fluorescens*. It is for topical use only.

Mupirocin is active against many Gram-positive and selected Gram-negative bacteria. It has good activity with MICs $\leq$ 1 µg/mL against *S. pyogenes* and methicillin-susceptible and methicillin-resistant strains of *S. aureus*. It is bactericidal at concentrations achieved with topical application.

Mupirocin inhibits bacterial protein synthesis by reversible binding and inhibition of isoleucyl transfer-RNA synthetase. There is no cross-resistance with other classes of antibiotics. Low-level resistance, which is not clinically significant, is due to mutations of the host gene encoding **isoleucyl transfer-RNA synthetase** or an extra chromosomal copy of a gene encoding a modified isoleucyl transfer-RNA synthetase. High-level resistance (MIC > 1 mg/ml) is mediated by a plasmid or chromosomal copy of *mupA*, which encodes a "bypass" synthetase that binds mupirocin poorly.

Systemic absorption through intact skin or skin lesions is minimal. Any **mupirocin** that is absorbed is rapidly metabolized to inactive monic acid.

Mupirocin is available as a 2% cream and a 2% ointment for dermatologic use, and as a 2% ointment for intranasal use. The dermatologic preparations are indicated in treatment of traumatic skin lesions and impetigo secondarily infected with *S. aureus* or *S. pyogenes*.

The nasal ointment is approved for eradication of *S. aureus* nasal carriage. **Mupirocin** is highly effective in eradicating *S. aureus* carriage. Because *S. aureus* colonization often precedes infection, eradication of carriage by intranasal application of mupirocin might reduce the risk of later infection. However, two clinical trials failed to demonstrate that **mupirocin** prophylaxis reduces nosocomial *S. aureus* infections.

A third large study found that *S. aureus* nasal carriers had fewer S. aureus nosocomial infections of any site, but failed to show a reduction in *S. aureus* surgical site infections, the primary end point of the study. The accumulated evidence indicates that patients who stand to benefit from **mupirocin** prophylaxis are those with proven *S. aureus* nasal colonization plus risk factors for distant infection or a history of skin or soft tissue infections. General in-patient populations and individuals lacking specific risk factors for *S. aureus* infection are not likely to benefit from mupirocin prophylaxis.

Mupirocin may cause irritation and sensitization at the site of application. Contact with the eyes should be avoided because it causes tearing, burning, and irritation that may take several days to resolve. Systemic reactions to mupirocin occur rarely, if at all. Polyethylene glycol present in the ointment can be absorbed from damaged skin. Application of the ointment to large surface areas should be avoided in patients with moderate to severe renal failure to avoid accumulation of polyethylene glycol.

Mupirocin (2% ointment) is used as a topical treatment of impetigo due to *S. aureus*, beta-hemolytic *Streptococcus*, and *S. pyogenes*.

MUROMONAB-CD3
(Orthoclone OKT3)

Muromonab-CD3, a monoclonal antibody, is used in the treatment of acute allograft rejection in renal transplant patients.

MUROMONAB-CD3
(Orthoclone OKT3 injection 5 mg per 5 mL)

Muromonab-CD3 is an immunosuppressive agent that blocks T-cell function, which plays a major role in graft rejection, by reacting with and blocking the T3 (CD3) molecule on the membrane of human T-cells associated with antigen recognition. Serum levels are measured with an enzyme-linked immunosorbent assay (ELISA). It is indicated in the treatment of renal, steroid resistant cardiac, or hepatic allograft rejection.

MUZOLIMINE

Ethacrynic acid, bumetanide, furosemide, and muzolimine are loop diuretics. The most often used and the major loop diuretics are furosemide (Lasix) and ethacrynic acid (Edecrin). Furosemide is chemically related to the thiazide diuretics, but ethacrynic acid is not. These agents inhibit the active resorption of chloride (and sodium) in the thick, ascending medullary portion of the loop of Henle and also in the cortical portion of the loop or the distal tubule. The diuresis they produce, which is similar to that seen with the thiazides, predominantly causes a loss of chloride, sodium, and potassium, but HCO_3 excretion is not increased. Although large volumes of fluid can be excreted with the use of these agents, the ability of the kidney to produce either a dilute or concentrated urine is greatly diminished. These agents are the most efficacious of all the diuretics now on the market, usually producing about a 20% loss in the filtered load of sodium (furosemide, 15 to 30%; ethacrynic acid, 17 to 23%).

Loop diuretics are ordinarily taken orally but can be given intravenously if a very rapid onset of action is sought, as when used in combination with antihypertensive medications in the management of a hypertensive crisis. Furosemide and ethacrynic acid undergo some active renal tubular secretion as well as glomerular filtration. A minor portion is excreted by the liver.

Loop diuretics are used for treating the following conditions:

- In edema of cardiac, hepatic, or renal origin, including acute pulmonary edema and hypertensive crisis
- In acute renal failure, to maintain urine flow, though an excessive loss of extracellular fluid volume can cause a decrease in the GFR
- In hypercalcemia

Excessive volume depletion, hyponatremia, and hypotension are major risks associated with the use of loop diuretics, and the side effects of hypokalemia, hyperuricemia, and hyperglycemia are always present. Loop diuretics should not be used concurrently with ototoxic aminoglycoside antibiotics (i.e., streptomycin, gentamicin, kanamycin, tobramycin) (see also Table 25).

MYASTHENIA GRAVIS: Treatment of

Myasthenia gravis is a neurological disease of autoimmune origin. The basic defect is the reduction of nicotinic acetylcholine receptors (AChR) at the neuromuscular junction, resulting in inadequate transmission through the neuromuscular junction and hence the clinical syndrome of weakness, frequently worsened by exercise or effort.

There are two basic strategies in treating myasthenia gravis. One is to treat it symptomatically by increasing the available amount of acetylcholine (ACh) at the neuromuscular junction with a cholinesterase inhibitor compound that inhibits the enzyme acetylcholinesterase, responsible for the breakdown of acetylcholine. This in turn raises the amount of ACh at the neuromuscular junction to stimulate whatever AChR are available. Other strategies include increasing ACh release or its effect.

Immunomodulation is the other important way to treat patients with myasthenia gravis. Corticosteroid drugs are the most widely used and some of the most effective agents currently available to treat myasthenic patients. Azathioprine is a prodrug that is converted into mercaptopurine, a purine analog that in turn is incorporated into nucleotides. These abnormal nucleotides affect synthesis of RNA and DNA, and thus preferentially affect the more actively multiplying cells. Azathioprine can be used in the treatment of generalized myasthenia gravis that is not responding to conventional therapy with cholinesterase inhibitors, thymectomy, and steroid drugs, or when the response is limited by side effects of these agents. Cyclosporin A and cyclophosphamide are used in cases of malignant thymoma with or without myasthenia gravis.

MYCOPHENOLATE MOFETIL/MYCOPHENOLIC ACID

(Cellcept capsules 250 mg, tablets 500 mg, powder for oral suspension 200 mg/mL (reconstituted), powder for injection 500 mg as hydrochloride, myfortic tablets, delayed release 180 mg tablets, delayed release 360 mg)

Myocphenolate mofetil is an immunosuppressive agent that inhibits immune-mediated inflammatory responses. **Cellcept**: is used in combination with cyclosporine and corticosteroids for prophylaxis of organ rejection in patients receiving allogeneic renal, cardiac, or hepatic transplants. **Myfortic**: is used in combination with cyclosporine and corticosteroids for prophylaxis of organ rejection in patients receiving allogeneic renal transplants.

Mycophenolate mofetil (Cellcept) is the 2-morpholinoethyl ester of mycophenolic acid (MPA).

Mycophenolate mofetil is a prodrug that is rapidly hydrolyzed to the active drug, **MPA**, a selective, noncompetitive, and reversible inhibitor of **inosine monophosphate dehydrogenase** (MPDH), an important enzyme in the *de novo* pathway of guanine nucleotide synthesis. B- and T-lymphocytes are highly dependent on this pathway for cell proliferation, whereas other cell types can use salvage pathways; MPA, therefore, selectively inhibits lymphocyte proliferation and functions, including antibody formation, cellular adhesion, and migration.

Mycophenolate mofetil undergoes rapid and complete metabolism to MPA after oral or intravenous administration. MPA, in turn, is metabolized to the inactive phenolic glucuronide MPAG. The parent drug is cleared from the blood within a few minutes. The half-life of MPA is about 16 hours. Negligible (<1%) amounts of MPA are excreted in the urine. Most (87%) is excreted in the urine as MPAG. Plasma concentrations of MPA and MPAG are increased in patients with renal insufficiency. In early renal transplant patients (<40 days posttransplant), plasma concentrations of MPA after a single dose of **mycophenolate mofetil** are about half of those found in healthy volunteers or stable renal transplant patients. Studies in children are limited, and safety and effectiveness have not been established.

Mycophenolate mofetil is indicated in prophylaxis of transplant rejection, and it typically is used in combination with glucocorticoids and a calcineurin inhibitor but not with azathioprine. Combined treatment with sirolimus is possible, although potential drug interactions necessitate careful monitoring of drug levels. For renal transplants, 1 g is administered orally or intravenously (over 2 hours) twice daily (2 g per day). A higher dose, twice daily (3 g per day) is recommended for African-American renal transplant patients and all cardiac transplant patients. Use of mycophenolate mofetil in other clinical settings is under investigation.

The principal toxicities of mycophenolate are gastrointestinal and hematologic. These include leukopenia, diarrhea, and vomiting. There also is an increased incidence of some infections, especially sepsis associated with cytomegalovirus. Tacrolimus in combination with mycophenolate mofetil has been associated with devastating viral infections including polyoma nephritis.

Potential drug interactions between mycophenolate mofetil and several other drugs commonly used by transplant patients have been studied. There appear to be no untoward effects produced by combination therapy with **cyclosporine**, **trimethoprimsulfamethoxazole**, or oral contraceptives. Unlike cyclosporine, tacrolimus delays elimination of mycophenolate mofetil by impairing the conversion of MPA to MPAG. This may enhance GI toxicity. Mycophenolate mofetil has not been tested with azathioprine. Coadministration with antacids containing aluminum or magnesium hydroxide leads to decreased absorption of mycophenolate mofetil; thus, these drugs should not be administered simultaneously. **Mycophenolate mofetil** should not be administered with cholestyramine or other drugs that affect enterohepatic circulation. Such agents decrease plasma MPA concentrations, probably by binding free MPA in the intestines. Acyclovir and ganciclovir may compete with MPAG for tubular secretion, possibly resulting in increased concentrations of both MPAG and the antiviral agents in the blood, an effect that may be compounded in patients with renal insufficiency.

Mycophenolate mofetil (Cellcept) is an immunosuppressant approved for prophylaxis of organ rejection in patients with renal, cardiac, and hepatic transplants. Mycophenolic acid, the active derivative of **mycophenolate mofetil**, inhibits the enzyme inosine monophosphatase dehydrogenase (IMPDH), thereby depleting guanosine nucleotides essential for DNA and RNA synthesis. Moreover, mycophenolic acid is a fivefold more potent inhibitor of the type II isoform of IMPDH found in activated B- and T-lymphocytes and thus functions as a specific inhibitor of T- and B-lymphocyte activation and proliferation. The drug also may enhance apoptosis.

Mycophenolate mofetil is used increasingly to treat inflammatory and autoimmune diseases in dermatology in doses ranging from 1 to 2 g/day orally. It is particularly useful as a corticosteroid-sparing agent in the treatment of **autoimmune blistering disorders**, including **pemphigus vulgaris**, **bullous pemphigoid**, cicatricial pemphigoid, and **pemphigus foliaceus**. It also has been used effectively in the treatment of inflammatory diseases such as **psoriasis**, **atopic dermatitis**, and **pyoderma gangrenosum**.

Imiquimod (Aldara) is a synthetic imidazoquinoline amine believed to exert immunomodulatory effects by acting as a ligand at toll-like receptors in the innate immune system and inducing the cytokines interferon-α (IFN-α), tumor necrosis factor-α (TNF-α), and IL-1, IL-6, IL-8, IL-10, and IL-12.

MYCOSES: Treatment of Deep-Seated Organisms

Aspergillosis, invasive	
Immunosuppressed	Amphotericin B
Nonimmunosuppressed	Amphotericin B, itraconazole
Blastomycosis	
Rapidly progressive or CNS	Amphotericin B
Indolent, non-CNS	Itraconazole, ketoconazole
Coccidioidomycosis	
Rapidly progressing	Amphotericin B
Indolent	Itraconazole, ketoconazole, fluconazole
Meningeal	Fluconazole, intrathecal amphotericin B
Cryptococcosis	
Non-AIDS and initial AIDS	Amphotericin B ± flucytosine
Maintenance, AIDS	Fluconazole
Histoplasmosis	
Chronic pulmonary	Itraconazole
Disseminated	
Rapidly progressing or CNS	Amphotericin B
Indolent, non-CNS	Itraconazole
Maintenance, AIDS	Itraconazole
Mucormycosis	Amphotericin B
Pseudallescheriasis	Itraconazole, IV miconazole
Sporotrichosis	
Cutaneous	Iodide, itraconazole
Extracutaneous	Amphotericin B

MYOCLONUS: Treatment of

Myoclonic jerks are sudden, rapid, twitch-like muscle contractions. They can be classified according to their distribution, relationship to precipitating stimuli, or etiology. Generalized myoclonus has a widespread distribution, while focal or segmental myoclonus is restricted to a particular part of the body. Myoclonus can be spontaneous, or it can be brought on by sensory stimulation, arousal, or the initiation of movement (action myoclonus). It may occur as a normal phenomenon (physiologic myoclonus) in healthy persons, as an isolated abnormality (essential myoclonus), or as a manifestation of epilepsy (epileptic myoclonus). It can also occur as a feature of a variety of degenerative infections, and metabolic disorders (symptomatic myoclonus).

Treatments of first choice for cortical myoclonus are valproic acid (sodium valproate) and clonazepam. Primidone and phenobarbital may also be useful. Piracetam has advantages in these circumstances, as its addition to existing treatments is rarely accompanied by sedation.

In patients with brain-stem reticular-reflex myoclonus, valproic acid and clonazepam are the most useful agents. In hyperreflexia, treatment is directed against the disabling tonic spasms, rather than jerks. Carbamazepine, phenytoin, and clonazepam are useful agents in this respect. Ballistic overflow myoclonus may improve with anticholinergic drugs such as benztropine or trihexyphenidyl.

Treatment of palatal myoclonus is often unsuccessful, but phenytoin, carbamazepine, clonazepam, trihexyphenidyl, and baclofen have been effective in some patients. Clonazepam is effective in over half of patients with propriospinal myoclonus, but other anticonvulsants are usually not helpful. Segmental spinal myoclonus is often resistant to drug treatment, but diazepam, carbamazepine, tetrabenazine and, particularly, clonazepam are sometimes effective.

N

NABUMETONE

(Relafen tablets 500 mg)

Nabumetone is a NSAID that decreases inflammation, pain and fever, probably through inhibition of cyclooxygenase activity and prostaglandin synthesis.

Nabumetone (1000 mg as a single dose) is indicated for the acute and chronic treatment of osteoarthritis and rheumatoid arthritis. **Nabumetone**, which has analgesic, antipyretic, and antiinflammatory properties, exerts its effects in part by inhibiting the synthesis of prostaglandin. **Nabumetone** is absorbed from the gastrointestinal (GI) tract, metabolized to an active metabolite, 6-methoxy 2-naphthylacetic acid, and excreted in the urine. **Nabumetone** and its metabolite, which are extensively bound to plasma proteins, are able to alter the binding of other drugs such as warfarin possessing the inherent potential to cause toxicity (see also Table 3).

Nabumetone and other antiinflammatory agents impair the synthesis of renal prostaglandin, decreasing reversibly the blood flow, which may become detrimental in individuals with renal impairment. Therefore, individuals with cardiovascular problems taking diuretics and nabumetone should be monitored carefully. The adverse reactions to nabumetone that have been reported, especially in higher than therapeutic doses, include CNS dizziness, headache, fatigue, increased sweating, nervousness, somnolence, pruritis, rash, diarrhea, dyspepsia, abdominal pain, gastric pain, flatulence, and mild gastric bleeding.

Nabumetone is an antiinflammatory agent approved in 1991 for use in the United States.

Clinical trials with **nabumetone** (Relafen) have indicated substantial efficacy in the treatment of rheumatoid arthritis and osteoarthritis, with a relatively low incidence of side effects. The dose typically is 1000 mg given once daily. The drug also has off-label use in the short-term treatment of soft-tissue injuries.

Nabumetone is a prodrug; thus it is a weak inhibitor of COX *in vitro* but a potent COX inhibitor *in vivo*.

Nabumetone is absorbed rapidly and is converted in the liver to one or more active metabolites, principally **6-methoxy-2-naphthylacetic acid**, a potent nonselective inhibitor of COX. This metabolite, inactivated by *O*-demethylation in the liver, is then conjugated before excretion, and is eliminated with a half-life of about 24 hours.

Nabumetone is associated with crampy lower abdominal pain and diarrhea, but the incidence of gastrointestinal ulceration appears to be lower than with other tNSAIDs, although randomized, controlled studies directly comparing tolerability and clinical outcomes have not been performed. Other side effects include rash, headache, dizziness, heartburn, tinnitus and pruritus.

Pyrazolon derivatives include **phenylbutazone**, **oxyphenbutazone**, **antipyrine**, **aminopyrine**, and **dipyrone**; currently, only antipyrine otic drops are available in the United States. These drugs were used clinically for many years but have essentially been abandoned because of their propensity to cause irreversible agranulocytosis. Dipyrone was reintroduced in Europe approximately 10 years ago because epidemiological studies suggested that the risk of adverse effects was similar to that of acetaminophen and lower than that of aspirin. However, its use remains limited.

The therapeutic use of the tNSAIDs has been limited by poor tolerability. Chronic users are prone to experience gastrointestinal irritation in up to 20% of cases. However, the incidence of these adverse events had been falling sharply in the population prior to the introduction of the coxibs, perhaps reflecting a move away from use of high-dose aspirin as an antiinflammatory drug strategy. Studies of the immediate early genes induced by inflammation led to the discovery of a gene with significant homology to the original COX enzyme, now designated COX-2. Because expression of this second COX enzyme was regulated by cytokines and mitogens, it was proposed to be the dominant source of prostaglandin formation in inflammation and cancer. It further was proposed that the original, constitutively expressed COX was the predominant source of cytoprotective prostaglandins formed by the gastrointestinal epithelium. Thus, selective inhibition of COX-2 was postulated to afford efficacy similar to tNSAIDs but with better tolerability. Subsequent crystallization of COX-1 and COX-2 revealed remarkable conservation of tertiary structure. However, one difference was in the hydrophobic channel by which the AA substrate gains access to the COX active site, buried deep within the molecule. This channel is more accommodating in the COX-2 structure and consequently exhibits wider substrate specificity than in COX-1, It also contains a side pocket that in retrospect affords a structural explanation for the identification in screens of the two enzymes *in vitro* of small molecule inhibitors that are differentially specific for COX-2. Although there were differences in relative hierarchies, depending on whether screens were performed using recombinantly expressed enzymes, cells, or whole blood assays, most NSAIDs expressed similar selectivity for inhibition of the two enzymes.

NADOLOL

(Corgard)

Nadolol is a nonselective beta-adrenergic-receptor-blocking agent that possesses no intrinsic sympathomimetic activity. It is indicated in angina pectoris (120 mg/day) and in combination with other antihypertensive medications in the management of hypertension (80 to 600 mg/day) (see also Figure 37).

Nadolol is absorbed modestly (30%) after oral administration, becomes bound to plasma protein to the extent of 20%, and is excreted mostly unchanged (70%) in the urine and feces.

The major hemodynamic effect of nadolol is a decrease in sinus node frequency causing a reduction in the heart rate and cardiac output, and the said effects are more pronounced during exercise. Nadolol decreases sinoatrial impulse formation but does not impair atrial conduction or that of accessory pathways. Similar to propranolol, nadolol causes a mild increase in plasma volume.

Unlike the $beta_1$ selective blockers, nadolol prevents the epinephrine-induced decrease in serum potassium level, an effect that is mediated by $beta_2$-adrenergic stimulation. Like all other beta-adrenergic-receptor blockers, nadolol antagonizes the thyroxine-mediated stimulation of beta-adrenergic receptors. Unlike most beta-adrenergic-receptor-blocking agents, nadolol preserves renal blood flow.

Because of its low lipid solubility, nadolol does not cross the blood–brain barrier, and hence is devoid of any CNS effects seen following administration of propranolol.

Nadolol is contraindicated in severe bradyarrhythmias or bronchospasm. It should be used cautiously in overt congestive heart failure (CHF), severe peripheral vascular disorder with claudication, and severe diabetes mellitus. As nadolol is largely excreted by the kidneys, decreased renal function affects the clearance of the drug. Nadolol concentrates fivefold in human breast milk and that should be taken into consideration in prescribing the drug for a mother nursing an infant.

NAFARELIN ACETATE

(Synarel)

Nafarelin, a synthetic decapeptide and a gonadotropin-releasing-hormone (GnRH) analog (200 mcg spray into one nostril in a.m. and in p.m.), is used in the management of endometriosis, pain relief, and reduction of endometriotic lesions (see also Table 15).

NAFCILLIN SODIUM

(Nafcillin sodium injection 1 g (as base), injection 2 g (as base))

Nafcillin sodium is a penicillinase-resistant penicillin that inhibits bacterial cell wall mucopeptide synthesis.

Nafcillin (IV 3 to 6 g/24 hours in severe infections) is indicated for the treatment of infections due to penicillinase-producing staphylococci. It may be used to initiate therapy when a staphylococcal infection is suspected (see also Table 23). Like penicillins, nafcillin, inhibits the formation of cell walls and hence is bactericidal in nature. Penicillin binds to cellular receptors, now identified as transpeptidation enzymes, and, by binding to and inhibiting the transpeptidation reactions, the synthesis of cell wall peptidoglycan is interrupted. In addition, penicillin removes or inactivates an inhibitor of the lytic enzymes (autolysin), resulting in the lysis of microorganisms in an isotonic environment. In general, penicillins are more active against Gram-positive organisms.

Nafcillin resists the effects of penicillinases—enzymes that inactivate penicillin—and is thus active against many strains of penicillinase-producing bacteria. This activity is most important against penicillinase-producing staphylococci; some strains may remain resistant. Nafcillin is also active against a few Gram-positive aerobic and anaerobic bacilli but has no significant effect on Gram-negative bacilli (see also Table 23).

Nafcillin is absorbed erratically from the GI tract and distributes poorly into cerebrospinal fluid, but this passage is enhanced by meningeal inflammation. Nafcillin, which is bound to plasma protein to the extent of 90%, crosses the placenta and is found in breast milk.

Nafcillin and aminoglycosides are chemically inactivated and should not be mixed together. Probenecid blocks renal tubular secretion of penicillins; however, this interaction has only a small effect on the excretion of nafcillin.

Nafcillin should be given with water only, as acid in fruit juices or carbonated water may inactivate it. Furthermore, it should be given on an empty stomach because food decreases its absorption. Clinical signs of overdose include neuromuscular irritability or seizures (see Table 23).

It is useful to classify the penicillins according to their spectra of antimicrobial activity.

Penicillin G and its close congener **penicillin V** are highly active against sensitive strains of Gram-positive cocci, but they are readily hydrolyzed by penicillinase. Thus they are ineffective against most strains of *S. aureus*.

The penicillinase-resistant penicillins [**methicillin**, **nafcillin**, **oxacillin**, **cloxacillin**, and **dicloxacillin**] have less potent antimicrobial activity against microorganisms that are sensitive to penicillin G, but they are the agents of first choice for treatment of penicillinase-producing *S. aureus* and *S. epidermidis* that are not methicillin-resistant.

Ampicillin, **amoxicillin**, and others make up a group of penicillins whose antimicrobial activity is extended to include such Gram-negative microorganisms as *Haemophilus influenzae*, *E. coli*, and *Proteus mirabilis*. Frequently, these drugs are administered with a β-lactamase inhibitor such as **clavalanate** or **salbactam** to prevent hydrolysis by broad-spectrum β-lactamases that are found with increasing frequency in clinical isolates of these Gram-negative bacteria.

The antimicrobial activity of carbenicillin, its indanyl ester (**carbenicillin indanyl**), and **ticarcillin** is extended to include *Pseudomonas*, *Enterobacter*, and *Proteus* spp. These agents are inferior to ampicillin against Gram-positive cocci and *Listeria* monocytogenes and are less active than piperacillin against *Pseudomonas*.

Mezlocillin, **azlocillin**, and **piperacillin** have excellent antimicrobial activity against *Pseudomonas*, *Klebsiella*, and certain other Gram-negative microorganisms. Piperacillin retains the activity of ampicillin against Gram-positive cocci and *L. monocytogenes*.

Nafcillin, a semisynthetic penicillin is highly resistant to penicillinase and has proven effective against infections caused by penicillinase-producing strains of *S. aureus*.

Nafcillin is slightly more active than oxacillin against penicillin-G-resistant *S. aureus* (most strains are inhibited by 0.06 to 2 μg/mL). Although it is the most active of the penicillinase-resistant penicillins against other microorganisms it is not as potent as penicillin G.

Nafcillin is variably inactivated in the acidic medium of the gastric contents. Its oral absorption is irregular regardless of whether the drug is taken with meals or on an empty stomach; injectable preparations therefore should be used. The peak plasma concentration is about 8 μg/mL 60 minutes after a 1-g intramuscular dose. **Nafcillin** is about 90% bound to plasma protein. Peak concentrations of nafcillin in bile are well above those found in plasma. Concentrations of the drug in CSF appear to be adequate for therapy of staphylococcal meningitis.

NAFTIFINE HYDROCHLORIDE

(Naftin)

Naftifine (1% cream once a day) is indicated for topical treatment of tinea pedis (athlete's foot), tinea cruris (jock itch), and tinea corporis (ringworm) caused by the organisms *T. rubrum*, *T. mentagrophytes*, *T. tonsurans*, and *E. floccosum*.

Naftifine, a broad-spectrum antifungal agent, is a synthetic allylamine derivative that interferes with sterol biosynthesis by inhibiting the enzyme squalene 2,3-epoxidase. This inhibition of enzyme activity results in decreased amounts of sterols, especially ergosterol, and a corresponding accumulation of squalene in the cells.

Naftifine penetrates the stratum corneum to inhibit the growth of dermatophytes. Following a single application of 1% naftifine to the skin, systemic absorption was 5%. Naftifine or its metabolites are excreted via the urine and feces with a half-life of approximately 2 to 3 days.

NALBUPHINE HYDROCHLORIDE

(Nubain injection 10 mg/mL)

Nalbuphine hydrochloride is an opioid agonist–antagonist analgesic that has both narcotic agonist and antagonist actions. Analgesic potency is about equal to that of morphine, and antagonist potency is about 1/25 that of naloxone. It may cause sphincter of Oddi spasm. It does not increase pulmonary artery pressure, systemic vascular resistance, or myocardial work load. It is indicated in the management of moderate to severe pain; as a preoperative and postoperative analgesia; as a supplement to balanced anesthesia; and obstetrical analgesia during labor and delivery.

Nalbuphine, a narcotic agonist-antagonist (10 mg in adult administered SC, IM, or IV every 3 to 6 hours) is indicated for the relief of moderate to severe pain, for preoperative analgesia, as a supplement to balanced analgesia and to surgical anesthesia, and for obstetrical analgesia during labor and delivery.

Nalbuphine is structurally related to both naloxone and oxymorphone. It is an agonist–antagonist opioid possessing a spectrum of effects that resemble those of pentazocine; however, nalbuphine is a more potent antagonist at mu receptors and is less likely to produce dysphoria than is pentazocine.

Its analgesic potency is essentially equivalent to that of morphine and about three times that of pentazocine on a milligram basis. Unlike the other agonist–antagonists, nalbuphine does not significantly increase pulmonary artery pressure, systemic vascular resistance, or cardiac work.

Nalbuphine's abuse potential is less than for codeine and propoxyphene. The most common effects of nalbuphine are sleepiness and mild dysphoria. Barbiturate anesthetics increase the respiratory and CNS-depressant effects of nalbuphine.

The drugs described in this section differ from clinically used μ-opioid receptor agonists. Drugs such as **nalbuphine** and **butorphanol** are competitive μ-receptor antagonists but exert their analgesic actions by acting as agonists at receptors. **Pentazocine** qualitatively resembles these drugs, but it may be a weaker μ-receptor antagonist or partial agonist although retaining its κ-agonist activity. Buprenorphine, on the other hand, is a partial agonist at μ receptors. The stimulus for the development of mixed agonist–antagonist drugs was a need for analgesics with less respiratory depression and addictive potential. The clinical use of these compounds is limited by undesirable side effects and limited analgesic effects.

Nalbuphine is related structurally to **naloxone** and **oxymorphone**. It is an agonist–antagonist opioid with a spectrum of effects that qualitatively resembles that of **pentazocine**; however, nalbuphine is a more potent antagonist at μ receptors and is less likely to produce dysphoric side effects than is pentazocine.

An intramuscular dose of 10 mg **nalbuphine** is equianalgesic to 10 mg morphine, with a similar onset and duration of analgesic and subjective effects. Nalbuphine depresses respiration as much as do equianalgesic doses of morphine. However, nalbuphine exhibits a ceiling effect such that increases in dosage beyond 30 mg produce no further respiratory depression. However, a ceiling effect for analgesia also is reached at this point. In contrast to pentazocine and butorphanol, 10 mg nalbuphine given to patients with stable coronary artery disease does not produce an increase in cardiac index, pulmonary arterial pressure, or cardiac work, and systemic blood pressure (BP) is not significantly altered; these indices also are relatively stable when nalbuphine is given to patients with acute myocardial infarction (MI). Its gastrointestinal effects probably are similar to those of pentazocine. **Nalbuphine** produces few side effects at doses of 10 mg or less; sedation, sweating, and headache are the most common. At much higher doses (70 mg), psychotomimetic side effects (e.g., dysphoria, racing thoughts, and distortions of body image) can occur. **Nalbuphine** is metabolized in the liver and has a half-life in plasma of 2 to 3 hours.

Given orally, nalbuphine is 20 to 25% as potent as when given intramuscularly.

In subjects dependent on low doses of morphine (60 mg/day), **nalbuphine** precipitates an abstinence syndrome. Prolonged administration of nalbuphine can produce physical dependence. The withdrawal syndrome is similar in intensity to that seen with pentazocine. The potential for abuse of parenteral **nalbuphine** in subjects not dependent on μ-receptor agonists probably is similar to that for parenteral pentazocine.

Nalbuphine hydrochloride (nubain) is used to produce analgesia. Because it is an agonist–antagonist, administration to patients who have been receiving morphine-like opioids may create difficulties unless a brief drug-free interval is interposed. The usual adult dose is 10 mg parenterally every 3 to 6 hours; this may be increased to 20 mg in nontolerant individuals.

NALIDIXIC ACID

(NegGram caplets 250 mg)

Nalidixic acid is a quinolone antibiotic, which interferes with DNA formation of certain bacteria. It is indicated in the treatment of UTIs caused by susceptible Gram-negative bacteria, including most *Proteus* strains, *Klebsiella* and *Enterobacter* species, and *E. coli*.

The quinolones include: nalidixic acid, cinoxacin (Cinobac), norfloxacin (Noroxin), and ciprofloxacin (Cipro). Other members of the quinolone family are pefloxacin, ofloxacin, enoxacin, and fleroxacin (see also Figure 85).

The bacterial enzyme DNA gyrase is responsible for the continuous introduction of negative supercoils into DNA, and the quinolones inhibit this gyrase-mediated DNA supercoiling.

Nalidixic acid and cinoxacin are bactericidal against Gram-negative organisms that cause urinary tract infections. The fluoroquinolones are bactericidal and considerably more potent against *E. coli* and various species of *Salmonella, Shigella*, *Enterobacter*, *Campylobacter*, and *Neisseria*. Ciprofloxacin also has good activity against staphylococci, including methicillin-resistant strains.

The quinolones and fluoroquinolones may produce arthropathy, and hence should not be used in prepubertal children or pregnant women.

Nalidixic acid and cinoxacin are useful only for treating urinary tract infections. Ciprofloxacin is useful for both urinary tract infections and prostatitis.

The first quinolone, **nalidixic acid**, was isolated as a byproduct of the synthesis of chloroquine. It has been available for the treatment of urinary tract infections for many years. The introduction of **fluorinated 4-quinolones**, such as **ciprofloxacin** (Cipro), **moxifloxacin** (Avelox), and **gatifloxacin** (Tequin) represents a particularly important therapeutic advance because these agents have broad antimicrobial activity and are effective after oral administration for the treatment of a wide variety of infectious diseases. Relatively few side effects appear to accompany the use of these fluoroquinolones, and microbial resistance to their action does not develop rapidly. Rare and potentially fatal side effects, however, have resulted in the withdrawal from the market of temafloxacin (immune hemolytic anemia), trovafloxacin (hepatotoxicity), grepafloxacin (cardiotoxicity), and clinafloxacin (phototoxicity). In all these cases, the side effects were so infrequent as to be missed by prerelease clinical trials and detected only by postmarketing surveillance.

The quinolone antibiotics target bacterial **DNA gyrase and topoisomerase IV**. For many Gram-positive bacteria (such as *S. aureus*), topoisomerase IV is the primary activity inhibited by the quinolones. In contrast, for many Gram-negative bacteria (such as *E. coli*), DNA gyrase is the primary quinolone target. The individual strands of double-helical DNA must be separated to permit DNA replication or transcription. However, anything that separates the strands results in "overwinding" or excessive positive supercoiling of the DNA in front of the point of separation. To combat this mechanical obstacle, the bacterial enzyme DNA gyrase is responsible for the continuous introduction of negative supercoils into DNA. This is an ATP-dependent reaction requiring that both strands of the DNA be cut to permit passage of a segment of DNA through the break; the break then is resealed.

The DNA gyrase of *E. coli* is composed of two 105,000-dalton A subunits and two 95,000-dalton B subunits encoded by the gyrA and gyrB genes, respectively. The A subunits, which carry out the strand-cutting function of the gyrase, are the site of action of the quinolones. The drugs inhibit gyrase-mediated DNA supercoiling at concentrations that correlate well with those required to inhibit bacterial growth (0.1 to 10 μg/mL). Mutations of the gene that encodes the A subunit polypeptide can confer resistance to these drugs.

Topoisomerase IV also is composed of four subunits encoded by the parC and parE genes in *E. coli*. Topoisomerase IV separates interlinked (catenated) daughter DNA molecules that are the product of DNA replication. Eukaryotic cells do not contain DNA gyrase. However, they do contain a conceptually and mechanistically similar type II DNA topoisomerase that removes positive supercoils from eukaryotic DNA to prevent its tangling during replication. This enzyme is the target for some antineoplastic agents. Quinolones inhibit eukaryotic type II topoisomerase only at much higher concentrations (100 to 1000 μg/mL).

Certain generic or metabolic abnormalities must be considered when prescribing antibiotics. A number of drugs (e.g., **sulfonamides**, **nitrofurantoin**, **chloramphenicol**, and **nalidixic acid**) may produce acute hemolysis in patients with glucose-6-phosphate dehydrogenase deficiency. Patients who acetylate isoniazid rapidly may have subtherapeutic concentrations of the drug in plasma.

Pregnancy may impose an increased risk of reaction to antimicrobial agents for both mother and fetus. Hearing loss in the child has been associated with administration of

streptomycin to the mother during pregnancy. **Tetracyclines** can affect the bones and teeth of the fetus. Pregnant women receiving tetracycline may develop fatal acute fatty necrosis of the liver, pancreatitis, and associated renal damage. Pregnancy also may affect the pharmacokinetics of various antibiotics.

The lactating female can pass antimicrobial agents to her nursing child. Both **nalidixic acid** and the sulfonamides in breast milk have been associated with hemolysis in children with **glucose-6-phosphate dehydrogenase deficiency**. In addition, sulfonamides, even in the small amounts received from breast milk, may predispose the nursing child to **kernicterus**.

Antibiotics, especially β-lactams, are notorious for provoking allergic reactions. Patients with a history of atopy seem particularly susceptible to the development of these reactions. Sulfonamides, trimethoprim, nitrofurantoin, and erythromycin also have been associated with hypersensitivity reactions, especially rash. A history of anaphylaxis (immediate hypersensitivity reaction) or hives and laryngeal edema (accelerated reaction) precludes use of the drug in all but extreme, life-threatening situations. Skin testing, particularly of the penicillins, may be of value in predicting life-threatening reactions. Antimicrobial agents, like other drugs, can cause drug fever, which can be mistaken for a sign of continued infection.

Patients predisposed to seizures are at risk for localized or major motor seizures while taking high doses of penicillin G. This neurotoxicity of penicillin and other β-lactam antibiotics correlates with high concentrations of drug in the CSF and typically occurs in patients with impaired renal function who are given large doses of the drugs. Isoniazid causes a peripheral neuropathy that is preventable and reversible by administration of pyridoxine. Diabetics and HIV-infected patients, who are prone to neuropathy because of their underlying diseases, and alcoholics, who often are malnourished, are particularly predisposed. Oncology and HIV-infected patients often have bone marrow suppression, which makes them particularly susceptible to hematologic side effects of antibiotics. Patients with myasthenia gravis or other neuromuscular problems are susceptible to the neuromuscular-blocking effect of the aminoglycosides.

NALORPHINE

(Nalline)

Nalorphine, a narcotic antagonist, differs from morphine in having an allyl (CH_2–CH=CH_2) group instead of a CH_2 group attached to the N atom. It and levallorphan, which is the corresponding allyl homolog of levorphanol, are effective antagonists against a wide variety of potent analgesics related pharmacologically to morphine. They antagonize many times their molecular equivalent of such narcotics as methadone, isomethadone, heptazone, codeine, dihydromorphinone, metopon, methomorphinan, and meperidine. This antagonism is so complete that administration of nalorphine during addiction leads to an acute abstinence syndrome.

Nalorphine in doses of 5 mg produces side effects that are comparable to those produced by 10 mg of morphine, unaccompanied by any significant analgesic effect. In higher doses, however, particularly in postoperative pain, it exerts analgesic action comparable to that of morphine without the addictive properties of the latter. However, it induces disturbing mental effects and other unpleasant side effects that preclude its use as an analgesic.

NALOXONE HYDROCHLORIDE

(Naloxone hydrochloride neonatal injection 0.02 mg/mL, Narcan injection 0.4 mg/mL, injection 1 mg/mL)

Naloxone hydrochloride is an antidote to narcotics. Evidence suggests that naloxone antagonizes opioid effects by competing for opiate receptor sites in the CNS. It is used for complete or partial reversal of opioid depression, including respiratory depression, induced by natural and synthetic opioids, including propoxyphene; diagnosis of suspected or known opioid overdosage; and as an adjunctive agent to increase BP in management of septic shock.

Naloxone, a pure narcotic antagonist (0.4 to 2.0 mg IV), is indicated for the complete or partial reversal of respiratory and CNS depression caused by naturally occurring and synthetic narcotics, including morphine, meperidine, methadone, nalbuphine, butorphanol, and pentazocine.

Naloxone differs from other narcotic analgesics in several respects. It does not cause respiratory depression, pupillary constriction, sedation, or analgesia. However, it does antagonize the actions of pentazocine. Naloxone neither antagonizes the respiratory-depressant effects of barbiturates and other hypnotics nor aggravates their depressant effects on respiration. Similar to nalorphine and naltrexone, naloxone precipitates an abstinence syndrome when administered to patients addicted to opiate-like drugs.

Naloxone is also therefore indicated for the diagnosis of acute opiate overdosage. As naloxone antagonizes the effects of beta-endorphin, it has been used to improve circulation in refractory shock, allowing prostaglandins and catecholamine to reestablish the control of circulation.

Intravenously administered naloxone is distributed widely, exerts its effects within 2 minutes, is metabolized in the liver by conjugation with glucuronic acid, and has a short duration of action of 1 to 4 hours, depending on the dosage given. Abrupt reversal of narcotic depression may result in nausea, vomiting, sweating, tachycardia, increased blood pressure, and tremulousness.

NALTREXONE HYDROCHLORIDE

(ReVia tablets 50 mg)

Naltrexone hydrochloride is a narcotic antidote. It is an opioid receptor antagonist, markedly attenuating or completely blocking, reversibly, the subjective effects of IV-administered opioids. It is indicated in the treatment of alcohol dependence and as a blockade of exogenously administered opioids.

Naltrexone (25 mg initially), a pure narcotic antagonist, is indicated for the treatment of the opioid-free state in formerly opioid-dependent individuals who have undergone a methadone detoxification program. Patients taking naltrexone may not benefit from opioid-containing medicines, such as cough and cold preparations, antidiarrheal preparations, and opioid analgesics.

Naltrexone, in a dose of 50 mg, will block the pharmacological effects of 25-mg heroin given intravenously for 24 hours, and the duration of blockade is dose-dependent. Naltrexone undergoes extensive first-pass metabolism, becoming converted to a 6-beta naltrexol, which is an active and pure narcotic-receptor antagonist and is excreted by the kidneys. Naltrexone can cause a dose-related hepatic injury.

Naltrexone was approved by the FDA for treatment of alcoholism in 1994. It is chemically related to the highly selective opioid-receptor antagonist **naloxone** (Narcan) but has higher oral bioavailability and a longer duration of action. Neither drug has appreciable opioid-receptor agonist effects. These drugs were used initially in the treatment of opioid overdose and dependence because of their ability to antagonize all the actions of opioids. Animal research and clinical experience suggested that **naltrexone** might reduce alcohol consumption and craving; this was confirmed in clinical trials. There is evidence that naltrexone blocks activation by alcohol of dopaminergic pathways in the brain that are thought to be critical to reward.

Naltrexone helps to maintain abstinence by reducing the urge to drink and increasing control when a "slip" occurs. It is not a "cure" for alcoholism and does not prevent relapse in all patients. **Naltrexone** works best when used in conjunction with some form of psychosocial therapy, such as cognitive behavioral therapy. It typically is administered after detoxification and given at a dose of 50 mg/day for several months. Adherence to the regimen is important to ensure the therapeutic value of naltrexone and has proven to be a problem for some patients. The most common side effect of **naltrexone** is nausea, which is more common in women than in men and subsides if the patients abstain from alcohol. When given in excessive doses, naltrexone can cause liver damage. It is contraindicated in patients with liver failure or acute hepatitis and should be used only after careful consideration in patients with active liver disease.

Nalmefene (Revex) is another opioid antagonist that appears promising in preliminary clinical tests. It has a number of advantages over **naltrexone**, including greater oral bioavailability, longer duration of action, and lack of dose-dependent liver toxicity.

NANDROLONE DECANOATE

(Deca-Durabolin)

Nandrolone decanoate is an anabolic steroid, which suppresses gonadotropic functions of the pituitary and may exert a direct effect upon the testes. Nandrolone decanoate (women: 50 to 100 mg/week; men: 100 to 200 mg/week) is indicated for the management of anemia of renal insufficiency by increasing hemoglobin and red call mass. Nandrolone stimulates the kidney's production of erythropoietin, leading to increases in red blood cells. Testosterone replacement therapy increases bone mass in hypogonadal men. Androgens also improve bone mass in osteoporotic women, but therapy is limited by virilizing side effects. Nandrolone decanoate (50 mg by injection every three weeks) increases peripheral and axial bone mass without bothersome side effects in osteoporotic women (see also Figure 95).

Nandrolone phenpropionate has antineoplastic action by exerting inhibitory actions on hormone-responsive breast tumors and metastases. Nandrolone decanoate is slowly released from the intramuscular depot following injection, and is hydrolyzed to free nandrolone by plasma esterase; peak serum levels of nandrolone are usually observed 8 to 24 hours following intramuscular injection of the decanoate. Nandrolone is subsequently metabolized in the liver; both unchanged nandrolone and its metabolites are excreted in the urine. The elimination half-life of nandrolone is 6 to 8 days after IM administration of nandrolone decanoate.

Androgens such as nandrolone are contraindicated in patients with severe renal or cardiac disease because fluid and electrolyte retention caused by this agent may aggravate these disorders; in patients with hepatic disease because impaired elimination of the drug may cause toxic accumulation; in male patients with prostatic or breast cancer or benign prostatic hypertrophy with obstruction and in patients with undiagnosed abnormal genital bleeding because this drug can stimulate the growth of cancerous breast or prostate tissue in males; and in pregnant or breast-feeding women because animal studies have shown that administration of anabolic steroids during pregnancy causes masculinization of the female fetus. The drug also is contraindicated in females with carcinoma of the breast and with hypercalcemia.

NAPHAZOLINE HYDROCHLORIDE

(Ak-Con, Albalon, Liquifilm, Allerest, Allergy drops, Clear Eyes, Comfort eye drops, Degest 2, 1-Naphline, Forte, Muro's Opcon, Naphcon A, Naphcon, Privine Hydrochloride, VasoClear, Vasocon)

Naphazoline, a sympathomimetic agent with decongestant properties, is used in nasal congestion and in ocular congestion, irritation, and itching.

NAPROXEN SODIUM

(Aleve)

Naproxen (200 mg every 8 to 12 hours with a full glass of liquid) is indicated for the relief of mild to moderate pain, treatment of primary dysmenorrhea, rheumatoid arthritis, osteoarthritis, ankylosing spondylitis, tendinitis, bursitis, and acute gout. Naproxen (Naprosyn) is used in juvenile arthritis. Naproxen, a nonsteroidal antiinflammatory agent, has analgesic and antipyretic actions. It should be used cautiously in patients with a history of angioedema or of

GI disease, peptic ulcer, or renal or cardiovascular disease, because the drug may worsen these conditions (see also Table 3).

Concomitant use of naproxen with anticoagulants and thrombolytic drugs (coumarin derivatives, heparin, streptokinase, or urokinase) may potentiate anticoagulant effects. Bleeding problems may occur if used with other drugs that inhibit platelet aggregation such as azlocillin, parenteral carbenicillin, dextran, dipyridamole, mezlocillin, piperacillin, sulfinpyrazone, ticarcillin, valproic acid, cefamandole, cefoperazone, moxalactum, plicamycin, aspirin, or other antiinflammatory agents. Alcohol, corticotropin, or steroids may cause increased GI-adverse reactions, including ulceration and hemorrhage. Aspirin may decrease the bioavailability of naproxen.

Because of the influence of prostaglandins on glucose metabolism, concomitant use with insulin or oral hypoglycemic agents may potentiate hypoglycemic effects. Naproxen may displace highly protein-bound drugs from binding sites. Toxicity may occur with coumarin derivatives, phenytoin, verapamil, or nifedipine. Increased nephrotoxicity may occur with gold compounds, other antiinflammatory agents, or acetaminophen. Naproxen may decrease the renal clearance of methotrexate and lithium. Naproxen may decrease the clinical effectiveness of antihypertensive agents and diuretics. Concomitant use may increase risk of nephrotoxicity.

Naproxen is absorbed fully when administered orally. Food delays the rate but not the extent of absorption. Peak concentrations in plasma occur within 2 to 4 hours and are somewhat more rapid after the administration of naproxen sodium. Absorption is accelerated by the concurrent administration of sodium bicarbonate but delayed by magnesium oxide or aluminum hydroxide. Naproxen also is absorbed rectally, but more slowly than after oral administration. The half-life of naproxen in plasma is variable. It is about 14 hours in the young, but it may increase about twofold in the elderly because of age-related decline in renal function.

Metabolites of **naproxen** are excreted almost entirely in the urine. About 30% of the drug undergoes 6-demethylation, and most of this metabolite, as well as naproxen itself, is excreted as the glucuronide or other conjugates.

Naproxen is almost completely (99%) bound to plasma proteins after normal therapeutic doses. Naproxen crosses the placenta and appears in the milk of lactating women at approximately 1% of the maternal plasma concentration.

Typical gastrointestinal adverse effects with **naproxen** occur at approximately the same frequency as with **indomethacin**, but perhaps with less severity. CNS side effects range from drowsiness, headache, dizziness, and sweating, to fatigue, depression, and ototoxicity. Less common reactions include pruritus and a variety of dermatological problems. A few instances of jaundice, impairment of renal function, angioedema, thrombocytopenia and agranulocytosis have been reported.

NARATRIPTAN

(Amerge tablets 1 mg (as hydrochloride))

Naratriptan is a serotonin 5-HT_1-receptor agonist that binds to serotonin (5-HT) 1_B and 1_D receptors in intracranial arteries leading to vasoconstriction and subsequent relief of migraine headache. It is indicated in the treatment of acute migraine attacks with or without aura.

Direct-acting 5-HT-receptor agonists have widely different chemical structures, as well as diverse pharmacological properties. This diversity is not surprising in light of the number of 5-HT-receptor subtypes. 5-HT_{1A}-receptor-selective agonists have helped elucidate the functions of this receptor in the brain and have resulted in a new class of antianxiety drugs including **buspirone**, **gepirone**, and **ipsapirone**. 5-HT_{1D}-receptor-selective agonists, such as **sumatriptan**, have unique properties that result in constriction of intracranial blood vessels. Sumatriptan was first in a series of new serotonin-receptor agonists available for treatment of acute migraine attacks. Other such agents now FDA approved in the United States for the acute treatment of migraine include zolmitriptan (Zomig), **naratriptan** (Aerge), and **rizatriptan** (Maxalt), all of which are selective for 5-HT_{1D} and 5-HT_{1B} receptors. A number of 5-HT_4 receptor-selective agonists have been developed or are being developed for the treatment of disorders of the GI tract.

The introduction of **sumatriptan** (Imitrex), **zolmitriptan** (Zomig), **naratriptan** (Amerge), and **rizatriptan** (Maxalt and Maxalt-MLT) in the therapy of migraine has led to significant progress in preclinical and clinical research on migraine. The selective pharmacological effects of these agents, dubbed the triptans, at 5-HT_1 receptors have led to insights into the pathophysiology of migraine. Clinically, the drugs are effective, acute antimigraine agents. Their ability to decrease, rather than exacerbate, the nausea and vomiting of migraine is an important advance in the treatment of the condition.

In contrast to ergot alkaloids, the pharmacological effects of the triptans appear to be limited to the 5-HT_1 family of receptors, providing evidence that this receptor subclass plays an important role in the acute relief of a migraine attack. The triptans are much more selective agents than are ergot alkaloids in that they interact potently with 5-HT_{1D} and 5-HT_{1B} receptors and have a low or no affinity for other subtypes of 5-HT receptors. The triptans are essentially inactive at α_1- and α_2-adrenergic, β-adrenergic, dopaminergic, muscarinic cholinergic, and benzodiazepine receptors. Clinically effective doses of the triptans do not correlate well with their affinity for either 5-HT_{1A} or 5-HT_{1E} receptors, but do correlate well with their affinities for both 5-HT_{1B} and 5-HT_{1D} receptors. Current data are thus consistent with the hypothesis that 5-HT_{1B} and/or 5-HT_{1D} receptors are the most likely receptors involved in the mechanism of action of acute antimigraine drugs.

The triptans are contraindicated in patients who have a history of ischemic or vasospastic coronary artery disease,

NARCOLEPSY: Treatment of

Narcolepsy is characterized by excessive daytime sleepiness that is typically associated with cataplexy and other rapid-eye-movement (REM) sleep phenomena such as sleep paralysis and hypnagogic hallucinations. Sleepiness, the main symptom in narcolepsy, leads to repeated daily episodes of naps or lapses into sleep of short duration.

The other main symptom, cataplexy, is characterized by a sudden loss of bilateral muscle tone provoked by strong emotion, typically by laughter. Cataplexy is usually of short duration, ranging from a few seconds to several minutes, and recovery is fast and complete.

The majority of patients need medication for the two main symptoms. Drugs with CNS-stimulating effects, mostly of the amphetamine type, are used to alleviate excessive sleepiness and sleep attacks. The resulting increased level of vigilance also decreases or abolishes cataplexy in a number of patients. If this is not achieved, tricyclic antidepressants, in the first instance, and selective serotonin (5-hydroxytryptamine; 5-HT) reuptake inhibitors, in the second instance, can be used to control cataplexy and other rapid-eye-movement sleep-related symptoms.

Stimulatory drugs used in the treatment of narcolepsy are:
Dexamphetamine
Mazindol
Methamphetamine
Methylphenidate
Modafinil
Pemoline
Selegiline

Anticataplectic drugs used in the treatment of narcolepsy are:
Clomipramine
Femoxetine
Fluoxetine
Imipramine
Protriptyline

cerebrovascular or peripheral vascular disease, or other significant cardiovascular diseases. Because triptans may cause an acute, usually small, increase in blood pressure, they also are contraindicated in patients with uncontrolled hypertension. **Naratriptan** is contraindicated in patients with severe renal or hepatic impairment. Rizatriptan should be used with caution in patients with renal or hepatic disease but is not contraindicated in such patients. Sumatriptan, rizatriptan, and zolmitriptan are contraindicated in patients who are taking monoamine oxidase inhibitors.

NATAMYCIN

(Natacyn suspension 5%)

Natamycin is an ophthalmic antifungal agent, which binds to fungal cell membrane, altering membrane permeability and depleting essential cellular constituents. A polyene macrolide antibiotic (instill 1 drop of 5% solution in conjunctival sac), natamycin is used in conjunctivitis, keratitis, and blepharitis caused by susceptible fungi.

The currently available topical ophthalmic antifungal preparation is a polyene, **natamycin** (Natacyn).

Other antifungal agents may be extemporaneously compounded for topical, subconjunctival, or intravitreal routes of administration. As with systemic fungal infections, the incidence of ophthalmic fungal infections has risen with the growing number of immunocompromised hosts. Ophthalmic indications for antifungal medications include fungal keratitis, scleritis, endophthalmitis, mucormycosis, and canaliculitis. Risk factors for fungal keratitis include trauma, chronic ocular surface disease, and immunosuppression (including topical steroid use). When fungal infection is suspected, samples of the affected tissues are obtained for smears, cultures, and sensitivities, and this information is used for drug selection.

Parasitic infections involving the eye usually manifest themselves as a form of uveitis, an inflammatory process of either the anterior or posterior segments, and less commonly as conjunctivitis, keratitis, and retinitis.

In the United States, the most commonly encountered protozoal infections include *Acanthamoeba* and *Toxoplasma gondii*. In contact-lens wearers who develop keratitis, physicians should be highly suspicious of the presence of *Acanthamoeba*. Additional risk factors for *Acanthamoeba* keratitis include poor contact lens hygiene, wearing contact lenses in a pool or hot tub, and ocular trauma. Treatment usually consists of a combination topical antibiotic, such as **polymyxin B sulfate**, **bacitracin zinc**, and **neomycin sulfate** (e.g., neosporin), and sometimes an **imidazole** (e.g., clotrimazole, miconazole, or ketoconazole). In the United Kingdom, the **aromatic diamidines** (i.e., propamidine isethionate in both topical aqueous and ointment forms, brolene) have been used successfully to treat this relatively resistant infectious keratitis. The cationic antiseptic agent **polyhexamethylene biguanide** (PHMB) also is typically used in drop form for *Acanthamoeba* keratitis, although this is not an FDA-approved antiprotozoal agent. Topical **chlorhexidine** can be used as an alternative to PHMB. Oral itraconazole or ketoconazole often are used in addition to the topical medications. Resolution of *Acanthamoeba* keratitis may require many months of treatment.

Toxoplasmosis may present as a posterior (e.g., focal retinochoroiditis, papillitis, vitritis, or retinitis) or occasionally as an anterior uveitis. Treatment is indicated when inflammatory lesions encroach upon the macula and threaten central visual acuity. Several regimens have been recommended with concurrent use of systemic steroids: (1) **pyrimethamine, sulfadiazine**, and **folinic acid** (leucovorin); (2) **pyrimethamine, sulfadiazine, clindamycin**, and **folinic acid**; (3) **sulfadiazine** and **clindamycin**; (4) **clindamycin**; and (5) **trimethoprim-sulfamethoxazole** with or without clindamycin.

Other protozoal infections (e.g., giardiasis, leishmaniasis, and malaria) and helminths are less common eye pathogens in the United States. Systemic pharmacological management as well as vitrectomy may be indicated for selected parasitic infections.

NATEGLINIDE

(Starlix tablets 60 mg)

Nateglinide is a meglitinide, which lowers blood glucose levels by stimulating insulin secretion from the pancreas. It is used as monotherapy to lower blood glucose in patients with type 2 diabetes mellitus (non-insulin-dependent diabetes mellitus) whose hyperglycemia cannot be adequately controlled by diet and exercise and who have not been chronically treated with other antidiabetic agents; in combination with metformin or a thiazolidinedione, in patients whose hyperglycemia is inadequately controlled with metformin, or after a therapeutic response to a thiazolidinedione. Do not use as a substitute for those drugs.

Nateglinide (Starlix) is an orally effective **insulin secretagogue** derived from D-phenylalanine. Like **sulfonylureas** and **repaglinide**, nateglinide stimulates insulin secretion by blocking ATP-sensitive potassium channels in pancreatic β cells. **Nateglinide** promotes a more rapid but less sustained secretion of insulin than do other available oral antidiabetic agents. The drug's major therapeutic effect is reducing postprandial glycemic elevations in type 2 diabetes mellitus patients. **Nateglinide** is approved by the FDA for use in type 2 diabetes mellitus and is most effective if administered in a dose of 120 mg 1 to 10 minutes before a meal. Nateglinide is metabolized primarily by the liver and thus should be used cautiously in patients with hepatic insufficiency. About 16% of an administered dose is excreted by the kidney as unchanged drug. Dosage adjustment is unnecessary in renal failure. **Nateglinide** therapy may produce fewer episodes of hypoglycemia than most other currently available oral insulin secretagogues including repaglinide.

NEDOCROMIL SODIUM

(Tilade, Alocril solution, ophthalmic 2% (20 mg/mL))

Nedocromil sodium is a mast-cell stabilizer that inhibits release of mediators from inflammatory cell types associated with asthma, including histamine from mast cells and beta-glucuronidase from macrophages. It may also suppress local production of leukotrienes and prostaglandins and inhibit development of bronchoconstriction responses to inhaled antigen and other challenges such as cold air. It is indicated in the maintenance of mild to moderate bronchial asthma and treatment of itching caused by allergic conjunctivitis.

Nedocromil, a well-tolerated drug (2 inhalations 4 times a day at regular intervals to provide 14 mg/day), is indicated for maintenance therapy in the management of patients with mild to moderate bronchial asthma. Nedocromil has no intrinsic bronchodilating, glucocorticoid, or antihistaminic properties. Therefore, it should not be used in status asthmaticus (see also Figure 94).

It inhibits the *in vitro* activation of, and mediator release from, a variety of inflammatory cell types associated with asthma, including eosinophils, neutrophils, macrophages, mast cells, monocytes and platelets. *In vitro*, nedocromil inhibits the release of mediators including histamine, leukotriene C_4 and prostaglandin D_2. Similar studies with human bronchoalveolar cells showed inhibition of histamine release from mast cells and beta-glucuronidase release from macrophages.

Nedocromil inhibits the development of early and late bronchoconstriction responses to inhaled antigen. The development of airway hyperresponsiveness to nonspecific bronchoconstrictors was also inhibited in airway microvasculature leakage. Nedocromil is bound to plasma proteins to the extent of 89%, is not metabolized, and is excreted unchanged.

Cromolyn was synthesized in 1965 in an attempt to improve on the bronchodilator activity of **khellin**. This chromone, derived from the plant ***Ammi visnaga***, had been used by the ancient Egyptians for its spasmolytic properties. Although devoid of the bronchodilating effect of the parent compound, cromolyn was found to inhibit antigen-induced bronchospasm as well as the release of histamine and other autacoids from sensitized rat mast cells. Cromolyn has been used in the United States for the treatment of asthma since 1973. The initial clinical results were disappointing, in retrospect largely owing to a misplaced hope that cromolyn would reduce or eliminate the need for systemic glucocorticoids in the treatment of patients with relatively severe asthma. However, its therapeutic role has been reevaluated in recent years, and cromolyn has emerged as one of the first-line agents in the treatment of mild to moderate asthma. **Nedocromil**, a compound with similar chemical and biological properties, became available in 1992.

Cromolyn and **nedocromil** have a variety of activities that may relate to their therapeutic efficacy in asthma. These include inhibiting mediator release from bronchial mast cells; reversing increased functional activation in leukocytes obtained from the blood of asthmatic patients; suppressing the activating effects of chemotactic peptides on human neutrophils, eosinophils, and monocytes; inhibiting parasympathetic and cough reflexes and inhibiting leukocyte trafficking in asthmatic airways.

For asthma, cromolyn is given by inhalation using either solutions (delivered by aerosol spray or nebulizer) or, in some countries but not in the United States, powdered drug (mixed with lactose and delivered by a special turboinhaler).

The pharmacological effects result from the topical deposition of the drug in the lung, since only about 1% of an oral dose of cromolyn is absorbed. Once absorbed, the drug is excreted unchanged in the urine and bile in about equal proportions. Peak concentrations in plasma occur within 15 minutes of inhalation, and excretion begins after some delay such that the biological half-life ranges from 45 to 100 minutes. The terminal half-time of elimination following intravenous administration is about 20 minutes.

Cromolyn and **nedocromil** generally are well tolerated by patients. Adverse reactions are infrequent and minor and include bronchospasm, cough or wheezing, laryngeal edema, joint swelling and pain, angioedema, headache, rash, and nausea. Such reactions have been reported at a frequency of less than 1 in 10,000 patients. Very rare instances of anaphylaxis also have been documented. Nedocromil and cromolyn can cause a bad taste.

The main use of **cromolyn** (Intal) and **nedocromil** (Tilade) is to prevent asthmatic attacks in individuals with mild to moderate bronchial asthma. These agents are ineffective in treating ongoing bronchoconstriction. When inhaled several times daily, cromolyn inhibits both the immediate and the late asthmatic responses to antigenic challenge or to exercise. With regular use for more than 2 to 3 months, bronchial hyperreactivity is reduced, as measured by response to challenge with histamine or methacholine. **Nedocromil** generally is more effective than cromolyn in animal models and human beings. **Nedocromil** is approved for use in asthmatic patients 12 years of age and older; cromolyn is approved for all ages.

Cromolyn and **nedocromil** generally are less effective than inhaled glucocorticoids in controlling asthma. Cromolyn (2 mg inhaled four times daily) was less effective than 200 μg twice daily of **beclomethasone** or 4 mg four times daily of **nedocromil**. Although nedocromil was roughly comparable with 200 μg **beclomethasone** inhaled twice daily, nedocromil was not as effective in controlling symptoms, reducing bronchodilator use, or improving bronchial hyperreactivity. In a second study, 4 mg nedocromil four times daily was as effective as 100 μg beclomethasone four times daily. **Nedocromil** is useful in patients with mild to moderate asthma as added therapy, as an alternative to regularly administered oral and inhaled β-adrenergic agonists and oral methylxanthines, and possibly as an alternative to low-dose inhaled glucocorticoids.

The addition of cromolyn to inhaled glucocorticoid therapy yields no additional benefit in moderately severe asthma. **Nedocromil** may allow a reduction of steroids in patients receiving high doses of inhaled steroids.

In patients with **systemic mastocytosis** who have GI symptoms owing to an excessive number of mast cells in the GI mucosa, an oral preparation of cromolyn (Gastrocrom) is effective in reducing symptoms. The benefits reflect local action rather than systemic absorption; cromolyn is poorly absorbed, and only the GI symptoms are improved in the treated patients.

NEFAZODONE HYDROCHLORIDE

(Serzone tablets 50 mg)

Nefazodone hydrochloride is an antidepressant that inhibits neuronal uptake of serotonin and norepinephrine; and antagonizes alpha$_1$-adrenergic receptors. It is indicated in the treatment of depression. Most antidepressants are fairly well absorbed after oral administration. A notable exception is that the bioavailability of **nefazodone** is only about 20%. The MAO inhibitors are absorbed readily when given by mouth. High doses of the strongly anticholinergic tricyclic antidepressants can slow GI activity and gastric emptying time, resulting in slower or erratic drug absorption and complicating management of acute overdosages. Serum concentrations of most tricyclic antidepressants peak within several hours. Intravenous administration of some tricyclic antidepressants (notably clomipramine) or intramuscular injection (amitriptyline) was used at one time, particularly with severely depressed, anorexic patients who refused oral medication, but injectable formulations are no longer commercially available in the United States.

NELFINAVIR MESYLATE

(Viracept tablets 250 mg)

Nelfinavir mesylate is a protease inhibitor that inhibits human immunodeficiency virus (HIV) protease, the enzyme required to form functional proteins in HIV-infected cells. It is indicated in the treatment or HIV infection in combination with other antiretroviral agents. **Nelfinavir** is a nonpeptidic protease inhibitor that is active against both HIV-1 and HIV-2 and is formulated as the mesylate salt of a basic amine. The mean IC_{95} for HTV-l in various *in vitro* assays is 59 nM. Like most drugs in this class, nelfinavir was a product of rational drug design.

Nelfinavir reversibly binds to the active site of the HIV protease, preventing polypeptide processing and subsequent virus maturation.

Viral replication in the presence of **nelfinavir** selects for drug resistance. The primary nelfinavir resistance mutation is unique to this drug and occurs at HIV protease codon 30 (aspartic acid-to-asparagine substitution); this mutation results in a sevenfold decrease in susceptibility. Isolates with only this mutation retain full sensitivity to other HIV protease inhibitors. Less commonly, a primary resistance mutation occurs at position 90, which can confer cross-resistance. In addition, secondary resistance mutations can accumulate at codons 35, 36, 46, 71, 77, 88, and 90, and these are associated with further resistance to nelfinavir, as well as cross-resistance to other HIV protease inhibitors.

Nelfinavir is absorbed more slowly than other HIV-1 protease inhibitors, with peak concentrations achieved in 2 to 4 hours. As a result, drug concentrations continue to fall for 2 to 3 hours after taking the next dose of drug. **Nelfinavir** absorption is very sensitive to food effects; a moderate-fat meal increases the AUC two- to threefold, and higher concentrations are achieved with high-fat meals. Intraindividual and interindividual variabilities in plasma nelfinavir concentrations are considerable, largely as a consequence of variable absorption. Originally approved at a dose of 750 mg three times daily, nelfinavir is now administered at a dose of 1250 mg twice daily using a reduced-volume 625-mg tablet.

Nelfinavir undergoes oxidative metabolism in the liver primarily by CYP2C19 but also by CYP3A4 and CYP2D6. Its major hydroxy-*t*-butylamide metabolite-M8, is formed by CYP2C19 and has *in vitro* antiretroviral activity similar to that of the parent drug. This is the only known active metabolite of an HIV protease inhibitor. M8 concentrations are 30 to 40% those of the parent drug. Nelfinavir and its metabolites are eliminated primarily in feces, with less than 2% of drug excreted unchanged in the urine. Moderate or severe liver disease may prolong the half-life and increase plasma concentrations of parent drug while lowering plasma concentrations of M8. Nelfinavir induces its own metabolism, and average trough concentrations after 1 week of therapy are approximately one-half those at day 2 of therapy.

Nelfinavir is greater than 98% bound to plasma proteins, mostly to albumin and α_1-acid glycoprotein. It is present in CSF at less than 1% of plasma concentrations at least in part owing to its extensive binding to plasma proteins and possibly to export by P-gp at the blood–brain barrier.

The most important side effect of **nelfinavir** is diarrhea or loose stools, which resolve in most patients within the first 4 weeks of therapy. Up to 20% of patients report chronic occasional diarrhea lasting more than 3 months, although fewer than 2% of patients discontinue the drug because of diarrhea. Nelfinavir augments intestinal calcium-dependent chloride channel secretory responses *in vitro*, and electrolyte analysis of stool is most consistent with a secretory diarrhea. Otherwise, **nelfinavir** is generally well tolerated but has been associated with glucose intolerance, elevated cholesterol levels, and elevated triglycerides.

Because **nelfinavir** is metabolized by CYP2C19 and CYP3A4, concomitant administration of agents that induce these enzymes may be contraindicated (as with rifampin) or may necessitate an increased nelfinavir dose (as with **rifabutin**). **Nelfinavir** is a moderate inhibitor of CYP3A4 and may alter plasma concentrations of other CYP3A4 substrates. Nelfinavir inhibits CYP3A4 less than does ritonavir and does not appear to inhibit other CYP isoforms. **Nelfinavir** is also an inducer of hepatic drug-metabolizing enzymes, reducing the AUC of ethinyl estradiol by H 47% and norethindrone by 18%. Combination oral contraceptives therefore should not be used as the sole form of contraception in patients taking **nelfinavir**. Nelfinavir reduces the zidovudine AUC by 35%, suggesting induction of glucuronosyl S-transferase.

Nelfinavir is indicated for the treatment of HIV infection in adults and children in combination with other antiretroviral drugs. Large clinical trials have demonstrated both virologic and clinical benefit when patients naive to HIV protease inhibitors and lamivudine received nelfinavir in combination with zidovudine and lamivudine. Recent large randomized, comparative trials have found that long-term virologic suppression with nelfinavir-based combination regimens is statistically significantly inferior to those using **lopinavir-ritonavir**, atazanavir, or efavirenz. This could reflect the unpredictable nature of nelfinavir absorption. **Nelfinavir** is well tolerated in pregnant HIV-infected women and shows no evidence of teratogenesis. The drug also has been used in HIV-infected patients with significant hepatic dysfunction without evidence of untoward toxicity despite higher drug concentrations.

NEOMYCIN SULFATE

(Neomycin sulfate tablets 500 mg)

Neomycin sulfate is an aminoglycoside antibiotic that inhibits production of protein in bacteria, causing bacterial cell death. It is used as adjunctive treatment for suppression of normal bacterial flora of the bowel (tablet); and as adjunctive therapy in hepatic coma to reduce ammonia-forming bacteria in the intestinal tract (tablet and solution).

Neomycin is indicated for the suppression of intestinal bacteria of the bowel as a preoperative prophylaxis for elective colorectal surgery. The treatment begins 3 days prior to surgery with liquid diets with minimum residue, oral capsule of bisacodyl, magnesium sulfate, enema, and repeated oral administration of neomycin and erythromycin (1 gram of each). Neomycin has been used as an adjunctive therapy in hepatic coma by reduction in the ammonia-forming bacteria in the intestinal tract. The subsequent reduction in blood ammonia has resulted in neurologic improvement. Neomycin combined with niacin reduces the cholesterol level.

Neomycin is a broad-spectrum antibiotic. Susceptible microorganisms usually are inhibited by concentrations of 5 to 10 μg/mL or less. Gram-negative species that are highly sensitive are *E. coli*, *Enterobacter aerogenes*, *K. pneumoniae*, and *Proteus vulgaris*.

Neomycin sulfate is available for topical and oral administration.

Neomycin and polymyxin B have been used for irrigation of the bladder. For this purpose, 1 ml of a preparation (Neosporin G.U. Irrigant) containing 40 mg neomycin and 200,000 units polymyxin B per milliliter is diluted in 1 L of 0.9% sodium chloride solution and is used for continuous irrigation of the urinary bladder through appropriate catheter systems. The goal is to prevent bacteriuria and bacteremia associated with the use of indwelling catheters. The bladder usually is irrigated at the rate of 1 L every 24 hours.

Neomycin currently is available in many brands of creams, ointments, and other products alone and in combination with **polymyxin**, **bacitracin**, other antibiotics and a variety of corticosteroids. There is no evidence that these topical preparations shorten the time required for healing of wounds or that those containing a steroid are more effective.

Neomycin has been used widely for topical application in a variety of infections of the skin and mucous membranes caused by microorganisms susceptible to the drug. These include infections associated with burns, wounds, ulcers, and infected dermatoses. However, such treatment does not eradicate bacteria from the lesions.

The oral administration of **neomycin** (usually in combination with **erythromycin** base) has been employed primarily for preparation of the bowel for surgery. For therapy of **hepatic encephalopathy**, a daily dose of 4 to 12 g (in divided doses) by mouth is given, provided that renal function is normal. Because renal insufficiency is a complication of hepatic failure and **neomycin** is nephrotoxic, it is used rarely for this indication. **Lactulose** is a much less toxic agent and is preferred.

Neomycin is poorly absorbed from the gastrointestinal tract and is excreted by the kidney, as are the other aminoglycosides. An oral dose of 3 g produces a peak plasma concentration of 1 to 4 μg/ml; a total daily intake of 10 g for 3 days yields a blood concentration below that associated with systemic toxicity if renal function is normal. Patients with renal insufficiency may accumulate the drug. About 97% of an oral dose of neomycin is not absorbed and is eliminated unchanged in the feces.

Hypersensitivity reactions, primarily skin rashes, occur in 6 to 8% of patients when **neomycin** is applied topically. Individuals sensitive to this agent may develop cross-reactions when exposed to other aminoglycosides. The most important toxic effects of neomycin are renal damage and nerve deafness; this is why the drug is no longer available for parenteral administration. Toxicity has been reported in patients with normal renal function after topical application or irrigation of wounds with 0.5% neomycin solution. Neuromuscular blockade with respiratory paralysis also has occurred after irrigation of wounds or serosal cavities.

The most important adverse effects resulting from the oral administration of neomycin are intestinal malabsorption and superinfection. Individuals treated with 4 to 6 g/day of the drug by mouth sometimes develop a spruelike syndrome with diarrhea, steatorrhea, and azotorrhea. Overgrowth of yeasts in the intestine also may occur; this is not associated with diarrhea or other symptoms in most cases.

NEOMYCIN/POLYMYXIN B SULFATES/BACITRACIN ZINC

(Neosporin ophthalmic ointment 10,000 units/g polymyxin B sulfate, 3.5 mg/g neomycin, and 400 units/g bacitracin zinc, Neosporin ophthalmic solution 10,000 units/g polymyxin B sulfate, 1.75 mg/g neomycin, and 0.025 mg/mL gramicidin)

Neomycin/polymyxin B sulfates are antibiotics that depress formation, release, and activity of endogenous mediators or inflammation including prostaglandins, kinins, histamine, liposomal enzymes, and complement system. **Neomycin** inhibits protein synthesis by binding to ribosomal RNA, causing bacterial genetic code misreading. **Polymyxin B** interacts with phospholipid components of bacterial cell membrane, increasing cell wall permeability. It is used in treatment of steroid-responsive inflammatory ocular conditions for which a corticosteroid is indicated and where bacterial infection or a risk of bacterial ocular infection exists; inflammatory conditions of the palpebral and bulbar conjunctiva, cornea, and anterior segment of the globe where the inherent risk of steroid use in certain infective conjunctivitis is accepted to obtain a diminution in edema and inflammation; chronic anterior uveitis and corneal injury from chemical, radiation, or thermal burns or penetration of foreign bodies; when risk of infection is high or where there is expectation that potentially dangerous numbers of bacteria will be present in the eye.

NEOMYCIN SULFATE/POLYMYXIN B SULFATE/GRAMICIDIN

(Neosporin ophthalmic solution 10,000 units/mL Polymyxin B sulfate, 1.75 mg/mL neomycin, and 0.025 mg/mL gramicidin)

Neomycin is an antibiotic that inhibits protein synthesis by binding to ribosomal RNA, causing bacterial genetic-code misreading. **Polymyxin B** interacts with phospholipid components of bacterial cell membranes, increasing cell wall permeability. Gramicidin increases the permeability of the bacterial cell wall to inorganic cations by forming a network of channels through the normal lipid bilayer of the membrane. It is used in topical treatment of superficial infections of the external eye and its adnexa caused by susceptible bacteria.

NEOSTIGMINE

(Prostigmin)

Neostigmine, a cholinesterase inhibitor which is unable to penetrate the blood–brain barrier, does not cause CNS toxicity. However, it may produce a dose-dependent and full range of muscarinic effects, characterized by miosis, blurring of vision, lacrimation, salivation, sweating, increased bronchial secretion, bronchoconstriction, bradycardia, hypotension, and urinary incontinence. Atropine can oppose these muscarinic effects. In addition, neostigmine, which has both a direct action and an indirect action that is mediated by acetylcholine on end-plate nicotinic receptors, may produce muscular fasciculation, muscular cramps, weakness, and even paralysis. These effects are not countered by atropine. Furthermore, neostigmine enhances gastric contraction and secretion. Neostigmine itself is metabolized by plasma acetylcholinesterase.

The therapeutic uses of neostigmine include the treatment of atony of the urinary bladder and postoperative abdominal distention. In addition, it antagonizes the action of *d*-tubocurarine and curariform drugs. Edrophonium, neostigmine, or pyridostigmine may be used to diagnose myasthenia gravis. Because edrophonium has the shortest duration of action, it is most often used for this purpose.

Neostigmine methylsulfate (2.5 mg) and atropine sulfate (1.2 mg) are given intravenously as an antidote to d-tubocurarine overdosage. The patient should be well ventilated and a patent airway maintained until complete recovery of normal respiration is assured. The optimum time to administer neostigmine methylsulfate is when the patient is being hyperventilated and the carbon dioxide level of the blood is low.

NESIRITIDE

(Natrecor powder for injection, lyophilized 1.58 mg)

Nesiritide is a human B-type natriuretic peptide, which binds to the particulate guanylate cyclase receptor of vascular smooth muscle and endothelial cells, leading to dose-dependent reductions in pulmonary capillary wedge pressure and systemic arterial pressure in patients with heart failure. It is indicated in the treatment of patients with acutely decompensated CHF who have dyspnea at rest or with minimal activity.

NETILMICIN SULFATE

(Netromycin)

Netilmicin, an aminoglycoside, is similar to gentamicin and tobramycin in its pharmacokinetic properties. It has broad antibacterial activity against aerobic Gram-negative bacilli and causes less ototoxicity and nephrotoxicity (see also Figure 88).

Netilmicin (1.3 to 2 mg/kg IM or IV q. 12 hours in serious systemic infections) is indicated for the short-term treatment of patients with serious or life-threatening bacterial infections caused by susceptible strains of the following organisms:

- **Complicated urinary tract infections** caused by *Escherichia coli*, *Klebsiella pneumoniae*, *Pseudomonas aeruginosa*, *Enterobacter* sp., *Proteus mirabilis*, *Proteus* sp., *Serratia* and *Citrobacter* sp., and *Staphylococcus aureus*
- **Septicemia** caused by *E. coli*, *K. pneumoniae*, *P. aeruginosa*, *Enterobacter* sp., *Serratia* sp., and *P. mirabilis*
- **Skin and skin structure infections** caused by *E. coli, K. pneumoniae, P. aeruginosa, Enterobacter* sp., *Serratia* sp., *P. mirabilis, Proteus* sp., and *S. aureus* (penicillinase- and nonpenicillinase-producing strains)
- **Intra-abdominal infections including peritonitis and intra-abdominal abscess** caused by *E. coli, K. pneumoniae, P. aeruginosa, Enterobacter* sp., *P. mirabilis*, *Proteus* sp., and *S. aureus* (penicillinase- and nonpenicillinase-producing strains)
- **Lower respiratory tract infections** caused by *E. coli, K. pneumoniae, P. aeruginosa, Enterobacter* sp., *Serratia* sp., *P. mirabilis, Proteus* sp., and *S. aureus* (penicillinase- and nonpenicillinase-producing strains)

NEUROLEPTICS

Neuroleptics (see Table 23) are also called neuroplegics, psychoplegics, psycholeptics, antipsychotics, and major tranquilizers. These agents are classified as follows:

- Phenothiazine derivatives (e.g., chlorpromazine)
- Thioxanthene derivatives (e.g., thiothixene)
- Butyrophenone derivatives (e.g., haloperidol)
- Dihydroindolone derivatives (e.g., molindone)
- Dibenzoxazepine derivatives (e.g., loxapine)
- Atypical neuroleptics (e.g., sulpiride, pimozide, and clozapine)

NEUROTRANSMITTERS AND THEIR RECEPTOR SUBTYPES

Types	Subtypes	Endogenous Transmitters	Ion Channel
Acetylcholine	Nicotinic	Acetylcholine	Yes
	Muscarinic: M_1, M_2, M_3, M_4, M_5	Acetylcholine	
Adrenergic	α_1, α_2	Epinephrine and norepinephrine	
	β_1, β_2, β_3	Epinephrine and norepinephrine	
GABA	A	GABA	Yes
	B	GABA	
Acidic amino acids	NMDA, kainate, quisqualate	Glutamate or aspartate	Yes
Opiate	μ, μ_1, κ, δ, ε	Enkephalins	
*Serotonin	5-HT_1, 5-HT_2, 5-HT_3 (14 of them)	5-HT	
Dopamine	D_1, D_2, D_3, D_4, D_5	Dopamine	
Adenosine	A_1, A_2	Adenosine	
Glycine	—	Glycine	Yes
Histamine	H_1, H_2, H_3	Histamine	
Insulin	—	Insulin	
Glucagon	—	Glucagon	
ACTH	—	ACTH	
Steroids	—	Several	

*See Serotonin Receptor Subtypes.

NEVIRAPINE

(Viramune tablets 200 mg, oral solution 50 mg/mL (as hemihydrate))

Nevirapine is a nonnucleoside reverse-transcriptase inhibitor that inhibits replication of retroviruses, including HIV. In combination with other antiretroviral agents it is used for treatment of HIV-1 infection.

Nevirapine is a dipyridodiazepinone NNRTI with potent activity against HIV-1. The *in vitro* IC_{50} of this drug ranges from 10 to 100 nM. Like other compounds in this class, nevirapine does not have significant activity against HIV-2 or other retroviruses.

Nevirapine is a noncompetitive inhibitor that binds to a site on the HIV-1 reverse transcriptase that is distant from the active site, inducing a conformational change that disrupts catalytic activity. As the target site is HIV-1-specific and is not essential for the enzyme, resistance can develop rapidly. A single mutation at either codon 103 or codon 181 of reverse transcriptase decreases susceptibility more than a hundredfold. **Nevirapine** resistance is also associated with mutations at codons 100, 106, 108, 188, and 190, but either the K103N or the Y181C mutation is sufficient to produce clinical treatment failure. Cross-resistance extends to all FDA-approved NNRTIs with the most common mutations. Therefore, any patient who fails treatment with one NNRTI because of a specific resistance mutation should be considered to have failed the entire class.

Nevirapine is well absorbed, and its bioavailability is not altered by food or antacids. The drug readily crosses the placenta and has been found in breast milk, a feature that has encouraged use of nevirapine for prevention of mother-to-child transmission of HIV.

Nevirapine is eliminated mainly by oxidative metabolism involving CYP3A4 and CYP2B6. Less than 3% of the parent drug is eliminated unchanged in the urine. Nevirapine has a long elimination half-life of 25 to 30 hours at steady state. The drug is a moderate inducer of CYPs, including CYP3A4; thus, the drug induces its own metabolism, which decreases the half-life from 45 hours following the first dose to 25 to 30 hours after 2 weeks. To compensate for this, it is recommended that the drug be initiated at a dose of 200 mg once daily for 14 days, with the dose then increased to 200 mg twice daily if no adverse reactions have occurred. Because of its long half-life, current clinical research is investigating once-daily dosing of nevirapine.

The most frequent adverse event associated with nevirapine is rash, which occurs in approximately 16% of patients. Mild macular or papular eruptions commonly involve the trunk, face, and extremities and generally occur within the first 6 weeks of therapy. Pruritus is also common. In the majority of patients, the rash resolves with continued administration of drug. Up to 7% of patients discontinue therapy owing to rash, and administration glucocorticoids may cause a more severe rash. Life-threatening Stevens–Johnson syndrome is rare but occurs in up to 0 3% of recipients.

Elevated hepatic transaminases occur in up to 14% of patients. Clinical hepatitis occurs in up to 1% of patients. Severe and fatal hepatitis has been associated with nevirapine use, and this may be more common in women, especially during pregnancy. Other reported side effects include fever, fatigue, headache, somnolence, and nausea.

Because **nevirapine** induces CYP3A4, this drug may lower plasma concentrations of coadministered CYP3A4 substrates. **Methadone** withdrawal has been reported in patients receiving nevirapine, presumably as a consequence of enhanced methadone clearance. Plasma **ethinyl estradiol** and **norethindrone** concentrations decrease by 20% with nevirapine, and alternative methods of birth control are advised. Nevirapine also can reduce concentrations of some coadministered HIV protease inhibitors.

Nevirapine is FDA approved for the treatment of HIV-1 infection in adults and children in combination with other antiretroviral agents. In original monotherapy studies, a rapid fall in plasma HIV RNA concentrations of 99% or greater was followed by a return toward baseline within 8 weeks because of rapid emergence of resistance. Nevirapine therefore never should be used as a single agent or as the sole addition to a failing regimen. The three-drug regimen of **nevirapine**, **zidovudine**, and **didanosine** reduced the plasma HIV RNA concentration to undetectable levels (<400 copies/ml) in 52% of antiretroviral-naive adults.

Single-dose nevirapine has been used commonly in pregnant HIV-infected women to prevent mother-to-child transmission. A single oral intrapartum dose of 200 mg nevirapine followed by a single dose given to the newborn reduced neonatal HIV infection to 13% compared with 21.5% infection with a more complicated zidovudine regimen. Although this regimen is very inexpensive and generally well tolerated, the high prevalence of nevirapine resistance following the single oral dose, coupled with the recent recognition of fatal nevirapine hepatitis, has prompted reexamination of the role this regimen should play in the prevention of vertical transmission.

NIACIN

(Vitamin B_3, nicotinic acid) (NIAC, NICO-400, Nicobid, Nicolar, Nicotinex, Span-Niacin)

Niacin, a B-complex vitamin, is used in the treatment of pellagra, peripheral vascular disease, and circulatory disorders, and as an adjunctive treatment of hyperlipidemias, especially those associated with hypercholesterolemia. Niacin, nicotinic acid (pyridine-3-carboxylic acid), is one of the oldest drugs used to treat dyslipidemia and favorably affects virtually all lipid parameters.

Niacin is a water-soluble B-complex vitamin that functions as a vitamin only after its conversion to NAD or NADP, in which it occurs as an amide. Both niacin and its amide may be given orally as a source of niacin for its functions as a vitamin but only niacin affects lipid levels. The hypolipidemic effects of niacin require larger doses than are required for its vitamin effects. Niacin is the best agent available for increasing high-density lipoprotein (HDL)-cholesterol (C) (increments of 30 to 40%); it also lowers triglycerides by 35 to 45% (as effectively as fibrates and the more potent statins) and reduces low-density lipoprotein (LDL)-cholesterol (C) levels by 20 to 30%. **Niacin** also is the only lipid-lowering drug that reduces lipoprotein (Lp) (a) levels significantly, by about 40%; however, adequate control of other lipid abnormalities renders an elevation of Lp(a) harmless. Estrogen and neomycin also significantly lower Lp(a) levels. Despite its salutary effect on lipids, niacin has side effects that limit its use.

In adipose tissue, niacin inhibits the lipolysis of triglycerides by hormone-sensitive lipase, which reduces transport of free fatty acids to the liver and decreases hepatic triglyceride synthesis. **Niacin** and related compounds (e.g., 5-methylpyrazine-2-carboxylic-4-oxide, acipimox) may exert their effects on lipolysis by inhibiting adipocyte adenylyl cyclase. A GPCR for niacin has been identified and designated as HM74A; its mRNA is highly expressed in the adipose tissue and spleen, sites of high-affinity nicotinic

NEWBORNS: Undeveloped Pharmacokinetic Profile

The pharmacokinetic and pharmacodynamic parameters are affected by developmental alterations that require critical evaluation. A few examples are cited to illustrate this concept.

At birth, the gastric pH ranges between 6 and 8, but declines within hours after birth. The most important factor influencing gastric acid secretion is the initiation of enteral feedings. The gastric emptying time in newborns approaches adult values within the first 6 to 8 months of life.

The activities of all pancreatic enzymes are lower at birth, hence decreasing the bioavailability of drugs (e.g., ester formulation of clindamycin or chloramphenicol palmitate) requiring hydrolysis prior to absorption.

The volume of distribution of drugs in newborns is different from that of adults. The percentage of fat that makes up the total body weight is 0.5% in the young fetus, increases to 15% at birth, and 20% by the age of 6 months, and then gradually declines until adolescence. The serum albumin and total protein concentrations are lower in infancy and increase to adult values by the age of 10 to 12 months. The concentration of bilirubin in neonates is much higher than the adult level, due to both increased red cell destruction and the limited capacity of the liver to conjugate bilirubin. Therefore, substantial differences exist in the binding of ampicillin, benzylpenicillin, phenobarbital, and phenytoin to plasma proteins of fetal, neonatal, and adult patients.

Postnatally, the hepatic P450 monooxygenase system matures rapidly, with metabolic capacities similar to those in adults achieved by approximately 5 months of age. On the other hand, alcohol dehydrogenase is detectable by 2 months of age (3 to 4% of adult activity) and approaches adult values after 5 years of age.

The hepatic metabolism of certain drugs has also been found to be different in neonates versus children and adults. The N-methylation of theophylline to caffeine occurs in preterm and full-term infants, whereas in adults theophylline is primarily N-demethylated and C-oxidated to monomethylxanthines and methyluric acid, respectively.

A glomerular filtration rate of 2 to 4 mL per minute in full-term infants increases to 8 to 20 mL per minute by 2 to 3 days of life and approaches adult values by 3 to 5 months of age. Tubular secretory function matures at a much slower rate.

---

acid binding. Niacin stimulates the HM74A (HM74b)-G_i-adenylyl cyclase pathway in adipocytes, inhibiting cAMP production and decreasing hormone-sensitive lipase activity, triglyceride lipolysis, and release of free fatty acids. **Niacin** may also inhibit a rate-limiting enzyme of triglyceride synthesis, diacylglycerol acetyltransferase 2. Identification of the nicotinic acid receptor may permit the development of new compounds that may affect fatty acid metabolism, dyslipidemia, and ultimately, atherogenesis.

Regular or crystalline niacin in doses of 2 to 6 g per day reduces triglycerides by 35 to 50%, and the maximal effect occurs within 4 to 7 days. Reductions of 25% in LDL-C levels are possible with doses of 4.5 to 6 g per day, but 3 to 6 weeks are required for maximal effect. HDL-C increases less in patients with low HDL-C levels (<35 mg/dL) than in those with higher levels. Average increases of 15 to 30% occur in patients with low HDL-C levels; greater increases may occur in patients with normal HDL-C levels at baseline. Combination therapy with resins can reduce LDL-C levels by as much as 40 to 60%.

The pharmacological doses of regular (crystalline) **niacin** used to treat dyslipidemia are almost completely absorbed, and peak plasma concentrations (up to 0.24 mmol) are achieved, within 30 to 60 minutes. The half-life is about 60 minutes, which accounts for the necessity of twice- or thrice-daily dosing. At lower doses, most niacin is taken up by the liver; only the major metabolite, **nicotinuric acid**, is found in the urine. At higher doses, a greater proportion of the drug is excreted in the urine as unchanged nicotinic acid.

Two of **niacin's** side effects, flushing and dyspepsia, limit patient compliance. The cutaneous effects include flushing and pruritus of the face and upper trunk, skin rashes, and acanthosis nigricans. Flushing and associated pruritus are prostaglandin mediated. Flushing is worse when therapy is initiated or the dosage is increased, but ceases in most patients after 1 to 2 weeks of a stable dose. Taking an aspirin each day alleviates the flushing in many patients. Flushing recurs if only one or two doses are missed, and the flushing is more likely to occur when niacin is consumed with hot beverages (coffee, tea) or with ethanol-containing beverages. Flushing is minimized if therapy is initiated with low doses (100 to 250 mg twice daily) and if the drug is taken after breakfast or supper. Dry skin, a frequent complaint, can be dealt with by using skin moisturizers, and **acanthosis nigricans** can be dealt with by using lotions or creams containing salicylic acid. Dyspepsia and rarer episodes of nausea, vomiting, and diarrhea are less likely to occur if the drug is taken after a meal. Patients with any history of peptic ulcer disease should not take niacin because it can reactivate ulcer disease.

The most common, medically serious side effects are hepatotoxicity, manifested as elevated serum transaminases, and hyperglycemia. Both regular (crystalline) niacin and sustained-release niacin, which was developed to reduce flushing and itching, have been reported to cause severe liver toxicity, and sustained-release niacin can cause fulminant hepatic failure. An extended-release **niacin** (Niaspan), appears to be less likely to cause severe hepatotoxicity, perhaps simply because it is administered once daily instead of more frequently. The incidence of flushing and pruritus with this preparation is not substantially different from that with regular niacin. Severe hepatotoxicity is more likely to occur when patients take more than 2 g of sustained-release, over-the-counter preparations. Affected patients experience flu-like fatigue and weakness. Usually, aspartate transaminase and ALT are elevated, serum albumin levels decline, and total cholesterol and LDL-C levels decline substantially. In fact, reductions in LDL-C of 50% or more in a patient taking niacin should be viewed as a sign of niacin toxicity.

In patients with diabetes mellitus, niacin should be used cautiously, as niacin-induced insulin resistance can cause hyperglycemia. **Niacin** use in patients with diabetes mellitus often mandates a change to insulin therapy. In a study of patients with type 2 diabetes taking Niaspan, 4% stopped taking the drug because of inadequate glycemic control. If niacin is prescribed for patients with known or suspected diabetes, blood glucose levels should be monitored at least weekly until proven to be stable. **Niacin** also elevates uric acid levels and may reactivate gout. A history of gout is a relative contraindication for niacin use. Rarer reversible side effects include toxic **amblyopia** and toxic **maculopathy**. Atrial tachyarrhythmias and atrial fibrillation have been reported, more commonly in elderly patients. Niacin at doses used in humans, has been associated with birth defects in experimental animals and should not be taken by pregnant women.

Niacin is indicated for hypertriglyceridemia and elevated LDL-C; it is especially useful in patients with both hypertriglyceridemia and low HDL-C levels. There are two commonly available forms of niacin. Crystalline niacin (immediate-release or regular) refers to niacin tablets that dissolve quickly after ingestion. Sustained-release niacin refers to preparations that continuously release niacin for 6 to 8 hours after ingestion. Niaspan is the only preparation of niacin that has been approved by the FDA for treating dyslipidemia and that requires a prescription.

Crystalline **niacin** tablets are available over the counter in a variety of strengths from 50- to 500-mg tablets. To minimize the flushing and pruritus, it is best to start with a low dose (e.g., 100 mg twice daily taken after breakfast and supper). The dose may be increased stepwise every 7 days by 100 to 200 mg to a total daily dose of 1.5 to 2 g. After 2 to 4 weeks at this dose, transaminases, serum albumin, fasting glucose, and uric acid levels should be measured. Lipid levels should be checked and the dose increased further until the desired effect on plasma lipids is achieved. After a stable dose is attained, blood should be drawn every 3 to 6 months to monitor for the various toxicities.

Because concurrent use of **niacin** and a statin can cause myopathy, the statin should be administered at no more than 25% of its maximal dose. Patients also should be instructed to discontinue therapy if flu-like muscle aches occur. Routine measurement of creatine kinase (CK) in patients taking niacin and statins does not assure that severe myopathy will be detected before onset of symptoms, as patients have developed myopathy after several years of concomitant use of niacin with a statin.

Over-the-counter, sustained-release niacin preparations and Niaspan are effective up to a total daily dose of 2 g per day. All doses of sustained-release niacin, but particularly doses above 2 g per day, have been reported to cause hepatotoxicity, which may occur soon after beginning therapy or after several years of use. The potential for severe liver damage should preclude its use in most patients, including those who have taken an equivalent dose of crystalline niacin safely for many years and are considering switching to a sustained-release preparation. Niaspan may be less likely to cause hepatotoxicity.

NIACIN/LOVASTATIN

(Advicor tablets 500/20 mg, tablets 1000/20 mg)

Niacin is an antihyerlipidemic combination. **Niacin** is necessary for lipid metabolism, tissue respiration, and glycogenolysis; reduces total cholesterol, LDL-C, and triglycerides (TG) while increasing HDL-C. **Lovastatin** increases the rate at which the body removes cholesterol from blood and reduces production of cholesterol in the body by inhibiting the enzyme that catalyses an early rate-limiting step in cholesterol synthesis; increases HDL; and reduces LDL, VLDL, and TG. They are indicated in the treatment of primary hypercholesterolemia (heterozygous familial and nonfamilial) and mixed dyslipidemia (Frederickson types IIa and IIb) in patients treated with lovastatin who require further TG lowering or HDL raising who may benefit from having niacin added to their regimen; and patients treated with niacin who require further LDL lowering who may benefit from having lovastatin added to their regimen

NIACINAMIDE

(Nicotinamide)

Niacinamide, a B-complex vitamin (150 to 500 mg p.o. daily), is used in the treatment of pellagra.

NICARDIPINE HYDROCHLORIDE

(Cardene capsules 20 mg)

Nicardipine is a calcium-channel-blocking agent that inhibits movement of calcium ions across cell membrane in systemic and coronary vascular smooth muscle and myocardium. It is indicated in the treatment of chronic stable (effort-associated) angina (immediate-release capsules); management of hypertension (immediate and sustained-release capsules; and by IV when oral therapy is not feasible or desirable).

Verapamil, nifedipine, diltiazem, and nicardipine are used in the treatment of arrhythmias, ischemic heart disease,

TABLE 21
Comparison of the Hemodynamic Effects of Calcium-Channel Antagonists

Effects	Nifedipine	Nicardipine	Verapamil	Diltiazem
Vasodilation	+++	+++	++	+
Negative inotropic effect	0	0	++	+
Negative chronotropic effect	0	0	+++	+++
Positive chronotropic effect[a]	+	+	0	0
Negative dromotropic effect (AV conduction)	0	0	+++	+++
Cardiac output increases[a]	+	+	0	0

Note: AV = atrioventricular; 0 = no effects; + = minor effects; ++ = moderate effects; and +++ = major side effects.
[a] Due to reflex stimulation.

hypertrophic cardiomyopathy, and hypertension. The hemodynamic effects of these agents are shown in Table 21.

Nicardipine inhibits the transmembrane flux of calcium ions into cardiac and smooth-muscle cells. The drug appears to act specifically on vascular muscle and may cause a smaller decrease in cardiac output than other calcium-channel blockers because of its vasodilatory effect (see Figure 84).

Nicardipine is contraindicated in patients with advanced aortic stenosis because the decrease in afterload produced by the drug may worsen myocardial oxygen balance in these patients. Some patients experience worsened severity, frequency, or duration of angina upon initiation of therapy.

Nicardipine should be used cautiously in patients with hepatic dysfunction or with CHF because the drug has a negative inotropic effect.

Concomitant administration of cimetidine results in higher plasma levels of nicardipine. Serum levels of dioxin should be carefully monitored because some calcium-channel antagonists may increase plasma levels of digitalis preparations.

Concomitant administration of cyclosporine results in increased plasma levels of cyclosporine. Careful monitoring is recommended.

Severe hypotension has been reported in patients taking calcium-channel-blocking agents who undergo fentanyl anesthesia. Overdosage with nicardipine may produce hypotension, bradycardia, drowsiness, confusion, and slurred speech.

Voltage-sensitive Ca^{2+} channels (L-type or slow channels) mediate the entry of extracellular Ca^{2+} into smooth muscle and cardiac myocytes and sinoatrial (SA) and atrioventricular (AV) nodal cells in response to electrical depolarization. In both smooth muscle and cardiac myocytes, Ca^{2+} is a trigger for contraction, albeit by different mechanisms. Ca^{2+}-channel antagonists, also called **Ca^{2+}-entry blockers**, inhibit Ca^{2+}-channel function. In vascular smooth muscle, this leads to relaxation, especially in arterial beds. These drugs also may produce negative inotropic and chronotropic effects in the heart.

An increased concentration of cytosolic Ca^{2+} causes increased contraction in cardiac and vascular smooth muscle cells. The entry of extracellular Ca^{2+} is more important in initiating the contraction of cardiac myocytes (Ca^{2+}-induced Ca^{2+} release). The release of Ca^{2+} from intracellular storage sites also contributes to contraction of vascular smooth muscle, particularly in some vascular beds. Cytosolic Ca^{2+} concentrations may be increased by various contractile stimuli. Thus, many hormones and neurohormones increase Ca^{2+} influx through so-called receptor-operated channels, whereas high external concentrations of K^+ and depolarizing electrical stimuli increase Ca^{2+} influx through voltage-sensitive, or "potential operated," channels. The Ca^{2+}-channel antagonists produce their effects by binding to the α_1 subunit of the L-type Ca^{2+} channels and reducing Ca^{2+} flux through the channel.

The 10 Ca^{2+}-channel antagonists that are approved for clinical use in the United States have diverse chemical structures. Five classes of compounds have been examined: phenylalkylamines, dihydropyridines, benzothiazepines, diphenylpiperazines and a diarylaminopropylamine. At present, **verapamil** (a phenylalkylamine); **diltiazem** (a benzothiazepine); **nifedipine**, **amlodipine**, **felodipine**, **isradipine**, **nicardipine**, **nisoldipine**, and **nimodipine** (dihydropyridines); and **bepridil** (a diarylaminopropylamine ether used only for refractory angina) are approved for clinical use in the United States.

Nicardipine has antianginal properties similar to those of **nifedipine** and may have selectivity for coronary vessels. **Isradipine** also produces the typical peripheral vasodilation seen with other dihydropyridines, but because of its inhibitory effect on the sinoatrial (SA) node, little or no rise in heart rate is seen. This inhibitory effect does not extend to the cardiac myocytes, however, because no cardiodepressant effect is seen. Despite the negative chronotropic effect, **isradipine** appears to have little effect on the atrioventricular (AV) node, so it may be used in patients with AV block or combined with a β-adrenergic-receptor antagonist.

In general, because of their lack of myocardial depression and, to a greater or lesser extent, lack of negative chronotropic effect, dihydropyridines are less effective as monotherapy in stable angina than are verapamil, diltiazem, or a β-adrenergic-receptor antagonist. **Nisoldipine** is more than 1000 times more potent in preventing contraction of human vascular smooth muscle than in preventing contraction of human cardiac muscle *in vitro*, suggesting a high degree of vascular selectivity. Although nisoldipine has a short elimination half-life, a sustained-release preparation has been developed that is efficacious as an antianginal agent. **Nimodipine** has high lipid solubility and was developed as an agent to relax the cerebral vasculature. It is effective in inhibiting cerebral vasospasm and has been used primarily to treat patients with neurological defects associated with cerebral vasospasm after subarachnoid hemorrhage.

Bepridil has been demonstrated to reduce blood pressure and heart rate in patients with stable exertional angina. It also produces an increase in left-ventricular performance in patients with angina, but its side-effect profile limits its use to truly refractory patients.

Verapamil is a less potent vasodilator *in vivo* than are the dihydropyridines. Like the latter agents, verapamil causes little effect on venous resistance vessels at concentrations that produce arteriolar dilation. With doses of verapamil sufficient to produce peripheral arterial vasodilation, there are more direct negative chronotropic, dromotropic, and inotropic effects than with the dihydropyridines. Intravenous verapamil causes a decrease in arterial blood pressure owing to a decrease in vascular resistance, but the reflex tachycardia is blunted or abolished by the direct negative chronotropic effect of the drug. This intrinsic negative inotropic effect is partially offset by both a decrease in afterload and the reflex increase in adrenergic tone. Thus, in patients without CHF, ventricular performance is not impaired and actually may improve, especially if ischemia limits performance. In contrast, in patients with CHF, intravenous verapamil can cause a marked decrease in contractility and left ventricular function. Oral administration of verapamil reduces peripheral vascular resistance and blood pressure, often with minimal changes in heart rate. The relief of pacing-induced angina seen with verapamil is due primarily to a reduction in myocardial oxygen demand.

Intravenous administration of diltiazem can result initially in a marked decrease in peripheral vascular resistance and arterial blood pressure, which elicits a reflex increase in heart rate and cardiac output. Heart rate then falls below initial levels because of the direct negative chronotropic effect of the agent. Oral administration of diltiazem decreases both heart rate and mean arterial blood pressure. Although diltiazem and verapamil produce similar effects on the SA and AV nodes, the negative inotropic effect of diltiazem is more modest.

The effects of Ca^{2+}-channel blockers on diastolic ventricular relaxation (the lusitropic state of the ventricle) are complex. The direct effect of several of these agents, especially when given into the coronary arteries, is to impair relaxation. Although several clinical studies have suggested an improvement in peak left ventricular filling rates when verapamil, nifedipine, nisoldipine, or nicardipine was given, one must be cautious in extrapolating this change in filling rates to enhancement of relaxation. Because ventricular relaxation is so complex, the effect of even a single agent may be pleiotropic. If reflex stimulation of sympathetic tone increases cyclic AMP levels in myocytes, increased lusitropy will result that may outweigh a direct negative lusitropic effect. Likewise, a reduction in afterload will improve the lusitropic state. In addition, if ischemia is improved, the negative lusitropic effect of asymmetrical left ventricular contraction will be reduced. The sum total of these effects in any given patient cannot be determined *a priori*. Thus caution should be exercised in the use of Ca^{2+}-channel blockers for this purpose; the ideal is to determine the end result objectively before committing the patient to therapy.

NICLOSAMIDE

(Yomesan)

Niclosamide, which is not absorbed from the gastrointestinal tract, is the safest effective drug in cestode infestations. It inhibits anaerobic metabolism and glucose uptake in *Taenia solium*, against which it is highly effective. As lethal doses of niclosamide in adult worms do not destroy the ova, purgation 1 to 2 hours after niclosamide is essential, or the risk of cysticercosis is likely.

NICOTINE POLACRILEX

(Nicorette)

Nicotine transdermal system or nicotine gum is indicated as a temporary aid to the cigarette smoker seeking to give up smoking while participating in a behavior modification program under medical supervision. In general, the smoker with the "physical" type of nicotine dependence is the most likely to benefit from the use of nicotine chewing gum or transdermal system.

Nicotine polacrilex contains nicotine bound to an ion exchange resin in a chewing-gum base. The nicotine transdermal system is a multilayered unit containing nicotine as the active agent that provides systemic delivery of nicotine for 24 hours following its application to intact skin.

Nicotine, the chief alkaloid in tobacco products, binds stereoselectively to acetylcholine receptors at the autonomic ganglia, in the adrenal medulla, at neuromuscular junctions, and in the brain. Two types of CNS effects are believed to be the basis of nicotine's positively reinforcing properties. A stimulating effect, exerted mainly in the cortex via the locus ceruleus, produces increased alertness and cognitive performance. A "reward" effect via the "pleasure system" in the brain is exerted in the limbic system. At low doses the stimulant effects predominate, whereas at high doses the reward effects predominate.

The cardiovascular effects of nicotine include peripheral vasoconstriction, tachycardia, and elevated BP. Nicotine is contraindicated during the immediate post-MI period, in life-threatening arrhythmias, and in severe or worsening angina pectoris.

Smoking causes enzyme induction accelerating the metabolism of acetaminophen, caffeine, imipramine, oxazepam, pentazocine, propranolol, and theophylline. Smoking cessation may reverse these actions. Smoking and nicotine can increase circulating cortisol and catecholamines. Therapy with adrenergic agonists or with adrenergic blockers may need to be adjusted according to changes in nicotine therapy or smoking status.

Smoking may reduce diuretic effects of furosemide and decrease cardiac output. Smoking cessation may reverse these actions.

NICOTINE TRANSDERMAL SYSTEM

(Habitrol, Nicoderm, Nicotrol, Prostep)

Transdermal nicotine is used in the relief of nicotine withdrawal symptoms in patients attempting smoking cessation. Two natural alkaloids, **nicotine** and **lobeline**, exhibit peripheral actions by stimulating autonomic ganglia. Nicotine was first isolated from leaves of tobacco, *Nicotiana tabacum*. Nicotine is of considerable medical significance because of its toxicity, presence in tobacco, and propensity for conferring a dependence on its users.

The complex and often unpredictable changes that occur in the body after administration of nicotine are due not only to its actions on a variety of neuroeffector and chemosensitive sites but also to the fact that the alkaloid can stimulate and desensitize receptors. The ultimate response of any one system represents the summation of stimulatory and inhibitory effects of nicotine. For example, the drug can increase heart rate by excitation of sympathetic or paralysis of parasympathetic cardiac ganglia, and it can slow heart rate by paralysis of sympathetic or stimulation of parasympathetic cardiac ganglia. In addition, the effects of the drug on the chemoreceptors of the carotid and aortic bodies and on brain centers influence heart rate, as do also the cardiovascular compensatory reflexes resulting from changes in blood pressure caused by nicotine. Finally, nicotine elicits a discharge of epinephrine from the adrenal medulla, which accelerates heart rate and raises blood pressure.

The major action of nicotine consists initially of transient stimulation and subsequently of a more persistent depression of all autonomic ganglia. Small doses of nicotine stimulate the ganglion cells directly and may facilitate impulse transmission. When larger doses of the drug are applied, the initial stimulation is followed very quickly by a blockade of transmission. Whereas stimulation of the ganglion cells coincides with their depolarization, depression of transmission by adequate doses of nicotine occurs both during the depolarization and after it has subsided. **Nicotine** also possesses a biphasic action on the adrenal medulla; small doses evoke the discharge of catecholamines, and larger doses prevent their release in response to splanchnic nerve stimulation.

Nicotine markedly stimulates the CNS. Low doses produce weak analgesia; with higher doses, tremors leading to convulsions at toxic doses are evident. The excitation of respiration is a prominent action of nicotine; although large doses act directly on the medulla oblongata, smaller doses augment respiration by excitation of the chemoreceptors of the carotid and aortic bodies. Stimulation of the CNS with large doses is followed by depression, and death results from failure of respiration owing to both central paralysis and peripheral blockade of muscles of respiration.

Nicotine induces vomiting by both central and peripheral actions. The central component of the vomiting response is due to stimulation of the emetic chemoreceptor trigger zone in the area postrema of the medulla oblongata. In addition, nicotine activates vagal and spinal afferent nerves that form the sensory input of the reflex pathways involved in the act of vomiting. Studies in isolated higher centers of the brain and spinal cord reveal that the primary sites of action of nicotine in the CNS are prejunctional, causing the release of other transmitters.

Reinforcing properties of drugs are associated with their capacity to increase neuronal activity in critical brain areas. Cocaine, amphetamine, ethanol, opioids, cannabinoids, and **nicotine** all reliably increase extracellular fluid dopamine levels in the ventral striatum, specifically the nucleus accumbens region. Because **nicotine** provides the reinforcement for cigarette smoking, the most common cause of preventable death and disease in the United States, it is arguably the most dangerous dependence-producing drug. The dependence produced by nicotine can be extremely durable, as exemplified by the high failure rate among smokers who try to quit. Although more than 80% of smokers express a desire to quit, only 35% try to stop each year, and fewer than 5% are successful in unaided attempts to quit.

Cigarette (**nicotine**) addiction is influenced by multiple variables. Nicotine itself produces reinforcement; users compare nicotine to stimulants such as cocaine or amphetamine, although its effects are of lower magnitude. Although there are many casual users of alcohol and cocaine, few individuals who smoke cigarettes smoke a small enough quantity (5 cigarettes or fewer per day) to avoid dependence. **Nicotine** is absorbed readily through the skin, mucous membranes, and lungs. The pulmonary route produces discernible CNS effects in as little as 7 seconds. Thus, each puff produces some discrete reinforcement. With 10 puffs per cigarette, the one-pack-per-day smoker reinforces the habit 200 times daily. The timing, setting, situation, and preparation all become associated repetitively with the effects of nicotine.

The **nicotine** withdrawal syndrome can be alleviated by nicotine-replacement therapy, available with (e.g., Nicotrol inhaler and Nicotrol nasal spray) or without (e.g., Nicorette gum and others and Nicoderm transdermal patch, Nicotrol transdermal patch, and others) a prescription. Because nicotine gum and a nicotine patch do not achieve the peak levels seen with cigarettes, they do not produce the same magnitude of subjective effects as **nicotine**. These methods do, however, suppress the symptoms of nicotine withdrawal. Thus, smokers should be able to transfer their dependence to the alternative delivery system and gradually reduce the daily nicotine dose with minimal symptoms. Although this results in more smokers achieving abstinence, most resume smoking over the ensuing weeks or months. Comparisons with placebo treatment show large benefits of nicotine replacement at 6 weeks, but the effect diminishes with time. The nicotine patch produces a steady blood level and seems to have better patient compliance than that observed with nicotine gum. Verified abstinence rates at 12 months are reported to be in the range of 20%, which is worse than the success rate for any other addiction. The necessary goal of complete abstinence contributes to the poor success rate; when ex-smokers "slip" and begin smoking a little, they usually relapse quickly to their prior level of dependence. A sustained-release preparation of the antidepressant bupropion improves abstinence rates among smokers. Newer agents such as the cannabinoid (CB-1) receptor antagonist rimonabant also have been reported to increase abstinence rates in clinical trials and are progressing through the FDA approval process. A combination of behavioral treatment with **nicotine** replacement to ease withdrawal and an anti-craving medication to reduce relapse is currently considered the treatment of choice.

NICOTINIC ACID

Nicotinic acid inhibits the release of free fatty acids, followed by a fall in the VLDL, and then the LDL level. Nicotinic acid may cause intense flushing and itching (vasodilation and histamine release), and tolerance develops to these effects.

NIFEDIPINE

(Procardia)

Nifedipine (10 to 20 mg t.i.d.) is indicated in vasospastic (Prinzmetal's or variant) angina. It may also be used in chronic stable angina (classical effort-associated angina) without vasospasm. Sustained release nifedipine (30 to 60 mg once daily) is used in hypertension.

The most common cause of hypertensive crises is an abrupt increase in blood pressure in patients with chronic hypertension. Other causes include renovascular hypertension, parenchymal renal disease, scleroderma, and other collagen–vascular diseases, the ingestion of drugs such as sympathomimetic agents (cocaine, amphetamines, phencyclidine hydrochloride, lysergic acid diethylmide, and diet pills) and tricyclic antidepressants, withdrawal from antihypertensive drugs (centrally acting agents and beta antagonists), preeclampsia, eclampsia, pheochromocytoma, acute glomerulonephritis, head injury, the ingestion of tyramine in conjunction with the use of a monoamine oxidase inhibitor, a renin-secreting tumor, vasculitis, and autonomic hyperactivity in patients with Guillain–Barré or other spinal cord syndromes. The parenteral and oral medications used in the treatment of hypertensive emergencies, including nicardipine and nifedipine, are all listed in Table 21.

NIFEDIPINE

(Adalat CC tablets)

Nifedipine is a calcium-channel-blocking agent that inhibits movement of calcium ions across cell membrane in systemic and coronary vascular smooth muscle and myocardium. It decreases peripheral vascular resistance; reduces myocardial oxygen demand; and relaxes and prevents coronary artery spasm. It is indicated in chronic stable angina (except Adalat CC, Afeditab CR, Nifediac CC); vasospastic angina (except Adalat CC, Afeditab CR, Nifediac CC); hypertension (except Procardia) (see also the description of Nicardipine).

NIFURTIMOX

(Lampit)

Trypanosomiasis is produced by the protozoa of the genus *Trypanosoma* and leads to Gambian or mid-African sleeping sickness (*T. gambiense*), Rhodesian or East African sleeping sickness (*T. rhodesiense*), and Chagas' disease, which is seen in the populations of Central and South America (*T. cruzi*).

Agents effective in the treatment of trypanosomiasis are the aromatic diamidines (pentamidine, stilbamidine, and propamidine). Pentamidine is the preferred drug for the prevention and early treatment of *T. gambiense* infections; however, it cannot penetrate the CNS. Melarsoprol is the drug recommended for *T. gambiense* infections that do not respond to pentamidine or for managing the late meningoencephalitic stages of infection. It does reach the CNS. Nifurtimox is the drug of choice for treating the acute form of Chagas' disease. Suramin (Naphuride) is effective only in the therapy for African sleeping sickness.

NILUTAMIDE

(Nilandron tablets 50 mg)

Nilutamide is an antiandrogen that blocks the effects of testosterone at the androgen-receptor (AR) level. The drug is rapidly and completely absorbed. There is moderate binding of the drug to plasma proteins. It is extensively metabolized. The majority is eliminated in the urine. Fecal elimination is negligible. The mean half-life, ranged from 38 to 59.1 hours. Metabolic enzyme inhibition may occur for this drug.

Compounds that competitively inhibit the natural ligands of the AR are called AR blockers, often referred to simply as antiandrogens. When given with GnRH agonists, the combination therapy is called CAB, as androgens from the adrenals are blocked, in addition to gonad-derived androgens. Currently, AR blockers as monotherapy are not indicated as routine, first-line treatment for patients with advanced prostate cancer, although some evidence points to reduced adverse effects of AR blockers relative to GnRH agonists on bone density and body composition.

From a structural standpoint, AR blockers are classified as steroidal, including **cyproterone** (Androcur) and megestrol, or nonsteroidal, including flutamide (Eulexin, others), **nilutamide** (Nilandron), and **bicalutamide** (Casodex). The nonsteroidal AR blockers are more commonly used in clinical practice. They inhibit ligand binding and consequent AR translocation from the cytoplasm to the nucleus. Unlike the steroidal agents, nonsteroidal AR blockers interrupt the negative feedback of testosterone to the pituitary–hypothalamic axis, resulting in increased serum testosterone levels, thus attenuating the **loss of libido and potency**. These drugs inhibit the binding of androgens to the androgen receptor or inhibit 5α-reductase.

Flutamide, **bicalutamide**, and **nilutamide**, potent AR antagonists, have limited efficacy when used alone because the increased LH secretion stimulates higher serum testosterone concentrations. They are used primarily in conjunction with a GnRH analog in the treatment of metastatic prostate cancer. In this situation, they block the action of adrenal androgens, which are not inhibited by GnRH analogs. Survival rates in groups of patients with metastatic prostate cancer treated with a combination of a GnRH agonist and flutamide (Eulexin), bicalutamide (Casodex), or **nilutamide** (Nilandron) are similar to one another and to survival rates in those treated by castration. Bicalutamide is replacing flutamide for this purpose because it appears to have less hepatotoxicity and is taken once a day instead of three times a day. **Nilutamide** appears to have worse side effects than flutamide and bicalutamide. Flutamide also has been used to treat **hirsutism** in women, and it appears to be as effective as any other treatment for this purpose. However, the association with hepatotoxicity warrants cautions against its use for this cosmetic purpose.

NIMODIPINE

(Nimotop capsules, liquid 30 mg)

Nimodipine is a calcium-channel-blocking agent that inhibits movement of calcium ions across cell membrane in systemic and coronary vascular smooth muscle and myocardium. It has greater effect on cerebral arteries than on other arteries. Nimodipine, a calcium-channel-blocking agent with cerebrovasodilating properties, is used for improvement of neurological deficits after subarachnoid hemorrhage from ruptured congenital aneurysms. Nimodipine is a calcium-channel-blocking agent of the 1,4-dihydropyridine family that produces relaxation of smooth muscle. It is marketed as an intravenous infusion for subarachnoid hemorrhage only. Nimodipine exerts its cytoprotective influence by reducing calcium influx into nerve cells. Therefore, it may be useful in stroke, severe head injury, cerebral resuscitation after cardiac arrest, impaired brain functions in old age, and senile dementia.

NIRIDAZOLE

(Ambilhar)

Niridazole possesses both schistosomicidal and amebicidal properties. In addition, it has antiinflammatory properties and is a potent inhibitor of cell-mediated responses. It destroys the vitellogenic gland and egg production in the female and spermatogenesis in the male *Schistosoma haematobium*, against which it is highly effective. Niridazole is extensively metabolized in the liver, and numerous toxicities do occur, especially in patients with impaired liver function. It causes hemolytic anemia in patients with glucose-6-phosphate dehydrogenase deficiency. It should be used cautiously in diseases involving the CNS, such as epilepsy.

NISOLDIPINE

(Sular tablets, extended-release 10 mg)

Nisoldipine is a calcium-channel-blocking agent that inhibits movement of calcium ions across cell membrane in systemic and coronary vascular smooth muscle and myocardium. It is indicated in the treatment of hypertension, alone or in combination with other antihypertensive agents.

NITAZOXANIDE

(Alinia tablets 500 mg)

Nitazoxanide is an antiprotozoal agent that interferes with pyruvate:ferredoxin oxidoreductase enzyme-dependent electron transfer reaction, which is essential to anaerobic energy metabolism. It is indicated in the treatment of diarrhea caused by *Giardia lamblia* or *Cyrptosporidium parvum*.

Nitazoxanide and its active metabolite, **tizoxanide** (desacetyl-nitazoxanide), inhibit the growth of sporozoites and oocytes of *C. parvum* and inhibit the growth of the trophozoites of *G. intestinalis, E. histolytica*, and *T. vaginalis in vitro*. Activity against other protozoans, including *Blastocystis hominis*, *Isospora belli*, and *Cyclospora cayetanensis* also has been reported. **Nitazoxanide** also demonstrated activity against the intestinal helminths: *Hymenolepsis nana, Trichuris trichura, Ascaris lumbricoides, Enterobius vermicularis, Ancylostoma duodenale, Strongyloides stercoralis*, and the liver fluke *Fasciola hepatica*. Effects against some anaerobic or microaerophilic bacteria, including *Clostridium* spp. and *H. pylori*, also have been reported.

Nitazoxanide appears to interfere with the PFOR enzyme-dependent electron-transfer reaction. This reaction is essential in anaerobic metabolism. **Nitazoxanide** does not appear to produce DNA mutations, suggesting that its mode of action is different from that of the nitroimidazoles (e.g., metronidazole). No resistance to nitazoxanide in infectious agents previously known to be susceptible to the drug has yet been reported.

Following oral administration, **nitazoxanide** is hydrolyzed rapidly to its active metabolite tizoxanide, which undergoes conjugation primarily to tizoxanide glucuronide. Bioavailability after an oral dose is excellent, and maximum plasma concentrations of the metabolites are detected within 1 to 4 hours of administration of the parent compound. Tizoxanide is greater than 99.9% bound to plasma proteins. Tizoxanide is excreted in the urine, bile and feces, whereas tizoxanide glucuronide is excreted in the urine and bile.

The pharmacokinetics of **nitazoxanide** in individuals with impaired hepatic or renal function have not been studied.

In the United States, **nitazoxanide** is currently available only as an oral suspension. It is approved for the treatment of *G. intestinalis* infection in children under the age of 12 (therapeutic efficacy of 85 to 90% for clinical response) and for the treatment of diarrhea in children under 12 caused by cryptosporidia (therapeutic efficacy ranging from 56 to 88% for clinical response). The efficacy of **nitazoxanide** in children (or adults) with cryptosporidia infection and AIDS has not been clearly established. For children between the ages of 12 and 47 months, the recommended dose is 100 mg **nitazoxanide** every 12 hours for 3 days; for children between 4 and 11 years of age, the dose is 200 mg nitazoxanide every 12 hours for 3 days. A 500-mg tablet, suitable for adult dosing (every 12 hours), is not yet available in the United States.

Nitazoxanide has been used as a single agent to treat mixed infections with intestinal parasites (protozoa and helminths) in several trials. Effective parasite clearance (based on negative follow-up fecal samples) after **nitazoxanide** treatment was shown for *G. intestinalis, E. histolytica/E. dispar, B. hominis, C. parvum, C. cayetanensis, I. belli, H. nana, T. trichura, A. lumbricoides*, and *E. vermicularis*, although more than one course of therapy was required in some cases. **Nitazoxanide** may have some efficacy against *Fasciola hepatica* infections, and has been used to treat infections with *G. intestinalis* that is resistant to metronidazole and albendazole.

To date, adverse effects appear to be rare with **nitazoxanide**. Abdominal pain, diarrhea, vomiting, and headache have been reported, but rates were no different from those in patients receiving placebo. A greenish tint to the urine is seen in most individuals taking nitazoxanide. **Nitazoxanide** is considered a category B agent for use in pregnancy based on animal teratogenicity and fertility studies, but there is no clinical experience with its use in pregnant women or nursing mothers.

NITRATES AND NITRITES

The mechanism underlying the therapeutic actions of nitrates and nitrites may be their ability to relax vascular smooth muscle and consequently reduce cardiac preload and afterload. The nitrates and nitrites bring about arterial dilation, and hence reduce BP and the work of the heart. These agents also produce venous dilation, thereby decreasing the venous return and ventricular volume, which in turn diminishes wall tension. The end result of these events is a reduction in the work of the heart. By decreasing BP, the heart rate is increased through the activation of carotid sinus reflexes. However, the extent of the reduction in wall tension is actually of greater benefit than the elevated heart rate (see Figure 69). The nitrate-induced tachycardia may be blocked by the administration of propranolol, a beta-adrenergic-receptor-blocking agent (see Figure 70).

Collateral vessels are silent blood vessels that become functional during hypoxic emergencies. By dilating, they permit greater blood flow to the ischemic areas, and nitrates accentuate this response. This effect of nitrates, which is greater than that of dipyridamole, seems to be potentiated by propranolol.

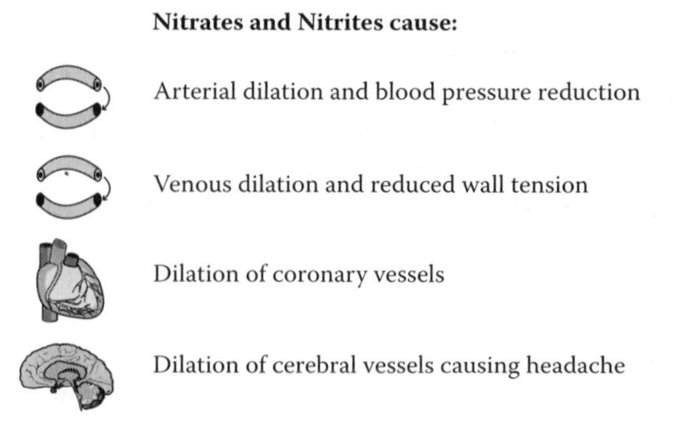

FIGURE 69 Nitroglycerin relaxes vascular smooth muscle of both the venous and arterial beds, resulting in a net decrease in myocardial oxygen consumption. The mechanism underlying the therapeutic actions of nitrates and nitrites may be their ability to relax vascular smooth muscle and consequently **reduce cardiac preload** and **afterload**.

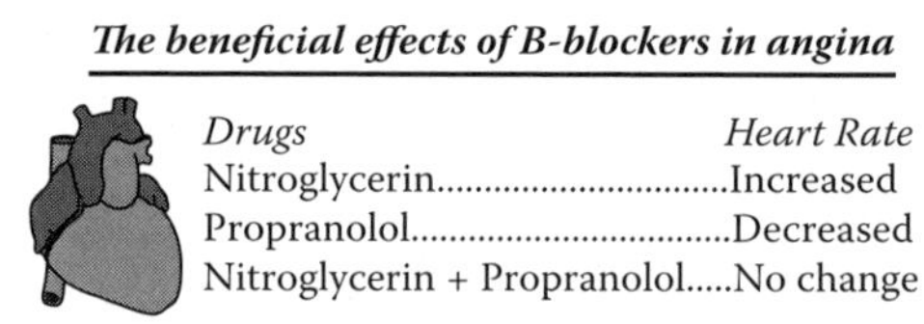

FIGURE 70 Propranolol is also frequently combined with nitrates to combat nitrate-induced reflex tachycardia.

Nitrites and nitrates dilate blood vessels in all smooth muscles. When they dilate the cutaneous blood vessels, they cause blushing. When they dilate the cerebral vessels, they cause headache. Thus, the appearance of headache and blushing is an indication of the efficacy of these medications (see Figures 69 and 70).

The nitrates and nitrites are best absorbed through the mucous membrane lining the mouth and nose. Therefore, they are usually administered sublingually or buccally. They may also be inhaled. When administered by these routes, the active ingredient is absorbed into the venous circulation and travels via the vena cava to the heart, aorta, and coronary arteries. If these agents are taken orally, they are metabolized to inactive compounds by nitrate reductase in the liver.

NITRENDIPINE

Calcium-entry blockers include those agents that are selective for slow calcium channels in the myocardium (slow-channel blockers), and consist of the following categories of substances:

Phenylalkylamines—verapamil, gallopamil, anipamil, desmethoxyverapamil, emopamil, falipamil, and ronipamil

Dihydropyridines—nifedipine, nicardipine, niludipine, nimodipine, nisoldipine, nitrendipine, ryosidine, amlodipine, azodipine, dazodipine, felodipine, flordipine, iodipine, isradipine, mesudipine, oxodipine, and riodipine

NITRATE PRODUCTS

Isosorbide dinitrate, sublingual and chewable

Isosorbide dinitrate	Isosorbide dinitrate	Isosorbide	Sorbitrate
Isonate 2.5 mg SL	Isonate 5 mg SL	Isordil	Isordil
Isordil	Isordil	Sorbitrate	Sorate-10
Sorate-2.5	Sorate-5	Onset-5	Sorbitrate
Sorbitrate	Sorbitrate	Sorate-5	

Isosorbide dinitrate, oral

Isosorbide dinitrate	Sorbitrate	Sorbitrate	Sorbitrate SA
Isonage	Isosorbide dinitrate	Isosorbide dinitrate	Isosorbide dinitrate
Isordil Titradose	Isonate	Isordil Titradose	Dilatrate-SR
Sorbitrate	Isordil Titradose	Sorbitrate	Iso-Bid
Isosorbide dinitrate	Sorbitrate	Isosorbide dinitrate	Isordil Tembids
Isonate	Isosorbide dinitrate	Isosorbide dinitrate	Isotrate Timecelles
Isordil Titradose	Isordil Titradose	Isordil Tembids	Sorate-40

Erythritol tetranitrate

Cardilate

Pentaerythritol tetranitrate (PETN)

PETN	Naptrate	Duotrate Plateau caps
Pentylan	Pentylan	Pentritol Tempules
Peritrate	Peritrate	Peritrate SA

Nitroglycerin, intravenous

Tridil	Nitrostat IV	Nitro-Bid IV	Nitrostat IV
Nitrol IV	Nitroglycerin	Nitrol IV concentrate	Tridil

Nitroglycerin, sublingual

Nitroglycerin	Nitroglycerin	Nitroglycerin	Nitroglycerin
Nitrostat	Nitrostat	Nitrostat	Nitrostat

Nitroglycerin, translingual

Nitrolingual

Nitroglycerin, transmucosal

Nitrogard

Nitroglycerin, sustained release

Nitroglycerin	Niong	Nitroglyn	Nitrong
Nitro-Bid Plateau caps	Nitronet	Nitrolan	Nitroglycerin
Nitrocap T.D.	Nitrong	Nitrospan	Nitro-Bid Plateau caps
Nitroglyn	Nitroglycerin	Klavikordal	Nitroglyn
Nitrolan	Nitro-Bid Plateau caps	Niong	Nitrolan
Nitrospan	Nitrocap 6.5	Nitronet	Nitrong
Klavikordal			

Nitroglycerin, transdermal

Nitro-Dur II 2.5 mg/24 hours	NTS 5 mg/24 hours	Nitrodisc 10 mg/24 hours	Nitro-Dur II 15 mg/24 hours
Transderm-Nitro 2.5	Transderm-Nitro 5	Nitro-Dur 10 mg/24 hours	NTS 15 mg/24 hours
Nitrodisc 5 mg/24 hours	Nitrodisc 7.5 mg/24 hours	Nitro-Dur II 10 mg/24 hours	NTS 15 mg/24 hours
Nitro-Dur 5 mg/24 hours	Nitro-Dur II 7.5 mg/24 hours	Transderm-Nitro 10	Transderm-Nitro 15
Nitro-Dur 5 mg/24 hours			

Nitroglycerin, topical

Nitroglycerin	Nitrong
Nitro-Bid	Nitrostat
Nitrol	

Nitrendipine is a 1,4-dihydropyridine derivative calcium-entry blocker structurally similar to nifedipine. It is further classified as a type II calcium antagonist because, at usual doses and concentrations, it is devoid of electrophysiologic effects, but is a potent peripheral vasodilator. Relaxation of peripheral vascular smooth muscle occurs as a result of inhibition of calcium influx across cellular membranes.

Nitrendipine is a potent vasodilator that effectively reduces blood pressure when given 1 to 3 times daily. The drug appears most useful in low-renin hypertensives. Biochemical abnormalities common to other currently used antihypertensives (e.g., hypokalemia, hyperglycemia, increased uric acid and lipids) are not seen with this class of drugs and may represent an advantage over beta-blockers and diuretics. Although most patients will require twice-daily dosing, the only other available dihydropyridine (nifedipine) usually requires dosing 3 to 4 times a day (see Table 26).

NITRIC OXIDE

A number of vasodilators, such as acetylcholine, bradykinin, adenine nucleosides, thrombin, histamine, or serotonin, need an intact vascular endothelium in order to exert their effects. For example, stimulation of endothelial cholinergic receptors causes the release of endothelium-derived relaxing factors (EDRF), which may involve arachidonic acid formation and compartmentalization via the lipoxygenase pathway. EDRF, which is identical to nitric oxide, activates guanylate cyclase and enhances the formation of cyclic guanosine monophosphate (cyclic GMP) in smooth muscle. Tetranoic acid (a vasoconstrictor), thromboxane A_2 (a vasoconstrictor), and prostacyclin (a vasodilator) are formed through the lipoxygenase pathway (Figure 30).

The vasodilating properties of captopril or hydralazine (antihypertensive agents) are mediated by the formation of EDRF or prostaglandin, or both. On the other hand, the vasodilating properties of nitroprusside (an antihypertensive agent) result directly from the formation of cyclic GMP.

NITROFURANTOIN

(Furadantin)

Nitrofurantoin (50 to 100 mg q.i.d.) is indicated in the treatment of urinary tract infections due to susceptible strains of *E. coli,* enterococci, *S. aureus*, and certain strains of *Klebsiella, Enterobacter*, and *Proteus* species.

Nitrofurantoin is a synthetic nitrofuran that is bacteriostatic in low concentrations (5 to 10 mcg/mL) and bactericidal in higher concentrations. Nitrofurantoin may inhibit acetyl-coenzyme A, interfering with bacterial carbohydrate metabolism. It may also disrupt bacterial cell wall formation.

Nitrofurantoin may cause pulmonary reactions manifested by sudden onset of dyspnea, chest pain, cough, fever, and chills. These reactions may occur rapidly (few hours) or slowly (few weeks). Chest X-rays show alveolar infiltrates or effusions; an elevated sedimentation rate and eosinophilia are also present. Resolution of clinical and radiological abnormalities occurs within 24 to 48 hours after discontinuation.

Hemolytic anemia of the primaquine sensitivity type has been induced by nitrofurantoin. The hemolysis appears to be linked to a glucose 6-phosphate dehydrogenase (G-6-PD) deficiency in the red blood cells of affected patients.

Peripheral neuropathy may occur and may become severe or irreversible. Prolonged or repeated therapy with nitrofurantoin may cause superinfection resulting in bacterial or fungal overgrowth of nonsusceptible organisms. Such overgrowth may lead to a secondary infection. *Pseudomonas* is the organism most commonly implicated in superinfections.

Anticholinergic drugs and food increase nitrofurantoin bioavailability by delaying gastric emptying and increasing absorption. Administration of high doses of probenecid with nitrofurantoin decreases renal clearance and increases serum levels of nitrofurantoin. The result could be increased toxic effects. Magnesium trisalicylate may delay or decrease the absorption of nitrofurantoin.

NITROFURANTOIN MACROCRYSTALS

(Macrodantin, Macrobid)

NITROFURANTOIN MICROCRYSTALS

(Furadantin, Furalan, Furan, Furanite, Nitrofan)

Nitrofurantoin, a nitrofuran urinary tract antiinfective agent (50 to 100 mg p.o. q.i.d. with meals), is indicated in initial or recurrent urinary tract infections caused by susceptible organisms, or as a long-term suppression therapy.

NITROGEN MUSTARDS

The activity of nitrogen mustards depends on the presence of a bis-(2-chloroethyl) grouping:

$$N\begin{cases} CH_2\text{-}CH_2Cl \\ CH_2\text{-}CH_2Cl \end{cases}$$

This is present in mechlorethamine (Mustargen), which is used in patients with Hodgkin's disease and other lymphomas, usually in combination with other drugs, such as in MOPP therapy (mechlorethamine, Oncovin [vincristine], procarbazine, and prednisone). It may cause bone marrow depression.

NITROGLYCERIN

(Transderm-Nitro)

Nitroglycerin is indicated for initial relief of acute angina pectoris and for prophylaxis to prevent or minimize anginal attacks when taken immediately before stressful events. Nitroglycerin has the following molecular structure:

$$\begin{array}{l} CH_2 - O - NO_2 \\ | \\ CH - O - NO_2 \\ | \\ CH_2 - O - NO_2 \end{array}$$

Nitroglycerin dilates the coronary arteries rapidly (1 to 2 minutes), but the coronary dilatation does not last as long as its antianginal effects (30 minutes). Nitroglycerin also dilates blood vessels in the bronchi, the uterus, and the gastrointestinal tract (see Figure 69). It has a pronounced effect on the meningeal vessels, and blushing and headache are common following administration. Nitroglycerin may also be provided on a continuous 24-hour basis through a transdermal therapeutic system called Transderm-Nitro. This system releases 5 to 10 mg of nitroglycerin over the course of 24 hours. Using this route of administration, nitroglycerin is absorbed through the skin into the systemic circulation. The beneficial effect is apparent 30 minutes after the pad is applied and ceases 30 minutes after it is removed. Therefore, sublingual nitroglycerin should be used for achieving an immediate effect, followed by Transderm-Nitro as a prophylactic measure.

Nitroglycerin may be applied topically (2% ointment). Its hemodynamic and beneficial effects appear as early as 15 minutes after application and last up to 4 hours. Nitroglycerin ointment may be especially useful for the management of angina decubitus, which may develop 3 hours after patients go to sleep.

Due to the first-pass effect, the orally administered nitrates such as isosorbide dinitrite are effective only when given in large doses (30 to 40 mg q.i.d.). Isosorbide is effective in low doses (5 mg) when given sublingually.

NITROPRUSSIDE

(Nipride, Nitropress)

Nitroprusside (3 mcg/kg/min) is indicated for immediate reduction of BP in patients in hypertensive crisis. It has also been used to produce controlled hypotension in order to reduce bleeding during surgery (see Table 22).

Nitroprusside, either alone or in combination with dopamine, has been used in patients with severe refractory CHF. Coadministration of these two agents has also been used in patients with acute MI.

The hypotensive effect of nitroprusside is seen within 1 to 2 minutes after the start of an adequate infusion, and it dissipates almost as rapidly after an infusion is discontinued. The effect is augmented by ganglionic-blocking agents

TABLE 22
Parenteral Medications Used in the Treatment of Hypertensive Emergencies

Drugs	Administration by IV	Onset	Duration of Action	Dosage	Adverse Effects and Comments
Sodium Nitroprusside	Infusion	Immediate	2–3 min	0.5–10 mcg/kg/min, initial dose; 0.25 mcg/kg/min for eclampsia and renal insufficiency	Hypotension, nausea, vomiting apprehension; risk of thiocyanate and cyanide toxicity is increased in renal and hepatic insufficiency, respectively; levels should be monitored; must shield from light
Diazoxide	Bolus	1–5 min	6–12 hr	50–100 mg every 5–10 min. up to 600 mg	Hypotension, tachycardia, nausea, vomiting, fluid retention, hyperglycemia; may exacerbate myocardial ischemia, heart failure, or aortic dissection
	Infusion			10–30 mg/min	May require concomitant use of a beta-antagonist
Labetalol	Bolus	5–10 min	3–6 hr	20–80 mg every 5–10 min	Hypotension, heart block, heart failure, bronchospasm, nausea, scalp tingling, paradoxical pressor response; may not be effective in patients receiving alpha- or beta-antagonists
	Infusion			0.5–2 mg/min	
Nitroglycerin	Infusion	1–2 min	3–5 min	5–100 mcg/min	Headache, nausea, vomiting; tolerance may develop with prolonged use
Phentolamine	Bolus	1–2 min	3–10 min	5–10 mg every 5–15 min	Hypotension, tachycardia, headache, angina, paradoxical pressor response
Trimethaphan	Infusion	1–5 min	10 min	0.5–5 mg/min	Hypotension, urinary retention, ileus, respiratory arrest, mydriasis, cycloplegia, dry mouth
Hydralazine (for treatment of eclampsia)	Bolus	10–20 min	3–6 hr	5–10 mg every 20 min	Hypotension, fetal distress, tachycardia, headache, nausea, vomiting, local thrombophlebitis; infusion site should be changed after 12 hr
Nicardipine	Infusion	1–5 min	3–6 hr	5 mg/hr	Hypotension, headache, tachycardia, nausea, vomiting

Note: IV = intravenous.

and inhaled anesthetics. Injudicious use of nitroprusside may cause precipitous decreases in BP leading to irreversible ischemic injuries or death.

Nitroprusside is given by infusion, and its BP-lowering effect is directly related to the rate at which it is administered. When it is discontinued, the BP rises rapidly. Lethal cyanide poisoning may occur in patients with rhodanase deficiency, and thiocyanate may accumulate in patients with renal failure, thus inhibiting iodine uptake and causing hypothyroidism (see Figure 71).

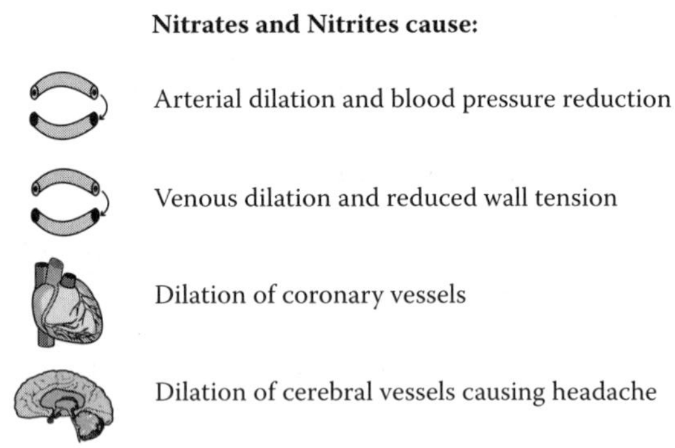

FIGURE 71 Nitroprusside is used exclusively in the management of **malignant hypertension** and a **hypertensive crisis**. It is given by infusion, and its blood pressure-lowering effect is directly related to the rate at which it is administered. When it is discontinued, blood pressure rises rapidly. Lethal cyanide poisoning may occur in patients with **rhodanase deficiency**, and thiocyanate may accumulate in patients with renal failure, thus inhibiting **iodine uptake** and causing **hypothyroidism**.

Nitroprusside is a potent IV antihypertensive agent. The principal pharmacological action of nitroprusside is relaxation of vascular smooth muscle and consequent dilation of peripheral arteries and veins. Other smooth muscle (e.g., uterus, duodenum) is not affected. Nitroprusside is more active on veins than on arteries, but this selectivity is much less marked than that of nitroglycerin. Dilation of the veins promotes peripheral pooling of blood and decreases venous return to the heart, thereby reducing left-ventricular end-diastolic pressure and pulmonary capillary wedge pressure (preload). Arteriolar relaxation reduces systemic vascular resistance, systolic arterial pressure, and mean arterial pressure (afterload). Dilation of the coronary arteries also occurs.

In association with the decrease in BP, nitroprusside administered by IV to hypertensive and normotensive patients produces slight increases in heart rate and a variable effect on cardiac output. In hypertensive patients, moderate doses induce renal vasodilation roughly proportional to the decrease in systemic BP, so there is no appreciable change in renal blood flow or glomerular filtration rate.

In normotensive subjects, acute reduction of mean arterial pressure to 60 to 75 mmHg by infusion of nitroprusside causes a significant increase in renin activity.

Nitroprusside infusions at rates >2 mcg/kg/min generate CN^- faster than the body can normally dispose of it. As cyanide is metabolized by hepatic enzymes, it may accumulate in patients with severe liver impairment. Nitroprusside infusions can cause sequestration of hemoglobin as methemoglobin. Like other vasodilators, nitroprusside can cause increases in intracranial pressure (see Figure 71).

The adverse reactions of nitroprusside are due to rapid reduction of BP. Abdominal pain, apprehension, diaphoresis, dizziness, headache, muscle twitching, nausea, palpitations, restlessness, retching, and retrosternal discomfort have been noted when the BP was reduced too rapidly. These symptoms quickly disappeared when the infusion was slowed or discontinued, and they did not reappear with a continued (or resumed) slower infusion (see Figure 71).

NITROUREAS

Carmustine (BCNU), lomustine (CCNU), and semustine (methyl-CCNU) generate alkyl carbonium ions and isocyanate molecules and hence are able to interact with DNA and other macromolecules. These agents, which are lipid soluble, cross the blood–brain barrier and are therefore effective in treating brain tumors. They are bone marrow depressants.

NITROUS OXIDE

Nitrous oxide (N_2O) is an inert, colorless, odorless, and tasteless gas. When a mixture of about 40% nitrous oxide and air is inhaled for a few seconds, a condition resembling alcoholic intoxication is produced with much hilarity and laughter so that the oxide is known popularly as "laughing gas."

The inhalation of 35 to 70% of nitrous oxide causes, after a few seconds, a rushing, drumming, hammering in the ears, indistinct sight, staggering gait, and swaying of the body from side to side. The patient seems brighter and more lively and often bursts into laughter.

When pure nitrous oxide is inhaled without the admixture of oxygen, the patient loses consciousness completely. The face is cyanotic, the respiration becomes stertorous and dyspneic, and ceases after a weak convulsion, while the heart continues to beat for some time afterward. If the mask through which the patient has been inhaling the gas is removed when the cyanosis becomes marked, complete anesthesia lasts for 30 to 60 seconds, and the patient then recovers within a few minutes. The pharmacology of nitrous oxide and that of halothane is compared in Table 16.

NIZATIDINE

(Axid)

Nizatidine, a histamine-receptor antagonist (300 mg once daily at bedtime), is indicated in the management of duodenal ulcer, benign gastric ulcer, and gastroesophageal reflux disease (see also Table 10).

Stimulation of H_2 receptors elicits a variety of responses, the most widely studied of which is gastric acid secretion from the parietal cells of the gastric glands. However, many other effects mediated by the H_2 receptors are manifested in peripheral tissues. These include the positive chronotropic action in the auricular muscle, the inotropic action in the ventricular muscle, and the lipolytic effect in fat cells. In addition, the extensive use of cimetidine has led to the synthesis and marketing of more specific and efficacious analogs with pharmacologic properties that are outlined in Table 10. Examples of the various H_2-receptor-blocking agents are:

Imidazole derivatives
Cimetidine and etintidine
Furan derivatives
Ranitidine and nizatidine
Guanidinothiazole derivatives
Famotidine
Piperidinomethylphenoxy derivatives
Roxatidine acetate and roxatidine

NONDEPOLARIZING NEUROMUSCULAR BLOCKING DRUGS

Drugs	Formulations	Comments
	Long-acting	
Doxacurium	Solution	Minimal cardiovascular effects; duration of action prolonged in renal failure
Metocurine	Solution	Histamine release may cause hypotension, bronchoconstriction
Pancuronium	Solution	Vagal blocking properties may cause tachycardia
Pipecuronium	Powder	Minimal cardiovascular effects; duration of action prolonged in renal failure
Tubocurarine	Solution	Histamine release may cause hypotension, bronchoconstriction
	Intermediate-acting	
Atracurium	Solution	Short duration of action may require repeated doses; no renal excretion; histamine release may cause hypotension, bronchoconstriction
Vecuronium	Powder	Similar to atracurium, but virtually no histamine release; some renal excretion

Halothane, enflurane, and isoflurane potentiate the activity of doxacurium, and phenytoin and carbamazepine shorten the duration of doxacurium block.

NONSTEROIDAL ANTIINFLAMMATORY AGENTS

Salicylates and allied compounds have analgesic, antipyretic, uricosuric, and antiinflammatory properties. Their mechanisms of action differ from those of the antiinflammatory steroids and the opioid analgesics. They are classified into the following categories (see Table 3).

Salicylate derivatives
Acetylsalicylic acid (aspirin)
Diflunisal (Dolobid)
Salsalate (Arthra-G, Disalcid, Mono-Gesic)
Pyrazolone derivatives
Phenylbutazone (Butazolidin)
Oxyphenbutazone (Oxalid, Tandearil)
Sulfinpyrazone (Anturane)
Paraaminophenol derivatives
Acetaminophen (Tylenol, Datril)
Phenacetin (Acetophenetidin)
Propionic acid derivatives
Ibuprofen (Motrin)
Naproxen (Naprosyn)
Fenoprofen (Nalfon)
Flurbiprofen (Ansaid)
Ketoprofen (Orudis)
Others
Indomethacin (Indocin)
Sulindac (Clinoril)
Mefenamic acid (Ponstel)
Tolmetin (Tolectin)
Piroxicam (Feldene)
Diclofenac sodium (Voltaren)
Etodolac
Nabumetone

In the following, the pharmacology of acetylsalicylic acid (aspirin) is discussed in detail as a prototype drug, and all the other drugs are compared to it.

Arachidonic acid, which is stored as a cellular membrane phospholipid, is the precursor for series 2 prostaglandins. Aspirin selectively acetylates the hydroxyl group of a single serine residue at position 530 within the polypeptide chain of prostaglandin G/H synthase, the enzyme that converts arachidonate into prostaglandin cyclic endoperoxide. Aspirin thereby reduces the synthesis of the eicosanoids—prostaglandins, prostacyclin, and thromboxane A.

Unlike the narcotic analgesics such as morphine, aspirin does not depress respiration, is relatively nontoxic, and lacks addiction liability. Aspirin is a weak or mild analgesic that is effective for ameliorating short, intermittent types of pain such as neuralgia, myalgia, and toothache. It does not have the efficacy of morphine and cannot relieve the severe, prolonged, and lancinating types of pain associated with trauma such as burns or fractures. Like morphine, it produces analgesia by raising the pain threshold in the thalamus, but, unlike morphine, it does not alter the patient's reactions to pain. Because aspirin does not cause hypnosis or euphoria, its site of action has been postulated to be subcortical. In addition to raising the pain threshold, the antiinflammatory effects of aspirin may contribute to its analgesic actions. However, no direct association between the antiinflammatory and analgesic effects of these compounds should be expected. For example, aspirin has both analgesic and antiinflammatory properties, whereas acetaminophen has analgesic but not antiinflammatory properties. Furthermore, potent antiinflammatory agents such as phenylbutazone have only weak analgesic effects.

Aspirin does not alter the normal body temperature, which is maintained by a balance between heat production and dissipation. In a fever associated with infection, increased oxidative processes enhance heat production. Aspirin acts by causing cutaneous vasodilation, which prompts perspiration and enhances heat dissipation. This effect is mediated via the hypothalamic nuclei, as proved by the fact that a lesion in the preoptic area suppresses the mechanism through which aspirin exerts its antipyretic effects. The antipyretic effects of aspirin may be due to its inhibition of hypothalamic prostaglandin synthesis. Although aspirin-induced diaphoresis contributes to its antipyretic effects, it is not an absolutely necessary process, as antipyresis takes place in the presence of atropine.

Numerous agents cause thermoregulatory dysfunction. This dysfunction may occur as the result of decreased sweating (antihistamines and tricyclic depressants), decreased cardiac output (diuretics causing volume depletion and beta-adrenergic-receptor-blocking agents causing myocardial depression), decreased vasodilation (sympathomimetic agents and alpha-adrenergic receptor agonists), depression of the hypothalamic centers (neuroleptics such as chlorpromazine or other alpha-adrenergic-receptor antagonists), or behavioral dysfunctions (sedatives and opioids).

Small doses (600 mg) of aspirin cause hyperuricemia, but large doses (>5 gm) have a uricosuric effect. Aspirin inhibits uric acid resorption by the tubules in the kidneys. However, because of the availability of more effective uricosuric agents, aspirin is no longer used for this purpose.

Aspirin has an antiinflammatory action as well as antirheumatic and antiarthritic effects, and may therefore be used in the treatment of rheumatic fever. However, it cannot alter the cardiac lesion and other visceral effects of the disease. Aspirin is extremely effective in managing rheumatoid arthritis and allied diseases involving the joints, such as ankylosing spondylitis and osteoarthritis. It is thought that aspirin and indomethacin exert their antiinflammatory effects by inhibiting prostaglandin synthesis through the inhibition of cyclooxygenase. The presynthesized prostaglandins are released during a tissue injury that fosters inflammation and pain. Furthermore, aspirin reduces the formation of prostaglandin in the platelets and leukocytes, which is responsible for the reported hematologic effects associated with aspirin (see also Figure 13).

The current thinking concerning the role of aspirin in the prevention of cardiovascular disease is that it is beneficial in the event of MI and stroke. It is effective because, in platelets, small amounts of aspirin acetylate irreversibly bind to the active site of thromboxane A_2, a potent promoter of platelet aggregation (see also Figure 14).

The menstrual cycle is associated with two potentially incapacitating events: dysmenorrhea and the premenstrual syndrome. Substantial evidence indicates that the excessive production of prostaglandin F_{2a} is the major source of painful menstruation. The nonsteroidal antiinflammatory drugs approved for the treatment of dysmenorrhea are aspirin, ibuprofen, mefenamic acid, and naproxen (see also Table 3).

Aspirin stimulates respiration both directly and indirectly. In analgesic doses, aspirin increases oxygen consumption and carbon dioxide production. However, increased alveolar ventilation balances the increased carbon dioxide production, thus the partial pressure of CO_2 (PCO_2) in plasma does not change. In the event of salicylate intoxication (e.g., 10 to 12 grams of aspirin given in 6 to 8 hours in adults, and an even smaller dosage in children, whose brains are far more sensitive to salicylate intoxication), salicylate stimulates the medullary centers directly, and this causes hyperventilation characterized by an increase in the depth and rate of respiration. The PCO_2 level declines, causing hypocapnia, and the blood pH increases, causing respiratory alkalosis. The low PCO_2 then decreases the renal tubular resorption of bicarbonate and compensates for the alkalosis.

If the salicylate level continues to rise, the respiratory centers become depressed, the PCO_2 becomes elevated, and the blood pH becomes more acidic, causing respiratory acidosis. Dehydration, reduced bicarbonate levels, and the accumulation of salicylic acid, salicyluric acid resulting from metabolism of aspirin, and lactic and pyruvic acid resulting from deranged carbohydrate metabolism may cause metabolic acidosis.

The supportive treatment of aspirin poisoning may include gastric lavage (to prevent the further absorption of salicylate), fluid replenishment (to offset the dehydration and oliguria), alcohol and water sponging (to combat the hyperthermia), the administration of vitamin K (to prevent possible hemorrhage), sodium bicarbonate administration (to combat acidosis), and, in extreme cases, peritoneal dialysis and exchange transfusion.

Although innocuous in most subjects, the therapeutic analgesic doses of aspirin may cause epigastric distress, nausea, vomiting, and bleeding. Aspirin can also exacerbate the symptoms of peptic ulcer, characterized by heartburn, dyspepsia, and erosive gastritis. An extensive number of salts have been synthesized from salicylate (e.g., calcium carbaspirin, choline salicylate, alloxiprin, and numerous buffered derivatives), and each has shown some ability to reduce the gastrointestinal toxicity of aspirin. However, other unknown factors may contribute to this undesirable GI property of aspirin. In experimental animals, the intravenous administration of sodium salicylate or subcutaneous administration of methyl salicylate has produced petechial hemorrhage of the gastric mucosa. Furthermore, compounds possessing antiinflammatory properties (aspirin, phenylbutazone, and oxyphenbutazone) are associated with a higher incidence of gastrointestinal toxicity than those compounds devoid of antiinflammatory properties (phenacetin and acetaminophen).

Aspirin reduces the leukocytosis associated with acute rheumatic fever. When given on a long-term basis, it also reduces the hemoglobin level and the hematocrit. Aspirin use can cause reversible hypoprothrombinemia by interfering with the function of vitamin K in prothrombin synthesis. Therefore, aspirin should be used with caution in patients with vitamin K deficiency, preexisting hypoprothrombinemia, or hepatic damage; in patients taking anticoagulants; and in patients scheduled for surgery. Aspirin leads to hemolytic anemia in individuals with glucose 6-phosphate dehydrogenase deficiency. An aspirin tolerance test is used diagnostically in von Willebrand's disease, because it will further prolong the bleeding time if the disease exists. Aspirin prevents platelet aggregation and may be helpful in the treatment of thromboembolic disease. In addition to aspirin, indomethacin, phenylbutazone, sulfinpyrazone, and dipyridamole prevent platelet aggregation, whereas epinephrine, serotonin, and prostaglandins promote platelet aggregation and hence are procoagulants. The erythrocyte sedimentation rate is often elevated in infections and inflammations, but aspirin therapy will yield a false negative.

NONSTEROIDAL ANTIINFLAMMATORY DRUGS

Chemical Classifications	Generic
Salicylates	**Acetylated**
	Aspirin
	Aspirin, buffered
	Enteric coated
	Sustained release
	Nonacetylated
	Choline salicylate
	Choline magnesium trisalicylate
	Diflunisal
	Salsalate
	Magnesium salicylate
	Sodium salicylate
Fenamates	Meclofenamic acid
	Mefenamic acid
Acetic acids	Diclofenac
	Etodolac
	Indomethacin
	Oxaprozin
	Sulindac
	Tolmetin
Propionic acids	Fenoprofen
	Flurbiprofen
	Ibuprofen
	Ketoprofen
	Naproxen
Pyrazolones	Phenylbutazone
Oxicam	Piroxicam
Nonacidic	Nabumetone

NOREPINEPHRINE BITARTRATE

(Levophed)

Norepinephrine (8 to 12 mcg/min by IV infusion), an alpha-adrenergic-receptor stimulant and vasopressor, is indicated for maintaining BP in acute hypotensive states.

Dopamine, norepinephrine, and epinephrine are classified as catecholamines. Tyrosine is converted to dopa by the rate-limiting enzyme, tyrosine hydroxylase, which requires tetrahydrobiopterin, and is inhibited by alpha-methyltyrosine. Dopa is decarboxylated to dopamine by L-aromatic amino acid decarboxylase, which requires pyridoxal phosphate (vitamin B_6) as a coenzyme. Carbidopa, which is used with L-dopa in the treatment of parkinsonism, inhibits this enzyme. Dopamine is converted to norepinephrine by dopamine beta-hydroxylase, which requires ascorbic acid (vitamin C), and is inhibited by diethyldithiocarbamate. Norepinephrine is converted to epinephrine by phenylethanolamine *N*-methyltransferase (PNMT), requiring *S*-adenosylmethionine. The activity of PNMT is stimulated by corticosteroids.

The catecholamine-synthesizing enzymes are not only able to synthesize dopamine and norepinephrine from a physiologically occurring substrate such as L-dopa, but also from exogenous substrates such as alpha-methyldopa, which is converted to alpha-methyldopamine and in turn to alpha-methylnorepinephrine. Alpha-methyldopamine and alpha-methylnorepinephrine are called "false transmitters" and, in general (except for alpha-methylnorepinephrine), are weaker agonists. Alpha-methyldopa is used in the management of hypertension.

In addition to being synthesized in the peripheral nervous system, dopamine is also synthesized in the corpus striatum and in the mesocortical, mesolimbic, and tuberoinfundibular systems. Norepinephrine is synthesized and stored primarily in sympathetic noradrenergic nerve terminals, as well as in the brain and the adrenal medulla. Epinephrine is synthesized and stored primarily in the adrenal medulla, and, to a certain extent, in the hypothalamic nuclei.

In sympathetic nerve terminals, as well as the brain, the adrenal medulla, and sympathetic postganglionic terminals, there are osmophilic granules (synaptic vesicles) that are capable of storing high concentrations of catecholamine (a complex with adenosine triphosphate [ATP] and protein). The stored amines are not metabolized by the intersynaptosomal mitochondrial enzyme (monoamine oxidase).

Besides releasing norepinephrine (through exocytosis), the stimulation of sympathetic neurons also releases ATP, storage protein, and dopamine beta-hydroxylase. The released norepinephrine interacts with receptor sites located postsynaptically ($alpha_1$) to produce the desired effects.

The action of norepinephrine is terminated by reuptake mechanisms, two of which have been identified: Uptake 1 is located in the presynaptic membrane, requires energy for the transport, is sodium and temperature dependent, and is inhibited by ouabain (a cardiac glycoside), cocaine (a local anesthetic), and imipramine (an antidepressant). Uptake 2 is located extraneuronally in various smooth muscles and glands, requires energy, and is temperature dependent. Approximately 20% of the amine is either taken up by the Uptake 2 mechanism or is metabolized.

There are two enzymes capable of metabolizing catecholamines. The first is monoamine oxidase (MAO), a mitochondrial enzyme that oxidatively deaminates catecholamines, tyramine, serotonin, and histamine. MAO is further subclassified as either monoamine oxidase A, which metabolizes norepinephrine and is inhibited by tranylcypromine, and monoamine oxidase B, which metabolizes dopamine and is inhibited by L-deprenyl. Catechol-*O*-methyltransferase (COMT), a soluble enzyme present mainly in the liver and kidney, is also found in postsynaptic neuronal elements. About 15% of norepinephrine is metabolized postsynaptically by COMT.

Epinephrine acts on both alpha and beta receptors. Norepinephrine acts on both alpha receptors and primarily on beta receptors. Isoproterenol is a pure beta agonist. The functions associated with alpha receptors are vasoconstriction, mydriasis, and intestinal relaxation.

The functions associated with beta receptors are vasodilation, cardioacceleration, bronchial relaxation, positive inotropic effect, intestinal relaxation, and glycogenolysis and fatty acid release. The $beta_1$ receptors are responsible for cardiac stimulation and lipolysis. $Beta_2$ receptors are responsible for bronchodilation and vasodepression. $Beta_2$ agonists are especially useful in the treatment of asthma because they produce bronchodilation without causing much cardiac acceleration.

The actions of norepinephrine and epinephrine on the cardiovascular system may be quite different when both drugs are administered in small doses (0.1 to 4.0 μg/kg/min in a slow intravenous infusion), but are essentially the same when given in large doses.

Following are the effects of small doses of norepinephrine in humans:

Systolic pressure—increased
Diastolic pressure—increased
Mean pressure—increased
Heart rate—slightly decreased
Cardiac output—slightly decreased
Peripheral resistance—increased

The effects of small doses of epinephrine in humans are:

Systolic pressure—increased
Diastolic pressure—decreased (increased by large dose)
Mean pressure—unchanged
Cardiac output—increased
Peripheral resistance—decreased

Epinephrine increases the heart rate, force of contraction, irritability, and coronary blood flow.

The inherent chronotropic effect of norepinephrine is opposed by reflex slowing that is secondary to vasoconstriction and elevated BP.

Epinephrine is a dilator of bronchial smooth muscle ($beta_2$ receptor), whereas norepinephrine is a weak dilator. Isoproterenol is more active than epinephrine.

NORETHINDRONE
(Micronor, Norlutin)

Norethindrone, a progestin with contraceptive properties, is indicated also in amenorrhea, abnormal uterine bleeding, or endometriosis. Norethindrone suppresses ovulation, thickens cervical mucus, and induces sloughing of the endometrium. Norethindrone is contraindicated in patients with a history of thromboembolic disorders, severe hepatic disease, breast cancer, or undiagnosed abnormal vaginal bleeding, and in pregnant and breast-feeding women.

Norethindrone should be used cautiously in patients with existing conditions that might be aggravated by fluid and electrolyte retention, such as cardiac or renal disease; epilepsy or migraine; and in patients with a history of mental depression because norethindrone may worsen this condition. Concomitant use with bromocriptine causes amenorrhea or galactorrhea, thus interfering with the action of bromocriptine.

NORETHINDRONE ACETATE
(Aygestin, Norlutate)

NORFLOXACIN
(Chibroxin solution 3 mg/mL, Noroxin)

Norfloxacin is a fluoroquinolone that interferes with microbial DNA synthesis. It is indicated as an oral treatment of urinary tract infections (UTIs) caused by susceptible organisms; treatment of sexually transmitted diseases (STDs) caused by *Neisseria gonorrhoeae*; ocular solution for treatment of superficial ocular infections due to strains of susceptible organisms; and prostatitis caused by *E. coli*.

The fluoroquinolones are potent bactericidal agents against *E. coli* and various species of *Salmonella, Shigella, Enterobacter, Campylobacter*, and *Neisseria*. Minimal inhibitory concentrations of the fluoroquinolones for 90% of these strains (MIC_{90}) usually are less than 0.2 μg/mL. Ciprofloxacin is more active than **norfloxacin** (Noroxin) against *P. aeruginosa*; values of MIC_{90} range from 0.5 to 6 μg/mL. Fluoroquinolones also have good activity against staphylococci, but not against methicillin-resistant strains (MIC_{90} = 0.1 to 2 μg/mL).

Activity against streptococci is limited to a subset of the quinolones, including **levofloxacin** (Levaquin), **gatifloxacin** (Tequin), and **moxifloxacin** (Avelox). Several intracellular bacteria are inhibited by fluoroquinolones at concentrations that can be achieved in plasma; these include species of *Chlamydia, Mycoplasma, Legionella, Brucella*, and *Mycobacterium* (including *Mycobacterium tuberculosis*. Ciprofloxacin, ofloxacin (FLOXIN), and pefloxacin have MIC_{90} values from 0.5 to 3 μg/mL for *M. fortuitum, M. kansasii*, and *M. tuberculosis*; ofloxacin and pefloxacin are active in animal models of leprosy. However, clinical experience with these pathogens remains limited.

Several of the new fluoroquinolones have activity against anaerobic bacteria, including **garenoxacin** and **gemifloxacin**.

Resistance to quinolones may develop during therapy via mutations in the bacterial chromosomal genes encoding DNA gyrase or topoisomerase IV or by active transport of the drug out of the bacteria. No quinolone-modifying or quinolone-inactivating activities have been identified in bacteria. Resistance has increased after the introduction of fluoroquinolones, especially in *Pseudomonas* and staphylococci. Increasing fluoroquinolone resistance also is being observed in *C. jejuni*, *Salmonella*, *N. gonorrhoeae*, and *S. pneumoniae*.

Norfloxacin (400 mg once daily for 1 to 20 days depending on the nature of the problem) is indicated for UTIs: uncomplicated (including cystitis), caused by *Enterococcus faecalis, E. coli, K. pneumoniae, P. mirabilis, P. aeruginosa, S. epidermidis, S. saprophyticus, C. freundii, Enterobacter aerogenes, Enterobacter cloacae, P. vulgaris, S. aureus*, or *S. agalactiae*; and complicated by *Enterococcus faecalis, E. coli, K. pneumoniae, P. mirabilis, P. aeruginosa*, or *Serratia marcescens*. STDs: Uncomplicated urethral and cervical gonorrhea caused by *N. gonorrhoeae*.

The quinolones include: nalidixic acid, cinoxacin (Cinobac), norfloxacin (Noroxin), and ciprofloxacin (Cipro). Other members of the quinolone family are pefloxacin, ofloxacin, enoxacin and fleroxacin. The bacterial enzyme DNA gyrase is responsible for the continuous introduction of negative supercoils into DNA, and the quinolones inhibit this gyrase-mediated DNA supercoiling.

Nalidixic acid and cinoxacin are bactericidal against Gram-negative organisms that cause urinary tract infections. The fluoroquinolones are bactericidal and considerably more potent against *E. coli* and various species of *Salmonella, Shigella, Enterobacter, Campylobacter*, and *Neisseria*. Ciprofloxacin also has good activity against staphylococci, including methicillin-resistant strains. The quinolones and fluoroquinolones may produce arthropathy, and hence should not be used in prepubertal children or pregnant women. Nalidixic acid and cinoxacin are useful only for treating urinary tract infections. Ciprofloxacin is useful for both urinary tract infections and prostatitis.

NORGESTREL

(Ovrette)

Norgestrel (0.075 mg p.o. daily) exerts its contraceptive activity by suppressing ovulation and causing the thickening of cervical mucus (also see Figure 56). Norgestrel is contraindicated in patients with a history of thromboembolic disorders because the drug may induce thromboembolic disorders; in patients with severe hepatic disease because it may worsen liver damage; in patients with breast or genital cancer or undiagnosed abnormal vaginal bleeding because the drug may stimulate growth of hormone-sensitive tumors; and in pregnant and breast-feeding women.

Norgestrel should be used cautiously in patients with existing conditions that might be aggravated by fluid and electrolyte retention, such as in cardiac or renal disease, epilepsy, or migraine. Caution is also advised in administering this agent to diabetic patients (because decreased glucose tolerance may occur) or to patients with a history of mental depression (because norgestrel may worsen this condition). Concomitant use with bromocriptine may cause amenorrhea or galactorrhea, thus interfering with the action of bromocriptine. Concurrent use of these drugs is not recommended.

NORTRIPTYLINE HYDROCHLORIDE

(Aventyl, Pamelor)

Nortriptyline, a tricyclic antidepressant (25 mg p.o. t.i.d. gradually increasing to a dose of 150 mg daily), is indicated in the relief of symptoms of endogenous depression. Nortriptyline blocks the uptake of norepinephrine and to a lesser extent that of serotonin. It blocks cholinergic muscarinic receptors and to a lesser extent, those of alpha$_1$-adrenergic receptor and H$_1$-histamine receptors. Nortriptyline causes mild sedation and possesses anticholinergic properties. Concomitant use of nortriptyline with sympathomimetics, including epinephrine, phenylephrine, phenylpropranolamine, and ephedrine (often found in nasal sprays), may increase BP. Concomitant use with warfarin may increase prothrombin time and cause bleeding. Concomitant use with thyroid medication, pimozide, or antiarrhythmic agents (quinidine, disopyramide, procainamide) may increase incidence of cardiac arrhythmias and conduction defects.

Nortriptyline may decrease hypotensive effects of centrally acting antihypertensive drugs, such as guanethidine, guanabenz, guanadrel, clonidine, methyldopa, and reserpine. Concomitant use with disulfiram or ethchlorvynol may cause delirium and tachycardia.

Additive effects are likely after concomitant use of nortriptyline with CNS depressants, including alcohol, analgesics, barbiturates, narcotics, tranquilizers, and anesthetics (oversedation); atropine and other anticholinergic drugs, including phenothiazines, antihistamines, meperidine, and antiparkinsonian agents (oversedation, paralytic ileus, visual changes, and severe constipation); and metrizamide (increased risk of convulsions).

Barbiturates and heavy smoking induce nortriptyline metabolism and decrease therapeutic efficacy; phenothiazines and haloperidol decrease its metabolism, decreasing therapeutic efficacy; methylphenidate, cimetidine, oral contraceptives, propoxyphene, and beta-blockers may inhibit nortriptyline metabolism, increasing plasma levels and toxicity (see Tables 5 through 7).

NOSCAPINE

(Nectadon)

Noscapine is a naturally occurring opium alkaloid with a structure and function similar to that of papaverine. It is antitussive and has no analgesic or additive properties. Diphenhydramine and chlorcyclizine are antihistaminic agents that also have antitussive properties. Dimethoxanate (Cothera) and pipazethate (Theratuss) are phenothiazine derivatives without analgesic but with weak antitussive and local anesthetic properties.

NYSTATIN

(Mycostatin)

Nystatin (500,000 to 1,000,000 units three times daily) is indicated in the treatment of intestinal candidiasis. Nystatin, a polyene antibiotic with antifungal activity, is poorly absorbed from the gastrointestinal tract. It is both fungistatic

NURSING INFANTS: Pharmacology of

Many drugs are excreted in breast milk, but the actual amount of a drug that appears in the milk depends on many factors. The higher the maternal plasma concentration of a drug, the more drug is likely to appear in the milk. Atropine poisoning has occurred in nursing infants when the mother has taken larger than therapeutic doses of the agent. Unionized and nonprotein-bound drugs are excreted more rapidly, and ionized drugs are excreted more slowly. The longer a drug stays in maternal plasma, due to diminished metabolism and excretion, or both, the more it will be excreted in the milk. Because the pH of milk is more acidic (6.7) than that of plasma, a proportionately greater amount of basic drugs than of acidic drugs will accumulate in milk. So, in most cases, when drugs are used in recommended amounts, the drug concentrations in milk and hence the infant's plasma are lower than those in the maternal plasma, causing no interference with breast-feeding. However, toxicity in the infant has been known to occur, and so the injudicious use of drugs should be avoided. For example, heavy smokers who intend to breast-feed should expect gastrointestinal, cardiovascular, and CNS disturbances (anorexia, vomiting, diarrhea, tachycardia, restlessness, and irritability) in their infants. Lactating mothers who are taking medications such as anticonvulsants, neuroleptics, or anxiolytic agents on an ongoing basis should perhaps refrain from breast-feeding their infants. The developing brain is far more susceptible to toxicity than is the developed one. For example, the methylmercury-contaminated fish ingested by lactating Japanese mothers has been the prime source of neurologic deficits in the infants of these women (Minamata disease).

Mercury has also been implicated in the etiology of acrodynia (pink disease) in children when mercury-containing teething powder was used. The methyl mercury contained in fungicides has been responsible for toxicity in children in Iraq. This toxicity is characterized by phalangeal erythema, muscular weakness, ataxia, hyperirritability, sensory impairment, visual disturbances, involuntary movement, and sometimes unconsciousness.

and fungicidal but has no effect on bacteria, viruses, or protozoa. It exerts its effect by binding to the sterol moiety and hence damaging the fungal membrane. It is used also as a topical agent to treat candidal infections of the skin and mucous membranes (paronychia, vaginitis, and stomatitis), and so causes no major toxicities.

NYSTATIN/TRIAMCINOLONE ACETONIDE

(Mycogen II cream 100,000 units/g nystatin, 0.1% triamcinolone, ointment 100,000 units/g nystatin, 0.1% triamcinolone, Mycolog II cream, 100,000 units/g nystatin, 0.1% triamcinolone, Mytrex cream 100,000 units/g nystatin, 0.1% triamcinolone, ointment 100,000 units/g nystatin, 0.1% triamcinolone)

Nystatin is a corticosteroid/antifungal combination. The antifungal binds to fungal cell membrane, changing membrane permeability and allowing leakage of intracellular components; the corticosteroid adds antiinflammatory, antipuritic, and vasoconstrictive action. It is indicated in cutaneous candidiasis. **Nystatin** was discovered in the New York State Health Laboratory and was named accordingly; it is a tetraene macrolide produced by *Streptomyces noursei.* Nystatin is structurally similar to **amphotericin B** and has the same mechanism of action. Nystatin is not absorbed from the gastrointestinal tract, skin, or vagina. A liposomal formulation (Nyotran) is in clinical trials for candidemia.

Nystatin (Mycostatin, Nilstat, others) is useful only for candidiasis and is supplied in preparations intended for cutaneous, vaginal, or oral administration for this purpose. Infections of the nails and hyperkeratinized or crusted skin lesions do not respond. Topical preparations include ointments, creams, and powders, all of which contain 100,000 units/g. Powders are preferred for moist lesions and are applied two or three times a day. Creams or ointments are used twice daily. Combinations of nystatin with antibacterial agents or corticosteroids also are available. Allergic reactions to nystatin are very uncommon.

Vaginal tablets containing 100,000 units of the drug are inserted once daily for 2 weeks. Although the tablets are well tolerated, imidazoles or triazoles are more effective agents than **nystatin** for vaginal candidiasis.

An oral suspension that contains 100,000 units/ml of **nystatin** is given four times a day. Premature and low-birth-weight neonates should receive 1 mL of this preparation, infants 2 mL, and children or adults 4 to 6 mL per dose. Older children and adults should be instructed to swish the drug around the mouth and then swallow. If not otherwise instructed, the patient may expectorate the bitter liquid and fail to treat the infected mucosa in the posterior pharynx or esophagus. **Nystatin** suspension is usually effective for oral candidiasis of the immunocompetent host. Other than the bitter taste and occasional complaints of nausea, adverse effects are uncommon. A 200,000-unit troche (mycostatin pastilles) is available for the treatment of oral candidiasis, and a 500,000-unit oral tablet is sold for the treatment of nonesophageal membrane GI candidiasis.

O

OBESITY: Treatment of

Obesity is defined as an excess of fat tissue in comparison with normal values for age and sex. In order to compare studies, standard definitions of overweight have been proposed. The most frequently used methods of calculation are ideal body weight and body mass index. The former takes height and sex into account and the individual is said to be obese when the actual weight exceeds 120% of the ideal weight. The latter is calculated with the ratio weight/height^2, and normal values are 23 kg/m^2 for men and 21 kg/m^2 for women.

Individual susceptibility to obesity is recognized to be influenced significantly by genetic inheritance. Recently, candidate obesity genes, such as the β_3-adrenergic receptor leptin, have been identified that may contribute to the inheritance of body fat mass and the partitioning of fat between central and peripheral fat depots. Nevertheless, overeating and inactive lifestyles are the direct causes of overweight and obesity.

Drugs that safely control food intake by correcting aberrant hunger and satiety signals, drugs that decrease energy efficiency or increase energy expenditure, and drugs that affect emotional states that have an effect on energy balance are being developed.

Agents Known to Enhance Food Intake

Antidepressants	Glucocorticoids	Neuropeptide Y
Bendorphin	Growth-hormone-releasing hormone	Opioid peptides
Dynorphin	Insulin	Testosterone
Galanin	Low serotonin levels	Thyroxine

Agents Known to Suppress Food Intake

Anorectic	High blood glucose	Phenylethylamines
Bombesin	High-fat diet	Satietin
Cholecystokinin	High-protein diet	Serotonin
Corticotropin-releasing hormone	Histidine	Somatostatin
Estrogen	Mazindol	Substance P
Fluoxetine	Neurotensin	Thyrotropin-releasing hormone
Glucagon	Pain	Tryptophane

OCTREOTIDE ACETATE

(Sandostatin injection 0.05 mg/mL)

Octreotide acetate is an endocrine and metabolic agent, whose actions mimic those of natural hormone somatostatin. It suppresses secretion of serotonin and gastroenteropancreatic peptides (e.g., gastrin, insulin, glucagon, secretin, and motilin), and also suppresses the growth hormone. It is indicated in the symptomatic treatment of diarrhea associated with carcinoid tumors, treatment of profuse watery diarrhea associated with vasoactive intestinal peptide tumors (VIPoma), and to reduce blood levels of growth hormone and IGF-1 in acromegaly patients who have had inadequate response to or cannot be treated with resection, pituitary irradiation, and bromocriptine at maximally tolerated doses.

Octreotide (200 to 300 mcg/day in divided doses) is indicated for the treatment of the following tumors:

Carcinoid tumors—Symptomatic treatment of patients with metastatic carcinoid tumors, where it suppresses or inhibits the associated severe diarrhea and flushing episodes.

Vasoactive intestinal peptide tumors (VIPomas)—Treatment of the profuse watery diarrhea associated with VIP-secreting tumors. Significant improvement has been noted in the overall condition of these otherwise therapeutically unresponsive patients. Therapy with octreotide results in improvement in electrolyte abnormalities (e.g., hypokalemia), often enabling reduction of fluid and electrolyte support.

Somatostatin, a cyclic tetradecapeptide with a disulfide bond between the third and fourteenth amino acid residue, has the following structure:

H-Ala-Gly-Cys-Lys-Asn-Phe-Phe-Trp-Lys-Thr-Phe-Thr-Ser-Cys-OH

The administration of somatostatin inhibits the secretion of a variety of peptides, including

- **Hypothalamic hormones**
  - GHRH (see also Table 15)
- **Anterior pituitary hormones**
  - GH
  - Thyrotropin (see Figure 70)
- **Pancreatic hormones**
  - Insulin (see Table 19)
  - Glucagon
  - Gastrin
  - Cholecystokinin
  - Secretin
  - Pepsin
  - Motilin
  - Pancreatic polypeptide
  - Gastrointestinal peptide
  - Vasoactive intestinal polypeptide
- **Kidney hormones**
  - Renin

Octreotide, a long-acting somatostatin analog, has been approved for the management of secretory carcinoid tumors and VIP-secreting tumors. Octreotide therapy, like the natural hormone, somatostatin, may be associated with cholelithiasis, presumably by altering fat absorption and possibly by decreasing the motility of the gallbladder.

In patients with severe renal failure requiring dialysis, the half-life of the octreotide may be increased, necessitating adjustment of the maintenance dosage. Octreotide acetate therapy is occasionally associated with mild transient hypo- or hyperglycemia due to alterations in the balance between the counterregulatory hormones insulin, glucagon, and growth hormone.

Currently, the most widely used somatostatin analog is octreotide (Sandostatin), an 8-amino-acid synthetic derivative of somatostatin, which has a longer half-life and binds preferentially to SSTR-2 and SSTR-5 receptors. Typically, octreotide (100 μg) is administered subcutaneously three times daily; bioactivity is virtually 100%, peak effects are seen within 30 minutes, serum half-life is approximately 90 minutes, and duration of action is approximately 12 hours. The goal of treatment is to decrease growth hormone (GH) levels to less than 2 ng/mL after an oral glucose tolerance test and to bring insulin-like growth factor 1 (IGF-1) levels to within the normal range for age and gender. Depending on the biochemical response, higher or lower octreotide doses may be used in individual patients.

In addition to its effect on GH secretion, octreotide can decrease tumor size—although tumor growth generally resumes after **octreotide** treatment is stopped. Octreotide also has significant inhibitory effects on thyrotropin secretion, and it is the treatment of choice for patients who have thyrotrope adenomas that oversecrete thyroid-stimulating hormone (TSH) and who are not good candidates for surgery.

Gastrointestinal (GI) side effects—including diarrhea, nausea, and abdominal pain—occur in up to 50% of patients receiving octreotide. In most patients these symptoms diminish over time, and do not require cessation of therapy. Approximately 25% of patients receiving octreotide develop gallstones, presumably due to the decreased gallbladder contraction and gastrointestinal transit time. In the absence of symptoms, gallstones are not a contraindication to the continued use of **octreotide**. Compared to somatostatin, octreotide reduces insulin secretion to a lesser extent and only infrequently affects glycemic control.

The need to inject octreotide three times daily poses a significant obstacle to patient compliance. A long-acting, slow-release form (**Sandostatin LAR**) is a more convenient alternative that can be administered intramuscularly, once every 4 weeks; the recommended dose is 20 or 30 mg. The long-acting preparation is at least as effective as the regular formulation and is used in patients who have responded favorably to a trial of the shorter-acting formulation of **octreotide**. Like the shorter-acting formulation, the longer-acting formulation of **octreotide** generally is well tolerated and has a similar incidence of side effects (predominantly GI and/or discomfort at the injection site) that do not require cessation of therapy.

Lanreotide (Somatuline La) is another long-acting octapeptide analog of somatostatin that causes prolonged suppression of GH secretion when administered in a 30-mg dose, intramuscularly. Although its efficacy appears comparable to that of the long-acting formulation of **octreotide**, its duration of action is shorter; thus it must be administered either at 10- or 14-day intervals. A 60-mg formulation of lanreotide (Somatuline autogel) has recently been introduced that reduces the required dosing frequency to once every 4 weeks; current results are comparable to those with the slow-release octreotide formulation, as are the incidence and severity of side effects. Lanreotide has not been approved by the FDA for use in the United States.

Somatostatin blocks not only GH secretion but also the secretion of other hormones, growth factors, and cytokines. Thus, octreotide and the delayed-release somatostatin analogs have been used to treat symptoms associated with metastatic carcinoid tumors (e.g., flushing and diarrhea) and adenomas secreting VIP (e.g., watery diarrhea). **Octreotide** also is used for treatment of acute variceal bleeding, for perioperative prophylaxis in pancreatic surgery, and for TSH-secreting adenomas in patients who are not candidates for surgery. Novel uses under evaluation currently include the treatment of eye diseases associated with excessive proliferation and inflammation (e.g., Graves' orbitopathy and diabetic retinopathy), diabetic nephropathy, and various systemic diseases associated with inflammation (e.g., rheumatoid arthritis, inflammatory bowel disease, and psoriasis). Finally, modified forms of **octreotide** labeled with indium or technetium have been used for diagnostic imaging of neuroendocrine tumors such as pituitary adenomas and carcinoids; modified forms labeled with β emitters such as ^{90}Y have been used in selective destruction of SSTR-2-positive tumors.

OCULOTOXICITY: Drug-induced

Antiinflammatory Agents

Corticosteroids	Ibuprofen	Ketoprofen	Piroxicam
Cyclosporine	Indomethacin	Phenylbutazone	Salicylates
Gold salts, auranofin			

Antimicrobial Agents

Amiodaquine	Ethambutol	Nalidixic acid	Sulfonamides
Clofazimine	Gentamicin	Nitrofurantoin	Suramin
Chloramphenicol	Griseofulvin	Quinine	Tetracycline
Chloroquine/hydroxychloroquine	Isoniazid	Rifampin	Vaccinations
Diethylcarbamazine	Minocycline	Streptomycin	

Antineoplastic Agents

BCNU/CCNU/MeCCNU	Cyclophosphamide	Ifosfamide	Nitrogen mustard
Busulfan	Cytosine arabinoside	Methotrexate	Procarbazine
Carmustine	Doxorubicin	Mitotane	Tamoxifen
Chlorambucil	Fludarabine	Mitoxanthrone	Vinca alkaloids
Cisplatin	5-fluorouracil		

Cardiovascular Agents

Amiodarone	Ergot alkaloids	Metoprolol	Propranolol
Diazoxide	Flecainide	Minoxidil	Quinidine
Digitalis glycoside	Guanethidine	Nifedipine	Reserpine

Central Nervous System Agents

Amantadine	Ethchlorvynol	Phenytoin
Barbiturates	Lithium	Protriptyline
Bromocriptine	Narcotic analgesics	Trimethadione
Carbamazepine	Phenothiazine	

Miscellaneous Agents

Allopurinol	Dantrolene	Disulfiram	Penicillamine
Amantadine	Deferoxamine	Ganiumnitrate	Thiazide
Clomiphene	Diphenhydramine	Isotretinoin	diuretics

Adverse effects of drugs may involve external ocular functions and structures, such as oculomotor function, eyelids, lacrimation, conjunctiva, and cornea; or internal structures, such as trabecular meshwork, ciliary body, iris, lens, retina, and optic nerve. Higher-than-therapeutic doses and long duration of administration enhance the incidence of drug-induced oculotoxicity.

OFLOXACIN

(Floxin tablets 200 mg, tablets 300 mg, tablets 400 mg, injection 200 mg, injection 400 mg, Ocuflox ophthalmic solution 3 mg/mL)

Ofloxacin interferes with microbial DNA synthesis. It is indicated in the treatment of acute bacterial exacerbations of chronic bronchitis, community acquired pneumonia, uncomplicated skin and skin structure infections, acute uncomplicated urethral and cervical gonorrhea, nongonococcal urethritis, cervicitis, acute pelvic inflammatory disease, uncomplicated cystitis, complicated urinary tract infections (UTI), and prostatitis caused by *Escherichia coli*. Ophthalmic use: for treatment of conjunctivitis and corneal ulcer infections caused by susceptible organisms; otic use: for treatment of otitis externa, chronic suppurative otitis media in patients with perforated tympanic membranes, and acute otitis media in pediatric patients with tympanostomy tubes.

Ofloxacin (400 mg p.o.) is indicated for acute bacterial exacerbations of chronic bronchitis and pneumonia caused by susceptible organisms; sexually transmitted diseases, such as acute uncomplicated urethral and cervical gonorrhea, nongonococcal urethritis and cervicitis, and mixed infections of urethra and cervix; mild to moderate skin and skin-structure infections; complicated UTI; and prostatitis. The quinolones include nalidixic acid (NegGram), cinoxacin (Cinobac), norfloxacin (Noroxin), and ciprofloxacin (Cipro). Other members of the quinolone family are pefloxacin, ofloxacin, enoxacin, and fleroxacin. The bacterial enzyme DNA gyrase is responsible for the continuous introduction of negative supercoils into the DNA, and the quinolones inhibit this gyrase-mediated DNA supercoiling.

Nalidixic acid and cinoxacin are bactericidal against Gram-negative organisms that cause UTI. The fluoroquinolones are bactericidal and considerably more potent against

Escherichia coli and various species of *Salmonella, Shigella, Enterobacter, Campylobacter*, and *Neisseria*. Ciprofloxacin also has good activity against staphylococci, including methicillin-resistant strains.

The quinolones and fluoroquinolones may produce arthropathy, and hence should not be used in prepubertal children or pregnant women.

Nalidixic acid and cinoxacin are useful only for treating UTI. Ciprofloxacin is useful for both UTI and prostatitis.

OLANZAPINE

(Zyprexa tablets 2.5 mg, tablets 5 mg, tablets 7.5 mg, tablets 10 mg, tablets 15 mg, tablets 20 mg, Zyprexa Zydis tablets, orally disintegrating 5 mg, tablets, orally disintegrating 10 mg, tablets, orally disintegrating 15 mg, tablets, orally disintegrating 20 mg, Zyprexa intramuscular powder for injection 10 mg)

Olanzapine is an antipsychotic that controls psychotic symptoms through antagonism of selected dopamine and serotonin receptors in the central nervous system (CNS). It is indicated in the treatment of schizophrenia (oral); short-term treatment of acute mixed or manic episodes with bipolar I disorder (oral); in combination with lithium or valproate, for short-term treatment of acute episodes associated with bipolar I disorder (oral); and treatment of agitation associated with schizophrenia and bipolar I mania (IM).

Olanzapine, a novel atypical antipsychotic, has properties similar to those exhibited by clozapine (see also Table 2).

Clozapine (Clozaril), a 5-$HT_{2A/2C}$-receptor antagonist, represents a class of atypical antipsychotic drugs with reduced incidence of extrapyramidal side effects compared to the classical neuroleptics, and possibly a greater efficacy for reducing negative symptoms of schizophrenia. Clozapine also has a high affinity for subtypes of dopamine receptors.

One of the newest strategies for the design of additional atypical antipsychotic drugs is to combine 5-$HT_{2A/2C}$-and dopamine D_2-receptor-blocking actions in the same molecule. **Risperidone** (Risperdal), for example, is a potent 5-HT_{2A}- and D_2-receptor antagonist. Low doses of risperidone have been reported to attenuate negative symptoms of schizophrenia with a low incidence of extrapyramidal side effects. Extrapyramidal effects are commonly seen, however, with doses of risperidone in excess of 6 mg/day. Other atypical antipsychotic agents—**quetiapine** (Seroquel) and **olanzapine** (Zyprexa)—act on multiple receptors, but their antipsychotic properties are thought to be due to antagonism of dopamine and serotonin.

The term **neuroleptic** is often applied to drugs that have relatively prominent experimental and clinical evidence of antagonism of D_2-dopamine-receptor activity, with substantial risk of adverse extrapyramidal neurological effects and increased release of prolactin. The term **atypical antipsychotic** is applied to agents that are associated with substantially lower risks of such extrapyramidal effects. Representative examples include **aripiprazole**, **clozapine**, **quetiapine**, **ziprasidone**, and low doses of **olanzapine** and **risperidone**.

Although the antipsychotic drugs have had a revolutionary, beneficial impact on medical and psychiatric practice, their liabilities, especially the adverse effects of the older typical or neuroleptic agents, must be emphasized. Newer antipsychotics are atypical in having less risk of extrapyramidal side effects, but these agents present their own spectrum of adverse effects, including hypotension, seizures, weight gain, and increased risk of type 2 diabetes mellitus and hyperlipidemia.

Several cognitive functions, including auditory processing and attention, spatial organization, verbal learning, semantic and verbal memory, and executive functions are impaired in schizophrenia patients and are a major source of social and occupational dysfunction and disability. Potent D_2-antagonist neuroleptics have very limited beneficial effects on such functions. Some atypical antipsychotic agents with mixed D_2/5-HT_{2A} activity (including clozapine, quetiapine, **olanzapine**, and risperidone), as well as the D_2 partial agonist, aripiprazole, seem to improve cognitive functioning in psychotic patients. Nevertheless, significant long-term gains in social and occupational functions during long-term treatment of chronically psychotic patients with these drugs are not well documented.

Many neuroleptic drugs can lower the seizure threshold and induce discharge patterns in the electroencephalogram (EEG)—effects associated with epileptic seizure disorders. Clozapine, **olanzapine**, and aliphatic phenothiazines with low potency (such as chlorpromazine) seem particularly able to do this, whereas the more potent piperazine phenothiazines and thioxanthenes (notably fluphenazine and thiothixene), risperidone, and quetiapine are much less likely to have this effect. The butyrophenones and molindone variably and unpredictably rarely cause seizures. Clozapine has a clearly dose-related risk of inducing EEG abnormalities and seizures in nonepileptic patients. Antipsychotic agents, especially clozapine, olanzapine, and low-potency phenothiazines and thioxanthenes, should be used with extreme caution, if at all, in untreated epileptic patients and in patients undergoing withdrawal from CNS depressants, such as alcohol, barbiturates, or benzodiazepines. Most antipsychotic drugs, especially the piperazines as well as the newer atypical agents, aripiprazole, quetiapine, risperidone, and ziprasidone, can be used safely in epileptic patients, if moderate doses are attained gradually and concomitant anticonvulsant drug therapy is maintained.

OLANZAPINE/FLUOXETINE HYDROCHLORIDE

(Symbyax capsules olanzapine 6 mg/fluoxetine hydrochloride 25 mg, capsules olanzapine 6 mg/fluoxetine hydrochloride 50 mg, capsules olanzapine 12 mg/fluoxetine hydrochloride 25 mg, capsules olanzapine 12 mg/fluoxetine hydrochloride 50 mg)

Olanzapine/fluoxetine hydrochloride is an antidepressant. It is thought that activation of 3 monoaminergic neural systems (dopamine, norepinephrine, and serotonin) is responsible for an enhancement of the antidepressant effect.

It is indicated in the treatment of depressive episodes associated with bipolar disorder. A combination of an antipsychotic drug and an antidepressant may be useful in some cases, especially in depressed psychotic patients, or in cases of agitated major depression with psychotic features. The first combination antipsychotic/antidepressant (**olanzapine**/fluoxetine; Symbyax) was recently FDA approved in the United States for treatment of depressive episodes associated with bipolar disorder. However, antidepressants and stimulants are unlikely to reduce apathy and withdrawal in schizophrenia, and they may induce clinical worsening in some cases. Adjunctive addition of **lithium** or an **antimanic anticonvulsant**, such as carbamazepine, may add benefit in some psychotic patients with prominent affective, aggressive, or resistant symptoms.

OLMESARTAN MEDOXOMIL

(Benicar tablets 5 mg, tablets 20 mg, tablets 40 mg)

Olmesartan medoxomil is an angiotensin-II-receptor antagonist that blocks vasoconstrictor effects of angiotensin II by selectively blocking the binding of angiotensin II to the AT_1 receptor in vascular smooth muscle. It is indicated in the treatment of hypertension.

Olmesartan medoxomil (Benicar) is an inactive ester prodrug that is completely hydrolyzed to the active form, **olmesartan**, during absorption from the GI tract. Peak plasma levels are obtained 1.4 to 2.8 hours after oral administration, and the plasma half-life is between 10 and 15 hours. Plasma clearance of olmesartan is through both renal elimination and biliary excretion. Although renal impairment and hepatic disease decrease the plasma clearance of olmesartan, no dose adjustment is required in patients with mild to moderate renal or hepatic impairment. The oral dosage of olmesartan medoxomil is 20 to 40 mg, once daily.

Angiotensin-II-receptor antagonists (ARBs) are approved for the treatment of hypertension. In addition, **irbesartan** and **losartan** are approved for diabetic nephropathy, **losartan** is approved for stroke prophylaxis, and **valsartan** is approved for heart failure patients who are intolerant of angiotensin-converting enzyme (ACE) inhibitors. The efficacy of ARBs in lowering blood pressure (BP) is comparable with that of other established antihypertensive drugs, with an adverse-effect profile similar to that of placebo. ARBs also are available as fixed-dose combinations with hydrochlorothiazide.

OLOPATADINE HYDROCHLORIDE

(Patanol solution 0.1%)

Olopatadine hydrochloride is an ophthalmic antihistamine that inhibits release of histamine from mast cells and is a relatively selective histamine H_1 antagonist. It inhibits type 1 immediate hypersensitivity reactions. Olopatadine hydrochloride is indicated in the temporary relief of itching caused by allergic conjunctivitis. H_1 antagonists have an established and valued place in the symptomatic treatment of various immediate hypersensitivity reactions. In addition, the central properties of some of the series are of therapeutic value for suppressing motion sickness or for sedation.

H_1 antagonists are most useful in acute types of allergy that present with symptoms of rhinitis, urticaria, and conjunctivitis. Their effect is confined to the suppression of symptoms attributable to the histamine released by the antigen–antibody reaction. In bronchial asthma, histamine antagonists have limited efficacy and are not used as sole therapy. In the treatment of systemic anaphylaxis, in which autacoids other than histamine play major roles, the mainstay of the therapy is epinephrine; histamine antagonists have only a subordinate and adjuvant role. The same is true for severe angioedema, in which laryngeal swelling constitutes a threat to life.

Other allergies of the respiratory tract are more amenable to therapy with H_1 antagonists. The best results are obtained in seasonal rhinitis and conjunctivitis (**hay fever**, **pollinosis**), in which these drugs relieve the sneezing, rhinorrhea, and itching of eyes, nose, and throat. A gratifying response is obtained in most patients, especially at the beginning of the season when pollen counts are low; however, the drugs are less effective when the allergens are most abundant, when exposure to them is prolonged, and when nasal congestion is prominent. Topical preparations of antihistamines such as **levocabastine** (Livostin), **azelastine** (Astelin), **ketotifen** (Zaditor), and **olopatadine** (Patanol) have been shown to be effective in allergic conjunctivitis and rhinitis. Nasal sprays or topical ophthalmic preparations of these agents are available in the United States. Histamine causes the release of inflammatory cytokines and eicosanoids and increases expression of endothelial adhesion molecules. In addition, H_1 receptors can, either via constitutive activity or after stimulation by agonists, activate the proinflammatory transcription factor NF-κB. Thus, H_1 antihistamines have been investigated for potential antiinflammatory properties. Although H_1 antihistamines do exhibit a variety of antiinflammatory effects *in vitro* and in animal models, in many cases the doses required are higher than those normally achieved therapeutically, and clinical effectiveness has not yet been proven.

Cromolyn sodium (Crolom), which prevents the release of histamine and other autacoids from mast cells, has found limited use in treating conjunctivitis that is thought to be allergen-mediated, such as vernal conjunctivitis. **Lodoxamide tromethamine** (Alomide) and **pemirolast** (Alamast), mast-cell stabilizers, are also available for ophthalmic use. Nedocromil (Alocril) also is primarily a mast-cell stabilizer with some antihistamine properties. Olopatadine hydrochloride (Patanol), **ketotifen fumarate** (Zaditor), and **azelastine** (Optivar) are H_1 antagonists with mast-cell-stabilizing properties. **Epinastine** (Elestat) antagonizes H_1 and H_2 receptors and exhibits mast-cell-stabilizing activity.

OLSALAZINE SODIUM

(Dipentum capsules 250 mg)

Olsalazine sodium is a G_1 agent, which becomes bioconverted to 5-aminosalicylic acid (mesalamine) in the colon. Although the mechanism of action is unknown, it probably reduces inflammation of the colon topically by preventing production of substances involved in the inflammatory process, such as arachidonic acid.

Olsalazine (1 g/day in 2 divided doses) is indicated for maintenance of remission of ulcerative colitis in patients intolerant to sulfasalazine (see Figure 91). Olsalazine sodium is a sodium salt of a salicylate compound that is effectively bioconverted to 5-aminosalicylic acid (mesalamine; 5-ASA), which has antiinflammatory activity in ulcerative colitis. Approximately 98 to 99% of an oral dose will reach the colon where each molecule is rapidly converted into two molecules of 5-ASA by colonic bacteria and the low prevailing redox potential found in this environment. More than 0.9 g mesalamine would usually be made available in the colon from 1 g olsalazine. The liberated 5-ASA is absorbed slowly, resulting in very high local concentrations in the colon.

The mechanism of action of mesalamine is unknown, but appears to be topical rather than systemic. It is possible that mesalamine diminishes colonic inflammation by blocking cyclooxygenase and inhibiting colon prostaglandin production in the bowel mucosa.

Symptoms of acute toxicity from olsalazine include diarrhea, vomiting, and decreased motor activity.

OMALIZUMAB

(Xolair powder for injection, lyophilized 202.5 mg (150 mg/l.2 mL after reconstruction))

Omalizumab is a monoclonal antibody that selectively binds to human IgE, inhibiting the binding of IgE to the high-affinity IgE receptor on the surface of mast cells and basophils, and limiting the degree of release of mediators of the allergic response. It is indicated in the treatment of moderate to severe persistent asthma in patients who have a positive skin test or *in vitro* reactivity to a perennial aeroallergen and whose symptoms are inadequately controlled with inhaled corticosteroids.

Omalizumab (Xolair) is the first "biological drug" approved for the treatment of asthma. **Omalizumab** is a recombinant humanized monoclonal antibody targeted against IgE. IgE bound to omalizumab cannot bind to IgE receptors on mast cells and basophils, thereby preventing the allergic reaction at a very early step in the process.

Omalizumab is a DNA-derived humanized monoclonal antibody of the IgG1κ subclass. It has a molecular weight of approximately 149,000 kDa. The antibody is produced in Chinese hamster ovary cells in cell culture. It is sold as a preservative-free powder. A vial of Xolair contains 202 mg **omalizumab**, as well as sucrose, L-histidine, and polysorbate 20.

Omalizumab is delivered as a single subcutaneous injection every 2 to 4 weeks. It has a bioavailability of about 60%, reaching peak serum levels after 7 to 8 days. The serum elimination half-life is 26 days, with a clearance rate of about 2.5 mL/kg per day. The elimination of **omalizumab**-IgE complexes occurs in the liver reticuloendothelial system at a rate somewhat faster than that of free IgG. Some intact omalizumab is also excreted in the bile. There is little evidence of specific uptake of **omalizumab** by any tissue.

The safety of **omalizumab** so far has been evaluated in only three large, randomized, placebo-controlled, multicenter studies. Omalizumab generally was well tolerated in several large, placebo-controlled, trials. The most frequent adverse effect was injection-site reactions (e.g., redness, stinging, bruising, and induration), but these reactions also were seen at comparable frequencies with placebo. Low titers of antibodies against omalizumab developed in 1 of 1723 treated patients, whereas anaphylaxis was seen in 0.1% of treated patients. Malignancies of various types were observed in 20 of 4127 patients taking omalizumab, a higher frequency than the five malignancies in 2236 patients taking other asthma and allergy drugs. Additional studies are needed to determine if **omalizumab** does indeed cause cancers.

Omalizumab is indicated for adults and adolescents older than 12 years of age with allergies and moderate to severe persistent asthma. In this population, it has proven to be effective in reducing the dependency on inhaled and oral corticosteroids and in decreasing the frequency of asthma exacerbations. **Omalizumab** is not an acute bronchodilator and should not be used as a rescue medication or as a treatment of status asthmaticus.

Based on its mechanism of action, **omalizumab** has been used in the treatment of other allergic disorders, such as nasal allergy and food allergy, but large-scale clinical trials are limited to asthma.

OMEGA-CONOTOXIN

Under normal conditions, the extracellular concentration of calcium is in the millimolar range (10^{-3} M), whereas its intracellular concentration is less than 10^{-7} M. The cytoplasmic concentration of calcium is increased through the actions of receptor-operated channels, voltage-activated channels, or ionic pumps. In addition, calcium can be released from internal stores.

There are two types of voltage-activated channels:

1. Low-voltage-activated channels or low-threshold channels, which are also termed T-type channels.
2. High-voltage-activated channels, which are further subdivided into L-type, N-type, and P-type channels.

T-Type Channels

T-type calcium channels (with the T standing for "transient") require only a weak depolarization for activation and

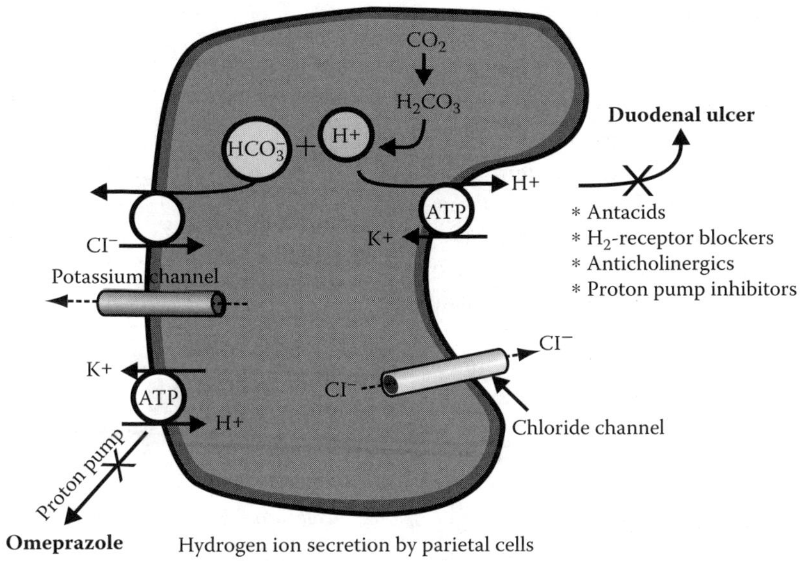

FIGURE 72 Omeprazole inhibits the activity of the acid (proton) pump H^+/K^+ adenosine triphosphate (ATPase) located at the secretory surface of the gastric parietal cells.

carry a transient current at negative membrane potentials that inactivates rapidly during a prolonged pulse. In neurons, the T-type channel is responsible for neuronal oscillatory activity and is thought to play a role in the regulation of wakefulness and motor coordination. The pyrazine diuretic, amiloride, inhibits the T-type calcium channel.

L-Type Channels

L-type calcium channels (with the L standing for "long lasting") exist in high numbers in the skeletal muscle and require a large depolarization for activation to take place. The channels are phosphorylated prior to opening. Each channel is composed of five subunits: $alpha_1$, (molecular weight [MW] = 175 kDa), $alpha_2$ (MW = 143 kDa), beta (MW = 54 kDa), gamma (MW = 30 kDa), and delta (MW = 27 kDa). The $alpha_1$ and beta subunits contain phosphorylation sites for cyclic adenosine monophosphate (AMP)-dependent protein kinase. The $alpha_1$ subunit contains the dihydropyridine-binding sites. The L-type calcium channel is involved in the generation of action potentials and in signal transduction at the cell membrane.

N-Type Channels

The N-type calcium channel (with the N standing for "neither T nor L" or "neuronal") appears to convey most of the whole-cell calcium current; it is insensitive to dihydropyridine and is blocked by omega-conotoxin. The N-type channel is involved in the release of transmitter in some, but not all, tissues, with the CNS neurons being the exception.

P-Type Channels

The P-type channels were first observed in the Purkinje cells and are inhibited by a toxin derived from a funnel-web spider poison, but not by other calcium-channel-blocking agents. P-type channels are widely distributed throughout the CNS and are thought to participate in the generation of intrinsic activity as well as serve as modulators of neuronal integration and transmitter release.

OMEPRAZOLE

(Prilosec capsules, delayed-release 10 mg, capsules, delayed-release 20 mg, capsules, delayed-release 40 mg, Prilosec OTC tablets, delayed-release 20 mg, Zegerid powder for oral suspension 20 mg, powder for oral suspension 40 mg)

Omeprazole is a GI agent/proton pump inhibitor/*H. pylori* agent that suppresses gastric acid secretion by blocking the acid (proton) pump within the gastric parietal cell (Figure 72). It is indicated in the short-term treatment of active duodenal ulcer and gastroesophageal reflux disease (GERD) including erosive esophagitis and symptomatic GERD; long-term treatment of pathologic hypersecretory conditions (e.g., Zollinger–Ellison syndrome, multiple endocrine adenomas, and systemic mastocytosis) (except Zegerid); to maintain healing of erosive esophagitis; in combination with clarithromycin to eradicate *Helicobacter pylori* (except Zegerid) (use clarithromycin and amoxicillin in combination with omeprazole in patients with a 1-year history of duodenal ulcers or active duodenal ulcers to eradicate *H. pylori*); for short-term treatment of active benign gastric ulcer; in heartburn; and to reduce the risk of upper GI bleeding in critically ill patients (Zegerid only).

Omeprazole (20 mg daily for 4 to 8 weeks) is indicated for active duodenal ulcer, GERD, and pathological hypersecretory conditions, such as Zollinger–Ellison syndrome, multiple endocrine adenomas, and systemic mastocytosis.

Omeprazole belongs to a new class of antisecretory compounds, the substituted benzimidazoles, that do not exhibit anticholinergic or H_2-histamine-antagonistic properties but suppress gastric acid secretion by specific inhibition of the H^+/K^+ ATPase enzyme system at the secretory surface of the gastric parietal cell. Because this enzyme system is the "acid (proton) pump" within the gastric mucosa, omeprazole has been characterized as a gastric acid pump inhibitor; it blocks the final step of acid production. This effect is dose-related, and inhibits both basal and stimulated acid secretion irrespective of the stimulus.

Omeprazole increases the half-life of diazepam by inhibiting its metabolism and reduces the plasma clearance of phenytoin and warfarin.

ONCOGENES

Tumor markers have been used for screening, diagnosing, establishing prognosis, monitoring treatment, and detecting the recurrence of tumors. For example, the measurement of human chorionic gonadotropin is used as a marker in patients with high-risk gestational trophoblastic tumors, alpha-fetoprotein for hepatocellular carcinoma, carcinoembryonic antigen for colon cancer, and prostatic acid phosphatase and prostate-specific antigen for prostate cancer. In addition, the application of monoclonal antibodies, DNA content analysis, DNA hybridization techniques, and cytogenic analysis have added new dimensions to the diagnosis and classification of hematologic malignancies.

Biotechnological innovations have fostered the exploitation of oncogenes as novel therapeutic targets for the diagnosis, prognosis, and treatment of cancer. The advent of magnetic resonance imaging (MRI) has also advanced the ability to noninvasively visualize smaller pituitary adenomas, and the introduction of computed tomography has led to improvements in the chemotherapy of malignant mesothelioma.

ONDANSETRON HYDROCHLORIDE

(Zofran)

Ondansetron, a serotonin ($5\text{-}HT_3$)-receptor antagonist (0.15 mg/kg IV with the first dose taken infused every 15 minutes before the start of chemotherapy), is used in the prevention of nausea and vomiting associated with initial and repeat courses of emetogenic cancer chemotherapy, including high-dose cisplatin (see Figure 73).

Ondansetron, granisetron, tropisetron, and batanopride are antagonists of the $5\text{-}HT_3$ receptor and are considered effective in controlling cancer chemotherapy-induced emesis.

Ondansetron is not a dopamine-receptor antagonist. Because serotonin receptors of the $5\text{-}HT_3$ type are present both peripherally on vagal nerve terminals and centrally in the chemoreceptor trigger zone, it is not certain if ondansetron's antiemetic action is mediated centrally, peripherally, or in both sites (see Figure 73).

Ondansetron is metabolized by cytochrome P450; thus, inducers or inhibitors of this enzyme may change the clearance and half-life of ondansetron; however, no dosage adjustment is required. Cisplatin, carmustine, and etoposide do not affect ondansetron's pharmacokinetics.

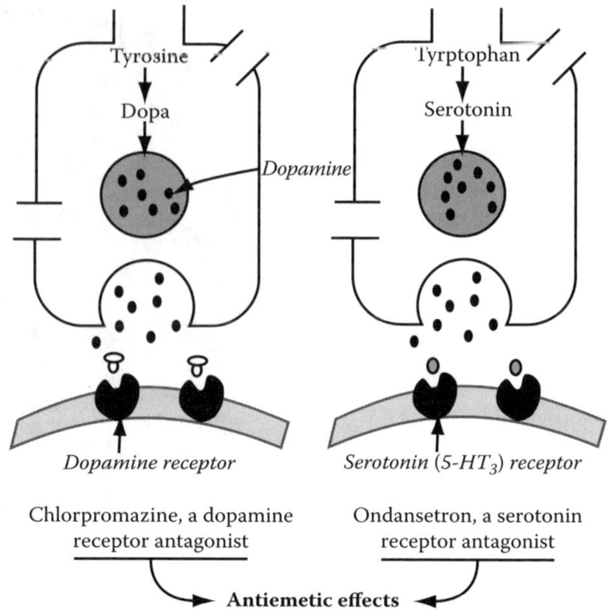

FIGURE 73 Selective antagonists of the serotonin type 3 ($5\text{-}HT_3$) receptor, such as **batanopride**, **granisetron**, **ondansetron**, or **zacopride**, have been shown to be potent antiemetic agents in patients receiving cytotoxic chemotherapy, with efficacy comparable to or superior to that of conventional antiemetics.

OPIUM ALKALOIDS

The opium alkaloids, which are obtained from *Papaver somniferum*, contain two groups of compounds: compounds with phenanthrene derivatives, consisting of morphine (1 to 10%), codeine (0.7 to 2.5%), and thebaine (0.5 to 1.5%); and compounds with isoquinoline derivatives, consisting of papaverine (1%) and noscapine (5 to 10%).

Narcotics are divided into naturally occurring, semisynthetic, and synthetic derivatives. The naturally occurring analgesics consist of morphine and codeine (methylmorphine); the semisynthetic analgesics include hydromorphine (Dilaudid) and hydrocodone (Dicodid); and the synthetic analgesics consist of meperidine (Demerol), alphaprodine (Nisentil), methadone (Dolophine), propoxyphene (Darvon), and pentazocine (Talwin).

The narcotic antagonists are nalorphine (Nalline), naloxone (Narcan), and naltrexone (Trexan). Dextromethorphan (Romilar) is used as an antitussive preparation; apomorphine is used as an emetic agent.

Narcotic analgesics may have either a high potency (morphine, hydromorphone, oxymorphone, methadone, meperidine, fentanyl, and levorphanol) or low potency (codeine, oxycodone, hydrocodone, propoxyphene, and diphenoxylate). These agents may be a pure agonist

OPIOID PEPTIDES

Endogenous Opioid Peptides

[Leu⁵]enkephalin	Tyr-Gly-Gly-Phe-Leu
[Met⁵]enkephalin	Tyr-Gly-Gly-Phe-Met
Dynorphin A	Tyr-Gly-Gly-Phe-Leu-Arg-Arg-Ile-Arg-Pro-Lys-Leu-Lys-Trp-Asp-Asn-Gln
Dynorphin B	Tyr-Gly-Gly-Phe-Leu-Arg-Arg-Gln-Phe-Lys-Val-Val-Thr
A-Neoendorphin	Tyr-Gly-Gly-Phe-Leu-Arg-Lys-Tyr-Pro-Lys
B-Neoendorphin	Tyr-Gly-Gly-Phe-Leu-Arg-Lys-Tyr-Pro
β_h-Endorphin	Tyr-Gly-Gly-Phe-Met-Thr-Ser-Glu-Lys-Ser-Gln-Thr-Pro-Leu-Val-Thr-Leu-Phe-Lys-Asn-Ala-Ile-Ile-Lys-Asn-Ala-Tyr-Lys-Lys-Gly-Glu

Synthetic Opioid Peptides

DAMGO	[D-Ala^2,MePhe^4,Gly(ol)^5]enkephalin
DPDPE	[D-Pen^2,D-Pen^5]enkephalin
DSLET	[D-Ser^2,Leu^5]enkephalin-Thr6
DADL	[D-Ala^2,D-Leu^5]enkephalin
CTOP	D-Phe-Cys-Tyr-D-Trp-Orn-Thr-Pen-Thr-NH_2
FK-33824	[D-Ala^2,N-MePhe^4,Met(O)^5-ol]enkephalin
[D-Ala^2]Deltorphin I	Tyr-D-Ala-Phe-Asp-Val-Val-Gly-NH_2
[D-Ala^2,Glu^4]Deltorphin (Deltorphin II)	Tyr-D-Ala-Phe-Glu-Val-Val-Gly-NH_2
Morphiceptin	Tyr-Pro-Phe-Pro-NH_2
PL-017	Tyr-Pro-MePhe-D-Pro-NH_2
DALCE	[D-Ala^2,Leu^5,Cys6]enkephalin

OPIOIDS: Receptor Agonists and Antagonists

Receptor Agonists

Buprenorphine	Hydromorphine	Nalmefene
Butorphanol	Levallorphan	Nalorphine
Codeine	Levorphanol	Oxycodone
Drocode	Meperidine	Oxymorphone
Fentanyl	Methadone	Pentazocine
Heroin	Morphine	Propoxyphene
Hydrocodone	Nalbuphine	

Receptor Antagonists

Naloxone
Naltrexone

(morphine), pure antagonist (naloxone), or mixed agonist–antagonist (pentazocine).

OPIUM TINCTURE

(Laudanum)

Powdered opium, U.S.P., is a light brown, bitter, fine powder, supplied for clinical use in capsule, tablet, or pill form. The average adult dose is 0.06 gram taken orally. This is equivalent to 6 mgm of morphine, the official morphine content of opium being 10% by weight. Opium tincture (**Laudanum**, deodorized opium tincture), U.S.P., is a hydroalcoholic solution containing 10% of opium (1.0% of morphine). The average adult dose is 0.6 to 1.5 mL (equivalent to 6 to 15 mgm of morphine), taken orally.

Opium (gum opium) and granulated opium are also official in the U.S.P. The dose of either is the same as for the powder. These preparations are infrequently employed. **Camphorated opium tincture** (paregoric), U.S.P., contains 4% of opium tincture, that is, 0.04% morphine. Also included are benzoic acid, camphor, and anise oil. The average adult dose is 4 mL, which corresponds to 16 mgm of opium or 1.6 mgm of morphine. Paregoric, by tradition, is used especially for children, but represents a needlessly complex therapeutic survival of a former day. It may have some value as an expectorant, especially when old. **Ipecac and opium powder** (Dover's powder), N.F., contains 10% each of ipecac and powdered opium; it is a very pale brown, coarse powder. The average adult dose is 0.3 to 0.6 g, the equivalent of 3 to 6 mgm of morphine, respectively. The powder has been employed especially as a diaphoretic, but it is no longer extensively used. Compound **opium and glycyrrhiza mixture** (Brown Mixture), N.F., is another therapeutic relic. It contains 12% paregoric, some tartar emetic, and a little ethyl nitrite spirit. The mixture is needlessly complex and little employed today, although it still is sometimes prescribed as a cough medicine for children. The average adult dose is 4 mL, taken orally.

OPIUM TINCTURE/PAREGORIC

(Opium tincture, deodorized liquid 10 mg anhydrous morphine equiv./mL, Paregoric liquid 2 mg anhydrous morphine equiv./5 mL)

Opium tincture/paregoric is an opioid analgesic that enhances tone in long segments of longitudinal muscle and inhibits propulsive contraction of both circular and longitudinal muscles. Opium tincture is used in acute and nonspecific diarrhea.

Opioids used for diarrhea include codeine (in doses of 30 mg given three or four times daily) and opium-containing compounds.

Paregoric (camphorated opium tincture) contains the equivalent of 2 mg of morphine per 5 mL (0.4 mg/mL); **deodorized tincture of opium**, which is 25 times stronger, contains the equivalent of 50 mg of morphine per 5 mL (10 mg/mL). The two tinctures sometimes are confused in prescribing and dispensing, resulting in dangerous overdoses. The antidiarrheal dose of opium tincture for adults is 0.6 mL (equivalent to 6 mg morphine), four times daily; the adult dose of paregoric is 5 to 10 mL (equivalent to 2 to 4 mg morphine), one to four times daily. **Paregoric** is used in children at a dose of 0.25 to 0.5 mL/kg (equivalent to 0.1 to 0.2 mg morphine/kg), one to four times daily.

Enkephalins are endogenous opioids that are important enteric neurotransmitters. Enkephalins inhibit intestinal secretion without affecting motility. **Racecadotril** (acetorphan), a dipeptide inhibitor of enkephalinase, reinforces the effects of endogenous enkephalins on the δ-opioid receptor to produce an antidiarrheal effect.

OPRELVEKIN

(Neumega powder for injection 5 mg)

Oprelvekin is an interleukin. Interleukin 11 (IL-11) is a thrombopoietic growth factor that directly stimulates the proliferation of hematopoietic stem cells and megakaryocyte progenitor cells and induces megakaryocyte maturation, resulting in increased platelet production. It prevents severe thrombocytopenia and reduces the need for platelet transfusions following myelosuppressive chemotherapy in patients with nonmyeloid malignancies.

IL-11 was cloned based on its activity to promote proliferation of an IL-6-dependent myeloma cell line. The 23,000-dalton cytokine contains 178 amino acids, stimulates hematopoiesis, intestinal epithelial cell growth, and osteoclastogenesis, and inhibits adipogenesis. IL-11 enhances megakaryocyte maturation *in vitro*, and its *in vivo* administration to animals modestly increases peripheral blood platelet counts. Clinical trials in patients who previously demonstrated significant chemotherapy-induced thrombocytopenia demonstrated that administration of the recombinant cytokine was associated with less severe thrombocytopenia and reduced use of platelet transfusion, resulting in its approval for clinical use by the FDA.

Recombinant human IL-11 **oprelvekin** (Neumega) is a bacterially derived, 19,000-dalton polypeptide of 177 amino acids that differs from the native protein only because it lacks the amino terminal proline residue and is not glycosylated. The recombinant protein has a 7-hour half-life after subcutaneous injection. In normal subjects, daily administration of oprelvekin leads to a thrombopoietic response in 5 to 9 days.

The drug is available in single-use vials containing 5 mg and is administered to patients at 25 to 50 μg/kg per day subcutaneously. **Oprelvekin** is approved for use in patients undergoing chemotherapy for nonmyeloid malignancies that displayed severe thrombocytopenia (platelet count <20,000/μl) on a prior cycle of the same chemotherapy and is administered until the platelet count returns to more than 100,000/μl. The major complications of the therapy are fluid retention and other associated cardiac symptoms, such as tachycardia, palpitation, edema, and shortness of breath; this is a significant concern in elderly patients and often requires concomitant therapy with diuretics. Fluid retention reverses upon drug discontinuation, but volume status should be carefully monitored in elderly patients, those with a history of heart failure, or those with preexisting fluid collections in the pleura, pericardium, or peritoneal cavity. Also reported are blurred vision, injection-site rash or erythema, and paresthesias.

ORAL HYPOGLYCEMIC AGENTS

First-Generation Agents
- Acetohexamide
- Chlorpropamide
- Tolazamide
- Tolbutamide

Second-Generation Agents
- Glipizide
- Glyburide

ORGANOPHOSPHOROUS COMPOUNDS

The cholinesterase inhibitors are divided into two categories: organophosphorous compounds, such as parathion, malathion, and tetraethyl pyrophosphate (TEPP), and the carbamates, such as naphthyl-*N*-methyl carbamate (carbaryl and Sevin).

The clinical manifestations of acute and severe poisoning from the organophosphorous insecticides include cholinergic crisis, resulting from the stimulation of muscarine cholinergic receptors (bronchoconstriction, salivation, sweating, lacrimation, bradycardia, hypotension, and urinary and fecal incontinence), from the stimulation of nicotinic cholinergic receptors (muscular fasciculation), and from CNS effects (with initial restlessness, tremors, ataxia, and convulsions, followed by CNS depression and respiratory and circulatory depression). The treatment of a cholinergic crisis caused by organophosphorous compounds includes the administration of a cholinesterase reactivator such as pralidoxine (2-PAM) together with atropine. The poisoning stemming from antidoting with 2-PAM can be avoided in the event of carbaryl toxicity, because this agent is a reversible cholinesterase inhibitor (see Figure 79).

ORLISTAT

(Xenical capsules 120 mg)

Orlistat is a lipase inhibitor that acts as a reversible lipase inhibitor for obesity management by inhibiting absorption of dietary fats. It is indicated for obesity management, including weight loss and weight maintenance when used in combination with a reduced-calorie diet; it reduces the risk for weight regain after weight loss.

Orlistat, a GI lipase inhibitor used for weight loss, was administered over a 4-year period that resulted in a 37% reduction in the progression of type 2 diabetes mellitus in a group of insulin-resistant obese patients. Finally, although the mechanisms are poorly understood, there are reports that **ACE inhibitors** are associated with a decreased incidence of diabetes mellitus in high-risk patients.

Based on the evidence that a variety of pharmacological agents can delay—and perhaps prevent—the onset of type 2 diabetes mellitus, multiple studies are under way investigating the effects of a range of pharmacologic agents in the prevention of type 2 diabetes mellitus.

ORPHAN DRUGS: Proposed Uses of

Acetylcysteine	for	Acetaminophen overdose
N-Acetylprocainamide	for	Arrhythmia
Aconiazide	for	Tuberculosis
Adenosine with BCNU	for	Treatment of brain tumors
Aldesleukin	for	Metastatic renal cell carcinoma
Alglucerase	for	Gaucher's disease type 1
Allopurinol riboside	for	Chagas' disease
Allopurinol sodium	for	Leukemia and lymphoma
L-Alpha-acetyl-methadol (LAAM)	for	Addiction to narcotics
Alpha-1-antitrypsin (recombinant DNA origin)	for	Alpha-1 antitrypsin deficiency
Alpha-galactosidase A (FABRase)	for	Fabry's disease
Alpha-1-proteinase inhibitor	for	Replacement therapy in alpha-1-proteinase inhibitor congenital deficiency state
Altretamine	for	Ovarian adenocarcinoma
Amiloride HCL	for	Cystic fibrosis
4-Aminopyridine	for	Multiple sclerosis
Aminosalicylate sodium	for	Crohn's disease
4-Aminosalicylic acid	for	Ulcerative colitis
Aminosidine	for	*Mycobacterium avium* complex
Amiodarone	for	Ventricular tachycardia
Ammonium tetrathimolybdate	for	Wilson's disease
Amphotericin B lipid complex	for	Cryptococcal meningitis
Amsacrine	for	Leukemia
Anagrelide	for	Polycythemia vera
Ananain, Comosain	for	Enzymatic debridement of severe burns
Anaritide acetate	for	Improving renal functions following transplantation
Ancrod	for	Antithrombotic effects
Antiepilepsirine	for	Epilepsy
Antihemophilic factor	for	von Willebrand's disease
Antihemophilic factor	for	Hemophilia
Autolymphocyte therapy; ALT	for	Renal cancer
Antimelanoma antibody	for	Imaging melanoma metastasis
Anti-pan T-lymphocyte monoclonal antibody (Anti-T)	for	Bone marrow recipients
Antipyrine	for	Diagnostic agent for hepatic function
Anti-Tac	for	Bone marrow transplantation
Anti-TAP-72 immunotoxin	for	Colorectal cancer
Antithrombin III	for	Thromboembolic episodes in genetic AT-III deficiency
Anti-thymocyte serum	for	Transplantation
Antivenin	for	Treatment of snake envenomations
Apomorphine HCl	for	Parkinson's disease
Aprotinin	for	Patients undergoing repeat coronary artery bypass graft (CABG) surgery
Arginine butyrate	for	Treatment of beta-hemoglobinopathies
Atovaquone	for	AIDS-associated *Pneumocystis carinii* pneumonia (PCP)
Bacitracin	for	Pseudomembranous entercolitis
Baclofen, L-Baclofen	for	Spasticity
Benzoate and phenylacetate	for	Prevention of hyperammonemia
Benzylpenicillin	to	Test hypersensitivity to penicillin
Beractant	to	Prevent respiratory distress syndrome in the newborn
Beta-glucocerebrosidase	for	Gaucher's disease

ORPHAN DRUGS: Proposed Uses of (Continued)

Betaine	for	Homocystinuria
Bethanidine sulfate	for	Prevention of ventricular fibrillation
Biodegradable polymer implant containing carmustine	for	Treatment of malignant glioma
Bispecific antibody 520C9x22	for	Ovarian cancer
Bleomycin sulfate	for	Pleural effusion
Botulinum toxin type A	for	Dystonia
Botulinum toxin type B	for	Cervical dystonia
Botulinum toxin type F	for	Torticollis and blepharospasm
Botulism immune globulin	for	Botulism
Bovine colostrum	for	AIDS-related diarrhea
Bovine whey protein concentrate (Immuno-C)	for	Cryptosporidiosis
Branched chain amino acids	for	Amyotrophic lateral sclerosis
Bromhexine	for	Keratoconjunctivitis sicca in Sjogren's syndrome
Busulfan	for	Malignancies
Butyrylcholinesterase	for	Cocaine toxicity
BW 12 C	for	Sickle cell disease
C1-Esterase inhibitor	for	Hereditary angioedema
Caffeine	for	Apnea
Calcitonin	for	Paget's disease
Calcium acetate	for	Hyperphosphatemia
Calcium carbonate	for	Hyperphosphatemia
Calcium gluconate gel	for	Treatment of hydrogen fluoride (hydrofluoric acid) burns
Carbovir	for	AIDS
CCD 1042	for	Infantile spasms
CD4 human truncated 369 AA polypeptide	for	AIDS
CD4 immunoglobulin G, recombinant human	for	AIDS
CD5-T-lymphocyte immunotoxin	for	Bone marrow tranplants
CD45 monoclonal antibodies	for	Organ transplants
Ceramide trihexosidase alpha-galactosidase A	for	Fabry's disease
Chenodiol	for	Gallbladder stones
Chimeric M-T412 IgG monoclonal anti-CD4	for	Multiple sclerosis
Chimeric (murine variable, human constant) Mab to CD20	for	Non-Hodgkin's B-cell lymphoma
Chlorhexidine gluconate mouth rinse	for	Oral mucositis
Choline chloride	for	Choline deficiency
Ciliary neurotrophic factor	for	Amyotrophic lateral sclerosis
Citric acid, glucono-delta-lactone and mag carbonate	for	Renal and bladder calculi
Cladribine	for	Hairy-cell and chronic lymphocytic leukemias; non-Hodgkin's lymphoma; chronic multiple sclerosis
Clindamycin	for	*Pneumocystis carinii* pneumonia associated with AIDS
Clofazimine	for	Lepromatous leprosy
Clonidine HCl	for	Treating pain in cancer
Coagulation factor IX	for	Hemophilia B
Colchicine	for	Multiple sclerosis
Colfosceril palmitate, cetyl alcohol, tyloxapol	for	Hyaline membrane disease
Copolymer 1, (COP 1)	for	Multiple sclerosis
Corticorelin ovine triflutate	to	Diagnose ACTH-dependent Cushing's syndrome
Cromolyn sodium	for	Mastocytosis
Cromolyn sodium 4% ophthalmic solution	for	Vernal keratoconjunctivitis
Cryptosporidium hyper immune bovine colostrum IgG concentrate	for	Diarrhea in AIDS
Cryptosporidium parvum bovine immunoglobulin concentrate	for	Treatment of *Cryptosporidium parvum* infection of the GI tract in immunocompromised patients
CY-1503	for	Postischemic pulmonary reperfusion edema
CY-1899	for	Hepatitis B infection
L-Cycloserine	for	Gaucher's disease
Cyclosporine ophthalmic	for	Keratoconjunctivitis sicca with Sjogren's syndrome
Cyclosporine 2% ophthalmic ointment	following	Keratoplasty
Cyproterone acetate	for	Hirsutism
Cysteamine	for	Nephrophatic cystinosis
L-Cysteine	in	Erythropoietic protoporphyria
Cystic fibrosis gene therapy	in	Cystic fibrosis
Cytarabine	for	Neoplastic meningitis
Cytomegalovirus immune globulin	for	Immunosuppressed recipients of organ transplants

ORPHAN DRUGS: Proposed Uses of (Continued)

Cytomegalovirus immune globulin (human) IV with ganciclovir sodium	for	Treatment of CMV pneumonia in bone marrow transplant patients
Dapsone	for	Prophylaxis of *Pneumocystis carinii* pneumonia
Defibrotide	for	Thrombocytopenic purpura
Dehydrex	for	Corneal erosion
Deoxyadenosine, 2-chloro-2′	for	Acute myeloid leukemia
Deoxycytidine, 5-AZA-2′	for	Acute leukemia
Deslorelin	for	Precocious puberty
Desmopressin acetate	for	Hemophilia A and von Willebrand's disease
Dexrazoxane	for	Prevention of doxorubicin-induced cardiomyopathy
Dextran and deferoxamine	for	Iron poisoning
Dextran sulfate	for	Cystic fibrosis
Dextran sulfate sodium	for	AIDS
3,4-Diaminopyridine	for	Lambert–Eaton myasthenic syndrome
Dianeal PD-2 peritoneal dialysis solution. with 1.1% amino acid	for	Malnutrition in peritoneal dialysis
Diazepam	for	Status epilepticus
Dibromodulcitol	for	Metastatic squamous cervical carcinoma
Dichloroacetate sodium	for	Lactic acidosis
Diethyldithiocarbamate	for	AIDS
Digoxin immune fab	for	Digitalis intoxication
Dihematoporphyrin ether	for	Therapy of transitional cell carcinoma
24,25-Dihydroxycholecalciferol	for	Uremic osteodystrophy
Dipalmitoylphosphatidylcholine/phosphatidyl glycerol	for	Neonatal respiratory distress syndrome
Disaccharide tripeptide glycerol dipalmitoyl	for	Pulmonary and hepatic metastases in colorectal adenocarcinoma
Disodium clodronate	for	Hypercalcemia of malignancy
Disodium clodronate tetrahydrate	for	Malignancy-induced bone resorption
Disodium silibinin dihemisuccinate	for	Mushroom poisoning
Dornase (deoxyribonuclease, recombinant human; rhDNase)	for	Cystic fibrosis
Dronabinol	to	Stimulate appetite in AIDS
Dynamine	for	Lambert–Eaton myasthenic syndrome and Charcot–Marie tooth disease
Eflornithine HCl	for	*Trypanosoma brucei gambiense* (sleeping sickness); *Pneumocystis carinii* pneumonia in AIDS
Enisoprost with cyclosporine	in	organ transplant recipients
Epidermal growth factor	for	Corneal epithelial regeneration and healing
Epoetin alfa	for	Anemia associated with end-stage renal disease
Epoetin beta	for	Anemia associated with end-stage renal disease
Epoprostenol	for	Primary pulmonary hypertension
Erwinia L-asparaginase	for	Acute lymphocytic leukemia
Erythropoietin	for	Anemia related to HIV infection or anemia associated with end-stage renal disease; anemia of premature infants
Ethanolamine oleate	for	Esophageal varices
Ethinyl estradiol	for	Turner's syndrome
Ethiofos	as	Chemoprotective agent for cisplatin and cyclophosphamide
Etidronate disodium	for	Hypercalcemia of malignancy
Factor VII-a recombinant, DNA origin	for	Hemophilia A and B
Factor XIII	for	Congenital factor XIII deficiency
Felbamate	for	Lennox-Gastaut syndrome
FGN-1	for	Colonic adenomatous polyps
FIAU	for	Treatment of hepatitis B
Fibronectin	for	Corneal ulcers
Filgrastim	for	Myelodysplastic syndrome
Fire ant venom	for	Diagnosing allergy to fire ant
Fludarabine phosphate	for	Non-Hodgkin's lymphoma
Flumecinol	for	Hyperbilirubinemia in newborns unresponsive to phototherapy

ORPHAN DRUGS: Proposed Uses of (Continued)

Flunarizine	for	Hemiplegia
Fluorouracil with interferon alpha-2a	for	Esophageal colorectal carcinoma
Fluorouracil with leucovorin	for	Metastatic adenocarcinoma of the colon and rectum
Fosphenytoin	for	Status epilepticus
Gallium nitrate injection	for	Hypercalcemia of malignancy
Gangliosides	for	Retinitis pigmentosa
Gelsolin	for	Cystic fibrosis
Gentamicin	for	Osteomyelitis
Glucocerebrosidase	for	Gaucher's disease
L-Glutathione	for	Cachexia
Gonadorelin acetate	to	Induce ovulation
Gossypol	for	Cancer of the adrenal cortex
Granulocyte macrophage colony-stimulating factor	for	AIDS
Growth hormone releasing factor	for	Children who have failed to grow
Guanethidine monosulfate	for	Sympathetic dystrophy and causalgia
Halofantrine	for	Malaria
Heme arginate	for	Acute porphyria; myelodysplastic syndromes
Hemin	for	Porphyria variegata and heredita coproporphyria
Hemin and zinc mesoporphyrin	for	Acute porphyric syndromes
Heparin, 2-0-desulfated	for	Cystic fibrosis
Herpes simplex virus gene	for	Primary and metastatic brain tumors
Histrelin	for	Treatment of acute intermittent porphyria, hereditary coproporphyria, and variegata porphyria
Histrelin acetate	for	Precocious puberty
HIV-neutralizing antibodies	for	AIDS
HIV immune globulin	for	AIDS
Hydroxocobalamin/sodium thiosulfate	for	Cyanide poisoning
L-5 Hydroxytryptophan	for	Myoclonus
Hydroxyurea	for	Sickle-cell anemia
I-131 radiolabeled B1 monoclonal antibody	for	Non-Hodgkin's B-cell lymphoma
Idarubicin HCl	for	Myelodysplastic syndromes
Ifosfamide	for	Germ-cell testicular cancer; bone sarcomas; soft tissue sarcomas
Iloprost infusion solution	for	Raynaud's phenomenon secondary to systemic sclerosis
Imciromab pentetate	for	Cardiac transplants
Immune globulin IV	for	Juvenile rheumatoid arthritis; polymyositis/dermatomyositis; infection prophylaxis in pediatric patients with HIV; acute myocarditis
Indium in 111 altumomab pentetate	for	Tumor detection
Indium in 111 murine monoclonal antibody fab to myosin	for	Diagnosis of myocarditis
Inosine pranobex	for	Subacute sclerosing panencephalitis
Insulin-like growth factor-1	for	Amyotrophic lateral sclerosis
Interferon alfa-2a	for	Chronic myelogenous leukemia
Interferon alfa-2a with fluorouracil	for	Advanced colorectal cancer and esophageal carcinoma
Interferon alfa-2a with teceleukin	for	Metastatic malignant melanoma and renal-cell carcinoma
Interferon alfa-2b	for	AIDS-related Kaposi's sarcoma; acute hepatitis B; chronic myelogenous leukemia
Interferon alfa-NL	for	AIDS-related Kaposi's sarcoma
Interferon beta	for	Multiple sclerosis
Interferon beta	for	Cutaneous T-cell lymphoma; malignant melanoma; metastatic renal-cell carcinoma
Interferon gamma 1-B	for	Chronic granulomatous disease
Interleukin-1 alpha	for	Bone marrow transplantation
Interleukin-1 receptor antagonist	for	Juvenile rheumatoid arthritis
Interleukin-2	for	Cancers of the kidney
Interleukin-3	for	Promotion of erythropoiesis
Iodine I-123 murine monoclonal antibody to alpha-fetoprotein	to	Detect alpha-fetoprotein-producing germ-cell tumors
Iodine I-123 murine monoclonal antibody to hCG	for	Detection of hCG-producing tumors
Iodine I-131 6B-iodomethyl-19-norcholesterol	for	Adrenal cortical imaging
Iodine I-131 metaiodobenzylguanidine sulfate	for	Diagnosis of pheochromocytoma

ORPHAN DRUGS: Proposed Uses of (Continued)

Iodine I-131 murine monoclonal antibody IgG2a to B-cell	for	B-cell lymphoma and B-cell leukemia
Isobutyramide	for	Sickle cell disease; beta-thalassemia; beta-hemoglobinopathies; beta-thalassemia syndromes
Ketoconazole with cyclosporine	in	Organ transplantation
Lactobin	in	AIDS-associated diarrhea
Leucovorin with methotrexate	in	Treatment of osteosarcoma
Leucovorin with 5-Fluorouracil	for	Metastatic colorectal cancer
Leukocyte protease inhibitor	for	Congenital alpha-1 antitrypsin deficiency; cystic fibrosis
Leukocyte protease inhibitor	for	Bronchopulmonary dysplasia
Leupeptin	to	Repair peripheral nerve
Leuprolide acetate	for	Precocious puberty
Levocarnitine	for	Carnitine deficiency
Levomethadyl acetate HCl	for	Addiction to narcotics
Liothyronine sodium injection	for	Myxedema coma
Lodoxamide tromethamine	for	Vernal keratoconjunctivitis
Loxoribine	for	Immunodeficiency
Mafenide acetate solution	for	Prevention of graft loss
Matrix metalloproteinase inhibitor	for	Corneal ulcers
Mazindol	for	Duchenne muscular dystrophy
Mefloquine HCl	for	Malaria
Megestrol acetate	for	Anorexia, cachexia or significant weight loss due to AIDS
Melanoma vaccine	for	Melanoma
Melatonin	for	Sleep disorders in blind people
Melphalan	for	Multiple myeloma
Mesna	for	Reducing ifosfamide-induced hemorrhagic cystitis
Methotrexate	for	Juvenile rheumatoid arthritis
Methotrexate sodium	for	Osteogenic sarcoma
Methotrexate with laurocapram	for	Topical treatment of Mycosis fungoides
8-Methoxsalen in conjunction with UVAR	to	Diffuse systemic sclerosis; for prevention of acute rejection of cardiac allografts
6-Methylenandrosta-1,4-diene-3,17-dione	for	Metastatic carcinoma of the breast
4-Methylpyrazole	for	Ethylene glycol poisoning
Metronidazole (topical)	for	Decubitus ulcers; acne rosacea; perioral dermatitis
Microbubble contrast agents	for	Diagnosing intracranial tumors
Midodrine HCl	for	Orthostatic hypotension
Minocycline HCl	for	Malignant pleural effusion
Mitoguazone	for	Non-Hodgkin's lymphoma
Mitoxantrone HCl	for	Acute myelogenous leukemia
Modafinil	for	Narcolepsy
Monoclonal antibodies B-cell lymphoma	for	B-cell lymphoma
Monoclonal antibodies PM-81	for	Acute myelogenous leukemia
Monoclonal antibody 17-1A	for	Pancreatic cancer
Monoclonal antibody to CD4, 5a8	for	Prophylaxis for exposure to HIV
Monoclonal antibody against hepatitis B virus	for	Prophylaxis of hepatitis B reinfection
Monoclonal antibody for lupus nephritis	for	Immunization against lupus nephritis
Monolaurin	for	Congenital primary ichthyosis
Monomercaptoundecahydrocloso-DO decaborate sodium	for	Glioblastoma multiforme
Monoctanoin	for	Dissolution of cholesterol gallstones
Morphine sulfate concentrate	for	Intraspinal administration for intractable chronic pain
Multivitamin infusion	for	Parenteral nutrition in low-birth-weight infants
Myelin	for	Multiple sclerosis
Mytomycin-C	for	Refractory glaucoma
Nafarelin acetate	for	Precocious puberty
Naltrexone HCl	for	Opioid addiction
Nebacumab	for	Opioid dependence
NG-29	for	Diagnosis of pituitary function
Nifedipine	for	Interstitial cystitis
Nitric oxide	for	Pulmonary hypertension
Ofloxacin solution	for	Bacterial corneal ulcers
OM 401	for	Sickle-cell disease
OncoRad OV103	for	Ovarian cancer
Oxaliplatin	for	Ovarian cancer

ORPHAN DRUGS: Proposed Uses of (Continued)

Oxandrolone	for	Turner's syndrome
L-2-Oxothiazolidine-4-carboxylic acid	for	Respiratory distress syndrome
Oxymorphone HCl	for	Relief of severe intractable pain in narcotic-tolerant patients
Papaverine topical gel	for	Sexual dysfunction in spinal cord injury patients
Paraaminosalicylic acid	for	Tuberculosis
Pegademase bovine	for	Severe combined immunodeficiency (SCID)
Pegaspargase	for	Acute lymphocytic leukemia
PEG-Glucocerebrosidase	for	Gaucher's disease
PEG-interleukin-2	for	Immunodeficiencies associated with T-cell defects
PEG-L-asparaginase	for	Acute lymphocytic leukemia
Pentamidine isethionate	for	*Pneumocystis carinii* pneumonia (PCP)
Pentamidine isethionate (inhalation)	for	PCP prevention in high-risk patients
Pentastarch	as	Adjunct in leukapheresis
Pentosan sodium polysulfate	for	Interstitial cystitis
Pentostatin	for	Chronic lymphocytic leukemia
Perfosfamide	in	Bone marrow transplants
Phenylbutyrate sodium	for	Sickling disorders; urea cycle disorders: Carbamylphosphate synthetase deficiency, ornithine transcarbamylase deficiency, and argininosuccinic acid synthetase deficiency
Phosphocysteamine	for	Cystinosis
Physostigmine salicylate	for	Friedreich's ataxias
Pilocarpine HCl	for	Xerostomia and keratoconjunctivitis
Piracetam	for	Myoclonus
Piritrexim isethionate	for	Infection caused by *P. carinii, Toxoplasma gondii*, and *Mycobacterium avium-intracellulare*
Poloxamer 188	for	Sickle-cell crisis
Poloxamer 331	for	Toxoplasmosis
Poly I: Poly C12U	for	Renal-cell carcinoma; invasive metastatic melanoma
Polymeric oxygen	for	Sickle-cell anemia
Potassium citrate	for	Uric acid nephrolithiasis; calcium renal stones
PPI-002	for	Malignant mesothelioma
PR-122 (Redox-phenytoin)	for	Status epilepticus
PR-225 (Redox-acyclovir)	for	Herpes simplex encephalitis
PR-239 (Redox-penicillin G)	for	Neurosyphilis
PR-320 (Molecusolcarbamazepine)	for	Status epilepticus
Pramiracetam sulfate	for	Cognitive dysfunction
Prednimustine	for	Malignant non-Hodgkin's lymphomas
Primaquine phosphate with clindamycin	in	Treatment of PCP associated with AIDS
Propamidine isethionate 0.1% ophthalmic solution.	for	Acanthamoeba keratitis
Prostaglandin E1 alpha-cyclodextrin	for	Peripheral arterial occlusive disease
Protein C concentrate	for	Congenital or acquired protein C deficiency
Protirelin	for	Respiratory distress syndrome associated with prematurity
Pseudomonas hyperimmune globulin (mucoid exopolysaccharide) (MEPIG)	for	Pulmonary *Pseudomonas aeruginosa* infections in cystic fibrosis
Pulmonary surfactant replacement	for	Infant respiratory distress syndrome
9-[3-pyridylmethyl]-9-deazaguanine	for	Cutaneous T-cell lymphoma
Respiratory syncytial virus immune globulin	for	Respiratory syncytial virus lower respiratory tract infections
Retinoic acid all-trans	for	Acute promyelocytic leukemia
Retinoic acid, 9-cis	for	Acute promyelocytic leukemia
Rho(D) immune globulin	for	Immune thrombocytopenic purpura
Ribavirin	for	Hemorrhagic fever with renal syndrome
Ricin conjugated murine MCA (anti-MY9)	for	Acute myelogenous leukemia; myeloid leukemia
Rifabutin	for	Disseminated *Mycobacterium avium* complex disease
Rifampin	for	Tuberculosis
Rifampin, isoniazid, pyrazinamide	for	Tuberculosis
Riluzole	for	Amyotrophic lateral sclerosis
Roquinimex	for	Bone marrow transplantation in leukemic patients
Sargramostim	for	Neutropenia associated with bone marrow transplant
Satumomab pendetide	for	Diagnosis of ovarian carcinoma
SDZ MSL-109	for	Cytomegalovirus disease
Secalciferol	for	Familial hypophosphatemic rickets

ORPHAN DRUGS: Proposed Uses of (Continued)

Selegiline HCl	for	Neuroprotection in Parkinson's disease
Sermorelin acetate	for	Growth-hormone deficiency
Serratia marcescens extract (polyribosomes)	for	Brain malignancies
Short chain fatty acid solution	for	Ulcerative colitis
SK&F 110679	for	Growth-hormone deficiency
Sodium benzoate/sodium phenylacetate	for	Urea cycle disorders: Carbamylphosphate synthetase deficiency, ornithine transcarbamylase deficiency, and argininosuccinic acid synthetase deficiency
Sodium/gamma hydroxybutyrate	for	Narcolepsy
Sodium tetradecyl sulfate	for	Bleeding esophageal varices
Somatostatin	for	Nonoperative management of secreting cutaneous fistulas of the stomach, duodenum, small intestine, or pancreas
Somatropin	for	Growth-hormone deficiency
Sotalol HCl	for	Ventricular tachyarrhythmias
Streptococcus immune globulin group B	for	Disseminated Group B streptococcal infection
ST1-RTA immunotoxin (SR 44163)	for	Lymphocytic leukemia
Succimer	for	Kidney stones
Sucralfate	for	Oral mucositis and stomatitis
Sucrase	for	Sucrase-isomaltase deficiency
Sulfadiazine with pyrimethamine	for	*Toxoplasma gondii*
Superoxide dismutase	for	Protection of donor organ during operative procedures
T4 endonuclease V	for	Cutaneous neoplasma
Teceleukin with interferon alfa-2a	for	Metastatic renal-cell carcinoma and malignant melanoma
Technetium TC-99M antimelanoma murine monoclonal antibody	for	Imaging, metastases of malignant melanoma
Teniposide	for	Acute lymphocytic leukemia
Teriparatide	for	Hypocalcemia due to hypoparathyroidism
Terlipressin	for	Bleeding esophageal varices
Testosterone ointment 2%	for	Vulvar dystrophies
Testosterone sublingual	for	Constitutional delay of growth and puberty in boys
Thalidomide	for	Bone marrow transplantation
L-Threonine	for	Spasticity associated with familial spastic paraparesis; amyotrophic lateral sclerosis
Thymosin alpha-1	for	Active hepatitis B
Thyroid stimulating hormone (TSH)	for	Diagnosis of thyroid cancer
Tiopronin	for	Cystine nephrolithiasis
Tiratricol with levothyroxine	to	suppress TSH in patients with thyroid cancer
Tizanidine HCl	for	Spasticity associated with multiple sclerosis and spinal cord injury
T-lymphotropic virus type III gp 160 antigens	for	AIDS
Topiramate	for	Lennox–Gastaut syndrome
Toremifene	for	Metastatic breast carcinoma
Tranexamic acid	for	Angioneurotic edema
Transforming growth factor-beta 2	for	Macular holes
Treosulfan	for	Ovarian cancer
Tretinoin	for	Squamous metaplasia of ocular surface epithelia
Tretinoin LF, IV	for	Leukemia
Trientine HCl	for	Wilson's disease
Trifluoroacetyladriamycin-14 valerate	for	Carcinoma of the urinary bladder
Trimetrexate glucuronate	for	Advanced non-small-cell carcinoma of the lung
Triptorelin pamoate	for	Ovarian carcinoma
Trisaccharides A and B	for	Hemolytic disease of the newborn
Troleandomycin	for	Asthma
Tumor necrosis factor-binding protein I and II	for	AIDS
Urofollitropin	to	Induce ovulation
Urogastrone	for	Corneal transplant surgery
Ursodeoxycholic acid	for	Cirrhosis
Ursodiol	for	Cirrhosis
Zalcitabine	for	AIDS
Zidovudine	for	AIDS
Zinc acetate	for	Wilson's disease

ORPHENADRINE CITRATE

(Banflex injection 30 mg/mL, Flexoject injection 20 mg/mL, Flexon injection 20 mg/mL, Norflex tablets, sustained-release 100 mg, injection 30 mg/mL)

Orphenadrine is a skeletal muscle relaxant. Its mechanism of action is unknown; it may be related to analgesic properties, as the drug acts on brain stem and does not act directly on muscles; possesses anticholinergic actions. It is used as an adjunctive treatment for acute, painful musculoskeletal conditions.

ORPHENADRINE CITRATE/ASPIRIN/CAFFEINE

(Norgesic tablets 25 mg orphenadrine citrate per 385 mg aspirin per 30 mg caffeine, Norgesic Forte tablets 50 mg orphenadrine citrate per 770 mg aspirin per 60 mg caffeine)

Orphenadrine citrate/aspirin/caffeine is a skeletal muscle relaxant. **Orphenadrine's** action may be related to its analgesic properties. **Aspirin** inhibits prostaglandin synthesis, resulting in analgesia, antiinflammatory activity, and inhibition of platelet aggregation. **Caffeine** is thought to produce constriction of cerebral blood vessels. It is indicated in symptomatic relief of mild to moderate pain of acute musculoskeletal disorders; and as an adjunct to rest, physical therapy, and other measures for the relief of discomfort with acute painful musculoskeletal conditions.

Orphenadrine citrate, which possesses analgesic and anticholinergic actions (100 mg each morning and evening), is indicated as an adjunct to rest, physical therapy, and other measures for relief of discomfort associated with acute, painful musculoskeletal conditions, including leg cramps. Because of its anticholinergic properties, orphenadrine is contraindicated in glaucoma, pyloric or duodenal obstruction, stenosing peptic ulcers, prostatic hypertrophy, obstruction of the bladder neck, cardiospasm (megaesophagus), and myasthenia gravis.

Orphenadrine's anticholinergic property is potentiated by amantadine. Orphenadrine antagonizes the effectiveness of haloperidol or chlorpromazine in managing schizophrenia. The adverse reactions, usually seen with higher-than-therapeutic doses, are primarily related to orphenadrine's anticholinergic properties, and include dry mouth, tachycardia, palpitations, transient syncope, weakness, headache, dizziness, light-headedness, confusion (in elderly patients), hallucinations, agitation, tremor, drowsiness, vomiting, nausea, constipation, gastric irritation, urinary hesitancy and retention, blurred vision, pupil dilation, and increased ocular tension.

OSELTAMIVIR PHOSPHATE

(Tamiflu capsules 75 mg, powder for oral suspension 12 mg/mL)

Oseltamivir phosphate is an antiviral agent that acts to inhibit influenza virus neuraminidase with possible alteration of virus particle aggregation and release. It is indicated in the treatment of uncomplicated acute illness caused by influenza infection in patients older than 1 year who have been symptomatic for 2 days or less; and for prophylaxis of influenza in patients 13 years and older.

Oseltamivir carboxylate [(3R, 4R, 5S)-4-acetylamino-5-amino-3(l-ethylpropoxyl)-l-cyclohexene-l-carboxylic acid] is a transition-state analog of sialic acid that is a potent selective inhibitor of influenza A and B virus neuraminidases.

Oseltamivir phosphate is an ethyl ester prodrug that lacks antiviral activity. Oseltamivir carboxylate has an antiviral spectrum and potency similar to that of **zanamivir**. It inhibits amantadine- and rimantadine-resistant influenza A viruses and some zanamivir-resistant variants.

Influenza neuraminidase cleaves terminal sialic acid residues and destroys the receptors recognized by viral hemagglutinin, which are present on the cell surface, in progeny virions, and in respiratory secretions. This enzymatic action is essential for release of virus from infected cells. Interaction of oseltamivir carboxylate with the neuraminidase causes a conformational change within the enzyme's active site and inhibits its activity. Inhibition of neuraminidase activity leads to viral aggregation at the cell surface and reduced virus spread within the respiratory tract.

Influenza variants selected *in vitro* for resistance to oseltamivir carboxylate contain hemagglutinin and/or neuraminidase mutations. The most commonly recognized variants (mutations at positions 292 in N2 and 274 in N1 neuraminidases) have reduced infectivity and virulence in animal models. Outpatient **oseltamivir** therapy has been associated with recovery of resistant variants in about 0.5% of adults and 5.5% of children; a higher frequency (~18%) occurs in hospitalized children.

Oral **oseltamivir phosphate** is absorbed rapidly and cleaved by esterases in the GI tract and liver to the active carboxylate. Low levels of the phosphate are detectable, but exposure is only 3 to 5% of that of the metabolite. The bioavailability of the carboxylate is estimated to be approximately 80%. The time to maximum plasma concentrations of the carboxylate is about 2.5 to 5 hours. Food does not decrease bioavailability but produces the risk of GI intolerance. After 75-mg doses, peak plasma concentrations average 0.07 μg/mL for **oseltamivir phosphate** and 0.35 μg/mL for the carboxylate. The carboxylate has a volume of distribution similar to extracellular water. Bronchoalveolar lavage levels in animals and middle-ear fluid and sinus concentrations in humans are comparable with plasma levels. Following oral administration, the plasma half-life of **oseltamivir phosphate** is 1 to 3 hours and that of the carboxylate ranges from 6 to 10 hours. Both the prodrug and active metabolite are eliminated primarily unchanged through the kidney. Probenecid doubles the plasma half-life of the carboxylate, which indicates tubular secretion by the anionic pathway.

OSTEOPOROSIS: Treatment of

Osteoporosis is a systemic skeletal disease characterized by a low bone mass and microarchitectural deterioration of bone tissue, with a consequent increase in bone fragility and susceptibility to fracture. It is a major cause of mortality, morbidity, and medical expense worldwide.

In the last few years, the concept of whole-life prevention has emerged. Before menopause, the prevention of osteoporosis may be achieved by increasing the bone mass at maturity. As peak bone mass is influenced by environmental as well as genetic factors, the bone mass at skeletal maturity might be improved during childhood and adolescence and, later in the young adult, by exercise, calcium intake, avoidance of smoking, and/or alcohol, and correction of estrogen-deficiency states.

The treatment of established osteoporosis includes two different approaches in order to prevent the worsening of the bone loss. One uses therapeutic agents that reduce bone resorption, and the other consists in using compounds that can stimulate bone formation. Ideally, these treatments should not only stimulate bone formation and increase bone mass, but also restore a normal bone microarchitecture in order to decrease the occurrence of new fractures. Selective analogs of estrogen, such as raloxifen and droloxifen, might be alternatives to estrogen in the prevention of late postmenopausal bone loss.

Oral **oseltamivir** is associated with nausea, abdominal discomfort, and, less often, emesis, probably owing to local irritation. GI complaints usually are mild to moderate in intensity, typically resolve in 1 to 2 days despite continued dosing, and are preventable by administration with food. The frequency of such complaints is about 10 to 15% when oseltamivir is used for the treatment of influenza illness and less than 5% when used for prophylaxis. An increased frequency of headache was reported in one prophylaxis study in elderly adults.

Oseltamivir phosphate and the carboxylate do not interact with the cytochrome P450 enzymes (CYPs) *in vitro*. Their protein binding is low. No clinically significant drug interactions have been recognized to date. Oseltamivir does not appear to impair fertility or to be teratogenic in animal studies, but safety in pregnancy is uncertain (pregnancy category C). Very high doses have been associated with increased mortality, perhaps related to increased brain concentrations, in unweaned rats, and **oseltamivir** is not approved for use in children younger than 1 year of age.

Oral oseltamivir is effective in the treatment and prevention of influenza A and B virus infections. Treatment of previously healthy adults (75 mg twice daily for 5 days) or children aged 1 to 12 years (weight-adjusted dosing) with acute influenza reduces illness duration by about 1 to 2 days, speeds functional recovery, and reduces the risk of complications leading to antibiotic use by 40 to 50%. Treatment is associated with approximate halving the risk of subsequent hospitalization in adults. When used for prophylaxis during the influenza season, oseltamivir (75 mg

OTITIS MEDIA: Treatment of

Antibiotics*	*Streptococcus pneumoniae*	*Haemophilus influenzae* β-Lactamase Negative	*Haemophilus influenzae* β-Lactamase Positive	*Moraxella catarrhalis* β-Lactamase Negative	*Moraxella catarrhalis* β-Lactamase Positive
Penicillin V	+++++	0	0	0	0
Amoxicillin	++++++	++	0	++++++	0
Ampicillin	++++++	+	0	+++	0
Trimethoprim	+	++	+++	0	0
Sulfamethoxazole	+	++++	++	+	0
Cefaclor	+	+	+	+	+
Erythromycin					
estolate	+++	0	0	+	+
ethylsuccinate	+	0	0	+	+

* Spectrum of activity.

OTOTOXICITY: Drug-Induced

		Antimicrobials	
Aminoglycosides	Clindamycin	Furazolidone	Rifampin
Antimalarials	Colistin	Metronidazole	Sulfonamides
Ampicillin	Cortimoxazole	Minocycline	Tetracycline
Capreomycin	Doxycycline	Paromomycin	Thiabendazole
Chloramphenicol	Erythromycin	Polymyxin B	Vancomycin
		Salicylates and NSAIDs	
		Loop diuretics	
		Antitumor agents	
		Miscellaneous	
Aminophylline	Haloperidol	Morphine	Propylthiouracil
Antihistamines	Levodopa	Penicillamine	Quinidine
Carbamazepine	Lidocaine	Pentazocine	Tocainide
Deferoxamine	Metaproterenol	Propranolol	Tricyclic antidepressants
Diazoxide	Molindone	Propoxyphene	Verapamil

The primary symptoms of drug-induced ototoxicity are the occasional to frequent cochlear signs of tinnitus and, in most cases, reversible hearing loss; and the vestibular signs of light-headedness, nystagmus, ataxia, and vertigo.

once daily) is effective (approximately 70 to 90%) in reducing the likelihood of influenza illness in both unimmunized working adults and in immunized nursing home residents; short-term use (7 to 10 days) protects against influenza in household contacts.

OSMOTIC DIURETICS

The osmotic diuretics and related agents consist of mannitol (Osmitrol), urea (Ureaphil), glycerin (glycerol, Osmoglyn), and isosorbide (Hydronol). Mannitol and urea are nonelectrolytes, which are freely filterable, and undergo very little or no metabolism or renal tubular resorption.

When given in sufficient quantities, these drugs increase the osmolarity of plasma, and the amount of glomerular filtrate and renal tubular fluid. The presence of such a drug in the lumen prevents the resorption of much of the water, hence the urine volume is increased. They do not prevent the active resorption of sodium from the tubular fluid, but some additional sodium is excreted as a normal constituent of the increased volume of urine. Osmotic diuretics are not effective in removing the edematous fluid caused by sodium retention but can maintain the flow of urine even when the glomerular filtration rate (GFR) is decreased. Osmotic diuretics are given by intravenous infusion in a hypertonic solution and they are excreted by glomerular filtration.

The osmotic diuretics may be used for any of the following conditions:

In congestive glaucoma, to reduce intraocular pressure
In neurosurgery, to reduce the pressure and volume of cerebrospinal fluid and hence decrease the intracranial pressure
In acute renal failure, to maintain urine flow
In drug poisoning, to prevent nephrotoxicity

These agents should not be used in edematous states associated with diminished cardiac reserve because any increase in the extracellular fluid volume constitutes a hazard.

OUABAIN

The most important and often-used drugs in the treatment of congestive heart failure (CHF) are the cardiac glycosides, which may exist and occur naturally in the body. Unfortunately, the margin of safety for these drugs is very narrow (therapeutic index, 3.0). Toxicity can develop readily, and careful attention to the pharmacokinetic principles is absolutely crucial. The cardiac glycosides are obtained from numerous natural sources, including *Digitalis lanata* and *Digitalis purpurea* (white and purple foxglove), squill (Mediterranean sea onion), oleander, lily of the valley, and other plants. Among the useful available cardiac glycosides are the following:

Digitalis purpurea	*Digitalis lanata*	*Strophanthus gratus*
Digitoxin	Digoxin	Ouabain
Digoxin	Lanatoside C	
Digitalis leaf	Deslanoside	

Of these, only digoxin, digitoxin and, to a certain extent, ouabain are used extensively (see Table 12 and Figure 42). Ouabain is a crystalline powder, slowly soluble in water (1:75) and alcohol (1:100), and is available in ampules.

There are only quantitative and no qualitative differences in the actions of any of the above-listed digitalis preparations; i.e., they vary only in the rate, intensity, and duration of their action and not in its kind.

OVULATION: Drugs to Induce

Categories	Contents
Menotropin	FSH and LH
Urofollitropin	FSH
Estrogen agonist/antagonist	Clomiphene citrate
Human chorionic gonadotropin (HCG)	HCG from human placenta
Synthetic GnRH	Gonadorelin acetate
	Gonadorelin HCl
Synthetic GnRH agonist/analog	Nafarelin acetate
	Leuprolide acetate
	Buserelin
	Goserelin acetate

OXACILLIN SODIUM

(Bactocill)

Oxacillin (500 mg every 4 to 6 hours for a minimum of 5 days) is indicated in the treatment of infections due to penicillinase-producing staphylococci. Furthermore, it may be used to initiate therapy when a staphylococcal infection is suspected (see Table 23).

Oxacillin is bactericidal; it adheres to bacterial penicillin-binding proteins, thus inhibiting bacterial cell wall synthesis. Oxacillin resists the effects of penicillinases— enzymes that inactivate penicillin—and is thus active against many strains of penicillinase-producing bacteria. This activity is most important against penicillinase-producing staphylococci; some strains may remain resistant. Oxacillin is also active against a few Gram-positive aerobic and anaerobic bacilli but has no significant effect on Gram-negative bacilli (see also Figure 74).

Oxacillin is absorbed rapidly, but incompletely from the GI tract; it is stable in an acid environment. Peak serum concentrations occur within 1/2 to 2 hours after an oral dose and 30 minutes after an IM dose. Food decreases absorption.

Oxacillin is distributed widely. CSF penetration is poor but enhanced by meningeal inflammation. Oxacillin crosses the placenta and is 89 to 94% protein-bound. Oxacillin is partially metabolized. Oxacillin and metabolites are excreted primarily in urine by renal tubular secretion and glomerular filtration; it is also excreted in breast milk and in small amounts in bile. Elimination half-life in adults is 1/2 to 1 hour, extending to 2 hours in severe renal impairment. Dosage adjustments are not required in patients with renal impairment. Concomitant use of oxacillin with aminoglycosides produces synergistic bactericidal effects against *Staphylococcus aureus*. However, the drugs are physically and chemically incompatible and are inactivated when mixed or given together. *In vivo* inactivation has been reported when aminoglycosides and penicillins are used concomitantly. Probenecid blocks renal tubular secretion of penicillins, raising their serum levels. Clinical signs of overdose include neuromuscular sensitivity or seizures.

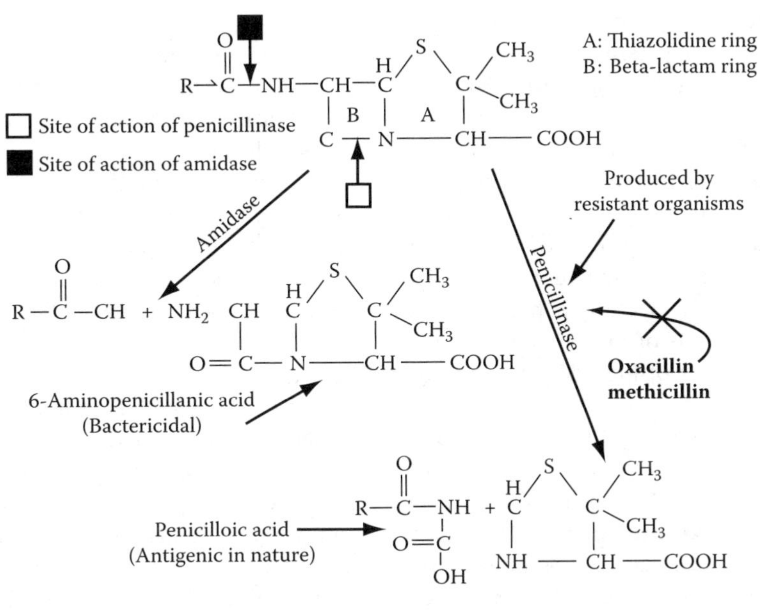

FIGURE 74 The **penicillinase-resistant penicillins** are **oxacillin**, **cloxacillin**, **dicloxacillin**, **methicillin**, and **nafcillin**. These agents are the drugs of choice for treating infections caused by penicillinase-producing *Staphylococcus aureus*.

OXAMNIQUINE

(Vansil)

Oxamniquine, a tetrahydroquinolone with antihelmintic properties, is used in schistosomiasis caused by *Schistosoma mansoni*.

Oxamniquine, which is absorbed following oral administration, is very effective only in *Schistosoma mansoni*. Following treatment, the *S. mansoni* shifts from the mesenteric veins to the liver, where it is destroyed. The male *S. mansoni* is more susceptible to this killing effect than the female, but this will prevent the production of eggs at any rate.

OXANDROLONE

(Oxandrin tablets 2.5 mg)

Oxandrolone (2.5 mg 2 to 4 times daily) is an anabolic steroid that suppresses gonadotropic functions of the pituitary and may exert a direct effect upon the testes. It is indicated as an adjunctive therapy to promote weight gain after weight loss following extensive surgery, chronic infections, or severe trauma, and in some individuals who, without definite pathophysiologic reasons, fail to gain or maintain normal weight; to offset protein catabolism associated with prolonged administration of corticosteroids; and for relief of bone pain frequently accompanying osteoporosis (see also Table 8).

In addition, oxandrolone has been used in short stature associated with Turner's syndrome, constitutional delay of growth and puberty; as adjunctive therapy for AIDS patients with HIV-wasting syndrome; and in moderate/severe acute alcoholic hepatitis and moderate protein calorie malnutrition. The side effects associated with anabolic steroids include cholestatic jaundice; prepubertal phallic enlargement and increased frequency or persistence of erections; postpubertal inhibition of testicular function; testicular atrophy and oligospermia; impotence; chronic priapism; epididymitis and bladder irritability; clitoral enlargement and menstrual irregularities; insomnia, depression, and changes in libido; nausea; vomiting, diarrhea; gynecomastia; potentiation of anticoagulant actions; deepening of voice and hirsutism in female subjects; acne; premature closure of epiphyses in children; disturbed electrolyte balance and edema, and increased serum levels of low-density lipoproteins (LDL) and decreased levels of high-density lipoproteins (HDL).

Several strategies to treat alcoholic liver disease have been evaluated. **Prednisolone** may improve survival in patients with hepatic encephalopathy. Nutrients such as **S-adenosylmethionine** and **polyunsaturated lecithin** have been found to have beneficial effects in nonhuman primates and are undergoing clinical trials. Other medications that have been tested include **oxandrolone**, **propylthiouracil**, and **colchicine**. At present, however, none of these drugs is approved for use in the United States for the treatment of alcoholic liver disease. The current primary treatment for liver failure is transplantation in conjunction with abstinence from ethanol. Long-term outcome studies suggest that patients who are alcohol-dependent have survival rates similar to those of patients with other types of liver disease. Alcoholics with hepatitis C may respond to **interferon-2α**.

OXAPROZIN

(Daypro caplets 600 mg)

Oxaprozin is a nonsteroidal antiinflammatory drug (NSAID) that decreases inflammation, pain, and fever, probably through inhibition of cyclooxygenase activity and prostaglandin synthesis. It is indicated in the relief of symptoms of rheumatoid arthritis and osteoarthritis.

Oxaprozin, an NSAID with analgesic and antipyretic properties (1200 mg p.o. daily), is used in the management of acute or chronic osteoarthritis or rheumatoid arthritis (see also Table 3).

Oxaprozin (Daypro) has similar pharmacological properties, adverse effects, and therapeutic uses to those of other **propionic acid** derivatives. However, its pharmacokinetic properties differ considerably. Peak plasma levels are not achieved until 3 to 6 hours after an oral dose, whereas its half-life of 40 to 60 hours allows for once-daily administration.

OXAZEPAM

(Serax tablets 15 mg)

Oxazepam (10 to 25 mg t.i.d.) is a benzodiazepine that potentiates action of gamma-aminobutyric acid (GABA), an inhibitory neurotransmitter, resulting in increased neuronal inhibition and CNS depression, especially in the limbic system and reticular formation. It is indicated in the control of anxiety, anxiety associated with depression; control of anxiety, tension, agitation, and irritability in the elderly; and in the treatment of alcoholic patients with acute tremulousness, inebriation, or anxiety associated with alcohol withdrawal.

Oxazepam (10 to 25 mg t.i.d.) is indicated for the management of anxiety disorders, for the symptoms of anxiety associated with depression, for the symptoms of anxiety, tension, agitation, and irritability in older patients, and for the management of alcoholics with acute tremulousness anxiety associated with alcohol withdrawal (see Figure 50 and Table 9).

Oxazepam, which is available only in oral preparations, is metabolized rapidly, and hence has a relatively shorter disposition half-life of 5 to 14 hours. Oxazepam is absorbed less rapidly than diazepam after oral administration, limiting its usefulness in the treatment of insomnia. As with diazepam, when alcohol is taken at the same time, the rate of oxazepam absorption is slowed, but food does not affect either the rate or extent of absorption. In healthy subjects, oxazepam is relatively highly protein bound (about 90 to 95%), like other benzodiazepines. Unlike chlordiazepoxide and diazepam, the biotransformation of oxazepam involves only simple glucuronidation to an inactive metabolite. In contrast to chlordiazepoxide and diazepam, neither age nor liver disease alters the elimination half-life or plasma clearance of oxazepam, but the elimination half-life is prolonged to 24 to 91 hours in uremic patients. As might be expected, the elimination of the inactive glucuronide metabolite is greatly prolonged in these patients, its renal clearance being closely related to creatinine clearance. There is evidence that oxazepam may carry a lower abuse liability than diazepam.

The benzodiazepines are metabolized extensively by CPYs, particularly CYP3A4 and CYP2C19. Some benzodiazepines, such as **oxazepam**, are conjugated directly and are not metabolized by these enzymes. Erythromycin, clarithromycin, ritonavir, itraconazole, ketoconazole, nefazodone, and grapefruit juice are inhibitors of CYP3A4 and can affect the metabolism of benzodiazepines. Because active metabolites of some benzodiazepines are biotransformed more slowly than are the parent compounds, the duration of action of many benzodiazepines bears little relationship to the half-life of elimination of the drug that has been administered. For example, the half-life of **flurazepam** in plasma is 2 to 3 hours, but that of a major active metabolite (**N-desalkylflurazepam**) is 50 hours or more. Conversely, the rate of biotransformation of agents that are inactivated by the initial reaction is an important determinant of their duration of action; these agents include **oxazepam**, **lorazepam**, **temazepam**, **triazolam**, and **midazolam**. Metabolism of the benzodiazepines occurs in three major stages.

OXCARBAZEPINE

(Trileptal tablets 150 mg)

Oxcarbazepine is an anticonvulsant. The pharmacologic activity is primarily through the 10-monohydroxy metabolite (MHD) of oxcarbazepine, but the exact mechanism is unknown. It may block voltage-sensitive sodium channels resulting in stabilization of hyperexcited neural membranes, inhibition of repetitive neuronal firing, and diminution of propagation of synaptic impulses. It is indicated as a monotherapy or adjunctive therapy in the treatment of partial seizures in patients with epilepsy.

Oxcarbazepine (Trileptal) (10,11-dihydro-10-oxocarbamazepine) is a keto analog of carbamazepine. **Oxcarbazepine** functions as a prodrug, in that it is almost immediately converted to its main active metabolite, a 10-monohydroxy derivative, which is inactivated by glucuronide conjugation and eliminated by renal excretion. Its mechanism of action is similar to that of carbamazepine. **Oxcarbazepine** is a less potent enzyme inducer than is carbamazepine, and substitution of oxcarbazepine for carbamazepine is associated with increased levels of phenytoin and valproic acid, presumably because of reduced induction of hepatic enzymes. **Oxcarbazepine** does not induce the hepatic enzymes involved in its own degradation. Although oxcarbazepine does not appear to reduce the anticoagulant effect of warfarin, it does induce CYP3A, and it thus reduces plasma levels of steroid oral contraceptives. It has been approved for monotherapy or adjunct therapy for partial seizures in adults and as adjunctive therapy for partial seizures in children aged 4 to 16.

OXICONAZOLE NITRATE

(Oxistat)

Oxiconazole, an ergosterol synthesis inhibitor possessing antifungal activity, is used for topical treatment of dermal infections caused by *Trichophyton rubrum* and *T. mentagrophytes* (tinea pedis, tinea cruris, and tinea corporis).

OXTRIPHYLLINE

(Choledyl)

Oxtriphylline, a xanthine derivative with bronchodilating properties (200 mg p.o. q. 6 hours), is used to relieve bronchial asthma and reversible bronchospasm associated with chronic bronchitis and emphysema (see also Figure 94).

OXYBUTYNIN CHLORIDE

(Ditropan tablets 5 mg, syrup 5 mg/5 mL, Ditropan XL tablets, extended-release 5 mg, tablets, extended-release 10 mg, tablets, extended-release 15 mg, Oxytrol transdermal system 36 mg of oxybutynin delivering 3.9 mg or oxybutynin/day)

Oxybutynin chloride is an anticholinergic that increases bladder capacity, diminishes frequency of uninhibited contractions of detrusor muscle and delays initial desire to void. It is indicated in the treatment of symptoms of bladder instability associated with voiding in patients with uninhibited and reflex neurogenic bladder (e.g., urinary leakage, dysuria); and treatment of overactive bladder with symptoms of urge urinary incontinence, urgency, and frequency.

The class of drugs referred to here as muscarinic receptor antagonists includes (1) the naturally occurring alkaloids, **atropine** and **scopolamine**; (2) semisynthetic derivatives of these alkaloids, which primarily differ from the parent compounds in their disposition in the body or their duration of action; and (3) synthetic congeners, some of which show selectivity for particular subtypes of muscarinic receptors. Noteworthy agents among the synthetic derivatives are **homatropine** and **tropicamide**, which have a shorter duration of action than atropine, and **methylatropine**, **ipratropium**, and **tiotropium**, which are quaternized and do not cross the blood–brain barrier or readily cross membranes. The latter two agents are given by inhalation in the treatment of chronic obstructive pulmonary disease and are pending approval for use in bronchial asthma. Ipratropium also has a FDA-approved indication for perennial and common-cold-associated rhinorrhea. The synthetic derivatives possessing partial receptor selectivity include **pirenzepine**, used in the treatment of acid-peptic disease in some countries, and **tolterodine**, **oxybutynin**, and several others, used in the treatment of urinary incontinence.

Oxybutynin possesses anticholinergic and osmolytic properties, which together form the basis for its use as a therapeutic option in patients with overactive detrusor function—either idiopathic detrusor instability (DI) or detrusor hyperreflexia. Of the symptoms of detrusor overactivity, urge incontinence is often the most distressing to the patient. Adverse effects—dry mouth, constipation, and blurred vision—related to the anticholinergic activity of oxybutynin occur frequently and can be sufficiently troublesome to necessitate treatment discontinuation in up to 25% of patients depending on the dosage. Increases in residual urine volume suggesting urinary retention (undesirable in patients with idiopathic DI), also can develop in some oxybutynin recipients (see also Figure 60).

OXYCODONE HYDROCHLORIDE

(Roxicodone)

Oxycodone, an opioid analgesic (5 mg p.o. every 3 to 6 hours), is used in the treatment of moderate to severe pain.

OXYCODONE/ACETAMINOPHEN

(Percocet tablets 5 mg oxycodone hydrochloride/325 mg acetaminophen, tablets 7.5 mg oxycodone hydrochloride/500 mg acetaminophen, tablets 10 mg oxycodone hydrochloride/650 mg acetaminophen, Roxicet tablets 5 mg oxycodone hydrochloride/325 mg acetaminophen, solution, oral 5 mg oxycodone hydrochloride/325 mg acetaminophen, Roxicet 5/500 caplets 5 mg oxycodone/500 mg acetaminophen, Roxilox capsules 5 mg oxycodone hydrochloride/500 mg acetaminophen, Tylox capsules 5 mg oxycodone hydrochloride/500 mg acetaminophen)

Oxycodone/acetaminophen is an opioid analgesic combination. **Acetaminophen** inhibits synthesis of prostaglandins and peripherally blocks pain impulse generation, whereas oxycodone binds to opiate receptors in the CNS. Their combination has a synergistic effect in alleviating pain. It is indicated in the relief of moderate to moderately severe pain.

Many semisynthetic derivatives are made by relatively simple modifications of **morphine** or **thebaine**. Codeine is methylmorphine, the methyl substitution being on the phenolic hydroxyl group. Thebaine differs from morphine only in that both hydroxyl groups are methylated and that the ring has two double bonds ($\Delta^{6,7}$, $\Delta^{8,14}$). Thebaine has little analgesic action but is a precursor of several important 14-OH compounds, such as **oxycodone** and **naloxone**. Certain derivatives of thebaine are more than 1000 times as potent as morphine (e.g., **etorphine**). **Diacetylmorphine**, or heroin, is made from morphine by acetylation at the 3 and 6 positions. **Apomorphine**, which also can be prepared from morphine, is a potent emetic and dopaminergic agonist. **Hydromorphone**, **oxymorphone**, **hydrocodone**, and **oxycodone** also are made by modifying the morphine molecule.

Morphine is available for oral use in standard and controlled-release preparations. Owing to first-pass metabolism, morphine is two to six times less potent orally than it is parenterally. This is important to remember when converting a patient from parenteral to oral medication. There is wide variability in the first-pass metabolism, and the dose should be titrated to the patient's needs. In children who weigh less than 50 kg, morphine can be given at 0.1 mg/kg every 3 to 4 hours parenterally, or at 0.3 mg/kg orally.

Codeine is used widely owing to its high oral/parenteral potency ratio. Orally, codeine at 30 mg is approximately equianalgesic to 325 to 600 mg aspirin. Combinations of codeine with aspirin or acetaminophen usually provide additive actions and, at these doses, analgesic efficacy can exceed that of 60 mg codeine. Many drugs can be used instead of either morphine or codeine. Oxycodone, with its high oral/parenteral potency ratio, is used widely in combination with aspirin (**Percodan**, others) or acetaminophen (**Percocet** 2.5/325, others), although it is available alone (Roxicodine, others). **Oxycodone** also is available in a sustained-release formulation for chronic pain management (Oxycontin). Unfortunately, this formulation has been subject to widespread abuse leading to serious consequences, including death, and the FDA has strengthened warnings for this drug.

Acetaminophen (paracetamol; *N*-acetyl-p-aminophenol; Tylenol, others) is the active metabolite of **phenacetin**, a so-called **coal tar analgesic**. (Due to its association with analgesic nephropathy, hemolytic anemia and, perhaps, bladder cancer, phenacetin is no longer available for medicinal purposes.) **Acetaminophen** is an effective alternative to aspirin as an analgesic–antipyretic agent; however, its antiinflammatory effects are much weaker. Although it is indicated for pain relief in patients with noninflammatory osteoarthritis, it is not a suitable substitute for aspirin or other NSAIDs in chronic inflammatory conditions such as rheumatoid arthritis. Acetaminophen is well tolerated and has a low incidence of GI side effects. It is available without a prescription and is used as a common household analgesic. However, acute overdosage can cause severe hepatic damage, and the number of accidental or deliberate poisonings with acetaminophen continues to grow. Chronic use of less than 2 g/day is not typically associated with hepatic dysfunction.

Acetaminophen has analgesic and antipyretic effects similar to those of aspirin. However, as mentioned above, it has only weak antiinflammatory effects and has been thought to have a generally poor ability to inhibit cyclooxygenase (COX) in the presence of high concentrations of peroxides, as are found at sites of inflammation. However, this aspect of its action has not been addressed rigorously. Certainly, the most commonly consumed daily dose, 1000 mg, results in roughly 50% inhibition of both COX-1 and

COX-2 in whole blood assays *ex vivo* in healthy volunteers. It has been suggested that COX inhibition might be disproportionately pronounced in the brain, explaining its antipyretic efficacy. A COX-1 splice variant identified in canine brain, termed COX-3, shows some susceptibility for inhibition by **acetaminophen** *in vitro*. However, it is presently unknown if this splice variant exists in human brain or if its inhibition relates to the efficacy of acetaminophen in humans. Minor metabolites contribute significantly to the toxic effects of acetaminophen.

Single or repeated therapeutic doses of acetaminophen have no effect on the cardiovascular and respiratory systems, on platelets, or on coagulation. Acid-base changes and uricosuric effects do not occur, nor does the drug produce the gastric irritation, erosion, or bleeding that may occur after salicylate administration.

Acetaminophen is a suitable substitute for aspirin for analgesic or antipyretic uses; it is particularly valuable for patients in whom aspirin is contraindicated (e.g., in those with peptic ulcer, aspirin hypersensitivity, and in children with a febrile illness). The conventional oral dose of **acetaminophen** is 325 to 1000 mg (650 mg rectally); total daily doses should not exceed 4000 mg (2000 mg/day for chronic alcoholics). The most common daily dose is 1000 mg, the dose at which epidemiological studies suggest that GI adverse effects are less common than with therapeutic doses of NSAIDs. Higher doses that may accomplish complete inhibition of COXs may approach the adverse effect profile of NSAIDs. Single doses for children range from 40 to 480 mg, depending upon age and weight; no more than five doses should be administered in 24 hours. A dose of 10 mg/kg also may be used.

Acetaminophen usually is well tolerated at recommended therapeutic doses. Rash and other allergic reactions occur occasionally. The rash usually is erythematous or urticarial, but sometimes it is more serious and may be accompanied by drug fever and mucosal lesions. Patients who show hypersensitivity reactions to the salicylates only rarely exhibit sensitivity to acetaminophen. The use of acetaminophen has been associated anecdotally with neutropenia, thrombocytopenia, and pancytopenia.

The most serious acute adverse effect of overdosage of acetaminophen is a potentially fatal hepatic necrosis. Renal tubular necrosis and hypoglycemic coma also may occur. The mechanism by which overdosage with **acetaminophen** leads to hepatocellular injury and death involves its conversion to the toxic NAPQI metabolite. The glucuronide and sulfate conjugation pathways become saturated, and increasing amounts undergo CYP-mediated *N*-hydroxylation to form NAPQI. This is eliminated rapidly by conjugation with glutathione (GSH) and, then, further metabolized to a mercapturic acid and excreted into the urine. In the setting of acetaminophen overdose, hepatocellular levels of GSH become depleted. The highly reactive NAPQI metabolite binds covalently to cell macromolecules, leading to dysfunction of enzymatic systems and structural and metabolic disarray. Furthermore, depletion of intracellular GSH renders the hepatocytes highly susceptible to oxidative stress and apoptosis.

OXYCODONE HYDROCHLORIDE/ASPIRIN

(Percodan tablets 4.5 mg oxycodone hydrochloride/ 0.38 mg oxycodone terephthalate/325 mg aspirin)

Oxycodone hydrochloride/aspirin is an opioid analgesic combination. **Oxycodone** relieves pain by stimulating opiate receptors in CNS. **Aspirin** inhibits prostaglandin synthesis, resulting in analgesia, antiinflammatory activity, and inhibition of platelet aggregation. It is indicated for the relief of moderate to moderately severe pain.

OXYMETAZOLLINE HYDROCHLORIDE

(Afrin, Allerest 12-hour long lasting nasal, Coricidin nasal mist, Dristan long lasting nasal mist, Duramist Plus, Duration, 4-way long-acting nasal spray, Neo-Synephrine 12-hour nasal spray, Nostrilla long acting nasal decongestant, NTZ long acting nasal, Sinarest 12-hour, Sinex long-lasting)

Oxymetazolline, a sympathomimetic agent with decongestant properties, is used in nasal congestion.

OXYMETHOLONE

(Anadrol-50 tablets 50 mg)

Oxymetholone is an anabolic steroid that suppresses gonadotropic functions of the pituitary and may exert a direct effect upon the testes. It enhances the production and urinary excretion of erythropoietin in patients with anemias caused by bone marrow failure and stimulates erythropoiesis in anemias caused by deficient RBC production. Oxymetholone is indicated in the treatment of anemias caused by deficient RBC production. Acquired aplastic anemia, congenital aplastic anemia, myelofibrosis, and the hypoplastic anemias caused by administration of myelotoxic drugs often respond to the drug.

Oxymetholone, an anabolic steroid (1 to 5 mg/kg/day), is indicated for the treatment of anemias caused by deficient red cell production, acquired or congenital aplastic anemia, myelofibrosis, and hypoplastic anemias due to the administration of myelotoxic drugs. Oxymetholone stimulates the kidney production of erythropoietin, leading to increases in red blood cell number, mass, and volume (see also Figure 44). Oxymetholone is contraindicated in patients with severe renal or cardiac disease, which may be worsened by the fluid and electrolyte retention, and in patients with prostatic hypertrophy with obstruction or prostatic cancer. The side effects associated with anabolic steroids include cholestatic jaundice, prepubertal phallic enlargement, and increased frequency or persistence of erections; postpubertal inhibition of testicular function, testicular atrophy and oligospermia, impotence; chronic priapism, epididymitis, and bladder irritability; clitoral enlargement and menstrual irregularities; insomnia, depression, and changes in libido; nausea, vomiting, diarrhea; gynecomastia; potentiation of anticoagulant actions; deepening of voice and hirsutism in female subjects; acne; premature closure of epiphyses in children; disturbed electrolyte balance and edema; and increased serum levels of LDL and depressed levels of HDL.

OXYMORPHONE HYDROCHLORIDE

(Numorphan injection 1 mg/mL, injection 1.5 mg/mL, suppositories 5 mg)

Oxymorphone hydrochloride is an opioid analgesic that relieves pain by stimulating opiate receptors in the CNS. It is indicated in the relief of moderate to severe pain.

Many semisynthetic derivatives are made by relatively simple modifications of morphine or thebaine. Codeine is methylmorphine, the methyl substitution being on the phenolic hydroxyl group. Thebaine differs from morphine only in that both hydroxyl groups are methylated and that the ring has two double bonds ($\Delta^{6,7}$, $\Delta^{8,14}$). Thebaine has little analgesic action but is a precursor of several important 14-OH compounds, such as oxycodone and naloxone. Certain derivatives of thebaine are more than 1000 times as potent as morphine (e.g., etorphine). **Diacetylmorphine**, or **heroin**, is made from morphine by acetylation at the 3 and 6 positions. Apomorphine, which also can be prepared from morphine, is a potent emetic and dopaminergic agonist. **Hydromorphone**, **oxymorphone**, **hydrocodone**, and **oxycodone** also are made by modifying the morphine molecule.

Oxymorphone, an opioid analgesic (1 to 1.5 mg SC), is used in the management of moderate to severe pain (see also Figure 68).

OXYPHENBUTAZONE

(Oxalid)

Oxyphenbutazone, a NSAID (300 to 600 mg/day in divided doses), is indicated in pain and inflammation of arthritis and ankylosing spondylitis. Oxyphenbutazone, a metabolite of phenylbutazone, has analgesic, antipyretic, antiinflammatory, and uricosuric properties. Oxyphenbutazone is absorbed orally, is bound to plasma proteins to the extent of 98%, has a half-life of 50 to 100 hours, is metabolized in the liver, and is excreted by the kidneys. Oxyphenbutazone is contraindicated in patients with known hypersensitivity to phenylbutazone; in patients in whom aspirin or other NSAIDs induce symptoms of asthma, urticaria, or rhinitis; in patients under age 14 because safety has not been established; and in patients with senility, GI bleeding, blood dyscrasias, or renal, hepatic, cardiac or thyroid disease because the drug may mask symptoms associated with these disorders or worsen these conditions. The drug should not be used in patients on long-term anticoagulant therapy because of its potential for adverse hematologic effects. Serious GI toxicity, especially ulceration or hemorrhage, can occur at any time in patients on chronic NSAID therapy. Use with caution in patients with a history of GI disease (especially peptic ulcer disease). Patients with known "triad" symptoms (aspirin hypersensitivity, rhinitis/nasal polyps, and asthma) are at high risk of cross sensitivity to oxyphenbutazone with precipitation of bronchospasm. Because of the potential for serious blood dyscrasias, oxyphenbutazone is not recommended for initial therapy. When used concomitantly, anticoagulants and thrombolytic drugs may be potentiated by the platelet-inhibiting effect of oxyphenbutazone. Concomitant use of oxyphenbutazone with highly protein-bound drugs (phenytoin, sulfonylureas, warfarin) may cause displacement of either drug, and adverse effects. Concomitant use with other GI-irritating drugs (steroids, antibiotics, NSAIDs) may potentiate the adverse GI effects of oxyphenbutazone. Antacids and food delay decrease the absorption of oxyphenbutazone. NSAIDs are known to decrease renal clearance of lithium carbonate, thus increasing lithium serum levels and risks of adverse effects. Oxyphenbutazone is known to induce liver microsomal enzyme activity. Concomitant use with other NSAIDs increases the risk of nephrotoxicity and decreases uricosuric effects.

Clinical manifestations of overdose include nausea, abdominal pain, and drowsiness; vomiting, hematemesis, diarrhea, restlessness, dizziness, agitation, hallucinations, psychosis, coma, convulsions, hyperpyrexia, electrolyte disturbances, hyperventilation, respiratory arrest, and cyanosis (see also Table 3 and Figures 13 and 14).

OXYTETRACYCLINE

(Terramycin)

Oxytetracycline (250 mg/day) is bacteriostatic, has a broad spectrum of activity, and is effective against infections with Gram-positive and Gram-negative bacteria, *Rickettsia*, *Mycoplasma*, *Amoeba*, and *Chlamydia*. Tetracyclines are drugs of choice in brucellosis, glanders, cholera, relapsing fever, meloidosis, leptospirosis, and the early stages of Lyme disease. They are preferred drugs for chlamydial infections, granuloma inguinale, and urethritis due to *Ureaplasma urealyticum* (see also Figure 96).

Tetracyclines enter bacterial cells by both passive diffusion and active transport, and then accumulate intracellularly. This does not occur in mammalian cells. The tetracyclines bind to the 30S subunit of the bacterial ribosome in such a way that the binding of the aminoacyl-transfer RNA to the acceptor site on the messenger RNA ribosome complex is blocked.

The resistant mutant bacteria do not transport or accumulate tetracycline. This plasmid-controlled resistance is transmitted by transduction or by conjugation.

The absorption of tetracyclines from the GI tract is nonuniform. Up to 30% of chlortetracycline is absorbed. The absorption for tetracycline, oxytetracycline, and demeclocycline ranges between 60 and 80%, whereas as much as 90 to 100% of doxycycline and minocycline is absorbed. The absorption of tetracyclines is impaired by divalent cations (calcium, magnesium, and ferrous iron), by aluminum, and by extremely alkaline pHs. Tetracyclines are distributed widely throughout the body fluid, cross the placental barrier, and can accumulate in growing bones. The concentrations of chlortetracycline in spinal fluid are only one fourth of those in plasma. Minocycline, a more lipid-soluble tetracycline, reaches a high concentration in tears and saliva and can eradicate the meningococcal carrier state. The tetracyclines are metabolized in the liver and excreted mainly by the bile and urine. The concentrations of tetracyclines in the bile are ten times higher than those in serum.

Tetracyclines, in general, cause toxic and hypersensitivity reactions. These consist commonly of GI irritations that are disabling and may necessitate the discontinuation of the medications. With continuous use, tetracyclines may alter the normal flora, allowing the growth of *Pseudomonas*, *Proteus*, staphylococci-resistant coliforms, *Clostridium*, and *Candida* organisms. These superinfections should be recognized and treated appropriately with vancomycin and other drugs (see also Figure 100).

Tetracyclines have been known to cause hepatic necrosis, especially when given in large intravenous doses, or when taken by pregnant women or patients with preexisting liver impairment.

Tetracycline preparations whose potency has expired can cause renal tubular acidosis. With the exception of doxycycline, tetracyclines accumulate in patients with renal impairment. They also produce nitrogen retention, especially when given with diuretics.

Tetracyclines bind to calcium and then become deposited in bone, causing damage to developing bone and teeth. Intravenous administration of tetracyclines has been observed to cause venous thrombosis.

Oxytetracycline is contraindicated during the second half of pregnancy and in children under 8 years of age because of the risk of permanent discoloration of teeth, enamel defects, and retardation of bone growth.

Concomitant use of tetracycline with antacids containing aluminum, calcium, or magnesium decreases absorption of oxytetracycline (because of chelation); concomitant use with food, milk or other dairy products, oral iron products, or sodium bicarbonate also impairs oral absorption.

Tetracyclines may antagonize the bactericidal effects of penicillin, inhibiting cell growth through bacteriostatic action.

Oxytetracycline enhances the risk of nephrotoxicity from methoxyflurane; it also necessitates lowered dosage of oral anticoagulants because of enhanced effects and lowered dosage of digoxin because of increased bioavailability.

OXYTETRACYCLINE HYDROCHLORIDE/POLYMYXIN B SULFATE

(Terak with Polymyxin B sulfate ophthalmic ointment 10,000 units/g Polymyxin B sulfate and 5 mg/g oxytetracycline hydrochloride, Terramycin with Polymyxin B sulfate ophthalmic ointment 10,000 units/g Polymyxin B sulfate and 5 mg/g oxytetracycline hydrochloride)

Oxytetracycline hydrochloride is an antibiotic that inhibits bacterial protein synthesis. Polymyxin B interacts with phospholipid components of bacterial cell membrane, increasing cell wall permeability. It is indicated in the treatment of superficial ocular infections involving the conjunctiva and/or cornea caused by susceptible organisms.

OXYTOCIN

(Pitocin, Syntocinon, and Uteracon)

Oxytocin (0.5 milliunits/min) is indicated to induce term labor, to control postpartum hemorrhage, to prevent postpartum uterine atony, to expel the placenta, and to prevent postpartum breast engorgement.

Oxytocin is a single polypeptide with eight amino acids that are sequenced as follows:

Gln – Asn – Cys – Pro – Leu – Gly
| |
Ile - - - - - - - Tyr

Oxytocin is synthesized in the cell bodies of supraoptic and paraventricular neurons and, then, transported (complexed with neurophysin) in membrane-bound vesicles to the posterior lobe of the pituitary gland, where it may be released by a reflex mechanism or mechanisms, initiated or amplified by genital stimulation, coitus, parturition, or suckling of the infant. Suckling also releases prolactin. The action of oxytocin on the uterus (muscular contraction and parturition) and mammary glands (contraction of myoepithelial cells and milk secretion) is a direct one and is not influenced by the autonomic nervous system.

The uterus contains both alpha- and beta$_2$-adrenergic-receptor sites. Stimulation of the alpha-receptor site causes contraction; stimulation of the beta$_2$-receptor site causes relaxation. Therefore, beta$_2$-receptor agonists such as ritodrine hydrochloride (Yutopar) and terbutaline sulfate (Brethine) are used to suppress premature labor.

The promotion of mammary development, lactation, and galactopoiesis requires growth hormone, ovarian estrogen (duct formation), ovarian progesterone (lobule-alveolar development), and adrenal corticoids, as well as prolactin and oxytocin. The secretion of prolactin is modified by substances that stimulate or block dopamine-receptor sites. Agents such as neuroleptics (chlorpromazine) may cause lactation in a nonpregnant woman. On the other hand, dopamine-receptor agonists such as bromocriptine (Parlodel) are used to prevent postpartum lactation.

The direct stimulatory effect of oxytocin is prominent in the gravid uterus during the late stage of pregnancy. Its action is augmented by estrogen and inhibited by progesterone. Oxytocin's effect is specific for uterine muscle, as little effect is observed on intestinal muscle or coronary arteries.

P

PACLITAXEL

(Onxol solution for injection 6 mg/mL)

Paclitaxel is a taxoid. It is a novel antimicrotubule agent that promotes the assembly of microtubules from tubulin dimers and stabilizes them by preventing depolymerization. This stability inhibits the normal dynamic reorganization of the microtubule network that is essential for vital interphase and mitotic cellular functions. In addition, paclitaxel induces abnormal arrays or bundles of microtubules throughout the cell cycle and multiple asters of microtubules during mitosis, further disrupting cell function. **Abraxane**, **Onxol**, and **Taxol** are used in treatment of breast cancer after failure of combination chemotherapy for metastatic disease or relapse within 6 months of adjuvant chemotherapy. Prior therapy should have included an anthracycline unless clinically contraindicated. **Onxol** and **Taxol** are used in treatment of advanced carcinoma of the ovary. **Taxol** is used for adjuvant treatment of node-positive breast cancer administered sequentially to standard doxorubicin-containing combination chemotherapy; in combination with cisplatin for the treatment of non-small-cell lung cancer (NSCLC) in patients who are not candidates for potentially curative surgery and/or radiation therapy; and second-line treatment of AIDS-related Kaposi's sarcoma.

Paclitaxel, an antineoplastic agent, is used in the treatment of metastatic ovarian cancer after failure of first-line or subsequent chemotherapy (135 mg/m^2 IV over 24 hours q. 3 weeks) and breast carcinoma after failure of combination chemotherapy for metastatic disease or relapse within 6 months of adjuvant chemotherapy (175 mg/m^2 IV over 3 hours q. 3 weeks).

The first compound of the taxanes series, **paclitaxel** (Taxol), was isolated from the bark of the Western yew tree in 1971. It and its congenic, the semisynthetic **docetaxel** (Taxotere), exhibit unique pharmacological actions as inhibitors of mitosis, differing from the **vinca alkaloids** and **colchicine** derivatives in that they bind to a different site on β-tubulin and promote rather than inhibit microtubule formation. The drugs have a central role in the therapy of ovarian, breast, lung, esophageal, bladder, and head and neck cancers.

Interest in **paclitaxel** was stimulated by the finding that the drug possessed the unique ability to promote microtubule formation at cold temperatures and in the absence of guanosine triphosphate (GTP). It binds specifically to the β-tubulin subunit of microtubules and antagonizes the disassembly of this key cytoskeletal protein, with the result that bundles of microtubules and aberrant structures derived from microtubules appear in the mitotic phase of the cell cycle. Arrest in mitosis follows. Cell killing (CK) is dependent on both drug concentration and duration of cell exposure. Drugs that block cell-cycle progression prior to mitosis antagonize the toxic effects of taxanes.

Schedules for optimal use alone or in combination with other drugs, including **doxorubicin** and **cisplatin**, still are evolving. Drug interactions have been noted; the sequence of cisplatin preceding **paclitaxel** decreases paclitaxel clearance and produces greater toxicity than the opposite schedule. Paclitaxel decreases doxorubicin clearance and enhances cardiotoxicity, whereas docetaxel has no apparent effect on anthracycline pharmacokinetics.

In cultured tumor cells, resistance to taxanes is associated in some lines with increased expression of the mdr-1 gene and its product, the P-glycoprotein; other resistant cells have β-tubulin mutations, and these latter cells may display heightened sensitivity to vinca alkaloids. Other cell lines display an increase in survivin, an antiapoptotic factor or aurora kinase, an enzyme that promotes completion of mitosis. The basis of clinical drug resistance is not known. Cell death occurs by apoptosis, but the effectiveness of **paclitaxel** against experimental tumors does not depend on an intact p53 gene product.

Docetaxel and **paclitaxel** have become central components of regimens for treating metastatic ovarian, breast, lung, and head and neck cancers. Docetaxel has significant activity with **estramustine** for treatment of hormone-refractory prostate cancer. In current regimens, either drug is administered once weekly or once every 3 weeks, with comparable response rates and somewhat different patterns of toxicity. Docetaxel produces greater leukopenia and peripheral edema, whereas **paclitaxel** causes a higher incidence of hypersensitivity, muscle aching, and neuropathy (particularly when used in combination with a platinum analog). The optimal schedule of taxane administration, alone or in combination with other drugs, is still under evaluation.

Paclitaxel exerts its primary toxic effects on the bone marrow. Neutropenia usually occurs 8 to 11 days after a dose and reverses rapidly by days 15 to 21. Used with filgrastim (granulocyte-colony-stimulating factor; G-CSF), doses as high as 250 mg m^2 over 24 hours are well tolerated, and peripheral neuropathy becomes dose limiting. Many patients experience myalgias for several days after receiving **paclitaxel**. In high-dose schedules, or with prolonged use, a stocking-glove sensory neuropathy can be disabling, particularly in patients with underlying diabetic alcoholic neuropathy or concurrent cisplatin therapy. Mucositis is prominent in 72- or 96-hour infusions and in the weekly schedule.

Hypersensitivity reactions occurred in patients receiving **paclitaxel** infusions of short duration (1 to 6 hours), but have largely been averted by pretreatment with dexamethasone, diphenhydramine, and histamine H_2-receptor antagonists, as already noted. Premedication is not necessary with 96-hour infusions. Many patients experience asymptomatic bradycardia, and occasional episodes of silent ventricular tachycardia also occur and resolve spontaneously during 3- or 24-hour infusions.

PALIFERMIN

(Kepivance powder for injection, lyophilized 6.25 mg)

Palifermin is a keratinocyte growth factor that shows linear pharmcokinetics and has extravascular distribution. Steady-state Vd appears to be twofold higher in cancer patients compared with healthy volunteers. It decreases incidence and duration of severe oral mucositis in patients with hematologic malignancies receiving myelotoxic therapy requiring hematopoietic stem-cell support.

PALIVIZUMAB

(Synagis powder for injection, lyophilized 50 mg, powder for injection, lyophilized 100 mg)

Palivizumab is a monoclonal antibody that possess neutralizing and fusion-inhibitory activity against respiratory syncytial virus (RSV), inhibiting RSV replication. It is indicated in prevention of serious lower respiratory tract disease caused by RSV in pediatric patients at high risk of RSV disease.

PALONOSETRON

(Aloxi injection 0.25 mg)

Palonosetron is a 5-HT_3-receptor antagonist that is a selective antagonist for the 5-HT_3 receptor with a strong binding affinity for this receptor. It is indicated in prevention of acute nausea and vomiting associated with moderately and highly emetogenic cancer chemotherapy; and prevention of delayed nausea and vomiting associated with moderately emetogenic cancer chemotherapy.

Ondansetron (Zofran) is the prototypical drug in this class. Since their introduction in the early 1990s, the serotonin (5-HT_3)-receptor antagonists have become the most widely used drugs for chemotherapy-induced emesis. Other agents in this class include **granisetron** (Kytril), **dolasetron** (Anzemet), **palonosetron** (Aloxi; intravenous use only) and **tropisetron.** The differences among these agents are related mainly to their chemical structures, 5-HT_3 receptor affinities, and pharmacokinetic profiles.

There is evidence that effects at peripheral and central sites contribute to the efficacy of these agents. 5-HT_3 receptors are present in several critical sites involved in emesis, including vagal afferents, the STN (which receives signals from vagal afferents), and the area postrema itself. Serotonin is released by the enterochromaffin cells of the small intestine in response to chemotherapeutic agents, and may stimulate vagal afferents (via 5-HT_3 receptors) to initiate the vomiting reflex. Experimentally, vagotomy has been shown to prevent cisplatin-induced emesis. However, the highest concentrations of 5-HT_3 receptors in the CNS are found in the STN and chemoreceptor trigger zone (CTZ), and antagonists of 5-HT_3 receptors also may suppress nausea and vomiting by acting at these sites.

The antiemetic effects of these drugs persist long after they disappear from the circulation, suggesting their continuing interaction at the receptor level. In fact, all of these drugs can be administered effectively just once a day.

These agents are absorbed well from the gastrointestinal (GI) tract. Ondansetron is extensively metabolized in the liver by CYP1A2, CYP2D6, and CYP3A4, followed by glucuronide or sulfate conjugation. Patients with hepatic dysfunction have reduced plasma clearance, and some adjustment in the dosage is advisable. Although ondansetron clearance also is reduced in elderly patients, no adjustment in dosage for age is recommended. Granisetron also is metabolized predominantly by the liver, a process that appears to involve the CYP3A family, as it is inhibited by **ketoconazole**. Dolasetron is converted rapidly by plasma carbonyl reductase to its active metabolite, hydrodolasetron. A portion of this compound then undergoes subsequent biotransformation by CYP2D6 and CYP3A4 in the liver, whereas about one-third of it is excreted unchanged in the urine. **Palonosetron** is metabolized principally by CYP2D6 and excreted in the urine as the metabolized and the unchanged form in about equal proportions.

These agents are most effective in treating chemotherapy-induced nausea and in treating nausea secondary to upper abdominal irradiation, where all three agents appear to be equally efficacious. They also are effective against hyperemesis of pregnancy and, to a lesser degree, postoperative nausea, but not against motion sickness. Unlike other agents in this class, palonosetron also may be helpful in delayed emesis, perhaps a reflection of its long half-life.

These agents are available as tablets, oral solution, and intravenous preparations for injection. For patients on cancer chemotherapy, these drugs can be given in a single intravenous dose infused over 15 minutes, beginning 30 minutes before chemotherapy, or in two to three divided doses, with the first usually given 30 minutes before and with subsequent doses at various intervals after chemotherapy. The drugs also can be used intramuscularly or orally.

In general, these drugs are very well tolerated, with the most common adverse effects being constipation or diarrhea, headache, and light-headedness. As a class, these agents have been shown experimentally to induce minor electrocardiographic changes, but these are not expected to be clinically significant in most cases.

PAMIDRONATE DISODIUM

(Aredia powder for injection, lyophilized 30 mg)

Pamidronate disodium is a bisphosphonate that inhibits normal and abnormal bone resorption. It is indicated in the treatment of moderate to severe hypercalcemia associated with malignancy with or without bone metastases; treatment of moderate to severe Paget's disease of bone; treatment of osteolytic bone lesions of multiple myeloma and bone metastases of breast cancer in conjunction with standard chemotherapy.

Intravenous bisphosphonates (**pamidronate**, **zoledronate**) have proven very effective in the management of hypercalcemia. These agents potently inhibit osteoclastic bone resorption. Oral bisphosphonates are less effective for treating hypercalcemia. Therefore, **pamidronate** (Aredia) is given as an intravenous infusion of 60 to 90 mg over 4 to 24 hours. With **pamidronate**, resolution of hypercalcemia occurs over several days, and the effect usually persists for several weeks.

Oral sodium phosphate lowers plasma Ca^{2+} concentrations and may offer short-term calcemic control of some patients with primary hyperparathyroidism who are awaiting surgery. However, the risk of precipitating calcium phosphate salts in soft tissues throughout the body is of concern. In light of satisfactory responses to other agents, administration of intravenous sodium phosphate is not recommended as a treatment for hypercalcemia.

Several bisphosphonates are available in the United States. **Etidronate sodium** (Didronel) is used for treatment of **Paget's disease** and may be used parenterally to treat hypercalcemia. Because etidronate is the only bisphosphonate that inhibits mineralization, it has been supplanted largely by pamidronate and zoledronate for treating hypercalcemia. **Pamidronate** (Aredia) is approved for management of hypercalcemia but also is effective in other skeletal disorders. **Pamidronate** is available in the United States only for parenteral administration. For treatment of hypercalcemia, it may be given as an intravenous infusion of 60 to 90 mg over 4 to 24 hours.

Several newer bisphosphonates have been approved for treatment of Paget's disease. These include **tiludronate** (Skelid), **alendronate** (Fosamax), and **risedronate** (Actonel). Although the drug is approved only for treating hypercalcemia of malignancy, a single injection of zoledronate (Zometa) decreased bone turnover markers for 90 days in patients with Paget's disease. Tiludronate and the potent bisphosphonate ibandronate currently are under development for treatment of women with osteoporosis, with encouraging preliminary results.

The first-generation bisphosphonate etidronate was associated with osteomalacia. This adverse effect, coupled with its relatively low efficacy, has limited its current use. Although alendronate and risedronate were well tolerated in clinical trials, some patients experience symptoms of esophagitis. Symptoms often abate when patients fastidiously take the medication with water and remain upright. Esophageal complications are infrequent when the drug is taken as described. If symptoms persist despite these precautions, use of a proton-pump inhibitor at bedtime may be helpful. Both drugs may be better tolerated on a once-weekly regimen with no reduction of efficacy. Patients with active upper GI tract disease should not be given oral bisphosphonates.

Mild fever and aches may attend the first parenteral infusion of pamidronate, likely owing to cytokine release. These symptoms are short lived and generally do not recur with subsequent administration.

Zoledronate has been associated with renal toxicity, deterioration of renal function, and potential renal failure. Thus, the infusion should be given over at least 15 minutes, and the dose should be 4 mg. Patients who receive zoledronate should have standard laboratory and clinical parameters of renal function assessed prior to treatment and periodically after treatment to monitor for deterioration in renal function.

PANCREATIC ENZYME PREPARATIONS

	Contents (units)		
Agents	**Lipase**	**Protease**	**Amylase**
Cotazym	8,000	30,000	30,000
Cotazym-S	5,000	20,000	20,000
Creon	8,000	13,000	30,000
Entolase	4,000	25,000	20,000
Entolase-HP	8,000	50,000	40,000
Ilozyme	11,000	30,000	30,000
Pancrease	4,000	25,000	20,000
Pancrease MT4	4,000	12,000	12,000
Pancrease MT10	10,000	30,000	30,000
Pancrease MT16	16,000	48,000	48,000
Viokase	8,000	30,000	30,000
Viokase	16,800	70,000	70,000
Zymase	12,000	24,000	24,000

PANCREATIN

(Creon, Dizymes, Donnazyme, Entozyme, Hi-Vegi-Lip, 4X Pancrezyme, 8X Pancrezyme)

Pancreatin, a pancreatic enzyme, is indicated in exocrine pancreatic secretion insufficiency, as a digestive aid in cystic fibrosis, steatorrhea, and for other disorders of fat metabolism secondary to insufficient pancreatic enzymes.

PANCRELIPASE

(Cotazym, Cotazym-S, Ilozyme, Ku-Zyme HP, Pancrease, Pancrease MT4, Pancrease MT10, Pancrease MT16, Pancrelipase, Protilase, Ultrase MT12, Ultrase MT20, Ultrase UT24, Viokase, Zymase)

Pancrelipase, a pancreatic enzyme, is indicated in exocrine pancreatic secretion insufficiency, cystic fibrosis in adults and children, steatorrhea, and in other disorders of fat metabolism secondary to insufficient pancreatic enzymes.

Chronic pancreatitis is a debilitating syndrome that results in symptoms from loss of glandular function (exocrine and endocrine) and inflammation (pain). Because there is no cure for chronic pancreatitis, the goals of pharmacological therapy are prevention of malabsorption and palliation of pain. The cornerstone of therapy for malabsorption still is the use of pancreatic enzymes. Although also used for pain, these agents are much less effective for this symptom.

The two common preparations of pancreatic enzymes for replacement therapy are obtained from the pancreas of the hog (*Sus scrofa* Linne var. *domesticus* Gray). **Pancreatin** (Donnazyme, others) contains **amylase**, **lipase**, and **protease**, and has one-twelfth of the lipolytic activity of pancrelipase, on a weight-by-weight basis. Pancrelipase is more commonly used and is available in uncoated forms, as well as capsules containing enteric-coated microspheres and enteric-coated microtablets, which withstand gastric acid (lipase is inactivated by acid) and disintegrate at pH > 6. Familiarity with these two classes of preparations is important clinically.

Fat malabsorption (**steatorrhea**) and protein maldigestion occur when the pancreas loses more than 90% of its ability to produce digestive enzymes. The resultant diarrhea and malabsorption can be managed reasonably well if 30,000 USP units of pancreatic lipase are delivered to the duodenum during a 4-hour period with and after meals; this represents about 10% of the normal pancreatic output. Alternatively, one can titrate the dosage to the fat content of the diet, with approximately 8,000 USP units of lipase activity required for each 17 g of dietary fat. Available preparations of pancreatic enzymes contain up to 20,000 units of lipase and 75,000 units of protease, and the typical dose of pancrelipase is 1 to 3 capsules or tablets with or just before meals and snacks, adjusted until a satisfactory symptomatic response is obtained. The loss of pancreatic amylase does not present a problem because of other sources of this enzyme (e.g., salivary glands). Patients using uncoated preparations require concomitant pharmacological control of gastric acid production with a proton-pump inhibitor.

Pain is the other cardinal symptom of chronic pancreatitis. The rationale for its treatment with pancreatic enzymes is based on the principle of negative feedback inhibition of the pancreas by the presence of duodenal proteases. The release of **cholecystokinin** (CCK), the principal secretagogue for pancreatic enzymes, is triggered by CCK-releasing monitor peptide in the duodenum, which normally is denatured by pancreatic trypsin. In chronic pancreatitis, trypsin insufficiency leads to persistent activation of this peptide and an increased release of CCK, which is thought to cause pancreatic pain because of continuous stimulation of pancreatic enzyme output and increased intraductal pressure. Delivery of active proteases to the duodenum (which can be done reliably only with uncoated preparations) therefore is important for the interruption of this loop. Although enzymatic therapy has become firmly entrenched for the treatment of painful pancreatitis, the evidence supporting this practice is equivocal at best.

In general, pancreatic enzyme preparations are tolerated extremely well by patients. For patients with hypersensitivity to pork protein, bovine enzymes are available. Hyperuricosuria in patients with cystic fibrosis can occur, and malabsorption of folate and iron has been reported. In the past, products with higher lipase content were available, but these were withdrawn after reports associating their use with the development of colonic strictures in patients with cystic fibrosis

Octreotide also has been used, with questionable efficacy, to decrease refractory abdominal pain in patients with chronic pancreatitis.

PANCURONIUM BROMIDE
(Pavulon)

Pancuronium, a nondepolarizing neuromuscular blocker (initially 0.04 to 0.1 mg/kg IV), is indicated as an adjunct to anesthesia in order to induce skeletal muscle relaxation, to insure the management of patients undergoing mechanical ventilation and to facilitate tracheal intubation. Agents such as tubocurarine and pancuronium compete with acetylcholine for the cholinergic receptors at the end plate. They combine with the receptors but do not activate them. Competitive or nondepolarizing agents are antagonized by neostigmine (see also Figure 99).

Use of a peripheral nerve stimulator will usually be of value for monitoring the neuromuscular blocking effect, avoiding overdosage, and assisting in evaluation of recovery. Patients with severe obesity or neuromuscular disease may pose airway or ventilatory problems requiring special care before, during, and after the use of neuromuscular blocking agents such as pancuronium.

Electrolyte imbalance, and diseases that lead to electrolyte imbalance, such as adrenal cortical insufficiency, alter neuromuscular blockade. Depending on the nature of the imbalance, either enhancement or inhibition may be expected. Magnesium sulfate, used in the management of toxemia of pregnancy, enhances the skeletal-muscle-relaxing effects of pancuronium. Antibiotics such as aminoglycosides, tetracyclines, clindamycin, lincomycin, colistin, and sodium colistimethate augment the pancuronium-induced neuromuscular blockade. Anesthetics such as halothane, enflurane, and isoflurane enhance the action of pancuronium, whereas azathioprine will cause a reversal of neuromuscular blockade.

PANIC DISORDER: Treatment of

Antihypertensive Medication
Clonidine

Benzodiazepines
Alprazolam
Clonazepam
Diazepam

Monoamine Oxidase Inhibitors
Phenelzine

Tricyclic Antidepressants
Imipramine

PANTOPRAZOLE SODIUM

(Protonix tablets, delayed-release 40 mg)

Pantoprazole sodium is a proton-pump inhibitor that suppresses gastric-acid secretion by blocking acid (proton) pump within gastric parietal cells. **Oral**: used for short-term (no more than 8 weeks) treatment in the healing and symptomatic relief of erosive esophagitis associated with gastroesophageal reflux disease (GERD); long-term treatment of pathological hypersecretory conditions, including **Zollinger–Ellison syndrome**; and maintenance of healing of erosive esophagitis. **IV**: used in short-term (7- to 10-day) treatment of GERD, as an alternative to oral therapy in patients unable to continue oral pantoprazole; and hypersecretory conditions associated with Zollinger–Ellison syndrome or other neoplastic conditions.

Pantoprazole, a substituted benzimidazole sulphoxide, is a proton-pump inhibitor recommended for the treatment of acid-related GI diseases such as reflux esophagitis and duodenal and gastric ulcers (see also Figure 72).

The most potent suppressors of gastric-acid secretion are inhibitors of the gastric H^+,K^+-ATPase (proton pump). In typical doses, these drugs diminish the daily production of acid (basal and stimulated) by 80 to 95%. Five proton-pump inhibitors are available for clinical use: **omeprazole** (Prilosec, Rapinex, Zegerid) and its S-isomer, **esomeprazole** (Nexium), **lansoprazole** (Prevacid), **rabeprazole** (Aciphex), and **pantoprazole** (Protonix). These drugs have different substitutions on their pyridine and/or benzimidazole groups but are remarkably similar in their pharmacological properties. Omeprazole is a racemic mixture of R- and S-isomers; the S-isomer, esomeprazole (*S*-omeprazole), is eliminated less rapidly than *R*-omeprazole, which theoretically provides a therapeutic advantage because of the increased half-life. Despite claims to the contrary, all proton-pump inhibitors have equivalent efficacy at comparable doses.

Proton-pump inhibitors are prodrugs that require activation in an acid environment. After absorption into the systemic circulation, the prodrug diffuses into the parietal cells of the stomach and accumulates in the acidic secretory canaliculi. Here, it is activated by proton-catalyzed formation of a tetracyclic sulfenamide, trapping the drug so that it cannot diffuse back across the canalicular membrane. The activated form then binds covalently with sulfhydryl groups of cysteines in the H^+,K^+-ATPase, irreversibly inactivating the pump molecule. Acid secretion resumes only after new pump molecules are synthesized and inserted into the luminal membrane, providing a prolonged (up to 24- to 48-hour) suppression of acid secretion, despite the much shorter plasma half-lives (0.5 to 2 hours) of the parent compounds. Because they block the final step in acid production, proton-pump inhibitors are effective in acid suppression regardless of other stimulating factors.

To prevent degradation of proton-pump inhibitors by acid in the gastric lumen, oral dosage forms are supplied in different formulations: (1) enteric-coated drugs contained inside gelatin capsules (omeprazole, esomeprazole, and lansoprazole); (2) enteric-coated granules supplied as a powder for suspension (lansoprazole); (3) enteric-coated tablets (**pantoprazole**, rabeprazole, and omeprazole); and (4) powdered drug combined with sodium bicarbonate (omeprazole). The delayed-release and enteric-coated tablets dissolve only at alkaline pH, whereas the admixture of omeprazole with sodium bicarbonate simply neutralizes stomach acid; both strategies substantially improve the oral bioavailability of these acid-labile drugs. Until recently, the requirement for enteric coating posed a challenge to the administration of proton-pump inhibitors in patients for whom the oral route of administration is not available. These patients and those requiring immediate acid suppression now can be treated parenterally with **pantoprazole** or lansoprazole, both of which are approved for intravenous administration in the United States.

A single intravenous bolus of 80 mg of pantoprazole inhibits acid production by 80 to 90% within an hour, and this inhibition persists for up to 21 hours, permitting once-daily dosing to achieve the desired degree of hypochlorhydria. The FDA-approved dose of intravenous pantoprazole for gastroesophageal reflux disease is 40 m daily for up to 10 days. Higher doses (e.g., 160 to 240 m, in divided doses) are used to manage hypersecretory conditions such as the Zollinger–Ellison syndrome. Because an acidic pH in the parietal cell acid canaliculi is required for drug activation, and because food stimulates acid production, these drugs ideally should be given about 30 minutes before meals. Concurrent administration of food may reduce somewhat the rate of absorption of proton-pump inhibitors, but this effect is not thought to be clinically significant. Concomitant use of other drugs that inhibit acid secretion, such as H_2-receptor antagonists, might be predicted to lessen the effectiveness of the proton-pump inhibitors, but the clinical relevance of this potential interaction is unknown.

Once in the small bowel, proton-pump inhibitors are rapidly absorbed, highly protein bound, and extensively metabolized by hepatic CYPs, particularly CYP2C19 and CYP3A4. Several variants of CYP2C19 have been identified. Asians are more likely than Caucasians or African-Americans to have the CYP2C19 genotype that correlates with the slow metabolism of proton-pump inhibitors (23% vs. 3%, respectively), which has been suggested to contribute to heightened efficacy and/or toxicity in this ethnic group. Although the CYP2C19 genotype is correlated with the magnitude of gastric acid suppression by proton-pump inhibitors in patients with gastroesophageal reflux disease, there is no evidence that the CYP2C19 genotype predicts clinical efficacy of these drugs.

Because not all pumps or all parietal cells are active simultaneously, maximal suppression of acid secretion requires several doses of the proton-pump inhibitors. For example, it may take 2 to 5 days of therapy with once-daily dosing to achieve the 70% inhibition of proton pumps that is seen at steady state. More frequent initial dosing (e.g., twice daily) will reduce the time to achieve full inhibition but is not proven to improve patient outcome. Because the proton-pump inhibition is irreversible, acid secretion will be suppressed for 24 to 48 hours or more until new proton pumps are synthesized and incorporated into the luminal membrane of parietal cells.

Chronic renal failure does not lead to drug accumulation with once-a-day dosing of the proton-pump inhibitors. Hepatic disease substantially reduces the clearance of **esomeprazole** and **lansoprazole**. Thus, in patients with severe hepatic disease, dose reduction is recommended for esomeprazole and should be considered for lansoprazole.

Proton-pump inhibitors generally cause remarkably few adverse effects. The most common side effects are nausea, abdominal pain, constipation, flatulence, and diarrhea. Subacute myopathy, arthralgias, headaches, and skin rashes also have been reported. As noted previously, proton-pump inhibitors are metabolized by hepatic CYPs and therefore may interfere with the elimination of other drugs cleared by this route. Proton-pump inhibitors have been observed to interact with **warfarin** (esomeprazole, lansoprazole, omeprazole, and rabeprazole), **diazepam** (esomeprazole and omeprazole), and **cyclosporine** (omeprazole and rabeprazole). Among the proton-pump inhibitors, only omeprazole inhibits CYP2C19 (thereby decreasing the clearance of **disulfiram**, **phenytoin**, and other drugs) and induces the expression of CYP1A2 (thereby increasing the clearance of **imipramine**, several antipsychotic drugs, **tacrine**, and **theophylline**).

Chronic treatment with omeprazole decreases the absorption of vitamin B_{12}, but the clinical relevance of this effect is not clear. Loss of gastric acidity also may affect the bioavailability of such drugs as ketoconazole, ampicillin esters, and iron salts.

Hypergastrinemia is more frequent and more severe with proton-pump inhibitors than with H_2-receptor antagonists, and gastrin levels of >500 ng/L occur in approximately 5 to 10% of users with chronic omeprazole administration. This hypergastrinemia may predispose patients to rebound hypersecretion of gastric acid upon discontinuation of therapy.

PAPAVERINE HYDROCHLORIDE

(Cerebid, Cerespan, Delapav, Myobid, Papacon, Pavabid, Pavacap, Pavacen, Pavadur, Pavadyl, Pavagen, Pava-Par, Pava-Rx, Pavased, Pavasule, Pavatine, Paverolan, P-200, Pasal)

Papaverine hydrochloride is a peripheral vasodilator that directly relaxes the tone of all smooth muscle, especially when spasmodically contracted. It causes vasodilatation of blood vessels of the coronary, cerebral, pulmonary and peripheral arteries; and relaxes musculature of the bronchi, GI tract, ureters, and biliary system. **Oral form**: is used for relief of cerebral and peripheral ischemia associated with arterial spasm and myocardial ischemia complicated by arrhythmias. **Parenteral form**: is used for vascular spasm associated with acute myocardial infarction (MI) (coronary occlusion), angina pectoris, peripheral and pulmonary embolism, peripheral vascular disease in which there is a vasospastic element, certain cerebral angiospastic states, visceral spasm (e.g., ureteral, biliary, and GI colic).

Papaverine, a benzylisoquinoline derivative with peripheral vasodilating properties (300 mg p.o. t.i.d.), is indicated in the relief of cerebral and peripheral ischemia associated with arterial spasm and myocardial ischemia; it is used in the treatment of coronary occlusion and certain cerebral angiospastic states.

PARA-AMINOSALICYLATE SODIUM (PAS)

(Parasal sodium, Pasdium, P.A.S. sodium, Teebacin)

Para-aminosalicylate, an aminobenzoic acid analog with antituberculant activity (12 to 15 g p.o. daily), is indicated as adjunctive treatment of tuberculosis.

PARALDEHYDE

(Paral)

Paraldehyde (4 to 8 mL in iced fruit juice to mask taste) is used as a sedative and hypnotic, and to calm patients during delirium tremens and other states characterized by excitement. Paraldehyde is a polymer of acetaldehyde (CH_3CHO) in which three molecules of the latter are combined. It is a colorless and transparent liquid with a characteristic pungent odor and a hot burning taste that renders its administration difficult. Paraldehyde is one of the safest of the hypnotics, inducing sleep in moderate doses, which is unaccompanied by any marked change in the circulation, respiration, or sensibility. However, its unpleasant odor and hot burning taste militate against its wide use. Paraldehyde is useful in delirium tremens and other forms of delirium, and in head injuries with agitation.

PARAMETHADIONE

(Paradione)

Paramethadione, an oxazolidine derivative (300 mg p.o. t.i.d.), is indicated as an alternate drug in the treatment of refractory absence seizures. Paramethadione raises the threshold for cortical seizures but does not modify the seizure pattern. It decreases projection of focal activity and reduces both repetitive spinal cord transmission and spike-and-wave patterns of absence (petit mal) seizures.

Paramethadione is dimethylated to an active anticonvulsant. It is contraindicated in patients with severe hepatic or renal disease, severe blood dyscrasias, or diseases of the retina or optic nerve because the drug may exacerbate diseases of the optic nerve.

The concomitant use of mephenytoin and paramethadione, which may cause fatal hypersensitivity reactions, is discouraged.

Symptoms of overdose include nausea, drowsiness, ataxia, and visual disturbances; coma may follow a massive overdose.

PARAMETHASONE ACETATE (Haldrone)

Paramethasone (0.5 to 6 mg p.o. t.i.d.), a glucocorticoid, is used for its antiinflammatory and immunosuppressant properties. It possesses no mineralocorticoid actions.

Paramethasone stimulates the synthesis of enzymes needed to decrease the antiinflammatory response. It suppresses the immune system by reducing activity and volume of the lymphatic system, thus producing lymphocytopenia (primarily of T-lymphocytes), decreasing passage of immune complexes through basement membranes, and possibly by depressing reactivity of tissue to antigen–antibody interactions (see Table 11).

Paramethasone is contraindicated in patients with systemic fungal infections. Patients receiving paramethasone should not be given live-virus vaccines because paramethasone suppresses the immune response.

Paramethasone should be used with extreme caution in patients with GI ulceration, renal disease, hypertension, osteoporosis, diabetes mellitus, thromboembolic disorders, seizures, myasthenia gravis, congestive heart failure (CHF), tuberculosis, hypoalbuminemia, hypothyroidism, cirrhosis of the liver, emotional instability, psychotic tendencies, hyperlipidemias, glaucoma, or cataracts because the drug may exacerbate these conditions.

Because adrenocorticoids increase the susceptibility to mask symptoms of infection, paramethasone should not be used (except in life-threatening situations) in patients with viral or bacteria infections not controlled by antiinfective agents.

Glucocorticoids increase the metabolism of isoniazid and salicylates; they cause hyperglycemia, requiring dosage adjustment of insulin or oral hypoglycemic agents in diabetic patients; and they may enhance hypokalemia associated with diuretic or amphotericin B therapy. The hypokalemia may increase the risk of toxicity in patients concurrently receiving digitalis glycosides.

Barbiturates, phenytoin, and rifampin may cause decreased paramethasone effects because of increased hepatic metabolism. Cholestyramine, colestipol, and antacids decrease the corticosteroid effect by absorbing the corticosteroid, decreasing the amount absorbed.

Concomitant use with estrogens may reduce the metabolism of paramethasone by increasing the concentration of transcortin. The half-life of paramethasone is then prolonged because of increased protein binding. Concomitant administration of ulcerogenic drugs, such as nonsteroidal antiinflammatory agents, may increase the risk of GI ulceration (see Table 3).

PARASITIC INFECTIONS: Treatment of

Infections	Drugs
AMEBIASIS (*Entamoeba histolytica*)	
Asymptomatic	
Drugs of choice	Iodoquinol
	or
	Paromomycin
Alternative	Diloxanide furoate
Mild to moderate intestinal disease	
Drugs of choice	Metronidazole
	or
	Tinidazole
Alternative	Dehydroemetine
Hepatic abscess	
Drugs of choice	Metronidazole
	or
	Tinidazole
Alternatives	Dehydroemetine
	followed by
	Chloroquine phosphate
AMEBIC MENINGOENCEPHALITIS, PRIMARY	
Naegleria	
Drug of choice	Amphotericin B
Acanthamoeba	
Drugs of choice	Pentamidine
	or
	Ketoconazole
	or
	Flucytosine
Ancylostoma duodenale, see Hookworm	
ANGIOSTRONGYLIASIS	
Angiostrongylus cantonensis	
Drug of choice	Mebendazole
Angiostrongylus costaricensis	
Drug of choice	Thiabendazole
ANISAKIASIS (*Anisakis*)	
Treatment of choice	Surgical or endoscopic removal
ASCARIASIS (*Ascaris lumbricoides*, roundworm)	
Drugs of choice	Mebendazole
	or
	Pyrantel pamoate
	or
	Albendazole

PARASITIC INFECTIONS: Treatment of (Continued)

Infections	Drugs
BABESIOSIS (*Babesia microti*)	
Drugs of choice	Clindamycin plus Quinine
BALANTIDIASIS (*Balantidium coli*)	
Drug of choice	Tetracycline
Alternatives	Iodoquinol
	Metronidazole
BAYLISASCARIASIS (*Baylisascaris procyonis*)	
Drugs of choice	Diethylcarbamazine or Levamisole or Fenbendazole
***BLASTOCYSTIS hominis* infection**	
Drug of choice	Metronidazole
CAPILLARIASIS (*Capillaria philippinensis*)	
Drug of choice	Mebendazole
Alternatives	Albendazole
	Thiabendazole

Chagas' disease, see Trypanosomiasis
Clonorchis sinensis, see Fluke infection

CRYPTOSPORIDIOSIS (*Cryptosporidium*)	
Drug of choice	Infection is self-limited in immunocompetent patients. Octreotide controls diarrhea
CUTANEOUS LARVA MIGRANS (creeping eruption, dog and cat hookworm)	
Drugs of choice	Thiabendazole or Albendazole
***CYCLOSPORA* infection**	
Drug of choice	Trimethoprim-sulfamethoxazole

Cysticercosis, see Tapeworm infection

***DIENTAMOEBA fragilis* infection**	
Drugs of choice	Iodoquinol or Paromomycin or Tetracycline

Diphyllobothrium latum, see Tapeworm infection

***DRACUNCULUS medinensis* (guinea worm) infection**	
Drug of choice	Metronidazole
Alternative	Thiabendazole

Echinococcus, see Tapeworm infection
Entamoeba histolytica, see Amebiasis

***ENTAMOEBA polecki* infection**	
Drug of choice	Metronidazole
***ENTEROBIUS vermicularis* (pinworm) infection**	
Drugs of choice	Pyrantel pamoate or Mebendazole or Albendazole

Fasciola hepatica, see Fluke infection

FILARIASIS

Wuchereria bancrofti, Brugia malayi	
Drug of choice	Dimethylcarbamazine
Loa loa	
Drug of choice	Dimethylcarbamazine
Mansonella ozzardi	
Drug of choice	Ivermectin
Mansonella perstans	
Drug of choice	Mebendazole
Tropical pulmonary eosinophilia (TPE)	
Drug of choice	Diethylcarbamazine
Onchocerca volvulus	
Drug of choice	Ivermectin

FLUKE, hermaphroditic, infection

***Clonorchis sinensis* (*Chinese liver fluke*)**	
Drug of choice	Praziquantel
***Fasciola hepatica* (*sheep liver fluke*)**	
Drug of choice	Bithionol
***Fasciolopsis buski* (*intestinal fluke*)**	
Drugs of choice	Praziquantel or Niclosamide
***Heterophyes heterophyes* (*intestinal fluke*)**	
Drug of choice	Praziquantel
***Metagonimus yokogawai* (*intestinal fluke*)**	
Drug of choice	Praziquantel
Nanophyetus salmincola	
Drug of choice	Praziquantel
***Opisthorchis viverrini* (*liver fluke*)**	
Drug of choice	Praziquantel
***Paragonimus westermani* (*lung fluke*)**	
Drug of choice	Praziquantel
Alternative	Bithionol
GIARDIASIS (*Giardia lamblia*)	
Drug of choice	Metronidazole
Alternatives	Quinacrine HCl or Tinidazole or Furazolidone or Paromomycin

PARASITIC INFECTIONS: Treatment of

Infections | **Drugs**

GNATHOSTOMIASIS (*Gnathostoma spinigerum*)

Treatment of choice — Surgical removal plus Albendazole

HOOKWORM infection (*Ancylostoma duodenale, Necator americanus*)

Drugs of choice — Mebendazole or Pyrantel pamoate or Albendazole

Hydatid cyst, see Tapeworm infection
Hymenolepis nana, see Tapeworm infection

ISOSPORIASIS (*Isospora belli*)

Drug of choice — Trimethoprim-sulfamethoxazole

LEISHMANIASIS (*L. Mexicana, L. tropica, L. major, L. braziliensis, L. donovani* [*Kala-azar*])

Drugs of choice — Sodium stibogluconate or Meglumine antimonate
Alternative — Pentamidine isethionate

LICE infestation (*Pediculus humanus, capitis, Phthirus pubis*)

Drugs of choice — 1% Permethrin (topically) or 0.5% Malathion (topically)
Alternatives — Pyrethrins with piperonyl butoxide; Lindane (topically)

Loa loa, see Filariasis
MALARIA, treatment of (*Plasmodium falciparum, P. ovale, P. vivax*, and *P. malariae*)

Chloroquine-resistant P. falciparum

ORAL
Drugs of choice — Quinine sulfate plus Pyrimethamine-sulfadoxine or, plus Tetracycline or, plus Clindamycin
Alternatives — Mefloquine; Halofantrine

PARENTERAL
Drugs of choice — Quinidine gluconate or Quinine dihydrochloride

Prevention of relapses: P. vivax and P. ovale only

Drug of choice — Primaquine phosphate

MALARIA, Prevention of

Chloroquine-sensitive areas

Drug of choice — Chloroquine phosphate

Chloroquine-resistant areas

Drugs of choice — Mefloquine or Doxycycline
Alternatives — Chloroquine phosphate plus Pyrimethamine-sulfadoxine for presumptive treatment or, plus Proguanil (in Africa south of the Sahara)

MICROSPORIDIOSIS

Ocular (Encephalitozoon hellem, Nosema corneum)

Drug of choice — Fumagillin eyedrops

Intestinal (Enterocytozoon bieneusi, Septata intestinalis)

Drug of choice — Octreotide

Mites, see Scabies

MONILIFORMIS moniliformis infection

Drug of choice — Pyrantel pamoate

***Naegleria* species**, see Amebic Meningoencephalitis, Primary
Necator americanus, see Hookworm infection

Oesophagostomum bifurcum

Drugs of choice — Albendazole or Pyrantel pamoate

Onchocerca volvulus, see Filariasis
Opisthorchis viverrini, see Fluke infection
Paragonimus westermani, see Fluke infection
Pediculus capitis, humanus, Phthirus pubis, see Lice
Pinworm, see *Enterobius*

PNEUMOCYSTIS carinii pneumonia

Drugs of choice — Trimethoprim-sulfamethoxazole or Pentamidine
Alternatives — Trimethoprim plus Dapsone; Atovaquone; Primaquine plus Clindamycin; Trimetrexate plus Folinic acid

Primary and secondary prophylaxis

Drug of choice — Trimethoprim-sulfamethoxazole
Alternatives — Dapsone or Aerosol pentamidine

Roundworm, see Ascariasis
SCABIES (*Sarcoptes scabiei*)

PARASITIC INFECTIONS: Treatment of (Continued)

Infections	Drugs
Drug of choice	5% Permethrin (topically)
Alternatives	Lindane (topically) or 10% Crotamiton (topically)

SCHISTOSOMIASIS (Bilharziasis)

S. haematobium	
Drug of choice	Praziquantel
S. japonicum	
Drug of choice	Praziquantel
S. mansoni	
Drug of choice	Praziquantel
Alternative	Oxamniquine
S. mekongi	
Drug of choice	Praziquantel

Sleeping sickness, see Trypanosomiasis

STRONGYLOIDIASIS (*Strongyloidis stercoralis*)

Drugs of choice	Thiabendazole or Ivermectin

TAPEWORM infection—Adult (intestinal stage)

Diphyllobothrium latum (fish), Taenia saginata (beef), Taenia solium (pork), Dipylidium caninum (dog)	
Drugs of choice	Praziquantel or Niclosamide
Hymenolepis nana (dwarf tapeworm)	
Drug of choice	Praziquantel
Alternative:	Niclosamide
—Larval (tissue stage)	
Echinococcus granulosus (hydatid cyst)	
Drug of choice	Albendazole
Echinococcus multilocularis	
Treatment of choice	Surgical excision
Cysticercus cellulosae (cysticercosis)	
Drugs of choice	Albendazole or Praziquantel
Alternative	Surgery

Toxocariasis, see Visceral Larva Migrans

TOXOPLASMOSIS (*Toxoplasma gondii*)

Drugs of choice	Pyrimethamine plus Sulfadiazine
Alternative	Spiramycin

TRICHINOSIS (*Trichinella spiralis*)

Drugs of choice	Steroids for severe symptoms plus Mebendazole

TRICHOMONIASIS (*Trichomonas vaginalis*)

Drugs of choice	Metronidazole or Tinidazole

TRICHOSTRONGYLUS infection

Drug of choice	Pyrantel pamoate
Alternatives	Mebendazole or Albendazole

TRICHURIASIS (*Trichuris trichiura*, whipworm)

Drugs of choice	Mebendazole or Albendazole

TRYPANOSOMIASIS

T. cruzi (South American trypanosomiasis, Chagas' disease)	
Drug of choice	Nifurtimox
Alternative	Benznidazole
T. brucei gambiense; T.b. rhodesiense (African trypanosomiasis, sleeping sickness)	
Drugs of choice	Suramin or Eflornithine
Alternative	Pentamidine isethionate
Late disease with CNS involvement	
Drugs of choice	Melarsoprol or Eflornithine
Alternative	Tryparsamide plus Suramin

VISCERAL LARVA MIGRANS

Drug of choice	Diethylcarbamazine
Alternatives	Albendazole or Mebendazole

Whipworm, see Trichuriasis
***Wuchereria bancrofti*, see Filariasis**

PARATHYROID HORMONE

Four parathyroid glands are situated on the lateral lobes of the thyroid. These glands secrete parathyroid hormone in response to low serum calcium levels. Parathyroid hormone then increases the serum calcium levels through the functioning of several mechanisms: it stimulates bone resorption; it increases the intestinal absorption of calcium; it

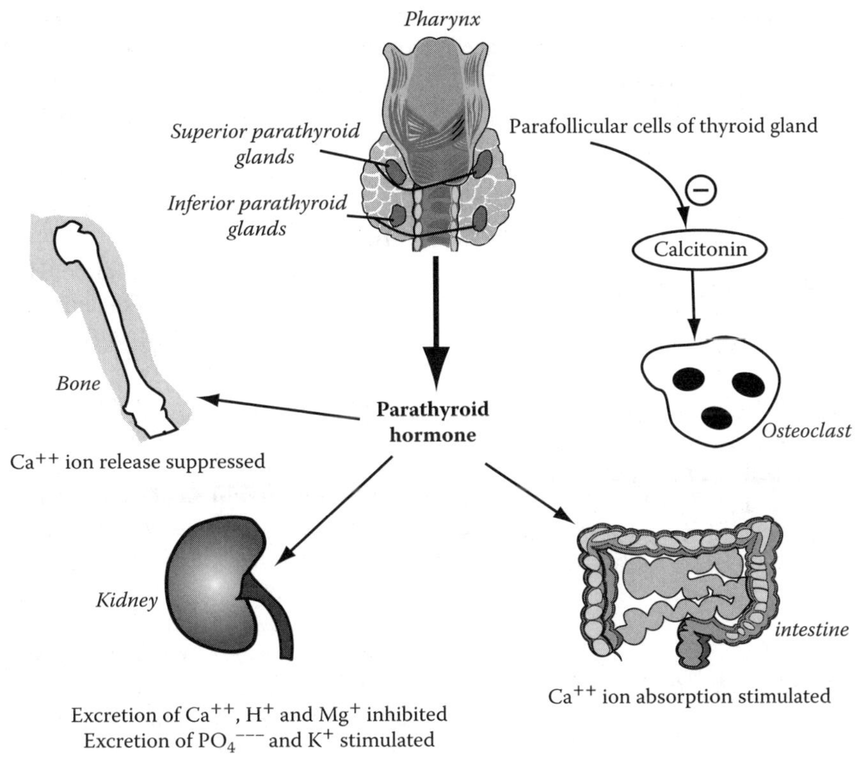

FIGURE 75 Four parathyroid glands are situated on the lateral lobes of the thyroid. These glands secrete parathyroid hormone in response to low serum calcium levels. Parathyroid hormone then increases the serum calcium levels by stimulating bone resorption, increasing the intestinal absorption of calcium, increasing the resorption of calcium by the renal tubules, and by acting on the kidney to decrease the tubular resorption of phosphate.

increases the resorption of calcium by the renal tubules; and it acts on the kidney to decrease the tubular resorption of phosphate.

A reciprocal relationship exists between the level of calcium and phosphorus, as shown by the following table:

	Serum Calcium	Serum Phosphate
Hyperparathyroidism	Elevated	Low
Hypoparathyroidism	Low	Elevated

Calcitonin is also involved in calcium homeostasis by inhibiting bone resorption and by preventing excess increases in the serum calcium concentration through its monitoring of parathyroid hormone's actions (see Figure 75).

Parathyroid hormone is a single-chain polypeptide composed of 84 amino acids. It has a molecular weight of 9500 and lacks an intrachain disulfide linkage. Parathyroid hormone is produced by means of two sequential enzymic cleavages from a larger precursor polypeptide, preparathyroid hormone.

The organs principally responsible for the peripheral metabolism of parathyroid hormone are the kidneys and liver, and possibly bone. When parathyroid hormones are lacking, the following events take place:

A decreasing serum calcium level (reduced bone resorption)
An increasing serum phosphorus level (increased tubular resorption)
Neuromuscular irritability and tonic–clonic convulsions (low calcium tetany)
Laryngeal stridor, asthma, and other muscular spasms (irritability due to low calcium levels)
Ectopic calcifications in the blood vessels, brain, subcutaneous tissue, muscles, and cartilage (calcium phosphate is an insoluble salt) (see Figure 75).

Other manifestations of hypoparathyroidism include lenticular cataracts, dental defects, dry scaly skin, tendency to monilial infections, impaired mental acuity, and psychiatric disturbances.

Hypocalcemic tetany is treated with the intravenous administration of calcium gluconate or calcium chloride (5 to 10 mL of 10% solution). The effects of these agents are rapid but transient. Furthermore, a 10-mL solution of calcium chloride and calcium gluconate contains 270 mg and 70 mg of calcium, respectively. Because calcium chloride is a highly irritating substance, it should not be administered intramuscularly. Parathyroid hormone (100 to 300 units) is injected subcutaneously after the initial administration of calcium salt, but its effect is transient and lasts only 3 to 4 weeks. Hypoparathyroidism is also treated with vitamin D (1 to 2 mg = 50,000 to 100,000 units per day) (see also Figure 75).

PAREGORIC

Paregoric (4 to 5 mL 1 tsp) is a camphorated tincture of opium. Opiate preparations, usually given as paregorics, are effective and fast-acting antidiarrheal agents. These agents are also useful postoperatively to produce solid stool following an ileostomy or colostomy. A meperidine derivative, diphenoxylate, is usually dispensed with atropine and sold as Lomotil. The atropine is added to discourage the abuse of diphenoxylate by narcotic addicts who are tolerant to massive doses of narcotic but not to the CNS stimulant effects of atropine.

PARKINSON'S DISEASE: Treatment of

Amantadine	100 mg twice a day
Bromocriptine	1.25 mg twice a day
Carbidopa/levodopa	25 to 100 mg three times a day
Carbidopa/levodopa, sustained release	50 to 200 mg twice a day
Pergolide	0.05 mg once a day
Selegiline	5.0 mg twice a day
Trihexyphenidyl HCl	1 mg twice a day

PAROMOMYCIN SULFATE

(Humatin capsules 250 mg)

Paromomycin sulfate is an amebicide/aminoglycoside that inhibits production of protein in bacteria, causing bacterial cell death. It is indicated in the treatment of acute and chronic intestinal amebiasis. It is adjunctive therapy in management of hepatic coma. The cornerstone of therapy for amebiasis is the **nitroimidazole** compound **metronidazole** or its analogs **tinidazole** and **omidazole**. Metronidazole and tinidazole are the only nitroimidazoles available in the United States and are the drugs of choice for the treatment of amebic colitis, amebic liver abscess, and any other extraintestinal form of amebiasis. Other agents, such as **dehydroemetine** and **chloroquine**, are now used rarely in the treatment of amebic colitis or amebic liver abscess, and are reserved for only very unusual cases where metronidazole is contraindicated. Because metronidazole is so well absorbed in the gut, levels may not be therapeutic in the colonic lumen, and it is less effective against cysts. Hence, patients with amebiasis (amebic colitis or amebic liver abscess) also should receive a luminal agent to eradicate any *E. histolytica* trophozoites residing within the gut lumen. Luminal agents are also used to treat asymptomatic individuals found to be infected with *E. histolytica*. The nonabsorbed aminoglycoside **paromomycin** and the **8-hydroxyquinoline** compound iodoquinol are two effective luminal agents. Diloxanide furoate, previously considered the luminal agent of choice for amebiasis, is no longer available in the United States. **Nitazoxanide** (Alinia), a drug approved in the United States for the treatment of cryptosporidiosis and giardiasis, is also active against *E. histolytica*.

Paromomycin (aminosidine, Humatin) is an aminoglycoside of the neomycin/kanamycin family that is used as an oral agent to treat *E. histolytica* infection. **Paromomycin** also has been used orally to treat cryptosporidiosis and giardiasis. A topical formulation has been used to treat trichomoniasis, and parenteral administration has been used for visceral leishmaniasis.

Paromomycin shares the same mechanism of action as **neomycin** and **kanamycin** (binding to the 30S ribosomal subunit) and has the same spectrum of antibacterial activity. Paromomycin is available only for oral use in the United States. Following oral administration, 100% of the drug is recovered in the feces, and even in cases of compromised gut integrity, there is little evidence for clinically significant absorption of paromomycin. Parenteral administration carries the same risks of nephrotoxicity and ototoxicity seen with other aminoglycosides.

Paromomycin has become the drug of choice for treating intestinal colonization with *E. histolytica*. It is used in combination with **metronidazole** to treat amebic colitis and amebic liver abscess, and can be used as a single agent for asymptomatic individuals found to have *E. histolytica* intestinal colonization. Recommended dosing for adults and children is 25 to 35 mg/kg per day orally in three divided doses. Adverse effects are rare with oral usage but include abdominal pain and cramping, epigastric pain, nausea and vomiting, steatorrhea, and diarrhea. Rarely, rash and headache have been reported. Paromomycin has been used to treat cryptosporidiosis in AIDS patients both as a single agent (oral doses of 500 mg three time daily or 1 g orally twice daily for 14 to 28 days followed by 500 mg orally twice daily) and in combination with azithromycin (paromomycin 1 g orally twice daily plus azithromycin 600 mg orally once daily for 4 weeks, followed by **paromomycin** alone for 8 weeks). Although still recommended by some authorities, in a randomized, controlled trial, paromomycin was no more effective than placebo in treating individuals with cryptosporidiosis and AIDS.

Paromomycin has been advocated as a treatment for giardiasis in pregnant women, especially during the first trimester, when metronidazole is contraindicated, and as an alternative agent for metronidazole-resistant isolates of *G. intestinalis*. Although there is limited clinical experience, response rates of 55 to 90% have been reported. Dosing in adults is 500 mg orally three times daily for 10 days, whereas children have been treated with 25 to 30 mg/kg per day in three divided oral doses. **Paromomycin** formulated as a 6.25% cream has been used to treat vaginal trichomoniasis in patients who had failed metronidazole therapy or could not receive metronidazole. Some cures have been reported, but vulvovaginal ulcerations and pain have complicated treatment.

Paromomycin as a topical formulation containing 15% paromomycin in combination with either a patented base from Walter Reed Army Institute of Research or 12% **methylbenzonium chloride** have shown variable efficacy in clinical trials for the treatment of **cutaneous leishmaniasis**. Paromomycin has been administered parenterally (doses of 16 to 18 mg/kg per day) alone or in combination with antimony to treat visceral leishmaniasis. In one study, cure rates of 89% with **paromomycin** alone were reported, and cure rates of 94% were seen with combination therapy. These results compared favorably with the cure rate for antimony alone (69% in this study) in an endemic area where antimony resistance is common.

Paromomycin, an aminoglycoside with antibacterial and amebicidal properties, is indicated in the treatment of acute and chronic intestinal amebiasis, of tapeworm (fish, beef, pork, and dog) infections in patients who cannot take praziquantel or niclosamide, and as an adjunctive regimen in the management of hepatic coma.

PAROXETINE

(Paxil tablets 10 mg, tablets 20 mg, tablets 30 mg, tablets 40 mg, oral suspension 10 mg/5 mL, Paxil CR tablets, controlled-release 12.5 mg, tablets, controlled-release 25 mg, tablets, controlled-release 37.5 mg)

Paroxetine is a selective serotonin reuptake inhibitor that blocks reuptake of serotonin, enhancing serotonergic function. It is used to treat panic disorder or social anxiety disorder (except Pexeva), as defined in the DSM-IV; major depressive disorder, as defined in DSM-III (immediate release) or DSM-IV (controlled release). Immediate release only: for obsessive–compulsive disorder (OCD); generalized anxiety disorder (GAD) (except Pexeva); posttraumatic stress disorder (PTSD), as defined in the DSM-IV (except Pexeva).

Controlled release only: is used for premenstrual dysphoric disorder (PMDD), as defined in the DSM-IV.

Paroxetine, a selective serotonin uptake inhibitor (20 mg p.o. daily), is indicated in the treatment of depression (see Tables 5 through 7 and Figure 78).

PEFLOXACIN

The quinolones include: nalidixic acid (NegGram), cinoxacin (Cinobac), norfloxacin (Noroxin), and ciprofloxacin (Cipro). Other members of the quinolone family are pefloxacin, ofloxacin, enoxacin, and fleroxacin. The bacterial enzyme DNA gyrase is responsible for the continuous introduction of negative supercoils into DNA, and the quinolones inhibit this gyrase-mediated DNA supercoiling (see Figure 86).

Nalidixic acid and cinoxacin are bactericidal against Gram-negative organisms that cause urinary tract infections. The fluoroquinolones are bactericidal and considerably more potent against *E. coli* and various species of *Salmonella*, *Shigella*, *Enterobacter*, *Campylobacter*, and *Neisseria*. Ciprofloxacin also has good activity against staphylococci, including methicillin-resistant strains.

The quinolones and fluoroquinolones may produce arthropathy, and hence should not be used in prepubertal children or pregnant women.

Nalidixic acid and cinoxacin are useful only for treating urinary tract infections. Ciprofloxacin is useful for both urinary tract infections and prostatitis.

PEGAPTANIB SODIUM

(Macugen injection 0.3 mg)

Pegaptanib sodium is a selective vascular endothelial growth factor antagonist that antagonizes effects of vascular endothelial growth factor, which are thought to contribute to the progression of the neovascular form of age-related macular degeneration. It is indicated in the treatment of neovascular (wet) age-related macular degeneration.

PEGASPARGASE

(Oncaspar injection 750 IU/mL)

Pegaspargase is an enzyme. Leukemic cells are unable to synthesize asparagine because of a lack of asparagine synthetase and are dependent on an exogenous source of asparagine for survival. Rapid depletion of asparagine, which results from treatment with the enzyme L-asparaginase, kills the leukemic cells. It is used in combination therapy of acute lymphocytic leukemia in patients who are hypersensitive to the native form of L-asparaginase; it may be used for single-agent therapy in these patients when combination therapy is inappropriate.

In 1953, it was reported that guinea pig serum had antileukemic activity, and L-asparaginase (L-asp) was identified as the source of this activity. Fifteen (15) years later, the enzyme was introduced into cancer chemotherapy in an effort to exploit a distinct, qualitative difference between normal and malignant cells. It remains a standard agent for treating **lymphocytic leukemia**.

Although most normal tissues are able to synthesize L-asparagine (L-as in amounts sufficient for protein synthesis, some types of lymphoid malignancies derive the required amino acid from plasma. L-asp, by catalyzing the hydrolysis of circulating asparagine to aspartic acid and ammonia, deprives these malignant cells of the asparagine necessary for protein synthesis, leading to cell death. L-asp is commonly used in combination with other agents, including **methotrexate**, **doxorubicin**, **vincristine**, and **prednisone** for the treatment of acute lymphoblastic leukemia (ALL) and for high-grade lymphomas. The sequence of drug administration in these combinations may be critical; for example, synergistic cytotoxicity results when methotrexate precedes the enzyme, but the reverse sequence leads to abrogation of methotrexate cytotoxicity. The latter outcome is a consequence of the inhibition of protein synthesis by L-asp, an effect that stops the progression of cells through the cell cycle and negates the effect of methotrexate, a drug that exerts its greatest effect during the DNA synthetic phase of the cell cycle.

Resistance arises through induction of asparagine synthetase in tumor cells. For unknown reasons, hyperdiploid ALL cells are particularly sensitive to L-asp.

L-Asparaginase (Elspar) is given parenterally. Three different preparations of L-asp are used clinically. Their pharmacokinetics and immunogenicity differ significantly. After intravenous administration, *E. coli*-derived L-asp has a clearance rate from plasma of 0.035 mL/minute per kg, a volume of distribution that approximates the volume of plasma in humans, and a half-life of 14 to 24 hours. It is given in doses of 6,000 to 10,000 international units (IU) every third day for 3 to 4 weeks, although doses up to 25,000 IUs once per week have been employed in experimental ALL protocols. Enzyme levels are maintained above 0.03 IU/mL in plasma to abolish asparagine in the bloodstream. An *Erwinia* preparation, used in patients hypersensitive to the enzyme from *E. coli*, has a shorter half-life of 16 hours and thus requires administration of higher doses. **Pegaspargase** (Peg-L-Asparaginase; Oncaspar) is a preparation in which the enzyme is conjugated to 5,000-dalton units of monomethoxy polyethylene glycol and is cleared much less rapidly. Its plasma half-life is 6 days, and it is administered in doses of 2500 IU/m^2 intramuscularly every week. **Pegaspargase** has much reduced immunogenicity (fewer than 20% of patients develop antibodies).

Intermittent dosage regimens have an increased risk of inducing anaphylaxis. In hypersensitive patients, circulating antibodies lead to immediate inactivation of the enzyme, and L-asp levels rapidly become immeasurable after drug administration. Not all patients with neutralizing antibodies experience hypersensitivity, although the enzyme may be inactivated and therapy may be ineffective. In previously untreated ALL, pegaspargase produces more rapid clearance of lymphoblasts from bone marrow than does the *E. coli* preparation and circumvents the rapid antibody-mediated clearance seen with *E. coli* enzyme in relapsed patients. Only partial depletion of CSF asparagine is achieved by the various asparaginase preparations in clinical use.

L-Asparaginase has minimal effects on bone marrow and GI mucosa. Its most serious toxicities result from its antigenicity as a foreign protein and its inhibition of protein synthesis. Hypersensitivity reactions occur in 5 to 20% of patients and may be fatal.

Pegaspargase, an antineoplastic agent with properties similar to those of L-asparaginase (2,500 IU/m^2 IM or IV q. 14 days), is indicated in the management of ALL in patients who require L asparaginase but have developed hypersensitivity to its native forms.

PEGFILGRASTIM

(Neulasta solution for injection 10 mg/mL)

Pegfilgrastim is a colony-stimulating factor (CSF) that stimulates neutrophil production within bone marrow. It decreases incidence of infection, manifested by febrile neutropenia, in patients with nonmyeloid malignancies receiving myelosuppressive anticancer drugs associated with febrile neutropenia.

Pegylated recombinant human G-CSP **pegfilgrastim** (Neulasta) is generated through conjugation of a 20,000-dalton polyethylene glycol moiety to the *N*-terminal methionyl residue of the 175-amino acid G-CSF glycoprotein produced in *E. coli*. The clearance of pegfilgrastim by glomerular filtration is minimized, thus making neutrophil-mediated clearance the primary route of elimination. Consequently the circulating half-life of **pegfilgrastim** is longer than that of **filgrastim**, allowing for more sustained duration of action and less frequent dosing. Clinical studies suggest that neutrophil-mediated clearance of **pegfilgrastim** may be self-regulating and therefore specific to each patient's hematopoietic recovery. As such, the recommended dose for pegfilgrastim is fixed at 6 mg administered subcutaneously.

The therapeutic roles of other growth factors still need to be defined, although IL-3 and IL-6 have been removed from testing due to poor efficacy and/or significant toxicity. Macrophage-colony stimulating factor (M-CSF) may play a role in stimulating monocyte and macrophage production, although with significant side effects, including splenomegaly and thrombocytopenia. Stem-cell factor (SCF) has been shown to augment peripheral blood mobilization of primitive hematopoietic progenitor cells.

PEGINTERFERON ALFA-2A

(PEGASYS injection 180 mcg/mL)

Peginterferon is an immunomodulator that binds to specific receptors on the cell surface and initiates a complex sequence of intracellular events (e.g., inhibition of viral replication and inhibition of cell proliferation). It is indicated in the treatment of chronic hepatitis C in patients with compensated liver disease and not treated previously with interferon alfa.

Two pegylated IFNs are available commercially: **peginterferon alfa-2a** and **peginterferon alfa-2b**. PegIFN alfa-2b has a straight-chain 12,000-dalton type of PEG that increases the plasma half-life from approximately 2 to 3 hours to approximately 30 to 54 hours. PegIFN alfa-2a consists of an ester derivative of a branched-chain 40,000-dalton PEG bonded to IPN-α2a and has a plasma half-life averaging about 80 to 90 hours. **PegIPN alfa-2a** is more stable and dispensed in solution, whereas pegIFN alfa-2b requires reconstitution prior to use. For **pegIFN alfa-2a**, peak serum concentrations occur up to 120 hours after dosing and remain detectable throughout the weekly dosing interval; steady-state levels occur 5 to 8 weeks after initiation of weekly dosing. For **pegIFN alfa-2a**, dose-related maximum plasma concentrations occur at 15 to 44 hours after dosing and decline by 96 to 168 hours. These differences in pharmacokinetics may be associated with differences in antiviral effects. Increasing PEG size is associated with longer half-life and less renal clearance. About 30% of pegIFN alfa-2b is cleared renally; pegIPN alfa-2a also is cleared primarily by the liver. Dose reductions in both pegylated IFNs are indicated in end-stage renal disease.

Recombinant, natural, and pegylated IFNs currently are approved in the United States, depending on the specific IFN type, for treatment of condyloma acuminatum, chronic HCV infection, chronic HBV infection, Kaposi's sarcoma in HIV-infected patients, other malignancies, and multiple sclerosis.

PEGVISOMANT

(Somavert injection 10 mg)

Pegvisomant is a pegvisomant that selectively binds to growth-hormone (GH) receptors on cell surfaces, where it blocks the binding of endogenous growth hormone, interfering with GH transduction. It is indicated in the treatment of **acromegaly** in patients who have had an inadequate response to surgery or radiation therapy or other medical therapies.

All of the effects of **GH** result from its interactions with the GH receptor, as evidenced by the severe phenotype of rare patients with homozygous mutations of the GH receptor gene (the **Laron syndrome** of **GH-resistant dwarfism**). The GH receptor is a widely distributed cell-surface receptor that belongs to the class I cytokine receptor superfamily and thus shares structural similarity with the receptors for prolactin, erythropoietin, granulocyte-macrophage CSF, and several of the ILs. Like other members of the cytokine receptor family, the GH receptor contains an extracellular domain that binds GH, a single membrane-spanning region, and an intracellular domain that mediates signal transduction. Receptor activation results from the binding of a single GH molecule to two identical receptor molecules, forming a ligand-occupied receptor dimer that presumably brings the intracellular domains of the receptor into close proximity to activate cytosolic components critical for cell signaling.

The mature human GH receptor contains 620 amino acids, ~250 of which are extracellular, 24 of which are transmembrane, and ~350 of which are cytoplasmic. The GH receptor exists as a dimer and forms a ternary complex with one molecule of GH. The formation of the GH–GH receptor ternary complex is initiated by high-affinity interaction of GH with one monomer of the GH receptor dimer (mediated by GH site 1), followed by a second interaction of GH with the GH receptor (mediated by GH site 2); these interactions induce a conformational change that activates downstream signaling. Guided by structure–function analyses, GH analogs have been engineered with a disrupted site 2; these analogs bind the receptor and induce its internalization but cannot induce a conformational change or stimulate downstream events in the signal transduction pathway. One such analog, **pegvisomant**, behaves as a GH antagonist and is used in the treatment of acromegaly.

The incidence and severity of side effects of lanreotide are comparable to those with the slow-release octreotide formulation. It has not been approved by the FDA for use in the United States.

Somatostatin blocks not only GH secretion but also the secretion of other hormones, growth factors, and cytokines. Thus, **octreotide** and the delayed-release somatostatin analogs have been used to treat symptoms associated with metastatic carcinoid tumors (e.g., flushing and diarrhea) and **adenomas secreting vasoactive intestinal peptide (VIP)** (e.g., watery diarrhea). Octreotide also is used in treatment of acute variceal bleeding, for perioperative prophylaxis in pancreatic surgery, and for TSH-secreting adenomas in patients who are not candidates for surgery. Novel uses under evaluation currently include the treatment of eye diseases associated with excessive proliferation and inflammation (e.g., **Graves' orbitopathy and diabetic retinopathy**), diabetic nephropathy, and various systemic diseases associated with inflammation (e.g., rheumatoid arthritis, inflammatory bowel disease, and psoriasis). Finally, modified forms of octreotide labeled with indium or technetium have been used for diagnostic imaging of neuroendocrine tumors such as pituitary adenomas and carcinoids; modified forms labeled with β emitters such as ^{90}Y have been used in selective destruction of SSTR-2-positive tumors.

Pegvisomant (Somavert) is a GH antagonist that is FDA approved for the treatment of acromegaly. It binds to the GH receptor but does not activate Jak-Stat signaling or stimulate IGF-1 secretion. **Pegvisomant** is administered subcutaneously as a 40-mg loading dose under a physician's supervision, followed by self-administration of 10 mg/day. Based on serum IGF-1 levels, the dose is titrated at 4- to 6-week intervals to a maximum of 40 mg/day. Liver function should be monitored in all patients, and **pegvisomant** should not be used in patients with elevated levels of liver transaminases. Because there are concerns that loss of negative feedback by GH and IGF-1 may increase the growth of GH-secreting adenomas, careful follow-up by pituitary MRI is mandatory. **Pegvisomant** differs structurally from native GH and induces the formation of specific antibodies in ~15% of patients despite the covalent coupling to lysine residues of 4 to 5 molecules of a polyethylene glycol polymer per modified GH molecule. Nevertheless, the development of tachyphylaxis due to these antibodies has not been reported.

In clinical trials, **pegvisomant** at higher doses significantly decreased serum IGF-1 to normal age- and sex-adjusted levels in >90% of patients, and significantly improved clinical parameters such as ring size, soft-tissue swelling, excessive perspiration, and fatigue. Thus, although its ultimate role in the management of acromegaly remains to be determined, pegvisomant is an exciting new pharmacologic agent, particularly for those acromegalic patients who do not respond to somatostatin analogs.

PEMETREXED

(Alimta injection 500 mg)

Pemetrexed is a folic-acid antagonist that disrupts folate-dependent metabolic processes essential for cell replication. It is indicated in combination with cisplatin for the treatment of **malignant pleural mesothelioma** in patients whose disease is unresectable or who are otherwise not candidates for curative surgery; and as a single agent for the treatment of locally advanced or metastatic non-small-cell lung cancer after prior chemotherapy.

Antifolate chemotherapy occupies a special place in the history of cancer treatment, as this class of drugs produced the first striking—although temporary—remissions in leukemia, and the first cure of a solid tumor, choriocarcinoma. These advances provided great impetus to the development of chemotherapy for cancer. Interest in folate antagonists further increased with the development of curative combination therapy for childhood acute lymphocytic leukemia; in this therapy, **methotrexate** played a critical role in both systemic treatment and intrathecal therapy. Introduction of high-dose regimens with "rescue" of host toxicity by the reduced folate, leucovorin (folinic acid, citrovorum factor, 5-formyl tetrahydrofolate, N^5-formyl FH_4), further extended the effectiveness of this drug to both systemic and CNS lymphomas, osteogenic sarcoma, and leukemias. Most recently, **pemetrexed**, an analog that differs from methotrexate in its transport properties and sites of action, has proven useful in treating mesothelioma and lung cancer.

Recognition that methotrexate, an inhibitor of dihydrofolate reductase, also directly inhibits the folate-dependent enzymes of *de novo* purine and thymidylate synthesis focused attention on the development of antifolate analogs that specifically target these other folate-dependent enzymes. Replacement of the N5 and/or N8 nitrogens of the pteridine ring and the N10 nitrogen of the bridge between the pteridine and benzoate rings of folate, as well as various side-chain substitutions, have generated a series of new inhibitors. These new agents have greater capacity for transport into tumor cells and exert their primary inhibitory effect on **thymidylate synthase** (raltitrexed, Tomudex), early steps in purine biosynthesis (lometrexol) or both (the multitargeted antifolate, **pemetrexed**).

Aside from its antineoplastic activity, methotrexate also has been used with benefit in the therapy of psoriasis. Additionally, it inhibits cell-mediated immune reactions and is employed as an immunosuppressive agent to suppress graft-versus-host disease in allogenic bone marrow and organ transplantation and for the treatment of dermatomyositis, rheumatoid arthritis, **Wegener's granulomatosis**, and **Crohn's disease**.

PEMOLINE

(Cylert tablets 18.75 mg)

Pemoline acts as a CNS stimulant but with minimal sympathomimetic effects. Pemoline, an oxazolidinedione derivative with possible analeptic and CNS-stimulating properties (37.5 mg p.o. daily), is indicated in the treatment of attention deficit/hyperactivity disorder (ADHD).

Pemoline (Cylert, others) is structurally dissimilar to **methylphenidate** but elicits similar changes in CNS function with minimal effects on the cardiovascular system. It is a schedule IV controlled substance in the United States and is employed in treating ADHD. It can be given once daily because of its long half-life. Clinical improvement may require treatment for 3 to 4 weeks. Use of **pemoline** has been associated with severe hepatic failure.

PENBUTOLOL SULFATE

(Levatol tablets 20 mg)

Penbutolol sulfate is a beta-adrenergic-blocking agent that nonselectively blocks beta-adrenergic receptors, primarily affecting the cardiovascular system (e.g., decreased heart rate, decreased cardiac contractility, decreased BP) and lungs (promotes bronchospasm). It is indicated in the management of mild to moderate hypertension.

Many β-receptor antagonists have been synthesized and evaluated to varying extents. **Oxprenolol** and **penbutolol** (Levatol) are non-subtype-selective β-blockers with intrinsic sympathomimetic activity. **Medroxalol** is a nonselective β-blocker with α_1-receptor-blocking activity. **Levobunolol** (Betagan liquifilm, others) is a non-subtype-selective β antagonist used as a topical agent in the treatment of glaucoma. **Betaxolol** (Betoptic), a β_1-selective antagonist, is available as an ophthalmic preparation for glaucoma and an oral formulation for systemic hypertension. Betaxolol may be less likely to induce bronchospasm than the ophthalmic preparations of the nonselective β-blockers timolol and levobunolol. Similarly, ocular administration of **carteolol** (Ocupress) may be less likely than timolol to have systemic effects, possibly because of its intrinsic sympathomimetic activity; cautious monitoring is required nonetheless. **Sotalol** (Betapace, Betapace AF, others) is a nonselective β antagonist that is devoid of membrane-stabilizing actions. However, it has antiarrhythmic actions independent of its ability to block β-adrenergic receptors. **Propafenone** (Rythmol) is a Na^+-channel-blocking drug that also is a β-adrenergic-receptor antagonist.

Penbutolol (20 mg p.o. daily) is a beta-adrenergic-receptor-blocking agent that is indicated in the treatment of mild to moderate hypertension. It blocks both $beta_1$- and $beta_2$-adrenergic receptors. Its antihypertensive effects may be related to its peripheral antiadrenergic effects that lead to decreased cardiac output, a central effect that leads to decreased sympathetic tone, or decreased renin secretion by the kidneys.

Penbutolol is absorbed well after oral administration, is bound to plasma proteins to the extent of 80 to 90%, and is metabolized in the liver to active and inactive metabolites that are excreted in the urine.

Penbutolol is contraindicated in patients with sinus bradycardia, cardiogenic shock, and bronchial asthma, and patients with greater than first-degree heart block. Beta-adrenergic-blocking agents should be avoided in patients with pheochromocytoma unless alpha-adrenergic-blocking agents are also used. Oral calcium antagonists may enhance the hypotensive effects of beta-adrenergic-blocking agents as well as predispose the patient to bradycardia and dysrhythmias. Clonidine may cause paradoxical hypertension when combined with beta-adrenergic-blocking agents. Also, beta-blockers may enhance rebound hypertension when clonidine is withdrawn. Beta-adrenergic-blocking agents may alter the hypoglycemic response to insulin or oral hypoglycemic agents. Beta-blockers may enhance the "first dose" orthostatic hypotension seen with prazocin and terazocin.

Penbutolol has been shown to increase the volume of distribution of lidocaine in normal patients, implying that it may increase the loading dose requirements in some patients. Clinical signs of overdose may include bradycardia, bronchospasm, heart failure, and severe hypotension.

PENCICLOVIR

(Denavir cream 10 mg/g)

Penciclovir is an antiviral agent that selectively inhibits herpes viral DNA synthesis and replication. It is indicated in the treatment of recurrent herpes labialis (cold sores) in adults.

Infection with herpes simplex virus type 1 (HSV-1) typically causes diseases of the mouth, face, skin, esophagus, or brain. Herpes simplex virus type 2 (HSV-2) usually causes infections of the genitals, rectum, skin, hands, or meninges. Both cause serious infections in neonates. HSV infection may be a primary one in a naive host, a nonprimary initial one in a host previously infected by other viruses, or the consequence of activation of a latent infection.

The first systemically administered antiherpesvirus agent, **vidarabine**, was approved by the Food and Drug Administration (FDA) in 1977. However, its toxicities restricted its use to life-threatening infections of HSV and varicella-zoster virus (VZV). The discovery and development of **acyclovir**, approved in 1982, provided the first effective treatment for less severe HSV and VZV infections in ambulatory patients. Intravenous acyclovir is superior to vidarabine in terms of efficacy and toxicity in HSV encephalitis and in VZV infections of immunocompromised patients. Acyclovir is the prototype of a group of antiviral agents that are phosphorylated intracellularly by a viral kinase and subsequently by host-cell enzymes to become inhibitors of viral DNA synthesis. Other agents employing this strategy include **penciclovir** and **ganciclovir**.

Famiciclovir is the diacetyl ester prodrug of 6-deoxy penciclovir and lacks intrinsic antiviral activity. **Penciclovir** (9-[4-hydroxy-3-hydroxymethylbut-1-yl] guanine) is an acyclic guanine nucleoside analog. The side chain differs structurally in that the oxygen has been replaced by a carbon, and an additional hydroxymethyl group is present.

Penciclovir is similar to acyclovir in its spectrum of activity and potency against HSV and VZV. The inhibitory concentrations of penciclovir depend on cell type but are usually within twofold of those of acyclovir for HSV and VZV. It also is inhibitory for HBV.

Penciclovir is an inhibitor of viral DNA synthesis. In HSV- or VZV-infected cells, penciclovir is phosphorylated initially by viral thymidine kinase. **Penciclovir** triphosphate serves as a competitive inhibitor of viral DNA polymerase. Although penciclovir triphosphate is approximately a hundred times as potent as acyclovir triphosphate in inhibiting viral DNA polymerase, it is present in much higher concentrations and for more prolonged periods in infected cells than acyclovir triphosphate. The prolonged intracellular $t_{1/2}$ of **penciclovir** triphosphate, 7 to 20 hours, is associated with prolonged antiviral effects. Because penciclovir has a 3′-hydroxyl group, it is not an obligate chain terminator but does inhibit DNA elongation.

Resistant variants owing to thymidine kinase or DNA polymerase mutations can be selected by passage *in vitro*, but the occurrence of resistance during clinical use is currently low. Thymidine kinase-deficient, acyclovir-resistant herpes viruses are cross-resistant to penciclovir.

Oral **penciclovir** has low (5%) bioavailability. In contrast, **famciclovir** is well absorbed orally and converted rapidly to penciclovir by deacetylation of the side chain and oxidation of the purine ring during and following absorption from the intestine. The bioavailability of **penciclovir** is 65 to 77% following oral administration of famciclovir. Food slows absorption but does not reduce overall bioavailability. After single 250- or 500-mg doses of famciclovir, the peak plasma concentration of penciclovir averages 1.6 and 3.3 μg/mL, respectively. A small quantity of the 6-deoxy precursor but no famciclovir is detectable in plasma. After intravenous infusion of **penciclovir** at 10 mg/kg, peak plasma levels average 12 μg/mL. The volume of distribution is about twice the volume of total-body water. The plasma $t_{1/2}$ of elimination of penciclovir averages about 2 hours, and over 90% is excreted unchanged in the urine, probably by both filtration and active tubular secretion. Following oral famciclovir administration, nonrenal clearance accounts for about 10% of each dose, primarily through fecal excretion, but penciclovir (60% of dose) and its 6-deoxy precursor (<10% of dose) are eliminated primarily in the urine. The plasma half-life averages 9.9 hours in renal insufficiency (Cl_{cr} < 30 ml/min); hemodialysis efficiently removes **penciclovir**. Lower peak plasma concentrations of penciclovir but no reduction in overall bioavailability occur in compensated chronic hepatic insufficiency.

Oral famciclovir is well tolerated but may be associated with headache, diarrhea, and nausea. Urticaria, rash, and hallucinations or confusional states (predominantly in the elderly) have been reported. Topical penciclovir, which is formulated in 40% propylene glycol and a cetomacrogol base, is associated infrequently with application-site reactions (~1%). The short-term tolerance of famciclovir is comparable with that of acyclovir.

Penciclovir is mutagenic at high concentrations. *In vitro* studies in laboratory animals indicate that chronic famciclovir administration is tumorigenic and decreases spermatogenesis and fertility in rodents and dogs; long-term administration (1 year) does not affect spermatogenesis in men. No teratogenic effects have been observed in animals, but safety during pregnancy has not been established.

No clinically important drug interactions have been identified to date with famciclovir or penciclovir.

Oral famciclovir, topical **penciclovir**, and intravenous penciclovir are approved for managing HSV and VZV infections in various countries. Oral famciclovir (250 mg three times a day for 7 to 10 days is as effective as acyclovir in treating first-episode genital herpes. In patients with recurrent genital HSV, patient-initiated famciclovir treatment (125 or 250 mg twice a day for 5 days) reduces healing time and symptoms by about 1 day. Famciclovir (250 mg twice a day for up to 1 year is effective for suppression of recurrent genital HSV, but single daily doses are less effective. Higher doses (500 mg twice a day) reduce HSV recurrences in HIV-infected persons. Intravenous penciclovir (5 mg/kg every 8 or 12 hours for 7 days) is comparable with intravenous acyclovir for treating mucocutaneous HSV infections in immunocompromised hosts. In immunocompetent persons with recurrent orolabial HSV, topical 1% penciclovir cream (applied every 2 hours while awake for 4 days) shortens healing time and symptoms by about 1 day.

In immunocompetent adults with herpes zoster of 3 days' duration or less, famciclovir (500 mg three times a day for 10 days) is at least as effective as acyclovir (800 mg five times daily) in reducing healing time and zoster-associated pain, particularly in those 50 years of age and older. Famciclovir is comparable with valacyclovir in treating zoster and reducing associated pain in older adults. Famciclovir (500 mg three times a day for 7 to 10 days) also is comparable with high-dose oral acyclovir in treating zoster in immunocompromised patients and in those with ophthalmic zoster.

Famciclovir is associated with dose-related reductions in HBV DNA and transaminase levels in patients with chronic HBV hepatitis, but is less effective than lamivudine. Famciclovir is also ineffective in treating lamivudine-resistant HBV infections owing to emergence of multiply-resistant variants.

PENICILLAMINE

(Cuprimine, Depen)

Penicillamine (250 mg p.o. q.i.d. 30 to 60 minutes before meals), a metal-chelating agent, is indicated in **Wilson's disease**, in cystinuria, in rheumatoid arthritis, and in heavy-metal poisoning. Penicillamine depresses circulating IgM rheumatoid factor (but not total circulating immunoglobulin levels) and depresses T-cell, but not B-cell, activity. It also depolymerizes some macroglobulins (for example, rheumatoid factors).

Penicillamine forms stable, soluble complexes with copper, iron, mercury, lead, and other heavy metals that are excreted in urine; it is particularly useful in chelating copper in patients with Wilson's disease. Penicillamine also combines with cystine alone, reducing free cystine below the level of urinary stone formation.

Penicillamine is contraindicated in patients with a history of penicillamine-related aplastic anemia or agranulocystosis; in patients with significant renal or hepatic insufficiency; in pregnant women; and in patients receiving gold salts, immunosuppressants, antimalarials, or phenylbutazone because of the increased risk of serious hematologic effects.

PENICILLIN G BENZATHINE

(Bicillin L-A, Megacillin suspension, Permapen)

PENICILLIN G BENZATHINE/PENICILLIN G PROCAINE

(Bicillin C-R injection 600,000 units/dose (300,000 units each penicillin G benzathine and penicillin G procaine), injection 1,200,000 units/dose (600,000 units each penicillin G benzathine and penicillin G procaine), injection 2,400,000 units/dose (1,200,000 units each penicillin G benzathine and penicillin G procaine), Bicillin C-R 900/300 injection 1,200,000 units/ dose (900,000 units penicillin G benzathine and 300,000 units penicillin G procaine))

Penicillin G benzathine/penicillin G procaine is a natural penicillin that inhibits mucopeptide synthesis of bacterial cell wall. It is indicated in the treatment of moderately severe infections caused by penicillin-G-susceptible microorganisms that are susceptible to serum levels common to this particular dosage form; moderately severe to severe infections of the upper respiratory tract, scarlet fever, erysipelas, and skin and soft-tissue infections caused by susceptible streptococci; and moderately severe pneumonia and otitis media caused by susceptible organisms. Severe pneumonia, empyema, bacteremia, pericarditis, meningitis, peritonitis, and arthritis of pneumococcal etiology are better treated with penicillin G sodium or potassium during the acute stage. When high, sustained serum levels are required, penicillin G sodium or potassium, either IM or IV, should be used. This drug should not be used in the treatment of venereal diseases, including syphilis, gonorrhea, yaws, bejel, and pinta.

The simultaneous use of two or more antimicrobial agents is recommended in specifically defined situations based on pharmacological rationale. However, selection of an appropriate combination requires an understanding of the potential for interaction between the antimicrobial agents. Interactions may affect either the microorganism or the patient. Antimicrobial agents acting at different targets may enhance or impair overall antimicrobial activity. A combination of drugs also may have additive or superadditive toxicities. For example, vancomycin given alone usually has minimal nephrotoxicity. However, when vancomycin is given with an aminoglycoside, the toxicity of the aminoglycoside is increased.

The international unit (IU) of penicillin is the specific penicillin activity contained in 0.6 μg of the crystalline sodium salt of **penicillin G**. One milligram of pure **penicillin G** sodium thus equals 1667 units; 1.0 mg of pure **penicillin G** potassium represents 1595 units. The dosage and the antibacterial potency of the synthetic penicillins are expressed in terms of weight.

The antimicrobial spectra of **penicillin G** (benzylpenicillin) and **penicillin V** (the phenoxymethyl derivative) are very similar for aerobic Gram-positive microorganisms. However, **penicillin G** is 5 to 10 times more active against *Neisseria* spp. that are sensitive to penicillins, and against certain anaerobes.

About one-third of an orally administered dose of penicillin G is absorbed from the intestinal tract under favorable conditions. Gastric juice at pH 2 rapidly destroys the antibiotic. The decrease in gastric-acid production with aging accounts for better absorption of **penicillin G** from the GI tract of older individuals. Absorption is rapid, and maximal concentrations in blood are attained in 30 to 60 minutes. The peak value is approximately 0.5 unit/mL (0.3 μg/mL) after an oral dose of 400,000 units (about 250 mg) in an adult. Ingestion of food may interfere with enteric absorption of all penicillins, perhaps by adsorption of the antibiotic onto food particles. Thus oral **penicillin G** should be administered at least 30 minutes before a meal or 2 hours after. Despite the convenience of oral administration of **penicillin G**, this route should be used only in infections in which clinical experience has proven its efficacy.

After intramuscular (IM) injection, peak concentrations in plasma are reached within 15 to 30 minutes. This value declines rapidly because the half-life of **penicillin G** is 30 minutes.

Many means for prolonging the sojourn of the antibiotic in the body and thereby reducing the frequency of injections have been explored. **Probenecid** blocks renal tubular secretion of penicillin, but it is used rarely for this purpose. More commonly, repository preparations of **penicillin G** are employed. The two such compounds currently favored are **penicillin G procaine** (Wycillin, others) and **penicillin G benzathine** (Bicillin L-A, Permapen). Such agents release penicillin G slowly from the area in which they are injected and produce relatively low but persistent concentrations of antibiotic in the blood.

Penicillin G procaine suspension is an aqueous preparation of the crystalline salt that is only 0.4% soluble in water. Procaine combines with penicillin mole for mole; a dose of 300,000 units thus contains approximately 120 mg procaine. When large doses of **penicillin G** procaine are given (e.g., 4.8 million units), procaine may reach toxic concentrations in the plasma. If the patient is believed to be hypersensitive to procaine, 0.1 mL of 1% solution of procaine should be injected intradermally as a test. The anesthetic effect of the procaine accounts in part for the fact that injections of **penicillin G** procaine are virtually painless.

The injection of 300,000 units of penicillin G procaine produces a peak concentration in plasma of about 0.9 μg/mL within 1 to 3 hours; after 24 hours, the concentration is reduced to 0.1 μg/mL, and by 48 hours it has fallen to 0.03 μg/mL. A larger dose (600,000 units) yields somewhat higher values that are maintained for as long as 4 to 5 days.

Penicillin G benzathine suspension is the aqueous suspension of the salt obtained by the combination of 1 mol of an ammonium base and 2 mol of **penicillin G** to yield *N,N′*-dibenzylethylenediamine dipenicillin G. The salt itself is 0.02% soluble in water. The long persistence of penicillin in the blood after a suitable IM dose reduces cost, the need for repeated injections, and local trauma. The local anesthetic effect of **penicillin G benzathine** is comparable with that of penicillin G procaine.

Penicillin G benzathine is absorbed very slowly from IM depots and produces the longest duration of detectable antibiotic of all the available repository penicillins. For example, in adults, a dose of 1.2 million units given intramuscularly produces concentration in plasma of 0.09 μg/mL on the first, 0.02 μg/mL on the fourteenth, and 0.002 μg/mL on the thirty-second day after injection. The average duration of demonstrable antimicrobial activity in the plasma is about 26 days.

PENICILLIN G POTASSIUM

(Cryspen, Deltapen, Lanacillin, Parcillin, Pensorb, Pentids, Pfizerpen)

PENICILLIN G PROCAINE

(Crysticillin A.S., Duracillin A.S., Fizerpen A.S., Wycillin)

PENICILLIN G SODIUM

Penicillin, a naturally occurring antibiotic, is indicated in the treatment of group A streptococcal upper respiratory infections, prophylaxis of poststreptococcal rheumatic fever, syphilis of less than one year's duration, moderate to severe systemic infections, uncomplicated gonorrhea, pneumococcal pneumonia, and endocarditis prophylaxis for dental surgery (see Table 23).

TABLE 23
Comparative Pharmacology of Penicillin Derivatives

	Properties		
Drugs	Acid Stability	Penicillinase Resistance	Spectrum of Activity
Penicillin G[a]	No	No	Narrow spectrum
Penicillin V[a]	Yes	No	Narrow spectrum
Oxacillin[a]	Yes	Yes	The isoxazolyl penicillins are potent inhibitors of the growth of most penicillinase-producing staphylococci
Cloxacillin[a]	Yes	Yes	
Dicloxacillin[a]	Yes	Yes	Slightly more active than oxacillin against penicillin G-resistant *S. aureus*
Nafcillin[b]	No	Yes	
Ampicillin[c]	Yes	No	Ampicillin and the related aminopenicillins are bactericidal for both Gram-positive and Gram-negative bacteria
Amoxicillin	Yes	No	

[a] Absorbed incompletely from the gastrointestinal tract, attains peak concentration in the plasma in 1 hr, and is excreted rapidly by the kidneys.

[b] Available for oral and parenteral uses.

[c] Appears in the bile, undergoes enterohepatic circulation, and is excreted in the feces.

PENICILLIN V (PHENOXYMETHYL PENICILLIN, PENICILLIN V POTASSIUM)

(Beepen-VK tablets 250 mg, tablets 500 mg, powder for oral solution 125 mg/5 mL, powder for oral solution 250 mg/5 mL, Pen-Vee K tablets 250 mg, tablets 500 mg, powder for oral solution 125 mg/5 mL, powder for oral solution 250 mg/5 mL, Penicillin VK tablets 250 mg, tablets 500 mg, powder for oral solution 125 mg/5 mL, powder for oral solution 250 mg/5 mL • Veetids tablets 250 mg, tablets 500 mg, powder for oral solution 125 mg/5 mL • Veetids '250' powder for oral solution 250 mg/5 mL)

Penicillin V is a natural penicillin that inhibits mucopeptide synthesis of bacterial cell wall. The antimicrobial spectra of penicillin G (benzylpenicillin) and penicillin V (the phenoxymethyl derivative) are very similar for aerobic Gram-positive microorganisms. However, penicillin G is 5 to 10 times more active against *Neisseria* spp. that are sensitive to penicillins, and against certain anaerobes.

The virtue of penicillin V in comparison with penicillin G is that it is more stable in an acidic medium and therefore is better absorbed from the GI tract. On an equivalent oral-dose basis, penicillin V (K^+ salt; Veetids) yields plasma concentrations two to five times greater than those provided by penicillin G. The peak concentration in the blood of an adult after an oral dose of 500 mg is nearly 3 μg/mL. Once absorbed, penicillin V is distributed in the body and excreted by the kidney in a manner similar to that of penicillin G.

After intramuscular injection, peak concentrations in plasma are reached within 15 to 30 minutes. This value declines rapidly because the half-life of penicillin G is 30 minutes.

Many means for prolonging the sojourn of the antibiotic in the body and thereby reducing the frequency of injections have been explored. Probenecid blocks renal tubular secretion of penicillin, but it is used rarely for this purpose. More commonly, repository preparations of penicillin G are employed. The two such compounds currently favored are **penicillin G procaine** (Wycillin, others) and **penicillin G benzathine** (Bicillin L-A, Permapen). Such agents release penicillin G slowly from the area in which they are injected and produce relatively low but persistent concentrations of antibiotic in the blood.

PENICILLIN V POTASSIUM

(Betapen-VK, Biotic-V powder, Bopen V-K, Cocillin V-K, Lanacillin VK, Ledercillin VK, LV, Penapar VK, Pen-Vee K, Pfizerpen VK, Robicillin-VK, Uticillin VK, V-Cillin K, Veetids)

Penicillin, a naturally occurring antibiotic, is indicated in the treatment of mild to moderate susceptible infections and endocarditis prophylaxis for dental surgery.

PENICILLINS

All penicillins (Figure 74) are composed of a thiazolidine ring attached to a beta-lactam, which in turn carries a free amide group (O=CNH) on which a substitution and an attachment (R) are made. In the case of benzylpenicillin, the R is a benzyl group. Penicillin may be metabolized by amidase to 6-aminopenicillanic acid, which has antibacterial activity, or by penicillinase (bacterial beta-lactamase), to penicilloic acid, which is devoid of antibacterial activity but is antigenic in nature and acts as a sensitizing structure. The main source of bacterial resistance to penicillin is in fact the production of penicillinase by the microorganisms.

Penicillin is an organic acid that is commonly supplied as sodium and potassium salts. Penicillin V (Pen-Vee K and V-cillin K) and phenethicillin (Syncillin and Maxipen) are different from penicillin G (benzylpenicillin) in that they are more acid resistant. In addition to the broad-spectrum penicillins such as ampicillin and amoxicillin, there is a newer group of anti-*Pseudomonas* penicillins that are effective against Gram-negative bacilli. These agents include carbenicillin, ticarcillin, azlocillin, and piperacillin. The latter two agents are also useful against *Klebsiella pneumoniae* and *Bacteroides fragilis* (see also Table 23).

The penicillinase-resistant penicillins are oxacillin, cloxacillin, dicloxacillin, methicillin, and nafcillin. These agents are the drugs of choice for treating infections caused by penicillinase-producing *Staphylococci aureus*.

One milligram of pure penicillin G sodium is equal to 1667 units.

Penicillins achieve their effect by inhibiting formation of cell walls, and hence are bactericidal. Penicillin binds to cellular receptors, now identified as transpeptidation enzymes, and, by binding to and inhibiting the transpeptidation reactions, the synthesis of cell-wall peptidoglycan is interrupted. In addition, penicillin removes or inactivates an inhibitor of the lytic enzymes (autolysin), resulting in the lysis of microorganisms in an isotonic environment. In general, penicillins are more active against Gram-positive organisms (see Figure 74).

The penicillin-susceptible organisms are nonpenicillinase-producing strains of most cocci, Gram-positive bacilli, and spirochetes.

Penicillin G may be used either actively or prophylactically in the following clinical settings:

- Streptococcal infections
  - Streptococcal pharyngitis (including scarlet fever)
  - Streptococcal pneumonia, arthritis, meningitis, and endocarditis
  - Streptococcal otitis media and sinusitis
  - Infectious endocarditis
- Pneumococcal infections
- Staphylococcal infections (generally resistant to penicillin G)
- Meningococcal disease
- Gonococcal infections
- Syphilis
- Actinomycosis, anthrax, and gas gangrene

Thirty percent (30%) of an oral dosage of penicillin is absorbed from the GI tract. Penicillin G is rapidly destroyed at pH 2 of gastric secretion. Penicillin is widely distributed throughout the body and, except in the case of meningitis, does not cross the blood–brain barrier. It is slightly metabolized by the liver but is mainly excreted by the kidney. Probenecid blocks the active tubular secretion of penicillin and hence prolongs its action. It is readily absorbed from intramuscular sites, and long-acting repository forms such as penicillin G procaine and penicillin G benzathine are available.

Penicillins, which are the safest of antibiotics, produce few direct toxic reactions, and most of the serious side effects are hypersensitivity reactions. Penicillins and their by-products, penicilloic acid and penicilloyl polylysine, are antigenic in susceptible individuals who develop immunoglobulin G antibodies to them. Furthermore, all penicillins cross-sensitize and cross-react. Allergic reactions, including anaphylactoid shock, occur in sensitized patients following the repeated administration of penicillin. Anaphylactoid reactions, which are more common following the parenteral administration of penicillin, may be reversed by the administration of corticosteroids.

The direct toxicity of penicillin following the administration of large doses may include phlebitis if it is given intravenously, injection site inflammatory reactions when given intramuscularly, degeneration of nerve tissue if injected into a nerve, and CNS excitability if given intrathecally.

The broad-spectrum penicillins, such as ampicillin and amoxicillin, may cause GI irritation. Occasionally, the overgrowth of staphylococci, *Pseudomonas*, *Proteus*, or yeasts may be responsible for causing enteritis. Methicillin and nafcillin may precipitate granulocytopenia, and methicillin has been known to cause nephritis. Carbenicillin may cause hypokalemic alkalosis. The properties of the various penicillins are shown in Table 23.

PENICILLINS

Amoxicillin	Dicloxacillin	Oxacillin
Ampicillin	Floxacillin	Penicillin G
Azlocillin	Methicillin	Penicillin V
Carbenicillin	Mezlocillin	Piperacillin
Cloxacillin	Nafcillin	Ticarcillin

PENTAERYTHRITOL TETRANITRATE (Peritrate)

Pentaerythritol (10 to 20 mg t.i.d.), a nitric acid ester of a tetrahydric alcohol, is indicated in the relief of angina pectoris and pain associated with coronary artery disease. It is not intended to abort the acute anginal episode but is widely regarded as useful in the prophylactic treatment of angina pectoris (see Figure 69).

The nitrates and nitrites bring about arterial dilation and hence reduce BP and the work of the heart. These agents also produce venous dilation, thereby decreasing the venous return and ventricular volume, which in turn diminishes wall tension. The end result of these events is a reduction in the work of the heart. By decreasing BP, the heart rate is increased through the activation of carotid sinus reflexes. However, the extent of the reduction in wall tension is actually of greater benefit than the elevated heart rate. The nitrate-induced tachycardia may be blocked by the administration of propranolol, a beta-adrenergic-receptor-blocking agent (see Figure 70).

Collateral vessels are silent blood vessels that become functional during hypoxic emergencies. By dilating, they permit greater blood flow to the ischemic areas, and nitrates accentuate this response. This effect of nitrates, which is greater than that of dipyridamole, seems to be potentiated by propranolol.

Nitrites and nitrates dilate blood vessels in all smooth muscles. When they dilate the cutaneous blood vessels, they cause blushing. When they dilate the cerebral vessels, they cause headache. Thus, the appearance of headache and blushing is an indication of the efficacy of these medications (see Figures 69 and 70).

PENTAMIDINE ISETHIONATE

(Pentam-300, NebuPent aerosol 300 mg, Pentacarinat injection 300 mg, Pentam 300 injection 300 mg)

Pentamidine isethionate is an antiprotozoal agent that interferes with synthesis of DNA, RNA, phospholipids, and proteins.

Pentamidine (4 mg/kg once a day for 14 days) is indicated in the treatment of *Pneumocystis carinii* pneumonia (PCP), prevention of PCP in high-risk, HIV-infected patients, and in the treatment of trypanosomiasis and visceral leishmaniasis.

Trypanosomiasis is produced by protozoa of the genus *Trypanosoma* and leads to Gambian or mid-African sleeping sickness (*T. gambiense*), Rhodesian or East African sleeping sickness (*T. rhodesiense*), and Chagas' disease, which is seen in the populations of Central and South America (*T. cruzi*).

Agents effective in the treatment of trypanosomiasis are the aromatic diamidines (pentamidine, stilbamidine, and propamidine). Pentamidine is the preferred drug for the prevention and early treatment of *T. gambiense* infections; however, it cannot penetrate the CNS. Melarsoprol is the drug recommended for *T. gambiense* infections that do not respond to pentamidine, or for managing the late meningoencephalitis stages of infection. It does reach the CNS. Nifurtimox (Lampit) is the drug of choice for treating the acute form of Chagas' disease. Suramin (Naphuride) is effective only in the therapy for African sleeping sickness.

Pentamidine is a positively charged aromatic diamine that was discovered in 1937 as a fortuitous consequence of the search for hypoglycemic compounds that might compromise parasite energy metabolism. Of the compounds tested, three were found to possess outstanding activity: **stilbamidine**, **pentamidine**, and **promamidine**. Pentamidine was the most useful clinically because of its relative stability, lower toxicity, and ease of administration. It is a broad-spectrum agent with activity against several species of pathogenic protozoa and some fungi. Alone or in combination with suramin, **pentamidine** is used in the treatment of early-stage *T. brucei gambiense* infection.

Pentamidine is an alternative agent for the treatment of antimony-resistant visceral leishmaniasis, although the availability of newer, less toxic agents (e.g., liposomal preparations of amphotericin and miltefosine) may decrease its use. **Pentamidine** is also used as an alternative agent in the treatment and prophylaxis of pneumocystis pneumonia caused by the ascomycetous fungus *Pneumocystis jiroveci* (formerly known as *Pneumocystis carinii*). *T. brucei rhodesiense* is refractory to treatment by **pentamidine** for unexplained reasons. **Diminazene** (Berenil) is a related diamidine that is used as an inexpensive alternative to pentamidine in the treatment of early African trypanosomiasis in some endemic areas despite the fact that it is approved for veterinary use only.

The positively charged aromatic diamidines are toxic to a number of different protozoa yet show rather marked selectivity of action. They are effective in the treatment of *T. brucei gambiense* sleeping sickness but not *T. brucei rhodesiense* or *T. cruzi* infections. Additionally, they are useful in the treatment of antimony-resistant leishmaniasis infections.

The diamidines also are fungicidal. Activity *in vitro* against *Blastomyces dermatitidis* led to the successful therapeutic trial of these drugs in systemic blastomycoses. The use of amphotericin B, however, has reduced the value of the diamidines in the treatment of this disease. At near-therapeutic levels, **pentamidine** kills nonreplicating forms of *P. jiroveci* in culture, but other evidence suggests that **pentamidine** exerts a biostatic rather than biocidal effect.

Pentamidine isethionate usually is given by IM injection or by slow IV infusion over 60 minutes in single doses of 1.7 to 4.5 mg/kg/day for a series of 10 days. However, alternative dosing schedules are common, and the coadministration of suramin on alternate days provides an alternative means of treating *T. brucei gambiense* infections. Because of failure to penetrate the CNS, **pentamidine** is not used to treat *T. brucei rhodesiense,* which affects the brain early in the course of infection. The drug is also ineffective in *T. brucei gambiense* infections once the CNS is involved.

Pentamidine has been used successfully in courses of 12 to 15 IM doses of 2 to 4 mg/kg either daily or every other day to treat visceral leishmaniasis (kala-azar caused by *L. donovani*). This compound provides an alternative to antimonials or lipid formulations of amphotericin B for patients who cannot tolerate the latter agents. **Pentamidine** isethionate given as four IM doses of 3 mg/kg every other day has enjoyed some success in the treatment of cutaneous leishmaniasis (Oriental sore caused by *L. tropica*) but is not used routinely to treat this infection.

PENTOBARBITAL SODIUM

(Nembutal)

Pentobarbital (200 to 300 mg 1 to 2 hours before surgery) may be used parenterally as a sedative, hypnotic, or preanesthetic medication. Oral pentobarbital may be used as a hypnotic for a short period of time because it loses its effectiveness after two weeks.

Pentobarbital acts throughout the CNS as a nonselective depressant with a fast onset of action and a short duration of action. Particularly sensitive to this drug is the reticular activating system that controls CNS arousal. Pentobarbital decreases both presynaptic and postsynaptic membrane excitability by facilitating the action of gamma-aminobutyric acid (GABA) (see also Figure 50).

Pentobarbital is contraindicated in patients with bronchopneumonia, status asthmaticus, or severe respiratory distress because of the potential for respiratory depression. It should not be used in patients who are depressed or have suicidal ideation because the drug can worsen depression; in patients with uncontrolled acute or chronic pain because exacerbation of pain and paradoxical excitement can occur; or in patients with porphyria because the drug can trigger symptoms of this disease. Pentobarbital should be used cautiously in patients who must perform hazardous tasks requiring mental alertness because the drug causes drowsiness.

Clinical manifestations of overdose include unsteady gait, slurred speech, sustained nystagmus, somnolence, confusion, respiratory depression, pulmonary edema, and coma.

PENTAZOCINE

(Talacen tablets 25 mg pentazocine (as hydrochloride)/650 mg acetaminophen, Talwin injection 30 mg/mL)

Pentazocine is an opioid agonist–antagonist analgesic. It produces analgesia by an agonistic effect at the kappa opioid receptor; it weakly antagonizes effects of opiates at the mu opioid receptor; it does not appear to increase biliary tract pressure. **Oral and parenteral forms**: are used for management of moderate to severe pain. **Parenteral form**: is used for preoperative or preanesthetic medication; and as a supplement to surgical anesthesia.

Pentazocine (50 to 100 mg every 3 to 4 hours) is indicated in relief of moderate to severe pain and for providing preoperative or preanesthetic medications. The analgesia produced by 30 mg of pentazocine, a mixed-narcotic agonist and a weak antagonist, is comparable to that elicited by 10 mg of morphine. Pentazocine will antagonize some of the respiratory depression and analgesia produced by morphine and meperidine. However, the analgesic action and respiratory depression produced by pentazocine can be reversed by a narcotic antagonist. Pentazocine causes tolerance and addiction, but they emerge very slowly compared to those induced by morphine (see Figure 68).

Mixed agonist–antagonist compounds were developed with the hope that they would have less addictive potential and less respiratory depression than morphine and related drugs. In practice, however, it has turned out that, for the same degree of analgesia, the same intensity of side effects will occur. A "ceiling effect," limiting the amount of analgesia attainable, is often seen with these drugs. Some mixed agonist–antagonist drugs, such as **pentazocine** and **nalorphine**, can produce severe psychotomimetic effects that are not reversible with **naloxone** (suggesting that these undesirable side effects are not mediated through classical opioid receptors). Also, **pentazocine** and nalorphine can precipitate withdrawal in opioid-addicted individuals.

The pattern of CNS effects produced by **pentazocine** generally is similar to that of the morphine-like opioids, including analgesia, sedation, and respiratory depression. The analgesic effects of **pentazocine** are due to agonistic actions at κ opioid receptors. Higher doses of **pentazocine** (60 to 90 mg) elicit dysphoric and psychotomimetic effects. The mechanisms responsible for these side effects are not known but might involve activation of supraspinal receptors because it has been suggested that these untoward effects may be reversible by naloxone.

The cardiovascular responses to pentazocine differ from those seen with typical μ-receptor agonists, in that high doses cause an increase in BP and heart rate. **Pentazocine** acts as a weak antagonist or partial agonist at opioid receptors. It does not antagonize the respiratory depression produced by morphine. However, when given to patients dependent on morphine or other μ-receptor agonists, **pentazocine** may precipitate withdrawal. Ceiling effects for analgesia and respiratory depression are observed above 50 to 100 mg pentazocine.

Tablets for oral use now contain **pentazocine** hydrochloride (equivalent to 50 mg of the base) and naloxone hydrochloride (equivalent to 0.5 mg of the base; Talwin NX), which reduces the potential use of tablets as a source of injectable **pentazocine**. After oral ingestion, naloxone is destroyed rapidly by the liver; however, if the material is dissolved and injected, the naloxone produces aversive effects in subjects dependent on opioids. An oral dose of about 50 mg pentazocine results in analgesia equivalent to that produced by 60 mg codeine orally.

PENTOSAN POLYSULFATE SODIUM

(Elmiron capsules 100 mg)

Pentosan polysulfate sodium is an interstitial cystitis agent that adheres to and may protect the mucosal membrane of the bladder. It is indicated in relief of bladder pain or discomfort associated with interstitial cystitis.

PENTOSTATIN

(2-Deoxycoformycin; DCF, Nipent powder for injection 10 mg/vial)

Pentostatin is a purine antimetabolite. It is a potent transition-state inhibitor of the enzyme adenosine deaminase (ADA) that leads to cytotoxicity because of elevated intracellular levels of dATP that can block DNA synthesis through inhibition of ribonucleotide reductase. Pentostatin can also inhibit RNA synthesis as well as cause increased DNA damage. It is indicated in the treatment for both untreated and alpha-interferon-refractory hairy-cell leukemia; and as palliative therapy of chronic lymphocytic leukemia, prolymphocytic leukemia, and cutaneous T-cell lymphoma.

Pentostatin, a transition-state analog of the intermediate type in the ADA reaction, is a potent inhibitor of ADA. Its effects mimic the phenotype of genetic ADA deficiency, which is associated with severe immunodeficiency affecting both T- and B-cell functions. It was isolated from fermentation cultures of *Streptomyces antibioticus*. Inhibition of ADA by pentostatin leads to accumulation of intracellular adenosine and deoxyadenosine nucleotides, which can block DNA synthesis by inhibiting ribonucleotide reductase. Deoxyadenosine also inactivates 5′-adenosyl homocysteine hydrolase. The resulting accumulation of 5′-adenosyl homocysteine is particularly toxic to lymphocytes. **Pentostatin** also can inhibit RNA synthesis, and its triphosphate derivative is incorporated into DNA, resulting in strand breakage. In combination with 2′-deoxyadenosine, it is capable of inducing apoptosis in human monocytoid leukemia cells. Although the precise mechanism of cytotoxicity is not known, it is probable that the imbalance in purine nucleotide pools accounts for its antineoplastic effect in hairy-cell leukemia and T-cell lymphomas.

Pentostatin is administered intravenously, and a single dose of 4 mg/m^2 has been reported to have a mean terminal half-life of 5.7 hours. The drug is eliminated almost entirely by renal excretion. Proportional reduction of dosage is recommended in patients with renal impairment as measured by reduced creatinine clearance.

Pentostatin (Nipent) is available for IV use. The recommended dosage is 4 mg/m^2 administered every other week. After hydration with 500 to 1000 mL of 5% dextrose in half-normal (0.45%) saline, the drug is administered by rapid IV injection or by infusion during a period of up to 30 minutes, followed by an additional 500 mL of fluids. Extravasation does not produce tissue necrosis.

Pentostatin is extremely effective in producing complete remissions in the hairy cell. Complete responses of 58% and partial responses of 28% have been reported, even in patients who were refractory to interferon-alfa. Activity also is seen against chronic lymphocytic leukemia (CLL), **chronic myelogenous leukemia** (CML), promyelocytic leukemia, cutaneous T-cell lymphoma, non-Hodgkin's lymphoma, and Langerhans cell histiocytosis. Pentostatin has no significant activity against solid tumors or multiple myeloma.

PENTOXIFYLLINE

(Trental)

Pentoxifylline (400 mg t.i.d. p.o. with meals) is indicated in the treatment of intermittent claudication on the basis of chronic occlusive arterial disease of the limbs.

Pentoxifylline, a dimethylxanthine derivative, and its metabolites improve blood flow by decreasing blood viscosity. It produces dose-related hemorrheologic effects, lowering blood viscosity and improving erythrocyte flexibility. In patients with chronic peripheral arterial disease, this increases blood flow to the affected microcirculation and enhances tissue oxygenation.

Pentoxifylline improves deformability of erythrocytes by increasing cellular ATP concentration via a membrane-metabolizing action, which in turn reduces the aggregation of erythrocytes and local hyperviscosity. It stimulates prostacyclin formation and release, and inhibits phosphodiesterase degradation of platelet cAMP. The increase of cAMP levels decreases the synthesis of thromboxane A_2, and the net result is reduced platelet aggregation. It increases blood fibrinolytic activity and decreases fibrinogen concentration.

The overdosage of pentoxifylline has caused flushing, hypotension, nervousness, agitation, tremors, convulsions, somnolence, loss of consciousness, fever, and agitation.

Most of the therapies shown to be efficacious in treatment of coronary artery disease also have a salutary effect on progression of peripheral artery disease. Reductions in cardiovascular morbidity and mortality in patients with peripheral arterial disease have been documented with antiplatelet therapy using aspirin or with ADP antagonists such as **clopidogrel** or **ticlopidine,** administration of ACE inhibitors, and treatment of hyperlipidemia. Interestingly, neither intensive treatment of diabetes mellitus nor antihypertensive therapy appears to alter the progression of symptoms of claudication. Other risk factor and lifestyle modifications remain cornerstones of therapy for patients with claudication: physical exercise, rehabilitation, and smoking cessation have proven efficacy. Drugs used specifically in the treatment of lower extremity claudication include **pentoxyfylline** and **cilastozol**. Pentoxyfylline is a methylxanthine derivative that has been termed a **rheologic modifier** for its effects on increasing the deformability of red blood cells. However, the effects of **pentoxifylline** on lower-extremity claudication appear to be modest. Cilastozol is an inhibitor of PDE3 and promotes accumulation of intracellular cAMP in many cells, including blood platelets. Cilastozol-mediated increases in cAMP inhibit platelet aggregation and promote vasodilation. The drug is metabolized by CYP3A4 and has important drug interactions with other drugs metabolized via this pathway. Cilastozol treatment improves symptoms of claudication but has no effect on cardiovascular mortality. As a PDE3 inhibitor, cilastozol is placed in the same drug class as milrinone, which had been used as an inotropic agent for patients with heart failure. **Milrinone** therapy was associated with an increase in sudden cardiac death, and the drug was withdrawn from the market. Cilastozol, therefore, is contraindicated in patients with heart failure.

PEPPERMINT OIL

The irritable bowel syndrome (IBS) is a functional bowel disorder exhibiting the following characteristics: abdominal pain, symptoms of disturbed defecation (urgency, straining, and feeling of incomplete evacuation), altered stool consistency, and altered stool frequency and timing. There are also symptoms of bloatedness (distention).

If diarrhea is the chief complaint, it is treated with loperamide or cholestyramine. Pain is treated with dicyclomine, amitriptyline, and peppermint oil. Bran and psyllium are used to treat the constipation that may occur in IBS. Flatulence is treated with simethicone.

Many volatile oils, on passing into the stomach, cause a sensation of warmth in the gullet accompanied by a sense of well-being and comfort; the appetite is often increased, and any feeling of distention after meals is relieved.

This is often attended by the eructation of gas. Substances that produce these effects are known as carminatives. They are used to relieve intestinal flatulence and distention, to lessen the spasms that cause colic, and as stimulants to the appetite. Those used for this purpose include camphor, cinnamon, fennel, peppermint, spearmint, wintergreen, bitter almond, and anise.

PEPTIC ULCER: Treatment of

The pathogenesis of peptic ulceration is not yet clear. It could be due to an imbalance between acid secretion and mucosal defensive and/or protective mechanisms, but the association between *H. pylori* and peptic ulceration has questioned this hypothesis. Therefore, drugs inhibiting acid secretion and/or eradicating *H. pylori* are of major interest.

Inhibition of Acid Secretion

Histamine H_2-receptor antagonists inhibit acid secretion by blocking the stimulation of H_2-receptors in the gastric parietal cell. They are:

- Cimetidine
- Nizatidine
- Ranitidine
- Roxatidine

Proton-Pump Inhibitors

They are:

- Lansoprazole
- Omeprazole
- Pantoprazole

Cytoprotective Agents

They are:

- Antacids
- Bismuth salts
- Prostaglandin derivatives (misoprostol)
- Sucralfate

Histamine H_2-receptor antagonists can still be considered as a kind of a "gold" standard for the treatment of peptic lesions based on their large therapeutic margins, extensive safety records, and well-documented clinical efficacy.

PERGOLIDE MESYLATE

(Permax)

Pergolide (0.05 mg initially in divided doses) is indicated as an adjunctive treatment to levodopa/carbidopa in the management of Parkinson's disease. Pergolide mesylate is a potent dopamine-receptor agonist at both D_1- and D_2-receptor sites. It is 10 to 1000 times more potent than bromocriptine on a milligram per milligram basis. In patients with Parkinson's disease, it exerts its therapeutic effect by directly stimulating postsynaptic dopamine receptors in the nigrostriatal system. In addition, pergolide inhibits the secretion of prolactin; it causes a transient rise in serum concentrations of growth hormone and a decrease in serum concentrations of luteinizing hormone (LH).

Pergolide is absorbed orally, is bound to plasma proteins to the extent of 90%, metabolized to *N*-despropylpergolide, pergolide sulfoxide, and pergolide sulfone, and the metabolites are excreted by the kidneys.

Dopamine-receptor antagonists having antipsychotic properties, such as phenothiazine, butyrophenone, and thioxanthene derivatives, and GI-stimulant drugs, such as metoclopramide, are contraindicated with pergolide. The most common side effects of pergolide, especially in higher-than-recommended doses, are dyskinesia, hallucinations, somnolence, insomnia, nausea, constipation, diarrhea, dyspepsia, and rhinitis.

PERINDOPRIL ERBUMINE

(Aceon tablets 2 mg)

Perindopril erbumine is an ACE inhibitor that competitively inhibits angiotensin-I-converting enzyme, resulting in prevention of angiotensin I conversion to angiotensin II, a potent vasoconstrictor that also stimulates aldosterone release. Clinical consequences are a decrease in BP, reduced sodium resorption, and potassium retention. It is indicated in the treatment of essential hypertension.

Perindopril erbumine is a prodrug, and 30 to 50% of systemically available perindopril is transformed to perindoprilat by hepatic esterases. Although the oral bioavailability of perindopril (75%) is not affected by food, the bioavailability of perindoprilat is reduced by approximately 35%. Perindopril is metabolized to perindoprilat and to inactive metabolites (glucuronides of **perindopril** and perindoprilat, dehydrated perindopril, and diastereomers of dehydrated perindoprilat) that are excreted predominantly by the kidneys. Peak concentrations of perindoprilat in plasma are achieved in 3 to 7 hours. Perindoprilat displays biphasic elimination kinetics with half-lives of 3 to 10 hours (the major component of elimination) and 30 to 120 hours (owing to slow dissociation of perindoprilat from tissue ACE). The oral dosage ranges from 2 to 15 mg daily (single or divided dosage).

Drugs that interfere with the renin–angiotensin system play a prominent role in the treatment of cardiovascular disease, the major cause of mortality in modern societies.

Inhibition of ACE lowers systemic vascular resistance and mean, diastolic, and systolic BPs in various hypertensive states. The effects are observed readily in animal models of renal and genetic hypertension. In human subjects with hypertension, ACE inhibitors commonly lower BP, except when high BP is due to **primary aldosteronism**. The initial change in BP tends to be positively correlated with plasma renin activity (PRA) and angiotensin II plasma levels prior to treatment. However, several weeks into treatment, additional patients show a sizable reduction in BP, and the antihypertensive effect then correlates poorly or not at all with pretreatment values of PRA. It is possible that increased local (tissue) production of angiotensin II and/or increased responsiveness of tissues to normal levels of angiotensin II in some hypertensive patients makes them sensitive to ACE inhibitors despite normal PRA. Regardless of the mechanisms, ACE inhibitors have broad clinical utility as antihypertensive agents.

The long-term fall in systemic BP observed in hypertensive individuals treated with ACE inhibitors is accompanied by a leftward shift in the renal pressure-natriuresis curve and a reduction in total peripheral resistance in which there is variable participation by different vascular beds.

The kidney is a notable exception to this variability because increased renal blood flow owing to vasodilation is a relatively constant finding. This is not surprising because the renal vessels are exceptionally sensitive to the vasoconstrictor actions of angiotensin II. Increased renal blood flow occurs without an increase in glomerular filtration rate (GFR); thus the filtration fraction is reduced. Both the afferent and efferent arterioles are dilated. Blood flows in the cerebral and coronary beds, where autoregulatory mechanisms are powerful, generally are well maintained.

Several large prospective, randomized clinical studies involving thousands of patients provide convincing evidence that ACE inhibitors reduce overall mortality when treatment is begun during the periinfarction period. The beneficial effects of ACE inhibitors in acute MI are particularly large in hypertensive and diabetic patients.

PERMETHRIN

(Elimite, Nix, Acticin cream 5%, Elimite cream 5%, Permethrin lotion 1%, Nix cream rinse liquid 1%)

Permethrin is a scabicide/pediculicide that acts on the nerve-cell membrane to disrupt the sodium-channel current by which the polarization of the membrane is regulated. Delayed repolarization and paralysis of the pests is the outcome. **Cream**: used for treatment of scabies (*Sarcoptes scabiei*) infestation. **Lotion/Cream rinse**: used for treatment of infestation with head lice (*Pediculus humanus capitis*) and its nits (eggs). **Liquid**: used for treatment of infestation with *Pediculus humanus* var. *capitis* (head louse) and its nits (eggs).

Permethrin is a synthetic derivative of the insecticide pyrethrum, which was obtained originally from *Chrysanthemum cinerariaefolium*. Neurotoxicity associated with this compound is extremely rare. A 5% cream (Acticin, Elimite, others) is available in the treatment of scabies. This is used as an 8- to 12-hour or overnight application. A 1% permethrin cream rinse (Nix) also is available in the treatment of lice.

PERPHENAZINE

(Trilafon)

Perphenazine, a phenothiazine (4 to 8 mg t.i.d.), is indicated in the management of psychotic disorders, in the control of nausea and vomiting in adults, and in the relief of intractable hiccups.

Perphenazine is thought to exert its antipsychotic effects by postsynaptic blockade of CNS dopamine receptors, thus inhibiting dopamine-mediated effects. The antiemetic effects of perphenazine are attributed to dopamine-receptor blockade in the medullary chemoreceptor trigger zone. Perphenazine has many other central and peripheral effects; it produces both alpha and ganglionic blockade and counteracts histamine- and serotonin-mediated functions. It produces a very high incidence of movement disorders including akathisia, dystonia, parkinsonism, tardive dyskinesia, and neuroleptic malignant syndrome. Perphenazine possesses anticholinergic properties and hence should be used cautiously in patients with arrhythmias, CHF, angina pectoris, valvular disease, heart block, encephalitis, Reye's syndrome, head injury, respiratory disease, epilepsy and other seizure disorders (the drug may lower the seizure threshold), glaucoma (the drug may raise intraocular pressure [IOP]), prostatic hypertrophy, Parkinson's disease, urinary retention (the drug may worsen these conditions), and hepatic or renal dysfunction (impaired metabolism and excretion may cause drug accumulation).

Concomitant use of perphenazine with sympathomimetics, including epinephrine, phenylephrine, phenylpropanolamine, and ephedrine (often found in nasal sprays), and with appetite suppressants may decrease their stimulatory and pressor effects. Phenothiazines can cause epinephrine reversal and a hypotensive response when epinephrine is used for its pressor effects.

Perphenazine may inhibit BP response to centrally acting antihypertensive drugs such as guanethidine, guanabenz, guanadrel, clonidine, methyldopa, and reserpine. Additive effects are likely after concomitant use of perphenazine with CNS depressants, including alcohol, analgesics, barbiturates, narcotics, tranquilizers, and general, spinal, or epidural anesthetics, or parenteral magnesium sulfate (oversedation, respiratory depression, and hypotension); antiarrhythmic agents, quinidine, disopyramide, and procainamide (increased incidence of cardiac dysrhythmias and conduction defects); atropine or other anticholinergic drugs, including antidepressants, monoamine oxidase inhibitors, phenothiazines, antihistamines, meperidine, and antiparkinsonian agents (oversedation, paralytic ileus, visual changes, and severe constipation); nitrates (hypotension) and metrizamide (increased risk of convulsions). Beta-blocking agents may inhibit perphenazine metabolism, increasing plasma levels and toxicity.

PERPHENAZINE/AMITRIPTYLINE

(Etrafon 2-10 tablets 2 mg perphenazine/10 mg amitriptyline, Etrafon tablets 2 mg perphenazine/25 mg amitriptyline, Etrafon-A tablets 4 mg perphenazine/ 10 mg amitriptyline, Etrafon-Forte tablets 4 mg perphenazine/25 mg amitriptyline)

Perphenazine/amitriptyline is a psychotherapeutic combination. **Amitriptyline** blocks reuptake of serotonin and norepinephrine in CNS. **Perphenazine** appears to block postsynaptic dopamine receptors.

Perphenazine/amitriptyline are indicated in the treatment of moderate to severe anxiety or agitation and depressed mood; moderate to severe depression and anxiety associated with chronic physical disease; treatment of patients in whom depression and anxiety cannot be clearly differentiated; and treatment of schizophrenia with associated depression.

PERTUSSIS TOXIN

The secretory product of *Bordetella pertussis* interferes with the ability of agonists to inhibit adenylate cyclase. It catalyzes the transfer of the ADP-ribose moiety of NAD^+ to a cysteine residue close to the carboxy terminus of G_{1a}.

Forskolin, which is isolated from *Coleus forskohlii*, stimulates adenylate cyclase. Choleragen, the secretory product of *Vibrio cholerae*, can persistently activate adenylate cyclase by catalyzing the transfer of the ADP-ribose moiety of nicotinamide adenine dinucleotide (NAD^+) to G_{sa} (see also Figure 52).

PHARMACOGENOMICS

Pharmacogenomics is a recent offspring of **pharmacogenetics**. Both sciences deal with **hereditary impacts upon** the action of drugs, and their goals are overlapping. Any proper account of the history of pharmacogenomics must include a look at the development of pharmacogenetics.

Adverse drug reactions (ADRs) are a major clinical problem. A rapidly growing body of evidence suggests that genetic factors, at least in part, determine individual susceptibility to ADRs. A large number of pharmacogenetic studies have identified several polymorphisms as predictors of drug efficacy and/or adverse events. These candidate markers should be investigated further to ascertain the underlying mechanism of action; for example, changes in the kinetic parameters of an enzyme, or transcriptional activity of a promoter region.

The analysis of gene differential expression is complicated by the potentially subtle differences associated with alterations in a single allele as well as by variations between individuals that arise from environmental or physiological factors. To circumvent these analytic problems, a method named **allele-specific differential expression analysis** was developed to compare the relative expression levels of two alleles of the same cellular sample. The studies of allele-specific expression revealed that differential expression is relatively common in the human population. Human variation is largely caused by DNA polymorphism and difference in gene expression. Common disease/common variant hypotheses suggest that quantitative differences among different alleles may be the basis for complex diseases. Quantitative difference in gene expression between alleles may affect most complex diseases.

Polymorphism and variation in gene expression provide the genetic basis for human variation. Mendelian diseases are caused by mutations in a single gene or a few genes. To date, mutations in more than 2000 genes have been identified (http://www.ncbi.nih.gov/entrez/query.fcgi?db=OMIM). Most of these mutations change the protein structure and function. Increasing efforts have been made toward understanding the genetic basis of common complex diseases.

The characterization of protein–DNA interactions occurring at an allele-specific level is important to resolving the functional consequences of genetic variation in noncoding DNA for gene expression and regulation. The approach of **haplo-type-specific chromatin immunoprecipitation** (i.e., haploChIP) resolves in living cells relative protein-DNA binding to a particular allele through immunoprecipitation of proteins cross-linked to DNA. Single-nucleotide polymorphisms present in a heterozygous form are used as markers to differentiate allelic origin. This in turn allows resolution of specific haplotypes showing differences in relative protein occupancy. The haploChIP approach allows testing of *in vitro* hypotheses that a transcription factor protein shows haplotype-specific occupancy. In addition, the haploChIP approach allows screening of haplotypes for differences in relative gene expression by immunoprecipitation using antibodies to phosphorylated Pol II.

The variety of genotyping methods currently available and the evolution of their capabilities have facilitated an expansion of the field of pharmacogenomics. Traditionally, limited genotyping capabilities have restricted the generation and application of genotyping data for pharmacogenomic studies. With the variety of platforms and chemistries available for flexible, high-throughput genotyping, it is important to keep in mind the limitations imposed by both the polymorphisms that are to be interrogated and the type of pharmacogenomics study for which the data are being generated.

Denaturing high-performance liquid chromatography (DHPLC) is an accurate and efficient screening technique used for detecting DNA sequence changes by heteroduplex analysis. It can also be used for genotyping of single-nucleotide polymorphisms. The high sensitivity of DHPLC has made this technique one of the most reliable approaches to mutation analysis, and it is used in various areas of genetics, both in the research and clinical arena.

The data generated from the Human Genome Project has led to an explosion of technology for low-, medium-, and high-throughput genotyping methods. **Pyrosequencing** is a genotyping assay based on sequencing by synthesis. Short runs of sequence around each polymorphism are generated, allowing for internal controls for each sample. Pyrosequencing can also be used to identify tri-allelic, indel, and short-repeat polymorphisms, as well as to determine allele percentages for methylation or pooled sample assessment. The analysis of human genetic variation, such as **single-nucleotide polymorphisms** (SNPs), has great applications in genome-wide association studies of complex genetic traits.

The successful application of **capillary electrophoresis technology** to the genotyping of various types of polymorphisms has been well documented. The flexibility and automation of the Applied Biosystems 3100 Genetic Analyzer make it an excellent capillary electrophoresis platform for the generation of high-quality genotype data. These data are readily applied to pharmacogenomic investigations of various types.

To undertake partial, or complete, genome screens by association-based methodology for quantitative trait loci, multiple individuals have to be screened for large numbers of genetic markers. Consequently, much recent interest has focused on methods enabling accurate allele quantification in pooled DNA samples. Microsatellites were the favored markers in initial studies, but the extraordinary wealth of data concerning SNPs has turned attention to the quantification of SNP alleles in pools. All such approaches require accurate estimation of DNA concentrations, followed by the preparation of replicate pools, validation, and application of procedures for determining allele frequencies.

The **Pharmacogenetics and Pharmacogenomics Knowledge Base** (PharmGKB) is an interactive tool for researchers investigating how genetic variation effects drug response. The PharmGKB Web site, www.pharmgkb.org, displays genotype, and molecular and clinical primary data integrated with literature, pathway representations, protocol information, and links to additional external resources. Users can search and browse the knowledge base by genes, drugs, diseases, and pathways. Registration is free to the entire research community but subject to an agreement to respect the rights and privacy of the individuals whose information is contained within the database. Registered users can access and download primary data to aid in the design of future pharmacogenetics and pharmacogenomics studies.

PHENACEMIDE

(Phenurone)

Phenacemide, a substituted acetylurea derivative with anticonvulsant properties (500 mg p.o. t.i.d.), is indicated in the treatment of refractory, complex-partial, generalized tonic–clonic, absence, and atypical absence seizures.

PHENACETIN

(Acetaphenetidin)

Phenacetin has analgesic and antipyretic but no antiinflammatory properties. Phenacetin and its deethylated metabolite, acetaminophen, are superior to aspirin in that they do not cause hypoprothrombinemia, GI irritation, or disturbances of acid-base balance. The serious, but rare, side effects of phenacetin are methemoglobinemia, hemolytic anemia, fatal hepatic necrosis, and hypoglycemic coma. Both interstitial nephritis and renal papillary necrosis can be caused by phenacetin and acetaminophen. The less toxic acetaminophen should be used only in patients who cannot tolerate aspirin or in whom aspirin is contraindicated (see also Table 3).

PHENAZOPYRIDINE HYDROCHLORIDE

(Azo-Standard tablets 95 mg, Baridium tablets 100 mg, Geridium tablets 100 mg, tablets 200 mg, Prodium tablets 95 mg, Pyridiate tablets 100 mg, Pyridium tablets 100 mg, tablets 200 mg, Pyridium Plus tablets 150 mg, Urodine tablets 100 mg, tablets 200 mg, Urogesic tablets 100 mg, UTI Relief tablets 97.2 mg)

Phenazopyridine hydrochloride is an interstitial cystitis agent that exerts a topical analgesic effect on urinary tract mucosa; and provides symptomatic relief of pain, burning, urgency, frequency and other discomforts arising from irritation of lower urinary tract mucosa.

Phenazopyridine hydrochloride (Pyridium, others) is not a urinary antiseptic. However, it does have an analgesic action on the urinary tract and alleviates symptoms of dysuria, frequency, burning, and urgency. The usual dose is 200 mg three times daily. The compound is an azo dye, which colors urine orange or red; the patient should be so informed. GI upset is seen in up to 10% of patients and can be reduced by administering the drug with food; overdosage may result in methemoglobinemia. **Phenazopyridine** has been marketed since 1925 and has had dual prescription/over-the-counter (OTC) marketing status since 1951. As part of their ongoing review of OTC drug products, the FDA is currently in the process of evaluating products containing less than 200 mg **phenazopyridine** to determine whether these products generally are recognized as safe and effective as urinary analgesics. The outcome of this evaluation will determine the continued availability of OTC **phenazopyridine** products in the United States. Products containing 200 mg **phenazopyridine** are sold by prescription, but their long-term availability in the marketplace also may be affected by the FDA's final OTC ruling.

Phenazopyridine (200 mg t.i.d.) is indicated in the symptomatic relief of pain, burning, urgency, frequency, and other discomforts arising from irritation of the lower urinary tract mucosa caused by infections, trauma, surgery, endoscopic procedures, or passage of sounds or catheters. Its analgesic action may reduce or eliminate the need for systemic analgesics or narcotics.

Overdosage of phenazopyridine is known to have caused headache, rash, pruritis, occasional GI disturbances; anaphylactoid-like reaction, methemoglobinemia, hemolytic anemia, and renal and hepatic toxicity.

PHENDIMETRAZINE HYDROCHLORIDE

(Adipost, Anorex, Bacarate, Bontril, Delcozine, Di-ap-trol, Obalan, Obezine, PDM, Phenzine, Prelu-2, SPRX-1, SPRX-2, SPRX-3, Statobex, Trimtabs, Wehless-105)

Phendimetrazine, an indirect-acting sympathomimetic agent with amphetamine-like action (35 mg p.o. b.i.d.), is indicated as a short-term adjunct in the treatment of obesity.

PHENDIMETRAZINE TARTRATE

(Bontril PDM tablets 35 mg, Bontril slow-release tablets 35 mg, Melfiat-105 Unicelles tablets 35 mg, Prelu-2 capsules, sustained release 105 mg)

Phendimetrazine tartrate is an anorexiant that may stimulate the satiety center in the brain, causing appetite suppression. It is indicated as a short-term (few weeks) adjunct to diet plans to reduce weight.

Obesity arises as a consequence of positive caloric balance. Optimally, weight loss is achieved by a gradual increase in energy expenditure from exercise combined with dieting to decrease the caloric intake. However, this obvious approach has a relatively low success rate. Consequently, alternative forms of treatment, including surgery or medications, have been developed in an effort to increase the likelihood of achieving and maintaining weight loss. Amphetamine was found to produce weight loss in early studies of patients with narcolepsy and was subsequently used in the treatment of obesity. The drug promotes weight loss by suppressing appetite rather than by increasing energy expenditure. Other anorexic drugs include **methamphetamine**, **dextroamphetamine**, **phentermine**, **benzphetamine**, **phendimetrazine**, **phenmetrazine**, **diethylpropion**, **mazindol**, **phenylpropanolamine**, and **sibutramine** (a mixed adrenergic/serotonergic drug).

PHENELZINE SULFATE

(Nardil)

Phenelzine, a monoamine oxidase (MAO) A inhibitor (15 mg t.i.d.), is indicated in treatment of depressed patients clinically characterized as "atypical," "nonendogenous," or "neurotic." These patients often have mixed anxiety and depression and phobic or hypochondriacal features (see also Tables 5 through 7).

Monoamine oxidase can metabolize monoamines by oxidative deamination and convert them to inactive acidic derivatives. MAO inhibitors seem to compete with physiologically active monoamine for the active site of the enzyme. In general, not only do these agents inhibit the oxidase that metabolizes amines but they also inhibit the oxidase that metabolizes drugs and essential nutrients. Hence, the incidence of drug–drug and drug–food interactions is extremely high with these agents. MAOs have various applications. They may be used as a local anesthetic (cocaine), as an antihistaminic (diphenylhydramine), or as an antidepressant (tranylcypromine, phenelzine). MAO inhibitors have been used in the treatment of hypertension (direct blockade of sympathetic ganglion), angina pectoris (coronary dilation), narcolepsy (stimulating the reticular activating system), and depression (increasing the brain's norepinephrine pool). Needless to say, these agents should be used with extreme caution in conjunction with sympathomimetic amines, ganglionic-blocking agents, procaine, and anesthetic agents. They are contraindicated in patients with hyperthyroidism and in combination with tricyclic antidepressants. In the event of poisoning, adrenergic-blocking agents such as phentolamine may be effective for combating the hypertensive crisis.

PHENINDAMINE TARTRATE

(Nolahist tablets 25 mg)

Phenindamine tartrate is an antihistamine that competitively antagonizes histamine at H_1-receptor sites. It is indicated in the temporary relief of runny nose, sneezing, itching of the nose or throat, and itchy, watery eyes caused by hay fever or other upper respiratory allergic rhinitis.

PHENOBARBITAL

(Luminal)

Phenobarbital is indicated as a hypnotic agent for the short-term treatment of insomnia, as an anticonvulsant in the treatment of partial and generalized tonic–clonic and cortical focal seizures; and in emergency control of certain acute convulsive episodes (e.g., those associated with status epilepticus, eclampsia, tetanus, and toxic reactions to strychnine or local anesthetics).

Phenobarbital is absorbed from the small intestine. As much as 50% binds to albumin, and it is metabolized in the liver to hydroxyphenobarbital. Approximately 20 to 25% of phenobarbital is excreted in the urine unchanged. It has a very long elimination half-life of up to 140 hours. Therefore, it is administered orally in a dose of 2 to 3 mg/kg once a day. The renal excretion of phenobarbital is enhanced by the alkalinization of urine, which favors its ionization and excretion. $NaHCO_3$ has been used in the management of phenobarbital toxicity.

Phenobarbital induces hepatic microsomal drug-metabolizing enzymes. The sudden withdrawal of phenobarbital may precipitate withdrawal seizures. Therefore, the doses should be tapered gradually whenever discontinuation is contemplated.

Phenobarbital inhibits posttetanic potentiation and especially raises the seizure threshold. The precise mechanism of action of phenobarbital is not known, though two dissimilar mechanisms have been advanced.

In the first, phenobarbital, by inhibiting aldehyde reductase, is thought to interfere with the metabolism of aldehyde generated by biogenic amines such as dopamine, norepinephrine, and serotonin. The accumulation of these aldehydes in the CNS has depressing properties, and this reduces the neuronal sensitivity to excitation.

In the second theory, phenobarbital is thought to enhance the presynaptic release of GABA and, at the same time, reduce the postsynaptic uptake of GABA (see also Figure 50).

Compared to phenytoin, phenobarbital is a relatively safe compound. Rarely, a morbilliform rash occurs. However, in some patients, heavy sedation, reduction in activity, and impairment in cognition may be pronounced.

Phenobarbital has a broad spectrum of antiepileptic activity and efficacy. It is often used by itself or in combination with phenytoin. Advantages of phenobarbital are:

- It has a long history of usage with few serious systemic and no dysmorphic side effects.
- It is inexpensive and widely available.
- It can be used both orally and parenterally.
- Its long elimination half-life allows simple single daily administration; missed doses have little clinical impact.
- It has broad-spectrum antiepileptic properties and is useful for febrile, toxic metabolic, and withdrawal seizures.
- The teratogenicity risk is less than that of phenytoin.

Disadvantages of phenobarbital are:

- It produces annoying sedative effects in many patients, even within the therapeutic range.
- Significant disturbance of cognitive function, mood, or behavior is seen in some patients, especially children and the elderly.
- Rapid manipulation to raise or lower serum levels is somewhat difficult due to slow accumulation and elimination.
- Accidental or purposeful overdose may be lethal.

PHENOLPHTHALEIN

Although often used interchangeably, the terms laxative and cathartic do have slightly different meanings. A laxative effect refers to the excretion of a soft, formed stool; catharsis implies a more fluid and complete evacuation.

Irritant agents used in the treatment of constipation include cascara, sagrada, castor oil, senna, rhubarb, phenolphthalein, and acetphenolisatin. Phenolphthalein is a constituent of many OTC preparations, including Ex-Lax and Feen-A-Mint. Most of these agents, with the exception of castor oil, are slow in their onset of action (24 hours). Castor oil is hydrolyzed to ricinoleic acid, the active cathartic. It has an onset of action of 2 to 6 hours.

Phenolphthalein is thought to exert its effect by inhibiting the movement of water and sodium from the colon into the blood and by stimulating mucus secretion. If misused on a prolonged basis, a consequential loss of mucus may lower the plasma protein level.

The misuse of any of these agents has been shown to cause hypokalemia, dehydration, and a cathartic colon (resembling ulcerative colitis). Phenolphthalein-containing products may color alkaline urine red.

PHENOTHIAZINE DERIVATIVES

The phenothiazine-derivative antipsychotics are classified according to their chemical structures. These are (see Table 2):

- Propylamine derivatives, which include chlorpromazine (Thorazine), promazine (Sparine), and triflupromazine (Vesprin)
- Propylpiperazine derivatives, which include fluphenazine (Permitil, Prolixin), perphenazine (Trilafon), prochlorperazine (Compazine), trifluoperazine (Stelazine), and acetophenazine (Tindal)
- Methylpiperidyl derivatives, which include thioridazine (Mellaril)

These agents differ in their potency but not their efficacy. Long-acting injectable drugs such as fluphenazine decanoate or fluphenazine enanthate, which need to be given only once every two or three weeks, are increasingly used in outpatients and in those patients who are uncooperative and noncompliant. Phenothiazine derivatives devoid of neuroleptic activity also exist. Promethazine (Phenergan) is an antihistaminic; ethopropazine (Parsidol) has a muscle relaxant effect and, because of its anticholinergic action, may be used in parkinsonism. Methotrimeprazine (Levoprome) is claimed to be a nonaddictive analgesic that does not cause respiratory depression (see Table 2).

PHENOXYBENZAMINE HYDROCHLORIDE

(Dibenzyline)

Phenoxybenzamine (5.0 to 60.0 mg/day) is used in order to control episodes of hypertension and sweating. If tachycardia is excessive, it may also be necessary to use a beta-blocker concomitantly. In addition, phenoxybenzamine has been tested for its efficacy in micturition disorders resulting from neurogenic bladder, functional outlet obstruction, and partial prostatic obstruction.

Phenoxybenzamine is a noncompetitive alpha-adrenergic-receptor blocker, and its action cannot be nullified by increasing the amount of agonist, or agonists. It causes epinephrine reversal in that the administration of epinephrine after pretreatment with phenoxybenzamine elicits vasodilation, and, conversely, phenoxybenzamine reverses epinephrine-mediated vasoconstriction to vasodilation (see also Figure 37).

The adverse effects of phenoxybenzamine include nasal congestion, miosis, postural hypotension, tachycardia, and inhibition of ejaculation.

PHENSUXIMIDE

(Milontin)

Phensuximide (500 to 1000 mg p.o. b.i.d.) suppresses the paroxysmal three-cycles-per-second spike-and-wave activity associated with lapses of consciousness common in absence (petit mal) seizures. The frequency of epileptiform attacks is reduced, apparently by motor cortex depression and elevation of the threshold of the CNS to convulsive stimuli.

Phensuximide may increase the incidence of generalized tonic–clonic seizures if used alone to treat mixed seizures; and abrupt withdrawal may precipitate petit mal seizures.

Concomitant use of phensuximide and other CNS depressants (alcohol, narcotics, anxiolytics, antidepressants, antipsychotics, and other anticonvulsants) may increase sedative effects.

Symptoms of overdose may include dizziness and ataxia, which may progress to stupor and coma.

PHENTERMINE HYDROCHLORIDE

(Adipex-P, Anoxine, Dapex, Fastin, Donamin, Ionamin, Obe-Nix, Obermine, Obiphen, Phentrol, Rolaphent, Unicelles, Wilpower)

Phentermine, an indirect-acting sympathomimetic agent with amphetamine-like actions (8 mg p.o. t.i.d.), is indicated as a short-term adjunct in the treatment of exogenous obesity.

Obesity arises as a consequence of positive caloric balance. Optimally, weight loss is achieved by a gradual increase in energy expenditure from exercise combined with dieting to decrease the caloric intake. However, this obvious approach has a relatively low success rate. Consequently, alternative forms of treatment, including surgery or medications, have been developed in an effort to increase the likelihood of achieving and maintaining weight loss. Amphetamine was found to produce weight loss in early studies of patients with narcolepsy and was subsequently used in the treatment of obesity. The drug promotes weight loss by suppressing appetite rather than by increasing energy expenditure. Other anorexic drugs include **methamphetamine**, **dextroamphetamine**, **phentermine**, **benzphetamine**, **phendimetrazine**, **phenmetrazine**, **diethylpropion**, **mazindol**, **phenylpropanolamine**, and **sibutramine** (a mixed adrenergic/serotonergic drug).

PHENTOLAMINE

(Regitine)

Phentolamine (5 mg IV or IM, 1 to 2 hours before surgery) is indicated in prevention or control of hypertensive episodes that may occur in a patient with pheochromocytoma as a result of stress or manipulation during preoperative preparation and surgical excision; and in prevention and treatment of dermal necrosis and sloughing following IV administration or extravasation of norepinephrine or dopamine. Phentolamine has been used to treat hypertensive crisis secondary to MAO inhibitors/sympathomimetic amine interactions and rebound hypertension on withdrawal of clonidine, propranolol, or other antihypertensives. It has also been used in combination with papaverine as an intracavernous injection for impotence.

Phentolamine is a competitive alpha-adrenergic blocker, and its action can be nullified by increasing the amount of agonist, or agonists. The vasoconstricting and hypertensive effects of epinephrine and ephedrine are antagonized by phentolamine (see also Figure 37).

The dose-dependent adverse effects of phentolamine include nausea, vomiting, diarrhea, nasal stuffiness, hypotension, tachycardia, dizziness, flushing, and weakness.

MI, cerebrovascular spasm, and cerebrovascular occlusion have followed phentolamine administration, usually in association with marked hypotensive episodes with shock-like states that occasionally follow parenteral use.

PHENYLBUTAZONE

(Butazolidin)

Phenylbutazone is indicated in relieving the symptoms of acute gouty arthritis, active rheumatoid arthritis, and active ankylosing spondylitis, acute attacks of degenerative joint disease of the hips and knees, and painful shoulder (peritendinitis, capsulitis, bursitis, and acute arthritis of that joint). However, because of the risk of agranulocytosis and aplastic anemia, it should be used only when other nonsteroidal antiinflammatory substances have proven unsatisfactory.

Phenylbutazone and its analog, oxyphenbutazone, are closely related chemically and pharmacologically to the pyrazolines, aminopyrine, and antipyrine. These drugs have antiinflammatory, antipyretic, analgesic, and mild uricosuric actions resulting in symptomatic relief only; the disease process is unaltered.

The exact mechanism of the antiinflammatory effect is unknown, but these agents inhibit factors believed to be involved in the inflammatory process, including prostaglandin synthesis, leukocyte migration, and release and activity of lysosomal enzymes.

The antiinflammatory effect of phenylbutazone is greater than aspirin's but less than that of the steroid antiinflammatory agents. Phenylbutazone causes sodium and chloride retention, and edema may result. In addition, fatal aplastic anemia and agranulocytosis have occurred following the use of phenylbutazone. The activation of and perforation of hemorrhagic ulcer can also take place, and hypersensitivity reactions are common. Consequently, phenylbutazone should be used only in the treatment of inflammatory conditions (rheumatoid arthritis, ankylosing spondylitis, or osteoarthritis) when the safer antiinflammatory agents are no longer effective.

Antiinflammatory agents, oral anticoagulants, oral antidiabetics, sulfonamides, sodium valproate, and phenytoin are competitively displaced by phenylbutazone from serum-binding sites. The activity, duration of effect, and toxicity of the displaced drugs may be increased.

Barbiturates, promethazine, chlorpheniramine, rifampin, and corticosteroids, inducers of microsomal enzymes, may decrease the half-life of phenylbutazone. Cholestyramine reduces the enteral absorption of phenylbutazone (see also Table 3).

PHENYLEPHRINE HYDROCHLORIDE

(Neo-Synephrine, Allerest, Sinex)

Phenylephrine is indicated in the treatment of vascular failure in shock, shock-like states, drug-induced hypotension, or hypersensitivity; to overcome paroxysmal supraventricular tachycardia; to prolong spinal anesthesia; as a vasoconstrictor in regional analgesia; and to maintain an adequate level of BP during spinal and inhalation anesthesia. Phenylephrine is a powerful postsynaptic alpha-receptor stimulant with little effect on the beta receptors of the heart (see also Figure 39).

The predominant actions of phenylephrine are on the cardiovascular system. Parenteral administration causes a rise in systolic and diastolic pressures due to peripheral vasoconstriction. Accompanying the pressor response to phenylephrine is a marked reflex bradycardia that can be blocked by atropine; after atropine, large doses of the peripheral resistance is considerably increased. Circulation time is slightly prolonged, and venous pressure is slightly increased; venous constriction is not marked. Most vascular beds are constricted; renal, splanchnic, cutaneous, and limb blood flows are reduced, but coronary blood flow is increased. Pulmonary vessels are constricted, and pulmonary arterial pressure is raised.

The drug is a powerful vasoconstrictor with properties very similar to those of norepinephrine but almost completely lacking the chronotropic and inotropic actions on the heart. Cardiac irregularities are seen only very rarely, even with large doses. In contrast to epinephrine and ephedrine, phenylephrine produces longer-lasting vasoconstriction, a reflex bradycardia, and increases the stroke output, producing no disturbance in the rhythm of the pulse.

In therapeutic doses, it produces little if any stimulation of either the spinal cord or cerebrum. An advantage is that repeated injections produce comparable effects.

PHENYLEPHRINE HYDROCHLORIDE/GUAIFENESIN

(Rescon-GG liquid 3 mg phenylephrine hydrochloride and 100 mg guaifenesin, Entex liquid 7.5 mg phenylephrine hydrochloride and 100 mg guaifenesin, Guaifed-PD capsules 7.5 mg phenylephrine hydrochloride and 200 mg guaifenesin, Entex ER capsules 10 mg phenylephrine hydrochloride and 300 mg guaifenesin, Guaifed capsules 15 mg phenylephrine hydrochloride and 400 mg guaifenesin, SINUvent PE tablets 15 mg phenylephrine hydrochloride and 600 mg guaifenesin, Endal nasal decongestant tablets 20 mg phenylephrine hydrochloride and 300 mg guaifenesin, GFN 600/ phenylephrine 20 tablets 20 mg phenylephrine hydrochloride and 600 mg guaifenesin, Liquibid-PD tablets 25 mg phenylephrine hydrochloride and 275 mg guaifenesin, Entex LA tablets 30 mg phenylephrine hydrochloride and 600 mg guaifenesin, Liquibid-D tablets 40 mg phenylephrine hydrochloride and 600 mg guaifenesin, Liquibid-D 1200 tablets 40 mg phenylephrine hydrochloride and 1200 mg guaifenesin)

Phenylephrine stimulates postsynaptic alpha receptors, resulting in vasoconstriction, which reduces congestion. **Guaifenesin** may enhance output of respiratory tract fluid by reducing adhesiveness and surface tension, enhancing removal of viscous mucus, and making nonproductive coughs more productive and less frequent. They are indicated in temporary relief of symptoms of upper respiratory tract disorders such as sinusitis, vasomotor rhinitis, and hay fever; in temporary relief of coughs associated with respiratory tract infections and related conditions such as sinusitis, pharyngitis, bronchitis, and asthma when tenacious mucus and/or mucus plugs and congestion complicate these conditions.

PHENYLEPHRINE TANNATE/ CHLORPHENIRAMINE TANNATE

(Rhinatate-NF pediatric suspension 5 mg phenylephrine tannate and 4.5 mg chlorpheniramine tannate, Nuhist suspension 5 mg phenylephrine tannate and 4.5 mg chlorpheniramine tannate, R-Tanna S pediatric suspension 5 mg phenylephrine tannate and 4.5 mg chlorpheniramine tannate, Rynatan pediatric suspension 5 mg phenylephrine tannate and 4.5 mg chlorpheniramine tannate)

Phenylephrine tannate is an antihistamine/decongestant/vasopressor used in shock.

Phenylephrine stimulates postsynaptic alpha receptors, resulting in vasoconstriction, which reduces nasal congestion. **Chlorpheniramine** competitively antagonizes histamine at H_1-receptor sites. They are indicated in the symptomatic relief of coryza and nasal congestion associated with common cold, sinusitis, allergic rhinitis, and other upper respiratory tract conditions.

PHENYLEPHRINE TANNATE/CHLORPHENIRAMINE TANNATE/PYRILAMINE TANNATE

(Triotann pediatric suspension 5 mg phenylephrine, 2 mg chlorpheniramine, 12.5 mg pyrilamine, Triotann-S pediatric suspension 5 mg phenylephrine, 2 mg chlorpheniramine, 12.5 mg pyrilamine)

Phenylephrine tannate is an antihistamine/decongestant/vasopressor used in shock. **Phenylephrine** stimulates postsynaptic alpha receptors, resulting in vasoconstriction, which reduces nasal congestion. **Chlorpheniramine and pyrilamine** competitively antagonizes histamine at H_1-receptor sites. They are indicated in symptomatic relief of coryza and nasal congestion associated with common cold, sinusitis, allergic rhinitis, and other upper respiratory tract conditions.

PHENYTOIN SODIUM

(Dilantin)

Phenytoin (2 to 3 mg/kg p.o. daily divided b.i.d.) is indicated in generalized tonic–clonic seizures, for status epilepticus, and for post-head-injury trauma.

Phenytoin, which has a pKa of 8.3 to 9.2, is insoluble at the pH of gastric juice and therefore is not absorbed to a significant degree from the stomach. On passage into the small intestine, where the pH is basic (7.0 to 7.5), phenytoin exists in a nonionized form that favors its absorption. Absorption is highest from the duodenum and decreases rapidly in the lower parts of the small intestine. Because phenytoin is not absorbed well from the large intestine, the rectal administration of phenytoin is of little therapeutic value and should not be encouraged.

When used on a long-term basis, phenytoin is always given orally. To abort status epilepticus, it is given intravenously. Because the injectable form of phenytoin has a pH of 12.0, it should not be injected intramuscularly.

After absorption, as much as 92 to 93% of phenytoin becomes bound to plasma proteins, allowing only 7 to 8% of the drug to remain free. Circumstances or drugs that alter the extent of protein binding will significantly affect phenytoin's therapeutic usefulness and may also precipitate phenytoin toxicity. For example, in uremic patients, whose free phenytoin levels may reach as high as 30%, the dosage of phenytoin should be reduced. Similarly, in patients with hypoalbuminemia resulting from numerous disorders, the doses of phenytoin should be adjusted downward.

Phenytoin becomes metabolized in the liver to hydroxyphenytoin, which is an inactive metabolite. Hydroxyphenytoin is then conjugated with glucuronic acid and excreted by the kidneys. Hydroxyphenytoin inhibits the metabolism of phenytoin, and the half-life of phenytoin may be altered if doses exceed the therapeutic level, as shown in the following example:

Oral Dose of Phenytoin (mg/kg)	Plasma Level of Phenytoin (μg/mL)	Half-Life (hour)
4	10–15	24
12	>25	60

Clinical evidence indicates that epileptic patients are either slow or rapid metabolizers of phenytoin. In the slow metabolizers, 4 mg/kg of phenytoin may produce toxicity, whereas, in the rapid metabolizers, this may be a subtherapeutic dose. In addition, the results of randomized, double-blind, controlled clinical trials of antiepileptic drugs conducted in adult patients with mostly partial onset or generalized tonic–clonic seizures, or both, have shown that there are considerable individual differences between patients' responses to the same drug. Side effects are common with all of the antiepileptic drugs.

The mode of action of phenytoin has been attributed to its membrane-stabilizing effects because it (1) limits the development of maximal seizure activity, and (2) reduces the spread of the seizure process from an epileptic focus. The precise mechanisms responsible for stabilization of the neuronal membrane are uncertain, though several concepts have been advanced (Figure 76).

One of these concerns phenytoin's interference with calcium action. Phenytoin inhibits the development of and reverses posttetanic potentiation, or posttetanic facilitation. It is thought that this is an important mechanism in the development of the high-frequency train of impulses that takes place in cerebral excitatory feedback circuits and in the spread of such activity to neighboring loops, resulting in maximal seizure activity. Phenytoin reduces calcium transport at the outer nerve membrane by blocking its high-affinity binding sites. This prevents the release of norepinephrine, which is necessary for the generation of posttetanic potentiation, and the spread of the impending seizure process is curtailed.

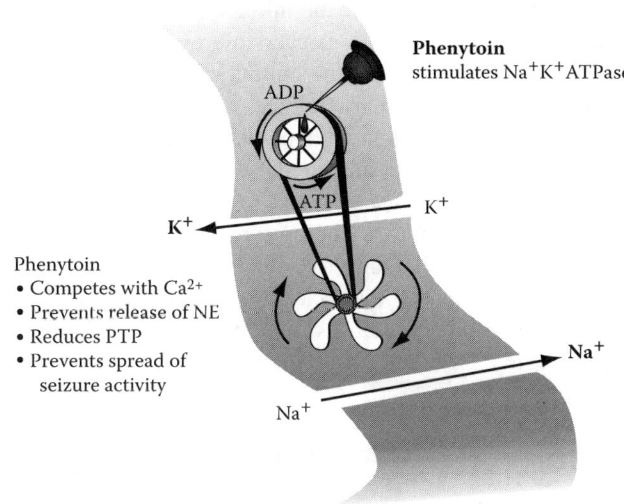

FIGURE 76 The mode of action of phenytoin has been attributed to its **membrane-stabilizing effects**, because it (1) limits the development of maximal seizure activity, and (2) reduces the spread of the seizure process from an epileptic focus.

A second concept that attempts to explain the mechanism of phenytoin's activity is its interference with sodium movement. In a hyperexcitable state, the intracellular concentration of sodium is elevated. Phenytoin decreases the inward sodium current. Furthermore, when the intracellular concentration of sodium is elevated, phenytoin is thought to stimulate Na^+K^+-ATPase to reestablish the ionic gradient. By the activity of Na^+, K^+-ATPase is reduced in the brains of epileptic patients (see Figure 76).

The membrane-stabilizing effect of phenytoin is not limited to neurons but is also seen in other excitable tissues, such as skeletal muscle and heart. Furthermore, phenytoin is effective in treating myotonia and cardiac arrhythmias.

A third concept is that phenytoin enhances GABAergic transmission. Chloride ions enhance the binding of phenytoin to a specific but unknown receptor site in the brain. It has been postulated that this binding may enhance GABA-mediated chloride conductance in the postsynaptic membrane.

Phenytoin may cause nystagmus, diplopia, staggering, and ataxia. These side effects are generally regarded as dose-dependent, and usually appear whenever the plasma concentration of phenytoin exceeds 20 μg/mL. These side effects are reversible with dose reduction.

Phenytoin causes gingival hyperplasia, which occurs with much greater frequency in children (60%) than in adults (40%), shows no race or sex predilection, and may appear 2 to 3 months after the initiation of therapy. Gingival hyperplasia, which does not occur in the toothless portion of the gum, regresses gradually on discontinuation of the medication. Other medications causing gingival hyperplasia include cyclosporin, nifedipine, diltiazem, verapamil, and nitrendipine (see also Table 10).

Phenytoin causes hypertrichosis in 5% of patients, which occurs several months after the initiation of therapy and is either slowly reversible, or irreversible even after discontinuation of medication. Phenytoin may also cause a hypersensitivity reaction, characterized by rashes, Stevens–Johnson syndrome, lymphoid hyperplasia, blood dyscrasias, and serum sickness. If any of these reactions occur, the medications must be discontinued.

Long-term phenytoin therapy carries several drawbacks. It may impair cognitive functions, cause bilateral peripheral neuropathy that is characterized by decreased reflexes and sensory deficits, and produce hypokalemia and osteomalacia, resulting in accelerated vitamin D metabolism.

Advantages of phenytoin are:

It is relatively nonsedating.
Serious toxicity is rare.
Parenteral administration is possible.
A loading dose may be given by the oral or IV route.
It only needs to be taken once a day by most adults.
It is relatively inexpensive.

Disadvantages of phenytoin are:

It may cause some sedation and/or impairment of higher intellectual function.
There is a relatively high incidence of annoying side effects with long-term administration, including gingival hyperplasia, hypertrichosis, acne, and coarsening of the facial features.

PHOTOSENSITIVITY: Medication-induced

Anticancer Drugs

Dacarbazine	Methotrexate
Fluorouracil	Vinblastine
Flutamide	

Antidepressants

Amitriptyline	Desipramine	Maprotiline	Protriptyline
Amoxapine	Doxepin	Nortriptyline	Trazodone
Clomipramine	Imipramine	Phenelzine	Trimipramine

Antihistamines

Cyproheptadine
Diphenhydramine

Antihypertensives

Captopril	Minoxidil
Diltiazem	Nifedipine
Methyldopa	

Antimicrobials

Ciprofloxacin	Enoxacin	Nalidixic acid	Pyrazinamide
Clofazimine	Flucytosine	Norfloxacin	Sulfonamides
Dapsone	Griseofulvin	Ofloxacin	Tetracycline
Demeclocycline	Lomefloxacin	Oxytetracycline	Trimethoprim
Doxycycline	Minocycline		

Antiparasitic Drugs

Chloroquine
Quinine
Thiabendazole

Antipsychotic Drugs

Chlorpromazine	Perphenazine	Thioridazine	Trifluoperazine
Fluphenazine	Prochlorperazine	Thiothixene	Triflupromazine
Haloperidol			

Diuretics

Acetazolamide	Chlorothiazide	Hydroflumethiazide	Polythiazide
Amiloride	Furosemide	Methyclothiazide	Triamterene
Bendroflumethiazide	Hydrochlorothiazide	Metolazone	Trichlormethiazide
Benzthiazide			

Hypoglycemics

Acetohexamide	Glipizide	Tolazamide
Chlorpropamide	Glyburide	Tolbutamide

PHOTOSENSITIVITY: Medication-induced (Continued)

Nonsteroidal Antiinflammatory Drugs

Diflunisal	Ketoprofen	Naproxen	Piroxicam
Ibuprofen	Nabumetone	Phenylbutazone	Sulindac
Indomethacin			

Others

Alprazolam	Chlordiazepoxide	Fluorescein	Promethazine
Amantadine	Clofibrate	Gold salts	Quinidine sulfate and gluconate
Amiodarone	Desoximetasone	Hexachlorophene	Tretinoin
Benzocaine	Disopyramide	Isotretinoin	Trimeprazine
Carbamazepine	Etretinate		

The frequency of photosensitivity reactions is nonuniform and may not be related either to the structure or the functions of the drugs. For example, the highest incidence of photosensitivity reactions have occurred following administration of amiodarone, chlorpromazine, chlorothiazide, demeclocycline, doxycycline, furosemide, hydrochlorothiazide, piroxicam, promethazine, or tolbutamide. Many chemicals are activated to toxic metabolites by enzymatic biotransformation. However, some chemicals can be activated in the skin by ultraviolet and/or visible radiation. In photoallergy, radiation absorbed by the drug, such as sulfonamide, results in its conversion to a product that is a more potent allergen than the parent compound. The clinical manifestations may range from acute urticarial reactions, which develop a few minutes after exposure to sunlight, to eczematous or papular lesions, which appear after 24 hours or more. Phototoxic reactions to drugs, in contrast to photoallergic ones, do not have an immunological component. Drugs, either absorbed locally into the skin or that have reached the skin through the systemic circulation, may be the object of photochemical reactions within the skin. This can lead directly either to chemically induced photosensitivity reactions or to enhancement of the usual effects of sunlight. Tetracyclines, sulfonamides, chlorpromazine, and nalidixic acid are examples of phototoxic chemicals; generally, they are innocuous to skin if not exposed to light.

PHYSOSTIGMINE SULFATE

(Eserine)

Physostigmine sulfate and physostigmine salicylate (Antilirium) are cholinesterase inhibitors that are indicated as antidotes to poisoning from substances possessing anticholinergic properties such as imipramine, a tricyclic antidepressant. In addition, it has been used in open-angle glaucoma.

Physostigmine competitively blocks acetylcholine hydrolysis by cholinesterase, resulting in acetylcholine accumulation at cholinergic synapses that antagonizes the muscarinic effects of overdose with antidepressants and anticholinergics. With ophthalmic use, miosis and ciliary-muscle contraction increases aqueous humor outflow and decreases IOP.

The reversible inhibitors, which have a short to moderate duration of action, fall into two categories. Type one, exemplified by edrophonium, forms an ionic bond at the anionic site and a weak hydrogen bond at the esteratic site of acetylcholinesterase. Type two, exemplified by neostigmine, forms an ionic bond at the anionic site and a hydrolyzable covalent bond at the esteratic site.

The irreversible inhibitors, exemplified by organophosphorous compounds (diisopropyl fluorophosphate [DFP], parathion, malathion, diazinon), have long durations of action and form a covalent bond with acetylcholinesterase, which is hydrolyzed very slowly and negligibly, but the inhibition may be overcome by cholinesterase activators such as pralidoxime.

Cholinesterase inhibitors may also be classified according to agents that possess tertiary nitrogens (e.g., physostigmine and most organophosphorous compounds) and those that contain quaternary nitrogens (e.g., neostigmine, pyridostigmine, and some organophosphorous compounds such as echothiphate). The following summarizes the comparative properties of these agents.

	Physostigmine	Neostigmine
Oral absorption	Good	Poor
Crosses the blood–brain barrier	Well	No
Stimulates nicotinic receptors (skeletal muscle)	Yes	Yes
Used to combat the CNS toxicity of numerous anticholinergic drugs	Yes	No

Physostigmine causes miosis and spasm of accommodation; it also lowers IOP and hence can be used in the treatment of wide-angle glaucoma (Figure 77). Being lipid soluble, it penetrates into the brain rapidly, raises the acetylcholine concentration, and, in toxic amounts, may cause cholinergic CNS toxicity, which is characterized by restlessness, insomnia, tremors, confusion, ataxia, convulsions, respiratory depression, and circulatory collapse. These effects are reversed by atropine.

Neostigmine, which is unable to penetrate the blood–brain barrier, does not cause CNS toxicity. However, it may produce dose-dependent and full-range muscarinic effects, characterized by miosis, blurring of vision, lacrimation, salivation, sweating, increased bronchial secretion, bronchoconstriction, bradycardia, hypotension, and urinary incontinence.

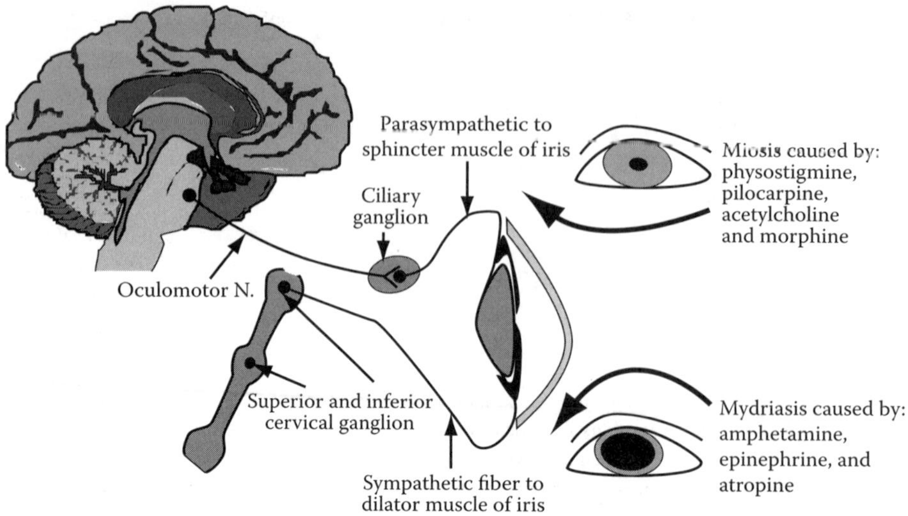

FIGURE 77 Physostigmine causes miosis and spasm of accommodations; it also lowers intraocular pressure and hence can be used in the treatment of wide-angle glaucoma.

Atropine is able to oppose these muscarinic effects. In addition, neostigmine, which has both a direct action as well as an indirect action that is mediated by acetylcholine on end-plate nicotinic receptors, may produce muscular fasciculation, muscular cramps, weakness, and even paralysis. These effects are not countered by atropine. Furthermore, neostigmine enhances gastric contraction and secretion. Neostigmine itself is metabolized by plasma acetylcholinesterase.

The therapeutic uses of neostigmine include the treatment of atony of the urinary bladder and postoperative abdominal distention. In addition, it antagonizes the action of *d*-tubocurarine and curariform drugs. Edrophonium, neostigmine, or pyridostigmine may be used to diagnose myasthenia gravis. Because edrophonium has the shortest duration of action, it is most often used for this purpose.

PHYTONADIONE (METHYLPHYTYL NAPHTHOQUINONE)

(AquaMEPHYTON injection (aqueous colloidal solution) 2 mg/mL, injection (aqueous dispersion) 10 mg/mL, Mephyton tablets 5 mg)

Phytonadione is a blood modifier/vitamin K. It promotes hepatic synthesis of active prothrombin (factor II), proconvertin (factor VII), plasma thromboplastin component (factor IX) and Stuart factor (factor X). It is indicated in the management of coagulation disorders due to faulty formation of factors II, VII, IX, and X due to vitamin K deficiency or interference with vitamin K activity. Oral/parenteral: used for treatment of anticoagulant-induced prothrombin deficiency; treatment of hypoprothrombinemia secondary to salicylates or antibacterial therapy, or secondary to obstructive jaundice and biliary fistulas, provided bile salts are also given. Parenteral: used for treatment of hypoprothrombinemia secondary to conditions limiting absorption or synthesis of vitamin K prophylaxis and therapy of hemorrhagic disease of the newborn.

Vitamin K activity is associated with at least two distinct natural substances, designated as vitamin K_1 and vitamin K_2. Vitamin K_1, or **phylloquinone** (phytonadione) is 2-methyl-3-phytyl-1,4-naphthoquinone; it is found in plants and is the only natural vitamin K available for therapeutic use. Vitamin K is actually a series of compounds (the **menaquinones**) in which the phytyl side chain of phylloquinone has been replaced by a side chain built up of 2 to 13 prenyl units. Considerable synthesis of menaquinones occurs in Gram-positive bacteria; indeed, intestinal flora synthesize the large amounts of vitamin K contained in human and animal feces. In animals menaquinone-4 can be synthesized from the vitamin precursor menadione (2-methyl-1,4-naphthoquinone), or vitamin K_3. Depending on the bioassay system used, menadione is at least as active on a molar basis as phylloquinone.

PILOCARPINE NITRATE

(Pilagan)

Pilocarpine (1 to 2 drops of 2% solution 2 to 4 times daily) is used to control IOP in glaucoma. In addition, it is used in emergency relief of mydriasis in an acutely glaucomatous situation or to reverse mydriasis caused by cycloplegic agents. It may be applied topically in the form of a drug reservoir (Ocusert) (see Figure 78).

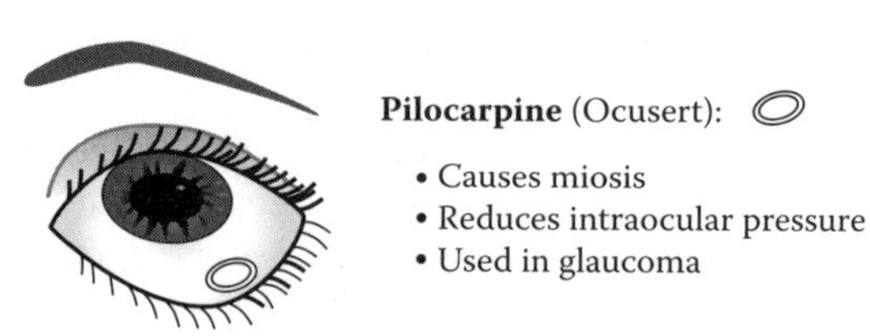

FIGURE 78 Pilocarpine is a naturally occurring cholinomimetic agent possessing both muscarinic and nicotinic properties. It causes miosis, reduces intraocular pressure, and is used in the treatment of wide-angle glaucoma. In addition, it may be applied topically in the eye in the form of a drug reservoir.

Pilocarpine is a naturally occurring (active ingredient of poisonous mushrooms, *Amanita muscaria*) cholinomimetic agent possessing both muscarinic and nicotinic properties (stimulates autonomic ganglia).

PIMECROLIMUS

(Elidel cream 1%)

Pimecrolimus is a topical immunomodulater. It inhibits T-cell activation by blocking the transcription of early cytokines. It is indicated in short-term and intermittent long-term treatment of mild to moderate atopic dermatitis in nonimmunocompromised patients.

Pimecrolimus 1% cream (Elidel), a macrolide derived from ascomycin, is FDA approved for the treatment of atopic dermatitis in patients older than 2 years of age.

Its mechanism of action and side-effect profile are similar to those of tacrolimus. Burning, although occurring in some patients, appears to be less common with pimecrolimus than with tacrolimus. In addition, pimecrolimus has less systemic absorption. Similar precautions with regard to UV exposure should be taken during treatment with pimecrolimus.

PIMOZIDE

(ORAP)

Pimozide (diphenylbutylpiperidine, an antipsychotic, 1 to 2 mg daily in divided doses) is indicated in suppression of severe motor and phonic tics in patients with Gilles de la Tourette's syndrome. Pimozide's mechanism of action in Gilles de la Tourette's syndrome is unknown. It is thought to exert its effects by postsynaptic and/or presynaptic blockade of CNS dopamine receptors, thus inhibiting dopamine-mediated effects. Pimozide also has anticholinergic, antiemetic, and anxiolytic effects, and produces alpha blockade.

Because pimozide has anticholinergic properties, it is contraindicated in patients with arrhythmias because the drug may cause ventricular arrhythmias or aggravate existing arrhythmias; in patients with congenital Q-T syndrome because it may cause conduction defects and sudden death; and in comatose states and CNS depression because of the risk of addictive effects.

Concomitant use of pimozide with quinidine, procainamide, disopyramide, and other antiarrhythmics, phenothiazines (other antipsychotics), and antidepressants may further depress cardiac conduction and prolong the Q-T interval, resulting in serious arrhythmias.

Concomitant use with anticonvulsants (phenytoin, carbamazepine, or phenobarbital) may induce seizures even in patients previously stabilized on anticonvulsants; an anticonvulsant dosage increase may be required.

Concomitant use with amphetamines, methylphenidate, or pemoline may induce Tourette-like tics and may exacerbate existing tics.

Concomitant use with CNS depressants, including alcohol, analgesics, barbiturates, narcotics, anxiolytics, parenteral magnesium sulfate, tranquilizers, and general, spinal, or epidural anesthetics may cause oversedation and respiratory depression because of additive CNS-depressant effects.

Clinical signs of overdose include severe extrapyramidal reactions, hypotension, respiratory depression, coma, and ECG abnormalities, including prolongation of the Q-T interval, inversion or flattening of T waves, and/or new appearance of U waves.

PINACIDIL

(Pindac)

Pinacidil (12.5 to 25.0 mg daily) appears to be a promising alternative agent for the treatment of moderate to severe hypertension.

Pinacidil is three- and tenfold more potent than hydralazine and minoxidil, respectively. It does not interact with alpha, beta, cholinergic, or histaminergic receptors, and also does not produce vasodilation via an indirect effect that is mediated by adenosine, prostaglandin, or endothelial-derived relaxant factor. Its vasodilating activity does not resemble that brought about by the conventional calcium-channel antagonists. Thus, pinacidil-induced vascular relaxation is a direct effect mediated by a novel mechanism.

PINDOLOL

(Visken)

Pindolol, a beta-adrenergic-receptor-blocking agent (15 to 40 mg daily in three divided doses), is indicated in the management of hypertension. The beta-blocking potency of pindolol is 10 to 40 times that of propranolol, and it is about 10 times more potent that propranolol in its efficacy as an antihypertensive agent. However, its membrane-stabilizing activity is lower than that of propranolol. Pindolol is not cardioselective, and induces significantly less impairment of bronchial function than propranolol.

As for nearly all beta antagonists, the main cardiovascular indications for pindolol are hypertension, angina pectoris, and arrhythmias. The usual warnings and precautions for beta antagonists also apply to pindolol (see also Figure 69).

PIOGLITAZONE

(Actos tablets 15 mg)

Pioglitazone is a thiazolidinedione that increases insulin sensitivity in muscle and adipose tissue, and inhibits hepatic gluconeogenesis. It is indicated in type 2 diabetes, as an adjunct to diet and exercise; it also may be used in conjunction with a sulfonylurea, metformin, or insulin when diet, exercise, and a single agent alone does not result in adequate glycemic control in patients with type 2 diabetes mellitus.

Three thiazolidinediones have been used in clinical practice (**troglitazone**, **rosiglitazone**, and **pioglitazone**); however, troglitazone was withdrawn from use because it was associated with severe hepatic toxicity. Rosiglitazone and pioglitazone can lower hemoglobin A_{1c} levels by 1 to 1.5% in patients with type 2 diabetes mellitus. These drugs can be combined with insulin or other classes of oral glucose-lowering agents. The thiazolidinediones tend to increase high-density lipoprotein cholesterol (HDL-C) but have variable effects on triglycerides and low-density lipoprotein cholesterol (LDL-C).

Thiazolidinediones are selective agonists for nuclear peroxisome proliferator-activated receptor-γ (PPARγ). These drugs bind to PPARγ, which activates insulin-responsive genes that regulate carbohydrate and lipid metabolism. Thiazolidinediones require insulin to be present for their action. Thiazolidinediones exert their principal effects by increasing insulin sensitivity in peripheral tissue but also may lower glucose production by the liver. Thiazolidinediones increase glucose transport into muscle and adipose tissue by enhancing the synthesis and translocation of specific forms of the glucose transporters. The thiazolidinediones also can activate genes that regulate fatty-acid metabolism in peripheral tissue. Although muscle is a major insulin-sensitive tissue, PPARγ is virtually absent in skeletal muscle. This has provoked questions as to how thiazolidinediones can reduce peripheral insulin resistance. One suggestion is that activation of PPARγ in adipose tissue reduces the flux of fatty acids into muscle, thereby lowering insulin resistance. Other suggestions include the activation of adipocyte hormones and/or adipokines, the most promising of which is adiponectin. Adiponectin is associated with increased insulin sensitivity and reportedly increases insulin sensitivity by elevating AMP kinase, which stimulates glucose transport into muscle and increases fatty-acid oxidation. Because the actions of both metformin and the thiazolidinediones apparently converge on AMP kinase, it has emerged as an attractive target for drug development.

Rosiglitazone (Avandia) and pioglitazone (Actos) are taken once a day. Both agents are absorbed within about 2 hours, but the maximum clinical effect is not observed for 6 to 12 weeks. The thiazolidinediones are metabolized by the liver and may be administered to patients with renal insufficiency, but should not be used if there is active hepatic disease or significant elevations of serum liver transaminases.

Rosiglitazone is metabolized by hepatic cytochrome P450 (CYP) 2C8, whereas pioglitazone is metabolized by CYP3A4 and CYP2C8. Other drugs that induce or inhibit these enzymes can cause drug interactions

Liver function should be monitored in patients receiving thiazolidinediones, even though **pioglitazone** and rosiglitazone rarely have been associated with hepatotoxicity. This lower hepatotoxicity has been attributed to the lack of the tocopherol side chain that was included in the troglitazone molecule. Additionally, the rare cases of hepatotoxicity occurring with second-generation thiazolidinediones appear to be less severe than those occurring with troglitazone. Hepatotoxicity can occur several months after initiation of the drugs. Any patient who has suffered any hepatotoxicity (even abnormal liver function tests) while on thiazolidinediones should not receive any drugs in this class. Thiazolidinediones also have been reported to cause anemia, weight gain, edema, and plasma volume expansion. Edema is more likely to occur when these agents are combined with insulin.

PIPAZETHATE

(Theratuss)

Noscapine (Nectadon) is a naturally occurring opium alkaloid with a structure and function similar to papaverine's. It is antitussive and has no analgesic or addictive properties.

Diphenhydramine and chlorcyclizine are antihistaminic agents that also have antitussive properties. Dimethoxanate (Cothera) and pipazethate are phenothiazine derivatives without analgesic but with weak antitussive and local anesthetic properties.

PIPECURONIUM BROMIDE

(Arduan)

Pipecuronium, a long-acting nondepolarizing neuromuscular-blocking agent, is indicated to provide skeletal muscle relaxation during surgery. Pipecuronium can also be used to provide skeletal muscle relaxation for endotracheal intubation. It is only recommended for procedures anticipated to last 90 minutes or longer. Pipecuronium, like other long-acting neuromuscular-blocking agents, displays a great deal of variability in the clinical duration of its effect. Pipecuronium competes for cholinergic receptors at the motor end plate, and this action is antagonized by acetylcholinesterase inhibitors such as neostigmine.

Pipecuronium should not be used in patients with myasthenia gravis. Muscle relaxants with short durations of action are more suitable. Aminoglycosides, tetracyclines, bacitracin, polymyxin B, colistin, and sodium colistimethate are apt to prolong the duration of action of pipecuronium. The most frequent side effect of nondepolarizing blocking agents is an extension of the drug's pharmacological action beyond the time period needed for surgery and anesthesia. Clinical signs may vary from skeletal muscle weakness to skeletal muscle paralysis resulting in respiratory insufficiency or apnea (see also Figure 99).

PIPERACILLIN SODIUM

(Pipracil)

Piperacillin (for serious infections 3 to 4 g every 4 to 6 hours as a 20- to 30-minute IV infusion) is indicated for the treatment of:

- Intra-abdominal infections (including hepatobiliary and surgical infections), caused by *E. coli*, *Pseudomonas aeruginosa*, enterococci, *Clostridium* sp., anaerobic cocci, *Bacteroides* sp. including *B. fragilis*
- Urinary tract infections caused by *E. coli, Klebsiella* sp., *P. aeruginosa*, *Proteus* sp., including *P. mirabilis*, and enterococci
- Gynecologic infections (including endometritis, pelvic inflammatory disease, pelvic cellulitis), caused by *Bacteroides* sp., including *B. fragilis*, anaerobic cocci, *Neisseria gonorrhoeae*, enterococci (*Streptococcus faecalis*)
- Septicemia (including bacteremia), caused by *E. coli*, *Klebsiella* sp., *Enterobacter* sp., *Serratia* sp.,

P. mirabilis, *S. pneumoniae*, enterococci, *P. aeruginosa*, *Bacteroides* sp., and anaerobic cocci

Lower respiratory tract infections caused by *E. coli*, *Klebsiella* sp., *Enterobacter* sp., *P. aeruginosa*, *Serratia* sp., *Haemophilus influenzae*, *Bacteroides* sp., and anaerobic cocci

Skin and skin-structure infections caused by *E. coli*, *Klebsiella* sp., *Serratia* sp., *Acinetobacter* sp., *Enterobacter* sp., *P. aeruginosa*; indole-positive *Proteus* sp., *P. mirabilis*, *Bacteroides* sp., including *B. fragilis*, anaerobic cocci, enterococci

Bone and joint infections caused by *P. aeruginosa*, enterococci, *Bacteroides* sp., and anaerobic cocci

Gonococcal infections, treatment of uncomplicated gonococcal urethritis

Streptococcal infections, infections caused by *Streptococcus* species including group A beta-hemolytic Streptococcus and *S. pneumoniae*; however, these infections are ordinarily treated with more narrow-spectrum penicillins.

Carbenicillin cures serious infections caused by *Pseudomonas* species and *Proteus* strains resistant to ampicillin. It is not absorbed from the GI tract, and therefore must be administered intraperitoneally. Carbenicillin indanyl is acid stable and hence can be given orally. Ticarcillin is four times more potent than carbenicillin in treating a *Pseudomonas aeruginosa* infection, and azlocillin is ten times more potent than carbenicillin against *Pseudomonas*. Mezlocillin and piperacillin are more active against *Klebsiella* infection than is carbenicillin.

PIPERACILLIN SODIUM/TAZOBACTAM SODIUM

(Zosyn powder for injection 2 g piperacillin, 0.25 g tazobactam, powder for injection 3 g piperacillin, 0.375 g tazobactam, powder for injection 4g piperacillin, 0.5 g tazobactam, powder for injection 36 g piperacillin, 4.5 g tazobactam (bulk), solution 2 g piperacillin, 0.25 g tazobactam, solution 3 g piperacillin, 0.375 g tazobactam, solution 4 g piperacillin, 0.5 g tazobactam)

Piperacillin sodium is an antibiotic/extended-spectrum penicillin that inhibits bacterial cell wall mucopeptide synthesis. It is indicated in the treatment of moderate to severe infections caused by piperacillin-resistant piperacillin/tazobactam-susceptible, β-lactamase-producing strains of microorganisms in the following conditions: appendicitis (complicated by rupture or abscess); uncomplicated and complicated skin and skin-structure infections; postpartum endometritis or pelvic inflammatory disease; community-acquired pneumonia (moderate severity only); nosocomial pneumonia (moderate to severe).

Piperacillin (Pipracil) extends the spectrum of ampicillin to include most strains of *P. aeruginosa*, *Enterobacteriaceae* (non-β-lactamase-producing), many *Bacteroides* spp., and *E. faecalis*. In combination with a β-lactamase inhibitor (piperacillin-tazobactam, Zosyn) it has the broadest antibacterial spectrum of the penicillins. Pharmacokinetic properties are reminiscent of the other ureidopenicillins. High biliary concentrations are achieved.

Piperacillin and related agents are important agents in the treatment of patients with serious infections caused by Gram-negative bacteria. Such patients frequently have impaired immunological defenses, and their infections often are acquired in the hospital. Therefore, these penicillins find their greatest use in treatment by mouth, and they can also be given parenterally. Piperacillin has been combined with amoxicillin as an oral preparation (Augmentin) and with ticarcillin as a parenteral preparation (Timentin).

Tazobactam is a penicillanic acid sulfone β-lactamase inhibitor. In common with the other available inhibitors, it has poor activity against the inducible chromosomal β-lactamases of *Enterobacteriaceae*, but has good activity against many of the plasmid β-lactamases, including some of the extended-spectrum class. It has been combined with piperacillin as a parenteral preparation (Zosyn).

The combination of piperacillin and tazobactam does not increase the activity of piperacillin against *P. aeruginosa* because there is resistance due to either chromosomal β-lactamases or decreased permeability of piperacillin into the periplasmic space. Because the currently recommended dose (3 g piperacillin per 375 mg tazobactam every 4 to 8 hours) is less than the recommended dose of piperacillin when used alone for serious infections (3 to 4 g every 4 to 6 hours), concern has been raised that **piperacillin-tazobactam** may prove ineffective in the treatment of some *P. aeruginosa* infections that would have responded to piperacillin. The combination of piperacillin plus tazobactam should be equivalent in antimicrobial spectrum to ticarcillin plus clavulanate.

PIPERAZINE CITRATE

(Antepar)

Piperazine (single dose of 3.5 g for two consecutive days) is indicated in the treatment of enterobiasis (pinworm infection) and ascariasis (roundworm infection).

Piperazine blocks the response of *Ascaris* muscle to acetylcholine, causing flaccid paralysis of the worm. The paralyzed *Ascaris* are dislodged and expelled via peristalsis. Piperazine affects all stages of the parasite in the gut but has little effect on larvae in the tissues. Toxic doses of piperazine cause convulsion, and hence the drug should be used cautiously in patients with epilepsy.

PIPOBROMAN

(Vercyte)

Pipobroman, an alkylating agent with antineoplastic properties, is indicated in the treatment of polycythemia vera and chronic myelocytic leukemia (see also Figure 15).

PIRBUTEROL ACETATE

(Maxair)

Pirbuterol, a beta-adrenergic agonist with bronchodilating properties (1 to 2 inhalations every 4 to 6 hours), is indicated in the prevention and reversal of bronchospasm and asthma (see also Figure 94).

PIRENZEPINE

Vagal impulses elicit the release of acetylcholine in the parietal cells and in the gastric mucosal cells containing gastrin, a peptide hormone. Both the directly released acetylcholine and the indirectly released gastrin then stimulate the parietal cells to secrete hydrogen ions into the gastric lumen.

The most useful anticholinergic drugs are propantheline (Pro-Banthine), pirenzepine, and telenzepine, which antagonize muscarinic cholinergic receptors (M_1 receptors). All three agents depress gastric motility and secretion. The production of pepsin is also reduced. Propantheline may be used as adjunctive therapy with antacids but not as a sole agent. The side effects and contraindications of propantheline use are identical to those of atropine (prostatic hypertrophy, urinary retention, glaucoma, and cardiac arrhythmias).

The timing of medication is critical in ulcer therapy. Anticholinergic drugs should be given about 30 minutes before meals, and antacids about 1 hour after meals. A double dose of an antacid is often taken just before bedtime.

PIROXICAM

(Feldene)

Piroxicam (25 mg p.o. daily) is indicated in the treatment of osteoarthritis and rheumatoid arthritis. Piroxicam, a nonsteroidal antiinflammatory agent (NSAID), has analgesic and antiinflammatory properties. It has a long half-life of 50 hours. Piroxicam should be used cautiously in patients with a history of peptic ulcer disease, angioedema, or cardiac disease because the drug may worsen these conditions, and in patients with decreased renal function because it may cause a further reduction in renal function (see also Table 3).

Patients with known "triad" symptoms (aspirin hypersensitivity, rhinitis/nasal polyps, and asthma) are at high risk for bronchospasm. NSAIDs may mask the signs and symptoms of acute infection, fever, myalgia, and erythema.

Concomitant use of piroxicam with anticoagulants and thrombolytic drugs (coumarin derivatives, heparin, streptokinase, or urokinase) may potentiate anticoagulant effects. Bleeding problems may occur if used with other drugs that inhibit platelet aggregation, such as azlocillin, parenteral carbenicillin, dextran, dipyridamole, mezlocillin, piperacillin, sulfinpyrazone, ticarcillin, valproic acid, cefamandole, cefoperazone, moxalactam, plicamycin, aspirin, or other antiinflammatory agents. Concomitant use with salicylates, antiinflammatory agents, alcohol, corticotropin, or steroids may cause increased GI adverse effects, including ulceration and hemorrhage. Aspirin may decrease the bioavailability of piroxicam. Because of the influence of prostaglandins on glucose metabolism, concomitant use with insulin or oral hypoglycemic agents may potentiate hypoglycemic effects.

Piroxicam may displace highly protein-bound drugs from binding sites. Toxicity may occur with coumarin derivatives, phenytoin, verapamil, or nifedipine. Increased nephrotoxicity may occur with gold compounds, other antiinflammatory agents, or acetaminophen. It may decrease the renal clearance of methotrexate and lithium. Piroxicam may decrease the effectiveness of antihypertensive agents and diuretics. Concomitant use with diuretics may increase risk of nephrotoxicity.

PLAGUE VACCINE

This bacterial vaccine is used primarily for immunization and as a booster.

PLASMA PROTEIN FRACTION

(Plasmanate, Plasma-Plex, Plasmatein, Protenate)

Plasma protein fraction, a plasma volume expander, is indicated in hypoproteinemia and shock.

PLATELET-ACTIVATING FACTOR

A platelet-activating factor, 1-0-alkyl-2(R)acetyl-sn-glyceryl-3-phosphocholine, is released in the presence of shock and ischemia. The platelet-activating factor antagonist can protect the heart and brain against ischemic injury.

Advances in medical practice, including the aggressive use of catheters and other invasive equipment, the implantation of prosthetic devices, the administration of chemotherapy to cancer patients, and the administration of immunosuppressive agents and corticosteroids to patients with organ transplants, have increased the risk of sepsis, septic syndrome, and septic shock.

The initiating event in the sepsis cascade is the release of endotoxin, which prompts the release of tumor necrosis factor alpha, interleukin-1, interleukin-6, interleukin-8, and platelet-activating factor from mononuclear phagocytes and endothelial cells.

Neonates with sepsis are treated with ampicillin, which is effective against group B streptococci, *Listeria monocytogenes*, enterococci, and some Gram-negative rods, and by gentamicin, which provides broader coverage against the Enterobacteriaceae.

PLICAMYCIN

(Formerly Mithramycin—Mithracin)

Plicamycin, an antineoplastic agent with hypocalcemic effect, is used in hypercalcemia and testicular cancer.

PNEUMOCOCCAL 7-VALENT CONJUGATE VACCINE

(Prevnar injection 2 mcg each of 6 polysaccharide isolates, 4 mcg of 1 polysaccharide isolate per 0.5 mL dose)

This is a bacterial vaccine that induces antibodies against (4, 6B, 9V, 14, 18C, 19F, and 23F) serotypes of *Streptococcus pneumoniae*, which are directly conjugated to the protein carrier CRM_{197} to form glycoconjugate. It is indicated in active immunization of infants and toddlers against *Streptococcus pneumoniae*; and in active immunization of infants and toddlers against otitis media caused by serotypes included in the vaccine.

PNEUMOCOCCAL VACCINE, POLYVALENT

(Pneumovax 23, Pnu-Imune 23)
(Pneumovax 23 injection 25 mcg each of 23 polysaccharide isolates/0.5 mL dose, Pnu-Imune 23 injection 25 mcg each of 23 polysaccharide isolates/0.5 mL dose)

Pneumococcal vaccine is a bacterial vaccine that induces antibodies against 23 capsular types of *Streptococcus pneumoniae*. The type-specific antibody facilitates bacterial destruction by complement-mediated lysis. It is indicated in protection against pneumococcal pneumonia, pneumococcal bacteremia, and other pneumococcal infections. This bacterial vaccine is used for pneumococcal immunization.

PODOFILOX

(Condylox)

Podofilox, a keratolytic agent with antimimetic properties (0.5% in 95% alcohol to be applied q. 12 hours for three days), is used in the treatment of external genital warts.

POLIOVIRUS VACCINE, INACTIVATED (IPV)

(IPOL injection suspension of 3 types of poliovirus (types 1, 2, and 3) grown in monkey kidney cell cultures)

Poliovirus vaccine, inactivated, is a viral vaccine that induces protective antipoliovirus antibodies, reducing pharyngeal excretion of poliovirus types 1, 2, and 3.

Its routine use in infants and children is not recommended; oral poliovirus vaccine (OPV) is generally preferred. It is given as prophylaxis to individuals traveling to regions where poliomyelitis is endemic or epidemic (e.g., developing countries), who routinely are exposed to patients who may be excreting polioviruses or to laboratory specimens that may contain polioviruses, and to members of communities with disease caused by wild polioviruses. Offer IPV to individuals who decline OPV or in whom OPV is contraindicated. In households with an immunocompromised member or close contacts, or in households with an unimmunized adult, use only IPV for all those requiring poliovirus immunization. Previous clinical poliomyelitis (usually because of single poliovirus type) or incomplete immunization with OPV are not contraindications to completing primary series of immunization with IPV.

POLIOVIRUS VACCINE, LIVE, ORAL, TRIVALENT (OPV)

(TOPV, Sabin, Orimune Trivalent, Orimune suspension, oral mixture or 3 viruses (types 1, 2, and 3) propagated in monkey kidney tissue culture)

Poliovirus vaccine, live, oral, trivalent, is a live virus vaccine that induces protective antibodies, reducing intestinal and pharyngeal excretion of poliovirus. OPV administration simulates natural infection, inducing active mucosal and systemic immunity against poliovirus types 1, 2, and 3.

It is indicated in the prevention of poliomyelitis. Infants as young as 6 to 12 weeks and all unimmunized children and adolescents up to 18 years are usual candidates for routine OPV prophylaxis. OPV is also recommended for control of epidemic poliomyelitis. If less than 4 weeks remain before protection is needed, a single dose of OPV is recommended, with remaining vaccine doses given later if the person remains at increased risk. Immunization with IPV may be indicated for unimmunized parents and those in other special situations in which protection may be needed. In households with immunocompromised members or other close contacts, or in a household with an unimmunized adult, use only IPV for all those requiring poliovirus immunization. Adults: Primary immunization with inactivated polio vaccine is recommended, whenever feasible, for unimmunized adults subject to increased risk of exposure, such as by travel to or contact with epidemic or endemic areas (e.g., developing countries), and for those employed in medical and sanitation facilities. This viral vaccine is used for the primary series of poliovirus immunizations.

POLY-L-LACTIC ACID

(Sculptra powder for injection, freeze dried)

Poly-L-Lactic acid is a physical adjunct that is an injectable implant of microparticles of poly-L-lactic acid. It is indicated in restoration and/or correction of signs of facial fat loss (lipoatrophy) in people with HIV.

POLYETHYLENE GLYCOL (PEG)

(MiraLax powder for oral solution 255 g PEG 3350, powder for oral solution 527 g PEG 3350)

Polyethylene glycol is a bowel evacuant that acts as an osmotic agent by causing water to be retained with the stool. It is used in the treatment of occasional constipation; use should be limited to 14 days or less.

POLYETHYLENE GLYCOL-ELECTROLYTE SOLUTION (PEG-ES)

(CoLyte powder for oral solution 1 gal: 227.1 g PEG 3350, 21.5 g sodium sulfate, 6.36 g sodium bicarb, 5.53 g NaCl, 2,82 g KCl, powder for oral solution 4L: 240 g PEG 3350, 22.72 g sodium sulfate, 6.72 g sodium bicarb, 5.84 g NaCl, 2.98 g KCl • GoLYTELY powder for oral suspension 236 g PEG 3350, 22.74 g sodium sulfate, 6.74 g sodium bicarb, 5.86 g NaCl, 2.97 g KCl, powder for oral suspension 227.1 g PEG 3350, 21.5 sodium sulfate, 6.36 g sodium bicarb, 5.53 g NaCl, 2.82 g KCl • NuLYTELY powder for reconstitution 420 g PEG 3350, 5.72 g sodium bicarb, 11.2 g NaCl, 1.48 g KCl • OCL oral solution 146 mg NaCl, 168 mg sodium bicarb, 1.29 g sodium sulfate decahydrate, 75 mg KCl, 6 g PEG 3350, 30 mg polysorbate 80/100 mL)

Polyethylene glycol–electrolyte solution is a bowel evacuant that induces diarrhea and rapidly cleanses the bowel, usually within 4 hours. It is used for bowel cleaning prior to GI examination.

Polyethylene glycol–electrolyte solutions: Long-chain polyethylene glycols (PEGs; molecular weight –3350 daltons) are poorly absorbed, and **PEG** solutions are retained in the lumen by virtue of their high osmotic nature. When used in high volume, aqueous solutions of **PEGs** (Colyte, Golytely, others) produce an effective catharsis and are used widely for colonic cleansing for radiological, surgical, and endoscopic procedures (4 L of this solution taken over 3 hours, beginning at least 4 hours before the procedure). To avoid net transfer of ions across the intestinal wall, these preparations contain an isotonic mixture of sodium sulfate, sodium bicarbonate, sodium chloride, and potassium chloride. The osmotic activity of the **PEG** molecules retains the added water, and the electrolyte concentration assures little or no net ionic shifts.

PEGs are also increasingly being used in smaller doses (250 to 500 mL daily) for the treatment of constipation in difficult cases. A powder form of polyethylene glycol 3350 (Miralax) is now available for the short-term treatment (2 weeks or less) of occasional constipation, although the agent has been prescribed safely for longer periods in clinical practice. The usual dose is 17 g of powder per day in 8 ounces of water. This preparation does not contain electrolytes, so larger volumes may represent a risk for ionic shifts. As with other laxatives, prolonged, frequent, or excessive use may result in dependence or electrolyte imbalance.

POLYMYXIN B SULFATE

(Aerosporin)

Polymyxin B, a polypeptide antibiotic (500,000 units in 300 to 500 mL of 5% dextrose in water for continuous IV drip), is used in acute infections caused by susceptible strains of *Pseudomonas aeruginosa*. It may be used topically and subconjunctivally in the treatment of infections of the eye caused by susceptible strains of *P. aeruginosa*.

Polymyxin B may be indicated (when less toxic drugs are ineffective or contraindicated) in serious infections caused by susceptible strains of the following organisms: *Haemophilus influenzae* (meningeal infections); *Escherichia coli* (urinary tract infections); *Enterobacter aerogenes* (bacteremia); *Klebsiella pneumoniae* (bacteremia). In meningeal infections, polymyxin B sulfate must be administered only intrathecally.

The polymyxins consist of polymyxin B (Aerosporin) and polymyxin E, or colisten (Coly-Mycin). These agents, which are bactericidal, are effective in the management of Gram-negative bacterial infections, especially *Pseudomonas*. Polymyxins are cationic detergent peptides, possessing both lipophilic and lipophobic groups that are able to bind and subsequently damage the bacterial cell membranes. They are not absorbed orally and must be administered parenterally for the treatment of systemic infections. Reversible nephrotoxicity (proteinuria, hematuria, and cyclindruria) can occur with their use, as well as neurotoxicity, which is characterized by giddiness, numbness, paresthesia, neuromuscular blockade, confusion, ataxia, and convulsions.

POLYTHIAZIDE

(Renese)

Polythiazide, a thiazide diuretic (2 to 4 mg p.o. daily), is used in the treatment of hypertension.

PORACTANT ALFA

(Curosurf suspension, intratracheal 80 mg phospholipids/mL)

Poractant alfa is a lung surfactant. It is an extract of natural procine lung surfactant that restores lung surfactant in premature infants with lung surfactant deficiency, which causes **respiratory distress syndrome** (RDS). It is indicated in the treatment of RDS in premature infants.

PORFIMER SODIUM

(Photofrin cake or powder for injection (freeze-dried 75 mg))

Porfimer sodium is an antineoplastic agent. Porfimer is a photosensitizing agent used in the photodynamic therapy (PDT) of tumors. Cellular damage caused by porfimer PDT is a consequence of the propagation of radical reactions. Tumor death also occurs through ischemic necrosis secondary to vascular occlusion that appears to be partly mediated by thromboxane A_2 release. The laser treatment induces a photochemical, not a thermal, effect. It is indicated in esophageal cancer; endobronchial non-small-cell lung cancer; and Barrett esophagus.

POTASSIUM CHANNELS

Calcium-activated potassium channels increase their permeability to potassium ions in response to increases in the intracellular calcium concentration. These potassium channels couple the membrane potential to the intracellular calcium concentration of calcium, in that a rise in the intracellular calcium levels leads to an efflux of potassium ions and hence hyperpolarization of the membrane.

POTASSIUM CITRATE/SODIUM CITRATE/ CITRIC ACID

(Polycitra syrup 550 mg potassium citrate, 500 mg sodium citrate, 334 mg citric acid/5 mL (1 mEq K, 1 mEq Na/mL; equiv. to 2 mEq bicarbonate), Polycitra-LC solution 550 mg potassium citrate, 500 mg sodium citrate, 334 mg citric acid/5 mL (1 mEq K, 1 mEq Na/mL; equiv. to 2 mEq bicarbonate))

Potassium citrate is a systemic alkalinizer/urinary alkalinizer. Potassium citrate and sodium citrate are metabolized to potassium bicarbonate and sodium bicarbonate, thus acting as systemic alkalizers. It is indicated in the treatment of chronic metabolic acidosis, particularly when caused by renal tubular acidosis; conditions when long-term maintenance of an alkaline urine is desirable, in treatment of patients with uric acid and cystine calculi of the urinary tract, and in conjunction with uricosurics in gout therapy to prevent uric acid nephropathy.

POTASSIUM ACETATE

POTASSIUM BICARBONATE

(Klor-Con, EF, K-Lyte, Quic-K)

POTASSIUM CHLORIDE

(Cena-K, Kalium, Kaochlor, Kaochlor S-F, Kaon-CL, Kato, Kay Ciel, K-Dur, K-Lor, Klor-10%, Klor-Con, Klor-Con/25, Klorvess, Klotrix, K-Lyte/Cl powder, K-Tab, Micro-K, Potachlor, Potage, Potasalan, Potassine, Rum-K, Slow-K, Ten-K)

POTASSIUM GLUCONATE

Potassium salts are used in hypokalemic states.

POTASSIUM IODIDE

(K1, SSK1) (Losat, Pima, Thyro-Block)

Potassium iodide is used as an expectorant, in preoperative thyroidectomy, nuclear radiation protection, and in the management of thyrotoxic crisis.

POTASSIUM SALTS, ORAL

POTASSIUM-SPARING DIURETICS

The potassium-sparing diuretics consist of spironolactone (Aldactone), which is an aldosterone antagonist, and triamterene (Dyrenium) and amiloride (Midamor), which exert their effects through a mechanism other than a mineralocorticoid action.

All act in the distal tubule, where the resorption of sodium is accompanied by the transfer of potassium into the lumen contents. When sodium resorption is hindered, potassium excretion is correspondingly reduced, such that more potassium is retained. The potassium-sparing diuretics are not very efficacious, as they affect only 1 to 2% of the filtered load of sodium. All are given orally and eliminated in the urine, mostly by glomerular filtration, though some active tubular secretion may also occur (see Figure 17).

A potassium-sparing diuretic can be given along with a thiazide or a loop diuretic to prevent hypokalemia. Spironolactone can also be beneficial in some patients with severe CHF or cirrhosis associated with ascites.

The potassium-sparing diuretics should not be used concurrently with potassium supplements, as this combination is likely to produce hyperkalemia. Poor renal function also heightens the risk of hyperkalemia. GI disturbances, rash, drowsiness, or dizziness are all associated with their use. Spironolactone can cause the blood urea nitrogen level to increase and lead to menstrual irregularities (see also Table 25).

PRALIDOXIME CHLORIDE

(2-Pam chloride, Pyridine-2-aldoxime methochloride, Protopam)

Pralidoxime, a quaternary ammonium oxime, is used to antidote poisoning from organophosphate pesticides (see also Figure 79).

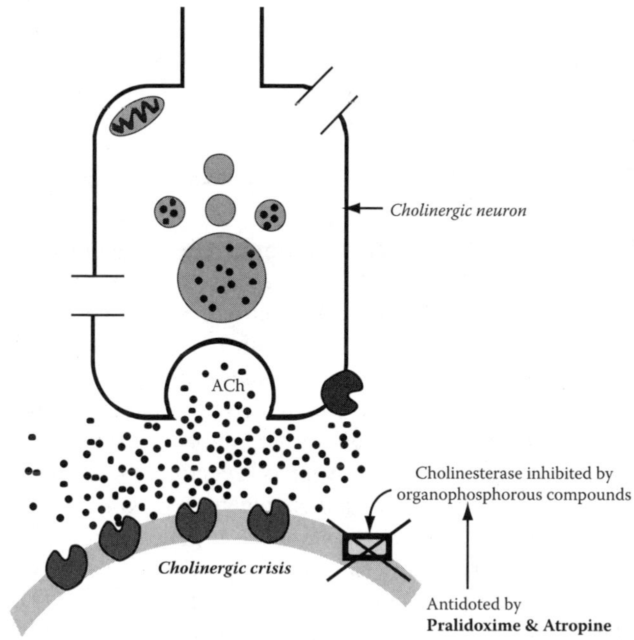

FIGURE 79 The clinical manifestations of acute and severe poisoning from the organophosphorous insecticides include cholinergic crisis, resulting from the stimulation of muscarinic cholinergic receptors (**bronchoconstriction**, **salivation**, **sweating**, **lacrimation**, **bradycardia**, **hypotension**, and **urinary and fecal incontinence**), from the stimulation of nicotinic cholinergic receptors (muscular fasciculation), and from central nervous system (CNS) effects (with initial restlessness, tremors, ataxia, and convulsions, followed by CNS depression and respiratory and circulatory depression). The treatment of a cholinergic crisis caused by organophosphorous compounds includes the administration of a cholinesterase reactivator such as **pralidoxime (2-PAM)**, **together with atropine**.

PRAMIPEXOLE

Pramipexole, a dopamine receptor agonist with activity at both autoreceptors and postsynaptic receptors, has shown efficacy in animal models of parkinsonism.

PRAMIPEXOLE DIHYDROCHLORIDE

(Mirapex tablets 0.125 mg, tablets 0.25 mg, tablets 1 mg, tablets 1.5 mg)

Pramipexole dihyrochloride is a non-ergot dopamine receptor agonist that stimulates dopamine receptors in the corpus striatum, relieving parkinsonian symptoms. It is used in the treatment of the signs and symptoms of idiopathic Parkinson's disease (PD). It may be used in conjunction with L-dopa.

An alternative to levodopa is the use of drugs that are direct agonists of striatal dopamine receptors, an approach that offers several potential advantages. Because enzymatic conversion of these drugs is not required for activity, they do not depend on the functional capacities of the nigrostriatal neurons. Most dopamine-receptor agonists in clinical use have durations of action substantially longer than that of levodopa and are often useful in the management of dose-related fluctuations in the motor state. Finally, if the hypothesis that free radical formation as a result of dopamine metabolism contributes to neuronal death is correct, then dopamine-receptor agonists may have the potential to modify the course of the disease by reducing endogenous release of dopamine as well as the need for exogenous levodopa.

Four orally administered dopamine-receptor agonists are available for treatment of PD: two older agents, **bromocriptine** (Parlodel) and **pergolide** (Permax); and two newer, more selective compounds, **ropinirole** (Requip) and **pramipexole** (Mirpex). Bromocriptine and pergolide both are ergot derivatives and share a similar spectrum of therapeutic actions and adverse effects. Bromocriptine is a strong agonist of the D_2 class of dopamine receptors and a partial antagonist of the D_1 receptors, whereas pergolide is an agonist of both classes. Ropinirole and **pramipexole** have selective activity at D_2 class sites (specifically at the D_2- and D_3-receptor proteins), and little or no activity at D_1-class sites. All four drugs are well absorbed orally and have similar therapeutic actions. Like levodopa, they can relieve the clinical symptoms of PD. The duration of action of the dopamine agonists (8 to 24 hours) is often longer than that of levodopa (6 to 8 hours), and they are particularly effective in the treatment of patients who have developed on–off phenomena. All four also may produce hallucinosis or confusion, similar to that observed with levodopa, and may worsen orthostatic hypotension.

PRAMLINTIDE ACETATE

(Symlin solution for injection 0.6 mg/mL)

Pramlintide acetate is an amylin analog. It is a synthetic analog of the naturally occurring neuroendocrine hormone amylin. Amylin is colocated with insulin in pancreatic beta cells and is cosecreted with insulin in response to food intake. Amylin slows gastric emptying, suppresses glucagon secretion, and regulates food intake by centrally mediated modulation of appetite. It is indicated as an adjunct treatment for type 1 diabetes in patients who use mealtime insulin therapy and who have failed to achieve desired glucose control despite optimal insulin therapy; as an adjunct treatment for type 2 diabetes in patients who use mealtime insulin therapy and who have failed to achieve desired glucose control despite optimal insulin therapy, with or without concurrent sulfonylurea and/or metformin therapy.

PRAVASTATIN

The hypolipidemic agent pravastatin differs from other HMG-CoA reductase inhibitors (e.g., lovastatin and simvastatin) because it has greater hydrophilicity as a result of the hydroxyl group attached to its decalin ring. The hydrophilic nature of pravastatin accounts for its minimal penetration into the intracellular space of nonhepatic tissues, including an apparent inability to cross the blood–brain barrier. The drug is also well tolerated because it is rapidly absorbed and excreted, and does not accumulate in plasma even with repeated administration.

PRAVASTATIN SODIUM

(Pravachol tablets 10 mg, tablets 20 mg, tablets 40 mg, tablets 80 mg)

Pravastatin sodium is a 3-hydroxy-3-methylglutaryl coenzyme A (HMG-CoA) reductase inhibitor that increases the rate at which the body removes cholesterol from blood and reduces production of cholesterol in the body by inhibiting enzyme that catalyzes an early rate-limiting step in cholesterol synthesis. It's used as an adjunct to diet for reduction of elevated total and LDL-C, apolipoprotein B, and triglyceride levels, and to increase HDL-C in patients with primary hypercholesterolemia and mixed dyslipidemia (Frederickson types IIa and IIb); as adjunctive therapy to diet for treatment of patients with elevated serum triglyceride levels (Frederickson type IV); treatment of primary dysbetalipoproteinemia (Frederickson type III) who do not respond adequately to diet; in hypercholesterolemic patients without clinically evident coronary heart disease (CHD) to reduce risk of MI or cardiovascular (CV) mortality with no increase in death from noncardiovascular causes; and in patients with clinically evident CHD, to reduce risk of total mortality by reducing coronary death, MI, undergoing myocardial revascularization procedures, stroke, and stroke/transient ischemic attack and slow progression of coronary arteriosclerosis.

The statins are the most effective and best-tolerated agents for treating dyslipidemia. These drugs are competitive inhibitors of HMG-CoA reductase, which catalyzes an early, rate-limiting step in cholesterol biosynthesis. Higher doses of the more potent statins (e.g., **atorvastatin** and **simvastatin**) also can reduce triglyceride levels caused by elevated very-low-density lipoprotein (VLDL) levels. Some statins also are indicated for raising HDL-C levels, although the clinical significance of these effects on HDL-C remains to be proven.

Multiple well-controlled clinical trials have documented the efficacy and safety of simvastatin, **pravastatin**, **lovastatin**, and **atorvastatin** in reducing fatal and nonfatal CHD events, strokes, and total mortality. Rates of adverse events in statin trials were the same in the placebo groups and in the groups receiving the drug. This was true with regard to noncardiac illness and the two laboratory tests, hepatic transaminases and creatine kinase (CK), that are commonly monitored in patients taking statins.

Statins exert their major effect—reduction of LDL levels—through a mevalonic acid-like moiety that competitively inhibits HMG-CoA reductase. By reducing the conversion of HMG-CoA to mevalonate, statins inhibit an early and rate-limiting step in cholesterol biosynthesis.

Pravastatin, an inhibitor of HMG-CoA reductase (5 to 10 mg daily), is used in reduction of LDL and total cholesterol levels in patients with primary hypercholesterolemia (types IIa and IIb).

PRAZEPAM

(Centrax)

Prazepam, a benzodiazepine derivative (30 mg p.o. daily in divided doses), is indicated in the management of anxiety disorders and for the short-term relief of the symptoms of anxiety. It depresses the CNS at the limbic and subcortical levels of the brain. It produces an antianxiety effect by enhancing the effect of the neurotransmitter GABA on its receptor in the ascending reticular activating system, which increases inhibition and blocks both cortical and limbic arousal.

Prazepam is metabolized to desmethyldiazepam and oxazepam, which is a pharmacologically short-acting anxiety agent. The half-life of demethyldiazepam ranges from 30 to 200 hours, and that of oxazepam ranges from 5 to 15 hours.

Prazepam potentiates the CNS depressant effects of phenothiazines, narcotics, antihistamines, monoamine oxidase inhibitors, barbiturates, alcohol, general anesthetics, and antidepressants.

Concomitant use with cimetidine and possibly disulfiram causes diminished hepatic metabolism of prazepam, which increases its plasma concentration.

Heavy smoking accelerates prazepam's metabolism, thus lowering its clinical effectiveness.

Antacids may delay the absorption of prazepam. Prazepam may antagonize levodopa's therapeutic effects. Clinical manifestations of overdose include somnolence, convulsion, coma, hypoactive reflexes, dyspnea, labored breathing, hypotension, bradycardia, slurred speech, and unsteady gait or impaired coordination (see also Table 4).

PRAZIQUANTEL

(Biltricide)

Praziquantel (three doses of 20 mg/kg as 1-day treatment only) is indicated in the treatment of infections due to *Schistosoma mekongi*, *S. japonicum*, *S. mansoni*, and *S. hematobium*; and for infections due to liver flukes, *Clonorchis sinensis*/*Opisthorchis viverrini*.

Praziquantel increases membrane permeability in susceptible worms, resulting in a loss of intracellular calcium, and massive contractions and paralysis of their musculature. The drug further results in vacuolization and disintegration of the schistosome tegument. This effect is followed by attachment of phagocytes to the parasite and death.

PRAZOSIN

(Minipress)

Prazosin, (1 mg t.i.d.) alone or in combination with other drugs such as a diuretic, is indicated in the management of moderate hypertension. It is a direct vasodilator and is used for long-term therapy. Its side effects are sedation, postural hypotension, and headache (due to vasodilation). As much as 97% of prazosin is bound to plasma protein. When used for the first time or in larger-than-recommended doses, prazosin may cause pronounced hypotension, faintness, dizziness, and palpitations. These effects, which have been labeled first-dose phenomena, are seen especially in salt- and water-depleted patients. Therefore, the initial dose of prazosin is small, and it is given at bedtime.

PREDNISOLONE

Prednisone, a glucocorticoid, is inactive and must be metabolized to prednisolone, which is available in the following preparations.

Nonproprietary and Proprietary Names	Oral Forms	Injectable Forms
Methylprednisolone (Medrol)	2–32 mg	—
Methylprednisolone acetate (Depo-Medrol, Medrol Acetate)	—	20–80 mg/mL (suspension)
Prednisolone (Delta-Cortef)	5 mg	—
Prednisolone acetate (Econopred)	3 mg/mL (syrup)	—
Prednisolone sodium phosphate (Hydeltra-T.B.A.)	1 mg/mL (liquid)	20 mg/mL (suspension)
Prednisone (Deltasone)	1–50 mg	—
	1 mg/mL (syrup)	—
	1,5 mg/mL (solution)	
	1–8 mg	

The administration of glucocorticoids to human subjects brings about lymphocytopenia, monocytopenia, and eosinopenia. In addition, glucocorticoids block a number of lymphocytic functions.

Although considered to be immunosuppressive, therapeutic doses of glucocorticoids do not significantly decrease the concentration of antibodies in the circulation. Furthermore, during glucocorticoid therapy, patients exhibit a nearly normal antibody response to antigenic challenge. Glucocorticoids are extensively used in medicine, and some of them are outlined in Table 11. For example, in bronchial asthma, prednisone is available in oral form, and beclomethasone may be used as an aerosol, especially in children. The corticosteroids may exert their effects through multiple mechanisms, including relaxing bronchospasm, decreasing mucus secretion, potentiating beta-adrenergic receptors, antagonizing cholinergic actions, stabilizing lysosomes possessing antiinflammatory properties, inhibiting antibody formation, and antagonizing histamine actions.

Corticosteroids do not inhibit the release of mediators from mast cells or block the early response to allergens, but they do block the late response and the subsequent bronchial hyperresponsiveness (see also Figure 28).

Steroids such as beclomethasone dipropionate, budesonide, triamcinolone acetonide, and flunisolide are active when given topically, and can control asthma without causing systemic effects or adrenal suppression. However, orally administered steroids such as prednisone, prednisolone, or methylprednisolone are still needed by some patients.

The side effects of high-dose inhalational steroids include oropharyngeal candidiasis and dysphonia. The orally administered steroids may produce osteoporosis, weight gain, hypertension, diabetes, myopathy, psychiatric disturbances, skin fragility, or cataracts.

PREDNISOLONE (SYSTEMIC)
(Cortalone, Delta-Cortef, Prelone)

PREDNISOLONE ACETATE
(Articulose, Key-Pred, Predaject, Predate, Predcor)

PREDNISOLONE ACETATE AND PREDNISOLONE SODIUM PHOSPHATE

PREDNISOLONE SODIUM PHOSPHATE
(Hydeltrasol, Key-Pred SP, PediaPred, Predate-S)

PREDNISOLONE TERBUTATE
(Hydeltra-T.B.A., Metalone T.B.A., Norpred T.B.A., Predate T.B.A., Predcor T.B.A., Predisol T.B.A.)

Prednisolone, a glucocorticoid–mineralocorticoid with antiinflammatory and immunosuppresant properties, is used for severe inflammation or immunosuppression (see also Tables 11 and 14).

PREDNISOLONE ACETATE (OPHTHALMIC)
(Ak-Tate, Econopred Ophthalmic, I-Prednicet, Ocu-Pred-A, Predair-A, Pred Forte, Pred mild ophthalmic)

PREDNISOLONE SODIUM PHOSPHATE
(Ak Pred, Inflamase, Inflamase mild ophthalmic, Inflamase Forte, I-Pred, Metreton, Ocu-Pred, Predair)

Prednisolone, a corticosteroid with ophthalmic antiinflammatory properties, is used in inflammation of the palpebral and bulbar conjunctiva, cornea, and the anterior segment of the globe.

PREDNISOLONE ACETATE/GENTAMICIN SULFATE
(Pred-G ophthalmic suspension 1% prednisolone acetate and gentamicin sulfate equiv. to 0.3% gentamicin base, Pred-G S.O.P. ophthalmic ointment 0.6% prednisolone acetate and gentamicin sulfate equiv to 0.3 gentamicin base)

Prednisolone acetate/gentamicin sulfate is a corticosteroid/antibiotic. **Prednisolone** depresses the formation, release, and activity of endogenous mediators of inflammation as well as modifying the body's immune response. **Gentamicin** inhibits production of bacterial protein, causing bacterial cell death. They are indicated in the treatment of steroid-responsive inflammatory ocular conditions for which a corticosteroid is indicated and when superficial bacterial ocular infection or a risk of bacterial ocular infection exists; inflammatory conditions of the palpebral and bulbar conjunctiva, cornea, and anterior segment of the globe where the inherent risk of steroid use in certain infective conjunctivitides is accepted to obtain a diminution in edema and inflammation; chronic anterior uveitis; corneal injury from chemical, radiation, or thermal burns or penetration of foreign bodies; high risk of superficial ocular infection; and the expectation that a potentially dangerous number of bacteria will be present.

PREDNISOLONE ACETATE/NEOMYCIN SULFATE/POLYMYXIN B SULFATE)
(Poly-Pred Liquifilm ophthalmic suspension 0.5% prednisolone acetate/neomycin sulfate equiv. to 0.35% neomycin base/10,000 units/mL polymyxin B sulfate)

Prednisolone acetate/neomycin sulfate/polymyxin B sulfate is a corticosteroid/antibacterial agent. **Prednisolone** depresses the formation, release, and activity of endogenous mediators of inflammation including prostaglandins, kinins, histamine, liposomal enzymes, and the complement system. **Neomycin** inhibits protein synthesis by binding to ribosomal RNA, causing bacterial genetic code misreading. **Polymyxin B** interacts with phospholipid components of bacterial cell membrane, increasing cell-wall permeability. They are indicated in the treatment of steroid- responsive inflammatory ocular conditions for which a corticosteroid is indicated and where bacterial infection or a risk of bacterial ocular infection exists; inflammatory conditions of the palpebral and bulbar conjunctiva, cornea, and anterior segment of the globe where the inherent risk of steroid use in certain infective conjunctivitis is accepted to obtain a diminution in edema and inflammation; chronic anterior uveitis and corneal injury from chemical, radiation, or thermal burns or penetration of foreign bodies; and when risk of infection is high or where there is expectation that potentially dangerous numbers of bacteria will be present in the eye.

PREDNISONE

(Meticorten, Orasone, Panasol, Prednicen-M, SK-Prednisone)

Prednisone, an adrenocorticoid with antiinflammatory and immunosuppressant properties, is used in severe inflammation or immunosuppression, and in acute exacerbations of multiple sclerosis. In addition, prednisone has been used as an adjunct to antiinfective therapy in the treatment of moderate to severe *Pneumocystis carinii* pneumonia.

PREGABALIN

(Lyrica capsules 25 mg, capsules 50 mg, capsules 75 mg, capsules 100 mg, capsules 150 mg, capsules 200 mg, capsules 225 mg, capsules 300 mg)

Pregabalin is an anticonvulsant. The mechanism of pregabalin's antinociceptice and antiseizure effects is unknown. Effects may be related to high-affinity binding to the alpha$_2$-delta site (an auxiliary subunit of voltage-gated calcium channels) in CNS tissue.

It is indicated in management of neuropathic pain associated with diabetic peripheral neuropathy; adjunctive therapy for adults with partial-onset seizures; and management of postherpetic neuralgia.

PREPARATHYROID HORMONE

Parathyroid hormone is a single-chain polypeptide composed of 84 amino acids. It has a molecular weight of 9500 and lacks an intrachain disulfide linkage. Parathyroid hormone is produced by means of two sequential enzymic cleavages from a larger precursor polypeptide, preparathyroid hormone.

The organs principally responsible for the peripheral metabolism of parathyroid hormone are the kidney and liver, and possibly bone (see Figure 75).

PREVENTIVE MEDICINE THROUGH NUTRITION

Nutritional epidemiology is concerned with exploring the relationship between nutrition and health in human populations. It has developed out of an epidemiological approach, classically defined as the study of the distribution and determinants of health-related conditions or events in defined populations, and the application of this study to the control of health problems. Distribution refers to analysis of time, place, and classes of persons affected; determinants are all the physiological, biological, social, cultural, and behavioral factors that influence health.

Diet is a complex aggregate of foods and behaviors. The food is comprised of a wide variety of intended and unintended chemicals that may act singly on human metabolism, but more likely act as a group in a synergistic fashion. It is important to study foods, food groups, and food patterns, as well as nutrients and other chemicals contained in food. Food is what people eat. Where many chemical constituents of a food act synergistically, an association will be found with the food, but none will be found with individual constituents. The association of food patterns with risk provides feedback to policy makers on the likely success of nutritional pronouncements.

The speed of increases in the prevalence of **overweight and obesity** in the developing world is greater than the same changes in the prevalence rates among much higher-income, developed countries. The major dietary changes are: increased intake of edible oil (an increase that is affordable by the world's poor in the majority of low-income countries); increased intake of caloric sweetener (particularly in sweetened beverages in some countries but also in many other processed food sources); and also a rapid increase in the total intake of animal-source foods.

The prevalence of type 2 diabetes is increasing rapidly in all parts of the world. Obesity and physical inactivity are major modifiable risk factors. Long-term clinical trials have documented the importance of metabolic control of glucose, lipids, and BP in patients with diabetes. Although new medications and insulins are now available, medical nutrition therapy (MNT) is essential if medical goals are to be achieved. Successful MNT is an ongoing process. Lipids and lipoproteins play a key role in modulating risk of **CHD**. Elevated levels of **total cholesterol**, **LDL-C**, and **triglyceride** (TG) increase CHD risk, whereas high **HDL-C** levels exert a **cardioprotective effect**.

The blood lipid profile is adversely affected by dietary saturated fatty acids, trans-fatty acids, and cholesterol, whereas unsaturated fatty acids and soluble fiber have favorable effects. Many clinical studies have demonstrated that designer diets low in saturated fatty acids, trans-fatty acids, and cholesterol and high in fiber lower total cholesterol and LDL-C levels, whereas the effects they have on TG and HDL-C levels are diet specific. New dietary interventions that can be implemented to control blood lipids provide a variety of options for individualizing diets to maximize CHD risk reduction and promote overall diet adherence. Current guidelines to achieve and maintain a healthy body weight, a desirable cholesterol profile, and a desirable BP emphasize a diet including a variety of fruits, vegetables, grain products, including whole grains, low-fat or nonfat dairy products, fish, nuts, legumes, spices, poultry, and lean meats.

Much evidence from epidemiological and intervention studies indicates that sodium (salt) is related to elevated BP and that a reduced intake of sodium helps lower the BP. However, there is uncertainty regarding the degree of compliance and effectiveness of **low-sodium diets** for long-term use. The average intake of sodium in the United States is around 3310 mg/day (8.3 g/day salt). This should be reduced to about 1600 to 2000 mg/day (4 to 5 g/day salt). This requires avoiding adding salt to food, avoiding eating salt-rich processed foods, and also a reduction in the salt content of processed foods, such as bread. Other minerals are also involved in hypertension. There is strong evidence that **potassium** is effective in treating hypertension and apparently counters the effects of a high intake of sodium, especially in black people. **Calcium** may also help lower BP, although the effect is quite small. This might also be true for **magnesium**, but the evidence is not clear. A combination of nonpharmacological methods can reduce BP as much as some antihypertensive drugs. The **Dietary Approaches to Stop Hypertension diet** (which is rich in fruit, vegetables, and low-fat dairy products, with a reduced saturated and total fat intake), combined with a low-sodium intake and weight loss, can decrease BP by about 9/4.5 mmHg. Other factors linked to hypertension are alcohol consumption beyond moderation, being overweight, and lack of exercise.

n-3 Fatty acids are **long-chain polyunsaturated fatty acid** (PUFAs). The fish-based and fish-oil-based n-3 PUFAs consist of eicosapentaenioc acid (C20:5 n-3) and docosahexaenoic acid (C22:6 n-3). Studies suggest that n-3 fatty acids protect against **CHD** and **sudden cardiac death**. The results of clinical trials are awaited. Both U.S. and U.K. health agencies recommend an increase in consumption of fish and n-3 PUFA. In the general population, the benefits of **fish consumption** within recommended amounts outweigh the risk posed by environmental contaminants.

Overweight (body mass index [BMI] >25 kg/m^2) and obesity (BMI >30 kg/m^2) are associated with increased risk for many of the most **common cancers**. Epidemiological and preclinical (animal and cell culture) studies indicate that increased consumption of fruits, vegetables, and whole grains is associated with reduced cancer risk. Alcohol consumption has been associated with an increased risk of some cancers. Many **bioactive food components** can simultaneously influence multiple sites involved in the cancer process.

Regular consumption of fruit and vegetables, as well as whole grains, is strongly associated with reduced risk of developing chronic diseases, such as **cardiovascular disease** (CVD), **cancer**, **diabetes**, **Alzheimer's disease**, **cataracts**, and **age-related functional decline**. Phytochemicals are defined as bioactive nonnutrient plant compounds in fruit, vegetables, grains, and other plant foods, which have been linked to reducing the risk of major chronic diseases. Phytochemicals are classified into **carotenoids**, **phenolics**, **alkaloids**, **nitrogen-containing compounds**, and **organosulfur compounds**. **Oxidative stress** can cause **oxidative damage** to large biomolecules such as proteins, DNA, and lipids, resulting in an increased risk for cancer and CVD. To prevent or slow down the oxidative stress induced by free radicals, sufficient amounts of antioxidants need to be consumed. The additive and synergistic effects of phytochemicals in fruit and vegetables are responsible for their potent antioxidant and anticancer activities. The benefit of a diet rich in fruit, vegetables, and whole grains is attributed to the complex mixture of phytochemicals present in these and other whole foods. Dietary modification by increasing the consumption of a wide variety of fruit, vegetables, and whole grains daily is a practical strategy for consumers to optimize their health and reduce the risk of chronic diseases. Antioxidants are best acquired through whole-food consumption, not from expensive dietary supplements.

Ethnic dishes that have become popular in recent years use a variety of interesting herbs and spices that provide healthful substances in addition to their unique flavors. A variety of common herbal products are available for the treatment of cardiovascular problems, for improving glycemic control, **enhancing immune function**, and providing **cancer chemopreventive activity**.

More clinical trials are needed to validate the activity of those herbs that show promise for the prevention or treatment of chronic diseases. Some herbal products are not standardized and provide highly variable amounts of active components. Most of the herbs that are promoted to promote weight loss are ineffective, unreliable, or unsafe.

Because there are a number of herb–drug interactions, it is imperative that primary health-care providers be aware of these interactions, and that they know what herbal products their clients are taking, how much, and how often (see Ebadi, M. *Pharmacodynamic Basis of Herbal Medicine*. 2nd edition. Taylor and Francis, New York, 2007).

An **alcoholic drink** is generally considered to contain 12.5 to 13 g of alcohol (ethanol); this amount is found in 12 oz (356 g) of beer, 4 to 5 oz (118 to 148 g) of wine, or 1.5 oz (42 g) of distilled spirits. The U.S. Department of Agriculture defines moderate alcohol consumption as two drinks per day for men or one drink per day for women. **Diet composition** plays a critical role in total energy management; current thinking is that different diets might work better for some individuals than others. Fat is the most energy-dense macronutrient. One gram (1 g) of fat provides 9 kcal of energy compared with 4 kcal/g for carbohydrate and protein. **Fat intake** is poorly regulated, whereas food volume appears to be better regulated. Extensive studies show that it is difficult to gain weight if a low-fat diet is consumed, combined with a higher complex carbohydrate (high fiber) intake. A large body of animal, clinical, and epidemiological data shows that higher-fat foods are less expensive, palatable, and easily consumed in excess of needs. Recent clinical trials show that a low-carbohydrate, high-protein diet can reduce body weight in the short term, but longer-term results are equivocal.

All diets work by reducing calorie consumption. Low-fat and low-carbohydrate diets use different strategies to reach the same end of calorie reduction. Both low-fat and low-carbohydrate diets can be safe and effective strategies for short-term weight loss.

Given that greater weight loss is associated with greater adherence and longer duration of diet, and the lack of data on which diet works best, potential dieters should be encouraged to consider a variety of diet strategies and choose one that they can most easily integrate into their daily life for the long term.

Exercise will modestly enhance weight loss and weight maintenance, and, given its other demonstrated health benefits, should be recommended for everyone trying to lose weight.

Exercise programs should be started gradually and work toward recommended goals of at least 30 min of daily moderate activity for overall health benefits and toward an ultimate goal of 60 min of daily physical activity for weight loss and weight maintenance.

Low birth-weight, as a result of slow fetal growth, is associated with increased rates of CHD and the related disorders such as stroke, hypertension, and type 2 diabetes; these associations extend across the normal range of birth weight. They are thought to be consequences of **developmental plasticity**, the phenomenon by which one genotype can give rise to a range of different physiological or morphological states in response to environmental conditions during development. People who were small at birth may be vulnerable to later disease because they have reduced functional capacity in key organs, such as the kidney, altered settings of hormones and metabolism, or altered responses to adverse influences in the postnatal environment. Slow growth in infancy and rapid weight gain after the age of 2 years further increase the risk of later disease. Slow fetal growth is the product of the mother's body composition and diet before and during pregnancy, together with her metabolism.

Numerous countries have published food guides that provide advice on the overall diet for the general public. One example is the American Food Guide Pyramid.

Other dietary recommendations published in different countries are those focused on reducing the risk of chronic disease; they are usually intended for health professionals. A third type of dietary recommendations concerns nutrient intake. An example is the recommended dietary allowance used in the United States and Canada. These are intended for health professionals and play an important role in food labels.

There is evidence suggesting that certain dietary supplements may be beneficial, especially **folate**, **selenium**, **chromium**, **calcium**, **vitamin D**, and **fish oil**. The use of **dietary supplements** has increased rapidly in recent years, and around half of the people in North America now use supplements regularly. There is very little regulation of the marketing of supplements in the United States. However, Canada is now in the process of enforcing strict regulations.

Novel foods include those providing protein (soy and dairy), and those that are intended to improve cardiovascular health (stanol esters, β-glucan, bioactive peptides, and n-3 fatty acids), bone and joint health (calcium, glucosamine, and chondroitin), eye health (lutein), the immune system (milkmicronutrients, lactoferrin, lactoperoxidase, and colostrum), gut health (probiotics and prebiotics), body fitness (conjugated linoleic acid, amino acids, and glycomacropeptide), energy level, and for beauty.

PRILOCAINE HYDROCHLORIDE

(Citanest)

Prilocaine, a local anesthetic (4% with 1:200,000 epinephrine in 1 to 8 mL dental cartridge), is indicated for local anesthesia by nerve block or infiltration in dental procedures.

Prilocaine, which is equal in potency to lidocaine, has a longer duration of action. It is metabolized to *o*-toluidine, which in toxic doses may cause methemoglobinemia.

PRIMAQUINE PHOSPHATE

Primaquine, an 8 aminoquinoline (26.3 mg daily for 14 days), is recommended only for the radical cure of vivax malaria, the prevention of relapse in vivax malaria, or following the termination of chloroquine phosphate suppressive therapy in an area where vivax malaria is endemic.

Primaquine may disrupt the parasite's mitochondria and bind to native DNA. The resulting structural changes create a major disruption in the metabolic process. The gametocyte and exoerythrocyte forms are inhibited. Some gametocytes are destroyed, whereas others are rendered incapable of undergoing maturation division in the mosquito gut. By eliminating tissue (exoerythrocyte) infection, primaquine prevents development of blood (erythrocytic) forms responsible for relapses in vivax malaria.

Primaquine is rapidly metabolized to a carboxylic acid derivative and then to further metabolites that have varying degrees of activity; elimination half-life is around 4 hours. Approximately 1% is excreted unchanged in the urine. Primaquine may cause hemolytic anemia, especially in patients who are deficient in glucose 6-phosphate dehydrogenase.

PRIMARY AND SECONDARY PREVENTIVE NUTRITION

For the two out of three adult Americans who do not smoke and do not drink excessively, one personal choice seems to influence long-term health prospects more than any other: what we eat.

Preventive nutrition incorporates dietary practices and interventions directed towards the **reduction in disease risk** (**primary prevention**), **improvements in diseases already manifest** (**secondary prevention**), and/or improvement in health outcomes. Preventive nutrition is a critical component not only of preventive medicine but also of **therapeutic medicine**, and provides approaches to prevent disease and reduce its impact once it occurs.

This is an exciting time for research into genetic and environmental influences on obesity. Advances in molecular biology, pharmacology, and other fields are allowing rapid advances to be made in this arena. Knowledge that there is a genetic component to variations in body weight and composition is not new. Indeed, animal breeders and ranchers have known for centuries that animals could be selectively bred for traits related to body weight and composition. For example, the average pig used for pork production in the United States today has substantially more lean body mass and substantially less fat mass than its ancestors, thus demonstrating the influence of selective breeding. Many argue that the ability to induce species-wide changes in the average value of a trait by selective breeding provides the strongest evidence for a genetic effect on that trait, a phenomenon that has been demonstrated in livestock and laboratory animals.

Obesity is the consequence of an energy imbalance in which energy intake has exceeded energy expenditure over considerable time. The amount of stored energy equals the difference between energy intake and energy expenditure, i.e., resting metabolic rate and physical activity. Although it is evident that obese individuals eat more than they need, there is increasing evidence to support the idea that there are genetically determined metabolic differences between individuals who gain extensive weight and those who do not.

Obesity is an increasing health problem in both industrialized and developing countries. In developing countries, obesity coexists with undernutrition, with prevalence rates higher in urban than in rural populations. Women generally have higher rates of obesity than men in both developed and developing countries. In adults, obesity is associated with increased mortality and morbidity (M&M) in a number of diseases, the most common being CVD and non-insulin-dependent diabetes mellitus (NIDDM).

Obesity has reached epidemic proportions in the United States in the past several decades. Prevalence rates have increased sharply among adults, reflecting an average weight gain of 8 lb over a single decade. Recent national survey data (National Health and Nutrition Examination Survey III [NHANES III]) indicate that more than one-third of American adults are obese. The health implications of this mounting problem are significant because obesity is now considered to be a chronic disease that is associated with other chronic conditions such as CHD, type II diabetes mellitus, hypertension, dyslipidemia, gallbladder disease, respiratory disease, and some types of cancer, gout, and arthritis. As such, direct health-care costs related to obesity annually exceed $68 billion, or about 6% of total health-care expenditures in the United States.

National surveys also indicate that the prevalence of **childhood obesity** has increased even among preschool children less than 5 years of age. The problem is especially acute among minority preschoolers, with the highest prevalence rates among Mexican-American children, intermediate rates among non-Hispanic black children, and lowest rates in non-Hispanic white children. Obesity has also increased among low-income preschool children.

The increasing prevalence of childhood obesity has serious implications for child health because it is associated with comorbidity, even during early childhood. This includes elevated BP, abnormal blood lipid concentrations, insulin resistance, type 2 diabetes mellitus, orthopedic disorders, skin problems, and psychological problems.

Treatment of human obesity at any age is very difficult, rarely successful, and is characterized by repeated recidivism over time. Prevention of obesity must therefore be the cornerstone of a widespread public health campaign to control overweight and to reverse the growing epidemic. Such prevention efforts can be targeted simultaneously on several levels, with appropriately different goals: primordial prevention—to prevent children from becoming at risk of overweight; primary prevention—to prevent at-risk children from becoming overweight; and secondary prevention—to prevent the increasing severity of obesity and reduce comorbidity among overweight children.

Large numbers of Americans are taking **vitamin and mineral supplements** despite the limited number of methodologically sound studies on whether supplement use affects disease risk. Recent randomized controlled trials of supplements have yielded some unexpected findings. **β-Carotene**, which was believed to prevent cancer was found to actually increase the incidence of lung cancer. **Selenium** (Se), which was hypothesized to reduce risk of nonmelenomatous skin cancers, had no affect on skin cancer but instead reduced the risk of a broad range of other cancers. The widespread use of supplements can be viewed as a large, uncontrolled, natural experiment.

Considerable research has identified several potential health benefits associated with increased **soy consumption**, and soybeans, which contain trypsin inhibitors such as **phytic acid**, **saponins**, and phytoestrogens, are now looked upon for potential health benefits.

Alcohol and tobacco seem to play a synergistic role in carcinogenesis in the oral cavity, hypopharynx, and esophagus. The risk of developing a carcinoma of the larynx increases directly proportional to the amount smoked. After decades of rigorous investigation of countless cancer chemotherapy regimens, many cancers, including those of the lung, and head and neck cancer (HNC), still remain beyond clinical ability to control them. Despite therapeutic advances and intensive efforts in tobacco-cessation education and counseling, overall survival rates for patients with aerodigestive tract cancers have improved only marginally over the past 30 years. Of all patients initially "cured" of early-stage HNC, 3 to 5%/year will develop second primary tumors. **Vitamin A** (**retinyl palmitate** [RP]) exhibits a positive effect in the prevention of a second primary cancer in the head and neck region and in the lung.

The **primary cause of blinding,** malnutrition and **vitamin A-related mortality,** is a persistent, inadequate dietary intake of absorbable vitamin A, which should be sufficient to meet normal metabolic requirements and the periodically increased need imposed by stress. Protein-energy malnutrition, frequent febrile diseases, and malabsorption are pathophysiological factors contributing to the increased need for the vitamin. Increased need also occurs during physiological periods of rapid growth, such as fetal development and early childhood, and when there is a need to replace the maternal vitamin A transferred to breast milk during lactation.

Most nonpathophysiological factors contributing to **vitamin A deficiency** (VAD) in poorly developed countries are common to the problems associated with overall social, economical, and ecological deprivation. VAD in industrialized countries occasionally occurs among malabsorbers of fat who do not receive supplements, those with abnormal liver function, and those who may habitually consume **cereal-based diets low in vitamin A**. Irrespective of age, most people in the United States and other industrialized countries, however, consume diets sufficient in vitamin A to maintain adequate serum levels. Dietary and medical interventions that prevent or control conditions causally associated with deficiency are commonly available in the industrialized world, but access to adequate diets or supplements and disease-control measures are less available in the nonindustrialized world.

A large body of evidence suggests that the early stages of **atherosclerosis** (Athsc) are comprised of a series of oxidative processes. Studies suggest that oxidative damage may be involved with **atherogenic-promoting processes**, such as **endothelial damage**, and that **antioxidants** reduce oxidative damage.

Diabetes mellitus is a leading cause of morbidity and mortality mostly because of its vascular complications. Diabetic complications can be broadly classified into microvascular (**retinopathy**, **nephropathy**) and macrovascular (**coronary artery disease** [CAD], **cerebrovascular disease**, **peripheral vascular disease**.)

Type 2 diabetes causes oxidative stress, and the beneficial effects of **antioxidants** have been proposed. CVD, which accounts for more deaths globally than any other cause of death, is 2 to 4 times higher in type 2 diabetic patients than in nondiabetic subjects. The identification of risk factors that can explain the excess risk for CVD in diabetic patients may improve understanding of the pathophysiological mechanisms of Athsc and allow the development of new preventive or therapeutic measures.

Only recently has the importance of **hyperhomocysteinemia** as a risk factor for CVD been recognized. It is a strong predictor of CV risk that is independent of other well-established risk factors, such as hypertension (HT), hypercholesterolemia, smoking, and, probably, diabetes. Blood concentrations of homocysteine (Hey) are governed by both genetic and environmental determinants, among which inherited enzymatic defects and nutritional deficiencies are most important. Lowering serum total homocysteine (Hcy) levels by increasing the intake of **folate** (FOL) (a **B-vitamin**), probably the most important dietary determinant of Hcy levels, may be an effective means of decreasing CV risk.

The causes of **autoimmune disease** are yet unknown. The hypothesis that there is an abnormal immunological response to an altered antigen, either viral or bacterial, is supported by much scientific evidence. All of the diseases share an immunological pathogenesis, involving mostly T-cells and B-cells, the cytokine network, and the complement system, resulting in an inflammatory condition that becomes chronic and self-perpetuating.

AD may have pathological and clinical manifestations in any part of the body, and the pathogenesis of the chronic inflammation can be divided in two stages. The first stage is the initiating event of unknown cause that triggers the inflammatory response. The second stage is the amplification of the inflammatory response, which involves a number of inflammatory cells, including lymphocytes, mast cells, macrophages, and neutrophils. Soluble mediators control the amplification of this inflammatory response; a long list of mediators with putative roles in AD has been enumerated, including various eicosanoids, platelet-activating factor, kinins, complement-derived peptides, a long series of cytokines, and bacterial products, neuropeptides, and free radicals.

The second stage, the amplification of the inflammatory response, is important in the pathogenesis of AD for two reasons. It is more important than the initiating event in causing tissue destruction and histological and functional changes, and is characteristic of AD. Second, those drugs that are effective in the treatment of AD appear to have a therapeutical effect by modulating the production of these soluble mediators. As long as the initiating event remains unknown, it is likely that further advances in medical therapy will result only from pharmacological modulation of these inflammatory mediators.

The rationale for **n-3 and n-6 polyunsaturated long-chain fatty acid** (PUFA) supplementation in the treatment of AD resides in the antiinflammatory effects of these lipid compounds. Over the past few years, a growing body of evidence has demonstrated that n-3 and n-6 PUFAs alleviate a number of inflammatory diseases. Actually, the first evidence of the importance of dietary intake of these lipids was derived from epidemiological observations about the very low incidence of chronic inflammatory condition in **Eskimos**.

Dietary **eicosapentaenoic acid** (EPA) and **docosahexaenoic acid** (DHA), the two major components of **fish oil**, partially replace arachidonic acid (AA), which is the initiating component of the homonymous metabolic pathway, in a time- and dose-dependent manner, in plasma and cellular **phospholipids** (PLs). Being less readily released upon cell stimulation, these components reduce substrate availability for **eicosanoid generation**.

Osteoarthritis (OA) is the most common form of joint disease and is a leading cause of disability in the elderly. The disease commonly affects the hands, spine, knees, and hips. Multiple joints may be affected in any one individual. The disorder is strongly associated with increasing age, and has been estimated to affect 2 to 10% of all adults. It is responsible for approximately 68 million work-loss days/year, and for more than 5% of the annual retirement rate. Furthermore, OA is the most frequent reason for joint replacement, a cost to the community of billions of dollars per year.

Factors Associated with Osteoarthritis

Constitutional factors

- Increased age
- Female gender
- Obesity

Mechanical factors
- Heavy/repetitive occupations
- Heavy physical activity
- Major joint injury

Endocrine factors
- Hemochromatosis

Genetic factors
- Mutations in the type II collagen gene

Focal cartilage damage is the central feature of OA. This may range in severity from minor surface roughening to complete cartilage erosion. The process is generally noninflammatory and is often described as being degenerative or caused by wear and tear. The cartilage damage is usually accompanied by some form of reaction in surrounding bone. Osteophytes are an early bony response to cartilage damage, and consist of outgrowths of bone from the peripheral margin of the joint. They may confer some protection to an OA joint by reducing instability. The trabeculae in the bone adjacent to an area of OA cartilage become thickened and are susceptible to microscopic fracturing. This gives rise to the appearance of subchondral sclerosis on a radiograph. In severe disease, particularly when full-thickness cartilage has occurred, circumscribed areas of bony necrosis may develop in the subchondral bone. These may be filled with marrow fat or with synovial fluid that has tracked from the joint space through the cartilage defect into the subchondral bone. They give rise to the radiographic appearance of cysts. Ultimately, the subchondral bone itself may be eroded, or may collapse. In some cases, a low-level synovitis develops as the result of the presence of crystal or other cartilaginous detritus, which may contribute to damage in the joint.

Biochemically, cartilage consists of a network of **collagen fibrils** (predominantly type H) that constrain an interlocking mesh of **proteoglycans** (PG) that resist compressive forces through their affinity for water. The tissue is relatively avascular and acellular. Turnover in healthy cartilage is slow, and represents a balance between collagen and PG synthesis and degradation by enzymes, such as **metalloproteinases**. In early OA, the chondrocytes (cartilage cells) proliferate and become metabolically active. These hypertrophic chondrocytes produce **cytokines** (e.g., interleukin [IL-1], tumor necrosis factor α [TNF-α]), degradative enzymes (e.g., **metalloproteinases**), and other growth factors. PG production is increased in early OA but falls sharply at a later stage when the chondrocyte fails.

There is enormous public interest in the relationship between diet and arthritis. Questions about nutrition and supplements are among the most frequently posed by people with OA to their physicians. Speculative lay publications on this subject abound, and health food stores are full of nutritional supplements touted for their putative ability to help arthritis sufferers.

In contrast, there has been relatively little focus in traditional scientific studies on the relationship between nutritional factors (other than obesity) and OA. Furthermore, the traditional physician's stance on this question has been to assert the lack of evidence supporting any association between diet and OA. This gulf between the levels of interest among scientists and among the general public is surprising, given the large numbers of studies of osteoporosis, another widespread, age-related skeletal disorder that has shown widely accepted association with dietary factors. A more important reason to study the relationship between dietary factors and OA, however, is that there are many mechanisms by which certain **micronutrients** can be hypothesized to influence OA processes. Furthermore, there have been several recent studies that have shown apparent effects of various micronutrients on the natural history of this disorder.

There is accumulating evidence that **calcium (Ca) supplementation** of the diet may be useful, under certain circumstances, for the prevention of **osteoporosis** (OP) in postmenopausal women. Calcium intake is an important determinant of bone health. Several clinical trials of calcium supplementation in the prevention and treatment of OP have shown that calcium can decrease the rate of bone loss and risk of fracture in postmenopausal women. This effect is more clearly seen after the first 5 years of menopause, rather than in early menopause.

Intake of nutrients by individuals is customarily described with broad areas of acceptable choice between some average lower limit of needed supply and an average safe upper limit. Safe upper limits of **average alcohol consumption** by individuals have been a principal focus of national dialogue for 200 years. The Dietary Guidelines for Americans recommend no more than 1 drink/day for women, or 2 drinks/day for men (with a standard drink being either 12 oz regular beer, 5 oz wine, or 1.5 oz distilled spirits, each containing about 14 g [100 calories] of ethanol). At this time, no major scientific body recognizes a nutritional need for alcohol, or recommends that those who do not drink should begin doing so.

Nutrition can play a key and cost-effective role in decreasing risks of different chronic diseases. An increasing body of evidence suggests that there are far more commonalities relating to how nutrition reduces risk factors for varied chronic diseases than differences. Different diets are not required to decrease the risk of cancer, compared to CVD. For example, as preventive nutrition strategies, increasing intake of fruits and vegetables has been linked to decreased prevalence of CVD, stroke, and also cancer. Likewise, increased whole grain intake (compared to refined grains) has been associated with decreased prevalence of CVD, cancer, and also type II diabetes.

Decreased fat intake, particularly saturated fat intake, is clearly linked to decreased serum cholesterol levels and decreased prevalence of CV complications, such as CAD. Although recent studies place some doubt on the contribution of fat intake toward increasing the risk of breast cancer, high levels of fat intake are still associated with the risk of some cancers, and perhaps type II diabetes. Foods rich in other dietary components, including fiber, complex carbohydrates, and micronutrients, appear to decrease the risk of certain forms of cancer, as well as CHD and manifestations of diabetes.

The major chronic diseases also share a number of common cellular and biochemical mechanisms in their pathogenesis. For example, **cell proliferation** is common in both atherosclerosis and cancer, and is of importance to some of the complications associated with diabetes. Changes in signal transduction and gene expression relate to cancer, atherosclerosis, obesity, and diabetes. DNA modifications likely contribute mechanistically to each of these disease classes. In examining the sets of nutrition recommendations aimed at reducing the risk of a number of chronic diseases, and developed by a number of different private and government organizations, the different recommendations show far more common themes and commonalities than differences. The recommendations of most nutrition and public health groups are very similar to the 1995 U.S. Dietary Guidelines of the U.S. Department of Health and Human Services and U.S. Department of Agriculture, which include the following recommendations

- Eat a variety of foods.
- Balance the food you eat with physical activity.
- Maintain or improve your weight.
- Choose a diet with plenty of grain products, vegetables, and fruit.
- Choose a diet low in fat, saturated fat, and cholesterol.
- Choose a diet moderate in sugars.
- Choose a diet moderate in salt and sodium.
- If you drink alcoholic beverages, do so in moderation.

PRIMIDONE

(Mysoline)

An anticonvulsant, primidone is given at an initial dose of 100 to 125 mg/day at bedtime, increasing gradually to a maintenance dose of 125 to 250 mg three times daily. The most frequent side effect of primidone is heavy sedation, which seems to be due to primidone itself and not to its metabolite phenobarbital. Tolerance develops to this sedation within a few days or weeks of continuous administration.

Primidone is a nonbarbiturate compound that is structurally related to phenobarbital. It is absorbed well and does not bind to plasma proteins extensively. It is probably not advisable to administer this agent to subjects with a history of adverse reactions to phenobarbital.

Primidone is indicated in control of grand mal, psychomotor, or focal epileptic seizures, either alone or with other anticonvulsants. It may control grand mal seizures refractory to other anticonvulsants. Primidone raises electroshock or chemoshock seizure thresholds, or alters seizure patterns. The mechanism of its antiepileptic action is not known.

Primidone and its two metabolites, phenobarbital and phenylethyl-malonamide (PEMA), have anticonvulsant activity. In addition, PEMA potentiates the activity of phenobarbital. Abrupt withdrawal of primidone may cause status epilepticus. Acetazolamide, succinimides, and carbamazepine reduce the plasma level of primidone, whereas the coadministration of hydantoin, isoniazid, or nicotinamide increases it (see also Figure 32).

PROBENECID

(Benemid)

Probenecid, a uricosuric agent (initially 0.25 g t.i.d. for 1 week), is indicated in the treatment of hyperuricemia associated with gout and gouty arthritis. In addition, probenecid is used as an adjunct to therapy with penicillins or cephalosporins, and for elevation and prolongation of plasma levels of these antibiotics.

A uricosuric and renal tubular-blocking agent, probenecid inhibits the tubular resorption of urate, thus increasing the urinary excretion of uric acid and decreasing serum uric-acid levels. Effective uricosuria reduces the miscible urate pool, retards urate deposition, and promotes resorption of urate deposits.

Probenecid also inhibits the tubular secretion of most penicillins and cephalosporins, and usually increases plasma levels by any route the antibiotic is given. A twofold to fourfold plasma elevation has been demonstrated.

The most commonly used uricosuric agents are probenecid and sulfinpyrazone (Anturane). In low doses, these agents block tubular secretion, but, at higher doses, they also block the tubular resorption of uric acid. Because the solubility of uric acid is increased in alkaline urine, the administration of sodium bicarbonate may at times be advantageous for offsetting this condition. In addition, probenecid and sulfinpyrazone inhibit the excretion of agents such as aspirin, penicillin, ampicillin, and indomethacin. Although probenecid and sulfinpyrazone may be coadministered, neither should be given with aspirin, as their uricosuric effects will then be nullified.

On the other hand, probenecid increases the plasma level of acyclovir, allopurinol, barbiturate, benzodiazepines, clofibrate, dapsone, dyphylline, methotrexate, NSAIDs, penicillamine, sulfonylureas, and zidovudine.

PROBENECID/COLCHICINE

(Probenecid and colchicine tablets 500 mg probenecid and 0.5 mg colchicine)

Probenecid/colchicine agents are used in gout. **Probenecid** inhibits the tubular reabsorption of urate, thus increasing urinary excretion of uric acid. **Colchicine** inhibits inflammation and reduces pain and swelling associated with gouty arthritis. They are indicated in treatment of chronic gouty arthritis when complicated by frequent, recurrent, acute attacks of gout.

PROBUCOL

(Lorelco)

Probucol, an antihyperlipidemic agent (500 mg twice daily with meals), is indicated in the reduction of elevated serum cholesterol in patients with primary hypercholesterolemia (elevated LDL) who have not responded to diet, weight reduction, and control of diabetes mellitus. It may be useful to lower elevated cholesterol that occurs with combined hypercholesterolemia and hypertriglyceridemia, but it is not indicated when hypertriglyceridemia is the major concern.

Probucol lowers serum cholesterol with relatively little effect on serum triglycerides. Patients responding to probucol exhibit a decrease in LDL-C. Cholesterol is reduced not only in the LDL fraction but also in some HDL fractions with proportionately greater effect on the HDL portion in some patients. Epidemiological studies have shown that low HDL-C and high LDL-C are independent risk factors for CHD. The risk of lowering HDL-C while lowering LDL-C is unknown. Little or no effect is reported on VLDL.

Probucol increases the fractional rate of LDL catabolism. This effect may be linked to the increased excretion of fecal bile acids. Probucol also inhibits the early stages of cholesterol synthesis and slightly inhibits absorption of dietary cholesterol. There is no increase in the cyclic precursors of cholesterol; hence, probucol does not appear to affect later stages of cholesterol biosynthesis.

Prolongation of the QT interval can occur in patients on probucol, predisposing them to ventricular tachycardia (see also Figure 84).

PROCAINAMIDE HYDROCHLORIDE

(Pronestyl)

Procainamide (an initial total daily oral dose up to 50 mg/kg) is indicated in the treatment of documented ventricular arrhythmias, such as sustained ventricular tachycardia, which is judged to be life threatening. Because procainamide has the potential to produce serious hematologic disorders, particularly leukopenia or agranulocytosis, its use should be reserved for patients in whom the benefits of treatment clearly outweigh the risks.

Quinidine and procainamide decrease automaticity by reducing the rate of phase 4 diastolic depolarization, which is probably mediated by a diminished membrane permeability to sodium, and they decrease conduction velocity throughout the conducting system. They produce an indirect (vagolytic) effect that sometimes counteracts the direct effect at the AV node, producing a paradoxical tachycardia in some cases of atrial flutter or fibrillation. These agents terminate reentry arrhythmias by producing a bidirectional block in infarcted conducting tissues. They directly depress contractility, leading to a decline in cardiac output (see also Figure 84).

Quinidine and procainamide are potent vasodilators, especially when given intravenously. This effect is so great that quinidine is rarely given parenterally, and great care must be taken when it is given by this route. They depress BP by means of their dual effects on cardiac output and peripheral resistance.

These agents produce widening of the QRS complex (by depressing ventricular conduction) and lengthening of the PR interval (by slowing AV conduction). A 25 to 30% widening of the QRS complex is considered the therapeutic limit with these agents. They are excreted up to 50% unmetabolized in the urine. They commonly cause GI disturbances, and these constitute their major side effect. Emboli may be liberated from the atria during conversion of atrial flutter or fibrillation. Toxicity is manifested by a profound fall in BP that leads to a shock-like state accompanied by a variety of arrhythmias.

Quinidine and procainamide may also provoke some unique but uncommon side effects. Quinidine may produce cinchonism (tinnitus, dizziness, visual disturbances, and vertigo) and cutaneous hypersensitivity reactions. Procainamide may produce agranulocytosis during long-term therapy, and a dose-dependent (>2 gm/day) lupus erythematosus-like syndrome. These agents are mainly used in the management of atrial (supraventricular) arrhythmias, although procainamide is also of value in treating premature ventricular contractions and ventricular tachycardia. If either drug is used to convert atrial flutter or fibrillation, digitalis must be given first to protect against paradoxical tachycardia.

PROCAINE HYDROCHLORIDE

(Novocain)

Procaine is indicated in infiltration anesthesia (0.25 to 0.50% solution), peripheral nerve block (0.5 to 2% solution), and spinal anesthesia (10% solution). Procaine, which has a pKa of 8.9, is highly ionized at the physiologic pH and has a short duration of action. Because it causes vasodilation, a vasoconstricting substance is added to the procaine solution to delay systemic absorption (see Figure 80). Procainamide, a congener of procaine, is an effective oral antiarrhythmic agent. Procaine may prolong the effect of succinylcholine because both drugs are metabolized by the same enzyme. Cholinesterase inhibitors alter procaine's metabolism.

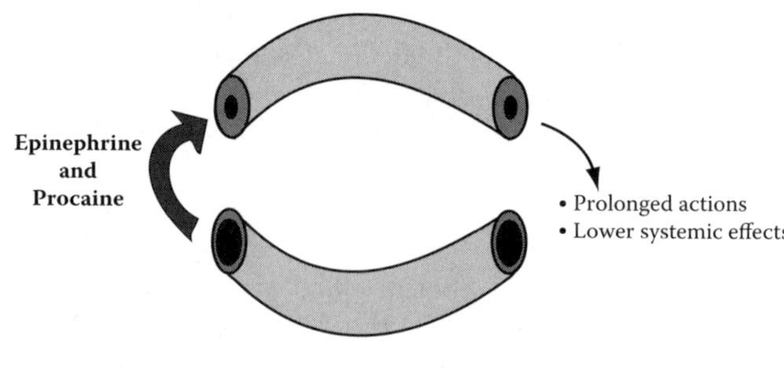

FIGURE 80 Procaine has a short duration of action. Because it causes vasodilation, a vasoconstricting substance is added to the procaine solution to delay systemic absorption.

PROCARBAZINE HYDROCHLORIDE

(Matulane)

Procarbazine, an antineoplastic agent (2 to 4 mg/kg/day for the first week) in combination with other antineoplastic agents (MOPP regimen—nitrogen mustard, vincristine, procarbazine, prednisone), is indicated in the treatment of stage III and IV Hodgkin's disease. Procarbazine inhibits the synthesis of protein RNA and DNA (see also Figure 15).

Procarbazine may inhibit transmethylation of methyl groups of methionine into tRNA. The absence of functional tRNA could cause the cessation of protein synthesis and consequently DNA and RNA synthesis. In addition, procarbazine may directly damage DNA. Hydrogen peroxide, formed during the autooxidation of the drug, may attack protein sulfhydryl groups contained in residual protein that is tightly bound to DNA.

Procarbazine is rapidly and completely absorbed from the GI tract and quickly equilibrates between plasma and CSF. Peak CSF levels occur in 30 to 90 minutes. Following oral administration, maximum peak plasma concentrations occur within 60 minutes.

Procarbazine is metabolized in the liver to cytotoxic products. The major portion of drug is excreted in the urine as *N*-isopropylterephthalamic acid (approximately 70% within 24 hours following oral and IV administration). Less than 5% is excreted in urine unchanged.

After IV injection, the plasma half-life is approximately 10 minutes. Procarbazine crosses the blood–brain barrier.

The most frequent adverse reactions of procarbazine are nausea, vomiting, leukopenia, anemia, and thrombocytopenia.

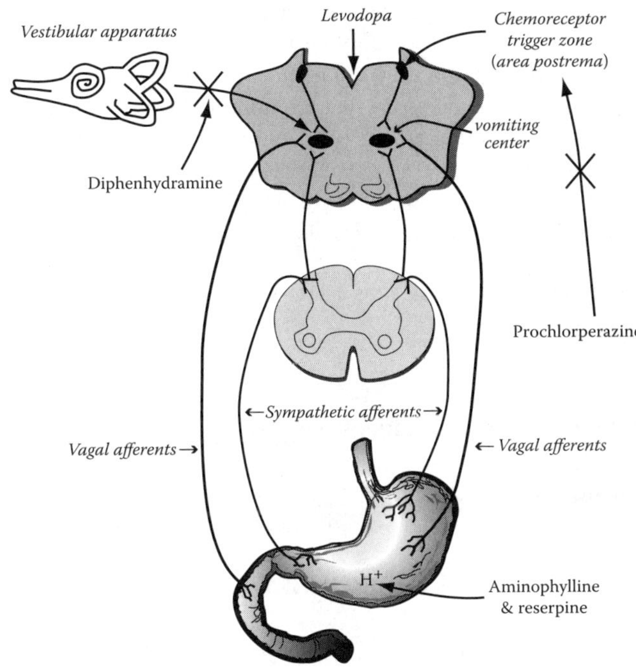

FIGURE 81 Phenothiazine derivatives such as chlorpromazine, perphenazine, **prochlorperazine**, promethazine, triethylperazine, and triflupromazine, exert their antiemetic effects by blocking the dopamine receptors in the **area postrema**.

PROCHLORPERAZINE

(Compazine)

Prochlorperazine, an antiemetic and antipsychotic agent, is indicated in controlling preoperative nausea (5 to 10 mg IM 1 to 2 hours before induction of anesthesia) and severe nausea and vomiting (5 to 10 mg p.o. t.i.d.) associated with circulating physical agents (radiation therapy and virus particles) and chemical agents (toxins and cancer chemotherapeutic agents) (see Figures 73 and 81).

Prochlorperazine is thought to exert its antipsychotic effects by postsynaptic blockade of CNS dopamine receptors, thus inhibiting dopamine-mediated effects. Its antiemetic effects are attributed to dopamine receptor blockade in the medullary chemoreceptor trigger zone (Figure 73).

Prochlorperazine causes sedation, has weak anticholinergic properties, and produces a high incidence of movement disorders.

Concomitant use of prochlorperazine with sympathomimetics, including epinephrine, phenylephrine, phenylpropranolamine, and ephedrine (often found in nasal sprays), and with appetite suppressants may decrease their stimulatory and pressor effects and may cause epinephrine reversal (hypotensive response to epinephrine).

Prochlorperazine may inhibit BP response to centrally acting antihypertensive drugs such as guanethidine, guanabenz, guanadrel, clonidine, methyldopa, and reserpine. Additive effects are likely after concomitant use of prochlorperazine with CNS depressants, including alcohol, analgesics, barbiturates, narcotics, tranquilizers, and anesthetics (general, spinal, or epidural), and parenteral magnesium sulfate (oversedation, respiratory depression, and hypotension); antiarrhythmic agents, quinidine, disopyramide, and procainamide (increased incidence of cardiac arrhythmias and conduction defects); atropine and other anticholinergic drugs, including antidepressants, monoamine oxidase inhibitors, phenothiazines, antihistamines, meperidine, and antiparkinsonian agents (oversedation, paralytic ileus, visual changes, and severe constipation); nitrates (hypotension); and metrizamide (increased risk of convulsions).

Beta-blocking agents may inhibit prochlorperazine metabolism, increasing plasma levels and toxicity.

Concomitant use with propylthiouracil increases the risk of agranulocytosis; concomitant use with lithium may result in severe neurologic toxicity with an encephalitis-like syndrome, and in decreased therapeutic response to prochlorperazine.

Pharmacokinetic alterations and subsequent decreased therapeutic response to prochlorperazine may follow concomitant use with phenobarbital (enhanced renal excretion); aluminum- and magnesium-containing antacids and antidiarrheals (decreased absorption); caffeine, or heavy smoking (increased metabolism).

Prochlorperazine may antagonize the therapeutic effect of bromocriptine on prolactin secretion; it also may decrease the vasoconstricting effects of high-dose dopamine and may decrease effectiveness and increase toxicity of levodopa (by dopamine blockade). Prochlorperazine may inhibit metabolism and increase toxicity of phenytoin.

PROCHLORPERAZINE EDISYLATE

(Compazine)

PROCHLORPERAZINE MALEATE

(Chlorazine, Compazine, Compazine Spansule)

Prochlorperazine, a phenothiazine derivative with antiemetic properties, is used to control preoperative nausea and severe nausea and vomiting.

PROCYCLIDINE HYDROCHLORIDE

(Kemadrin)

Procyclidine (2.5 mg t.i.d. with meals) is indicated in the treatment of Parkinson's disease at its early stage. In addition, it is effective in relieving the neuroleptic-induced extrapyramidal symptoms. Procycline is an anticholinergic agent that, by blocking central cholinergic receptors, helps to reestablish the proper cholinergic-dopaminergic transmission in the basal ganglion.

Procyclidine is contraindicated in patients with narrow-angle glaucoma because drug-induced cycloplegia and mydriasis may increase IOP. It should be administered cautiously in patients with tachycardia because the drug may block vagal inhibition of the sinoatrial node pacemaker, thus exacerbating tachycardia, and in patients with urinary retention or prostatic hypertrophy because the drug may exacerbate these conditions.

Procyclidine may reduce the antipsychotic effectiveness of haloperidol and phenothiazines, possibly by direct CNS antagonism related to its anticholinergic properties. Haloperidol and phenothiazine exert their effects in part by blocking the hyperactivity of dopaminergic transmission in the mesocortical and mesolimbic systems. Concomitant use with phenothiazine derivatives, especially thioridazine having pronounced anticholinergic effects, also increases the risk of anticholinergic adverse effects. Paralytic ileus may result from concomitant use with phenothiazines or tricyclic antidepressants. Concomitant use with alcohol and other CNS depressants increases procyclidine's sedative effects.

Antacids and antidiarrheals may decrease procyclidine's absorption, thus reducing its effectiveness.

Clinical symptoms of overdosage with procyclidine, which result primarily from its anticholinergic effects, include central stimulation followed by depression, and such psychotic symptoms as disorientation, confusion, hallucinations, delusions, anxiety, agitation, and restlessness. Peripheral effects may include dilated, nonreactive pupils; blurred vision; flushed, hot, dry skin; dry mucus membranes; dysphagia; decreased or absent bowel sounds; urinary retention; hyperthermia; tachycardia; hypertension; and increased respiration.

PROGESTERONE

(Bay Progest, Femotrone, Gesertol 50, Progestaject-50, Progestasert, Progesteronaq-LA)

Progesterone is synthesized in the ovaries, the adrenal glands, and the placenta. In a nonpregnant woman, it is produced by the corpus luteum during the latter part of the menstrual cycle under the influence of luteinizing and luteotropic hormones. In a pregnant woman, it is produced initially by the corpus luteum under the influence of chorionic gonadotropins, and is synthesized by the placenta after failure of the corpus luteum.

Progesterone is not only an important progestin but also an important precursor for androgen. It is synthesized according to the following scheme:

Acetate→ cholesterol → pregnenolone→ progesterone
testosterone→ estradiol

Progesterone is absorbed rapidly when given orally and has a plasma half-life of 5 minutes. It is completely metabolized in the liver and is cleared completely during first passage through the liver.

Progesterone initially prepares the uterus for implantation of the fertilized egg and prevents uterine contraction that would expel the fetus. Progesterone has been used in the past to prevent threatened abortion. In addition, it exerts effects on the secretory cells of the mammary glands. Progesterone competes with aldosterone and causes a decrease in sodium resorption; therefore, it antagonizes aldosterone-induced sodium retention. It increases the body temperature and decreases the plasma level of many amino acids.

In the treatment of progesterone-related disorders, progesterone, which must be injected and has a short duration of action, has been replaced by the progestins. These newer synthetic derivatives of progesterone are effective orally and have a longer duration of action. Unlike progesterone, some of these agents have androgenic, estrogenic, and even glucocorticoid-like effects.

Progestins are used as antifertility agents and in the treatment of dysfunctional uterine bleeding, which may occur as a result of insufficient estrogen or because of continued estrogen secretion in the absence of progesterone.

Progestins such as medroxyprogesterone are useful in the diagnosis and treatment of amenorrhea.

Because prostaglandin F_{2a} is capable of inducing contraction in the uterus, agents that are able to block the synthesis of prostaglandin, such as aspirin or aspirin-like substances, have been shown to be effective in easing dysmenorrhea. For sexually active women, oral contraceptives have been found to be effective in relieving dysmenorrhea.

Endometriosis, which was formerly treated by surgical removal of the ovaries and uterus, is now treated with the continuous administration of progestin, or with progestin combined with estrogen. In addition, progestin may be useful in the management of endometrial carcinoma.

Estrogen, progesterone, and bromocriptine (a dopamine-receptor agonist) are all effective in suppressing postpartum lactation.

PROMAZINE HYDROCHLORIDE

(Sparine)

Promazine (initially 50 to 150 mg IM) is indicated in the management of psychotic disorders. In addition, it has antiemetic and antivertigo properties and possesses antihistaminic actions, and hence may be used pre- or post-operatively (25 to 50 mg IM). The antiemetic effects of promazine may be due to its anticholinergic actions. Furthermore, promazine inhibits the medullary chemoreceptor trigger zone for emesis. The antipsychotic effects of promazine may be due in part to blockade of hyperactive dopaminergic transmission in the mesocortical and mesolimbic systems.

Like other antihistamines, promethazine has significant anticholinergic effects; it should be used with caution in patients with narrow-angle glaucoma, peptic ulcer, or pyloroduodenal obstruction or urinary bladder obstruction from prostatic hypertrophy or narrowing of the bladder neck. It also should be used with caution in patients with CVD or hypertension because of the risk of palpitations with acute or chronic respiratory dysfunction (especially children) as promazine may depress the cough reflex.

Clinical manifestations of overdose may include either CNS depression (sedation, reduction in mental alertness, apnea, and cardiovascular collapse) or CNS stimulation (insomnia, hallucinations, tremors, or convulsions). Atropine-like symptoms, such as dry mouth, flushed skin, fixed and dilated pupils, and GI symptoms are common, especially in children.

PROMETHAZINE HYDROCHLORIDE

(Phenergan tablets 12.5 mg, tablets 25 mg, tablets 50 mg, suppositories 12.5 mg, suppositories 25 mg, suppositories 50 mg, injection 25 mg/mL, injection 50 mg/mL (IM use only))

Promethazine hydrochloride is a nonselective phenothiazine that competitively antagonizes histamine at H_1-receptor sites. It produces sedative and antiemetic effects. **Oral/Rectal**: It is indicated for temporary relief of runny nose and sneezing caused by common cold; symptomatic relief of perennial and seasonal allergic rhinitis, vasomotor rhinitis, allergic conjunctivitis, allergic and nonallergic pruritic symptoms, mild, uncomplicated skin manifestations of urticaria, and angioedema; amelioration of allergic reactions to blood or plasma; treatment of dermographism; adjunctive therapy in anaphylactic reactions; preoperative, postoperative, or obstetric sedation; prevention and control of nausea and vomiting associated with certain types of anesthesia and surgery; adjunctive therapy to analgesics for postoperative pain; sedation and relief of apprehension; induction of light sleep; active and prophylactic treatment of motion sickness; and antiemetic therapy in postoperative patients. **Injection**: It is used in amelioration of allergic reactions to blood or plasma; as an adjunct to epinephrine and other standard measures after acute symptoms of anaphylaxis have been controlled; uncomplicated allergic conditions of the immediate type when other therapy is impossible or contraindicated; sedation and relief of apprehension and to produce light sleep from which a patient can be easily aroused; as an active treatment of motion sickness; prevention and control of nausea and vomiting associated with certain types of anesthesia and surgery; as an adjunct to analgesics for control of postoperative pain; preoperative, postoperative, and obstetric (during labor) sedation; and intravenously in special surgical situations (e.g., repeated bronchoscopy, ophthalmic surgery, poor-risk patients with reduced amounts of meperidine or other narcotic analgesic as an adjunct to anesthesia and analgesia).

Promethazine (25 mg 1 hour before travel) is indicated for acute and prophylactic treatment of motion sickness, and for prevention and control of nausea and vomiting associated with anesthesia and surgery.

Promethazine competes with histamine for the H_1 receptor, thereby suppressing allergic rhinitis and urticaria; the drug does not prevent the release of histamine.

The central anticholinergic and antihistaminic effects of promethazine causing inhibition of the medullary chemoreceptor trigger zone for emesis are responsible for its antiemetic and antivertigo effects (see also Figures 73 and 81).

Promethazine causes sedation by reducing stimuli to the brain stem reticular system. Like other antihistamines, promethazine has significant anticholinergic effects; it should be used with caution in patients with narrow-angle glaucoma, peptic ulcer, or pyloroduodenal obstruction or urinary bladder obstruction from prostatic hypertrophy or narrowing of the bladder neck. It also should be used with caution in patients with CVD or hypertension because of the risk of palpitations with acute or chronic respiratory dysfunction (especially children) because promazine may depress the cough reflex.

Concurrent administration of drugs such as promethazine or chlorpromazine may greatly enhance meperidine-induced sedation without slowing clearance of the drug.

Clinical manifestations of overdose may include either CNS depression (sedation, reduced mental alertness, apnea, and CV collapse) or CNS stimulation (insomnia, hallucinations, tremors, or convulsions). Atropine-like symptoms, such as dry mouth, flushed skin, fixed and dilated pupils, and GI symptoms, are common, especially in children.

PROMETHAZINE HYDROCHLORIDE/CODEINE PHOSPHATE

(Prometh with codeine syrup 10 mg codeine phosphate and 6.25 mg promethazine hydrochloride)

Promethazine competitively antagonizes histamine at H_1-receptor sites and produces sedative as well as antiemetic effects. **Codeine** stimulates opiate receptors in the CNS in addition to causing respiratory depression, peripheral vasodilation, inhibition of intestinal peristalsis, stimulation of the chemoreceptors that cause vomiting, increased bladder tone, and suppression of cough. They are indicated in the temporary relief of coughs and upper respiratory tract symptoms associated with allergy or the common cold.

PROMETHAZINE HYDROCHLORIDE/PHENYLEPHRINE HYDROCHLORIDE

(Prometh VC plain syrup 5 mg phenylephrine hydrochloride and 6.25 promethazine hydrochloride)

Promethazine hydrochloride is an antihistamine/decongestant. **Promethazine** competitively antagonizes histamine at H_1-receptor sites and produces sedative as well as antiemetic effects. **Phenylephrine** stimulates postsynaptic alpha receptors, resulting in a rise in arterial peripheral vasoconstriction. They are indicated in temporary relief of upper respiratory tract symptoms, including nasal congestion associated with allergy or the common cold.

PROMETHAZINE HYDROCHLORIDE/PHENYLEPHRINE HYDROCHLORIDE/CODEINE PHOSPHATE

(Prometh VC w/codeine syrup 6.25 mg promethazine hydrochloride/5 mg phenylephrine hydrochloride/10 mg codeine phosphate/5 mL)

It is an antihistamine/decongestant/antitussive/narcotic analgesic. **Promethazine** competitively antagonizes histamine at H_1-receptor sites and produces sedative as well as antiemetic effects.

Phenylephrine stimulates postsynaptic alpha receptors, resulting in a rise in arterial peripheral vasoconstriction. **Codeine** stimulates opiate receptors in the CNS in addition to causing respiratory depression, peripheral vasodilation, inhibition of intestinal peristalsis, stimulation of the chemoreceptors that cause vomiting, increased bladder tone, and suppression of cough, which are indicated in temporary relief of coughs and upper respiratory tract symptoms, including nasal congestion associated with allergy or the common cold.

PROPAFENONE HYDROCHLORIDE

(Rythmol)

Propafenone (150 mg every 8 hours) is indicated in the treatment of documented life-threatening ventricular arrhythmias such as sustained ventricular tachycardia. In addition, propafenone appears to be effective in the treatment of supraventricular tachycardias including atrial fibrillation and flutter, and arrhythmias associated with Wolff–Parkinson–White syndrome.

Propafenone is a class 1C antiarrhythmic drug with local anesthetic effects and a direct stabilizing action on myocardial membranes. The electrophysiological effect of propafenone manifests itself in a reduction of upstroke velocity (phase O) of the monophasic action potential. In Purkinje fibers, and to a lesser extent myocardial fibers, propafenone reduces the fast inward current carried by sodium ions. The diastolic excitability threshold is increased, and the effective refractory period prolonged. Propafenone reduces spontaneous automaticity and depresses triggered activity.

Propafenone, which has a weak beta-adrenergic-blocking effect (1/40 that of propranolol) causes a dose-related decrease in the rate of single and multiple PVCs and can suppress recurrence of ventricular tachycardia. Additionally, like other class 1C antiarrhythmic drugs, propafenone exerts a negative inotropic effect on the myocardium.

Propafenone is completely absorbed after oral administration, exhibits an extensive first-pass metabolism, and its clearance is reduced and the elimination half-life increased in patients with significant hepatic dysfunction.

Propafenone is metabolized into two active metabolites: 5-hydroxypropafenone and *N*-depropylpropafenone. It is contraindicated in CHF; cardiogenic shock; sinoatrial, AV, and intraventricular disorders of impulse generation or conduction (e.g., sick sinus node syndrome, AV block) in the absence of an artificial pacemaker; as well as in bradycardia, marked hypotension, bronchospastic disorders, and manifest electrolyte imbalance.

Cimetidine and quinidine increase, and rifampin decreases, the serum level of propafenone. Propafenone increases the plasma levels and hence the actions of anticoagulants, beta-adrenergic-receptor-blocking agents, cyclosporine, and digoxin. The adverse reactions occurring most often are headaches, dizziness, unusual taste, first-degree AV block, intraventricular conduction delay, nausea or vomiting, and constipation.

Symptoms of overdosage that are usually most severe within 3 hours of ingestion may include hypotension, somnolence, bradycardia, intra-atrial and intraventricular conduction disturbances, and rarely convulsions and high-grade ventricular arrhythmias.

PROPANIDID

Propanidid is a nonbarbiturate ultra-short-acting anesthetic agent that may cause hypotension and tachycardia. Unlike thiopental, which is redistributed, propanidid is metabolized rapidly by pseudocholinesterases.

PROPANTHELINE BROMIDE

(Pro-Banthine)

Propantheline (50 to 100 mg every 6 hours) is indicated as an adjunctive therapy in the treatment of peptic ulcer. In addition, it has been advocated for its antisecretory and antispasmodic effects for use in IBS and other GI disorders, and to reduce duodenal motility during diagnostic radiologic procedures.

Propantheline, a muscarinic cholinergic receptor antagonist, competitively blocks acetylcholine's actions at cholinergic neuroeffector sites, decreasing GI motility and inhibiting gastric acid secretion.

Like other anticholinergic agents, propantheline is contraindicated in patients with narrow-angle glaucoma because drug-induced cycloplegia and mydriasis may increase IOP; in patients with obstructive uropathy and obstructive GI-tract disease, severe ulcerative colitis, myasthenia gravis, paralytic ileus, intestinal atony, or toxic megacolon because the drug may exacerbate these conditions.

Propantheline should be administered cautiously in patients with autonomic neuropathy, hyperthyroidism, coronary artery disease, cardiac arrhythmias, CHF, or ulcerative colitis because the drug may exacerbate symptoms of these disorders; in patients with hepatic or renal disease because toxic accumulation may occur; in patients over age 40 because the drug increases glaucoma risk; in patients with hiatal hernia associated with reflux esophagitis because the drug may decrease lower esophageal sphincter tone; and in hot or humid environments because the drug may predispose the patient to heatstroke.

Overdosage with propantheline may cause curare-like symptoms and such peripheral effects as headache; dilated, nonreactive pupils; blurred vision; flushed, hot, dry skin; dryness of mucus membranes; dysphagia; decreased or absent bowel sounds; urinary retention; hyperthermia; tachycardia; hypertension; and increased respiration.

PROPARACAINE HYDROCHLORIDE

(Ak-Taine, Alcaine, Ophthaine Hydrochloride, Opthetic sterile ophthalmic solution)

Proparacaine, a local anesthetic (ophthalmic solution 0.5%), is used in anesthesia for tonometry, anesthesia for the removal of foreign bodies or sutures from the eye, and anesthesia for cataract extraction and glaucoma surgery.

PROPOFOL

(Diprivan)

Propofol, a rapidly acting IV anesthetic agent, is indicated in induction or maintenance of anesthesia as part of a balanced anesthetic technique for inpatient and outpatient surgery in adults, and children 3 years of age or under. Propofol can be used to initiate and maintain monitored anesthesia care (MAC) sedation during diagnostic procedures in adults, and it may also be used for MAC sedation in conjunction with local/regional anesthesia in patients undergoing surgical procedures (see Figure 82).

When nitrous oxide, oxygen, and propofol are used for maintenance of general anesthesia, supplementation with analgesics and neuromuscular-blocking agents is usually required. Induction of anesthesia with propofol is frequently associated with apnea. If spontaneous ventilation is maintained, a major cardiovascular effect is arterial hypotension.

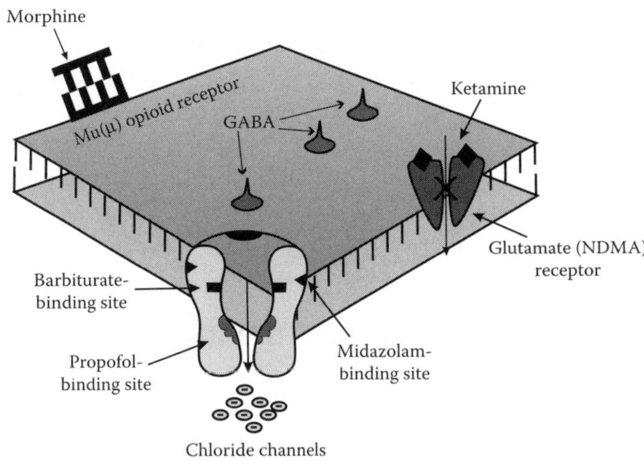

FIGURE 82 Propofol, like thiopental, induces anesthesia rapidly, but the maintenance of anesthesia may require nitrous oxide, inhalational anesthetics, and opioids. Propofol does not impair hepatic or renal functions.

Propofol is chiefly eliminated by hepatic conjugation to inactive metabolites, which are excreted by the kidney. A glucuronide conjugate accounts for about 50% of the administered dose. Following an IV bolus dose, plasma levels initially decline rapidly due to both high metabolic clearance and rapid drug distribution into tissues. Distribution accounts for about half of this decline following a bolus of propofol.

CNS depressants (e.g., hypnotics/sedatives, inhalational anesthetics, narcotics) can increase the CNS depression induced by propofol. Morphine premedication with nitrous oxide decreases the necessary propofol maintenance infusion rate and therapeutic blood concentrations when compared to nonnarcotic (e.g., lorazepam) premedication. In addition, the induction dose requirements of propofol may be reduced in patients with IM or IV premedication, particularly with narcotics alone or in combination with sedatives. These agents may increase the anesthetic effects of propofol and may also result in more pronounced decreases in systolic, diastolic, and mean arterial pressures and cardiac output.

PROPOXYPHENE/ACETAMINOPHEN

(Propoxyphene hydrochloride/Acetaminophen, Propoxyphene hydrochloride/acetaminophen tablets 65 mg propoxyphene hydrochloride/650 mg acetaminophen, propoxyphene napsylate/acetaminophen Darvocet-N 50 tablets 50 mg propoxyphene napsylate/325 mg acetaminophen, Darvocet A500 tablets 100 mg propoxyphene napsylate/500 mg acetaminophen, Darvocet-N 100 tablets 100 mg propoxyphene)

Propoxyphene is an opioid analgesic combination. It relieves pain by stimulating opiate receptors in the CNS; causes respiratory depression; causes peripheral vasodilation, inhibition of intestinal peristalsis, sphincter of hepatopancreatic ampulla spasm, stimulation of receptors that cause vomiting, and increased bladder tone. **Acetaminophen** inhibits synthesis of prostaglandins; it does not have significant antiinflammatory effects or antiplatelet effects; it produces antipyresis by direct action on the hypothalamic heat-regulating center. These agents are indicated in the relief of mild to moderate pain; as an analgesic–antipyretic in the presence of aspirin allergy, hemostatic disturbances, bleeding diatheses, upper-GI disease, and gouty arthritis.

PROPOXYPHENE HYDROCHLORIDE

(Dextropropoxyphene, Darvon)

Propoxyphene (65 mg every 4 hours as needed) is indicated in the relief of mild to moderate pain. It is structurally very similar to methadone and possesses four stereoisomers. Dextropropoxyphene is an analgesic with a potency two-thirds that of codeine. Levopropoxyphene is an antitussive but lacks analgesic properties.

Adverse reactions to dextropropoxyphene include nausea, vomiting, sedation, dizziness, constipation, and skin rash, with a frequency of incidence somewhat less than that seen with codeine use. Although respiratory depression is a cardinal sign of acute dextropropoxyphene poisoning, the drug apparently does not affect respiration in the usual therapeutic doses of 32 to 65 mg.

The symptoms of overdosage are usually somnolent but may be stuporous or comatose and convulsing. Respiratory depression is characteristic; the ventilatory rate or tidal volume is decreased, resulting in cyanosis and hypoxia. Pupils, initially pinpoint, may dilate as hypoxia increases. Cheyne–Stokes respiration and apnea may occur. BP falls, and cardiac performance deteriorates, resulting in pulmonary edema and circulatory collapse, unless corrected promptly. Cardiac arrhythmias and conduction delay may be present. A combined respiratory–metabolic acidosis occurs due to hypercapnia and lactic acid formation. Death may occur. Naloxone (0.4 to 2 mg IV) reverses the propoxyphene-induced respiratory depression.

PROPOXYPHENE HYDROCHLORIDE/ASPIRIN/CAFFEINE

(Darvon compound-65 pulvules 65 mg propoxyphene hydrochloride, 389 mg aspirin, 32.4 caffeine)

Propoxyphene hydrochloride is an opioid analgesic combination that relieves pain by stimulating opiate receptors in the CNS. **Aspirin** inhibits prostaglandin synthesis, resulting in analgesia, antiinflammatory activity, and inhibition of platelet aggregation. **Caffeine** is thought to produce constriction of cerebral blood vessels. These agents are indicated in the relief of mild to moderate pain.

PROPRANOLOL

(Inderal)

Propranolol, a noncardioselective beta-adrenoreceptor blocker (80 to 480 mg/day p.o.) is approved for more indications than any other beta-adrenergic-receptor-blocking drug. The three major areas of use in cardiovascular medicine are the management of CAD, the treatment of hypertension, and the treatment and prophylaxis of supraventricular and ventricular arrhythmias. In addition, propranolol has many other uses and has had a major impact on areas of medicine remote from cardiology and hypertension (see Figures 69, 70, and 83).

Propranolol has an oxypropanolamine side chain attached to the 1 position of naphthalene. All beta-adrenergic-blocking drugs, including propranolol, have asymmetric centers at the beta-carbon to which the –OH is attached.

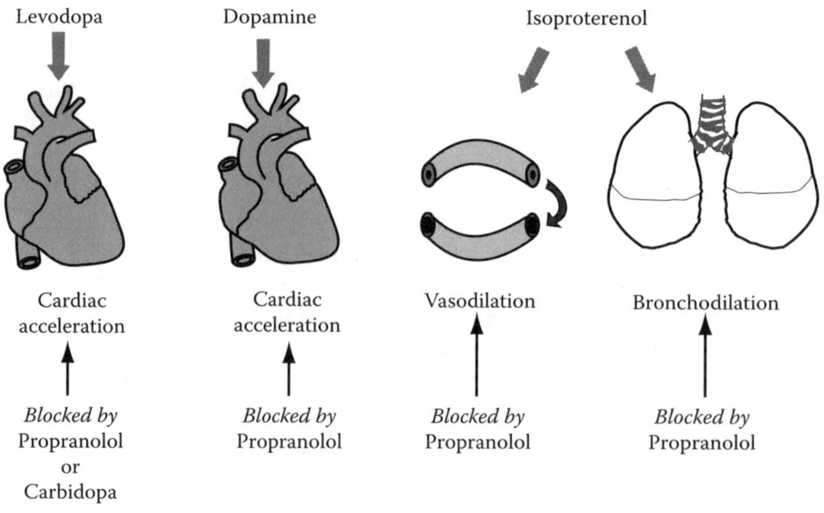

FIGURE 83 Therapeutic doses of levodopa produce cardiac stimulation by activating the $beta_1$-receptor site in the heart. The cardiac stimulation is blocked by **propranolol**, a beta-adrenergic-receptor-blocking agent, or carbidopa, a peripheral dopa decarboxylase inhibitor.

The major effect of propranolol is to antagonize the action of norepinephrine and epinephrine at all beta-adrenergic receptors. However, it does not distinguish between receptor subtypes, and is therefore called a nonselective beta-adrenergic blocker. The beta-adrenergic-receptor antagonism produced by propranolol is competitive in that it binds reversibly with high affinity to the beta-adrenergic receptor, but it can be displaced by a sufficiently high concentration of agonist. Although propranolol binds to the same site on the receptor as the agonists, the antagonist does not trigger any response, indicating that it does not have any agonist or intrinsic sympathomimetic activity.

Propranolol is converted to a large number of metabolites resulting from oxidation or conjugation of the aromatic ring, the side chain, or both. One metabolite, 4-hydroxypropranolol, is an active beta-adrenergic blocker having nearly the same activity as the parent compound and is formed in substantial quantities only after oral dosing. However, the metabolite has a half-life that is shorter than that of propranolol and thus accumulates less than the parent drug during multiple-dose therapy. For this reason, the metabolite does not make a substantial contribution to the beta-adrenergic blockade that is present during chronic therapy.

When given intravenously, propranolol is extracted approximately 90% from the blood on a single passage through the liver, resulting in a clearance of 1.0 to 1.2 L/min, which is close to hepatic blood flow.

Because of the high hepatic extraction of propranolol, changes in hepatic blood flow can alter the delivery of propranolol to the liver and affect the drug's clearance. Because beta-adrenergic blockade with propranolol reduces cardiac output and hepatic blood flow, the drug reduces its own clearance. This effect accounts for the fact that (+)-propranolol, which does not produce beta-adrenergic blockade, has a higher clearance than racemic propranolol, which reduces hepatic blood flow.

After the first dose of propranolol, cardiac output and heart rate are reduced with a reflex rise in peripheral vascular resistance such that arterial pressure is little changed. When given acutely, propranolol reduces renal blood flow because of the reduction in cardiac output and the reflex rise in vascular resistance. When given chronically, propranolol may continue to produce small reductions in renal blood flow and glomerular filtration rate. These effects are usually of no clinical consequence (Table 24).

Propranolol gains ready access to the brain because of its lipophilicity, and it can produce side effects attributable to CNS function. The genesis of these side effects is unclear. Do they occur because propranolol interacts with beta-adrenergic receptors in the brain, or are they related to nonspecific effects of the drug? It seems unlikely that propranolol dissolved in brain lipid would produce abnormalities in neuronal function, but it is conceivable that the drug could reach high enough concentrations to produce membrane-stabilizing effects. However, beta-adrenergic-receptor-blocking drugs that are less lipid soluble and do not have membrane-stabilizing effects also can produce symptoms attributable to action in the CNS, suggesting that blockade of beta-adrenergic receptors in the brain is likely to account for some of the side effects. Water-soluble drugs are claimed to have fewer side effects attributable to CNS dysfunction. However, it has been suggested recently that the magnitude of the CNS effects of the lipophilic and hydrophilic drugs is similar, but the time course of these effects varies.

Propranolol has spermicidal effects at high concentrations. Such concentrations are not achieved in sperm or seminal fluid but may be achieved in cervical mucus in women taking the drug. The clinical importance of this observation is unknown, but it should be kept in mind as a potential explanation for infertility in women receiving propranolol.

Stimulation of the beta$_2$-adrenergic receptors on skeletal muscle will cause a tremor that can be blocked by propranolol.

Propranolol has been shown to be effective in the management of angina pectoris, myocardial infarction, ventricular and supraventricular arrhythmias, hypertension, aortic dissection, hypertrophic cardiomyopathy, mitral valve prolapse, thyrotoxicosis, migraine, tremor, and performance anxiety (stage fright).

Patients with compensated heart failure often have increased sympathetic nervous activity as a compensatory mechanism. Propranolol can precipitate acute exacerbation of CHF in such patients.

Propranolol effectively blocks the beta$_2$-adrenergic receptors that mediate bronchodilation. Patients with bronchospastic pulmonary disease may develop exacerbations when given propranolol, and such attacks are resistant to therapy with beta-adrenergic-receptor agonists. Thus, propranolol should never be given to an asthmatic patient. Patients with bronchospastic pulmonary disease in remission also should not receive propranolol; however, if a beta-adrenergic-receptor blocker is required, a beta$_1$-selective drug should be chosen.

Hepatic dysfunction can decrease the clearance of propranolol because of reduced metabolic enzyme activity and reduced hepatic blood flow.

PROPRANOLOL HYDROCHLORIDE/HYDROCHLOROTHIAZIDE (HCTZ)

(Inderide tablets 40 mg propranolol/25 mg HCTZ, tablets 80 mg propranolol/25 mg HCTZ)

Propranolol hydrochloride is an antihypertensive combination. **Propranolol** blocks beta receptors, primarily affecting the cardiovascular system (decreases heart rate, cardiac contractility, and BP) and lungs (promotes bronchospasm). **HCTZ** increases chloride, sodium, and water excretion by interfering with transport of sodium ions across renal tubular epithelium. Both agents are indicated in the management of hypertension.

TABLE 24
Drugs Used in the Treatment of Chronic Postural Hypotension

Drugs	Routes	Doses	Likely Duration of Action (hr)
Mineralocorticoids			
Fludrocortisone acetate	Oral	0.1–1 mg	12–24
Prostaglandin synthetase inhibitors			
Indomethacin	Oral	25–50 mg	8–12
Flurbiprofen	Oral	50–200 mg	8–12
Beta-adrenergic-receptor agonists/antagonists			
Propranolol	Oral	10–80 mg	8–12
Pindolol	Oral	5–15 mg	8–12
Xamoterol	Oral	200 mg	12
Alpha-adrenergic-receptor agonists/antagonists			
Phenylpropanolamine	Oral	25–75 mg	203
Phenylephrine	Oral	30 mg	4–6
Ephedrine	Oral	30 mg	4–6
Clonidine	Oral	0.2–0.4 mg	6–8
Yohimbine	Oral	5 mg	8–12
Monoamine-oxidase inhibitors			
Tranylcypromine	Oral	10–20 mg	8–12
Phenelzine	Oral	15 mg	8
Vasopressors			
Dihydroergotamine	SC	10 mcg/kg	8–12
Ergotamine	Oral	1–4 mg	4–6
Desmopressin	Nasal	5–40 mcg	8–24
	IM	2–4 mcg	8–24
Somatostatin	SC	0.2–0.4 mcg/kg	12–24
Dopamine antagonists			
Domperidone	Oral	10 mg	8–12

Note: SC = subcutaneous; IM = intramuscular.

PROPYLTHIOURACIL (PTU)

Propylthiouracil, a thyroid hormone antagonist, is used in hyperthyroidism, in thyrotoxic crisis, and in preparation for thyroidectomy (see also Figure 66).

PROTAMINE SULFATE

Protamine sulfate, a heparin antagonist, is used in heparin overdose (see also Table 17).

PROTEASE INHIBITORS

Cellular proteases are required for processing many protein antigens. Protease inhibitors with specificities for cathepsin-like enzymes, such as leupeptin, block the presentation of protein antigens by antigen-presenting cells (APC). The function of proteases is to cleave native protein antigens into small peptides. These proteases also probably act on the invariant chain, promoting its dissociation from class II MHC (major histocompatability complex) molecules. Many cellular proteases function optimally at acid pH, and this is probably the reason antigen processing occurs best in acidic compartments.

Novel cysteine protease and serine protease inhibitors are being developed for respiratory and CV applications, for cancer and inflammation, and for viral targets. Indinovir and ritonavir are potent HIV inhibitors.

HIV-1 encodes an aspartate protease consisting, in its active form, of two symmetric subunits. This enzyme is required for cleavage of polypeptide precursors that generate the structural proteins and enzymes of the virus, including reverse transcriptase, integrase, and the protease itself.

Other inhibitors interact with catalytic residues and displace a structural water molecule. These protease inhibitors block viral maturation and are therefore active in both acutely and chronically infected cells. Resistance to these agents develops *in vitro* and in patients treated over a period of months, and may limit the usefulness of monotherapy. However, viruses with reduced susceptibility to structurally similar compounds may retain susceptibility to others. Some of these protease inhibitors lack *in vivo* activity because of high plasma-protein binding, particularly to alpha-1 acid glycoprotein, low oral bioavailability, and/or short plasma elimination half-lives. Most peptidomimetic inhibitors are cleared through cytochrome P450 metabolism in the liver and GI tract. However, saquinavir (600 mg three times a day) has been well tolerated and associated with antiretroviral effects despite low oral bioavailability (approximately 4%). About 50% of patients have emergence of resistance, generally of moderate degree (three- to tenfold) after 1 year.

PROTEASOME INHIBITORS IN CANCER THERAPY

A perfect cancer treatment in a world of perfectly treatable cancers would target only the unique features of malignant cells and leave normal cells untouched. In the real world of real cancers, cancer-specific alterations of common pathways have been identified that can offer opportunities for the development of targeted drugs. A recent successful example is STI 571, which has been used to target the deregulated tyrosine-kinase bcr-abl in **CML**. This is recognized as a key translocation in this disease. Unfortunately, most cancers have many mutations, and several molecules may have to be targeted for success. Furthermore, recent data provide strong evidence that this process is not exclusively determined by mutations of the genome but is also driven by the tumor microenvironment, and that, in principle, the process is reversible.

A key regulator of many molecular pathways in eukaryotic cells is the **ubiquitin/26S proteasome system**. It has the potential to take a unique position as a master controller that integrates multiple physiologic signals in a cell, and its interaction with pathways that are abnormal in cancer is an area of growing interest. Cancers and rapidly growing embryonic cells generally have higher levels of proteasome activity than their normal well-differentiated counterparts. The reason for this is unknown, but it may relate to the needs of rapidly proliferating cells, or to higher levels of oxidative stress, or to cytokines and growth factors. Proteasome structure and function appears to depend on the demands put on the cell and can be modulated by many factors. For example, the **cytokine interferon-γ** (IFN-γ) and **tumor necrosis factor-α** (TNF-α) affect proteasome structure as well as function, and we have evidence suggesting that autocrine **interleukin-3** (IL-3) production by cancer cells increases proteasome activity. Autocrine loops involving growth factors and their receptors, which are frequently overexpressed in cancer, may therefore drive alterations in proteasome structure and function. In addition, the proinflammatory tumor environment contains high levels of growth factors that might act through paracrine action to affect proteasomes. Also, hypoxia/reperfusion within the tumor microenvironment is known to affect the distribution and function of proteasomes. Differences in proteasomes between cancer and normal cells suggest that they may serve as a promising target for cancer therapy.

The proteasome field has exploded in the years since the proteasome's discovery in the early 1990s. The proteasome is a highly conserved multicatalytic protease that is responsible for cellular protein turnover, and by definition governs critical processes in cell biology. This field is no less complex and exciting than the more trodden path of transcription and protein synthesis. The unique biochemistry of the proteasome as one of nature's most fascinating proteases has allowed chemists to develop synthetic inhibitors of this most intriguing enzyme. Although chemists applied their skills to developing mechanism-based inhibitors, it was also revealed that Mother Nature had evolved her own inhibitors, natural products, secondary metabolites, all with origins in bacteria.

Although all these investigations represent an enzymologist's dreamscape for academic investigation, the development of "tool drugs" to inhibit the proteasome has allowed an even more impressive number of studies in cell biology to interrogate the function of the ubiquitin proteasome pathway in numerous cell lines. Such research has allowed the determination of the function, temporal presence of short-lived proteins, antigen presentation, cell-cycle regulation, transcriptional activation, cell adhesion, and apoptosis, to name a few processes.

The development of **proteasome inhibitors** in treatment of multiple myeloma and probably other cancers has followed an unusual course, but is clearly linked to recent basic advances in our understanding of intracellular protein breakdown. After the discovery of the ATP-dependent pathway for protein degradation in the 1970s, ATP was shown as necessary for the conjugation of ubiquitin to cell proteins, which marks them for degradation by the 26S proteasome. Its 19S regulatory complex uses ATP to unfold proteins and to inject them into the 20S core proteasome where proteins are digested to small peptides. The active sites in the 20S proteasome function by a novel threonine-based mechanism that allows their selective inhibition (e.g., by the boronate, Velcade). The availability of proteasome inhibitors has greatly advanced our understanding of the many functions of the proteasome, such as its key role in the activation of the transcription factor NF-KB, which led to a recognition that proteasome inhibitors might have antiinflammatory and antineoplastic actions. The unexpected discovery that these inhibitors cause apoptosis selectively in neoplastic cells led to systematic studies and clinical trials against cancer. Amongst their multiple actions, proteasome inhibitors cause the accumulation of abnormal proteins that can trigger apoptosis; stabilize tumor suppressors (p53, p27); and inhibit production of NF-κB, which is antiapoptic and generates important growth factors and cell adhesion molecules. However, the actual importance of these mechanisms *in vivo* in combating cancer remains uncertain.

The transcription factor nuclear factor kappa B (NF-κB) is a member of the Rel family of proteins that plays an important role in a variety of cellular response mechanisms including immunity, inflammation, cell growth, and apoptosis. Recent evidence suggests that this transcription factor is induced following exposure of cancer cells to apoptotic stimuli such as tumor necrosis factor (TNF), chemotherapy, and irradiation. The activation of NF-κB involves the proteasome-dependent degradation of an inhibitor of NF-κB and results in a cascade of events leading to the suppression of apoptosis.

The **ubiquitin-proteasome pathway** has emerged as a major player in regulating several important signaling processes such as cell proliferation and inflammation. As a result, proteasome inhibitors are being intensely pursued as both molecular probes of proteasome biology and as therapeutic agents. Thus far, many proteasome inhibitors have been synthesized or isolated from natural sources, some of which are in clinical trial for cancer therapy.

The **cyclin-dependent kinases** (CDKs) are essential for cell-cycle progression. Cyclins and CDK inhibitors regulate the activity of CDKs, and, in turn, the proteasome regulates these proteins. Destruction of proteins that prevent transition into anaphase or S phase is controlled by two dedicated multiprotein complexes—the anaphase-promoting complex (APC) and Skpl-cullin-F-box protein ligase complex. These gatekeepers include **ubiquitin E3 ligases** that specify the proteins that will be targeted for degradation by the proteasome. Proteasome activity is required for progression through the cell cycle; and when proteasome activity is disrupted by any of a number of small molecule inhibitors, cell-cycle arrest follows. The presence or absence of p53 affects proteasome inhibitor-induced cell-cycle arrest: in p53+ cells, proteasome inhibitors cause arrest at the G_1S boundary, whereas proteasome inhibition in p53 cells leads to G_2M phase arrest. In some instances, proteasome inhibition also culminates in cell death; however, proteasome inhibitor-induced apoptosis may be a consequence of effects on pathways not directly involved in cell-cycle progression, and may also be dependent on the specific proteasome inhibitor or cell line.

A series of peptidic boronic acids that inhibit the activity of the proteasome were screened by the NCI for activity against a panel of 60 human tumor cell lines. Comparison to data from approximately 80,000 other compounds demonstrated that these proteasome inhibitors exhibited a novel pattern of growth inhibition against these cell lines. The potency of these compounds in the cell-line screen correlated well with activity against purified proteasomes, indicating that proteasome inhibition was likely causing the growth inhibition. Comparison of **bortezomib** (formerly known as PS-341) sensitivity to expression levels of thousands of molecular targets within the 60-cell-line panel did not yield strong correlations with any single molecular target, consistent with the role of the proteasome in degradation of a multitude of proteins.

Radiation is an important modality of therapy for a variety of cancers, including squamous cell carcinomas (SCC) of the head and neck and skin. Cell survival and resistance following radiation are mediated by cytoprotective molecules that regulate cell-cycle progression and cell death. Constitutive and radiation-induced activation of the transcription factor nuclear factor-KB (NF-κB) and cell-cycle regulatory proteins have been shown to contribute to differences in resistance of SCC to radiation. NF-κB and one of its target genes, cyclin Dl, are regulated by signal activation and degradation of inhibitor-κBs by the proteasome. In addition, the proteasome degrades cyclin inhibitors. Scientists have investigated the effects of the proteasome inhibitor **bortezomib** (PS-341, Velcade) on NF-κB activation and cell-cycle regulatory protein expression, as well as cell-cycle and radiosensitizing effects in SCC. Bortezomib produced accumulation of cyclin inhibitor p21 and inhibited activation of NF-κB and cyclin Dl. Bortezomib had direct cytotoxic activity, and an accumulation of SCC cells in the radiosensitive G_2/M phase of the cell cycle was accompanied by further radiosensitization.

Anthracycline chemotherapeutics display activity against a broad range of cancers and are therefore in clinical use for therapy of patients with both hematologic malignancies and solid tumors. However, these drugs have the ability to activate pathways such as nuclear factor-κB and p44/42 mitogen-activated protein kinase that play roles in inductible chemoresistance and promote tumor-cell survival. Because proteasome inhibitors block activation of these pathways, it is possible that combinations of an anthracycline and a proteasome inhibitor could induce higher levels of tumor-cell apoptosis. Furthermore, other mechanisms of resistance to **anthracyclines**, such as P-glycloprotein expression and downregulation of topoisomerase II, may also be abrogated by proteasome inhibitors, further supporting the development of such a regimen. Furthermore, **bortezomib** has the potential to simultaneously enhance the anticancer efficacy of **cisplatin** and to prevent the emergence of DNA-repair **enzyme excision repair cross-complementation group 1**(ERCC-1)-dependent cisplatin resistance.

PROTRIPTYLINE HYDROCHLORIDE

(Triptil, Vivactil)

Protriptyline, a tricyclic antidepressant (15 to 40 mg p.o. daily), is used in the treatment of depression (see also Tables 5 through 7).

PRUSSIAN BLUE

(Radiogardase capsules 0.5 g)

Prussian blue is a chelating agent. It insolubly binds radioactive and nonradioactive cesium and thallium in the GI tract by ion-exchange, adsorption, and mechanical trapping within the crystal structure. It is indicated in the treatment of patients with known or suspected internal contamination with radioactive cesium and/or radioactive or nonradioactive thallium to increase the rate of their elimination.

PSEUDOEPHEDRINE HYDROCHLORIDE

PSEUDOEPHEDRINE SULFATE

(Afrinol, Cenafed, Decofed, Dorcol, Efidac 24, Myfedrine, NeoFed, Novafed, PediaCare, Pseudogest, Sudafed, Sinufed)

Pseudoephedrine, a sympathomimetic agent with decongestant properties (60 mg p.o. q. 4 to 6 hours), is used in nasal and eustachian tube decongestion.

PSEUDOEPHEDRINE HYDROCHLORIDE/ GUAIFENESIN/DEXTROMETHORPHAN HBR

(PanMist-DM syrup 15 mg dextromethorphan HBr, 100 mg guaifenesin, 40 mg pseudoephedrine hydrochloride per 5 mL, tablets 32 mg dextromethorphan HBr, 595 mg guaifenesin, 48 mg pseudoephedrine hydrochloride)

Pseudoephedrine hydrochloride/guaifenesin/dextromethorphan HBr is an antitussive and expectorant combination. **Pseudoephedrine** causes vasoconstriction and subsequent shrinkage of nasal mucous membranes by alpha-adrenergic stimulation, which promotes nasal drainage. **Guaifenesin** may enhance output of respiratory tract fluid by reducing adhesiveness and surface tension, enhancing removal of viscous mucus and making nonproductive coughs more productive and less frequent. **Dextromethorphan** suppresses cough by central action on the cough center in medulla. These agents are indicated in the temporary relief of nasal congestion and cough associated with respiratory tract infections and related conditions, such as sinusitis, pharyngitis, bronchitis, and asthma, when these conditions are complicated by tenacious mucus or mucus plugs and congestion.

PSYCHIATRIC SYMPTOMS CAUSED BY DRUGS

Drugs	Reactions
Acyclovir	Hallucinations, fearfulness, confusion, insomnia, hyperacusis, paranoia, depression
Albuterol	Hallucinations, paranoia
Alprazolam	See Benzodiazepines
Amantadine	Visual hallucinations, paranoid delusions, nightmares, mania, exacerbation of schizophrenia
Aminocaproic acid	Acute delirium, hallucinations
Amiodarone (Cordarone)	Delirium, hallucinations
Amitriptyline	See Antidepressants
Amphetamine-like drugs	Bizarre behavior, hallucinations, paranoia, agitation, anxiety, manic symptoms, depression
Amphotericin B	Delirium
Anabolic steroids	Aggression, mania, depression, psychosis
Anticholinergics and atropine	Confusion, memory loss, disorientation, depersonalization, delirium, auditory and visual hallucinations, fear, paranoia, agitation, bizarre behavior
	Sudden incoherent speech, delirium with high fever, flushed dry skin, hallucinations, retrograde amnesia
Anticonvulsants	Agitation, confusion, delirium, depression, psychosis, aggression, mania, toxic encephalopathy
Antidepressants, tricyclic	Mania or hypomania, delirium, hallucinations, paranoia
Antihistamines	Hallucinations
Asparaginase	Confusion, depression, paranoia
Atenolol	See Beta-adrenergic blockers
Atropine	See Anticholinergics and atropine
Baclofen	Hallucinations, paranoia, nightmares, mania, depression, anxiety, confusion
Barbiturates	Excitement, hyperactivity, visual hallucinations, depression, delirium-tremens-like syndrome
Belladonna alkaloids	See Atropine and Anticholinergics
Benzodiazepines	Rage, hostility, paranoia, hallucinations, delirium, depression, nightmares, anterograde amnesia, mania
Beta-adrenergic blockers	Depression, confusion, nightmares, hallucinations, paranoia, delusions, mania, hyperactivity
Betaxolol	See Beta-adrenergic blockers
Biperiden	See Anticholinergics and Atropine
Bromocriptine	Mania, delusions, hallucinations, paranoia, aggressive behavior, schizophrenic relapse, depression, anxiety
Desipramine	See Antidepressants, tricyclic
Diazepam	See Benzodiazepines
Diethylpropion	See Amphetamine-like drugs
Digitalis glycosides	Nightmares, confusion, paranoia, depression, visual hallucinations
Diltiazem	Depression, suicidal thoughts
Disopyramide	Hallucinations, paranoia, panic, depression
Disulfiram	Catatonia, delirium, depression, psychosis
Dronabinol	Anxiety, disorientation, psychosis
Enalapril	Agitation, depression, panic, hallucinations
Ephedrine	Hallucinations, paranoia
Ethchlorvynol	Agitation, hallucinations, paranoia
Ethionamide	Depression, hallucinations
Ethosuximide	See Anticonvulsants
Etretinate	Severe depression
Famotidine	See Histamine H_2-receptor antagonists
Fenfluramine	See Amphetamine-like drugs

PSYCHIATRIC SYMPTOMS CAUSED BY DRUGS (Continued)

Drugs	Reactions
Flecainide	Visual hallucinations
Fluoxetine	Mania, hypomania, depersonalization
Flurbiprofen	See Nonsteroidal antiinflammatory drugs
Fluvoxamine	Mania, hypomania
Ganciclovir	Hallucinations, delirium, confusion, agitation
Gentamicin	Confusion, disorientation, hallucinations
Histamine H_2-receptor antagonists	Hallucinations, paranoia, bizarre behavior, delirium, disorientation, depression, mania
Hydroxychloroquine	Irritability, difficulty concentrating, psychosis
Ibuprofen	See Nonsteroidal antiinflammatory drugs
Imipramine	See Antidepressants, tricyclic
Indomethacin	See Nonsteroidal antiinflammatory drugs
Iohexol	Confusion, disorientation
Iopamidol	Confusion, disorientation
Isocarboxazid	Mania, insomnia, anxiety, paranoid delusions
Isoniazid	Depression, agitation, hallucinations, paranoia
Isosorbide dinitrate	Hallucinations, depression, suicidal thoughts
Isotretinoin	Depression
Ketamine	Nightmares, hallucinations, crying, delirium
Ketoconazole	Hallucinations
Levodopa	Delirium, depression, agitation, hypomania, nightmares, night terrors, hallucinations, paranoia
Lidocaine	See Procaine
Loperamide	Delirium
Lorazepam	See Benzodiazepines
Lovastatin	Depression
Loxapine	Mania
Maprotiline	Hallucinations, agitation, disorientation
Mefloquine	Psychosis, panic attacks, depression
Methadone	See Narcotics
Methandrostenolone	See Anabolic steroids
Meperidine	See Narcotics
Methyldopa	Depression, amnesia, nightmares, psychosis
Methylphenidate	Hallucinations, paranoia
Methyltestosterone	See Anabolic steroids
Methysergide	Depersonalization, hallucinations, agitation
Metoclopramide	Mania, severe depression, crying, delirium
Metrizamide	Confusion, hallucinations, depression, anxiety
Metronidazole	Depression, agitation, uncontrollable crying, disorientation, hallucinations
Midazolam	See Benzodiazepines
Misoprostol	Delirium
Morphine	See Narcotics
Nalidixic acid	Confusion, depression, hallucinations
Nalorphine	See Narcotics
Naloxone	Violent behavior
Naproxen	See Nonsteroidal antiinflammatory drugs
Narcotics	Nightmares, anxiety, agitation, euphoria, dysphoria, depression, paranoia, hallucinations
Nifedipine	Irritability, agitation, panic, belligerence, depression
Niridazole	Confusion, hallucinations, mania, suicide
Nonsteroidal antiinflammatory drugs	Paranoia, depression, anxiety, disorientation, hallucinations
Norfloxacin	Depression, anxiety
Nortriptyline	See Antidepressants
Ofloxacin	Delirium, depression and mania, catatonia
Oxandrolone	See Anabolic steroids
Oxymetazoline	Hallucinations
Oxymetholone	See Anabolic steroids
Pargyline	Manic psychosis
Penicillin G procaine	See Procaine derivatives
Pentazocine	See Narcotics
Pergolide	Hallucinations, paranoia, confusion, anxiety, depression
Phenelzine	Paranoia, delusions, fear, mania, rage
Phenmetrazine	See Amphetamine-like drugs
Phentermine	See Amphetamine-like drugs
Phenylephrine	Depression, hallucinations, paranoia, delusions
Phenylpropanolamine	See Amphetamine-like drugs
Phenytoin	See Anticonvulsants
Podophyllin	Delirium, paranoia, bizarre behavior
Polythiazide	See Thiazides
Pravastatin	Depression
Prazosin	Hallucinations, depression, paranoia
Primidone	See Anticonvulsants
Procainamide	See Procaine derivatives
Procaine derivatives	Confusion, "doom" anxiety, psychosis, agitation, bizarre behavior, depression, panic
Procarbazine	Mania
Promethazine	Hallucinations, terror
Propafenone	Agitation, delusions, disorientation, mania, paranoia
Propoxyphene	See Narcotics
Propranolol	See Beta-adrenergic blockers
Pseudoephedrine	Hallucinations, paranoia
Quinacrine	Mania, paranoia, anxiety, hallucinations, delirium

PSYCHIATRIC SYMPTOMS CAUSED BY DRUGS (CONTINUED)

Drugs	Reactions
Quinidine	Confusion, agitation, psychosis
Ranitidine	See Histamine H_2-receptor antagonists
Reserpine	Depression, nightmares
Salicylates	Agitation, confusion, hallucinations, paranoia
Scopolamine	See Atropine and Anticholinergics
Selegiline	Hallucinations, mania, nightmares
Simvastatin	Depression
Sulfonamides	Confusion, disorientation, depression, euphoria, hallucinations
Sulindac	See Nonsteroidal antiinflammatory drugs
Tamoxifen	Delusions
Theophylline	Withdrawal, mutism, hyperactivity, anxiety, mania
Thiabendazole	Psychosis
Thiazides	Depression, suicidal ideation
Thyroid hormones	Mania, depression, hallucinations, paranoia
Timolol	See Beta-adrenergic blockers
Tobramycin	Delirium, hallucinations, agitation
Tocainide	See Procaine derivatives
Tranylcypromine	Mania or hypomania
Trazodone	Delirium, hallucinations, paranoia, mania
Triazolam	See Benzodiazepines
Trichlormethiazide	See Thiazides
Trihexyphenidyl	See Atropine and Anticholinergics
Trimethoprim-sulfamethoxazole	Psychosis, depression, disorientation, hallucinations, delusions
Valproic acid	See Anticonvulsants
Verapamil	Auditory, visual, and tactile hallucinations
Vincristine	Hallucinations
Zidovudine	Mania, paranoia, hallucinations

The drug-induced psychiatric symptoms are dose-dependent, of idiosyncratic nature, and reversible.

PSYCHOTROPIC MEDICATIONS: Side Effects of

ACETOPHENAZINE, see Phenothiazines, piperazine
ALPRAZOLAM, see Benzodiazepines
AMITRIPTYLINE, see Tricyclic antidepressants
AMOXAPINE, see Tricyclic antidepressants
BENZODIAZEPINES (alprazolam, chlordiazepoxide, clorazepate, diazepam, halazepam, lorazepam, oxazepam, prazepam, temazepam)
Frequent: Drowsiness; ataxia
Occasional: Confusion; amnesia; disinhibition; paradoxical excitement; depression; dizziness; withdrawal symptoms, including convulsions, on abrupt discontinuance (withdrawal may be especially difficult with alprazolam); rebound insomnia or excitement
Rare: Hypotension; blood dyscrasias; jaundice; allergic reactions; paradoxical rage reactions; stuttering with alprazolam
BUPROPION, Anxiety; agitation; insomnia; tremor; anorexia
BUSPIRONE, Dizziness; headache; nausea; paresthesias; diarrhea
CHLORDIAZEPOXIDE, see Benzodiazepines
CHLORPROMAZINE, see Phenothiazines, aliphatic
CHLORPROTHIXENE, similar to Phenothiazines
CLOMIPRAMINE, see Tricyclic antidepressants
CLORAZEPATE, see Benzodiazepines
CLOZAPINE
Frequent: Drowsiness; anticholinergic effects; postural hypotension; increase in body temperature; increased salivation; ECG changes
Occasional: Constipation; hypertension; granulocytopenia; agranulocytosis in 1 to 2%; seizures
DESIPRAMINE, see Tricyclic antidepressants
DIAZEPAM, see Benzodiazepines
DOXEPIN, see Tricyclic antidepressants
FLUOXETINE
Frequent: Nausea; nervousness; headache; insomnia; sexual dysfunction (anorgasmia)
Occasional: Akathisia; rash; fever; arthralgia; mania; aminotransferase elevations; abulia; alopecia
Rare: Extrapyramidal reactions; seizures in patients with preexisting seizure disorder; leukocytosis; bradycardia with syncope; respiratory distress
FLUPHENAZINE, see Phenothiazines, piperazine
HALAZEPAM, see Benzodiazepines
HALOPERIDOL
Extrapyramidal effects (especially in young patients); blood dyscrasias; postural hypotension; sedation; menstrual changes; galactorrhea; tardive dyskinesia; cholestatic jaundice; photosensitivity; rash; weight gain; convulsions; impotence; neurotoxicity in hyperthyroid patients; neuroleptic malignant syndrome
IMIPRAMINE, see Tricyclic antidepressants
ISOCARBOXAZID, see MAO inhibitors
LITHIUM
At therapeutic serum concentrations (0.6–1.2 mEq/L): Thirst; polyuria; fine tremor; GI irritation; mild diarrhea; weight gain; edema; acne; leukocytosis
At toxic serum concentrations (above 2 mEq/L): Confusion; vomiting; diarrhea; polyuria; muscle weakness; ataxia; lethargy; slurred speech; tinnitus; blurred vision; nystagmus; stupor; coma; convulsions; permanent neurologic impairment
Occasional: (at all serum concentrations): Goiter; hypothyroidism; nephrogenic diabetes insipidus; acne; renal tubular acidosis; metallic taste; induction or exacerbation of psoriasis; folliculitis; T-wave changes; nausea; extrapyramidal effects
Rare: (at all serum concentrations): Exophthalmos; cardiac arrhythmias; vomiting; acute renal failure; progressive decrease in renal function; Raynaud's phenomenon; hypoglycemia; hair loss; pseudotumor cerebri; hyperthyroidism; hyperparathyroidism; serum concentrations and toxic effects are increased by dehydration, diuretics, sweating, fever, protracted diarrhea, or diminished intake of sodium
LORAZEPAM, see Benzodiazepines
LOXAPINE, see Phenothiazines, piperazine

PSYCHOTROPIC MEDICATIONS: Side Effects of (Continued)

MAO INHIBITORS (isocarboxazid, phenelzine, tranylcypromine)
Hypotension; restlessness; insomnia; daytime sleepiness; mania; urinary retention; tremors; sexual disturbances; paresthesias; dry mouth; nausea; constipation; anorexia; weight gain; edema; rash; hepatitis; tinnitus; muscle spasm; lupus-like reaction; leukopenia; hyperthermia; hypertension; interactions with other drugs or foods may be severe

MAPROTILINE
Similar to tricyclics, but seizures occur more frequently (especially with more than 200 mg/day) and anticholinergic effects may occur less frequently

MESORIDAZINE, see Phenothiazines, piperidine

MOLINDONE
Extrapyramidal effects; akathisia; anticholinergic effects; drowsiness; dystonia; menstrual changes; anorexia; weight loss; rash; tardive dyskinesia; leukopenia; postural hypotension; ECG abnormalities; liver abnormalities; neuroleptic malignant syndrome

NORTRIPTYLINE, see Tricyclic antidepressants

OXAZEPAM, see Benzodiazepines

PERPHENAZINE, see Phenothiazines, piperazine

PHENELZINE, see MAO inhibitors

PHENOTHIAZINES, ALIPHATIC (chlorpromazine, triflupromazine)
Frequent: Drowsiness; anticholinergic effects; postural hypotension
Occasional: Extrapyramidal effects; galactorrhea; photosensitivity; menstrual changes; cholestatic jaundice; rashes; skin pigmentation; convulsions; ECG changes; tardive dyskinesia; weight gain; lenticular deposits and opacities; blood dyscrasias; gastritis, nausea and vomiting; dizziness and tremulousness following withdrawal of high-dose therapy; disturbed temperature regulation; lupus-like syndrome; neuroleptic malignant syndrome

PHENOTHIAZINES, PIPERAZINE (acetophenazine, fluphenazine, loxapine, perphenazine, prochlorperazine, trifluoperazine)
Frequent: Extrapyramidal effects
Occasional: Anticholinergic effects; photosensitivity; galactorrhea; menstrual changes; drowsiness; postural hypotension; anorexia; rash; tardive dyskinesia; weight gain
Rare: Cholestatic jaundice; blood dyscrasias; lenticular deposits and opacities; ECG abnormalities; convulsions; gastritis; neuroleptic malignant syndrome; nausea and vomiting; dizziness and tremulousness following withdrawal of high-dose therapy; disturbed temperature regulation

PHENOTHIAZINES, PIPERIDINE (mesoridazine, thioridazine)
Frequent: Drowsiness; anticholinergic effects; postural hypotension; weight gain; inhibition of ejaculation
Occasional: Extrapyramidal effects (but less than with aliphatic phenothiazines); menstrual changes; photosensitivity reactions; ECG abnormalities; galactorrhea; tardive dyskinesia
Rare: Pigmentary retinopathy (thioridazine has an 800 mg/day upper limit on recommended dosage because of a high incidence of pigmentary retinopathy); cholestatic jaundice; blood dyscrasias; dystonia; convulsions; rash; gastritis, nausea and vomiting; dizziness and tremulousness following withdrawal of high-dose therapy; disturbed temperature regulation; neuroleptic malignant syndrome; torsade de pointes; ventricular arrhythmia with thioridazine

PRAZEPAM, see Benzodiazepines

PROCHLORPERAZINE, see Phenothiazines, piperazine

PROTRIPTYLINE, see Tricyclic antidepressants

TEMAZEPAM, see Benzodiazepines

THIORIDAZINE, see Phenothiazines, piperidine

THIOTHIXENE
Frequent: Extrapyramidal effects; anticholinergic effects
Occasional: Galactorrhea; menstrual changes; drowsiness; postural hypotension; anorexia; rash; tardive dyskinesia
Rare: Blood dyscrasias; lenticular deposits and opacities (with long-term high dosage); ECG abnormalities; convulsions; neuroleptic malignant syndrome

TRANYLCYPROMINE, see MAO inhibitors

TRAZODONE
Frequent: Drowsiness; headaches; gastrointestinal upset
Occasional: Ventricular arrhythmias; peripheral edema
Rare: Priapism in men; increased libido

TRICYCLIC ANTIDEPRESSANTS (amitriptyline, amoxapine, clomipramine, desipramine, doxepin, imipramine, nortriptyline, protriptyline, trimipramine)
Frequent: Anticholinergic effects; hypotension (less with nortriptyline); drowsiness; weight gain; tachycardia
Occasional: Mania; psychosis; tremor; first-degree heart block; other ECG abnormalities; rash; sweating; confusion; insomnia; sexual disturbances, especially with clomipramine; increase in dental caries; gingivitis
Rare: Hepatic toxicity; tinnitus; bone marrow depression, including agranulocytosis; seizures; peripheral neuropathy; severe cardiovascular effects in patients with cardiac disease; photosensitivity; dysarthria; stuttering; withdrawal symptoms; nausea, tremor, anorgasmia, and seizures may be more common with clomipramine; tardive dyskinesia and neuroleptic malignant syndrome with amoxapine; renal failure with overdosage of amoxapine

TRIFLUOPERAZINE, see Phenothiazines, piperazine

TRIFLUPROMAZINE, see Phenothiazines, aliphatic

TRIMIPRAMINE, see Tricyclic antidepressants

PSYLLIUM

(e.g., Metamucil)

(Wafers: approximately 1.7 g psyllium mucilloid, 18 g carbohydrate, 18 mg sodium, 4.5 g fat, 96 calories per dose)

Psyllium, lignin, and pectin bind bile acids, reducing their intestinal reabsorption and promoting their excretion. The consequent enhancement of hepatic synthesis of bile acids from cholesterol may reduce plasma cholesterol in LDL. With several months of use, bulk-forming agents reduce intraluminal rectosigmoid pressure and relieve symptoms in patients with IBS and diverticular disease of the colon. The capacity of these agents to absorb water makes them useful in relieving the symptoms of mild diarrhea and in the regulation of effluent in patients with ileostomy or colostomy.

IBS is a functional bowel disorder exhibiting the following characteristics: abdominal pain, symptoms of disturbed defecation (urgency, straining, and feeling of incomplete evacuation), altered stool consistency, and altered stool frequency and timing. There are also symptoms of bloatedness (distention).

If diarrhea is the chief complaint, it is treated with loperamide or cholestyramine. Pain is treated with dicyclomine, amitriptyline, and peppermint oil. Bran and psyllium are used to treat the constipation that may occur in IBS. Flatulence is treated with simethicone.

PULMONARY TOXICITY: Drug-Induced

Drugs	Reactions
Amiodarone	Acute pneumonitis, fibrosis, hypersensitivity pneumonitis
Aspirin	see Salicylates
Atracurium	see Neuromuscular blockers
Azathioprine	Hypersensitivity pneumonitis
Beta-adrenergic blockers	Bronchospasm
Bleomycin	Acute pneumonitis, fibrosis, bronchiolitis obliterans, hypersensitivity pneumonitis
Bromocriptine	Pleuritis, fibrosis
Busulfan	Fibrosis
Captopril	Cough
Carbamazepine	Hypersensitivity pneumonitis
Carmustine	Acute pneumonitis, fibrosis
Chlorambucil	Acute pneumonitis, fibrosis
Cocaine	Edema, hemorrhage
Cyclophosphamide	Hypersensitivity pneumonitis, edema, fibrosis
Cytarabine	Edema
Dantrolene	Pleuritis, pneumonitis
Diclofenac	see NSAIDs
Enalapril	Cough
Ethchlorvynol	Edema
Gold salts	Hypersensitivity pneumonitis, fibrosis, bronchiolitis obliterans
Hydrochlorothiazide	Edema
Ibuprofen	see NSAIDs
Indomethacin	see NSAIDs
Interleukin-2 (Proleukin)	Edema
Lidocaine	Edema
Lisinopril	Cough
Lomustine	Fibrosis
Melphalan	Fibrosis
Methadone	see Opiates
Methotrexate	Pleuritis, hypersensitivity pneumonitis, edema, fibrosis
Methysergide	Pleuritis
Mitomycin	Acute pneumonitis, fibrosis
Naloxone	Edema
Naproxen	see NSAIDs
Neuromuscular blockers	Bronchospasm
Nitrofurantoin	Hypersensitivity pneumonitis, fibrosis
NSAIDs	Bronchospasm, hypersensitivity pneumonitis, edema, fibrosis
Opiates	Edema
Pancuronium	see Neuromuscular blockers
Penicillamine	Bronchiolitis obliterans, hypersensitivity pneumonitis, fibrosis, pulmonary–renal syndrome
Phenylbutazone	see NSAIDs
Phenytoin	Hypersensitivity pneumonitis
Pilocarpine	Bronchospasm
Pindolol	see Beta-adrenergic blockers
Piroxicam	see NSAIDs
Procarbazine	Hypersensitivity pneumonitis
Propafenone	Bronchospasm
Propoxyphene	see Opiates
Propranolol	see Beta-adrenergic blockers
Protamine	Edema
Pyrimethamine-chloroquine	Hypersensitivity pneumonitis
Pyrimethamine-dapsone	Hypersensitivity pneumonitis
Pyrimethamine-sulfadoxine	Hypersensitivity pneumonitis
Salicylates	Edema, bronchospasm
Semustine	Fibrosis
Sulfasalazine	Hypersensitivity pneumonitis, bronchiolitis obliterans, fibrosis
Sulindac	see NSAIDs
Suxamethonium	see Neuromuscular blockers
Terbutaline	Edema
Timolol	see Beta-adrenergic blockers
Tocainide	Pneumonitis, fibrosis
Ritodrine	Edema
Tryptophan	Pneumonitis
Tubocurarine	see Neuromuscular blockers
Vecuronium	see Neuromuscular blockers
Vinblastine	Acute pneumonitis, bronchospasm
Vindesine	Acute pneumonitis, bronchospasm

PYRANTEL PAMOATE

(Antiminth)

Pyrantel, a pyrimidine derivative with antihelmintic properties (single dose of 11 mg/kg p.o.), is used in the treatment of roundworm and pinworm infections.

PYRAZINAMIDE

(Pyrazinamide tablets 500 mg)

Pyrazinamide is an antituberculosis agent. Pyrazine analog of nicotinamide may be bacteriostatic or bactericidal against *Mycobacterium tuberculosis*. It is indicated in an initial treatment of active tuberculosis in adults and selected children when combined with other antituberculosis agents.

PYRIDOSTIGMINE BROMIDE

(Mestinon, Regonol)

Pyridostigmine, a cholinesterase inhibitor, is used as an antagonist for curariform paralysis and in myasthenia gravis.

PYRIDOXINE HYDROCHLORIDE

(Vitamin B_6) (Beesix, Hexa-Betalin, Nestrex)

Pyridoxine, a water-soluble vitamin, is used in dietary vitamin B_6 deficiency, seizures related to vitamin B_6 deficiency or dependency, vitamin B_6-responsive anemias or dependency syndrome (inborn errors of metabolism), prevention of vitamin B_6 deficiency during isoniazid therapy, and treatment of vitamin B_6 deficiency secondary to isoniazid.

PYRILAMINE MALEATE

(Nisaval)

Pyrilamine, an ethylenediamine antihistaminic substance, has mild sedative and antihistaminic properties with no anticholinergic and antiemetic actions. Pyrilamine (25 to 50 mg p.o. t.i.d.) is indicated in relief of symptoms associated with perennial and seasonal allergic rhinitis, vasomotor rhinitis, allergic conjunctivitis, temporary relief of runny nose and sneezing due to the common cold, allergic and nonallergic pruritic symptoms, mild, uncomplicated urticaria and angioedema, amelioration of allergic reactions to blood or plasma, dermatographism, and adjunctive therapy in anaphylactic reactions.

Pyrilamine competitively antagonizes histamine at the H_1-receptor site but does not bind with histamine to inactivate it. Terfenadine and astemizole, the most specific H_1 antagonists available, bind preferentially to peripheral rather than central H_1 receptors. Antihistamines do not block histamine release, antibody production, or antigen–antibody interactions. They antagonize in varying degrees most of the pharmacological effects of histamine.

PYRIMETHAMINE

(Daraprim)

Pyrimethamine (25 mg once weekly) is indicated in chemoprophylaxis of malaria due to susceptible strains of plasmodia. Fast-acting schizonticides (chloroquine or quinine) are preferable for treatment of acute attacks. However, concurrent pyrimethamine will initiate transmission control and a suppressive cure.

In addition, sulfadoxine and pyrimethamine (Fansidar) are indicated in prophylaxis of malaria in individuals traveling to areas where chloroquine-resistant *P. falciparum* malaria is endemic. However, resistant strains may be encountered. Regardless of the prophylactic regimen used, it is still possible to contract malaria. Moreover, this combination has been used as a prophylactic agent in the prevention of *Pneumocystis carinii* pneumonia in patients with AIDS.

Pyrimethamine is a folic-acid antagonist; its therapeutic action is based on differential requirements between host and parasite for nucleic acid precursors involved in growth as it selectively inhibits plasmodial dihydrofolate reductase. Pyrimethamine inhibits the enzyme dihydrofolate reductase that catalyzes the reduction of dihydrofolate to tetrahydrofolate. This activity is highly selective against plasmodia and *Toxoplasma gondii*. It does not destroy gametocytes but arrests sporogony in the mosquito. Pyrimethamine possesses a blood schizonticidal, and some tissue schizonticidal activity may be slower than that of 4-amino-quinoline compounds.

Overdose effects of pyrimethamine may include abdominal pain, nausea, and severe and repeated vomiting, possibly including hematemesis. CNS toxicity may be manifest by initial excitability, and generalized and prolonged convulsions that may be followed by respiratory depression, circulatory collapse, and death within a few hours. Neurological symptoms, including convulsive seizures, appear rapidly (30 minutes to 2 hours after drug ingestion), suggesting that in gross overdosage, pyrimethamine has a direct toxic effect on the CNS.

Q

QUAZEPAM

(Doral tablets 7.5 mg)

Quazepam is a benzodiazepine that potentiates action of GABA, an inhibitory neurotransmitter, resulting in increased neuronal inhibition and CNS depression, especially in the limbic system and reticular formation. It is indicated for short-term management of insomnia (see Table 9).

The physicochemical and pharmacokinetic properties of the benzodiazepines greatly affect their clinical utility. They all have high lipid–water distribution coefficients in the nonionized form; nevertheless, lipophilicity varies more than 50-fold according to the polarity and electronegativity of various substituents.

All the benzodiazepines are absorbed completely, with the exception of **clorazepate**; this drug is decarboxylated rapidly in gastric juice to ***N*-desmethyldiazepam** (nordazepam), which subsequently is absorbed completely. Some benzodiazepines (e.g., **prazepam** and **flurazepam**) reach the systemic circulation only in the form of active metabolites.

Drugs active at the benzodiazepine receptor may be divided into four categories based on their elimination half-lives: (1) ultra-short-acting benzodiazepines, (2) short-acting agents, with half-lives less than 6 hours, including **triazolam**, the nonbenzodiazepine **zolpidem** (half-life approximately 2 hours), and **zopiclone** (half-life 5 to 6 hours), (3) intermediate-acting agents, with half-lives of 6 to 24 hours, including estazolam and **temazepam**, and (4) long-acting agents, with half-lives of greater than 24 hours, including **flurazepam**, **diazepam**, and **quazepam**.

The benzodiazepines and their active metabolites bind to plasma proteins. The extent of binding correlates strongly with lipid solubility and ranges from about 70% for **alprazolam** to nearly 99% for diazepam. The concentration in the cerebrospinal fluid is approximately equal to the concentration of free drug in plasma. Competition with other protein-bound drugs may occur, but no clinically significant examples have been reported.

The plasma concentrations of most benzodiazepines exhibit patterns that are consistent with two-compartment models, but three-compartment models appear to be more appropriate for the compounds with the highest lipid solubility. Accordingly, there is rapid uptake of benzodiazepines into the brain and other highly perfused organs after intravenous (IV) administration (or oral administration of a rapidly absorbed compound); rapid uptake is followed by a phase of redistribution into tissues that are less well perfused, especially muscle and fat. Redistribution is most rapid for drugs with the highest lipid solubility. In the regimens used for nighttime sedation, the rate of redistribution sometimes can have a greater influence than the rate of biotransformation on the duration of CNS effects. The kinetics of redistribution of diazepam and other lipophilic benzodiazepines are complicated by enterohepatic circulation. The volumes of distribution of the benzodiazepines are large and in many cases are increased in elderly patients. These drugs cross the placental barrier and are secreted into breast milk.

The benzodiazepines are metabolized extensively by cytochrome P450 enzymes, particularly CYP3A4 and CYP2C19. Some benzodiazepines, such as **oxazepam**, are conjugated directly and are not metabolized by these enzymes. **Erythromycin**, **clarithromycin**, **ritonavir**, **itraconazole**, **ketoconazole**, **nefazodone**, and **grapefruit juice** are inhibitors of CYP3A4 and can affect the metabolism of benzodiazepines. Because active metabolites of some benzodiazepines are biotransformed more slowly than are the parent compounds, the duration of action of many benzodiazepines bears little relationship to the half-life of elimination of the drug that has been administered. For example, the half-life of **flurazepam** in plasma is 2 to 3 hours, but that of a major active metabolite (***N*-desalkylflurazepam**) is 50 hours or more. Conversely, the rate of biotransformation of agents that are inactivated by the initial reaction is an important determinant of their duration of action; these agents include **oxazepam**, **lorazepam**, **temazepam**, **triazolam**, and **midazolam**.

An ideal hypnotic agent would have a rapid onset of action when taken at bedtime, a sufficiently sustained action to facilitate sleep throughout the night, and no residual action by the following morning. Among the benzodiazepines that are used commonly as hypnotic agents, triazolam theoretically fits this description most closely. Because of the slow rate of elimination of **desalkylflurazepam**, **flurazepam** (or **quazepam**) might seem to be unsuitable for this purpose. In practice, there appear to be some disadvantages.

At the time of peak concentration in plasma, hypnotic doses of benzodiazepines can be expected to cause varying degrees of lightheadedness, lassitude, increased reaction time, motor incoordination, impairment of mental and motor functions, confusion, and anterograde amnesia. Cognition appears to be affected less than motor performance. All these effects can greatly impair driving and other psychomotor skills, especially if combined with ethanol. When the drug is given at the intended time of sleep, the persistence of these effects during the waking hours is adverse. These dose-related residual effects can be insidious because most subjects underestimate the degree of their impairment. Residual daytime sleepiness also may occur, even though successful drug therapy can reduce the daytime sleepiness resulting from chronic insomnia. The intensity and incidence of CNS toxicity generally increase with age; both pharmacokinetic and pharmacodynamic factors are involved.

Other relatively common side effects of benzodiazepines are weakness, headache, blurred vision, vertigo, nausea and vomiting, epigastric distress, and diarrhea; joint pains, chest pains, and incontinence are much more rare.

QUETIAPINE FUMARATE

(Seroquel tablets 25 mg)

Quetiapine fumarate is a dibenzapine derivative that has antipsychotic effects, apparently caused by dopamine and serotonin receptor blockade in the CNS. It is indicated in the treatment of schizophrenia; and as short-term treatment of acute manic episodes associated with bipolar I disorder, as either monotherapy or adjunct therapy to lithium or divalproex.

The term **neuroleptic** is often applied to drugs that have relatively prominent experimental and clinical evidence of antagonism of D_2-dopamine-receptor activity, with substantial risk of adverse extrapyramidal neurological effects and increased release of prolactin. The term atypical antipsychotic is applied to agents that are associated with substantially lower risks of such extrapyramidal effects. Representative examples include **aripiprazole**, **clozapine**, **quetiapine**, **ziprasidone**, and low doses of **olanzapine** and **risperidone**.

Although the antipsychotic drugs have had a revolutionary, beneficial impact on medical and psychiatric practice, their liabilities, especially the adverse effects of the older typical or neuroleptic agents, must be emphasized. Newer antipsychotics are atypical in having less risk of extrapyramidal side effects, but these agents present their own spectrum of adverse effects, including hypotension, seizures, weight gain, and increased risk of type 2 diabetes mellitus and hyperlipidemia.

QUINAPRIL HYDROCHLORIDE

(Accupril tablets 5 mg)

The angiotensin-converting enzyme (ACE) inhibitor competitively inhibits angiotensin-I-converting enzyme, resulting in prevention of angiotensin I conversion to angiotensin II, a potent vasoconstrictor that also stimulates aldosterone release. Clinical consequences are a decrease in blood pressure (BP), reduced sodium resorption, and potassium retention.

Quinapril, an ACE inhibitor with antihypertensive properties, is used in hypertension and in hypertension in patients receiving diuretics (see also Figure 24).

QUINAPRIL HYDROCHLORIDE/HYDROCHLOROTHIAZIDE

(Accuretic tablets 10 mg quinapril/12.5 mg HCTZ, tablets 20 mg quinapril/12.5 mg HCTZ, tablets 20 mg quinapril/25 mg HCTZ)

Quinapril hydrochloride/hydrochlorothiazide are antihypertensive combinations. **Quinapril** competitively inhibits angiotensin-I-converting enzyme, resulting in the prevention of angiotensin I conversion to angiotensin II, a potent vasoconstrictor that stimulates aldosterone secretion. This action results in a decrease in sodium and fluid retention, an increase in diuresis, and a decrease in BP. **Hydrochlorothiazide** (HCTZ) increases chloride, sodium, and water excretion by interfering with transport of sodium ions across renal tubular epithelium. It is indicated in the treatment of hypertension.

Cleavage of the ester moiety by hepatic esterases transforms **Quinapril (Accupril)**, a prodrug, into quinaprilat, an ACE inhibitor that, *in vitro*, is about as potent as **benazeprilat**. **Quinapril** is absorbed rapidly (peak concentrations are achieved in 1 hour, but the peak may be delayed after food), and the rate but not extent of oral absorption (60%) may be reduced by food. It is metabolized to quinaprilat and to other minor metabolites, and quinaprilat is excreted in the urine (61%) and feces (37%). Peak concentrations of quinaprilat in plasma are achieved in about 2 hours.

Angiotensin II is an important regulator of cardiovascular function. The ability to reduce levels of angiotensin II with orally effective inhibitors of ACE represents an important advance in the treatment of hypertension. **Captopril** (Capoten) was the first such agent to be developed for the treatment of hypertension. Since then, **enalapril** (Vasotec), **lisinopril** (Prinivil), **quinapril** (Accupril) **ramipril** (Altace), **benazepril** (Lotensin), **moexipril** (Univasc), **fosinopril** (Monopril), **trandolapril** (Mavik), and **perindopril** (Aceon) also have become available. These drugs have proved to be very useful for the treatment of hypertension because of their efficacy and their very favorable profile of adverse effects, which enhances patient adherence.

The ACE inhibitors appear to confer a special advantage in the treatment of patients with diabetes, slowing the development and progression of diabetic glomerulopathy. They also are effective in slowing the progression of other forms of chronic renal disease, such as glomerulosclerosis, and many of these patients also have hypertension. An ACE inhibitor is the preferred initial agent in these patients. Patients with hypertension and ischemic heart disease are candidates for treatment with ACE inhibitors; administration of ACE inhibitors in the immediate post-myocardial infarction (MI) period has been shown to improve ventricular function and reduce morbidity and mortality.

The endocrine consequences of inhibiting the biosynthesis of angiotensin II are of importance in a number of facets of hypertension treatment. Because ACE inhibitors blunt the rise in aldosterone concentrations in response to Na^+ loss, the normal role of aldosterone in opposing diuretic-induced natriuresis is diminished. Consequently, ACE inhibitors tend to enhance the efficacy of diuretic drugs. This means that even very small doses of diuretics may substantially improve the antihypertensive efficacy of ACE inhibitors; conversely, the use of high doses of diuretics together with ACE inhibitors may lead to excessive reduction in BP and to Na^+ loss in some patients.

QUINESTROL

(Estrovis)

Quinestrol (100 mcg daily for 7 days), which mimics the action of endogenous estrogen, is indicated for the treatment of moderate to severe vasomotor symptoms associated with menopause, atrophic vaginitis, kraurosis vulvae, female hypogonadism, female castration, and primary ovarian failures. Quinestrol is stored in body fat, slowly released over several days, and metabolized to ethinyl estradiol.

Quinestrol is contraindicated in patients with thrombophlebitis or thromboembolism because it may induce thromboembolic disease; in patients with estrogen-responsive carcinoma (breast or genital tract cancer), because it may increase tumor growth; in patients with undiagnosed abnormal genital bleeding; and in pregnant or breast-feeding women.

Quinestrol should be administered cautiously to patients with disorders that may be aggravated by fluid and electrolyte accumulation, such as asthma, seizure disorders, migraine, or cardiac, renal, or hepatic dysfunction. Carefully monitor female patients who have breast nodules, fibrocystic breast disease, or a family history of breast cancer. Because of the risk of thromboembolism, therapy with this drug should be discontinued at least one week before elective surgical procedures associated with an increased incidence of thromboembolism.

Concomitant administration of drugs that induce hepatic metabolism, such as rifampin, barbiturates, pyrimidone, carbamazepine, and phenytoin, may result in decreased estrogenic effects from a given dose. These drugs are known to accelerate the rate of metabolism of certain other agents.

In patients with diabetes, this agent increases blood glucose levels, necessitating dosage adjustment of insulin or oral hypoglycemic drugs.

Quinestrol has the potential to decrease the effects of warfarin-type anticoagulants. Patients receiving this drug concurrently with an adrenocorticosteroid or adrenocorticotropic hormone are at greater risk for fluid and electrolyte accumulation.

QUINETHAZONE

(Hydromox)

Quinethazone, a quinazoline derivative with diuretic and antihypertensive properties (50 to 100 mg p.o. daily), is used in edema.

QUINIDINE GLUCONATE

(Duraquin, Quinaglute Dura-Tabs, Quinalan, Quinate)

QUINIDINE POLYGALACTURONATE

(Cardioquin)

QUINIDINE SULFATE

(Cin-Quin, Novoquinidin, Quinidex Extentabs, Quinora)

Quinidine (200 to 600 mg t.i.d.), a cinchona alkaloid with antiarrhythmic properties, is indicated in premature atrial, AV junctional, and ventricular contractions; paroxysmal atrial (supraventricular) tachycardia; paroxysmal AV junctional rhythm; atrial flutter; paroxysmal and chronic atrial fibrillation; established atrial fibrillation when therapy is appropriate; paroxysmal ventricular tachycardia not associated with complete heart block; and maintenance therapy after electrical conversion of atrial fibrillation or flutter (see Figure 103).

Quinidine, a class 1A antiarrhythmic, depresses myocardial excitability, conduction velocity, and contractility. Therapeutically, it prolongs the effective refractory period and increases conduction time, thereby preventing the reentry phenomenon. In addition, quinidine exerts an indirect anticholinergic effect; it decreases vagal tone and may facilitate conduction in the atrioventricular junction.

Quinidine and procainamide decrease automaticity by reducing the rate of phase 4 diastolic depolarization, which is probably mediated by a diminished membrane permeability to sodium, and they decrease conduction velocity throughout the conducting system (Figure 84). They produce an indirect (vagolytic) effect that sometimes counteracts

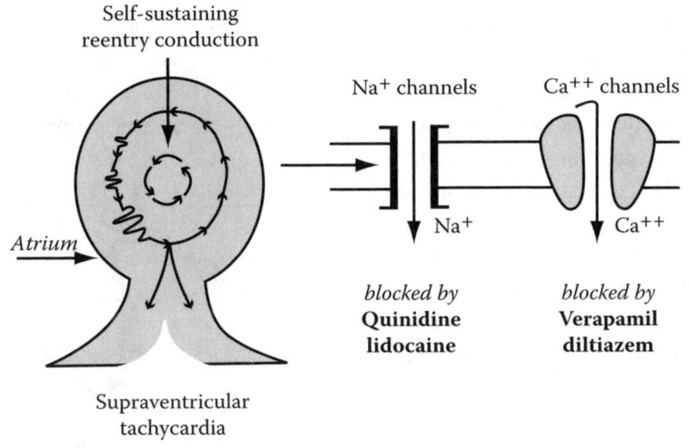

FIGURE 84 As antiarrhythmic drugs, quinidine and procainamide decrease automaticity by reducing the **rate of phase 4 diastolic depolarization**, which is probably mediated by a diminished membrane permeability to sodium, and they decrease conduction velocity throughout the conducting system.

the direct effect at the AV node, producing a paradoxical tachycardia in some cases of atrial flutter or fibrillation. These agents terminate reentry arrhythmias by producing a bidirectional block in infarcted conducting tissues. They directly depress contractility, leading to a decline in cardiac output.

These agents are potent vasodilators, especially when given intravenously. This effect is so great that quinidine is rarely given parenterally, and great care must be taken when it is given by this route. They depress blood pressure by means of their dual effects on cardiac output and peripheral resistance.

These agents produce widening of the QRS complex (by depressing ventricular conduction) and lengthening of the PR interval (by slowing AV conduction). A 25 to 30% widening of the QRS complex is considered the therapeutic limit with these agents. They are excreted up to 50% unmetabolized in the urine. These agents commonly cause gastrointestinal (GI) disturbances, and these constitute their major side effect. Emboli may be liberated from the atria during conversion of atrial flutter or fibrillation. Toxicity is manifested by a profound fall in blood pressure that leads to a shock-like state accompanied by a variety of arrhythmias.

Quinidine and procainamide may also provoke some unique but uncommon side effects. Quinidine may produce cinchonism (tinnitus, dizziness, visual disturbances, and vertigo) and cutaneous hypersensitivity reactions. Procainamide may produce agranulocytosis during long-term therapy, and dose-dependent (>2 gm/day) lupus erythematosus-like syndrome. These agents are mainly used in the management of atrial (supraventricular) arrhythmias, although procainamide is also of value in treating premature ventricular contractions and ventricular tachycardia. If either drug is used to convert atrial flutter or fibrillation, digitalis must be given first to protect against paradoxical tachycardia.

QUININE SULFATE

(Quinora)

Quinine (650 mg every 8 hours for 5 to 7 days) is indicated for the treatment of chloroquine-resistant falciparum malaria, either alone, with pyrimethamine and a sulfonamide, or with a tetracycline. It is also considered as an alternative therapy for chloroquine-sensitive strains of *P. falciparum*, *P. malariae*, *P. ovale*, and *P. vivax*. Mefloquine and clindamycin may also be used with quinine, depending on the geographical location in which the malaria was acquired.

Quinine, a cinchona alkaloid, acts primarily as a blood schizonticide. Quinine's antimalarial action is unclear. It was once believed to be due to the intercalation of the quinoline moiety into the DNA of the parasite, thereby reducing the effectiveness of DNA to act as a template, as well as depression of the oxygen uptake and carbohydrate metabolism of the plasmodia. Recently it has been thought that quinine's pH elevation in the intracellular organelles of the parasites plays a role in the mechanism.

Quinine has a skeletal muscle-relaxant effect, increasing the refractory period by direct action on the muscle fiber, decreasing the excitability of the motor end plate by a curariform action, and affecting the distribution of calcium within the muscle fiber. It also has analgesic, antipyretic, and oxytocic effects.

Quinine is contraindicated in patients with glucose-6-phosphate dehydrogenase (G-6-PD) deficiency, optic neuritis, tinnitus, or a history of blackwater fever and thrombocytopenia purpura. The symptoms of overdosage are tinnitus, dizziness, skin rash, and GI disturbance (intestinal cramping). With higher doses, cardiovascular and CNS effects may occur, including headache, fever, vomiting, apprehension, confusion, and convulsions.

Aluminum-containing antacids may decrease the absorption of quinine. Quinine may depress the hepatic enzyme system that synthesizes the vitamin-K-dependent clotting factors and thus may enhance the action of warfarin and other oral anticoagulants. Cimetidine may reduce quinine's oral clearance and increase its elimination half-life. Digoxin serum concentrations may be increased by concurrent quinine.

Quinine may potentiate the actions of neuromuscular-blocking agents causing respiratory depression.

QUINOLONE AND FLUOROQUINOLONE ANTIBIOTICS

Amifloxacin	Lomefloxacin	Ofloxacin
Cinoxacin	Nalidixic acid	Pefloxacin
Ciprofloxacin	Norfloxacin	Sparfloxacin
Fleroxacin		

QUINOLONE ANTIBIOTICS

The quinolones include nalidixic acid (NegGram), cinoxacin (Cinobac), norfloxacin (Noroxin), and ciprofloxacin (Cipro). Other members of the quinolone family are pefloxacin, ofloxacin, enoxacin, and fleroxacin. The bacterial enzyme DNA gyrase is responsible for the continuous introduction of negative supercoils into DNA, and the quinolones inhibit this gyrase-mediated DNA supercoiling.

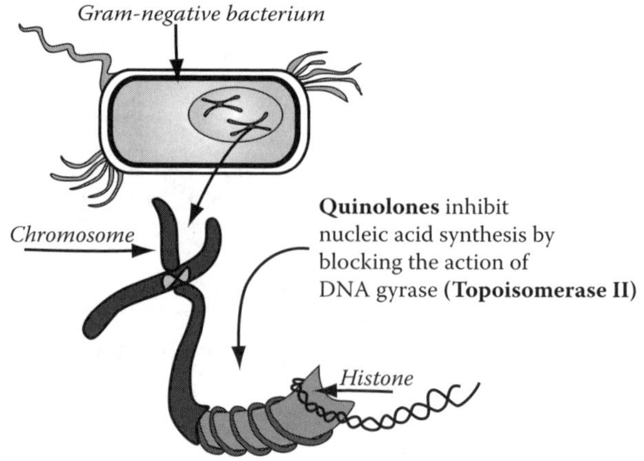

FIGURE 85 The quinolones include **nalidixic acid** (NegGram), **cinoxacin** (Cinobac), **norfloxacin** (Noroxin), and **ciprofloxacin** (Cipro). Other members of the quinolone family are **pefloxacin**, **ofloxacin**, **enoxacin**, and **fleroxacin**.

Nalidixic acid and cinoxacin are bactericidal against Gram-negative organisms that cause urinary tract infections. The fluoroquinolones are bactericidal and considerably more potent against *Escherichia coli* and various species of *Salmonella*, *Shigella*, *Enterobacter*, *Campylobacter*, and *Neisseria*. Ciprofloxacin also has good activity against staphylococci, including methicillin-resistant strains.

The quinolones and fluoroquinolones may produce arthropathy, and hence should not be used in prepubertal children or pregnant women.

Nalidixic acid and cinoxacin are useful only for treating urinary tract infections. Ciprofloxacin is useful for both urinary tract infections and prostatitis.

QUINUPRISTIN/DALFOPRISTIN

(Synercid injection, lyophilized 500 mg (150 mg quinupristin; 350 mg dalfopristin)/10 mL))

Quinupristin/dalfopristin is a streptogramin. Quinupristin inhibits the late phase of protein synthesis; dalfopristin inhibits the early phase of protein synthesis. It is indicated in the treatment of serious or life-threatening infections associated with VREF; treatment of complicated skin and skin-structure infections caused by *Staphylococcus aureus* (methicillin-susceptible) or *Streptococcus pyogenes*.

R

RABEPRAZOLE SODIUM

(Aciphex tablets, delayed-release 20 mg)

Rabeprazole sodium is a proton-pump inhibitor that suppresses gastric acid secretion by blocking acid (proton) pump within gastric parietal cells. It is indicated in short-term treatment in healing and symptomatic relief of duodenal ulcers and erosive or ulcerative **gastroesophageal reflux disease** (GERD); maintaining healing and reducing relapse rates of heartburn symptoms in patients with GERD; and treatment of daytime and nighttime heartburn and other symptoms associated with GERD; long-term treatment of pathological hypersecretory conditions, including **Zollinger–Ellison syndrome** and in combination with amoxicillin and clarithromycin to eradicate ***Helicobacter pylori***.

The most potent suppressors of gastric acid secretion are inhibitors of the gastric H^+K^+-ATPase (proton pump). In typical doses, these drugs diminish the daily production of acid (basal and stimulated) by 80 to 95%. Five proton pump inhibitors are available for clinical use: **omeprazole** (Prilosec, Rapinex, Zegerid) and its S-isomer, **esomeprazole** (Nexium); **lansoprazole** (Prevacid), **rabeprazole** (Aciphex); and **pantoprazole** (Protonix). These drugs have different substitutions on their pyridine and/or benzimidazole groups but are remarkably similar in their pharmacological properties. Omeprazole is a racemic mixture of R- and S-isomers; the S-isomer, esomeprazole (*S*-omeprazole), is eliminated less rapidly than *R*-omeprazole, which theoretically provides a therapeutic advantage because of the increased half-life. Despite claims to the contrary, all proton pump inhibitors have equivalent efficacy at comparable doses.

Proton-pump inhibitors are prodrugs that require activation in an acid environment. After absorption into the systemic circulation, the prodrug diffuses into the parietal cells of the stomach and accumulates in the acidic secretory canaliculi. Here, it is activated by proton-catalyzed formation of a **tetracyclic sulfenamide**, trapping the drug so that it cannot diffuse back across the canalicular membrane. The activated form then binds covalently with sulfhydryl groups of cysteines in the H^+K^+-ATPase, irreversibly inactivating the pump molecule. Acid secretion resumes only after new pump molecules are synthesized and inserted into the luminal membrane, providing a prolonged (up to 24- to 48-hour) suppression of acid secretion, despite the much shorter plasma half-lives (0.5 to 2 hours) of the parent compounds. Because they block the final step in acid production, the proton-pump inhibitors are effective in acid suppression regardless of other stimulating factors.

To prevent degradation of proton-pump inhibitors by acid in the gastric lumen, oral dosage forms are supplied in different formulations: (1) enteric-coated drugs contained inside gelatin capsules (**omeprazole**, **esomeprazole**, and **lansoprazole**); (2) enteric-coated granules supplied as a powder for suspension (**lansoprazole**); (3) enteric-coated tablets (**pantoprazole**, **rabeprazole**, and **omeprazole**); and (4) powdered drug combined with sodium bicarbonate (**omeprazole**). The delayed-release and enteric-coated tablets dissolve only at alkaline pH, whereas an admixture of omeprazole with sodium bicarbonate simply neutralizes stomach acid; both strategies substantially improve the oral bioavailability of these acid-labile drugs. Until recently, the requirement for enteric coating posed a challenge to the administration of proton-pump inhibitors in patients for whom the oral route of administration is not available. These patients and those requiring immediate acid suppression now can be treated parenterally with **pantoprazole** or **lansoprazole**, both of which are approved for intravenous administration in the United States. A single intravenous bolus of 80 mg of pantoprazole inhibits acid production by 80 to 90% within an hour, and this inhibition persists for up to 21 hours, permitting once-daily dosing to achieve the desired degree of hypochlorhydria. The FDA-approved dose of intravenous pantoprazole for gastroesophageal reflux disease is 40 mg daily for up to 10 days. Higher doses (e.g., 160 to 240 mg in divided doses) are used to manage hypersecretory conditions such as the Zollinger–Ellison syndrome.

The control of acid-peptic disease represents a major triumph for modern pharmacology. Proton pump inhibitors are considered superior for acid suppression in most clinically significant acid-peptic diseases, including gastroesophageal reflux disease, peptic ulcers, and nonsteroidal antiinflammatory drug (NSAID)-induced ulcers. Proton-pump inhibitors also are employed in combination with antibiotics to eradicate infection with *H. pylori* and thereby play a role in preventing recurrent peptic ulcers. These agents largely have replaced the use of misoprostol and sucralfate, although the latter still is a low-cost alternative for prophylaxis against stress ulcers. The delay in maximal inhibition of acid secretion with the proton-pump inhibitors (3 to 5 days) makes them less suited for use on an as-needed basis for symptom relief. In this setting, H_2-receptor antagonists, though less effective than proton pump inhibitors in suppressing acid secretion, have a more rapid onset of action that makes them useful for patient-directed management of mild or infrequent symptoms.

RABIES IMMUNE GLOBULIN, HUMAN (RIG)

(BayRab injection 150 units/mL, Imogam rabies-HT injection 150 units/mL)

Rabies immune globulin is an immune globulin that directly neutralizes rabies virus. It is indicated in passive, transient postexposure prevention of rabies infection in susceptible individuals.

RABIES VACCINE

(Imovax rabies vaccine (human diploid cell) powder for injection freeze-dried suspension of Wistar rabies virus strain PM-1503-3M grown in human diploid cell cultures (inactivated whole virus). Contains 2.5 IU or more rabies antigen/mL, Imovax rabies I.D. vaccine (human diploid cell) powder for injection freeze-dried suspension of Wistar rabies virus strain PM-1503-3M grown in human diploid cell cultures. Contains 0.25 IU rabies antigen/ 0.1 mL intradermal use. (For pre-exposure use only via intradermal route), RabAvert powder for injection freeze-dried fixed-virus strain Flury LEP grown in cultures of chicken fibroblasts. Contains 2.5 IU or more rabies antigen/mL IM dose, rabies vaccine (adsorbed) injection challenge virus standard (CVS) Kissling/MDPH strain)

Rabies vaccine is a viral vaccine that induces neutralizing antibodies and cellular immunity. It is used in induction of active immunity against rabies virus either before or after viral exposure.

RADIOACTIVE IODINE

(Sodium iodide)

^{131}I(Iodotope therapeutic, sodium iodide ^{131}I therapeutic)

Radioactive iodine, a thyroid hormone antagonist, is used in hyperthyroidism and in thyroid cancer (see also Table 20).

RADIOPAQUE AGENTS

Oral Cholecystographic Agents Containing Iodine

Iocetamic acid (62% iodine)	(Cholebrine)
Iopanoic acid (66.68% iodine)	(Telepaque)
Ipodate calcium (61.7% iodine)	(Oragrafin Calcium)
Ipodate sodium (61.4% iodine)	(Bilivist, Oragrafin Sodium)
Tyropanoate sodium (57.4% iodine)	(Bilopaque)

GI Contrast Agents Containing Iodine

Diatrizoate sodium 41.66% (24.9% iodine)	(Hypaque Sodium)
Diatrizoate sodium (59.87% iodine)	(Hypaque Sodium)
Diatrizoate meglumine 66% and diatrizoate sodium 10% (37% iodine)	(Gastrografin, MD-Gastroview)

GI Contrast Agents Containing Barium

Barium sulfate	(Baro-cat, Prepcat, Enecat, Tomocat, Entrobar, Liquid Barosperse, HD 85, Barobag, Liquipake, Flo-Coat, Epi-C, Barium Sulfate, USP, Baroflave, Tonopaque, Baricon, HD 200 Plus, Barosperse, Anatrast)

GI Contrast Agents (Miscellaneous)

Radiopaque polyvinyl chloride	(Sitzmarks)
Sodium bicarbonate	(Baros)

Radiopaque Agents Administered Parenterally

Diatrizoate meglumine 30% (14.1% iodine)	(Hypaque Meglumine 30%, Reno-M-Dip, Urovist Meglumine DIU/CT)
Diatrizoate meglumine 60% (28% iodine)	(Angiovist 282, Hypaque Meglumine 60%, Reno-M-60)
Diatrizoate meglumine 76% (35.8% iodine)	(Diatrizoate Meglumine 76%)
Diatrizoate sodium 25% (15% iodine)	(Hypaque Sodium 25%)
Diatrizoate sodium 50% (30% iodine)	(Hypaque Sodium 50%)
Gadopentetate dimeglumine 46.9%	(Magnevist)
Iodamide meglumine 24% (11.1% iodine)	(Renovue-Dip)
Iodamide meglumine 65% (30% iodine)	(Renovue-65)
Iodipamide meglumine 10.3% (5.1% iodine)	(Cholografin Meglumine)
Iodipamide meglumine 52% (25.7% iodine)	(Cholografin Meglumine)
Iohexol (46.36% iodine)	(Omnipaque)
Iopamidol 26% (12.8% iodine)	(Isovue-128)
Iopamidol 41% (20% iodine)	(Isovue-200)
Iopamidol 61% (30% iodine)	(Isovue-300)
Iopamidol 76% (37% iodine)	(Isovue-370)
Iothalamate meglumine 30% (14.1% iodine)	(Conray 30)
Iothalamate meglumine 43% (20.2% iodine)	(Conray 43)
Iothalamate meglumine 60% (28.2% iodine)	(Conray)
Iothalamate sodium 54.3% (32.5% iodine)	(Conray 325)
Iothalamate sodium 66.8% (40% iodine)	(Conray 400)
Iothalamate sodium 80% (48% iodine)	(Angio Conray)
Ioversol 34% (16% iodine)	(Optiray 160)
Ioversol 51% (24% iodine)	(Optiray 240)
Ioversol 68% (32% iodine)	(Optiray 320)
Ioversol 74% (35% iodine)	(Optiray 350)
Metrizamide (48.25% iodine)	(Amipaque)
Diatrizoate meglumine 28.5% and diatrizoate sodium 29.1% (31% iodine)	(Renovist II)
Diatrizoate meglumine 34.3% and diatrizoate sodium 35% (37% iodine)	(Renovist)
Diatrizoate meglumine 50% and diatrizoate sodium 25% (38.5% iodine)	(Hypaque-M, 75%)
Diatrizoate meglumine 52% and diatrizoate sodium 8% (29.3% iodine)	(Angiovist 292, MD-60, Renografin-60)
Diatrizoate meglumine 60% and diatrizoate sodium 30% (46.2% iodine)	(Hypaque-M, 90%)
Diatrizoate meglumine 66% and diatrizoate sodium 10% (37% iodine)	(Angiovist 370, Hypaque-76, MD-76, Renografin-76)
Iothalamate meglumine 52% and iothalamate sodium 26% (40% iodine)	(Vascoray)

Radiopaque Agents Administered Parenterally (continued)

Ioxaglate meglumine 39.3% and ioxaglate sodium 19.6% (32% iodine)	(Hexabrix)

Radiographic contrast media (radiopaques) increase the absorption of X-rays as they pass through the body and are used for delineating body structures. Magnetic resonance contrast agents enhance the images obtained from the absorption of radio waves by atomic nuclei.

RADIOSENSITIZERS

Malignant neoplastic diseases may be treated by various approaches: surgery, radiation therapy, immunotherapy, chemotherapy, or a combination of these. The extent of a malignant disease (staging) should be ascertained in order to plan an effective therapeutic intervention. Surgery is effective in eliminating localized tumors but is ineffective for metastasized or disseminated tumors. Often the treatment regimen for this type of tumor combines surgery with radiotherapy or chemotherapy. For example, soft-tissue sarcomas are initially treated by local excision, high-dose radiation, and adjuvant chemotherapy with doxorubicin, cyclophosphamide, or methotrexate. Radiation therapy is an effective alternative to surgery and is used in the locoregional, but not widely disseminated, treatment of a malignancy. Rapidly dividing malignant cells are especially sensitive to radiation. The beneficial effects of radiation therapy stem from its ability to cause the formation of ion pairs or reactive oxygen metabolites such as superoxide, H_2O_2, or hydroxyl radicals. These have the ability to cause breaks in the cancer cell DNA, which, if not repaired, will lead to cell death. Radiosensitizers such as metronidazole and bromodeoxyuridine are agents that enhance the effect of radiation; radioprotectors are designed to protect normal cells.

RALOXIFENE HYDROCHLORIDE

(Evista tablets 60 mg)

Raloxifene hydrochloride is a selective estrogen-receptor modulator. The biological actions of raloxifene are mediated largely through binding to estrogen receptors, which results in activation of certain estrogenic pathways and blockade of others. Raloxifene decreases resorption of bone and reduced biochemical markers of bone turnover to the premenopausal range. Effects on bone are manifested as reductions in the serum and urine levels of bone turnover markers, decreases in bone resorption based on radiocalcium kinetics studies, increases in bone mineral density, and decreases in incidence of fractures. Raloxifene also effects lipid metabolism, decreasing total and LDL cholesterol (LDL-C) levels but does not increase triglyceride levels or change total HDL cholesterol (HDL-C) levels. It is indicated for the prevention and treatment of osteoporosis in postmenopausal women.

Tamoxifen, **raloxifene**, and **toremifene** are selective estrogen-receptor modulators, or SERMs, that are compounds with tissue-selective actions. The pharmacological goal of these drugs is to produce beneficial estrogenic actions in certain tissues (e.g., bone, brain, and liver) during postmenopausal hormone therapy, but antagonist activity in tissues such as breast and endometrium, where estrogenic actions (e.g., carcinogenesis) might be deleterious. Currently approved drugs in the United States in this class are **tamoxifen citrate** (Nolvadex, others), **raloxifene hydrochloride** (Evista), and **toremifene** (Fareston), which is chemically related and has similar actions to tamoxifen. Tamoxifen and toremifene are used for treatment of breast cancer, and raloxifene is used primarily for prevention and treatment of osteoporosis.

Raloxifene acts as a partial agonist in bone but does not stimulate endometrial proliferation in postmenopausal women. Presumably this is due to some combination of differential expression of transcription factors in the two tissues and the effects of this SERM on ER conformation. **Raloxifene** induces a configuration in ER α that is distinct from that of tamoxifen-ER β, suggesting that a different set of coactivators/corepressors may interact with ER-**raloxifene** compared to ER-tamoxifen.

Raloxifene is adsorbed rapidly after oral administration and has an absolute bioavailability of about 2%. The drug has a half-life of about 28 hours and is eliminated primarily in the feces after hepatic glucuronidation; it does not appear to undergo significant biotransformation by cytochrome p450s (CYPs).

Raloxifene reduces the rate of bone loss and may increase bone mass at certain sites. In a large clinical trial, **raloxifene** increased spinal bone mineral density by more than 2% and reduced the rate of vertebral fractures by 30 to 50%, but did not significantly reduce nonvertebral fractures. **Raloxifene** does not appear to increase the risk of developing endometrial cancer. The drug has beneficial actions on lipoprotein metabolism, reducing both total cholesterol and LDL; however, HDL is not increased. Adverse effects include hot flashes, deep vein thrombosis, and leg cramps.

RAMELTEON

(Rozerem tablets 8 mg)

Ramelteon is a melatonin receptor agonist with high affinity for melatonin MT_1 and MT_2 receptors and selectivity over the MT_3 receptor. Activation of MT_1 and MT_2 receptors is believed to contribute to ramelteon's sleep-promoting properties. It is indicated in the treatment of insomnia characterized by sleep onset difficulty.

RAMIPRIL

(Altace)

Ramipril, an angiotensin-converting enzyme (ACE) inhibitor with antihypertensive properties (2 to 5 mg p.o. daily), is used in the treatment of hypertension, either alone or in combination with thiazide diuretics (see also Figure 24).

Ramipril is a long-acting nonsulfhydryl ACE inhibitor. It is a prodrug that undergoes de-esterification in the liver to form ramiprilat, its active metabolite. No clinically significant pharmacokinetic interactions between ramipril and other drugs have been reported. The drug has been generally well tolerated, with the most prevalent adverse effects being dizziness, headache, weakness, and nausea. Ramipril is an effective and well-tolerated drug for the treatment of hypertension and congestive heart failure (CHF) in all patients, including those with renal or hepatic dysfunction, and in the elderly.

RANITIDINE

(Zantac)

Ranitidine, a histamine$_2$ receptor antagonist (150 to 400 mg p.o. daily as a single or divided dose), is indicated in the treatment of duodenal ulcer, benign gastric ulcer, pathological hypersecretory conditions, gastroesophageal reflux disease, and erosive esophagitis. Ranitidine competitively inhibits histamine's action at H_2-receptors in gastric and parietal cells. This reduces basal and nocturnal gastric acid secretion, as well as that caused by histamine, food, amino acids, insulin, and pentagastrin. Antacids reduce the absorption of ranitidine and should not be administered concomitantly.

H_2-receptor blockers include **cimetidine** (Tagamet), **ranitidine** (Zantac), **famotidine** (Pepcid), and **nizatidine** (Axid). Besides their use in combination with H_1-receptor blockers for **pruritus**, the H_2-receptor blockers have immunomodulating effects, and this property has been exploited in children to treat **warts**.

RASBURICASE

(Elitek powder for injection, lyophilized 1.5 mg/vial)

Rasburicase is an antimetabolite that catalyzes enzymatic oxidation of uric acid into an inactive and soluble metabolite (allantoin). It is indicated in initial management of plasma uric acid levels in pediatric patients with leukemia, lymphoma, and solid tumor malignancies who are receiving anticancer therapy expected to result in tumor lysis and subsequent elevation of plasma uric acid.

Rasburicase (Elitek) is a recombinant urate-oxidase that catalyzes the enzymatic oxidation of uric acid into the soluble and inactive metabolite allantoin. It has been shown to lower urate levels more effectively than **allopurinol**. It is indicated in the initial management of elevated plasma uric acid levels in pediatric patients with **leukemia**, **lymphoma**, and solid tumor malignancies who are receiving anticancer therapy expected to result in tumor lysis and significant hyperuricemia.

Produced by a genetically modified *Saccharomyces cerevisiae* strain, the therapeutic efficacy may be hampered by the production of antibodies against the drug. Hemolysis in glucose-6-phosphate dehydrogenase (G6PD)-deficient patients, methemoglobinemia, acute renal failure, and anaphylaxis all have been associated with the use of **rasburicase**. Other frequently observed adverse reactions include vomiting, fever, nausea, headache, abdominal pain, constipation, diarrhea, and mucositis. **Rasburicase** causes enzymatic degradation of the uric acid in blood samples, and special handling is required to prevent spuriously low values for plasma uric acid in patients receiving the drug. The recommended dose of rasburicase is 0.15 mg/kg or 0.2 mg/kg as a single daily dose for 5 days, with chemotherapy initiated 4 to 24 hours after infusion of the first rasburicase dose.

RAUWOLFIA

(Raudixin, Rauval, Rauverid, Wolfina)

Rauwolfia alkaloid, a peripherally acting adrenergic blocking agent (200 to 400 mg p.o. daily), is used in the treatment of mild to moderate hypertension.

REMIFENTANIL HYDROCHLORIDE

(Ultiva powder for injection, lyophilized 1 mg/mL after reconstitution)

Remifentanil is an opioid analgesic that is indicated in analgesic use during the induction and maintenance of general anesthesia for inpatient and outpatient procedures and for continuation as an analgesic into the immediate postoperative period under supervision of an anesthesia practitioner; and as an analgesic component of monitored anesthesia care.

With the exception of **ketamine**, neither parenteral nor currently available inhalational anesthetics are effective analgesics. Thus, analgesics typically are administered with general anesthetics to reduce anesthetic requirement and minimize hemodynamic changes produced by painful stimuli. Nonsteroidal antiinflammatory drugs, cyclooxygenase-2 inhibitors, or **acetaminophen** sometimes provide adequate analgesia for minor surgical procedures. However, because of the rapid and profound analgesia produced, opioids are the primary analgesics used during the perioperative period.

Fentanyl (Sublimaze), **sufentanil** (Sufenta), **alfentanil** (Alfenta), **remifentanil** (Ultiva), **meperidine** (Demerol), and **morphine** are the major parenteral opioids used in the perioperative period. The primary analgesic activity of each of these drugs is produced by agonist activity at μ-opioid receptors. Their order of potency (relative to morphine) is: sufentanil (1000x) > **remifentanil** (300x) > fentanyl (100x) > alfentanil (15x) > morphine (1x) > meperidine (0.1x).

The choice of a perioperative opioid is based primarily on duration of action, given that at appropriate doses, all produce similar analgesia and side effects. **Remifentanil** has an ultra-short duration of action (~10 minutes) and accumulates minimally with repeated doses or infusion; it is particularly well suited for procedures that are briefly painful, but for which little analgesia is required postoperatively. Single doses of fentanyl, alfentanil, and sufentanil all have similar intermediate durations of action (30, 20, and 15 minutes, respectively), but recovery after prolonged administration varies considerably. Fentanyl's duration of action lengthens most with infusion, sufentanil's much less so, and alfentanil's the least. Except for **remifentanil**, all of the afore-mentioned opioids are metabolized in the liver followed by renal and biliary excretion of the metabolites. **Remifentanil** is hydrolyzed by tissue and plasma esterases. After prolonged administration, morphine metabolites have significant analgesic and hypnotic activity.

Although opioids are used clinically primarily for their pain-relieving properties, they produce a host of other effects. This is not surprising in view of the wide distribution of opioids and their receptors in the brain and the periphery. A brief summary of some of these effects is presented below. High doses of opioids can produce muscular rigidity in humans. Chest wall rigidity severe enough to compromise respiration is not uncommon during anesthesia with **fentanyl**, **alfentanil**, **remifentanil**, and **sufentanil**.

REPAGLINIDE

(Prandin tablets 0.5 mg, tablets 1 mg, tablets 2 mg)

Repaglinide is a meglitinide that decreases blood glucose by stimulating insulin release from the pancreas. It is indicated as an adjunct to diet and exercise to lower blood glucose in patients with non-insulin-dependent diabetes mellitus (NDDM) (type 2) whose hyperglycemia cannot be controlled by diet and exercise alone. It can be used with metformin or thiazolidinediones (e.g., rosiglitazone) when hyperglycemia cannot be controlled by exercise, diet, and monotherapy with metformin, sulfonylureas, repaglinide, or thiazolidinediones.

Repaglinide (Prandin) is an oral insulin secretagogue of the meglitinide class. This agent is a derivative of benzoic acid, and its structure is unrelated to that of the sulfonylureas.

Like sulfonylureas, repaglinide stimulates insulin release by closing ATP-dependent potassium channels in pancreatic β-cells. The drug is absorbed rapidly from the GI tract, and peak blood levels are obtained within 1 hour. The half-life of the drug is about 1 hour. These features of the drug allow for multiple preprandial use as compared with the classical once- or twice-daily dosing of sulfonylureas. **Repaglinide** is metabolized primarily by the liver to inactive derivatives. Repaglinide should be used cautiously in patients with hepatic insufficiency. Because a small proportion (about 10%) of repaglinide is metabolized by the kidney, increased dosing of the drug in patients with renal insufficiency also should be performed cautiously. As with sulfonylureas, the major side effect of repaglinide is hypoglycemia.

RESCINNAMINE

(Moderil)

Rescinnamine, a rauwolfia alkaloid with peripherally acting adrenergic-blocking effects (1 mg p.o. daily), is used in mild to moderate hypertension.

RESERPINE

(Sandril, Serpalan, Serpanray, Serpasil, Serpate, Zepine)

Reserpine, a rauwolfia alkaloid with peripherally acting antiadrenergic effects (0.5 mg p.o.), is used in mild to moderate essential hypertension. In addition, reserpine (0.1 to 1 mg p.o. daily) has been used as an antipsychotic.

RESERPINE/HYDRALAZINE HYDROCHLORIDE/HYDROCHLOROTHIAZIDE

(Hydrap-ES tablets 15 mg hydrochlorothiazide, 0.1 mg reserpine, and 25 mg hydralazine hydrochloride, Ser-Ap-Es tablets 15 mg hydrochlorothiazide, 0.1 mg reserpine, and 25 mg hydralazine hydrochloride)

Reserpine/hydralazine hydrochloride/hydrochlorothiazide is an antihypertensive combination. **Reserpine** depletes stores of catecholamines and 5-hydroxytryptamine, resulting in decreased heart rate and lowering of arterial BP. **Hydralazine** directly relaxes vascular smooth muscle to cause peripheral vasodilation, decreasing arterial BP, and peripheral vascular resistance. **Hydrochlorothiazide** increases chloride, sodium, and water excretion by interfering with the transport of sodium ions across renal tubular epithelium. It is indicated in the treatment of hypertension.

RESTACORIN

Restacorin, a novel class 1C antiarrhythmic drug, exerts a concentration-related negative inotropic effect. It has hemodynamic effects similar to other class 1 antiarrhythmic drugs.

RETEPLASE, RECOMBINANT

(Retavase powder for injection, lyophilized 10.4 U (18.1 mg))

Reteplase is a tissue plasminogen activator that aids in dissolution of blood clots. It is indicted in the management

---

RESTLESS LEGS SYNDROME: Treatment of

Restless legs syndrome is characterized by an unpleasant creeping discomfort that is perceived as arising deep within the legs and occasionally in the arms as well. Such symptoms tend to occur when patients are relaxed, especially while lying down or sitting, and lead to a need to move about. They are often particularly troublesome at night and may delay the onset of sleep. A sleep disorder associated with periodic movements during sleep may also occur and can be documented by polysonographic recording. The cause is unknown, although the disorder seems especially common among pregnant women and is not uncommon among uremic or diabetic patients with neuropathy. Most patients, however, have no obvious predisposing cause. Symptoms sometimes resolve following correction of coexisting iron-deficiency anemia, and they may respond to treatment with drugs such as levodopa, bromocriptine, diazepam, clonazepam, or opiates. When opiates are required, those with long half-lives or low addictive potential should be used.

---

of acute myocardial infarction (MI), to reduce incidence of congestive heart failure (CHF) and mortality associated with an acute MI.

Contraindications to thrombolytic therapy include:

- Surgery within 10 days, including organ biopsy, puncture of noncompressible vessels, serious trauma, cardiopulmonary resuscitation
- Serious GI bleeding within 3 months
- History of hypertension (diastolic pressure >110 mm Hg)
- Active bleeding or hemorrhagic disorder
- Previous cerebrovascular accident or active intracranial process
- Aortic dissection
- Acute pericarditis

RETINOIDS

The retinoids comprise a family of polyisoprenoid lipids that includes vitamin A (retinol) and structurally related compounds. The biological activity of retinoids can be modified, for example, by changes in the molecules' state of oxidation and cis/trans isomerization. Their activity is also dependent on the levels of specific types of retinoid-binding proteins that exist in extracellular, cytosolic, and nuclear compartments. The role of retinoids in gene expression represents an important biological function for this family of molecules. Retinoid-dependent modulation of gene expression is critical for normal cell and tissue function in mature as well as developing animals.

RETINOIDS

First Generation
- Retinol
- Tretinoin
- Isotretinoin

Second Generation
- Etretinate
- Acitretin

Third Generation
- Arotinoid

RH$_0$(D) IMMUNE GLOBULIN (RHIG)

(Gamulin Rh package vial of Rh$_0$(D) immune globulin dissolved in 0.3 M glycine with 0.01% thimersol, HypRh$_0$-D package syringe of Rh$_0$ (D) immune globulin dissolved in 0.21 to 0.32 M glycine with 80 to 120 mcg thimersol, HypRho-D mini-dose package syringe of Rh$_0$ (D) immune globulin microdose dissolved in 0.21 to 0.32 M glycine with 80 to 120 mcg thimerosal, MICRh$_0$GAM package syringe of Rh$_0$(D) immune globulin microdose dissolved in glycine 15 mg/mL with 0.003% thimersol, RH$_0$GAM package vial of Rh$_0$(D) immune globulin microdose dissolved in glycine 15 mg/mL with 0.003% thimersol, 2.9 mg sodium chloride, and 0.01% polysorbate 80)

Rh$_0$(D) immune globulin (RhIG) is an immune globulin. By binding Rh$_0$(D) antigen on red blood cells (RBCs), RhIG prevents production of anti-Rh$_0$(D) antibodies in Rh$_0$(D) antigen-negative people. Prevention of Rh sensitization, in turn, prevents hemolytic disease of the fetus and newborn in subsequent Rh$_0$(D) antigen-positive children.

Passive, transient protection against development of endogenous anti-Rh antibodies (isoimmunization) in non-sensitized Rh antigen-negative people who receive Rh antigen-positive blood. Such exposure may result from fetomaternal hemorrhage occurring during delivery, spontaneous or induced abortion, abdominal trauma, ectopic pregnancy, chorionic villus sampling (CVS), percutaneous umbilical cord blood sampling (PUBS), amniocentesis, fetal surgery or manipulation, or as result of transfusion accident. RhIG prevents hemolytic disease of the fetus and newborn (including erythroblastosis fetalis and hydrops fetalis) in subsequent Rh antigen-positive children. If Rh typing of the fetus is not possible, assume the fetus is Rh antigen-positive and give the mother RhIG. Do not perform a Rh cross-match prior to administration. **Term delivery**: to warrant RhIG administration, (1) the mother must be Rh antigen-negative, (2) the mother should not have been previously sensitized to Rh factor (and thus produce her own anti-Rh antibodies), and (3) the infant must be Rh antigen-positive and direct anti-globulin negative. (4) If the father can be determined to be Rh antigen-negative, RhIG need not be given. **Other obstetric conditions**: administer RhIG to all nonsensitized Rh antigen-negative women after spontaneous or induced abortions, after ruptured ectopic pregnancies amniocentesis, other abdominal trauma, CVS, PUBS, fetal surgery or manipulation, or any transplacental hemorrhage, unless the blood type of the fetus has been determined to be Rh antigen-negative. Sensitization occurs more frequently in women undergoing induced abortions than in those aborting spontaneously. Transfusion accidents: RhIG can be used to prevent Rh sensitization in Rh antigen-negative patients who accidentally receive transfusions with RBCs or blood components containing RBCs, platelets, or granulocytes prepared from Rh antigen-positive blood. Administer it within 72 hours following Rh-incompatible transfusion.

RH$_0$(D) IMMUNE GLOBULIN IV (HUMAN) (RHIVIG)

(WinRho SDF powder for injection lyophilized 600 IU (120 mcg) (2.5 mL 0.9% sodium chloride injection diluent), powder for injection, lyophilized 1500 IU (300mg) (2.5 mL 0.9% sodium chloride injection diluent), powder for injection, lyophilized 5000 IU (1000 mcg) (8.5 mL 0.9% sodium chloride injection diluent))

Rh$_0$(D) immune globulin IV (human) (RhIVIG) is an immune globulin. By binding Rh$_0$(D) antigen and red blood cells, RhIGIV prevents production of anti-Rho(D) antibodies in

$Rh_0(D)$ antigen-negative people, which prevents hemolytic disease of the fetus and newborn in subsequent $Rh_0(DP)$ antigen-positive children. It increases platelets in immune thrombocytopenia purpura (ITP) patients. **Treatment of ITP**: used in the treatment of nonsplenectomized $Rh_0(D)$-positive children with chronic or acute ITP, adults with chronic ITP, or children and adults with ITP secondary to HIV infection. **Suppression of Rh isoimmunization**: used in pregnancy and other obstetric conditions—suppression of Rh isoimmunization in nonsensitized, $Rh_0(D)$-negative women after spontaneous or induced abortions, amniocentesis, chorionic villus sampling, ruptured tubal pregnancy, abdominal trauma, or transplacental hemorrhage, or in the normal course of pregnancy unless the blood type of the fetus or father is known to be $Rh_0(D)$-negative. To warrant RhIGIV administration for an Rh-incompatible pregnancy, the mother must be $Rh_0(D)$-negative; carrying a child whose father is $Rh_0(D)$positive or $Rh_0(D)$ unknown; the baby is $Rh_0(D)$-positive or $Rh_0(D)$ unknown, and mother must not be previously sensitized to $Rh_0(D)$ factor. **Transfusion**: indicated in suppression of Rh isoimmunization in $Rh_0(D)$-negative female children and female adults in their childbearing years transfused with $Rh_0(D)$-positive RBCs or blood components containing $Rh_0(D)$-positive RBCs.

The commercial forms of $Rh_0(D)$ immune globulin consist of IgG containing a high titer of antibodies against the **Rh(D)** antigen on the surface of red blood cells. All donors are carefully screened to reduce the risk of transmitting infectious diseases. Fractionation of the plasma is performed by precipitation with cold alcohol followed by passage through a viral clearance system.

$Rh_0(D)$ immune globulin binds Rho antigens, thereby preventing sensitization. Rh-negative women may be sensitized to the "foreign" Rh antigen on RBCs via the fetus at the time of birth, miscarriage, ectopic pregnancy, or any transplacental hemorrhage. If the women go on to have a primary immune response, they will make antibodies to Rh antigen that can cross the placenta and damage subsequent fetuses by lysing RBCs. This syndrome, called hemolytic disease of the newborn, is life-threatening. The form due to Rh incompatibility is largely preventable by $Rh_0(D)$ immune globulin.

$Rh_0(D)$ immune globulin is indicated whenever fetal red blood cells are known or suspected to have entered the circulation of an Rh-negative mother unless the fetus is known also to be Rh-negative. The drug is given intramuscularly. The half-life of circulating immunoglobulin is approximately 21 to 29 days.

Injection-site discomfort and low-grade fever have been reported. Systemic reactions are extremely rare, but myalgia, lethargy, and anaphylactic shock have been reported. As with all plasma-derived products, there is a theoretical risk of transmission of infectious disease.

Intravenous immunoglobulin (IVIC): In recent years indications for the use of intravenous immunoglobulin (IVIG) have expanded beyond replacement therapy for agammaglobulinemia and other immunodeficiencies to include a variety of bacterial and viral infections, and an array of autoimmune and inflammatory diseases as diverse as **thrombocytopenic purpura**, **Kawasaki's disease**, and autoimmune skin, neuromuscular, and neurologic diseases. Although the mechanism of action of IVIG in immune modulation remains largely unknown, proposed mechanisms include modulation of expression and function of Fc receptors on leukocytes and endothelial cells, interference with complement activation and cytokine production, provision of antiidiotypic antibodies (Jerne network theory), and effects on the activation and effector function of T- and B-lymphocytes. Although IVIG is effective in many autoimmune diseases, its spectrum of efficacy and appropriate dosing (especially duration of therapy) are unknown. Additional controlled studies of IVIG are needed to identify proper dosing, cost-benefit, and quality-of-life parameters.

RIBAVIRIN

(Virazole)

Ribavirin is indicated in the treatment of carefully selected hospitalized infants and young children with severe lower respiratory tract infections due to respiratory syncytial virus (RSV). In addition, ribavirin (600 to 1800 mg/day for 10 to 14 days) has shown effectiveness in acute and chronic hepatitis, herpes genitalis, measles, and Lassa fever.

Ribavirin has antiviral inhibitory activity *in vitro* against respiratory syncytial virus, influenza virus, and herpes simplex virus.

The antiviral mechanism of action of ribavirin relates to alteration of cellular nucleotide pools and inhibition of viral messenger RNA synthesis. Intracellular phosphorylation to the mono-, di-, and triphosphate derivatives is mediated by host cell enzymes. In both uninfected and RSV-infected cells, the predominant derivative (>80%) is the triphosphate, which has an intracellular $t_{1/2}$ of elimination of less than 2 hours.

Ribavirin monophosphate competitively inhibits cellular inosine-5′-phosphate dehydrogenase and interferes with the synthesis of guanosine triphosphate (GTP) and, thus, nucleic acid synthesis in general. Ribavirin triphosphate also competitively inhibits the GTP-dependent 5′-capping of viral messenger RNA and, specifically, influenza virus transcriptase activity. Ribavirin appears to have multiple sites of action, and some of these (e.g., inhibition of GTP synthesis) may potentiate others (e.g., inhibition of GTP-dependent enzymes).

Ribavirin, which is teratogenic, gonadotoxic, embryotoxic, and oncogenic, has caused malformation of skull, palate, eye, jaw, skeleton, and GI tract, and hence is contraindicated in female subjects who are or intend to become pregnant during exposure to the drug.

Aerosolized ribavirin has been well tolerated but may cause mild conjunctival irritation, rash, transient wheezing, and occasional reversible deterioration in pulmonary function. When used in conjunction with mechanical ventilation, equipment modifications and frequent monitoring are required to prevent plugging of ventilator valves and tubing with ribavirin.

Systemic ribavirin causes dose-related anemia due to extravascular hemolysis and dose-related suppression of bone marrow. Reversible increases of serum bilirubin, serum iron, and uric acid concentrations occur during short-term oral administration. Bolus intravenous infusion may cause rigors. In HIV-infected patients, chronic oral therapy is also associated with dose-related lymphopenia and gastrointestinal and CNS complaints, including headache, lethargy, insomnia, and mood alteration.

RIBOFLAVIN (VITAMIN B_2)

(Riboflavin tablets 50 mg)

Riboflavin is a water-soluble vitamin that is converted in the body to coenzymes necessary in oxidation reduction. It is also necessary in maintaining integrity of RBCs. It is indicated in the prevention and treatment of riboflavin deficiency.

Pure red cell aplasia that responded to the administration of riboflavin was reported in patients with protein depletion and complicating infections. Nutritionists induced riboflavin deficiency in human beings and demonstrated that a hypoproliferative anemia resulted within a month. The spontaneous appearance in human beings of red cell aplasia due to **riboflavin** deficiency undoubtedly is rare, if it occurs at all. It has been described in combination with infection and protein deficiency, both of which are capable of producing a hypoproliferative anemia. However, it seems reasonable to include **riboflavin** in the nutritional management of patients with gross, generalized malnutrition.

RIFABUTIN

(Mycobutin)

Rifabutin is a newly marketed, semisynthetic antimycobacterial agent similar to rifampicin (rifampin) in structure and activity. However, rifabutin has important pharmacokinetic differences compared with rifampicin. The clinical effectiveness of rifabutin for prophylaxis of disseminated *Mycobacterium avium* complex infections has recently been demonstrated in HIV-positive patients with low CD4 counts.

Rifabutin is a derivative of **rifamycin** that shares a common mechanism of action (inhibition of mycobacterial **RNA polymerase**), but is more active than rifampin *in vitro* and in **experimental murine tuberculosis**.

Rifabutin has better activity against the minimum alveolar concentration (MAC) organisms than does rifampin. Rifabutin is active *in vitro* against MAC bacteria isolated from both HIV-infected (where the majority of MAC infections are *M. avium*) and non-HIV-infected individuals (in whom approximately 40% of MAC infections are *M. intracellulare*). **Rifabutin** inhibits the growth of most MAC isolates at concentrations ranging from 0.25 to 1 μg/mL. Rifabutin also inhibits the growth of many strains of *M. tuberculosis* at concentrations of 0.125 μg/mL.

Cross-resistance between rifampin and rifabutin is common in *M. tuberculosis*, although some strains have been identified that are resistant to rifampin yet sensitive to rifabutin. Of 225 *M. avium* strains that were resistant to 10 μg/mL of rifampin, 80% were sensitive to 1 μg/ml **rifabutin**.

The oral administration of 300 mg of rifabutin produces a peak plasma concentration of approximately 0.4 μg/mL at 2 to 3 hours. The drug is metabolized by hepatic CYPs and eliminated in a biphasic manner with a mean terminal half-life of 45 hours (range of 16 to 96 hours). Because **rifabutin** is a lipophilic drug, concentrations are substantially higher (five- to tenfold) in tissue than in plasma. Following absorption from the GI tract, rifabutin is eliminated in the urine and bile. Adjustment of dosage is not necessary in patients with impaired renal function. **Rifabutin** is a weaker inducer of hepatic CYPs than is rifampin.

Rifabutin is effective for the prevention of MAC infection in HIV-infected individuals. At a dose of 300 mg per day, rifabutin decreased the frequency of MAC bacteremia (2%). However, **azithromycin** or **clarithromycin** are more effective and less likely to interact with highly active antiretroviral therapy (HAART) drugs. **Rifabutin** also is commonly substituted for rifampin in the treatment of tuberculosis in HIV-infected patients, as it has a less profound CYP-dependent interaction with indinavir and nelfinavir. Rifabutin also is used in combination with **clarithromycin** and **ethambutol** for the therapy of MAC disease.

Rifabutin generally is well tolerated in persons with HIV infection; primary reasons for discontinuation of therapy include rash (4%), gastrointestinal intolerance (3%), and neutropenia (2%). Overall, neutropenia occurred in 25% of patients with severe HIV infection who received rifabutin. Uveitis and arthralgias have occurred in patients receiving rifabutin doses greater than 450 mg daily in combination with clarithromycin or fluconazole. Patients should be cautioned to discontinue the drug if visual symptoms (pain or blurred vision) occur. Like rifampin, the drug causes an orange-tan discoloration of skin, urine, feces, saliva, tears, and contact lenses. Rarely, thrombocytopenia, a flu-like syndrome, hemolysis, myositis, chest pain, and hepatitis have occurred in patients treated with rifabutin.

Although a less potent inducer of CYPs than rifampin, rifabutin does induce hepatic microsomal enzymes, with its administration decreasing the half-life of a number of different compounds, including zidovudine, prednisone, digitoxin, quinidine, ketoconazole, propranolol, phenytoin, sulfonylureas, and warfarin. It has less effect than does rifampin on serum levels of indinavir and nelfinavir.

RIFAMPIN

(Rifadin)

Rifampin (600 mg once daily) is indicated in the treatment of all forms of tuberculosis in conjunction with at least one other antituberculous drug. Frequently used regimens include: isoniazid and rifampin; ethambutol and rifampin; or isoniazid, ethambutol, and rifampin; or isoniazid, pyrazinamide, and rifampin. In addition, it is used in the treatment of asymptomatic carriers of *Neisseria* meningitis in order to eliminate meningococci from the nasopharynx. It is not indicated for treatment of meningococcal infection.

Rifampin inhibits DNA-dependent RNA polymerase of mycobacteria and other microorganisms by forming a stable drug–enzyme complex, leading to suppression of initiation of chain formation (but not chain elongation) in RNA synthesis. More specifically, the beta subunit of this complex enzyme is the site of action of the drug, although rifampin binds only to the holoenzyme. Nuclear RNA polymerase from a variety of eukaryotic cells does not bind rifampin, and RNA synthesis is correspondingly unaffected. Whereas rifampin can inhibit RNA synthesis in the mammalian mitochondria, considerably higher concentrations of the drug are required than for the inhibition of the bacterial enzyme. High concentrations of rifampin antibiotics also inhibit viral DNA-dependent RNA polymerases and reverse transcriptases. Rifampin is bactericidal for both intracellular and extracellular microorganisms.

Rifampin is absorbed well orally and is bound to plasma proteins to the extent of 80%. It penetrates and concentrates in many body tissues, including the cerebrospinal fluid, and is metabolized in the liver by deacetylation, which is active against *Mycobacterium tuberculosis*.

Rifampin induces the activity of the hepatic microsomal enzyme, metabolizing numerous drugs including acetaminophen, anticoagulants, barbiturates, benzodiazepines, beta-blockers, chloramphenicol, clofibrate, contraceptives, corticosteroids, cyclosporine, digitoxin, disopyramide, estrogens, hydantoins, methadone, mexiletine, quinidine, sulfones, sulfonylureas, theophyllines, tocainide, and verapamil. The plasma levels and effectiveness of these agents may be decreased.

Rifampin is generally well tolerated. When given in usual doses, fewer than 4% of patients with tuberculosis have significant adverse reactions; the most common are rash (0.8%), fever (0.5%), and nausea and vomiting (1.5%). The most notable problem is the development of jaundice.

Hepatitis from rifampin rarely occurs in patients with normal hepatic function; likewise, the combination of isoniazid and rifampin appears generally safe in such patients. However, chronic liver disease, alcoholism, and old age appear to increase the incidence of severe hepatic problems when rifampin is given alone or concurrently with isoniazid.

RIFAPENTINE

(Priftin tablets 150 mg)

Rifapentine is an antituberculosis agent that inhibits DNA-dependent RNA polymerase in susceptible strains of *Mycobacterium tuberculosis*. It is bactericidal for intracellular and extracellular *M. tuberculosis* organisms. It is indicated in the treatment of pulmonary tuberculosis in conjunction with one or more other antituberculosis drugs to which the isolate is susceptible.

The **rifamycins** (**rifampin**, **rifabutin**, **rifapentine**) are a group of structurally similar, complex macrocyclic antibiotics produced by *Amycolatopsis mediterranei*; rifampin (Rifadin, Rimactane) is a semisynthetic derivative of one of these—rifamycin B. Rifamycins were first isolated from cultures obtained from a pine forest near Nice, France.

Rifapentine (Priftin) has a longer half-life than rifampin and rifabutin, which allows once-weekly dosing. Compared to rifabutin and rifampin, it is intermediate in its induction of CYPs. Its use in the treatment of tuberculosis in HIV-infected patients was associated with the selection of rifamycin resistance; **rifabutin** is therefore preferred in this situation.

Combination therapy is almost always the desirable approach for myobacterial disease to ensure effective eradication and to prevent the emergence of resistance. **Isoniazid**, **rifampin**, **ethambutol**, **streptomycin**, and **pyrazinamide** are first-line agents for the treatment of tuberculosis. The use of immunomodulators such as interferon-γ to increase macrophage killing of the intracellular bacterium is a potentially interesting new avenue for treatment. Antimicrobial agents with excellent activity against *Mycobacterium avium* complex include **rifabutin**, **clarithromycin azithromycin**, and **fluoroquinolones**. Drug interactions and adverse drug reactions, however, are common with multiple-drug regimens, and clinical monitoring is important. Considerable progress has been achieved in eliminating leprosy through the use of multiple-drug chemotherapy including dapsone, rifampin, and clofazimine. Thalidomide also has been found to have activity in patients with leprosy.

RIFAXIMIN

(Xifaxan tablets 200 mg)

Rifaximin is an antiinfective agent that inhibits bacterial RNA synthesis. It is indicated in the treatment of traveler's diarrhea by noninvasive strains of *Escherichia coli*.

RILUZOLE

(Rilutek tablets 50 mg)

Riluzole is a CNS agent. It inhibits glutamate release; inactivates voltage-dependent sodium channels; and interferes with intracellular events following transmitter binding at excitatory amino acid receptors. These effects may protect neural tissues against degenerative changes. It is indicated in the treatment of patients with **amyotrophic lateral sclerosis** (ALS; **Lou Gehrig's disease**).

Riluzole (2-amino-6-[trifluoromethoxylbenzothiazole]; Rilutek) is an agent with complex actions in the nervous system.

Riluzole is absorbed orally and is highly protein bound. It undergoes extensive metabolism in the liver by both cytochrome P450-mediated hydroxylation and glucuronidation. Its half-life is about 12 hours. *In vitro* studies have shown that riluzole has both presynaptic and postsynaptic effects. It inhibits glutamate release, but it also blocks postsynaptic *N*-methyl-D-aspartate (NMDA)- and kainate-type glutamate receptors and inhibits voltage-dependent sodium channels. Some of the effects of **riluzole** *in vitro* are blocked by pertussis toxin, implicating the drug's interaction with an as-yet-unidentified GPCR. In clinical trials riluzole has modest but genuine effects on the survival of patients with ALS. In the largest trial conducted to date, with nearly 1000 patients, the median duration of survival was extended by about 60 days. The recommended dose is 50 mg every 12 hours, taken 1 hour before or 2 hours after a meal. Riluzole usually is well tolerated, although nausea or diarrhea may occur. Rarely, **riluzole** may produce hepatic injury with elevations of serum transaminases, and periodic monitoring of these is recommended. Although the magnitude of the effect of **riluzole** on ALS is small, it represents a significant therapeutic milestone in the treatment of a disease refractory to all previous treatments.

RIMANTADINE HYDROCHLORIDE

(Flumadine)

Rimantadine (100 mg t.i.d.) and amantadine are indicated in prophylaxis and treatment of illness caused by various strains of influenza A virus. Amantadine and rimantadine share two mechanisms of antiviral action. They inhibit an early step in viral replication, probably viral uncoating; for some strains, they have an effect on a late step in viral assembly probably mediated through altering hemagglutinin processing. The primary locus of action is the influenza A virus M2 protein, an integral membrane protein that functions as an ion channel. By interfering with this function of the M2 protein, the drugs inhibit the acid-mediated dissociation of the ribonucleoprotein complex early in replication and potentiate acidic pH-induced conformational changes in the hemagglutinin during its intracellular transport later in replication (see also Figure 19).

Resistant variants are selected readily by virus passage in the presence of drug and have been recovered from treated persons. Resistance with over 100-fold increases in inhibitory concentrations has been associated with single nucleotide changes leading to amino-acid substitutions in the transmembrane region of M2. Amantadine and rimantadine share cross-susceptibility and resistance (see Figure 19).

Following oral administration, rimantadine is extensively metabolized in the liver, with <25% of the dose excreted in the urine as unchanged drug. Three hydroxylated metabolites have been found in plasma. These metabolites, an additional conjugated metabolite, and parent drug account for 74% of a single 200 mg dose excreted in urine over 72 hours. Acetaminophen and aspirin reduce, whereas cimetidine increases, the plasma level of rimantadine.

The most common side effects related to amantadine and rimantadine are minor dose-related gastrointestinal and central nervous system (CNS) complaints. These include nervousness, lightheadedness, difficulty concentrating, insomnia, and loss of appetite or nausea. CNS side effects occur in approximately 5 to 33% of patients treated with amantadine at doses of 200 mg/day, but are significantly less frequent with rimantadine. Amantadine dose reductions are required in older adults (100 mg/day) because of decreased renal function, but 20 to 40% of infirm elderly patients will experience side effects even at this lower dose.

High amantadine plasma concentrations (1.0 to 5.0 μg/ml) have been associated with serious neurotoxic reactions, including delirium, hallucinosis, seizures or coma, and cardiac arrhythmias. Exacerbations of preexisting seizure disorders and psychiatric symptoms may occur with amantadine and possibly with rimantadine.

RIMEXOLONE

(Vexol ophthalmic suspension 1%)

Rimexolone is a corticosteroid that suppresses inflammatory response to stimuli of a mechanical, chemical, or immunological origin. It is indicated in the treatment of postoperative inflammation following ocular surgery; and in the treatment of **anterior uveitis**.

RINGER'S INJECTION

Ringer's solution is used in fluid and electrolyte replacement.

RISEDRONATE SODIUM

(Actonel tablets 30 mg)

Risedronate sodium is a bisphosphonate that inhibits normal and abnormal bone resorption. It is indicated in the treatment of osteoporosis in postmenopausal women; the prevention of osteoporosis in postmenopausal women at risk of developing osteoporosis; the prevention and treatment of glucocorticoid-induced osteoporosis in men and women; and in the treatment of **Paget's disease of the bone**.

Bisphosphonates are analogs of pyrophosphate that contain two phosphonate groups attached to a geminal (central) carbon that replaces the oxygen in pyrophosphate. Because they form a three-dimensional structure capable of chelating divalent cations such as Ca^{2+}, the bisphosphonates have a strong affinity for bone, targeting especially bone surfaces undergoing remodeling. Accordingly, they are used extensively in conditions characterized by **osteoclast-mediated bone resorption**, including **osteoporosis**, **steroid-induced osteoporosis**, **Paget's disease**, **tumor-associated osteolysis**, breast and prostate cancer, and hypercalcemia. Recent evidence suggests that second- and third generation bisphosphonates also may be effective anticancer drugs.

The clinical utility of bisphosphonates resides in their direct inhibition of bone resorption. First-generation bisphosphonates contain minimally modified side chains (Rl, R2) (**medronate**, **clodronate**, and **etidronate**) or contain a chlorophenyl group (tiludronate). They are the least potent and in some instances cause bone demineralization. Second- generation aminobisphosphonates (e.g., **alendronate** and **pamidronate**) contain a nitrogen group in the side chain. They are 10 to 100 times more potent than first-generation compounds. Third-generation bisphosphonates (e.g., **risedronate** and **zoledronate**) contain a nitrogen atom within a heterocyclic ring and are up to 10,000 times more potent than first-generation agents.

Bisphosphonates concentrate at sites of active remodeling. Because they are highly negatively charged, bisphosphonates are membrane impermeable but are incorporated into the bone matrix by fluid-phase endocytosis. Bisphosphonates remain in the matrix until the bone is remodeled and then are released in the acid environment of the resorption lacunae beneath the osteoclast as the overlying mineral matrix is dissolved. The importance of this process for the antiresorptive effect of bisphosphonates is evidenced by the fact that **calcitonin** blocks the antiresorptive action.

Although bisphosphonates prevent hydroxyapatite dissolution, their antiresorptive action is due to direct inhibitory effects on osteoclasts rather than strictly physiochemical effects. The antiresorptive activity apparently involves two primary mechanisms: osteoclast apoptosis and inhibition of components of the cholesterol biosynthetic pathway.

The current model is that apoptosis accounts for the antiresorptive effect of first-generation bisphosphonates, whereas the inhibitory action of aminobisphosphonates proceeds through the latter mechanism. Consistent with this view, the antiresorptive effect of aminobisphosphonates such as alendronate and risedronate, but not of clodronate or etidronate, persists when apoptosis is suppressed. First-generation bisphosphonates are metabolized into a nonhydrolyzable ATP analog ($AppCCl_2p$) that accumulates within osteoclasts and induces apoptosis. In contrast, the aminobisphosphonates such as alendronate and ibandronate directly inhibit multiple steps in the pathway from mevalonate to cholesterol and isoprenoid lipids, such as geranylgeranyl diphosphate, that are required for the prenylation of proteins that are important for osteoclast function. The potency of aminobisphosphonates for inhibiting farnesyl synthase correlates directly with their antiresorptive activity.

Much interest is focused on the role of bisphosphonates in the treatment of osteoporosis. Clinical trials show that treatment is associated with increased bone mineral density and protection against fracture.

Bisphosphonates also may act as anticancer drugs by inhibiting the activation of cancer-associated proteins, such as Ras, through suppression of geranylgeranylation and farnesylation. Second- and third-generation bisphosphonates inhibit the proliferation of some cancer cells by preventing posttranslational prenylation of Ras-related proteins. Zoledronate has been used successfully as an adjunct in treating **Philadelphia chromosome-positive chronic myelogenous leukemia**.

RISPERIDONE

(Risperdal tablets 0.25 mg, tablets 0.5 mg, tablets 1 mg, tablets 2 mg, tablets 3 mg, tablets 4 mg, oral solution 1 mg/mL, Risperdol Consta powder for injection 25 mg, powder for injection 37.5 mg, powder for injection 50 mg, Risperdal M-TAB tablets, orally disintegrating 0.5 mg, tablets, orally disintegrating 1 mg, tablets, orally disintegrating 2 mg)

Risperidone is a benzisoxazole derivative, and has antipsychotic effects, apparently caused by dopamine and serotonin receptor blocking in the CNS. A benzisoxazole derivative causing few movement disorders (1 mg p.o. b.i.d.), risperidone is used in psychosis (see also Table 2).

Clozapine (Clozaril), a $5\text{-}HT_{2A/2C}$-receptor antagonist, represents a class of atypical antipsychotic drugs with reduced incidence of extrapyramidal side effects compared to the classical neuroleptics, and possibly a greater efficacy for reducing negative symptoms of schizophrenia. Clozapine also has a high affinity for subtypes of dopamine receptors.

One of the newest strategies for the design of additional atypical antipsychotic drugs is to combine $5\text{-}HT_{2A/2C}$ and dopamine D_2-receptor-blocking actions in the same molecule. **Risperidone** (Risperdal), for example, is a potent $5\text{-}HT_{2A}$- and D_2-receptor antagonist. Low doses of **risperidone** have been reported to attenuate negative symptoms of schizophrenia with a low incidence of extrapyramidal side effects. Extrapyramidal effects are commonly seen, however, with doses of risperidone in excess of 6 mg/day. Other atypical antipsychotic agents—**quetiapine** (Seroquel) and **olanzapine** (Zyprexa)—act on multiple receptors, but their antipsychotic properties are thought to be due to antagonism of dopamine and serotonin.

Risperidone has prominent antiserotonergic ($5\text{-}HT_{2A}$), antidopaminergic (D_2-like), antiadrenergic (α_1), and antihistaminic (H_1) activity, as well as very low antimuscarinic activity. Although risperidone and clozapine share relatively high serotonin $5\text{-}HT_{2A}$ and lower dopamine D_2-receptor affinities, risperidone has much more potent antidopaminergic and much less potent antimuscarinic activity. Unlike clozapine, it can induce extrapyramidal symptoms and prominent hyperprolactinemia. Nevertheless, risperidone can be considered an "atypical" antipsychotic in that its adverse extrapyramidal neurological effects are limited at low daily doses (i.e., 6 mg or less), usually with adequate and antipsychotic effects.

Many **neuroleptic** drugs can lower the seizure threshold and induce discharge patterns in the electroencephalogram (EEG)—effects associated with **epileptic seizure disorders**. Clozapine, olanzapine, and aliphatic phenothiazines with low potency (such as chlorpromazine) seem particularly able to do this, whereas the more potent piperazine phenothiazines and thioxanthenes (notably fluphenazine and thiothixene), **risperidone**, and quetiapine are much less likely to have this effect. The butyrophenones and molindone variably and unpredictably rarely cause seizures. Clozapine has a clearly dose-related risk of inducing EEG abnormalities and seizures in nonepileptic patients. Antipsychotic agents, especially clozapine, olanzapine, and low-potency phenothiazines and thioxanthenes, should be used with extreme caution, if at all, in untreated epileptic patients and in patients undergoing withdrawal from CNS depressants such as alcohol, barbiturates, or benzodiazepines. Most antipsychotic drugs, especially the piperazines as well as the newer atypical agents **aripiprazole**, **quetiapine**, **risperidone**, and **ziprasidone**, can be used safely in epileptic patients if moderate doses are attained gradually and if concomitant anticonvulsant drug therapy is maintained.

RITODRINE HYDROCHLORIDE

(Yutopar)

Ritodrine (0.1 mg/min IV and 10 mg orally 30 min before termination of IV therapy) is indicated in the management of preterm labor. Ritodrine is a beta$_2$-adrenergic-receptor agonist influencing the uterine smooth muscle. Stimulation of the beta$_2$ receptors inhibits contractility of the uterine smooth muscle by stimulation of adenyl cyclase, which increases intracellular cyclic adenosine 3′-5′-monophosphate (cAMP); this leads to altering cellular calcium balance that affects smooth muscle contractility. In addition, ritodrine may directly affect the interaction between the actin and myosin of muscle through inhibition of myosin light-chain kinase.

Ritodrine is contraindicated in antepartum hemorrhage, which demands immediate delivery; eclampsia and severe preeclampsia; intrauterine fetal death; chorioamnionitis; maternal cardiac disease; pulmonary hypertension; maternal hyperthyroidism; and uncontrolled maternal diabetes mellitus. Overdosage with ritodrine may cause tachycardia (maternal and fetal), palpitations, cardiac arrhythmia, hypotension, dyspnea, nervousness, tremor, nausea, and vomiting.

RITONAVIR

(Norvir)

Ritonavir is an inhibitor of the human immunodeficiency virus (HIV) protease which, in combination with nucleoside analogs (600 mg/b.i.d. p.o.), is indicated in the treatment of HIV infection. Ritonavir is a peptidomimetic inhibitor of both the HIV-1 and HIV-2 proteases. Inhibition of HIV protease renders the enzyme incapable of processing the gag-pol polyprotein precursor, which leads to production of noninfectious immature HIV particles.

Ritonavir exhibits additive to synergistic effects against HIV when used in combination with reverse-transcriptase inhibitors such as zidovudine or zalcitabine. Ritonavir produces a large increase in the plasma concentration of amiodarone, astemizole, bepridil, bupropion, cisapride, clozapine, encainide, flecainide, meperidine, peroxicam, propafenone, propoxyphene, quinidine, rifabutin, and terfenadine.

RITONAVIR

(Norvir capsules 100 mg, oral solution 80 mg/mL)

Ritonavir is a protease inhibitor that inhibits human immunodeficiency virus (HIV) protease, the enzyme required to form functional proteins in HIV-infected cells. It is indicated in the treatment of HIV infections in combination with other antiretroviral agents.

Current treatment assumes that all aspects of disease derive from the direct toxic effects of HIV on host cells, mainly CD4+ T-lymphocytes. This viewpoint is based on studies demonstrating the importance of high plasma HIV RNA concentration and low CD4+ lymphocyte count as predictors of disease progression and mortality. Validation has come from evidence that treatment regimens associated with long-term suppression of HIV replication (as measured by decreased plasma HIV RNA) and repletion of peripheral CD4 cells are clinically beneficial. The goal of therapy is to suppress virus replication as much as possible for as long as possible.

Deciding when to start antiretroviral therapy has been a shifting target during the epidemic. **Zidovudine**, the first antiretroviral drug, was approved initially only for patients with advanced, symptomatic disease. In this population, zidovudine monotherapy dramatically reduced HIV-associated mortality after only 6 months of treatment compared with placebo. The clinical benefit of this drug in patients with less advanced disease or no symptoms was more difficult to demonstrate, and two large comparative trials showed no benefit.

Ritonavir is a peptidomimetic HIV protease inhibitor designed to complement the C_2- symmetry of the enzyme active site. **Ritonavir** is active against both HIV-1 and HIV-2, although it may be slightly less active against the latter. Its IC_{50} for wild-type HIV-1 variants in the absence of human serum ranges from 4 to 150 nM.

Ritonavir reversibly binds to the active site of the HIV protease, preventing polypeptide processing and subsequent virus maturation. Virus particles are produced in the presence of ritonavir but are noninfectious.

In patients treated with **ritonavir** as the sole protease inhibitor, virus replication in the presence of drug selects for drug-resistance mutations. The primary **ritonavir** resistance mutation is usually at protease codon 82 (several possible substitutions for valine) or codon 84 (isoleucine-to-valine substitution). Additional mutations associated with increasing resistance occur at codons 20, 32, 46, 54, 63, 71, 84, and 90. High-level resistance requires accumulation of multiple mutations.

Absorption of **ritonavir** is rapid and is only slightly affected by food, depending on the formulation. The overall absorption of **ritonavir** from the capsule formulation increases by 13% when the capsule is taken with meals, but the bioavailability of the oral solution decreases by 7%. Interindividual variability in pharmacokinetics is high, with a greater than sixfold variability in trough concentrations among patients given 600 mg **ritonavir** every 12 hours.

Ritonavir is metabolized primarily by CYP3A4 and to a lesser extent by CYP2D6. Ritonavir and its metabolites are mainly eliminated in feces (86% of parent drug and metabolites), with only 3% of drug eliminated unchanged in the urine. It is 98 to 99% bound to plasma proteins, mainly to α_1-acid glycoprotein. Physiological concentrations of α_1-acid glycoprotein increase the *in vitro* IC_{50} by a factor of 10, whereas albumin increases the 1050 by a factor of four.

The major side effects of ritonavir are GI and include nausea, vomiting, diarrhea, anorexia, abdominal pain, and taste perversion. These side effects are dose-dependent and are less common with lower doses. Gastrointestinal toxicity may be reduced if the drug is taken with meals. Peripheral and perioral paresthesias also are common. These side effects generally abate within a few weeks of starting therapy.

Ritonavir induces its own metabolism, and gradual dose escalation over the first 2 weeks may minimize early intolerance. When ritonavir is used as the sole protease inhibitor, it should be initiated at 300 mg every 12 hours and escalated gradually to 600 mg every 12 hours by day 14 of therapy. **Ritonavir** causes dose-dependent elevations in serum total cholesterol and triglycerides, as well as other signs of lipodystrophy, and could increase the long-term risk of atherosclerosis in some patients.

Ritonavir is one of the most potent known inhibitors of CYP3A4, markedly increasing the plasma concentration and prolonging the elimination of many drugs including amiodarone, propafenone, ergot derivatives, pimozide, triazolam, and midazolam. This drug should be avoided or used with caution in combination with any CYP3A4 substrate, especially those with a narrow therapeutic index. **Ritonavir** is also a weak inhibitor of CYP2D6. Potent inducers of CYP3A4 activity such as rifampin may lower ritonavir concentrations and should be avoided or dosage adjustments considered. The capsule and solution formulations of ritonavir contain alcohol and should not be administered with disulfiram or metronidazole.

Ritonavir is a moderate inducer of CYP3A4, glucuronosyl *S*-transferase, and possibly other hepatic enzymes. The concentrations of some drugs therefore will be decreased in the presence of ritonavir. Ritonavir reduces the ethinyl estradiol AUC by 40%, and alternative forms of contraception should be used.

Among patients with susceptible strains of HTV-1, ritonavir as a sole agent lowers plasma HTV-1 RNA concentrations by one hundred- to one thousandfold. In a double-blind, randomized, controlled trial in 1090 patients with advanced HIV disease, the addition of ritonavir to current therapy reduced HIV-related mortality and disease progression by about 50% over a median of 6 months of follow-up. **Ritonavir** is used infrequently as the sole protease inhibitor in combination regimens because of GI toxicity. However, numerous clinical trials have shown efficacy for **ritonavir** in various dual protease inhibitor combinations.

Ritonavir inhibits the metabolism of all current HIV protease inhibitors and is frequently combined with most of these drugs, with the exception of nelfinavir, to enhance their pharmacokinetic profile and allow a reduction in dose and dosing frequency of the coadministered drug. **Ritonavir** also overcomes the deleterious effect of food on indinavir bioavailability. Under most circumstances, low doses of ritonavir (100 or 200 mg twice daily) are just as effective at inhibiting CYP3A4 and are much better tolerated than the 600-mg twice-daily treatment dose. The positive impact of low-dose ritonavir on the pharmacokinetics of lopinavir made possible the development and eventual approval of that drug, which is a component of one of two preferred starting regimens recommended by the U.S. Department of Health and Human Services in 2004.

RITUXIMAB

(Rituxan solution for injection 10 mg/mL)

Rituximab is a monoclonal antibody directed against the CD20 antigen found on the surface of normal and malignant B-lymphocytes. The CD20 antigen is also expressed on more than 90% of B-cell **non-Hodgkin's lymphomas** (NHL). It is indicated as a relapsed or refractory low-grade or follicular, CD20-positive, B-cell non-Hodgkin's lymphoma.

Rituximab (Rituxan) is a chimeric monoclonal antibody that targets the CD20 B-cell antigen. CD20 is found on cells from the pre-B-cell stage through terminal differentiation to plasma cells and is expressed on 90% of B-cell neoplasms. The biological functions of CD20 are uncertain, although incubation of B-cells with anti-CD20 antibody has variable effects on cell-cycle progression, depending on the monoclonal antibody type. Monoclonal antibody binding to CD20 generates transmembrane signals that produce autophosphorylation and activation of serine/tyrosine protein kinases, and induction of *c-myc* oncogene expression and major histocompatibility complex class II molecules. Studies have shown that CD20 also is associated with transmembrane Ca_{2+} conductance, through its possible function as a Ca_{2+} channel. These studies demonstrate the importance of CD20 in B-cell regulation, but do not in themselves indicate how ligation of the receptor produces cell death independent of ADCC or complement-mediated pathways.

Rituximab is the first monoclonal antibody to receive FDA approval and initially was approved for relapsed indolent lymphomas. However, it has shown activity in a wide variety of clinical settings. In the initial phase II study of rituximab in 37 patients with relapsed low-grade lymphoma, 46% responded with a median time to progression of 10 months. Notably, rituximab also was shown to be effective in 40% of patients who had previously responded to rituximab, but has a longer median time to progression of 18 months. Recent studies also have demonstrated significant activity of rituximab in mantle cell lymphoma, relapsed aggressive B-cell lymphomas, and CLL. The use of maintenance rituximab has gained increased acceptance, based on demonstration of delayed time to progression, but effects on survival have not been demonstrated. Increasingly evident are the synergistic effects of rituximab and chemotherapy, suggesting it sensitizes lymphoma cells to the apoptotic effects of chemotherapy by directly acting on tumor cells. Based on *in vitro* studies showing synergistic effects of chemotherapy and rituximab, rituximab is being clinically combined with agents such as **fludarabine** and combinations such as CHOP (regimen with cyclophosphamide, doxorubicin, and prednisone). Of great importance is the recent finding that the addition of rituximab to CHOP chemotherapy significantly improves the event-free survival of diffuse large B-cell lymphoma.

Rituximab demonstrates dose-dependent pharmacokinetics. At a dose of 375 mg/m^2, the mean serum half-life was 76.3 hours (range, 32 to 153 hours) after one dose and

205.8 hours (range, 84 to 407 hours) after the last dose. The wide range of half-lives likely reflects differences in patient tumor burden and normal B-cell populations. Rituximab toxicities are mostly related to infusion reactions, although there are increasing reports of late-onset neutropenia and rare reports of severe skin toxicity.

RIVASTIGMINE TARTRATE

(Exelon capsules 1.5 mg (as base), capsules 3 mg (as base), capsules 4.5 mg (as base), capsules 6 mg (as base), solution 2 mg/mL (as base))

Rivastigmine tartrate is a cholinesterase inhibitor that increases acetylcholine by inhibiting acetylcholinesterase, thereby increasing cholinergic function. It is indicated in the treatment of mild to moderate dementia of the Alzheimer type. A major approach to the treatment of Alzheimer's disease (AD) has involved attempts to augment the cholinergic function of the brain. An early approach was the use of precursors of acetylcholine synthesis, such as **choline chloride** and **phosphatidyl choline** (lecithin). Although these supplements generally are well tolerated, randomized trials have failed to demonstrate any clinically significant efficacy.

A somewhat more successful strategy has been the use of inhibitors of acetylcholinesterase (AChE), the catabolic enzyme for acetylcholine. Physostigmine, a rapidly acting, reversible AChE inhibitor, produces improved responses in animal models of learning, and some studies have demonstrated mild transitory improvement in memory following physostigmine treatment in patients with AD. The use of physostigmine has been limited because of its short half-life and tendency to produce symptoms of systemic cholinergic excess at therapeutic doses.

Four inhibitors of AChE currently are approved by the FDA for treatment of AD: **tacrine** (1,2,3,4-tetrahydro-9-aminoacridine; Cognex), **donepezil** (Aricept), **rivastigmine** (Exelon), and **galantamine** (Razadyne). Tacrine is a potent centrally acting inhibitor of AChE. Studies of oral tacrine in combination with lecithin have confirmed that there is indeed an effect of tacrine on some measures of memory performance, but the magnitude of improvement observed with the combination of lecithin and tacrine is modest at best. The side effects of tacrine often are significant and dose-limiting; abdominal cramping, anorexia, nausea, vomiting, and diarrhea are observed in up to one-third of patients receiving therapeutic doses, and elevations of serum transaminases are observed in up to 50% of those treated. Because of significant side effects, tacrine is not used widely clinically. **Donepezil** is a selective inhibitor of AChE in the CNS with little effect on AChE in peripheral tissues. It produces modest improvements in cognitive scores in AD patients and has a long half-life, allowing once-daily dosing. Rivastigmine and galantamine are dosed twice daily and produce a similar degree of cognitive improvement. Adverse effects associated with donepezil, **rivastigmine**, and **galantamine** are similar in character but generally less frequent and less severe than those observed with tacrine; they include nausea, diarrhea, vomiting, and insomnia. Donepezil, rivastigmine, and galantamine are not associated with the hepatotoxicity that limits the use of tacrine.

RIZATRIPTAN BENZOATE

(Maxalt tablets 5 mg)

Rizatriptan benzoate is a serotonin 5-HT_1-receptor-agonist that binds to serotonin 1_B- and 1_D-receptors in intracranial arteries leading to vasoconstriction and subsequent relief of migraine headache. It is indicated in the treatment of acute migraine attacks with or without aura.

Direct-acting 5-HT-receptor agonists have widely different chemical structures, as well as diverse pharmacological properties. This diversity is not surprising in light of the number of 5-HT-receptor subtypes. 5-HT_{1A}-receptor-selective agonists have helped elucidate the functions of this receptor in the brain and have resulted in a new class of antianxiety drugs including **buspirone**, **gepirone**, and **ipsapirone**. 5-HT_{1D}-receptor-selective agonists, such as **sumatriptan**, have unique properties that result in constriction of intracranial blood vessels. Sumatriptan was first in a series of new serotonin-receptor agonists available for treatment of acute migraine attacks. Other such agents now FDA approved in the United States for the acute treatment of migraine include **zolmitriptan** (Zomig), **naratriptan** (Amerge), and **rizatriptan** (Maxalt), all of which are selective for 5-HT_{1D} and 5-HT_{1B} receptors. A number of 5-HT_4-receptor-selective agonists have been developed or are being developed for the treatment of disorders of the GI tract.

Migraine headache afflicts 10 to 20% of the population, producing a morbidity estimated at 64 million missed workdays per year in the United States. Although migraine is a specific neurological syndrome, the manifestations vary widely. The principal types are: migraine without aura (common migraine); migraine with aura (classic migraine), which includes subclasses of migraine with typical aura, migraine with prolonged aura, migraine without headache, and migraine with acute-onset aura; and several other rarer types. Auras also may appear without a subsequent headache. Premonitory aura may begin as long as 24 hours before the onset of pain and often is accompanied by photophobia, hyperacusis, polyuria, and diarrhea, and by disturbances of mood and appetite. A migraine attack may last for hours or days and be followed by prolonged pain-free intervals. The frequency of migraine attacks is extremely variable, but usually ranges from 1 to 2 a year to 1 to 4 per month.

The therapy of migraine headaches is complicated by the variable responses among and within individual patients and by the lack of a firm understanding of the pathophysiology of the syndrome. The efficacy of antimigraine drugs varies with the absence or presence of aura, duration of the headache, its severity and intensity, and as yet undefined environmental and genetic factors. A rather vague and inconsistent pathophysiological characteristic of migraine is the spreading depression of neural impulses from a focal point of vasoconstriction followed by vasodilation. However, it is unlikely that vasoconstriction followed by vasodilation (spreading depression) or vasodilation alone accounts for the local edema and focal tenderness often observed in migraine patients.

Consistent with the hypothesis that 5-HT is a key mediator in the pathogenesis of migraine, 5-HT-receptor agonists have become the mainstay for acute treatment of migraine headaches. This hypothesis is based on evidence obtained in laboratory experiments and on the following evidence obtained in human beings: (1) Plasma and platelet concentrations of 5-HT vary with the different phases of the migraine attack. (2) Urinary concentrations of 5-HT and its metabolites are elevated during most migraine attacks. (3) Migraine may be precipitated by agents such as reserpine and fenfluramine that release biogenic amines, including serotonin, from intracellular storage sites. New treatments for the prevention of migraines, such as botulinum toxin and newer antiepileptic drugs, have unique mechanisms of action, presumably unrelated to 5-HT.

The introduction of **sumatriptan** (Imitrex), **zolmitriptan** (Zomig), **naratriptan** (Amerge), and **rizatriptan** (Maxalt and Maxalt-MLT) in the therapy of migraine: The selective pharmacological effects of these agents, dubbed the triptans, at 5-HT_1 receptors have led to insights into the pathophysiology of migraine. Clinically, the drugs are effective, acute antimigraine agents. Their ability to decrease, rather than exacerbate, the nausea and vomiting of migraine is an important advance in the treatment of the condition.

Two hypotheses have been proposed to explain the efficacy of 5-HT_{1D}-receptor agonists in migraine. One hypothesis implicates the capacity of these receptors to cause constriction of intracranial blood vessels including arteriovenous anastomoses. According to a prominent pathophysiological model of migraine, unknown events lead to the abnormal dilation of carotid arteriovenous anastomoses in the head. As much as 80% of carotid arterial blood flow has been reported to be "shunted" via these anastomoses, located mainly in the cranial skin and ears, diverting blood from the capillary beds and thereby producing cerebral ischemia and hypoxia. Based on this model, an effective antimigraine agent would close the shunts and restore blood flow to the brain. Indeed, ergotamine, **dihydroergotamine**, and **sumatriptan** share the capacity to produce this vascular effect with a pharmacological specificity that mirrors the effects of these agents on 5-HT_{1B}- and 5-HT_{1D}-receptor subtypes.

An alternative hypothesis concerning the significance of one or more 5-HT_1 receptors in migraine pathophysiology relates to the observation that both 5-HT_{1DB} and 5-HT_{1D} receptors serve as presynaptic autoreceptors, modulating neurotransmitter release from neuronal terminals. 5-HT_1 agonists may block the release of proinflammatory neuropeptides at the level of the nerve terminal in the perivascular space. Indeed, **ergotamine**, **dihydroergotamine**, and **sumatriptan** can block the development of neurogenic plasma extravasation in dura mater associated with depolarization of perivascular axons following capsaicin injection or unilateral electrical stimulation of the trigeminal nerve. The ability of potent 5-HT_1-receptor agonists to inhibit endogenous neurotransmitter release in the perivascular space could account for their efficacy in the acute treatment of migraine.

When given subcutaneously, **sumatriptan** reaches its peak plasma concentration in approximately 12 minutes. Following oral administration, peak plasma concentrations occur within 1 to 2 hours. Bioavailability following the subcutaneous route of administration is approximately 97%; after oral administration or nasal spray, bioavailability is only 14 to 17%. The elimination half-life is approximately 1 to 2 hours. Sumatriptan is metabolized predominant-ly by MAO-A, and its metabolites are excreted in the urine.

Zolmitriptan reaches its peak plasma concentration 1.5 to 2 hours after oral administration. Its bioavailability is about 40% following oral ingestion. Zolmitriptan is converted to an active *N*-desmethyl metabolite, which has several-fold higher affinity for 5-HT_{1B} and 5-HT_{1D} receptors than does the parent drug. Both the metabolite and the parent drug have half-lives of 2 to 3 hours.

Naratriptan, administered orally, reaches its peak plasma concentration in 2 to 3 hours and has an absolute bioavailability of about 70%. It is the longest acting of the triptans, having a half-life of about 6 hours. Fifty percent (50%) of an administered dose of naratriptan is excreted unchanged m the urine, and about 30% is excreted as products of oxidation by CYPs.

Rizatriptan has an oral bioavailability of about 45% and reaches peak plasma levels within 1 to 1.5 hours after oral ingestion of tablets of the drug. An orally disintegrating dosage form has a somewhat slower rate of absorption aiding peak plasma levels of the drug 1.6 to 2.5 hours after administration. The principal route of metabolism of rizatriptan is via oxidative deamination by MAO-A.

Plasma-protein binding of the triptans ranges from about 14% (sumatriptan and rizatriptan) to 30% (naratriptan).

Rare but serious cardiac events have been associated with the administration of 5-HT_1 agonists, including coronary artery vasospasm, transient myocardial ischemia, atrial and ventricular arrhythmias, and myocardial infarction, predominantly in patients with risk factors for coronary artery disease (CAD). In general, however, only minor side effects are seen with the triptans in the acute treatment of migraine. As much as 83% of patients experience at least one side effect after subcutaneous injection of sumatriptan. Most patients report transient mild pain, stinging, or burning sensations at the site of injection. The most common side effect of sumatriptan nasal spray is a bitter taste. Orally administered triptans can cause paresthesias; asthenia and fatigue;

flushing; feelings of pressure, tightness, or pain in the chest, neck, and jaw; drowsiness; dizziness; nausea; and sweating.

The triptans are contraindicated in patients who have a history of ischemic or vasospastic CAD, cerebrovascular or peripheral vascular disease, or other significant cardiovascular diseases. Because triptans may cause an acute, usually small, increase in blood pressure (BP), they also are contraindicated in patients with uncontrolled hypertension. Naratriptan is contraindicated in patients with severe renal or hepatic impairment. **Rizatriptan** should be used with caution in patients with renal or hepatic disease but is not contraindicated in such patients. Sumatriptan, rizatriptan, and zolmitriptan are contraindicated in patients who are taking monoamine oxidase inhibitors.

The triptans are effective in the acute treatment of migraine (with or without aura), but are not intended for use in prophylaxis of migraine. Treatment with these agents should begin as soon as possible after onset of a migraine attack. Oral dosage forms of the triptans are the most convenient to use, but they may not be practical in patients experiencing migraine-associated nausea and vomiting. Approximately 70% of individuals report significant headache relief from a 6-mg subcutaneous dose of sumatriptan. This dose may be repeated once within a 24-hour period if the first dose does not relieve the headache. An oral formulation and a nasal spray of sumatriptan also are available. The onset of action is as early as 15 minutes with the nasal spray. The recommended oral dose of sumatriptan is 25 to 100 mg, which may be repeated after 2 hours up to a total dose of 200 mg over a 24-hour period. When administered by nasal spray, from 5 to 20 mg of sumatriptan is recommended. The dose can be repeated after 2 hours up to a maximum dose of 40 mg over a 24-hour period. **Zolmitriptan** is given orally in a 1.25- to 2.5-mg dose, which can be repeated after 2 hours, up to a maximum dose of 10 mg over 24 hours, if the migraine attack persists. Naratriptan is given orally in a 1- to 2.5-mg dose, which should not be repeated until 4 hours after the previous dose. The maximum dose over a 24-hour period should not exceed 5 mg. The recommended oral dose of **rizatriptan** is 5 to 10 mg. The dose can be repeated after 2 hours up to a maximum dose of 30 mg over a 24-hour period. The safety of treating more than 3 or 4 headaches over a 30-day period with triptans has not been established. Triptans should not be used concurrently with (or within 24 hours of) an **ergot derivative**, nor should one triptan be used concurrently or within 24 hours of another.

ROCURONIUM BROMIDE

(Zemuron injection 10 mg/mL)

Rocuronium bromide is a nondepolarizing neuromuscular blocker that binds competitively to cholinergic receptors on motor end plate to antagonize action of acetylcholine, resulting in block of neuromuscular transmission. It is indicated as an adjunct to general anesthesia for inpatients and outpatients to facilitate both rapid sequence and routine tracheal intubation and to provide skeletal muscle relaxation during surgery or mechanical ventilation.

At present, only a single depolarizing agent, **succinylcholine**, is in general clinical use, whereas multiple competitive or nondepolarizing agents are available. Therapeutic selection should be based on achieving a pharmacokinetic profile consistent with the duration of the interventional procedure and minimizing cardiovascular compromise or other side effects. Two general classifications are useful because they are helpful in distinguishing side effects and pharmacokinetic behavior. The first relates to the duration of drug action, and these agents are categorized as long-, intermediate-, and short-acting. The persistent blockade and difficulty in complete reversal after surgery with ***d*-tubocurarine**, **metocurine**, **pancuronium**, and **doxacurium** led to the development of **vecuronium** and **atracurium**, agents of intermediate duration. This was followed by the development of a short-acting agent, **mivacurium**. Often the long-acting agents are the more potent, requiring the use of low concentrations. The necessity of administering potent agents in low concentrations delays their onset. **Rocuronium** is an agent of intermediate duration but of rapid onset and lower potency. Its rapid onsets allows it to be used as an alternative to succinylcholine in rapid-induction anesthesia and in relaxing the laryngeal and jaw muscles to facilitate tracheal intubation.

The second useful classification is derived from the chemical nature of the agents and includes the natural alkaloids or their congeners, the ammonio steroids, and the benzylisoquinolines. The natural alkaloid *d*-tubocurarine and the semisynthetic alkaloid alcuronium seldom are used. Apart from a shorter duration of action, the newer agents exhibit greatly diminished frequency of side effects, chief of which are ganglionic blockade, block of vagal responses, and histamine release. The prototype ammonio steroid, pancuronium, induces virtually no histamine release; however, it blocks muscarinic receptors, and this antagonism is manifested primarily in vagal blockade and tachycardia. Tachycardia is eliminated in the newer ammonio steroids, vecuronium and rocuronium.

Rocuronium, a nondepolarizing neuromuscular-blocking agent (0.6 mg/kg IV bolus), is used as an adjunct to general anesthesia, facilitation of endotracheal intubation, or skeletal muscle relaxation during surgery or mechanical ventilation (see also Figure 99).

ROPINIROLE HYDROCHLORIDE

(Requip tablets 0.25 mg)

Ropinirole hydrochloride is a nonergot dopamine-receptor agonist. It stimulates dopamine receptors in the corpus striatum, relieving parkinsonian symptoms.

Ropinirole is an efficacious and highly selective nonergoline D_2 agonist. It has no significant alpha- or beta-adrenergic nor serotoninergic activity. Ropinirole has beneficial adjuvant effects in parkinsonian patients with moderate motor disability and motor fluctuations.

Four orally administered dopamine-receptor agonists are available for treatment of PD: two older agents, **bromocriptine** (Parlodel) and **pergolide** (Permax); and two newer, more selective compounds, **ropinirole** (Requip) and **pramipexole** (Mirpex). Bromocriptine and pergolide both are ergot derivatives and share a similar spectrum of therapeutic actions and adverse effects. Bromocriptine is a strong agonist of the D_2-class of dopamine receptors and a partial antagonist of the D_1 receptors, whereas pergolide is an agonist of both classes. **Ropinirole** and pramipexole have selective activity at D_2-class sites (specifically at the D_2-and D_3-receptor proteins) and little or no activity at D_1-class sites. All four of the drugs are well absorbed orally and have similar therapeutic actions. Like levodopa, they can relieve the clinical symptoms of PD. The duration of action of the dopamine agonists (8 to 24 hours) often is longer than that of levodopa (6 to 8 hours), and they are particularly effective in the treatment of patients who have developed on/off phenomena. All four also may produce hallucinosis or confusion, similar to that observed with levodopa, and may worsen orthostatic hypotension.

The principal distinction between the newer, more selective agents and the older ergot derivatives is in their tolerability and speed of titration. Initial treatment with bromocriptine or pergolide may cause profound hypotension, so they should be initiated at low dosage. The ergot derivatives also often induce nausea and fatigue with initial treatment. Symptoms usually are transient, but they require slow upward adjustment of the dose over a period of weeks to months. Ropinirole and pramipexole can be initiated more quickly, achieving therapeutically useful doses in a week or less. They generally cause less GI disturbance than do the ergot derivatives, but they can produce nausea and somnolence. The somnolence in some cases may be quite severe, and several instances of sudden attacks of irresistible sleepiness leading to motor vehicle accidents have been reported. This effect seems to be uncommon, but it is prudent to advise patients of this possibility and to switch to another treatment if sleepiness interferes with the activities of daily life. Recent reports have associated long-term use of pergolide with significant cardiac valvular disease. If these reports are confirmed, this may be another important factor favoring the use of the nonergot agents.

The introduction of pramipexole and ropinirole has led to a substantial change in the clinical use of dopamine agonists in PD. Because these selective agonists are well tolerated, they are used increasingly as initial treatment for PD rather than as adjuncts to levodopa. This change has been driven by two factors: (1) the belief that, because of their longer duration of action, dopamine agonists may be less likely than levodopa to induce on/off effects and dyskinesias, and (2) the concern that levodopa may contribute to oxidative stress, thereby accelerating loss of dopaminergic neurons. Two large controlled clinical trials comparing levodopa with pramipexole or ropinirole as initial treatment of PD have provided convincing evidence for a reduced rate of motor fluctuation in patients treated with these agonists.

It would be desirable to identify a treatment that modifies the progressive degeneration that underlies PD rather than simply controlling the symptoms. Current research strategies are based on the mechanistic approach (e.g., energy metabolism, oxidative stress, environmental triggers, and excitotoxicity) and on discoveries related to the genetics of PD. Some of the strongest evidence for a neuroprotective action has emerged from long-term studies of the effects of the dopamine agonists pramipexole and **ropinirole**. The therapeutic effects of these are related to actions at postsynaptic dopamine receptors, but they also can activate presynaptic autoreceptors found on dopamine terminals, which are principally of the D_2 class. By stimulating presynaptic receptors, **pramipexole** and **ropinerole** may reduce endogenous dopamine production and release, and thereby diminish oxidative stress. Two trials have attempted to examine the effect of pramipexole or ropinirole on neurodegeneration in PD. Both trials observed that in patients treated with one of these agonists, there was a reduced rate of loss of markers of dopaminergic neurotransmission measured by brain imaging compared with a similar group of patients treated with levodopa.

ROSIGLITAZONE MALEATE

(Avandia tablets 2 mg, tablets 4 mg, tablets 8 mg)

Rosiglitazone maleate is a thiazolidinedione that increases insulin sensitivity; improves sensitivity to insulin in muscles, adipose tissue; and inhibits hepatic gluconeogenesis. It is indicated in improving glycemic control of type 2 diabetes mellitus as monotherapy and as an adjunct to diet and exercise; and in combination with metformin, insulin, or a sulfonylurea when diet, exercise, and a single agent does not result in adequate glycemic control in patients with type 2 diabetes mellitus.

Three thiazolidinediones have been used in clinical practice (**troglitazone**, **rosiglitazone**, and **pioglitazone**); however, troglitazone was withdrawn from use because it was associated with severe hepatic toxicity. Rosiglitazone and pioglitazone can lower hemoglobin A_{1C} levels by 1 to 1.5% in patients with type 2 DM. These drugs can be combined with insulin or other classes of oral glucose-lowering agents. The thiazolidinediones tend to increase HDL-C but have variable effects on triglycerides and LDL-C.

Thiazolidinediones are selective agonists for nuclear peroxisome proliferator-activated receptor-γ (PPARγ). These drugs bind to PPARγ, which activates insulin-responsive genes that regulate carbohydrate and lipid metabolism. Thiazolidinediones require insulin to be present for their action. Thiazolidinediones exert their principal effects by increasing insulin sensitivity in peripheral tissue but also may lower glucose production by the liver. Thiazolidinediones increase glucose transport into muscle and adipose tissue by enhancing the synthesis and translocation of specific forms of the glucose transporters. The thiazolidinediones also can activate genes that regulate fatty acid metabolism in peripheral tissue. Although muscle is a major insulin-sensitive tissue, PPAR is virtually absent in skeletal muscle. This has provoked questions as to how thiazolidinediones can reduce peripheral insulin resistance. One suggestion is that activation of PPAR in adipose tissue reduces the flux of fatty acids into muscle, thereby lowering insulin resistance. Other suggestions include the activation of adipocyte hormones and/or adipokines, the most promising of which is adiponectin. Adiponectin is associated with increased insulin sensitivity and reportedly increases insulin sensitivity by elevating AMP kinase, which stimulates glucose transport into muscle and increases fatty acid oxidation. Because the actions of both metformin and the thiazolidinediones apparently converge on AMP kinase, it has emerged as an attractive target for drug development.

Rosiglitazone (Avandia) and **pioglitazone** (Actos) are taken once a day. Both agents are absorbed within about 2 hours, but the maximum clinical effect is not observed for 6 to 12 weeks. The thiazolidinediones are metabolized by the liver and may be administered to patients with renal insufficiency but should not be used if there is active hepatic disease or significant elevations of serum liver transaminases.

Rosiglitazone is metabolized by hepatic cytochrome P450 (CYP) 2C8, whereas **pioglitazone** is metabolized by CYP3A4 and CYP2C8. Other drugs that induce or inhibit these enzymes can cause drug interactions. Clinically significant interactions between the available thiazolidinediones and other drug classes have not yet been described, but further studies are in progress.

ROSIGLITAZONE MALEATE/METFORMIN HYDROCHLORIDE

(Avandamet tablets 1 mg/500 mg, tablets 2 mg/500 mg, tablets 2 mg/1000 mg, tablets 4 mg/500 mg, tablets 4 mg/1000 mg)

Rosiglitazone maleate/metformin hydrochloride is an antidiabetic combination. **Rosiglitazone** increases insulin sensitivity. **Metformin** decreases blood glucose by reducing hepatic glucose production, increases peripheral glucose uptake and utilization, and may decrease intestinal absorption of glucose. They are indicated as an adjunct to diet and exercise to improve glycemic control in patients with type 2 diabetes mellitus who are already treated with combination rosiglitazone and metformin or who are not adequately controlled on metformin alone.

ROSUVASTATIN CALCIUM

(Crestor tablets 5 mg)

Rosuvastatin is a 3-hydroxy-3-methylglutaryl coenzyme A (HMG-CoA) reductase inhibitor that inhibits HMG-CoA reductase, the rate-limiting enzyme that converts HMG-CoA to mevalonate, a precursor of cholesterol. It is indicated as an adjunct to diet to reduce elevated total cholesterol (C), LDL-C, non-HDL-C, ApoB, and TG levels and to increase HDL-C in patients with primary hypercholesterolemia and mixed dyslipidemia; as an adjunct to diet for the treatment of patients with elevated serum TG levels; and to reduce LDL-C, total C, and ApoB in patients with homozygous familial hypercholesterolemia as an adjunct to other lipid-lowering treatments or if such treatments are not available.

The statins are the most effective and best-tolerated agents for treating dyslipidemia. These drugs are competitive inhibitors of **HMG-CoA reductase**, which catalyzes an early, rate-limiting step in cholesterol biosynthesis. Higher doses of the more potent statins (e.g., **atorvastatin** and **simvastatin**) also can reduce triglyceride levels caused by elevated very-low-density lipoprotein (VLDL) levels. Some statins also are indicated for raising HDL-C levels, although the clinical significance of these effects on HDL-C remains to be proven.

Multiple well-controlled clinical trials have documented the efficacy and safety of simvastatin, pravastatin, lovastatin, and atorvastatin in reducing fatal and nonfatal coronary heart disease (CHD) events, strokes, and total mortality. Rates of adverse events in statin trials were the same in the placebo groups and in the groups receiving the drug. This was true with regard to noncardiac illness and the two laboratory tests, hepatic transaminases and creatine kinase (CK), that are commonly monitored in patients taking statins.

RUBELLA AND MUMPS VIRUS VACCINE, LIVE

(Biavax II)

This viral vaccine is used in rubella (German measles) and mumps immunization.

RUBELLA VIRUS VACCINE, LIVE, ATTENUATED

(Meruvax II)

This viral vaccine is used in rubella (German measles) immunization.

S

SACCHARIDE IRON OXIDE

Extensive numbers of oral preparations are available for the treatment of iron deficiency anemias. In general, the ferrous salts (ferrous sulfate, ferrous gluconate, and ferrous fumarate) are better absorbed than the ferric salts (ferric sulfate). Ferrous calcium citrate is used mostly in patients during pregnancy to provide iron as well as calcium.

The parenteral iron medications available include iron-dextran (ferric hydroxide and high-molecular-weight dextran) for intramuscular use, dextriferron (a complex of ferric hydroxide and partially hydrolyzed dextran) for intravenous use, and saccharated iron oxide (a complex of ferric hydroxide and sucrose) for intravenous use. These preparations are reserved for those cases in which oral preparations are not tolerated, absorbed, or rapid enough in their onset of action, or are otherwise not suitable for noncompliant patients.

SALICYLATES AND ALLIED MEDICATIONS

Salicylates and allied compounds have analgesic, antipyretic, uricosuric, and antiinflammatory properties. Their mechanisms of action differ from those of the antiinflammatory steroids and the opioid analgesics. They are classified into the following categories (see Table 3):

Salicylate derivatives
- Acetylsalicylic acid (aspirin)
- Diflunisal (Dolobid)
- Salsalate (Arthra-G, Disalcid, Mono-Gesic)

Pyrazolone derivatives
- Phenylbutazone (Butazolidin)
- Oxyphenbutazone (Oxalid, Tandearil)
- Sulfinpyrazone (Anturane)

Paraaminophenol derivatives
- Acetaminophen (Tylenol, Datril)
- Phenacetin (Acetophenetidin)

Propionic acid derivatives
- Ibuprofen (Motrin)
- Naproxen (Naprosyn)
- Fenoprofen (Nalfon)
- Flurbiprofen (Ansaid)
- Ketoprofen (Orudis)

Others
- Indomethacin (Indocin)
- Suldindac (Clinoril)
- Mefenamic acid (Ponstel)
- Tolmetin (Tolectin)
- Piroxicam (Feldene)
- Diclofenac sodium (Voltaren)
- Etodolac
- Nabumetone

Unlike the narcotic analgesics such as morphine, salicylates do not depress respiration, are relatively nontoxic, and lack addiction liability. They are weak or mild analgesics effective in ameliorating short, intermittent types of pain such as neuralgia, myalgia, and toothache.

They do not have the efficacy of morphine and cannot relieve the severe, prolonged, and lancinating types of pain associated with trauma such as burns or fractures. Like morphine, they produce analgesia by raising the pain threshold in the thalamus, but, unlike morphine, they do not alter the patient's reactions to pain. Because they do not cause hypnosis or euphoria, their sites of action have been postulated to be subcortical. In addition to raising the pain threshold, the antiinflammatory effects of salicylates may contribute to their analgesic actions. However, no direct association between the antiinflammatory and analgesic effects of these compounds should be expected. For example, aspirin has both analgesic and antiinflammatory properties, whereas acetaminophen has analgesic but not antiinflammatory properties. Furthermore, potent antiinflammatory agents such as phenylbutazone have only weak analgesic effects.

Salicylates, including aspirin, do not alter the normal body temperature, which is maintained by a balance between heat production and dissipation. In a fever associated with infection, increased oxidative processes enhance heat production.

Salicylates act by causing cutaneous vasodilation, which prompts perspiration and enhances heat dissipation. This effect is mediated via the hypothalamic nuclei, as proved by the fact that a lesion in the preoptic area suppresses the mechanism through which aspirin exerts its antipyretic effects. The antipyretic effects of aspirin and other salicylates may be due to their inhibition of hypothalamic prostaglandin synthesis. Although aspirin-induced diaphoresis contributes to its antipyretic effects, it is not an absolutely necessary process, since antipyresis takes place in the presence of atropine.

Salicylates, including aspirin, have an antiinflammatory action as well as antirheumatic and antiarthritic effects, and may therefore be used in the treatment of rheumatic fever. However, they cannot alter the cardiac lesion and other visceral effects of the disease. Aspirin is extremely effective in managing rheumatoid arthritic and allied diseases involving the joints, such as ankylosing spondylitis and osteoarthritis. It is thought that aspirin and indomethacin exert their antiinflammatory effects by inhibiting prostaglandin synthesis through the inhibition of cyclooxygenase. The presynthesized prostaglandins are released during a tissue injury that fosters inflammation and pain. Furthermore, aspirin reduces the formation of prostaglandin in the platelets and leukocytes, which is responsible for the reported hematologic effects associated with aspirin (see Figures 13 and 14).

SALMETEROL

(Serevent Diskus inhalation powder 50 mcg salmeterol (as salmeterol xinafoate salt))

Salmeterol is a sympathomimetic agent, which produces bronchodilation by relaxing bronchial smooth muscle through beta$_2$-receptor stimulation. It is indicated in the maintenance treatment of asthma and prevention of bronchospasm with reversible obstructive airway disease; prevention of exercise-induced bronchospasm; and maintenance treatment of bronchospasm associated with chronic obstructive pulmonary disease (COPD) (including emphysema and chronic bronchitis).

Salmeterol, a sympathomimetic (25 mcg salmeterol base/actuation t.i.d.), is indicated in the prevention of bronchospasm and in the maintenance treatment of those with obstructive airway disease including patients with symptoms of nocturnal asthma. In addition, salmeterol may be used in the prevention of exercise-induced bronchospasm.

The selective beta$_2$-adrenergic stimulants cause bronchodilation without cardiac acceleration. Metaproterenol and terbutaline are available in tablet form, and terbutaline is also available for subcutaneous injection. Metaproterenol and albuterol are available in metered-dose inhalers. Inhaled selective beta$_2$-adrenergic receptor agonists (albuterol, terbutaline, fenoterol, and bitolterol) have a rapid onset of action and are effective for 3 to 6 hours. Formoterol and salmeterol are longer-acting agents (12 hours) and may prove useful in treating nocturnal symptoms. The side effects of beta-adrenergic-receptor agonists are tremor, tachycardia, and palpitations (see also Figure 94).

SALSALATE

(Athra-G, Disalcid, Mono-Gesic)

Salsalate, a nonnarcotic analgesic, antipyretic, and antiinflammatory agent (3 g p.o. daily divided q.i.d. p.r.n.), is indicated in minor pain associated with arthritis. Unlike the narcotic analgesics such as morphine, salsalate does not depress respiration, is relatively nontoxic, and lacks addiction liability. It is a weak or mild analgesic that is effective for ameliorating short, intermittent types of pain such as neuralgia, myalgia, toothache, and minor pain associated with arthritis and related disorders. Salsalate does not have the efficacy of morphine and cannot relieve the severe, prolonged, and lancinating types of pain associated with trauma such as burns or fractures. Like morphine, it produces analgesia by raising the pain threshold in the thalamus, but, unlike morphine, it does not alter the patient's reactions to pain. Because salsalate does not cause hypnosis or euphoria, its sites of action have been postulated to be subcortical. In addition to raising the pain threshold, the antiinflammatory effects of salsalate may contribute to its analgesic actions. However, no direct association between the antiinflammatory and analgesic effects of salicylate should be expected. For example, aspirin has both analgesic and antiinflammatory properties, whereas acetaminophen has analgesic but not antiinflammatory properties. Furthermore, potent antiinflammatory agents such as phenylbutazone have only weak analgesic effects.

Salicylates including aspirin do not alter the normal body temperature, which is maintained by a balance between heat production and dissipation. In a fever associated with infection, increased oxidative processes enhance heat production.

Salicylates act by causing cutaneous vasodilation, which prompts perspiration and enhances heat dissipation. This effect is mediated via the hypothalamic nuclei, as proved by the fact that a lesion in the preoptic area suppresses the mechanism through which aspirin exerts its antipyretic effects. The antipyretic effects of aspirin and other salicylates may be due to their inhibition of hypothalamic prostaglandin synthesis. Although aspirin-induced diaphoresis contributes to its antipyretic effects, it is not an absolutely necessary process, since antipyresis takes place in the presence of atropine.

Salicylates including aspirin have an antiinflammatory action as well as antirheumatic and antiarthritic effects, and may therefore be used in the treatment of rheumatic fever. However, they cannot alter the cardiac lesion and other visceral effects of the disease. Aspirin is extremely effective in managing rheumatoid arthritis and allied diseases involving the joints, such as ankylosing spondylitis and osteoarthritis. It is thought that aspirin and indomethacin exert their antiinflammatory effects by inhibiting prostaglandin synthesis through the inhibition of cyclooxygenase. The presynthesized prostaglandins are released during a tissue injury that fosters inflammation and pain. Furthermore, aspirin reduces the formation of prostaglandin in the platelets and leukocytes, which is responsible for the reported hematologic effects associated with aspirin (see also Figures 13 and 14).

Salsalate is contraindicated in patients with known hypersensitivity to aspirin or other nonsteroidal antiinflammatory drugs (NSAIDs) and in the presence of gastrointestinal (GI) ulcer or GI bleeding because the drug may irritate the GI tract. It should be used cautiously in patients with hypothrombinemia, vitamin K deficiency, and bleeding disorders because of the potential for bleeding problems.

Patients with known "triad" symptoms (aspirin hypersensitivity, rhinitis/nasal polyps, and asthma) are at high risk of cross-sensitivity to salicylates with precipitation of bronchospasm.

Concomitant use of salsalate with drugs that are highly protein-bound (phenytoin, sulfonylureas, warfarin) may cause displacement of either drug, and adverse effects. Therapy must be monitored closely for both drugs. Concomitant use with other GI-irritating drugs (steroids, antibiotics, other NSAIDs) may potentiate adverse GI effects of salsalate.

Ammonium chloride and other urine acidifiers, as well as probenecid and sulfinpyrazone, increase salsalate blood levels. Antacids in high doses and other urine alkalizers decrease salsalate blood levels. Corticosteroids enhance salsalate elimination. Food and antacids delay and decrease absorption of salsalate.

Overdosage of salicylate causes metabolic acidosis with respiratory alkalosis; hyperpnea and tachypnea are caused by increased CO_2 production and direct stimulation of the respiratory center.

SAMARIUM SM 153 LEXIDRONAM

(Quadramet injection 1850 MBq/mL)

Samarium SM 153 lexidronam is a radiopharmaceutical, which provides relief of pain in patients with **osteoblastic metastatic bone lesions** that enhance on radionuclide bone scan.

SAQUINAVIR MESYLATE

(Fortovase capsules 200 mg, Invirase capsules 200 mg (as mesylate))

Saquinavir mesylate is a protease inhibitor that inhibits human immunodeficiency virus (HIV) protease, the enzyme required to form functional proteins in HIV-infected cells. It is indicated in the treatment of advanced HIV infection. Saquinavir is given in combination with nucleoside analogs (e.g., zidovudine).

Saquinavir is a peptidomimetic hydroxyethylamine HIV protease inhibitor. It is a transition-state analog of a phenylalanine-proline cleavage site in one of the native substrate sequences for the HIV aspartyl protease and was the product of a rational drug-design program. Saquinavir inhibits both HIV-1 and HIV-2 replication and has an *in vitro* IC_{50} in peripheral blood lymphocytes that ranges from 3.5 to 10 nM.

Saquinavir is selectively toxic by potently inhibiting the HTV-encoded protease but not host-encoded aspartyl proteases. Saquinavir reversibly binds to the active site of HIV protease, preventing polypeptide processing and subsequent virus maturation. Virus particles are produced in the presence of Saquinavir but are noninfectious.

Virus replication in the presence of Saquinavir selects for drug-resistant virus. The primary saquinavir resistance mutation occurs at HIV protease codon 90 (a leucine-to-methionine substitution), although primary resistance also has been reported with a glycine-to-valine substitution at codon 48. Secondary resistance mutations occur at codons 36, 46, 82, 84, and others, and these are associated with clinical saquinavir resistance as well as cross-resistance to other HIV protease inhibitors. As is typical of HIV protease inhibitors, high-level resistance requires accumulation of multiple-resistance mutations.

Saquinavir is marketed in two formulations, a hard-gelatin (**Invirase**) and a soft-gelatin (**Fortovase**) capsule. Fractional oral bioavailability of the original hard-gelatin capsule was only about 4% owing mainly to extensive first-pass metabolism. The soft-gelatin capsule formulation has threefold greater oral bioavailability, although the hard-gel capsule is used when this drug is combined with ritonavir. The bioavailability of saquinavir is increased up to sixfold with a high-calorie, high-fat meal. Saquinavir has nonlinear pharmacokinetics with increasing dose; for example, tripling the oral dose of saquinavir is associated with an eightfold increase in AUC. Substances that inhibit intestinal but not hepatic CYP3A4, such as grapefruit juice, increase the saquinavir AUC by threefold at most.

Saquinavir is metabolized primarily by intestinal and hepatic CYP3A4. Its metabolites are not known to be active against HIV-1. Saquinavir and its metabolites are eliminated through the biliary system and feces (>95% of drug), with minimal urinary excretion (<3%). Saquinavir's short half-life requires administration every 8 hours. However, saquinavir metabolism is exquisitely sensitive to inhibition by ritonavir, thus saquinavir is usefully combined with low doses of ritonavir to allow once- or twice-daily administration. Low doses of ritonavir increase the saquinavir steady-state AUC by 20- to 30-fold.

The most frequent side effects of saquinavir are gastrointestinal and include nausea, vomiting, diarrhea, and abdominal discomfort. Diarrhea and other GI side effects may be more prevalent with the soft-gelatin formulation. Most side effects of saquinavir are mild and short-lived, although long-term use is associated with lipodystrophy.

Of all the HIV protease inhibitors, saquinavir is the least potent inhibitor of **CYP3A4**. Nonetheless, it is recommended that the drug not be coadministered with ergot derivatives, **triazolam**, **midazolam**, or other **CYP3A4** substrates with a low therapeutic index. Saquinavir clearance is increased with CYP3A4 induction; thus coadministration of rifampin, nevirapine, or efavirenz lowers saquinavir concentrations and should be avoided. The effect of nevirapine or efavirenz on saquinavir may be partially or completely reversed with ritonavir.

In initial clinical trials, hard-gelatin capsules of saquinavir mesylate at the approved dose (600 mg three times daily) produced only modest virologic effect most likely because of poor oral bioavailability. Greater activity was achieved by increasing the dose fourfold, to 1200 mg six times daily. When combined with ritonavir and nucleoside analogs, saquinavir produces viral load reductions comparable with those of other HIV protease inhibitor regimens.

Saquinavir is an inhibitor of the HIV protease, which in combination with nucleoside analogs (three 200 mg capsules t.i.d.) is indicated for the treatment of HIV infection. HIV protease cleaves viral polyprotein precursors to generate functional proteins in HIV-infected cells. The cleavage of viral polyprotein precursors is essential for maturation of infectious virus. Saquinavir mesylate is a synthetic peptide-like substrate analog that inhibits the activity of HIV protease and prevents the cleavage of viral polyproteins. Saquinavir inhibits HIV activity in both acutely and chronically infected cells. Moreover, saquinavir exhibits additive to synergistic effects against HIV in double and triple combination regimens with reverse transcriptase inhibitors zidovudine, zalcitabine, and didanosine without enhanced cytotoxicity.

Rifampin, phenobarbital, phenytoin, or carbamazepine reduce the plasma concentration of saquinavir. On the other hand, agents which inhibit the activity of the cytochrome P450 3A pathway, such as terfenadine, astemizole, or cisapride, elevate the plasma concentration of saquinavir. The long-term adverse effects of saquinavir remain to be established. However, the low incidences of side effects of saquinavir are diarrhea (3.8%), abdominal discomfort, nausea, abdominal pain, buccal mucosal ulceration, headache, paresthesia, asthenia, rash, and musculoskeletal pain (0.6%).

SARAFOTOXIN

The endothelins belong to a family of potent vasoconstrictor peptides that were originally isolated from the supernatant of cultured aortic endothelial cells. Endothelins bear striking structural similarities to the sarafotoxins, which are potent cardiotoxic peptides isolated from the venom of the burrowing asp *Atractaspis engadensis*. Four endothelins and four sarafotoxin isopeptides, having different receptor subtypes, have been identified (see also Figure 44).

SARGRAMOSTIM

(Granulocyte macrophage-colony stimulating factor (GM-CSF) (Leukine, Prokine))

Sargramostim, a colony-stimulating factor (CSF), is used for acceleration of hematopoietic reconstitution after autologous BMT in patients with non-Hodgkin's lymphoma, acute lymphoblastic leukemia, or Hodgkin's disease undergoing autologous BMT; and for BMT failure or engraftment delay (see also Cytokines).

SARGRAMOSTIM

(Leukine powder for injection, lyophilized 250 mcg, powder for injection, lyophilized 500 mcg, liquid 500 mcg/mL)

Sargramostim is a CSF, which supports survival, proliferation, and differentiation of hematopoietic progenitor cells; induces partially committed progenitor cells to divide and differentiate in granulocyte-macrophage pathways; activates mature granulocytes and macrophages; promotes proliferation of megakaryocytic and erythroid progenitors. It is indicated in myeloid reconstitution after autologous BMT and after BMT failure or graft failure; promotion of early engraftment or engraftment delay; treatment of neutropenia associated bone marrow transplant; induction chemotherapy in **acute myelogenous leukemia** (AML); mobilization and following transplantation of autologous peripheral blood progenitor cell (PBPC); and myeloid reconstitution after allogeneic BMT.

Sargramostim (Leukine) is administered by subcutaneous injection or slow intravenous infusion at doses of 125 to 500 $\mu g/m^2$ per day. Plasma levels of GM-CSF rise rapidly after subcutaneous injection and then decline with a half-life of 2 to 3 hours. When given intravenously, infusions should be maintained over 3 to 6 hours. With the initiation of therapy, there is a transient decrease in the absolute leukocyte count secondary to margination and sequestration in the lungs. This is followed by a dose-dependent, biphasic increase in leukocyte counts over the next 7 to 10 days. Once the drug is discontinued, the leukocyte count returns to baseline within 2 to 10 days. When GM-CSF is given in lower doses, the response is primarily neutrophilic, while monocytosis and eosinophilia are observed at larger doses. After hematopoietic stem-cell transplantation or intensive chemotherapy, sargramostim is given daily during the period of maximum neutropenia until a sustained rise in the granulocyte count is observed. Frequent blood counts are essential to avoid an excessive rise in the granulocyte count. The dose may be increased if the patient fails to respond after 7 to 14 days of therapy. However, higher doses are associated with more pronounced side effects, including bone pain, malaise, flu-like symptoms, fever, diarrhea, dyspnea, and rash. An acute reaction to the first dose, characterized by flushing, hypotension, nausea, vomiting, and dyspnea, with a fall in arterial oxygen saturation due to granulocyte sequestration in the pulmonary circulation occurs in sensitive patients. With prolonged administration, a few patients may develop a capillary leak syndrome, with peripheral edema and pleural and pericardial effusions. Other serious side effects have included transient supraventricular arrhythmia, dyspnea, and elevation of serum creatinine, bilirubin, and hepatic enzymes.

SCOPOLAMINE

(Transderm Scop)

SCOPOLAMINE HYDROBROMIDE

(Isopto Hyoscine, Triptone)

Scopolamine, an anticholinergic agent, is used as an adjunct to anesthesia. In addition, scopolamine is indicated in cycloplegia and mydriasis in diagnostic procedures for preoperative and postoperative states in the treatment of iridocyclitis. For uveitis, 1 or 2 drops of 0.25% solution are instilled into the eye(s) up to 4 times daily. For refraction, 1 or 2 drops are instilled into the eye/eyes 1 hour before refraction.

Scopolamine (0.32 to 0.65 mg SC, IM, or IV) is indicated for producing preanesthetic sedation and obstetric amnesia in conjunction with analgesics. It may be used for calming delirium and for motion sickness.

Atropine and scopolamine, which are obtained from belladonna alkaloids, as well as other synthetic anticholinergic drugs, inhibit the actions of acetylcholine and cholinomimetic drugs at muscarinic receptors in smooth muscles, heart, and exocrine glands. In addition to these peripheral effects, anticholinergic drugs, by blocking the acetylcholine receptor sites in the CNS, have pronounced CNS effects such as restlessness, irritability, excitement, and hallucinations. Scopolamine, on the other hand, depresses the CNS and, in therapeutic doses, produces fatigue, hypnosis, and amnesia. Therefore, it is used extensively in numerous medications, often in combination with antihistamines (see also Figure 12).

The ability of scopolamine to prevent motion-induced nausea is believed to be associated with inhibition of vestibular input to the CNS, which results in inhibition of the vomiting reflex. In addition, scopolamine may have a direct action on the vomiting center within the reticular formation of the brain stem (see also Figure 81).

The transdermal system is a 0.2-mm-thick film with four layers. It is 2.5 cm^2 in area and contains 1.5 mg scopolamine, which is gradually released from an adhesive matrix of mineral oil and polyisobutylene following application to the postauricular skin. An initial priming dose released from the system's adhesive layer saturates the skin binding site for scopolamine and rapidly brings the plasma concentration to the required steady-state level. A continuous controlled release of scopolamine flows from the drug reservoir through the rate-controlling membrane to maintain a constant plasma level. Antiemetic protection is produced within several hours following application behind the ear.

The most common adverse reactions of scopolamine are dry mouth, drowsiness, transient impairment of accommodation including mydriasis and blurred vision. The infrequent adverse reactions of scopolamine, especially in higher-than-therapeutic doses, include disorientation, memory disturbances, dizziness, restlessness, hallucinations, confusion, difficulty urinating, rashes or erythema, acute narrow-angle glaucoma, and dry, itchy, or red eyes.

SCOPOLAMINE HBR (HYOSCINE HBR)

(Isopto Hyoscine ophthalmic solution 0.25%, Scopace tablets, soluble 0.4 mg, Transderm-Scop transdermal system 1.5 mg)

Scopolamine HBr is a belladonna alkaloid/cycloplegic mydriatic/anticholinergic, which supports survival, proliferation, and differentiation of hematopoietic progenitor cells; induces partially committed progenitor cells to divide and differentiate in granulocyte-macrophage pathways; activates mature granulocytes and macrophages; and promotes proliferation of megakaryocytic and erythroid progenitors. It is indicated as an anticholinergic CNS depressant, in symptomatic treatment of postencephalitic parkinsonism and paralysis agitans, in spastic states and locally, as a substitute for atropine in ophthalmology, to inhibit excessive motility and hypertonus of the GI tract in such conditions as irritable colon syndrome, mild dysentery, diverticulitis, pylorospasm, and cardiospasm, and may prevent motion sickness (oral); accomplishment of cycloplegia and mydriasis for diagnostic procedures and for preoperative and postoperative states in treatment of iridocyclitis (ophthalmic use); prevention of nausea and vomiting associated with motion sickness and recovery from anesthesia and surgery (transdermal); and antiemetic, preanesthetic sedation, antisecretory action, obstetric amnesia in conjunction with analgesics and to calm delirium (parenteral).

SECOBARBITAL

(Seconal)

Secobarbital, a barbiturate sedative–hypnotic and anticonvulsant (200 to 300 mg 1 to 2 hours before surgery), is used to cause preoperative sedation; secobarbital (100 to 200 mg p.o.) is used in short-term treatment of insomnia since it appears to lose its effectiveness after two weeks; secobarbital (5.5 mg/kg IM or slow IV) is indicated in treating acute tetanus convulsions; and secobarbital (50 mg/min IV) is indicated in treating acute psychotic agitation.

Secobarbital acts throughout the CNS as a nonselective depressant with a rapid onset of action and short duration of action. Particularly sensitive to this drug is the reticular activating system, which controls CNS arousal. Secobarbital decreases both presynaptic and postsynaptic membrane excitability by facilitating the action of gamma-aminobutyric acid (GABA) (see also Figure 50).

After oral administration, 90% of secobarbital is absorbed rapidly. After rectal administration, secobarbital is nearly 100% absorbed. Peak serum concentration after oral or rectal administration occurs between 2 and 4 hours. The onset of action is rapid, occurring within 15 minutes when administered orally. Peak effects are seen 15 to 30 minutes after oral and rectal administration, 7 to 10 minutes after IM administration, and 1 to 3 minutes after IV administration.

Secobarbital is distributed rapidly throughout body tissues and fluids; approximately 30 to 45% is protein bound. It is oxidized in the liver to inactive metabolites. Duration of action is 3 to 4 hours; 90% of a secobarbital dose is eliminated as glucuronide conjugates and other metabolites in urine. Secobarbital has an elimination half-life of about 30 hours.

Secobarbital is contraindicated in patients with bronchopneumonia, status asthmaticus, or other severe respiratory distress because of the potential for respiratory depression. Secobarbital should not be used in patients who are depressed or have suicidal ideation because the drug can worsen depression; in patients with uncontrolled acute or chronic pain, because exacerbation of pain and paradoxical excitement can occur; and in patients with porphyria, because this drug can trigger symptoms of this disease.

Secobarbital should be used cautiously in patients who must perform hazardous tasks requiring mental alertness, because this drug causes drowsiness.

Clinical manifestations of overdose with secobarbital include unsteady gait, slurred speech, sustained nystagmus, somnolence, confusion, respiratory depression, pulmonary edema, areflexia, and coma. Typical shock syndrome with tachycardia and hypotension, jaundice, hypothermia, followed by fever, and oliguria may occur.

SECRETIN

(SecreFlo powder for injection, lyophilized 16 mcg or purified secretin)

Secretin is a GI function test, which increases the volume and bicarbonate content of secreted pancreatic juices. It is indicated in stimulation of pancreatic secretions, including bicarbonate, to aid in diagnosis of pancreatic exocrine dysfunction; stimulation of gastrin secretion to aid in diagnosis of gastrinoma; stimulation of pancreatic secretions to facilitate the identification of ampulla of Vater and accessory papilla during endoscopic retrograde cholangiopancreatography.

Because of significant homology in amino acid sequences, families of related molecules can be defined as either ancestral or concurrent. The ancestral relationship is illustrated by peptides such as the tachykinin or the vasotocin (vasopressin/oxytocin) family, in which species' differences can be correlated with modest variations in peptide structure. The concurrent relationship is best exemplified by the endorphins and by the glucagon-**secretin** family. In the endorphin superfamily, three major systems of endorphin peptides (pro-opiomelanocortin, proenkephalin, and prodynorphin) and at least two populations of minor opioid peptides (the endomorphins and the orphanin/nociceptin peptides) exist in independent neuronal circuits. These natural opioid peptides arise from independent but homologous genes. The peptides all share some actions at receptors once classified generally as "opioid," but now are undergoing progressive refinement. In the glucagon family, multiple and somewhat homologous peptides are found simultaneously in different cells of separate organ systems: glucagon and vasoactive intestinal polypeptide (VIP) in pancreatic islets; secretin in duodenal mucosa; VIP and related peptides in enteric, autonomic, and central neurons, and growth hormone-releasing hormone (GHRH) only in central neurons. The general metabolic effects produced by this family can be viewed as leading to increased blood glucose. To some degree, ancestral and concurrent relationships are not mutually exclusive. For example, multiple members of the tachykinin/substance P family within mammalian brains and intestines may account for the apparent existence of subsets of receptors for these peptides. The mammalian terminus of the vasotocin family also shows two concurrent products, vasopressin and oxytocin, each having evolved to perform separate functions once executed by single vasotocin-related peptides in lower phyla.

SEDATIVE–HYPNOTICS

Sedatives, hypnotics, and alcohol are depressants of the central nervous system (CNS). The degree of this reversible depression depends on the amount of drug ingested, producing effects according to the following scheme:

$$\text{Sedation} \quad \text{Hypnosis} \quad \text{Anesthesia} \rightarrow \text{Death}$$

Sedation is defined as the act of calming or reducing the activity or excitement of an individual. Hypnosis represents a condition of artificially produced sleep or a trance resembling sleep. Anesthesia constitutes a loss of feeling or sensation.

The degree of CNS depression, including the loss of consciousness, may be assessed according to the response to painful stimuli, and is graded according to the following criteria.

Drowsy but responsive to vocal command
Unconscious but responsive to minimal stimuli
Unconscious and responsive only to maximal painful stimuli
Unconscious and no response is evident

Contrary to the general belief, the size and activity of the pupils and the limb reflexes are too variable to be useful indices of the degree of CNS depression. However, absent bowel sounds, when noted on auscultation of the abdomen, are often associated with pronounced CNS depression.

Sedatives and hypnotics may be divided into two categories: barbiturates and nonbarbiturates (see Table 9).

In the past, barbiturates were used extensively as hypnotic-sedatives but have been replaced by the much safer benzodiazepine derivatives. They do continue to be used as anesthetics and as anticonvulsants. The primary mechanism of action of barbiturates is to increase inhibition of neurons through the GABA system. Anesthetic barbiturates also decrease excitation via a decrease in calcium conductance (see also Figure 50).

The most commonly used barbiturates are:

Thiopental (Pentothal)
Methohexital (Brevital)
Secobarbital (Seconal)
Pentobarbital (Nembutal)
Amobarbital (Amytal)
Phenobarbital (Luminal)

Barbiturates are classified according to their duration of action. These are: ultra-short-acting (thiopental and methohexital), short- to intermediate-acting (pentobarbital, secobarbital, and amobarbital), and long-acting (phenobarbital).

In general, the more lipid soluble a barbiturate derivative is, the greater its plasma- and tissue-binding capacity, the extent of its metabolism, and its storage in adipose tissues. In addition, very lipid-soluble substances have a faster onset of action and a shorter duration of action.

Barbiturates do not raise the pain threshold and have no analgesic property. In anesthetic doses, they depress all areas of the CNS, including the hypothalamic thermoregulatory system, respiratory center, and vasomotor centers, as well as the polysynaptic pathways in the spinal column. In addition, some, such as phenobarbital, but not all are anticonvulsants. In toxic doses, barbiturates cause oliguria.

Barbiturates are absorbed orally and distributed widely throughout the body. They are metabolized in the liver by aliphatic oxygenation, aromatic oxygenation, and *N*-dealkylation.

The inactive metabolites are excreted in the urine. The administration of bicarbonate enhances the urinary excretion of barbiturates that have a pK_a of 7.4 (phenobarbital and thiopental). This generalization is not true of other barbiturates. The long-term administration of barbiturates activates the cytochrome P450 drug-metabolizing system.

Acute barbiturate toxicity is characterized by automatism, or a state of drug-induced confusion, in which patients lose track of how much medication they have taken and take more. Death results from respiratory failure. The treatment of poisoning consists of supporting the respiration, preventing hypotension, diuresis, hemodialysis, and in the event of phenobarbital poisoning, administering sodium bicarbonate. Tolerance does not develop to lethal doses.

The abrupt withdrawal from barbiturates may cause tremors, restlessness, anxiety, weakness, nausea and vomiting, seizures, delirium, and cardiac arrest.

The selection of a barbiturate is in part determined by the duration of action desired and by the clinical problems at hand. An ultra-short-acting drug is used for inducing anesthesia. For treating epilepsy, a long-acting drug is used, whereas in a sleep disorder, a short-acting or an intermediate-type drug is used, depending on whether patients have difficulty falling asleep or if they have difficulty staying asleep.

Flurazepam (Dalmane), temazepam (Restoril), and triazolam (Halcion) are all marketed as hypnotic agents, but other benzodiazepine derivatives are also effective hypnotic agents (see Table 9).

Chloral Hydrate

Chloral hydrate (Noctec and Somnos) lacks analgesic effects. It also has no effect on respiration or circulation when given in therapeutic doses. In toxic doses (10 mg), it causes hypotension and respiratory depression. Chloral hydrate is reduced to trichlorethanol.

Ethchlorvynol

Ethchlorvynol has a rapid onset and short duration of action. It has sedative, hypnotic, muscle relaxant, and anticonvulsant properties. It has a mint-like aftertaste and causes facial numbness.

Paraldehyde

The therapeutic uses of paraldehyde (Paral) resemble those of chloral hydrate.

Glutethimide

Glutethimide (Doriden) is used to cause daytime or preoperative sedation, or for the treatment of simple insomnia. Furthermore, it is useful in patients who cannot tolerate barbiturates.

Methaqualone

Methaqualone (Quaalude and Sopor) is used for daytime sedation and in patients with simple insomnia. It is useful for patients who cannot tolerate barbiturates.

Methyprylon

Methyprylon (Nodular) is used for the treatment of simple insomnia and is also useful in patients who cannot tolerate barbiturates.

SEIZURES: Treatment of

Seizure Disorders	Drugs
Primary Generalized Tonic-Clonic (Grand Mal)	
Drugs of Choice:	Carbamazepine or Phenytoin or Valproate
Alternatives:	Phenobarbital Primidone
Partial, Including Secondarily Generalized	
Drugs of Choice:	Carbamazepine or Phenytoin
Alternatives:	Phenobarbital Primidone
Absence (Petit Mal)	
Drugs of Choice:	Ethosuximide or Valproate
Alternative:	Clonazepam
Atypical Absence, Myoclonic, Atonic	
Drug of Choice:	Valproate
Alternative:	Clonazepam
Status Epilepticus	
Drugs of Choice: (adults and children)	Diazepam, IV Phenytoin, IV Phenobarbital, IV

SELECTINS

There is a variety of adhesion molecules which facilitate the adherence of formed elements in the blood (for example, platelets and leukocytes) to the vascular endothelium. These leukocyte-endothelial adhesion molecules belong to one of three major families of molecules: (1) the integrins, (2) the immunoglobulin superfamily, and (3) the selectin family. The adhesion molecules appear to act in concert in attracting leukocytes to the reperfused coronary endothelium and in promoting adherence, transendothelial migration, and activation of the leukocytes. One important property of selectins is that they appear to be the initial adhesion molecules to influence the properties of leukocytes at the start of the inflammatory process and hence in ischemia–reperfusion injury.

SELECTIVE SEROTONIN/NORADRENALINE REUPTAKE INHIBITORS

(SNRIs)

In recent years, potential new antidepressants have been developed that inhibit serotonin (5-hydroxytryptamine; 5-HT) and noradrenaline (norepinephrine) reuptake in a selective manner. Examples of these SNRIs are duloxetine, milnacipran, and venlafaxine. Controlled studies in depressed patients have shown an efficacy superior or comparable to tricyclic antidepressants (see Tables 5 through 7 and Figure 86).

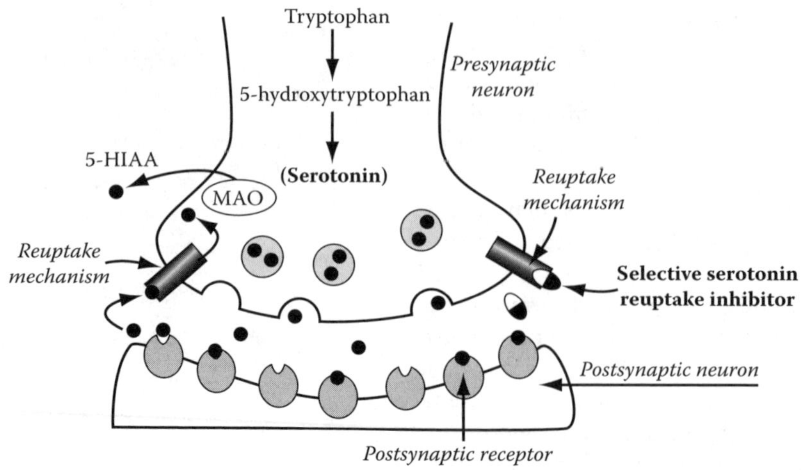

FIGURE 86 Selective serotonin reuptake inhibitors (SSRIs) such as citalopram, fluoxetin, fluvoxamine, paroxetine, and sertraline, are antidepressants.

SELEGILINE HYDROCHLORIDE

(L-Deprenyl, Eldepryl)

Selegiline, a monoamine oxidase B inhibitor (5 to 10 mg in divided doses), is indicated as an adjunct in the management of parkinsonian patients being treated with levodopa/carbidopa who exhibit deterioration in the quality of their response to this therapy. Selegiline is effective in the treatment of parkinsonism because it inhibits the catabolism of dopamine. Monoamine oxidase inhibitors are classified into A and B types. Monoamine oxidase A preferentially uses serotonin and norepinephrine as substrates and is inhibited by chlorgyline and harmaline. Monoamine oxidase B preferentially uses dopamine and is inhibited by selegiline (Figure 87). Clinical evidence indicates that 10 mg of selegiline in combination with levodopa and carbidopa is superior to levodopa–carbidopa therapy alone. There are indications that selegiline alone can slow the progression of the disease. Although the factors responsible for the loss of nigrostriatal dopaminergic neurons in Parkinson's disease are not understood, the findings from neurochemical studies have suggested that the surviving striatal dopamine neurons accelerate the synthesis of dopamine, thus enhancing the formation of H_2O_2 according to the scheme depicted in Figure 87.

The evidence suggesting that oxidative reactions may contribute to the pathogenesis of Parkinson's disease includes the following: In patients with Parkinson's disease, the iron content is increased in the substantia nigra; the ferritin level is decreased in the brain; and the glutathione concentration is decreased in the substantia nigra. Furthermore, although 1-methyl-4-phenyl-1,2,3,6-tetrahydropyridine (MPTP) is not in itself toxic, when oxidized by monoamine oxidase B to the methylphenylpyridium ion, it becomes a select nigral toxin that interferes with mitochondrial respiratory mechanisms. The toxicity of MPTP may be prevented by pretreatment with a monoamine oxidase B inhibitor such as selegiline. Therefore, it is thought that

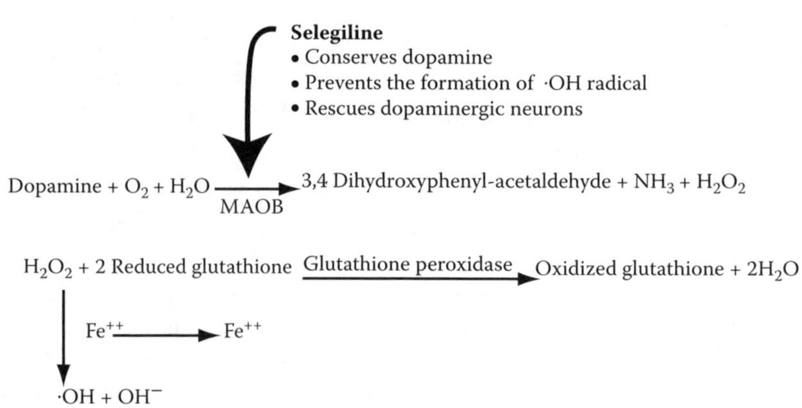

FIGURE 87 Monoamine oxidase B preferentially uses dopamine and is inhibited by selegiline. Clinical evidence indicates that 10 mg of selegiline in combination with levodopa and carbidopa is superior to levodopa–carbidopa therapy alone. There are indications that selegiline alone can slow the progression of Parkinson's disease, when taken in the early stages of the disease.

selegiline, by conserving dopamine and preventing the formation of ·OH radicals, rescues dopaminergic neurons.

SELENIUM (AS SELENIOUS ACID)

(Sele-Pak injection 40 mcg/mL (as 65.4 mcg selenious acid), Selepen injection 40 mcg/mL (as 65.4 mcg selenious acid))

Selenium is a trace metal, which is part of glutathione peroxidase, which protects cell components from oxidative damage caused by peroxidases produced in cellular metabolism. It is indicated for its use as a supplement to IV total parenteral nutrition (TPN) solutions to prevent depletion of endogenous stores and subsequent deficiency symptoms.

SEMILENTE INSULIN

Insulin preparations are fast-, intermediate-, or long-acting, as summarized in Table 19. Crystalline (regular) insulin may be used as a supplemental injection or for instituting corrective measures in the management of infection and trauma, for postoperative stabilization, and for the rehabilitation of patients recovering from ketoacidosis and coma. In addition, NPH contains regular insulin. Ultralente or semilente insulin is used to eliminate nocturnal and early morning hyperglycemia (see also Table 19).

SEMUSTINE

(Methy-CCNU)

The alkyl sulfonate busulfan (Myleran) is metabolized to an alkylating agent. Because it produces selective myelosuppression, it is used in cases of chronic myelocytic leukemia. It causes pronounced hyperuricemia stemming from the catabolism of purine.

SENNA

(Agoral liquid 25 mg, Black-Draught granules 20 mg/ 5 mL, tablets 6 mg, laxative tablets 15 mg, laxative chocolate tablets 15 mg, Fletcher Castoria liquid 33.3 mg/mL, Senexon tablets 8.5 mg, Senna-Gen tablets 8.6 mg, Senokot granules 15 mg/5 mL, syrup 8.8 mg/5 mL, tablets 8.6 mg, SenokotXTRA tablets 17 mg)

Senna is a laxative, which directly acts on intestinal mucosa by altering water and electrolyte secretion, inducing peristalsis and defecation. Senna, an **anthraquinone derivative** with laxative properties, is used in acute constipation and preparation for bowel examination.

Stimulant laxatives have direct effects on enterocytes, enteric neurons, and GI smooth muscle that only now are beginning to be understood. These agents probably induce a limited low-grade inflammation in the small and large bowel to promote accumulation of water and electrolytes and stimulate intestinal motility. Mechanisms include activation of prostaglandin–cyclic AMP(cAMP) and NO–cyclic GMP (cGMP) pathways, platelet-activating factor production, and perhaps inhibition of Na^+K^+-ATPase. Included in this group are **diphenylmethane derivatives**, **anthraquinones**, and **ricinoleic acid**.

Phenolphthalein, once among the most popular components of laxatives, has been withdrawn from the market in the United States because of potential carcinogenicity. **Oxyphenisatin**, another older drug, was withdrawn due to hepatotoxicity. **Sodium picosulfate** (Lubrilax, SUR-LAX) is a diphenylmethane derivative widely available outside of the United States. It is hydrolyzed by colonic bacteria to its active form, and hence acts locally only in the colon. Effective doses of the diphenylmethane derivatives vary as much as four- to eightfold in individual patients. Consequently, recommended doses may be ineffective in some patients but may produce cramps and excessive fluid secretion in others.

Anthraquinone laxatives: These derivatives of plants such as **aloe**, **cascara**, and **senna** share a tricyclic anthracene nucleus modified with hydroxyl, methyl, or carboxyl groups to form monoanthrones, such as rhein and frangula monoanthrones that are irritating to the oral mucosa; however the process of aging or drying converts them to more innocuous dimeric (dianthrones) or glycoside forms. This process is reversed by bacterial action in the colon to generate the active forms. Senna (**Senokot**, **Ex-lax**) is obtained from the dried leaflets on pods of ***Cassia acutifolia*** or ***Cassia angustifolia*** and contains the rhein dianthrone glycosides **sennoside A and B**. **Cascara sagrada** ("sacred bark"; Colamin, Sagrada-lax) is obtained from the bark of the buckthorn tree and contains the glycosides **barbaloin** and **chrysaloin**. Barbaloin is also found in aloe. The rhubarb plant also produces anthraquinone compounds that have been used as laxatives. Anthraquinones can also be synthesized; however, the synthetic monoanthrone danthron was withdrawn from the United States market because of concerns over possible carcinogenicity. In addition, all aloe and cascara sagrada products sold as laxatives have been withdrawn from the United States market because of failure to demonstrate scientific evidence of efficacy and safety.

Anthraquinone laxatives can produce giant migrating colonic contractions and induce water and electrolyte secretion. They are poorly absorbed in the small bowel, but because they require activation in the colon, the laxative effect is not noted until 6 to 12 hours after ingestion. Active compounds are absorbed to a variable degree from the colon and excreted in the bile, saliva, milk, and urine.

The adverse consequences of long-term use of these agents have limited their use. A melanotic pigmentation of the colonic mucosa (melanosis coli) has been observed in patients using anthraquinone laxatives for long periods (at least 4 to 9 months). Histologically, this is caused by the presence of pigment-laden macrophages within the lamina propria. The condition is benign and reversible on discontinuation of the laxative. These agents also have been associated with the development of "**cathartic colon**," which can be seen in patients (typically women) who have a long-standing history (typically years) of laxative abuse. Regardless of whether a definitive causal relationship can be demonstrated between the use of these agents and colonic pathology, it is clear that they should not be recommended for chronic or long-term use.

SERMORELIN ACETATE

(Geref)

Sermorelin, a growth-hormone-releasing hormone, is used as a diagnostic aid to determine the pituitary gland's ability to secrete growth hormone.

SEROTONIN

5-Hydroxytryptamine (serotonin) is metabolized according to the following scheme:

Tryptophan
↓ Tryptophan 5-hydroxylase
5-Hydroxytryptophan
↓ Aromatic L-amino acid decarboxylase
5-Hydroxytryptamine (serotonin)
↓ Monoamine oxidase
5-Hydroxyindoleactaldehyde
↓ Aldehyde dehydrogenase
5-Hyroxyindoleacetic acid

A large amount of 5-hydroxyindoleacetic acid is excreted by patients with malignant carcinoid.

Extensive ligand-binding studies and molecular biologic examination of membrane preparations have revealed that there are at least 14 types of serotonin receptors, including 5-HT_{1A}, 5-HT_{1B}, 5-HT_{1D}, 5-HT_3, and 5-HT_4.

Serotonin possesses many actions; it:

- Is involved in the neural network that regulates intestinal motility.
- Is released by a carcinoid.
- Is released by platelets (also ADP) during aggregation.
- Causes vasoconstriction by stimulating 5-HT_2 receptors, and this effect is blocked by ketanserine.
- Causes vasodilation by stimulating 5-HT_1 receptors.
- Causes positive inotropic and chronotropic effects by interacting with both 5-HT_1 and 5-HT_3 receptors.
- Increases the motility of the stomach as well as small and large intestines.
- Causes uterine contractions.
- Causes bronchial contractions.

Following are the serotonin-receptor agonist-antagonists:

Ketanserine, a 5-HT_2 and alpha$_1$-adrenergic-receptor antagonist, lowers blood pressure.

Methysergide, a 5-HT_{1C} antagonist, has been used for the prophylactic treatment of migraine and other vascular headache, including Horton's syndrome. Calcium-entry blockers such as flunarizine have been shown to be effective in treating migraine.

Cyproheptadine, a serotonin and histamine$_1$-receptor- and muscarinic cholinergic-receptor-blocking agent, has been used in the treatment of the postgastrectomy dumping syndrome and the intestinal hypermotility seen with carcinoid.

Sumatriptan, an agonist of the 5-HT_1-like receptor, is highly effective in the treatment of migraine (see Figure 93).

Ondansetron, granisetron, tropisetron, and batanopride are antagonists of the 5-HT_3 receptor and are considered effective in controlling cancer chemotherapy-induced emesis (see Figure 73).

Clozapine, an effective antipsychotic agent with little or no extrapyramidal side effects, blocks the 5-HT_2 receptor (see also Table 2).

SEROTONIN-RECEPTOR SUBTYPES

Subtypes	Drugs	Disorders
5-HT_{1A}	Buspirone, ipsaperone	Anxiety, depression
5-HT_{1B}		
5-HT_{1D}	Sumatriptan	Migraine
5-HT_{1E}		
5-HT_{1F}		
5-HT_{2A}	Ketanserin	Hypertension
5-HT_{2B}	Methysergide, risperidone	Migraine, depression, schizophrenia
5-HT_{2C}		
5-HT_3	Ondansetron	Chemotherapy-induced emesis
5-HT_4	Cisapride	GI disorders
5-HT_{5A}		
5-HT_{5B}		
5-HT_6		
5-HT_7		
5-HT transporter	Fluoxetine, sertraline	Depression, obsessive-compulsive disorder

Buspirone, ipsaperone, sumatriptan, and cisapride are agonists; whereas methysergide, risperidone, ketanserin, and ondansetron are antagonists at serotonin receptors.

SERTACONAZOLE NITRATE

(Ertaczo cream 2%)

Sertaconazole nitrate is an antifungal agent, which alters permeability of fungal cell membrane, leading to cell death. It is indicated in the topical treatment of interdigital tinea pedis caused by *Trichophyton rubrum*, *Trichophyton mentagrophytes*, and *Epidermophyton floccosum* in immunocompetent patients.

Tioconazole (Vagistat 1, others) is an imidazole that is marketed for treatment of *Candida* vulvovaginitis. A single 4.6-g dose of ointment (300 mg) is given at bedtime.

Oxiconazole, **Sulconazole**, and **Sertaconazole** are imidazole derivatives used for the topical treatment of infections caused by the common pathogenic dermatophytes. Oxiconazole nitrate (Oxistat) is available as a cream and lotion; sulconazole nitrate (Exelderm) is supplied as a solution and cream. Sertaconazole (Ertaczo) is a 2% cream marketed for tinea pedis.

SERTRALINE HYDROCHLORIDE
(Zoloft)

Sertraline (50 mg p.o. daily) is a nontricyclic, potent, and selective serotonin reuptake inhibitor (SSRI) which is currently approved in the treatment of depression. The role of serotonin in the etiology of obsessive compulsive disorder (OCD) has been established through considerable indirect evidence. The strongest evidence comes from the fact that drugs known to be SSRIs have been found to be useful in the pharmacotherapy of OCD (see also Figure 86 and Tables 5 through 7).

SEVELAMER HYDROCHLORIDE
(Renagel tablets 400 mg, tablets 800 mg)

Sevelamer hydrochloride is a phosphate binder, which decreases intestinal phosphate absorption by binding to phosphate in the GI tract. It is indicated in the reduction of serum phosphorus in patients with chronic kidney disease who are on hemodialysis.

Osteomalacia, distinguished by undermineralization of bone matrix, occurs commonly during sustained phosphate depletion. Patients with chronic renal disease are at risk for developing osteomalacia but also may develop a complex bone disease called **renal osteodystrophy**. In this setting, bone metabolism is stimulated by an increase in parathyroid hormone (PTH) and by a delay in bone mineralization that is due to decreased renal synthesis of calcitriol. In renal osteodystrophy, low bone mineral density may be accompanied by high-turnover bone lesions typically seen in patients with uncontrolled **hyperparathyroidism** or by low bone remodeling activity seen in patients with adynamic bone disease. The therapeutic approach to the patient with renal osteodystrophy depends on its specific type. In high-turnover (hyperparathyroid) or mixed high-turnover disease with deficient mineralization, dietary phosphate restriction, generally in combination with a phosphate binder, is recommended because phosphate restriction is limited by the need to provide adequate protein intake to maintain nitrogen balance. Although highly effective, **aluminum** is no longer used as a phosphate binder because it promotes adynamic bone disease, anemia, myopathy, and occasionally dementia. Calcium-containing phosphate binders along with calcitriol administration may contribute to oversuppression of PTH secretion and likewise result in adynamic bone disease and an increased incidence of vascular calcification. Highly effective non-calcium-containing phosphate binders have been developed. **Sevelamer hydrochloride** (Renagel), a nonabsorbable phosphate-binding polymer, effectively lowers serum phosphate concentration in hemodialysis patients, with a corresponding reduction in the calcium X phosphate product. Sevelamer hydrochloride consists of cross-linked poly[allylamine hydrochloride] that is resistant to digestive degradation. Partially protonated amines spaced one carbon from the polymer backbone chelate phosphate ions by ionic and hydrogen bonding. Side effects of sevelamer include vomiting, nausea, diarrhea, and dyspepsia. Sevelamer does not affect the bioavailability of digoxin, warfarin, enalapril, or metoprolol.

Renal osteodystrophy associated with low bone turnover (adynamic bone disease) is increasingly common and may be due to oversuppression of PTH with aggressive use of either calcitriol or other vitamin D analogs. While PTH levels generally are low (<100 pg/ml), a high PTH level does not exclude the presence of adynamic bone disease, especially with PTH assays that do not distinguish between biologically active and inactive PTH fragments. Current guidelines suggest that treatment with an active vitamin D preparation is indicated if serum 25-OHD levels are less than 30 ng/mL and serum calcium is less than 9.5 mg/dL (2.37 mM). However, if 25-OHD and serum calcium levels are elevated, vitamin D supplementation should be discontinued. If the serum calcium level is less than 9.5 mg/dl, treatment with a vitamin D analog is warranted irrespective of the 25-OHD level.

SEXUAL DYSFUNCTION CAUSED BY DRUGS

Drugs	Adverse Effects
Acetazolamide	Loss of libido; decreased potency
Alprazolam	Inhibition of orgasm; delayed or no ejaculation; decreased libido
Amiloride	Impotence; decreased libido
Amiodarone	Decreased libido
Amitriptyline	Loss of libido; impotence; no ejaculation
Amoxapine	Loss of libido; impotence; ejaculatory problems
Amphetamines and related anorexic drugs	Chronic abuse; impotence; delayed or no ejaculation in men; no orgasm in women
Anticholinergics	Impotence
Atenolol	Impotence
Baclofen	Impotence; inability to ejaculate
Barbiturates	Decreased libido; impotence
Bromocriptine	Painful clitoral tumescence; impotence
Buserelin	Loss of libido; impotence
Buspirone	Priapism
Carbamazepine	Impotence
Chlorpromazine	Decreased libido; impotence; no ejaculation; priapism
Chlorprothixene	Inhibition of ejaculation
Chlorthalidone	Decreased libido; impotence
Cimetidine	Decreased libido; impotence
Clofibrate	Decreased libido; impotence
Clomipramine	Decreased libido; impotence; retarded or no ejaculation or orgasm; orgasm precipitated by yawning; painful ejaculation
Clonidine	Impotence; delayed or retrograde ejaculation; decreased libido
Clozapine	Priapism
Cocaine	Priapism
Danazol	Increased or decreased libido
Desipramine	Decreased libido; impotence; painful orgasm

SEXUAL DYSFUNCTION CAUSED BY DRUGS (Continued)

Drugs	Adverse Effects
Diazepam	Decreased libido; delayed ejaculation; retarded or no orgasms in women; erection difficulties
Dichlorphenamide	Decreased libido; impotence
Digoxin	Decreased libido; impotence
Disopyramide	Impotence
Disulfiram	Impotence
Doxepin	Decreased libido; ejaculatory dysfunction
Ethosuximide	Increased libido
Ethoxzolamide	Decreased libido
Etretinate	Erection difficulties
Famotidine	Impotence
Fenfluramine	Loss of libido with large doses or long-term use; impotence
Fluoxetine	Anorgasmia; delayed orgasm; spontaneous orgasm; ejaculation difficulties; penile anesthesia; decreased libido
Fluphenazine	Changes in libido; erection difficulties; inhibition of ejaculation; priapism
Gemfibrozil	Impotence; loss of libido
Guanabenz	Impotence
Guanadrel	Decreased libido; delayed or retrograde ejaculation; impotence
Guanethidine	Decreased libido; impotence; delayed, retrograde, or no ejaculation
Guanfacine	Impotence
Haloperidol	Impotence; painful ejaculation
Hydralazine	Impotence; priapism
Imipramine	Decreased libido; impotence; painful, delayed ejaculation; delayed orgasm in women
Indapamide	Decreased libido; impotence
Indomethacin	Sexual dysfunction; impotence; decreased libido
Interferon alfa	Decreased libido; impotence
Isocarboxazid	Impotence; delayed ejaculation; no orgasm in women
Ketoconazole	Impotence; decreased libido
Labetalol	Priapism; impotence; delayed or no ejaculation; decreased libido
Leuprolide	Impotence
Levodopa	Increased libido
Lithium	Decreased libido; impotence
Lorazepam	Loss of libido
Maprotiline	Impotence; decreased libido
Mazindol	Impotence; spontaneous ejaculation; painful testes
Mecamylamine	Impotence; decreased libido
Mepenzolate bromide	Impotence
Mesoridazine	No ejaculation; impotence; priapism
Methadone	Decreased libido; impotence; no orgasm (men and women); retarded ejaculation
Methandrostenolone	Decreased libido
Methantheline bromide	Impotence
Methazolamide	Decreased libido; impotence
Methotrexate	Impotence; erection difficulties
Methyldopa	Decreased libido; impotence; delayed or no ejaculation or orgasm
Metoclopramide	Impotence; decreased libido
Metoprolol	Impotence
Metyrosine	Impotence; failure of ejaculation
Mexiletine	Impotence; decreased libido
Molindone	Priapism
Nafarelin	Impotence; loss of libido
Naltrexone	Delayed ejaculation; decreased potency
Naproxen	Impotence; no ejaculation
Nifedipine	Priapism
Nizatidine	Impotence
Norethandrolone	Decreased libido; impotence
Nortriptyline	Impotence; decreased libido
Omeprazole	Painful nocturnal erections
Papaverine	Priapism, especially with neurological disorders
Pargyline	No ejaculation; impotence
Pergolide	Hypersexuality; priapism; spontaneous ejaculation
Perphenazine	Decreased or no ejaculation
Phenelzine	Impotence; retarded or no ejaculation; delayed or no orgasm; priapism
Phenytoin	Decreased libido; impotence; priapism
Pimozide	Impotence; no ejaculation; decreased libido
Prazosin	Impotence; priapism
Primidone	Decreased libido; impotence
Propantheline bromide	Impotence
Propofol	Sexual disinhibition
Propranolol	Loss of libido; impotence
Protriptyline	Loss of libido; impotence; painful ejaculation
Ranitidine	Impotence; loss of libido
Reserpine	Decreased libido; impotence; decreased or no ejaculation
Sertraline	Sexual dysfunction
Spironolactone	Decreased libido; impotence
Sulfasalazine	Impotence
Tamoxifen	Priapism
Testosterone	Priapism
Thiazide diuretics	Impotence
Thioridazine	Impotence; priapism; delayed, decreased, painful, retrograde, or no ejaculation; anorgasmia
Thiothixene	Spontaneous ejaculations; impotence; priapism
Timolol	Decreased libido; impotence
Tranylcypromine	Impotence; painful ejaculation; retarded ejaculation
Trazodone	Priapism; clitoral priapism; increased libido; retrograde or no ejaculation; anorgasmia
Trifluperazine	Painful ejaculation; spontaneous ejaculations
Verapamil	Impotence

Drugs cause sexual dysfunctions by diversified mechanisms such as having peripheral sympatholytic actions (guanadrel), central sympatholytic actions (clonidine), anticholinergic actions (imipramine), or enhancing the concentration of prolactin (amoxapine). Drug-induced sexual dysfunctions are usually reversible with dose reduction or discontinuation of drugs.

SIBUTRAMINE

Sibutramine, a novel pharmacologic agent, is a specific reuptake inhibitor for norepinephrine and serotonin. Sibutramine and its two metabolites reduce food intake and hence show promise as antiobesity medications.

SEXUALLY TRANSMITTED DISEASES: Treatment of

Diseases	First Drug of Choice	Alternate Drug(s)
	Chlamydia trachomatis	
Urethritis, cervicitis, conjunctivitis, or proctitis	Azithromycin **or** Doxycycline	Ofloxacin Erythromycin
Infection in pregnancy	Erythromycin	Amoxicillin Azithromycin
	Neonatal	
Ophthalmia	Erythromycin	Sulfisoxazole
Pneumonia	Erythromycin	
Lymphogranuloma venereum	Doxycycline	Erythromycin
	Gonorrhea	
Urethral, cervical, rectal, or pharyngeal	Ceftriaxone	Cefixime Ciprofloxacin Ofloxacin Spectinomycin
Ophthalmia	Ceftriaxone	
Bacteremia, arthritis, and disseminated	Ceftriaxone	Ceftizoxime **or** Cefotaxime
	Neonatal	
Ophthalmia	Cefotaxime **or** Ceftriaxone	Penicillin G
Bacteremia, arthritis, and disseminated	Cefotaxime	Penicillin G
	Children	
Urogenital, rectal, and pharyngeal	Ceftriaxone	Spectinomycin Amoxicillin **plus** Probenecid
Bacteremia, arthritis, and disseminated	Ceftriaxone **or** Cefotaxime	Penicillin G
	Sexually Acquired Epididymitis	
	Ofloxacin	Ceftriaxone **followed by** Doxycycline
	Pelvic Inflammatory Disease	
Hospitalized patients	Cefoxitin **or** Cefotetan **either one plus** Doxycycline **followed by** Doxycycline	Clindamycin **plus** Gentamicin **followed by** Gentamicin **followed by** Doxycycline
Outpatients	Cefoxitin **plus** Probenecid **or** Cetriaxone **either one followed by** Doxycycline	Ofloxacin **plus** Metronidazole **or** Clindamycin
	Vaginal Infection	
Trichomoniasis	Metronidazole	Metronidazole
Bacterial vaginosis	Metronidazole or Clindamycin	Metronidazole Clindamycin
Vulvovaginal candidiasis	Topical butoconazole, clotrimazole, miconazole, terconazole, **or** tioconazole	Fluconazole
	Syphilis	
Early	Penicillin G benzathine	Doxycycline
Late	Penicillin G benzathine	Doxycycline
Neurosyphilis	Penicillin G	Penicillin G procaine **plus** Probenecid
Congenital	Penicillin G **or** Penicillin G procaine	
Chancroid	Erythromycin **or** Ceftriaxone **or** Azithromycin	Ciprofloxacin
	Herpes Simplex	
First episode genital	Acyclovir	Acyclovir
First episode proctitis	Acyclovir	Acyclovir
Recurrent	Acyclovir	
Severe (hospitalized patients)	Acyclovir	
Prevention of recurrence	Acyclovir	Acyclovir

SIBUTRAMINE HYDROCHLORIDE

(Meridia capsules 5 mg, capsules 10 mg, capsules 15 mg)
Sibutramine hydrochloride is an anorexiant that inhibits reuptake of norepinephrine, serotonin and dopamine. It may stimulate the satiety center in brain, causing appetite suppression. It is indicated as an adjunct to a reduced calorie diet for the management of obesity, including weight loss and maintenance of weight loss. Recommended for patients with an initial body mass index greater than 30 kg/m2 or greater than 27 kg/m^2 in the presence of other risk factors (e.g., hypertension, diabetes, dyslipidemia).

Obesity arises as a consequence of positive caloric balance. Optimally, weight loss is achieved by a gradual increase in energy expenditure from exercise combined with dieting to decrease the caloric intake. However, this obvious approach has a relatively low success rate. Consequently, alternative forms of treatment, including surgery or medications, have been developed in an effort to increase the likelihood of achieving and maintaining weight loss. **Amphetamine** was found to produce weight loss in early studies of patients with narcolepsy and was subsequently used in the treatment of obesity. The drug promotes weight loss by suppressing appetite rather than by increasing energy expenditure. Other anorexic drugs include **methamphetamine**, **dextroamphetamine**, **phentermine**, **benzphetamine**, **phendimetrazine**, **phenmetrazine**, **diethylpropion**, **mazindol**, **phenylpropanolamine**, and **sibutramine** (a mixed adrenergic/serotonergic drug).

SHINGLES: Treatment of

Varicella-zoster virus (VZV) is responsible for a primary infection (varicella) followed by a latency, eventually resulting in herpes zoster (shingles).

Treatment of herpes zoster primarily relies upon antiviral drugs and incidentally on immunomodulating agents, specific immunoglobulins, antimicrobial agents, antiviral enzymes, and corticosteroids. Drugs with a clinically relevant activity against varicella-zoster virus infections include acyclovir, adenosine monophosphate, bromodeoxyuridine, descyclovir, fiacitabine, idoxuridine, interferon-α, and vidarabine. Among them, acyclovir appears to be a first-line agent. Its efficacy has been well established by many clinical studies. Promising drugs for the future include famciclovir, pencyclovir, valacyclovir, and other molecules currently under investigation.

In short-term (up to 20 weeks), double-blind controlled studies, amphetamine-like drugs have been shown to be more effective than placebo in promoting weight loss; the rate of weight loss typically is increased by about 0.5 pound per week with these drugs. There is little to choose among these drugs in terms of efficacy. However, long-term weight loss has not been demonstrated unless these drugs are taken continuously. In addition, other important issues have not yet been resolved, including the selection of patients who might benefit from these drugs, whether the drugs should be administered continuously or intermittently, and the duration of treatment. Adverse effects of treatment include the potential for drug abuse and habituation, serious worsening of hypertension (although in some patients blood pressure actually may fall, presumably as a consequence of weight loss), sleep disturbances, palpitations, and dry mouth. These agents may be effective adjuncts in the treatment of obesity. However, available evidence does not support the isolated use of these drugs in the absence of a more comprehensive program that stresses exercise and modification of diet. β_3-Receptor agonists were found to have remarkable antiobesity and antidiabetic effects in rodents. However, pharmaceutical companies have not yet succeeded in developing β_3-receptor agonists for the treatment of these conditions in humans, perhaps because of important differences in β_3 receptors between humans and rodents. With the cloning of the human β_3 receptor, compounds with favorable metabolic effects have been developed. The use of β_3 agonists in the treatment of obesity remains a possibility for the future.

SILDENAFIL CITRATE

(Viagra tablets 25 mg, tablets 50 mg, tablets 100 mg)

Sildenafil citrate is a phosphodiesterase type 5 inhibitor that enhances the effect of nitric oxide by inhibiting phosphodiesterase type 5 in the **corpus cavernosum of the penis**. This results in vasodilation, increased inflow of blood into the corpora cavernosa, and ensuing penile erection upon sexual stimulation. It is indicated in the treatment of impotence related to erectile dysfunction of the penis.

PGE_1 (**alprostadil**) may be used in the treatment of impotence. Intracavernous injection of PGE_1 causes complete or partial erection in impotent patients who do not have disorders of the vascular system or cavernous body damage. The erection lasts for 1 to 3 hours and is sufficient for sexual intercourse. PGE_1 is more effective than **papaverine**. The agent is available as a sterile powder that is reconstituted with water for injections (**Caverject**), although it has been superseded largely by the use of PDE5 inhibitors, such as **sildenafil**, **tadalafil**, and **vardenafil**.

Erectile dysfunction is a frequently encountered problem whose risk factors parallel those of coronary artery disease (CAD). Thus many men desiring therapy for erectile dysfunction already may be receiving (or may require, especially if they increase physical activity) antianginal therapy. The combination of **sildenafil** and other phosphodiesterase 5 (PDE5) inhibitors with organic nitrate vasodilators can cause extreme hypotension.

Cells in the **corpus cavernosum** produce NO during sexual arousal in response to nonadrenergic, noncholinergic neurotransmission. NO stimulates the formation of cGMP, which leads to relaxation of smooth muscle of the corpus cavernosum and penile arteries, engorgement of the corpus cavernosum, and erection. The accumulation of cGMP can be enhanced by inhibition of the cGMP-specific PDE5 family. **Sildenafil** (Viagra) and congeners inhibit PDE5 and have been demonstrated to improve erectile function in patients with erectile dysfunction. Not surprisingly, PDE5 inhibitors have assumed the status of widely used recreational drugs. Since the introduction of sildenafil, two additional PDE5 inhibitors have been developed for use in therapy of erectile dysfunction. **Tadalafil** (Cialis) and **vardenafil** (Levitra) share similar therapeutic efficacy and side-effect profiles with sildenafil; tadalafil has a longer time to onset of action and a longer therapeutic half-life than the other PDE5 inhibitors. **Sildenafil** has been the most thoroughly characterized of these compounds, but all three PDE5 inhibitors are contraindicated for patients taking organic nitrate vasodilators or adrenergic receptor antagonists.

The side effects of **sildenafil** and other PDE5 inhibitors are largely predictable on the basis of their effects on PDE5. Headache, flushing, and rhinitis may be observed, as may dyspepsia owing to relaxation of the lower esophageal sphincter. **Sildenafil** and vardenafil also weakly inhibit

PDE6, the enzyme involved in photoreceptor-signal transduction, and can produce visual disturbances, most notably changes in the perception of color hue or brightness. Tadalafil inhibits PDE11, a widely distributed phosphodiesterase isoform, but the clinical importance of this effect is not clear. The most important toxicity of all these PDE5 inhibitors is hemodynamic. When given alone to men with severe coronary artery disease, these drugs have modest effects on blood pressure (BP), producing less than a 10% fall in systolic, diastolic, and mean systemic pressures and in pulmonary artery systolic and mean pressures. However, sildenafil, tadalafil, and vardenafil all have a significant and potentially dangerous interaction with organic nitrates, the therapeutic actions of which are mediated via their conversion to NO with resulting increases in cGMP. In the presence of a PDE5 inhibitor, nitrates cause profound increases in cGMP and can produce dramatic reductions in BP. Compared with controls, healthy male subjects pretreated with sildenafil or the other PDE5 inhibitors exhibit a much greater decrease in systolic BP when treated with sublingual glyceryl trinitrate, and in many subjects a fall of more than 25 mmHg was detected. This drug class toxicity is the basis for the warning that PDE5 inhibitors should not be prescribed to patients receiving any form of nitrate and dictates that patients should be questioned about the use of PDE5 inhibitors within 24 hours before nitrates are administered. A period of longer than 24 hours may be needed following administration of a PDE5 inhibitor for safe use of nitrates, especially with tadalafil because of its prolonged half-life. In the event that patients develop significant hypotension following combined administration of sildenafil and a nitrate, fluids and adrenergic receptor agonists, if needed, should be used for support.

Sildenafil, tadalafil, and vardenafil are metabolized via cytochrome P450 (CYP3A4), and their toxicity may be enhanced in patients who receive other substrates of this enzyme, including macrolide and imidazole antibiotics, some statins, and antiretroviral agents. PDE5 inhibitors also may prolong cardiac repolarization by blocking the I_{Kr}. Although these interactions and effects are important clinically, the overall incidence and profile of adverse events observed with PDE5 inhibitors, when used without nitrates, are consistent with the expected background frequency of the same events in the treated population. In patients with coronary artery disease whose exercise capacity indicates that sexual activity is unlikely to precipitate angina and who are not currently taking nitrates, the use of PDE5 inhibitors can be considered. Such therapy needs to be individualized, and appropriate warnings must be given about the risk of toxicity if nitrates are taken subsequently for angina; this drug interaction may persist for approximately 24 hours for sildenafil and vardenafil and for considerably longer with tadalafil. Alternative nonnitrate antianginal therapy, such as β-adrenergic receptor antagonists, should be used during these time periods.

SILVER NITRATE, SILVER NITRATE 1%

(Dey drops silver nitrate)

Silver nitrate, an ophthalmic antiseptic and topical cauterizing agent, is used in the prevention of gonorrheal ophthalmia neonatorum; and to treat indolent wounds, destroy exuberant granulations, freshen the edges of ulcers and fissures, provide styptic action, and treat vesicular bullous or aphthous lesions.

SILVER SULFADIAZINE

(Silvadene cream 10 mg/g in a water-miscible base, SSD cream 10 mg/g in a water-miscible base, SSD AF cream 10 mg/g in a water-miscible base, Thermazene cream 10 mg/g in a water-miscible base)

Silver sulfadiazine is a burn preparation, which inhibits bacteria by acting on cell membrane and cell wall. It is indicated as an adjunct in prevention and treatment of wound sepsis in patients with second- and third-degree burns.

Silver sulfadiazine (Silvadene, others) inhibits the growth *in vitro* of nearly all pathogenic bacteria and fungi, including some species resistant to sulfonamides. The compound is used topically to reduce microbial colonization and the incidence of infections of wounds from burns. It should not be used to treat an established deep infection. Silver is released slowly from the preparation in concentrations that are selectively toxic to the microorganisms. However, bacteria may develop resistance to **silver sulfadiazine**. Although little silver is absorbed, the plasma concentration of sulfadiazine may approach therapeutic levels if a large surface area is involved. Adverse reactions—burning, rash, and itching—are infrequent. Silver sulfadiazine is considered by most authorities to be one of the agents of choice for the prevention of burn infection.

SIMETHICONE

(Degas tablets, chewable 80 mg, extra strength Gas-X capsules, softgel 125 mg, tablets, chewable 125 mg, Flatulex drops 40 mg/0.6 mL, Genasyme tablets, chewable 80 mg, Genasyme drops 40 mg/0.6 mL, Gas-X tablets, chewable 80 mg, Maalox anti-gas tablets, chewable 80 mg, Mylanta gas tablets, chewable 40 mg, tablets, chewable 80 mg, maximum strength Mylanta gas tablets, chewable 125 mg, Mylicon drops 40 mg/0.6 mL, Phazyme drops 40 mg/0.6 mL, tablets 60 mg, Phazyme 95 tablets, chewable 95 mg, Phazyme 125 tablets, chewable 125 mg)

Simethicone is an antiflatulent that relieves flatulence by dispersing and preventing formation of mucus-surrounded gas pockets in the GI tract. It is indicated in relief of painful symptoms and pressure of excess gas in the digestive tract. It is an adjunct in treatment of many conditions in which gas retention may be a problem, such as postoperative gaseous distention and pain, endoscopic examination, air swallowing, functional dyspepsia, peptic ulcer, spastic or irritable colon, and diverticulosis.

SINUSITIS: Treatment of

Normal physiological functioning of the sinuses depends on ostial patency, mucociliary function, and the quantity and quality of secretions. Retention of sinus secretions may result if ostial diameter is compromised; if cilia are damaged, impairing mucociliary clearance of secretions; or if increased viscosity or volume of secretions exceeds the clearing capacity of the sinus mucociliary drainage system.

Factors predisposing to the development of sinusitis are:

Adenoidal hypertrophy	Dysmotile cilia syndrome
Allergic rhinitis	Immune deficiency
Barotrauma	Nasal polyps
Bone spurs	Overuse of topical decongestants
Bronchiectasis	Swimming and diving
Cigarette smoke	Tumors
Deviated nasal septum	Upper respiratory infection

The goal in treatment of sinusitis is eradication of infection with clearance of the infected material from the sinuses. While the use of an appropriate antibiotic is necessary, the use of ancillary therapy is also of utmost importance. Steam and nasal saline, decongestants, topical corticosteroids, and mucoevacuants are given in an attempt to reduce nasal obstruction, increase sinus ostia size, promote improved mucociliary function, decrease mucosal inflammation, and thin secretions. In selected patients who fail to respond to aggressive medical therapy, functional endoscopic surgery can often provide relief. In patients with poorly controlled asthma, treatment of underlying sinusitis has been shown to dramatically improve the asthmatic state.

SIMVASTATIN

(Zocor)

Simvastatin, an HMG-CO reductase inhibitor with antilipemic activity (5 to 10 mg daily), is used for reduction of low-density lipoprotein (LDL) and total cholesterol levels in patients with primary hypercholesterolemia (types IIa and IIb).

SIROLIMUS

(Rapamune solution, oral 1 mg/mL, tablets 2 mg)

Sirolimus is an immunosuppressive agent, which inhibits T-lymphocyte activation and proliferation that occurs in response to antigenic and cytokine stimulation; and inhibits antibody production. It is indicated for prophylaxis of organ rejection in patients receiving renal transplants.

Intracoronary stents can ameliorate angina and reduce adverse events in patients with acute coronary syndromes. However, the long-term efficacy of intracoronary stents is limited by subacute luminal restenosis within the stent, which occurs in a substantial minority of patients. The pathways that lead to "in-stent restenosis" are complex, but smooth muscle proliferation within the lumen of the stented artery is a common pathological finding. Local antiproliferative therapies at the time of stenting have been explored over many years, and the development of drug-eluting stents has had an important impact on clinical practice. Two drugs are currently being used in intravascular stents: **paclitaxel** (Taxol) and **sirolimus** (rapamycin). Paclitaxel is a tricyclic diterpene that inhibits cellular proliferation by binding to and stabilizing polymerized microtubules. **Sirolimus** is a hydrophobic macrolide that binds to the cytosolic immunophilin $FKBP_{12}$; the $FKBP_{12}$-sirolimus complex inhibits the mammalian kinase target of rapamycin (mTOR), thereby inhibiting cell-cycle progression. Paclitaxel and sirolimus differ markedly in their mechanisms of action but share common chemical properties as hydrophobic small molecules. Differences in the intracellular targets of these two drugs are associated with marked differences in their distribution in the vascular wall. Stent-induced damage to the vascular endotheial cell layer can lead to thrombosis; patients typically are treated with antiplatelet agents, including clopidogrel (for up to 6 months) and aspirin (indefinitely), sometimes in conjunction with intravenously administered GPIIb/IIIa inhibitors. The inhibition of cellular proliferation by paclitaxel and sirolimus not only affects vascular smooth muscle cell proliferation but also attenuates the formation of an intact endothelial layer within the stented artery. Therefore, antiplatelet therapy (typically with clopidogrel) is continued for several months after intracoronary stenting with drug-eluting stents. The rate of restenosis with drug-eluting stents is reduced markedly compared with "bare metal" stents, and the ongoing development of mechanopharmacological approaches likely will lead to novel approaches in intravascular therapeutics.

SMALLPOX VACCINE

(Dryvax powder for injection dried, calf lymph type live-virus preparation of vaccinia virus (Polymyxin B sulfate, dihydrostreptomycin sulfate, chlortetracycline hydrochloride, and neomycin sulfate are added in trace amounts). The reconstituted vaccine contains approximately 100 million infectious vaccinia viruses/mL)

Smallpox vaccine is a viral vaccine. Introduction of infectious vaccinia virus into superficial layers of the skin results in viral multiplication, immunity and cellular hypersensitivity. It is used in immunization against smallpox disease.

SODIUM BENZOATE-SODIUM PHENYLACETATE

(Ucephan)

Sodium benzoate sodium phenylacetate (25 mg/kg p.o. daily) is used as an adjunctive therapy for the prevention of hyperammonemia in patients with urea cycle enzymopathy.

SODIUM BICARBONATE

(Neut, Soda Mint)

Sodium bicarbonate, an alkalinizing agent (1 mEq/kg IV bolus), is used as an adjunct to advanced cardiac life support in metabolic acidosis, as a urinary alkalinization, and as an antacid.

SODIUM CELLULOSE PHOSPHATE

(Calcibind)

Sodium cellulose phosphate, an ion exchange resin with antiurolithic properties (15 g p.o. daily), is used for absorptive hypercalciuria type I and prophylaxis of calcium renal calculi.

SODIUM CHLORIDE

(Slo-Salt, Thermotab)

Sodium chloride is used for water and electrolyte replacement in hyponatremia from electrolyte loss or severe sodium chloride depletion.

SODIUM FERRIC GLUCONATE

(Ferrlecit injection 62.5 mg per 5 mL (12.5 mg/mL) of elemental iron)

Sodium ferric gluconate is a parenteral iron preparation, which provides iron to replenish hemoglobin and depleted iron stores. It is indicated in the treatment of iron deficiency anemia in patients undergoing chronic hemodialysis and supplemental erythropoietin.

SODIUM FLUORIDE

(Act, Fluorigard, Fluorinse, Fluoritabs, Flura, Flura-Drops, Flura-Loz, Gel II, Karidium, Karigel, Karigel-N, Listermint with fluoride, Luride, Luride Lozi-Tabs, Luride-SF Lozi Tabs, Pediaflor, Phos-Flur, Point Two, PreviDent, Thera-Flur, Thera-Flur-N)

Fluoride, a trace mineral, is used as an aid in the prevention of dental caries.

SODIUM IODIDE ^{131}I

(Iodotope capsules 1 to 50 mCi, oral solution 7.05 mCi, Sodium iodide 1 131 capsules 0.75 to 100 mCi, oral solution 3.5 to 150 mCi)

Sodium iodide ^{131}I is a radiopharmaceutical/antithyroid agent. After rapid GI absorption, iodine ^{131}I is primarily distributed within extracellular fluid. It is trapped and rapidly converted to protein-bound iodine by the thyroid; it is concentrated, but not protein bound, by the stomach and salivary glands. It is promptly excreted by kidneys. About 90% of the local irradiation is caused by beta radiation and 10% is caused by gamma radiation. ^{131}I has a physical half-life of 8.04 days. It is indicated in the treatment of **thyroid carcinoma, hyperthyroidism**.

Although iodine has several radioactive isotopes, greatest use has been made of ^{131}I. It has a half-life of 8 days; therefore, more than 99% of its radiation is expended within 56 days. Its radioactive emissions include both γ rays β and particles. The short-lived radionuclide of iodine, ^{123}I, is primarily a γ-emitter with a half-life of only 13 hours. This permits a relatively brief exposure to radiation during thyroid scans.

The chemical behavior of the radioactive isotopes of iodine is identical to that of the stable isotope, ^{127}I. ^{131}I is rapidly and efficiently trapped by the thyroid, incorporated into the iodoamino acids, and deposited in the colloid of the follicles, from which it is slowly liberated. Thus, the destructive β particles originate within the follicle and act almost exclusively upon the parenchymal cells of the thyroid, with little or no damage to surrounding tissue. The γ-radiation passes through the tissue and can be quantified by external detection. The effects of the radiation depend on the dosage. When small tracer doses of ^{131}I are administered, thyroid function is not disturbed. However, when large amounts of radioactive iodine gain access to the gland, the characteristic cytotoxic actions of ionizing radiation are observed. Pyknosis and necrosis of the follicular cells are followed by disappearance of colloid and fibrosis of the gland. With properly selected doses of ^{131}I, it is possible to destroy the thyroid gland completely without detectable injury to adjacent tissues. After smaller doses, some of the follicles, usually in the periphery of the gland, retain their function.

Radioactive iodine finds its widest use in the treatment of hyperthyroidism and in the diagnosis of disorders of thyroid function. **Sodium iodide** ^{131}I (Iodotope Therapeutic) is available as a solution or in capsules containing essentially carrier-free ^{131}I suitable for oral administration. Sodium iodide ^{123}I is available for scanning procedures. Discussion here is limited to the uses of ^{131}I.

Radioactive iodine is highly useful in the treatment of hyperthyroidism; in many circumstances it is regarded as the therapeutic procedure of choice for this condition. The use of stable iodide as treatment for hyperthyroidism, however, may preclude treatment and certain imaging studies with radioactive iodine for weeks after the iodide has been discontinued.

Dosage and technique; ^{131}I, 7000 to 10,000 rads per gram of thyroid tissue, is administered orally. The effective dose for a given patient depends primarily upon the size of the thyroid, the iodine uptake of the gland, and the rate of release of radioactive iodine from the gland subsequent to the nuclide's deposition in the colloid. Comparison studies have shown little advantage of a standard individualized dose, based on gland weight and radioactive iodine uptake, over a fixed dose. For these reasons, the optimal dose of ^{131}I, expressed in terms of microcuries taken up per gram of thyroid tissue, varies in different laboratories from 80 to 150 μCi. The usual total dose is 4 to 15 mCi. The incidence of hypothyroidism in the early years after doses on the lower side is reduced; however, many patients with late hypothyroidism may go undetected. Therefore, the ultimate incidence of hypothyroidism is probably no less than with the larger doses. In addition, relapse of the hyperthyroid state, or initial failure to alleviate the hyperthyroid state, is increased in patients receiving lower doses of ^{131}I. Thus, many endocrinologists recommend initial treatment with thyroid ablative doses of ^{131}I, with subsequent treatment for hypothyroidism. There also is evidence that pretreatment with propylthiouracil reduces the therapeutic efficacy of ^{131}I, necessitating a higher dose for a desired effect. **Methimazole** appears not to share this effect of **propylthiouracil**.

The course of hyperthyroidism in a patient who has received an optimal dose of ^{131}I is characterized by progressive recovery. Beginning a few weeks after treatment, the symptoms of hyperthyroidism gradually abate over a period of 2 to 3 months. If therapy has been inadequate, the necessity for further treatment is apparent within 6 to 12 months. It is not uncommon, however, for the serum thyroid-stimulating hormone (TSH) to remain low for several months after ^{131}I therapy, especially if the patient was not rendered euthyroid prior to receiving the radioactive iodine. Occasionally, this delayed recovery of the hypothalamic–pituitary–thyroid axis results in a picture of central hypothyroidism, with low-circulating thyroid hormones. Thus, assessing radioactive iodine failure based on TSH concentrations alone may be misleading and should always be accompanied by determination of free T_4 and serum T_3 concentrations. Furthermore, transient hypothyroidism, lasting up to 6 months, may occur in up to 50% of patients receiving a dose of ^{131}I calculated to result in euthyroidism. This is less of a problem if the patient receives a higher, ablative dose of ^{131}I, since hypothyroidism occurs far more frequently and persists.

Depending to some extent upon the dosage schedule adopted, one-half to two-thirds of patients are cured by a single dose, one-third to one-fifth require two doses, and the remainder require three or more doses before the disorder is controlled. Patients treated with larger doses of ^{131}I almost always develop hypothyroidism within a few months.

β-Adrenergic antagonists, antithyroid drugs, or both, or stable iodide, can be used to hasten the control of hyperthyroidism while awaiting the full effects of the radioactive iodine.

SODIUM LACTATE

Sodium lactate, an alkalinizing agent, is used to alkalinize urine and as treatment in mild to moderate metabolic acidosis.

SODIUM OXYBATE

(Xyrem oral solution 500 mg/mL)

Sodium oxybate is a CNS agent, which has anticatapletic activity in patients with narcolepsy. It is indicated in the treatment of cataplexy in patients with narcolepsy.

SODIUM PHOSPHATE P 32

(Sodium phosphate P 32 injection 0.67 mCi/mL)

Sodium phosphate P 32 is a radiopharmaceutical. Phosphorus is necessary to the metabolic and proliferative activity of cells. Radioactive phosphorus concentrates to a very high degree in rapidly proliferating tissue. Sodium phosphate P 32 decays by beta emission with a physical half-life of 14.3 days. The mean energy of the sodium phosphate P 32 beta particle is 695 keV. It is indicated in the treatment of **polycythemia vera**, **chronic myelocytic leukemia**, and **chronic lymphocytic leukemia**; and skeletal metastases.

SODIUM POLYSTYRENE SULFONATE

(Kayexalate powder finely powdered sodium polystyrene sulfonate, sodium content approximately 100 mg (4.1 mEq)/g, SPS suspension 15 g/60 mL, sodium content 1.5 g (65 mEq))

Sodium polystyrene sulfonate is a potassium-removing resin, which exchanges sodium ions for potassium in large intestine. Sodium polystyrene sulfonate, a cation exchange resin removing potassium (15 g p.o. daily), is used in hyperkalemia.

SODIUM SALICYLATE

(Uracel)

Sodium salicylate, a nonnarcotic analgesic, antipyretic, and antiinflammatory agent, is used in minor pain or fever, and in rheumatoid arthritis, osteoarthritis, or other inflammatory conditions (see also Table 3).

SODIUM SULFACETAMIDE/SULFUR

(Avar cleanser 10% sodium sulfacetamide and 5% sulfur, gel 10% sodium sulfacetamide and 5% sulfur, Cleria cream 10% sodium sulfacetamide and 5% sulfur, foam 10% sodium sulfacetamide and 5% sulfur, Rosula gel 10% sodium sulfacetamide and 5% sulfur, Sulfacet-R lotion 10% sodium sulfacetamide and 5% sulfur, Zetacet topical suspension 10% sodium sulfacetamide and 5% sulfur)

Sodium sulfacetamide/sulfur is a keratolytic agent. **Sulfacetamide** competitively antagonizes PABA, an essential component of folic acid synthesis. **Sulfur** inhibits the growth of *Propionibacterium acnes* and the formation of free fatty acids. It is indicated in the topical control of acne vulgaris, acne rosacea, and seborrheic dermatitis.

SODIUM TETRADECYL SULFATE

(Sotradecol injection 10 mg/mL, injection 30 mg/mL)

Sodium tetradecyl sulfate is a sclerosing agent, which causes venous intima inflammation and thrombus formation, which occludes the injected vein and subsequently forms fibrous tissue that results in partial or complete vein obliteration. It is indicated in the treatment of small uncomplicated varicose veins of the lower extremities that show simple dilation with competent valves.

SODIUM THIOSALICYLATE

(Arthrolate, Asproject, Rexolate, Thiocyl, Thiosal, Tusal)

Sodium thiosalicylate, a nonnarcotic analgesic, antipyretic, and antiinflammatory agent, is indicated for mild pain, in the treatment of rheumatic fever, or acute gouty arthritis (see also Table 3).

SOLIFENACIN SUCCINATE

(Vesicare tablets 5 mg, tablets 10 mg)

Solifenacin succinate is an anticholinergic agent, which is used in the treatment of overactive bladder with symptoms of urge urinary incontinence, urgency, and urinary frequency.

SOMATOSTATIN

Somatostatin, a cyclic tetradecapeptide with a disulfide bond between the third and fourteenth amino acid residues, has the following structure:

H-Ala-Gly-Cys-Lys-Asn-Phe-Phe-Tryp-Lys-
Thr-Phe-Thr-Ser-Cys-OH

The administration of somatostatin inhibits the secretion of a variety of peptides, including:

Hypothalamic hormones
- Growth-hormone-releasing hormone (GHRH) (see also Table 15)

Anterior pituitary hormones
- Growth hormone (GH)
- Thyrotropin

Pancreatic hormones
- Insulin
- Glucagon
- Gastrin
- Cholecystokinin
- Secretin
- Pepsin
- Motilin
- Pancreatic polypeptide
- GI peptide
- Vasoactive intestinal polypeptide

Kidney hormones
- Renin

Octreotide (Sandostatin), a long-acting somatostatin analog, has been approved for the management of secretory carcinoid tumors and vasoactive intestinal peptide-secreting tumors.

SOMATREM

(Protropin)

Somatrem, an anterior pituitary hormone, is used in long-term treatment of growth failure from lack of adequate endogenous growth hormone secretion.

SOMATROPIN

(Genotropin powder for injection, lyophilized 5.8 mg (approximately 17.4 IU)/vial, powder for injection, lyophilized 13.8 mg (approximately 41.4 IU)/vial, Genotropin Miniquick powder for injection, lyophilized 0.2 mg/vial, powder for injection, lyophilized 0.4 mg/vial, powder for injection, lyophilized 0.6 mg/vial, powder for injection, lyophilized 0.8 mg/vial, powder for injection, lyophilized 1 mg/vial, powder for injection, lyophilized 1.2 mg/vial, powder for injection, lyophilized 1.4 mg/vial, powder for injection, lyophilized 1.6 mg/vial, powder for injection, lyophilized 1.8 mg/vial, powder for injection, lyophilized 2 mg/vial, Humatrope powder for injection, lyophilized 5 mg (approximately 15 IU)/vial, powder for injection, lyophilized 6 mg (18 IU)/cartridge, powder for injection, lyophilized 12 mg (36 IU)/cartridge, powder for injection, lyophilized 24 mg (72 IU)/cartridge, Norditropin powder for injection, lyophilized 4 mg (approximately 12 IU)/vial, powder for injection, lyophilized 8 mg (approximately 24 IU)/vial, injection 5 mg/1.5 mL, injection 10 mg/ 1.5 mL, injection 15 mg/1.5 mL, Nutropin powder for injection, lyophilized 5 mg (approximately 15 IU)/vial, powder for injection, lyophilized 10 mg (approximately 26 ILJ)/vial, Nutropin AQ injection 10 mg (approximately 30 IU)/vial, Nutropin Depot powder for injection 13.5 mg, powder for injection 18 mg, powder for injection 22.5 mg, Saizen powder for injection, lyophilized 5 mg (approximately 15 IU)/vial, Serostim powder for injection, lyophilized 4 mg (approximately 12 IU)/ vial, powder for injection, lyophilized 5 mg (approximately 15 IU)/vial, powder for injection, lyophilized 6 mg (approximately 18 IU)/vial)

Somatropin is a growth hormone, which mimics actions of naturally occurring growth hormone to stimulate linear and skeletal growth; increases the number and size of skeletal muscle cells; increases RBC mass and internal organ size; increases cellular protein synthesis; reduces body fat stores and lipid mobilization, and increases plasma fatty acids. It is indicated in long-term treatment of children with growth failure caused by lack of adequate endogenous growth hormone secretion (except Serostim).

(Genotropin only) is indicated in long-term treatment of children with growth failure caused by Prader–Willi syndrome (PWS); (Genotropin, Nutropin, Nutropin AQ, and Humatrope only) in long-term replacement therapy in adults with growth hormone deficiency of either childhood- or adult-onset etiology; (Nutropin and Nutropin AQ only) in treatment of growth failure associated with chronic renal insufficiency up to the time of renal transplantation; (Nutropin, Nutropin AQ, and Humatrope only) in long-term treatment of short stature associated with Turner's syndrome; (Serostim only) in treatment of AIDS wasting or cachexia.

SOTALOL HYDROCHLORIDE

(Betapace tablets 80 mg, tablets 120 mg, tablets 160 mg, tablets 240 mg, Betapace AF tablets 80 mg, tablets 120 mg, tablets 160 mg)

Sotalol hydrochloride is a beta-adrenergic-blocking agent, which blocks beta receptors, which primarily affect heart (slows rate), vascular musculature (decreases BP), and lungs (reduces function). **Betapace**: is used in the management or prevention of life-threatening ventricular arrhythmias. **Betapace AF**: is used in the maintenance of normal sinus rhythm in patients with highly symptomatic atrial fibrillation/atrial flutter (AFIB/AFL) (Betapace AF).

Sotalol (80 mg t.i.d.) is indicated in the treatment of documented ventricular arrhythmias, such as sustained ventricular tachycardia.

Sotalol is a nonselective beta-adrenergic blocker that depresses sinus heart rate, slows AV conduction, increases AV nodal refractoriness, prolongs the refractory period of atrial and ventricular muscle and AV accessory pathways in both anterograde and retrograde directions, decreases cardiac output, and lowers systolic and diastolic blood pressure.

Sotalol is well absorbed after oral administration with a bioavailability of 90 to 100%. Peak-plasma concentrations are reached in 2.5 to 4 hours, and steady-state plasma concentrations are attained in 2 to 3 days. Sotalol does not bind to plasma proteins and crosses the blood–brain barrier poorly. Sotalol is not metabolized, and is excreted primarily in the urine and in unchanged form.

Sotalol is contraindicated in patients with bronchial asthma, sinus bradycardia, second- and third-degree AV block (unless a functioning pacemaker is present), congenital or acquired long QT syndromes, cardiogenic shock, or uncontrolled congestive heart failure.

Sotalol should be used cautiously in pregnant patients and patients with renal failure or diabetes mellitus. Sotalol should be used with extreme caution in patients with sick-sinus syndrome associated with symptomatic arrhythmias, because the drug can cause sinus bradycardia, sinus pauses, or sinus arrest.

Catecholamine-depleting drugs, such as reserpine and guanethidine, enhance the hypotensive effects of sotalol. Calcium-channel antagonists enhance myocardial depression and should not be given concomitantly with sotalol. Sotalol may enhance the rebound hypertensive effect seen after withdrawal of clonidine.

Sotalol may require dosage adjustments with insulin or oral antidiabetic agents because it may increase blood glucose. It also may mask symptoms of hypoglycemia.

Overdosage of sotalol may cause bradycardia, congestive heart failure, hypotension, hypoglycemia, and bronchospasm.

Because of the lack of protein binding, hemodialysis is useful in reducing sotalol plasma concentrations. Patients should be carefully observed until QT intervals are normalized.

In addition, atropine, another anticholinergic drug, a beta-adrenergic agonist, or transvenous cardiac pacing may be used to treat bradycardia; transvenous cardiac pacing may be employed to treat second- or third-degree heart block; epinephrine can be used to treat hypotension (depending on associated factors); aminophylline or an aerosol beta$_2$-receptor stimulant can be used to treat bronchospasm; and DC cardioversion, transvenous cardiac pacing, epinephrine, or magnesium sulfate can be used to treat torsade de pointes.

SPARFLOXACIN

Sparfloxacin is a recently developed fluoroquinolone. The drug has shown potent antimicrobial activity against a wide range of Gram-positive and Gram-negative bacteria, glucose nonfermenters, anaerobes, *Legionella* spp., *Mycoplasma* spp., *Chlamydia* spp., and *Mycobacterium* spp. Methicillin-resistant *Staphylococcus aureus* is also susceptible to sparfloxacin.

SPECTINOMYCIN

(Trobicin)

Spectinomycin (2 g IM into the upper outer quadrant of the gluteus) is indicated in the treatment of acute gonorrheal urethritis and proctitis in the male and acute gonorrheal cervicitis and proctitis in the female due to susceptible strains of *Neisseria gonorrhoeae*. The injection may be painful. A single injection of 2 g produces an average peak serum concentration of 160 mcg/ml at 2 hours.

Spectinomycin is not effective in the treatment of syphilis. Antibiotics used to treat gonorrhea may mask or delay the symptoms of incubating syphilis. All patients with gonorrhea should have a serologic test for syphilis at the time of diagnosis and a follow-up test after 3 months.

Spectinomycin is not effective in pharyngeal infections due to *N. gonorrhoeae*.

Spectinomycin selectively inhibits protein synthesis in Gram-negative bacteria. The antibiotic binds to and acts on the 30S ribosomal subunit (see also Figure 75). Its action has similarities to that of the aminoglycosides; however, spectinomycin is not bactericidal and does not cause misreading of polyribonucleotides. A high degree of bacterial resistance may develop as a result of mutation.

Spectinomycin, when given as a single intramuscular injection, produces few significant untoward effects.

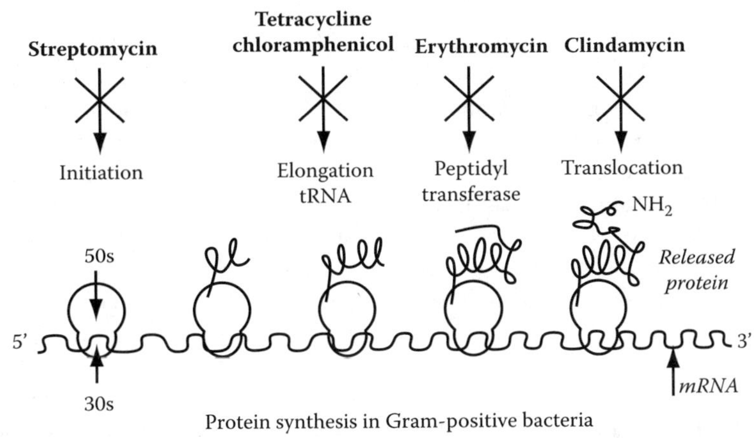

FIGURE 88 Streptomycin and other aminoglycosides are bactericidal and **inhibit protein synthesis** in susceptible microorganisms. They exert this effect by (1) interfering with the initiation complex of peptide formation, (2) inducing misreading of the code on the messenger RNA template, which causes the incorporation of inappropriate amino acid into peptide, and (3) rupturing the polysomes into monosomes that become nonfunctional.

Urticaria, chills, and fever have been noted after single doses, as have dizziness, nausea, and insomnia. The injection may be painful.

SPIRAMYCIN

Spiramycin is a macrolide antibiotic. However, in contrast to other macrolide derivatives such as erythromycin salts, ototoxicity, neurosensorial disorders, and cardiac rhythm disorders do not appear to have been described after spiramycin. Reported adverse effects of spiramycin include GI disorders, immune-allergic reactions, and liver injury (see also Figure 88).

SPIRONOLACTONE

(Aldactone)

The potassium-sparing diuretics consist of spironolactone, which is an aldosterone antagonist, and triamterene (Dyrenium) and amiloride (Midamor), which exert their effects through a mechanism other than a mineralocorticoid action (see also Figure 17).

All act in the distal tubule, where the resorption of sodium is accompanied by the transfer of potassium into the lumen contents (see also Figure 17). When sodium resorption is hindered, potassium excretion is correspondingly reduced, such that more potassium is retained. The potassium-sparing diuretics are not very efficacious, as they affect only 1 to 2% of the filtered load of sodium. All are given orally and eliminated in the urine, mostly by glomerular filtration, though some active tubular secretion may also occur.

A potassium-sparing diuretic can be given along with a thiazide or a loop diuretic to prevent hypokalemia. Spironolactone can also be beneficial in some patients with severe CHF or cirrhosis associated with ascites.

The potassium-sparing diuretics should not be used concurrently with potassium supplements, as this combination is likely to produce hyperkalemia. Poor renal function also heightens the risk of hyperkalemia. GI disturbances, rash, drowsiness, or dizziness are all associated with their use. Spironolactone can cause the blood urea nitrogen level to increase and lead to menstrual irregularities.

SPIRONOLACTONE/HYDROCHLOROTHIAZIDE

(Aldactazide tablets 25 mg spironolactone and 25 mg hydrochlorothiazide, tablets 50 mg spironolactone and 50 mg hydrochlorothiazide)

Spironolactone/hydrochlorothiazide is a diuretic combination. **Spironolactone** competitively inhibits aldosterone in distal tubules, resulting in increased excretion of sodium and water and decreased excretion of potassium. **Hydrochlorothiazide** increases chloride, sodium, and water excretion by interfering with transport of sodium ions across renal tubular epithelium. It is indicated in edematous conditions for patients with CHF, cirrhosis of the liver accompanied by edema or ascites, nephrotic syndrome, or essential hypertension.

STANOZOLOL

(Winstrol)

Stanozolol, an anabolic steroid (2 mg t.i.d.), is indicated as a prophylactic measure in reducing the frequency and severity of hereditary angioedema (see also Table 8).

It increases the concentration of C1 esterase inhibitor in patients with hereditary angioedema. This leads to an increased level of the C4 component of complement, which may be deficient in these patients, thus decreasing the number and severity of attacks of this disorder.

Stanozolol is contraindicated in patients with severe renal or cardiac disease, which may be worsened by the fluid and electrolyte retention that this drug may cause; in patients with hepatic disease because impaired elimination may cause toxic accumulation of the drug; in female patients with breast cancer, in male patients with benign prostatic hypertrophy with obstruction, or undiagnosed abnormal genital bleeding because this drug can stimulate the growth of cancerous breast or prostate tissues; and in pregnant women because studies have shown that administration of anabolic steroids during pregnancy causes masculinization of the fetus. Because of its hypercholesterolemic effects, stanozolol should be administered cautiously in patients with a history of coronary artery disease. In patients with diabetes, decreased blood glucose levels require adjustment of insulin or oral hypoglycemic drug dosage.

Stanozolol may potentiate the effects of warfarin-type anticoagulants, prolonging prothrombin time. The adverse reactions to stanozolol in female subjects include deepening of voice, clitoral enlargement, and changes in libido. The adverse effects in prepubertal male subjects include premature epiphyseal closure, priapism, phallic enlargement; in postpubertal males they are testicular atrophy, oligospermia, decreased ejaculatory volume, impotence, gynecomastia, and epididymitis.

STAVUDINE

(Zerit capsules 15 mg, capsules 20 mg, capsules 30 mg, capsules 40 mg, powder for oral solution 1 mg/mL solution after reconstitution (200 mL bottle), Zerit XR capsules, extended release 37.5 mg, capsules, extended release 50 mg, capsules, extended-release 75 mg, capsules, extended-release 100 mg)

Stavudine is a nucleoside reverse transcriptase inhibitor, which inhibits replication of HIV. It is indicated in the treatment of HIV-1 infection in combination with other antiretroviral agents.

STREPTOKINASE

(Kabikinase, Streptase)

Streptokinase (1,500,000 IU within 60 minutes by IV infusion) is indicated in lysis of coronary artery thrombosis after acute myocardial infarction; streptokinase (250,000 IU by IV infusion pump into each occluded limb of the cannula over 25 to 35 minutes) is indicated in arteriovenous cannula occlusion; and streptokinase (250,000 IU IV infusion over 30 minutes) is indicated in the treatment of venous thrombosis, pulmonary embolism, and arterial thrombosis and embolism.

Streptokinase is a 47-kDa protein produced by beta-hemolytic streptococci. It has no intrinsic enzymatic activity, but it forms a stable, noncovalent 1:1 complex with plasminogen. This produces a conformational change that exposes the active site on plasminogen that cleaves arginine 560 on free plasminogen molecules to form free plasmin.

A loading dose of streptokinase (250,000 U; 2.5 mg) must be given intravenously to overcome plasma antibodies that are directed against the protein. These inactivating antibodies result from prior streptococcal infections. The half-life of streptokinase (once antibodies are depleted) is about 40 to 80 minutes. The streptokinase-plasminogen complex is not inhibited by alpha$_2$-antiplasmin. Levels of antibodies differ greatly among individuals, but this variable probably is of little clinical significance when streptokinase is given in the large doses currently used for coronary thrombolysis.

Plasminogen activation begins promptly after infusion or instillation of streptokinase; adequate activation of the fibrinolytic system occurs in 3 to 4 hours. Streptokinase does not cross the placenta, but its antibodies do.

Streptokinase is removed from circulation by antibodies and the reticuloendothelial system. Its half-life is biphasic: initially it is 18 minutes (from antibody action) and then extends up to 83 minutes. Anticoagulant effects may persist for 12 to 24 hours after infusion is discontinued.

Concomitant use with anticoagulants may cause hemorrhage. It may also be necessary to reverse effects of oral anticoagulants before beginning therapy. Concomitant use with aspirin, indomethacin, phenylbutazone, or other drugs affecting platelet activity increases the risk of bleeding.

Streptokinase is contraindicated in patients with ulcerative wounds, active internal bleeding, recent trauma with possible internal injuries, visceral or intracranial malignancy, ulcerative colitis, diverticulitis, severe hypertension, acute or chronic hepatic or renal insufficiency, uncontrolled hypocoagulation, chronic pulmonary disease with cavitation, subacute bacterial endocarditis or rheumatic valvular disease, recent cerebral embolism, thrombosis, or hemorrhage, and diabetic hemorrhagic retinopathy, because excessive bleeding may occur.

Epsilon-aminocaproic acid inhibits the activator-mediated formation of plasmin and hence may be used as an antidote to streptokinase–urokinase, or in a defibrination syndrome when bleeding from a mucus membrane occurs (Figure 45).

STREPTOMYCIN SULFATE

Streptomycin, an aminoglycoside antibiotic (1 g IM q 12 hours for two weeks; then 500 mg IM q 12 hours for four weeks with penicillin), is indicated in primary and adjunctive treatment in tuberculosis, for enterococcal endocarditis, and for tularemia. Streptomycin and penicillin produce a synergistic bactericidal effect against strains of enterococci, group D streptococci, and the various oral streptococci of the viridans group.

However, gentamicin has almost entirely replaced streptomycin for treatment of endocarditis caused by these microorganisms. Penicillin G alone is ineffective in the therapy of enterococcal endocarditis, and either streptomycin (500 mg twice daily) or gentamicin (1 mg/kg three times daily) must also be given to ensure a cure. Gentamicin is preferred when the strain is resistant to streptomycin. Both penicillin G and the aminoglycoside are administered for 4 to 6 weeks.

Aminoglycosides are bactericidal and inhibit protein synthesis in susceptible microorganisms (see Figure 88).

They exert this effect by (1) interfering with the initiation complex of peptide formation, (2) inducing misreading of the code on the messenger RNA template, which causes the incorporation of inappropriate amino acid into peptide, and (3) rupturing the polysomes into monosomes, which become nonfunctional (see Figure 88).

Resistance to aminoglycosides may be due to one or a combination of the following mechanisms:

Interference with the transport of aminoglycoside into bacterial cells.
Deletion of receptors on the 30S ribosomal subunit, thus preventing the functioning of aminoglycosides.
The bacterial biotransformation of aminoglycosides to inactive forms.

In addition, because the initial transport of aminoglycosides into bacterial cells is an oxygen-dependent process, microorganisms that are able to grow under anaerobic conditions show or develop resistance.

The aminoglycosides are poorly absorbed from the GI tract, and, for this reason, they are administered intramuscularly. Furthermore, since they do not penetrate into the central nervous system, they may have to be given intrathecally or intraventricularly in the treatment of meningitis. Aminoglycosides are excreted by glomerular filtration, which is greatly reduced in the presence of renal impairment, thus leading to toxic blood levels.

The most serious toxic reactions following aminoglycoside therapy are cochlear damage and vestibular impairment, which lead to vertigo and disturb the ability to maintain postural equilibrium. Aminoglycosides given during pregnancy cause deafness in the newborn. Nephrotoxicity and reversible neuromuscular blockade causing respiratory paralysis have also been seen following the use of high doses.

STREPTOZOCIN

(Zanosar)

Streptozocin, a naturally occurring nitrosourea antibiotic derived from *Streptomyces acromogenes* (500 mg/m2 IV for 5 consecutive days q 4 to 6 weeks until maximum benefit or toxicity is observed), is indicated in metastatic islet cell carcinoma of the pancreas. Streptozocin is nephrotoxic causing azotemia, glycosuria and renal tubular acidosis, and mild proteinuria.

Streptozocin exerts its cytotoxic activity by selectively inhibiting DNA synthesis. The drug also causes cross-linking of DNA strands through an alkylation mechanism.

Streptozocin is not active orally; it must be given intravenously.

After an IV dose, streptozocin and its metabolites distribute mainly into the liver, kidneys, intestines, and pancreas. The drug has not been shown to cross the blood–brain barrier; however, its metabolites achieve concentrations in the cerebrospinal fluid equivalent to the concentration in the plasma.

Streptozocin is extensively metabolized in the liver and kidneys.

The elimination of streptozocin from the plasma is biphasic, with an initial half-life of 35 to 40 minutes. The plasma half-life of the metabolites is longer than that of the parent drug. The drug and its metabolites are excreted primarily in urine. A small amount of a dose may also be excreted in expired air.

When used concomitantly, other nephrotoxic drugs may potentiate the nephrotoxicity caused by streptozocin. Concomitant use with doxorubicin prolongs the elimination half-life of doxorubicin and requires a reduced dosage of doxorubicin. Concurrent use with phenytoin may decrease the effects of streptozocin on the pancreas.

Toxicity of streptozocin includes nausea, which is a frequent side effect. Renal or hepatic toxicity occurs in approximately two thirds of cases; although usually reversible, renal toxicity may be fatal, and proximal tubular damage is the most important toxic effect. Serial determinations of urinary protein are most valuable in detecting early renal effects. Hematological toxicity — anemia, leukopenia, or thrombocytopenia — occurs in 20% of patients.

STRONTIUM-89 CHLORIDE

(Metastron injection 148 MBq, 4 mCi)

Strontium-89, a radioisotope, is used in the relief of metastatic bone pain. Strontium-89 chloride is a radiopharmaceutical. Following IV injection, soluble strontium compounds behave like their calcium analogs, clearing rapidly from blood and selectively localizing in bone mineral. Uptake of strontium by bone occurs preferentially in sites of active osteogenesis. It selectively irradiates sites of primary metastatic bone involvement with minimal effect on soft tissues distant from bone lesions. It is indicated for painful skeletal metastases.

STRYCHNINE

Strychnine, a neurotoxin, is the chief alkaloid present in nux vomica, which is derived from special species of *Strychnos*, particularly *Strychnos nux vomica* and *Strychnos ignatia*. Strychnine is found chiefly in the seeds of these plants, accompanied usually by brucine. Strychnine poisoning causes muscular stiffness, increased reflex reactions, tremors, involuntary twitches, sudden convulsions, and opisthotonus (see Figure 89).

SUCCIMER

(Chemet capsules 100 mg)

Succimer, a heavy-metal-chelating agent, is used in the treatment of lead poisoning in children with blood levels about 45 mcg/dl. Succimer forms water soluble chelate with lead, increasing the urinary excretion.

Succimer is the first orally active lead chelator available for children, with a safety and efficacy profile that surpasses that of **D-penicillamine**. Succimer usually is given every

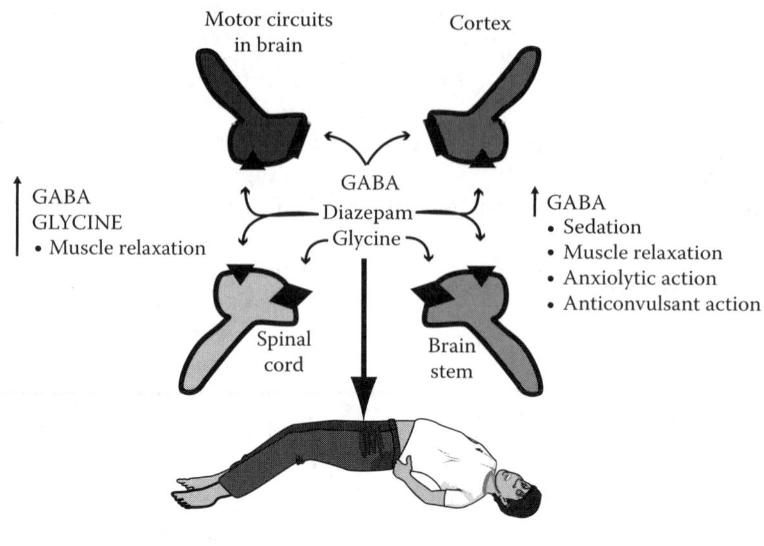

FIGURE 89 Strychnine is the chief alkaloid present in *nux vomica*. In cases of poisoning, it causes convulsions which are accompanied by strong contraction of the face muscles. The respiratory muscles are involved in the general paroxysm and the blood rapidly becomes deoxygenated.

8 hours (10 ng/kg) for 5 days and then every 12 hours for an additional 2 weeks.

Succimer (2,3-dimercaptosuccinic add, Chemet) is an orally effective chelator that is chemically similar to **dimercaprol** but contains two carboxylic acids that modify both the distribution and chelating spectrum of the drug.

After its absorption in humans, succimer is biotransformed to a mixed disulfide with cysteine.

Succimer produces a lead diuresis with a subsequent lowering of blood lead levels and attenuation of the untoward biochemical effects of lead, manifested by normalization of δ-ALA dehydrase activity. The **succimer-lead chelate** also is eliminated in bile; the fraction eliminated undergoes enterohepatic circulation.

A desirable feature of succimer is that it does not significantly mobilize essential metals such as zinc, copper, or iron. Animal studies suggest that **succimer** is effective as a chelator of arsenic, cadmium, mercury, and other metals.

Toxicity with **succimer** is less than that with dimercaprol perhaps because its relatively lower lipid solubility minimizes its uptake into cells. Nonetheless, transient elevations in hepatic transaminases are observed following treatment with succimer. The most commonly reported adverse effects of succimer treatment are nausea, vomiting, diarrhea, and loss of appetite. Rashes also have been reported that may necessitate discontinuation of therapy.

Succimer has been approved in the United States for treatment of children with blood lead levels in excess of 45 μg/dL.

SUCCINYLCHOLINE CHLORIDE, SUXAMETHONIUM CHLORIDE

(Anectine, Anectine Flo-Pack, Quelicin, Sucostrin)

Succinylcholine, a depolarizing neuromuscular blocking agent (0.3 to 1.1 mg/kg IV over 10 to 30 seconds), is used to induce skeletal muscle relaxation; to facilitate intubation, ventilation, or orthopedic manipulations; and to lessen muscular contraction in convulsions induced by physicians. A peripheral nerve stimulator may be used to monitor effects and degree of blockade.

STUTTERING: Treatment of

Stuttering is increasingly being recognized as a neurodevelopmental disorder. This has stimulated new interest in pharmacological approaches to the treatment of the condition. Psychosocial factors are also regarded as important to the course of the condition. Therefore, psychosocial interventions, such as psychotherapy and speech retraining, are important components of a comprehensive treatment program. A wide range of pharmacological agents are effective in reducing stuttering in selected patients. These include haloperidol, verapamil, bethanechol and some antidepressants. The agents are presumed to work through different mechanisms. Unilateral injection of botulinum toxin directly into the vocal folds is another promising treatment.

Succinylcholine, like acetylcholine, interacts with the cholinergic receptors at the end-plate region of the muscle, resulting in depolarization of the chemically excitable membrane. This, in turn, creates local action potentials, spreading them to and depolarizing the adjacent excitable membranes, finally culminating in a muscle contraction, or fasciculation, which is an uncoordinated muscle contraction. However, unlike acetylcholine, succinylcholine is not metabolized by acetylcholinesterase, and hence causes persistent depolarization of the end plate. The continuous presence of succinylcholine leads to inexcitability of the membrane adjacent to the end plate, resulting in neuromuscular blockade, which is not reversed by the administration of cholinesterase inhibitors. In fact, agents such as neostigmine may even prolong neuromuscular blockade.

Agents such as tubocurarine and pancuronium compete with acetylcholine for the cholinergic receptors at the end plate. They combine with the receptors but do not activate them. Competitive or nondepolarizing agents are antagonized by neostigmine (see also Figure 99).

Succinylcholine is an ultra-short-acting depolarizing skeletal muscle relaxant. Paralysis usually appears in the following muscles consecutively: levator muscles of the eyelids, muscles of mastication, limb muscles, abdominal muscles, muscles of the glottis, and finally, the intercostals, the diaphragm, and all other skeletal muscles. Recovery of normal muscle tone follows the reverse order.

Succinylcholine has no effect on consciousness, pain threshold, or cerebration. Although it has no direct effect upon the myocardium, changes in rhythm may result from vagal stimulation resulting from surgical procedures, or from potassium-mediated alterations in electrical conductivity. These effects are enhanced by halogenated anesthetics. Succinylcholine slightly increases intraocular pressure, which may persist after the onset of complete paralysis. Tachyphylaxis occurs with repeated doses. It has no direct effect on the uterus or other smooth muscles. Because the drug is highly ionized and has a low lipid solubility, it does not readily cross the placenta.

Succinylcholine is metabolized according to the following scheme:

$$\text{Succinylcholine} \xrightarrow{\text{Plasma cholinesterase}} \text{Succinylmonocholine}$$

$$\text{Succinylmonocholine} \xrightarrow[\text{Liver}]{} \text{Succinate and choline}$$

Because cholinesterase is synthesized in the liver, succinylcholine's duration of action is elevated in the presence of liver disease. Cholinesterase inhibitors dramatically increase succinylcholine's duration of action. In patients with atypical cholinesterase, the intensity and duration of succinylcholine's effects are enhanced.

Succinylcholine is contraindicated in patients with genetic disorders of plasma pseudocholinesterase because of the potential for impaired metabolism; in patients with personal or family history of malignant hyperthermia because the drug may induce the disorder; with myopathies associated with elevated serum creatine kinase values because the drug may exacerbate the damage associated with the disease; and in patients with narrow-angle glaucoma or penetrating eye injuries because the drug elevates intraocular pressure.

Succinylcholine should be used with extreme caution in patients with low plasma pseudocholinesterase and in those recovering from severe trauma. It also should be used with caution in patients with electrolyte imbalances; in those receiving quinidine or cardiac glycosides, in patients with preexisting hyperkalemia, paraplegia, extensive or severe burns, or extensive denervation of skeletal muscle from disease because the drug may raise potassium levels; and during ocular surgery, because the drug increases IOP.

Concomitant use of succinylcholine with aminoglycoside antibiotics (including amikacin, gentamicin, kanamycin, neomycin, streptomycin), polymyxin antibiotics (polymyxin B sulfate, colistin), clindamycin, lincomycin, general anesthetics, local anesthetics, antimalarial agents, cholinesterase inhibitors (echothiophate, demecarium, isoflurophate), cyclophosphamide, oral contraceptives, nondepolarizing neuromuscular-blocking agents, parenteral magnesium salts, lithium, phenelzine, hexafluorenium, quinidine, quinine, pancuronium, phenothiazines, thiotepa, and exposure to neurotoxic insecticides enhance or prolong succinylcholine's neuromuscular-blocking effects.

Clinical manifestations of overdose include apnea or prolonged muscle paralysis, which may be treated with controlled respiration.

SUCRALFATE

(Carafate tablets 1 g, suspension 1 g/10 mL)

Sucralfate is a GI agent that adheres to ulcer in acidic gastric juice, forming a protective layer that serves as a barrier against acid, bile salts, and enzymes present in the stomach and duodenum. It is indicated in short-term treatment of duodenal ulcer; and maintenance therapy of duodenal ulcer (tablets only).

In the presence of acid-induced damage, pepsin-mediated hydrolysis of mucosal proteins contributes to mucosal erosion and ulcerations. This process can be inhibited by sulfated polysaccharides. **Sucralfate** (Carafate) consists of the octasulfate of sucrose to which $Al(OH)_3$ has been added. In an acid environment ($pH < 4$), sucralfate undergoes extensive cross-linking to produce a viscous, sticky polymer that adheres to epithelial cells and ulcer craters for up to 6 hours after a single dose. In addition to inhibiting hydrolysis of mucosal proteins by pepsin, sucralfate may have additional cytoprotective effects, including stimulation of local production of **prostaglandins** and **epidermal growth factor**. Sucralfate also binds bile salts; thus, some clinicians use sucralfate to treat individuals with the syndromes of biliary esophagitis or gastritis.

The use of sucralfate to treat peptic acid disease has diminished in recent years. Nevertheless because increased gastric pH may be a factor in the development of nosocomial

SUICIDE: Prevention of

The assessment and management of suicidal patients are important issues that may be faced by any physician. Risk factors for suicidal behavior which have been identified are:

- Psychiatric diagnosis
- Psychosocial and environmental factors
- Personality disorders and traits
- Genetic and family variables
- Biochemical factors

Psychopharmacological agents such as antidepressants, antipsychotics (in patients with personality disorders) and lithium (in patients with bipolar disorders) have been shown to be effective in preventing suicidal behavior. The efficacy of electroconvulsive therapy (ECT) is more controversial. Another equally important aspect of the optimal clinical management of suicidal patients is the quality of the doctor–patient relationship.

pneumonia in critically ill patients, sucralfate may offer an advantage over **proton-pump inhibitors** and **H_2-receptor antagonists** for the prophylaxis of stress ulcers. Due to its unique mechanism of action, sucralfate also has been used in several other conditions associated with mucosal inflammation/ulceration that may not respond to acid suppression, including oral mucositis (radiation and aphthous ulcers) and bile reflux gastropathy. Administered by rectal enema, sucralfate also has been used for radiation proctitis and solitary rectal ulcers.

Since it is activated by acid, sucralfate should be taken on an empty stomach 1 hour before meals. The use of antacids within 30 minutes of a dose of sucralfate should be avoided. The usual dose of sucralfate is 1 g four times daily (for active duodenal ulcer) or 1 g twice daily (for maintenance therapy).

The most common side effect of **sucralfate** is constipation (about 2%). As some aluminum can be absorbed, sucralfate should be avoided in patients with renal failure who are at risk for aluminum overload. Likewise, aluminum-containing antacids should not be combined with **sucralfate** in these patients. **Sucralfate** forms a viscous layer in the stomach that may inhibit absorption of other drugs, including phenytoin, digoxin, cimetidine, ketoconazole, and fluoroquinolone antibiotics. **Sucralfate** therefore should be taken at least 2 hours after the administration of other drugs. The "sticky" nature of the viscous gel produced by sucralfate in the stomach also may be responsible for the development of bezoars in some patients, particularly in those with underlying gastroparesis.

SUFENTANIL CITRATE

(Sufenta)

Sufentanil, an opioid analgesic (8 mcg/kg IV administered with nitrous oxide and oxygen), is indicated in patients undergoing major surgical procedures, such as cardiovascular surgery or neurosurgical procedures in the sitting position, in order to provide favorable myocardial and cerebral oxygen balance or when extended postoperative ventilation is anticipated.

Alfentanil and sufentanil are newer and more potent opioid analgesics than either morphine or fentanyl. The potency of alfentanil (Alfenta) is one-third to one-fourth that of fentanyl, and its duration of action is about one-half as long, even after administration of large doses. These drugs can induce profound analgesia and, in sufficient doses, anesthesia; cardiovascular stability is impressive, and the desirability of reducing the duration of mechanical ventilation following cardiac surgery has led to an increasing use of these agents. All may be associated with increased intracranial pressure during spontaneous ventilation, so caution is necessary with head trauma. Remifentanil is a potent opioid selective for opioid receptors that produces intense analgesia very rapidly. It shares with other opioids respiratory depression, bradycardia, skeletal muscle rigidity, and reversibility by naloxone. In contrast to other short-acting opioids, remifentanil contains an ester linkage, and so it is metabolized by circulating and tissue-nonspecific esterases. As a result, recovery time from remifentanil is rapid and almost independent of dose or duration of infusion (see also Figure 68).

Sufentanil is contraindicated in patients with known hypersensitivity to phenylpiperidine opiates including alfentanil, diphenoxylate, fentanyl, or meperidine.

Sufentanil should be administered carefully to patients with supraventricular arrhythmias, recent head injuries or increased intracranial pressure, or pulmonary disease such as asthma.

Concomitant use with other CNS depressants (narcotic analgesics, general anesthetics, antihistamines, phenothiazines, barbiturates, benzodiazepines, sedative–hypnotics, tricyclic antidepressants, alcohol, and muscle relaxants) potentiates respiratory and CNS depression, sedation, and hypotensive effects.

SUICIDE GENE THERAPY

Gene therapy has expanded rapidly over the last decade. The area of gene therapy is vast, and both malignant and nonmalignant cells can be targeted. Gene therapy that targets malignant cells in a treatment has become known as "suicide gene therapy." Basically, this approach uses the transduction of cancer cells with a gene for a foreign enzyme that, when expressed, is able to activate a nontoxic prodrug into a highly cytotoxic drug able to kill the cancer cell population. This is a major area in cancer gene therapy.

Chemotherapy is widely used with surgery and radiotherapy for the treatment of malignant disease. Selectivity of most drugs for malignant cells remains elusive. Unfortunately, an insufficient therapeutic index, a lack of specificity, and the emergence of drug-resistant cell subpopulations often hamper the efficacy of drug therapies. Despite the significant progress achieved by chemotherapy in the treatment of disseminated malignancies, the prognosis for solid tumors remains poor. A number of specific difficulties are associated with the treatment of solid tumors, where the access of drugs to cancer cells is often limited by poor, unequal vascularization and areas of necrosis. The histological heterogeneity of the cell population within the tumor is another major drawback.

One approach aimed at enhancing the selectivity of cancer chemotherapy for solid tumors relies on the application of gene therapy technologies. Gene therapies are techniques for modifying the cellular genome for therapeutic benefit. In cancer gene therapy, both malignant and nonmalignant cells may be suitable targets. The possibility of rendering cancer cells more sensitive to drugs or toxins by introducing "suicide genes" has two alternatives: toxin gene therapy, in which the genes for toxic products are transduced directly into tumor cells, and enzyme-activating prodrug therapy, in which the transgenes encode enzymes that activate specific prodrugs to create toxic metabolites. The latter approach, known as suicide gene therapy, **gene-directed enzyme prodrug therapy** (GDEPT), **virus-directed enzyme prodrug therapy** (VDEPT), or **gene prodrug activation therapy** (GPAT) may be used, in isolation or combined with other strategies, to make a significant impact on cancer treatment.

In this chapter, the terms **GDEPT** and **suicide gene therapy** are used. The terms **suicide gene therapy** and **GDEPT** can be used interchangeably to describe a two-step treatment designed to treat solid tumors. In the first step, the gene for a foreign enzyme is delivered and targeted in a variety of ways to the tumor where it is to be expressed. In the second step, a prodrug is administered that is activated to the corresponding drug by the foreign enzyme expressed in the tumor. Ideally, the gene for the enzyme should be expressed exclusively in the tumor cells compared to normal tissues and blood. The enzyme must reach a concentration sufficient to activate the prodrug for clinical benefit. The catalytic activity of the expressed protein must be adequate to activate the prodrug under physiological conditions. Because expression of the foreign enzymes will not occur in all cells of a targeted tumor *in vivo*, a **bystander effect** (BE) is required, whereby the prodrug is cleaved to an active drug that kills not only the tumor cells in which it is formed but also neighboring tumor cells that do not express the foreign enzyme.

The main advantages of optimized suicide gene therapy systems are as follows:

- Increased selectivity for cancer cells, reducing side effects.
- Higher concentrations of active drug at the tumor, compared to the concentrations accessible by classical chemotherapy.
- Bystander effects generated.
- Tumor cell enzyme transduction and kill may induce immune responses that enhance the overall therapeutic response.
- Prodrugs are not required to exhibit intrinsic specificity for cancer cells; they are designed to be activated by the foreign enzymes, which is technically easier to achieve.

A number of hurdles are still to be overcome. The most important are the following:

- The vectors for gene transduction that target the tumor and achieve efficient infection of cancer cells
- Ideally, the vectors should be also nonimmunogenic and nontoxic
- The control of gene expression at the tumor

There are specific requirements of the enzymes used in GDEPT. They should have high catalytic activity (preferably without the need for cofactors), should be different from any circulating endogenous enzymes, and should be expressed in sufficient concentration for therapeutic efficacy. The enzymes proposed for suicide gene therapy can be characterized into two major classes. The first class comprise enzymes of nonmammalian origin with or without human counterparts. Examples include **viral thymidine kinase** (TK), **bacterial cytosine deaminase** (CD), **bacterial carboxypeptidase G2** (CPG2), **purine nucleotide phosphorylase** (PNP), **thymidine phosphorylase** (TP), **nitroreductase** (NR), **D-amino-acid oxidase** (DAAO), **xanthine-guanine phosphoribosyi transferase** (XGPRT), **penicillin-G amidase** (PGA), β-lactamase (β-L), **multiple-drug activation enzyme** (MDAE), β-galactosidase (β-Gal), **horseradish peroxidase** (HRP), and **deoxyribonucleotide kinase** (DRNK). Those enzymes that do have human homologs have different structural requirements with respect to their substrates in comparison to the human counterparts. Their main drawback is that they are likely to be immunogenic. The second class of enzymes for suicide gene therapy comprises enzymes of human origin that are absent from or are expressed only at low concentrations in tumor cells. Examples include **deoxycytidine kinase** (dCK), **carboxypeptidase A** (CPA), **β-glucuronidase** (β-Glu), and **cytochrome P450** (CYP). The advantages of such systems reside in the reduction of the potential for inducing an immune response. However, their presence in normal tissues is likely to preclude specific activation of the prodrugs only in tumors unless the transfected enzymes are modified for different substrate requirements.

The genes can be engineered to express their product either intracellularly or extracellularly in the recipient cells. The extracellularly expressed variants are either tethered to the outer cell membrane or secreted from cells. There are potential advantages to each approach. Where the enzyme is intracellularly expressed, the prodrug must enter the cells for activation and, subsequently, the active drug must diffuse through the interstitium across the cell membrane to elicit a BE. Cells in which the enzyme is expressed tethered to the outer surface are able to activate the prodrug extracellularly. A more substantial BE should therefore be generated in the latter system, but spread of the active drug into the general circulation is a possible disadvantage.

Good pharmacological properties, good pharmacokinetic properties of prodrugs, low cytoxicity of prodrugs with high cytotoxicity of the activated drugs, and effective activation of prodrugs by the expressed enzyme are all important features. Prodrugs should be chemically stable under physiological conditions and be highly diffusible in the tumor interstitium. The released drugs should be as potent as possible, highly diffusible, ideally active in both proliferative and quiescent cells, and induce BEs.

The activation of the prodrugs is a key step in suicide gene therapy. It is an advantage if the expressed enzyme can activate the prodrug directly to the drug, without the need for additional steps requiring further catalysis, because it is possible for the host endogenous enzymes needed for the latter steps to become defective or deficient in cancer cells.

Two basic types of prodrug have been used in GDEPT: the directly linked and the self-immolative prodrugs. The directly linked prodrugs can be defined as a pharmacological inactive derivative of a drug, which requires chemical transformation to release the active drug. In terms of anticancer activity, the conversion of the prodrug to an active drug results in a sharp increase in its cytotoxicity. In a directly linked prodrug, the active drug is released directly following the activation process.

A self-immolative prodrug can be defined as a compound generating an unstable intermediate which, following the activation process, will extrude the active drug in a number of subsequent steps. The most important feature is that the site of activation is normally separated from the site of extrusion. The activation process remains an enzymatic one. However, the extrusion of the active drug relies on a supplementary spontaneous fragmentation. Potential advantages of self-immolative prodrugs are the possibility of altering the lipophilicity of the prodrugs with minimal effect on the activation kinetics and the possibility to improve unfavorable kinetics of activation as a result of unsuitable electronic or steric features of the active drug. The range of drugs that can be converted to prodrugs is greatly extended and is restricted only by the structural substrate requirements for a given enzyme.

Some hurdles must be overcome before GDEPT will become a clinically efficient treatment of cancers.

The simultaneous release of active drugs that can act by different mechanisms, leading to a synergistic effect on tumor cells and the design of more effective new types of prodrug, is another way to progress. Modalities to enhance and to control the BE, particularly if cell-permeable and cell-impermeable active metabolites can be released together may be useful to improve the therapies. Also, the occurrence of resistant populations is less likely for drugs with different mechanisms of action.

GDEPT systems have already shown efficacy *in vivo*. Future developments in this technology should use mutagenesis to obtain more efficient activation of a given prodrug or to adapt the active site so that it binds better to prodrugs that are not substrates for endogenous enzymes. The prodrugs, too, could be redesigned to create better substrates for the enzymes, to maximize drug release or the BE, to take advantage of self-immolative strategies of activation, or to allow the active drug to accumulate more readily in tumor cells. Finally, it will also be useful to investigate the ways in which different prodrug systems synergize with each other or with other cancer treatments. The combination of GDEPT with radiotherapy or immunotherapy has previously been investigated. Such approaches may involve either a sequential treatment schedule (GDEPT/radiation therapy or GDEPT/immunotherapy) or the transfection of suicide gene/genes together with genes able to increase the sensitivity of the tumors to radiation or enhance the potential of the host immune system with cytokine genes.

Improvements are needed in the vector design area to enhance targeting and delivery of suicide genes. Multiple options are available, including nonviral vectors, more complex systems involving coexpression of suicide genes with immunological or tumor suppressor genes, and selectively replicating viruses.

SULCONAZOLE NITRATE

(Exelderm)

Sulconazole, an imidazole derivative with antifungal effectiveness, is used in the treatment of tinea cruris, tinea corporis, and tinea pedis caused by *Trichophyton mentagrophytes*, *Epidermophyton floccosum*, and *Microsporum canis*. It is also used in the treatment of tinea versicolor caused by *Malassezia furfur*.

SULFACETAMIDE SODIUM

(Ak-Sulf Forte, Ak-Sulf ointment, Bleph-10 S.O.P., Cetamide, Isopto Cetamide, Sodium Sulamyd 10%, Sodium Sulamyd 30%, Sulamyd, Sulf-10, Sulfair 15, Sulten-10)

Sulfacetamide, a sulfonamide antibiotic (instill 1 to 2 drops of 10% solution into lower conjunctival sac), is used in inclusion conjunctivitis, corneal ulcers, trachoma, and prophylaxis for ocular infection.

SULFADIAZINE

(Microsulfon)

Sulfadiazine, a sulfonamide antibiotic, is used in rheumatic fever prophylaxis, as an alternative to penicillin, as an adjunctive regimen in treatment of toxoplasmosis, and in uncomplicated attacks of malaria (see also Figure 90).

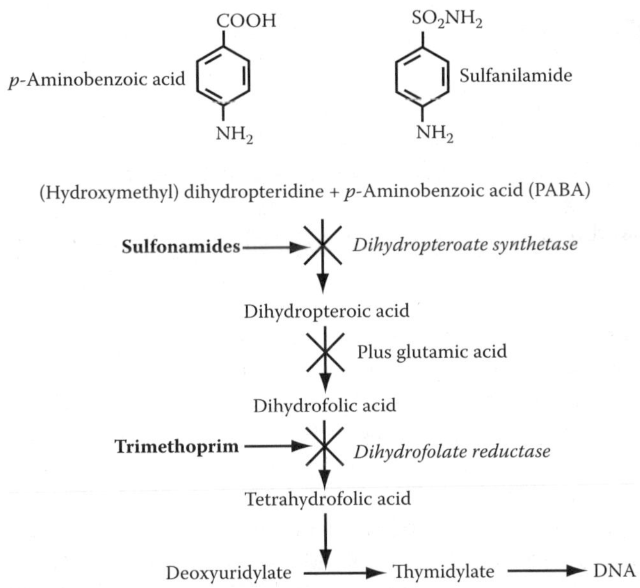

FIGURE 90 In acute and chronic urinary tract infection, the combination of **trimethoprim** and **sulfamethoxazole** exerts a truly synergistic effect on bacteria. The sulfonamide inhibits the utilization of **p-amino-benzoic acid** in the synthesis of folic acid, whereas trimethoprim, by inhibiting dihydrofolic acid reductase, blocks the conversion of dihydrofolic acid to **tetrahydrofolic acid**, which is essential to bacteria in the *de novo* synthesis of purines, pyrimidines, and certain amino acids.

SULFADOXINE AND PYRIMETHAMINE

(Fansidar tablets 500 mg sulfadoxine and 25 mg pyrimethamine)

Sulfadoxine/pyrimethamine is an antimalarial preparation. The two components sequentially block two enzymes involved in the biosynthesis of folinic acid within the parasites. It is indicated in the treatment of *Plasmodium falciparum* malaria for those patients in whom chloroquine resistance is suspected; and as prophylaxis of malaria for travelers to areas where chloroquine-resistant *P. falciparum* malaria is endemic.

Sulfadoxine (1500 mg) and pyrimethamine (75 mg) orally as a single dosage is indicated for the treatment of *P. falciparum* malaria in patients in whom chloroquine resistance is suspected. However, chloroquine remains the drug of choice for travelers to malarious areas. In addition, sulfadoxine-pyrimethamine has been used as a prophylactic agent for the prevention of *Pneumocystis carinii* pneumonia in patients with AIDS, usually as a second-line agent.

Sulfadoxine/pyrimethamine is an antimalarial agent that acts by reciprocal potentiation of its components, achieved by a sequential blockade of two enzymes involved in the biosynthesis of folinic acid within the parasites. The bacteriostatic action of sulfonamides occurs through competitive antagonism of para-aminobenzoic acid (PABA), an essential component in folic acid synthesis. Pyrimethamine inhibits the enzyme dihydrofolate reductase, which catalyzes the reduction of dihydrofolate to tetrahydrofolate and is important to cellular biosynthesis of purines, pyrimidines, and some amino acids.

Antifolic acid medications such as methotrexate should not be used in patients receiving sulfadoxine and pyrimethamine. The adverse reactions reported in susceptible patients taking sulfadoxine and pyrimethamine are headache, peripheral neuritis, mental depression, convulsions, ataxia, hallucinations, tinnitus, vertigo, insomnia, apathy, fatigue, muscle weakness, nervousness, glossitis, stomatitis, nausea, emesis, abdominal pains, hepatitis, hepatocellular necrosis, diarrhea, pancreatitis, agranulocytosis, aplastic, megaloblastic, or hemolytic anemia, thrombocytopenia, leukopenia, eosinophilia, purpura, hypoprothrombinemia, and methemoglobulinemia.

SULFAMETHOXAZOLE

(Gantanol)

Sulfamethoxazole (initially 2 g p.o.) is indicated in urinary tract and systemic infections, and in lymphogranuloma venereum (genital, inguinal, or anorectal infection) (1 g p.o. b.i.d. for 21 days).

Sulfamethoxazole like other sulfonamides is bacteriostatic. It acts by inhibiting formation of tetrahydrofolic acid from PABA, thus preventing bacterial cell synthesis of folic acid (see Figure 90).

Sulfamethoxazole's spectrum of action includes some Gram-positive bacteria: *Chlamydia trachomatis*, many Enterobacteriaceae, and some strains of *Toxoplasma* and *Plasmodium.*

Sulfamethoxazole is absorbed from the GI tract after oral administration, and is metabolized partially in the liver; peak serum levels occur at 3 to 4 hours.

Sulfamethoxazole is distributed widely into most body tissues and fluids, including cerebrospinal, synovial, pleural, amniotic, prostatic, peritoneal, and seminal fluids. Sulfamethoxazole crosses the placenta; it is 50 to 70% protein-bound.

Both unchanged drug and metabolites are excreted primarily in urine by glomerular filtration and, to a lesser extent, renal tubular secretion; some drug is excreted in breast milk. Urinary solubility of unchanged drug increases as urine pH increases. Plasma half-life in patients with normal renal function is 7 to 12 hours.

Sulfamethoxazole may inhibit hepatic metabolism of oral anticoagulants, displacing them from binding sites and enhancing anticoagulant effects. Concomitant use with PABA antagonizes sulfonamide effects. With oral hypoglycemics (sulfonylureas), the drug enhances their hypoglycemic effects, probably by displacing sulfonylureas from protein-binding sites; and with either trimethoprim or pyrimethamine (folic

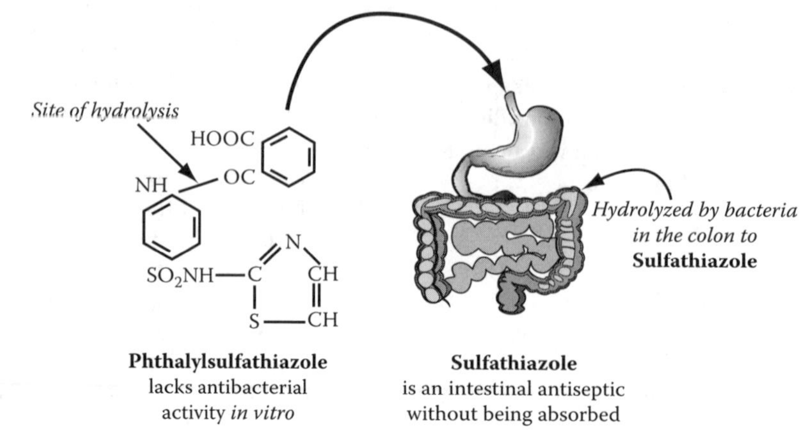

FIGURE 91 Sulfonamides that are **poorly absorbed** include succinylsulfathiazole, phthalylsulfathiazole, and sulfasalazine and they are used as **intestinal antiseptics**.

acid antagonists with different mechanisms of action), the drug results in synergistic antibacterial effects and delays or prevents bacterial resistance.

The sulfonamides are structurally related to p-aminobenzoic acid. The presence of a free *p*-amino group is essential for the antibacterial action. Succinylsulfathiazole (sulfasuxidine) and phthalysulfathiazole (sulfathalidine) are agents with a substituted *p*-amino group. These intestinal antiseptics are slowly hydrolyzed in the intestine, releasing sulfathiazole, which exerts antiseptic effects against the coliform and clostridial organisms.

SULFASALAZINE

(Azulfidine, Azulfidine En-tabs)

Sulfasalazine, a sulfonamide antibiotic (3 to 4 g p.o. daily in divided dosage), is indicated in the treatment of ulcerative colitis.

Sulfasalazine is cleaved in the colon by intestinal bacteria to form sulfapyridine and mesalamine (5-aminosalicylic acid; 5-ASA), both of which may act locally within the gut. Mesalamine, which is different from aminosalicylates used to treat tuberculosis, is thought to be the major active moiety. Mucosal production of arachidonic acid metabolites, both through the cyclooxygenase and the lipoxygenase pathways, is increased in patients with inflammatory bowel disease. Mesalamine appears to diminish inflammation by inhibiting cyclooxygenase and lipoxygenase, thereby decreasing the production of prostaglandins, and leukotrienes and hydroxyeicosatetraenoic acids (HETEs), respectively. It is also believed that mesalamine acts as a scavenger of oxygen-derived free radicals, which are produced in greater numbers in patients with inflammatory bowel disease.

Sulfasalazine is absorbed poorly from the GI tract after oral administration: 70 to 90% is transported to the colon where intestinal flora metabolize the drug to its active ingredients, sulfapyridine (antibacterial) and 5-aminosalicylic acid (antiinflammatory), which exert their effects locally. Sulfapyridine is absorbed from the colon, but only a small portion of 5-aminosalicylic acid is absorbed.

Systemically absorbed sulfasalazine is excreted chiefly in urine; some parent drug and metabolites are excreted in breast milk. Plasma half-life is about 6 to 8 hours.

Like all sulfonamides, sulfasalazine is contraindicated in patients with known hypersensitivity to other drugs containing sulfur (thiazides, furosemide, or oral sulfonylureas), in patients with known hypersensitivity to salicylates, in patients with severe renal or hepatic dysfunction, or porphyria, during pregnancy, and during lactation, and in infants and children under age 2. Sulfasalazine is also contraindicated in patients with intestinal or urinary tract obstructions because of the risk of local GI irritation and of crystalluria.

Sulfasalazine may inhibit hepatic metabolism of oral anticoagulants, displacing them from binding sites and enhancing anticoagulant effects.

Concomitant use with oral hypoglycemics (sulfonylureas) enhances hypoglycemic effects, probably by displacing sulfonylureas from protein-binding sites.

Sulfasalazine may reduce GI absorption of digoxin and folic acid.

Concomitant use of urine-acidifying agents (ammonium chloride, ascorbic acid) decreases urine pH and sulfonamide solubility, thus increasing risk of crystalluria. Concomitant use with antibiotics that alter intestinal flora may interfere with conversion of sulfasalazine to sulfapyridine and 5-aminosalicylic acid, decreasing its effectiveness.

Concomitant use of antacids may cause premature dissolution of enteric-coated tablets designed to dissolve in the intestines, thus increasing systemic absorption and hazard of toxicity.

SULFINPYRAZONE

(Anturane)

Sulfinpyrazone (200 to 400 mg daily in two divided doses) is indicated in the treatment of chronic and intermittent gouty arthritis (see also Table 3).

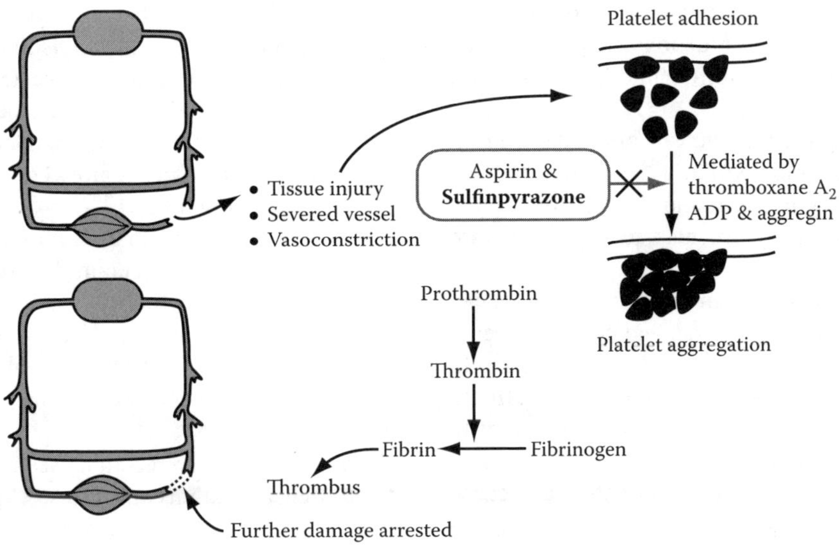

FIGURE 92 As an inhibitor of platelet aggregation, sulfinpyrazone is used in the prophylaxis of thromboembolic disorders.

Sulfinpyrazone, a pyrazolidine derivative, is a potent uricosuric agent which also has antithrombotic and platelet inhibitory effects (see Figure 92). It lacks antiinflammatory and analgesic properties. Sulfinpyrazone inhibits renal tubular reabsorption of uric acid. It reduces renal tubular secretion of other organic anions, e.g., paraaminohippuric acid and salicylic acid, and displaces other organic anions bound extensively to plasma proteins (e.g., sulfonamides, salicylates). It is not intended for the relief of an acute attack of gout.

Sulfinpyrazone competitively inhibits prostaglandin synthesis, which prevents platelet aggregation (Figure 92). It is well absorbed after oral administration; 98 to 99% is bound to plasma proteins. The plasma half-life is about 2.2 to 3 hours. Approximately one-half of the administered oral dose appears in the urine unchanged.

GI irritation occurs in 10 to 15% of all patients receiving sulfinpyrazone, and occasionally a patient may require discontinuance of its use. Gastric distress is lessened when the drug is taken in divided doses with meals. Sulfinpyrazone should be given cautiously to patients with a history of peptic ulcer. Hypersensitivity reactions, usually a rash with fever, do occur, but less frequently than with probenecid. The severe blood dyscrasias and salt and water retention, hazards of phenylbutazone therapy, have not been observed during sulfinpyrazone therapy. However, depression of hematopoiesis has been demonstrated, and periodic blood-cell counts should be examined during prolonged therapy.

Because it is a potent uricosuric agent, sulfinpyrazone may precipitate acute gouty arthritis, urolithiasis, and renal colic, especially in initial stages of therapy. Therefore, adequate fluid intake and alkalinization of the urine are recommended.

Sulfinpyrazone increases the effectiveness of anticoagulants (with a potential to cause hemorrhage) and of tolbutamide (with a potential to cause hypoglycemia). It increases the plasma clearance of theophylline and verapamil, hence decreasing their effectiveness.

SULFISOXAZOLE
(Gantrisin)

SULFISOXAZOLE DIOLAMINE
(Gantrisin ophthalmic ointment, Gantrisin ophthalmic solution)

Sulfisoxazole is used in urinary tract and systemic infections; in lymphogranuloma venereum (genital, inguinal, or anorectal infections); in uncomplicated urethral, endocervical, or rectal infections caused by *C. trachomatis*; in conjunctivitis, corneal ulcer, superficial ocular infections; and as an adjunct in systemic treatment of trachoma.

SULFONAMIDES

The sulfonamides are structurally related to PABA. Substances that resemble the sulfonamides but lack antibacterial activities are some of the oral hypoglycemic agents (tolbutamide) and some of the carbonic anhydrase inhibitors (acetazolamide). The presence of a free p-amino group is essential for the antibacterial action. Succinylsulfathiazole (Sulfasuxide) and phthalylsulfathiazole (Sulfathalidine) are agents with a substituted p-amino group. These intestinal antiseptics are slowly hydrolyzed in the intestine, releasing sulfathiazole, which exerts antiseptic effects against the coliform and clostridial organisms (see Figure 91).

As bacteriostatic agents, the sulfonamides are active against both Gram-positive and Gram-negative bacteria, including streptococci, Gram-negative bacilli, *Chlamydia*, *Nocardia*, and *Actinomyces*. Sulfonamides alone or in combination with trimethoprim are the drugs of choice in the management of urinary tract infections, nocardiosis, and toxoplasmosis (see Figure 91). Sulfonamides are also used topically in the treatment of burns.

By competing with PABA, the sulfonamides inhibit the synthesis of folic acid, which is essential for the production of purines by bacteria and their ultimate synthesis of nucleic acids. They are also incorporated into folic acid.

The widespread use of sulfonamides against gonococci, meningococci, hemolytic streptococci, and coliform organisms has resulted in the emergence of resistant strains. In general, organisms that are either impermeable to sulfonamides or produce large amounts of PABA are resistant to sulfonamides. Furthermore, resistance in a previously sensitive organism may arise as a result of mutation and cause either overproduction of PABA or an alteration in the folic-acid-synthesizing enzymes.

Except for those sulfonamides that exert their local effects in the bowel, most sulfonamides are absorbed orally, become bound to plasma proteins, are distributed widely throughout the body including the cerebrospinal fluid, pass readily through the placenta to reach the fetal circulation, and become metabolized in the liver by acetylation. The acetylated metabolites, which have no bacteriostatic activity, retain the toxic property of the parent compounds. The free sulfonamides undergo glomerular filtration and are not readily absorbed and excreted. The urinary concentration of acetylated derivatives is higher than the plasma level. The urinary solubility of the sulfonamides decreases when the pH of the urine decreases. Therefore, there is a tendency for crystalluria to increase in the presence of acidic pHs. Conversely, the solubility of the sulfonamides increases greatly when the pH is alkaline. The recently introduced sulfonamides are more soluble at the usual urinary pH. The incidence of crystalluria can be diminished by the following measures: enhancing fluid intake, alkalization of the urine, and taking a mixture of sulfonamides.

Based on their pharmacokinetic characteristics, the sulfonamides can be classified into four separate categories:

1. Sulfonamides that have a rapid rate of absorption and elimination. These consist of sulfisoxazole (Gantrisin), sulfamethoxazole (Gantanol), sulfacytine (Renoquid), and sulfamethiazole (Thiosulfil). The highly soluble and recently introduced sulfonamides have shown excellent antibacterial activity and lack, or show a minimal, renal toxicity, which is a problem with the older sulfonamides. In addition, sulfisoxazole acetyl is tasteless and hence is preferred for oral use in children.
2. Sulfonamides that have a rapid rate of absorption but a slow rate of elimination. These relatively toxic agents, which are no longer used in the United States, include sulfamethoxypyridazine and sulfadimethoxine.
3. Sulfonamides that are poorly absorbed. These agents include: succinylsulfathiazole (Sulfasuxide), phthalylsulfathiazole (Sulfathalidine), and sulfasalazine (Azulfidine); they are used as intestinal antiseptics. Sulfasalazine is used especially in the therapy of regional enteritis and ulcerative colitis (Figure 91).
4. Sulfonamides that are used topically. These consist of sulfacetamide (Sulamyd and Isopto Cetamide), which is used in ophthalmic infections, and sulfamylon (Mafenide) and silver sulfadiazine (Silvadene), which are used in infections associated with burns.

Many of the adverse reactions seen with sulfonamides are due to hypersensitivity reactions, which include dermatitis, leukopenia, hemolytic anemia, and drug fever. Stevens–Johnson syndrome is a very severe, but rare hypersensitivity reaction that occurs only with some of the long-acting sulfonamide preparations.

Renal lesions may be due to the precipitation of sulfonamides and their acetyl derivatives in the urinary tract. Renal damage may also be attributable to a direct toxic effect of sulfonamides on the kidney tubules.

Sulfonamides may also cause jaundice and kernicterus in newborns. This is due to the displacement of bilirubin from protein-binding sites. Therefore, sulfonamides should not be used during pregnancy.

The combination of trimethoprim and sulfamethoxazole (usually five parts sulfamethoxazole to one part trimethoprim) interferes with the synthesis of active folic acid by means of two separate reactions. In the first, sulfonamides compete with PABA and prevent its conversion to dihydrofolic acid. In the second, trimethoprim, by inhibiting the activity of dihydrofolic acid reductase, prevents the conversion of dihydrofolic acid into tetrahydrofolic acid, which is necessary for the synthesis of DNA. These reactions are summarized in Figure 90.

These drug combinations have the following therapeutic advantages:

They cause synergistic antibacterial effects.
They have bactericidal activity.
The emergence of bacterial resistance is decreased.
The spectrum of antibacterial activity is enhanced.
Toxicity is reduced.

Folic acid deficiency may occur either following prolonged usage of methotrexate or in patients with preexisting folic acid deficiency. Folinic acid may be administered to overcome the folic-acid-deficiency-related megaloblastic anemia.

Orally administered trimethoprim is used in the treatment of chronic recurring urinary tract infection. Oral forms of trimethoprim-sulfamethoxazole are used in *Shigella* and some *Salmonella* infections, particularly when they are resistant to ampicillin and chloramphenicol. High doses of oral trimethoprim-sulfamethoxazole are used in *Pneumocystis* pneumonia. This combination, along with polymyxin, has been shown to be effective in treating sepsis caused by *Serratia* or *Pseudomonas* organisms.

Intravenously administered trimethoprim-sulfamethoxazole is indicated in severe cases of *Pneumocystis carinii* pneumonia, Gram-negative bacterial sepsis, and shigellosis.

Oral trimethoprim in combination with sulfonamide has been used in the treatment of leishmaniasis, toxoplasmosis, and falciparum malaria.

SULFONAMIDES

Sulfacetamide	Sulfamethoxine
Sulfadiazine	Sulfamethoxypyrazine
Sulfaguanidine	Sulfamethoxypyridazine
Sulfamerazine	Sulfanilamide
Sulfamethazine	Sulfisomidine
Sulfamethizole	Sulfisoxazole
Sulfamethoxazole	Sulformethoxine

SULFONES

Agents such as primaquine destroy exoerythrocytic tissue schizonts such as those developing in the liver.

Other pharmacologic agents are sometimes used in combination with the antimalarial agents for greater effect. These include:

- Sulfonamides — Sulfadoxine or sulfadiazine is used with pyrimethamine.
- Sulfones — Dapsone (DDS) is used in place of or in addition to the sulfonamides and pyrimethamine.
- Acridines — Quinacrine (Atabrine) has an action similar to chloroquine's.
- Biguanides — Chlorguanide (Proguanil and Paludrine) has suppressive as well as prophylactic actions.

SULFONYLUREAS

Oral hypoglycemic agents have advantages over insulin, because, by releasing insulin and by decreasing the release of glucagon, they mimic physiologic processes and cause fewer allergic reactions. Furthermore, they are effective in an oral form, thus eliminating the need for daily injections. The properties of these agents are described in Table 1.

The mechanisms that underlie the hypoglycemic actions of sulfonylureas are:

Pancreatic
- Improved insulin secretion
- Reduced glucagon secretion

Extrapancreatic
- Improved tissue sensitivity to insulin
  - Direct
    - Increased receptor binding
    - Improved post-binding action
  - Indirect
    - Reduced hyperglycemia
    - Decreased plasma free fatty-acid concentrations
    - Reduced hepatic insulin extraction

Sulfonylureas such as glyburide and glipizide bind to sulfonylurea receptors located on the surface of beta cells and trigger insulin releases at nanomolar concentrations (Figure 54). Sulfonylureas bind to ATP-sensitive potassium channels and inhibit potassium efflux through these channels. The inhibition of ATP-sensitive potassium channels then leads to depolarization of the beta cell.

SULFOXONE SODIUM

Leprosy (Hansen's disease) is a chronic granulomatous disease that attacks superficial tissues such as the skin, nasal mucosa, and peripheral nerves. There are two types of leprosy: lepromatous and tuberculoid. The sulfones, which are derivatives of 4,4'-diamino-diphenylsulfone, are bacteriostatic. DDS and sulfoxone sodium are the most useful and effective agents currently available. They should be given in low doses initially, and then the dosage should be gradually increased until a full dose of 300 to 400 mg per week is reached. During this period, the patient must be monitored carefully. With adequate precautions and appropriate doses, sulfones may be used safely for years. Nevertheless, side effects such as anorexia, nervousness, insomnia, blurred vision, paresthesia, and peripheral neuropathy do occur. Hemolysis is common, especially in patients with glucose 6-phosphate dehydrogenase deficiency. A fatal exacerbation of lepromatous leprosy and an infectious mononucleosis-like syndrome rarely occur. Clofazimine (Lamprene) may be effective in patients who show resistance to the sulfones and may also dramatically reduce an exacerbation of leprosy. Red discoloration of the skin and eosinophilic enteritis have occurred following clofazime therapy.

Not all mycobacterial infections are caused by *Mycobacterium tuberculosis* or *Mycobacterium leprae*. These atypical mycobacteria require treatment with secondary medications as well as other chemotherapeutic agents. For example, *Mycobacterium maninum* causes skin granulomas, and effective drugs in the treatment of such infections are rifampin or minocycline. *Mycobacterium fortuitum* cause skin ulcers, and the medications recommended for treatment are ethambutol, cycloserine, and rifampin in combination with amikacin.

SULFURIC ACID/SULFONATED PHENOLICS

(Debacterol liquid 30% sulfuric acid and 22% sulfonated phenolics)

Sulfuric acid/sulfonated phenolics is a mouth-and-throat product. **Sulfuric acid** is a tissue denaturant and sterilizing agent. **Sulfonated phenolics** are antiseptic agents with

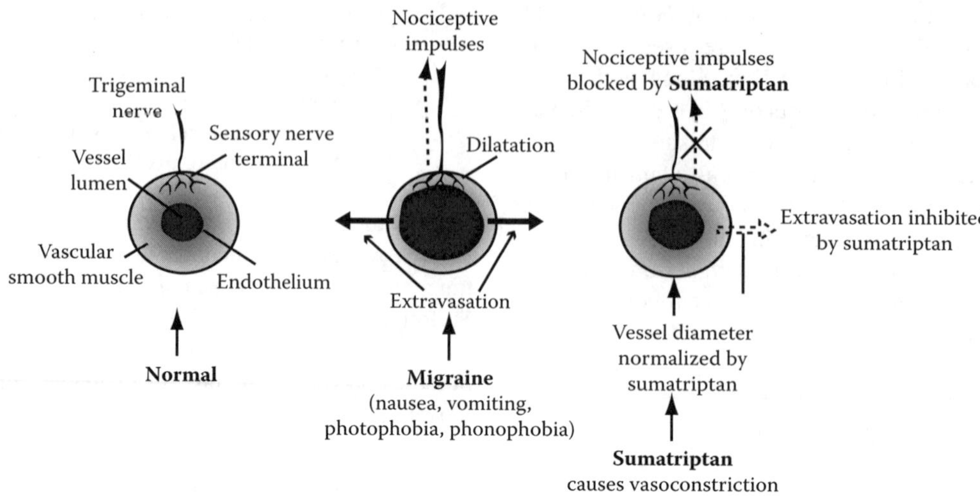

FIGURE 93 **Sumatriptan**, an agonist of the $5HT_1$-like receptor, is highly effective in the treatment of **migraine**.

topical analgesic properties. It is indicated for topical treatment of ulcerating lesions of the oral cavity (e.g., recurrent aphthous stomatitis [canker sores]); relief of pain and discomfort of oral mucosal ulcers; and decrease risk of infection of ulcerated tissue.

SULINDAC
(Clinoril)

Sulindac, a nonsteroidal antiinflammatory agent, is used in osteoarthritis, rheumatoid arthritis, ankylosing spondylitis, acute subacromial bursitis or supraspinatus tendinitis, and acute gouty arthritis (see also Table 3).

SUMATRIPTAN SUCCINATE
(Imitrex)

Sumatriptan, a selective serotonin ($5\text{-}HT_1$) receptor agonist (6 mg SC), is used in acute migraine attack with or without aura (see Figure 93).

SURAMIN
(Naphuride)

Trypanosomiasis is produced by protozoa of the genus *Trypanosoma* and leads to Gambian or mid-African sleeping

SYPHILIS: Treatment of

Stage/Type of Syphilis	Medications
Primary, secondary, or latent syphilis of less than 1 year's duration	Benzathine penicillin G 2.4 million units IM in a single dose
Syphilis of more than 1 year's duration (except neurosyphilis)	Benzathine penicillin G 2.4 million units IM once a week for three successive weeks
Neurosyphilis	Aqueous crystalline penicillin G 12-24 million units IV (2-4 million units every 4 hours) for 10–14 days, followed by benzathine penicillin G 2.4 million units IM weekly for three doses or
	Aqueous procaine penicillin G 2.4 million units IM daily plus probenecid 500 mg PO four times daily, both for 10–14 days, followed by benzathine penicillin G 2.4 million units IM weekly for three doses
Congenital syphilis	Aqueous crystalline penicillin G 50,000 units/kg IV every 8–12 hours for 10–14 days or
	Aqueous procaine penicillin G 50,000 U/kg IM daily for 10–14 days
Penicillin-allergic patients	
Primary, secondary, or latent syphilis of less than 1 year's duration	Doxycycline 100 mg PO two times a day for 2 weeks or Tetracycline 500 mg PO four times daily for 2 weeks or Erythromycin 500 mg PO four times daily for 2 weeks
Syphilis of more than 1 year's duration (except neurosyphilis)	Tetracycline 500 mg PO four times daily for 4 weeks or Doxycycline 100 mg PO two times a day for 4 weeks

sickness (*T. gambiense*), Rhodesian or East African sleeping sickness (*T. rhodesiense*), and Chagas' disease, which is seen in the populations of Central and South America (*T. cruzi*).

Agents effective in the treatment of trypanosomiasis are the aromatic diamidines (pentamidine, stilbamidine, and propamidine). Pentamidine is the preferred drug for the prevention and early treatment of *T. gambiense* infections; however, it cannot penetrate the CNS. Melarsoprol is the drug recommended for *T. gambiense* infections that do not respond to pentamidine or for managing the late meningoencephalitic stages of infection. It does reach the central nervous system either. Nifurtimox (Lampit) is the drug of choice for treating the acute form of Chagas' disease. Suramin (Naphuride) is effective only as therapy for African sleeping sickness.

SUTILAINS

(Travase)

Sutilains, a topical proteolytic enzyme, is used in debridement of major burns, decubitus ulcers, ulcers in peripheral vascular disease, and incisional, traumatic, and pyrogenic wounds.

SYRUP OF IPECAC

Ipecac is a mixture of the alcohol-soluble alkaloid which is obtained from the South American plant *Cephaelis ipecacuanha*, and is used solely in the form of syrup of ipecac. Apomorphine hydrochloride and copper sulfate are also emetics.

Syrup of ipecac and copper sulfate cause emesis by locally irritating the stomach, whereas apomorphine stimulates the chemoreceptor trigger zone for emesis located in the caudal portion of the fourth ventricle (area postrema), which in turn stimulates the vomiting center in the lateral reticular formation of the medulla (see also Figure 73).

T

TACRINE HYDROCHLORIDE
(Cognex)

Tacrine (initially 10 mg p.o. q.i.d.) is indicated in the treatment of mild to moderate dementia of the Alzheimer's type. Although many neuronal systems are affected in Alzheimer's disease, the decline in central cholinergic activity is one of the most pronounced neurotransmitter deficits. Tacrine's primary effect is the reversible inhibition of cholinesterase—butyrylcholinesterase more than acetylcholinesterase. This inhibition increases the level of acetylcholine in the central nervous system. In fact, increased levels of acetylcholine have been detected in the cerebrospinal fluid of patients receiving tacrine (see also Figure 12).

Tacrine may also block potassium channels, increasing the duration of the action potential and augmenting acetylcholine release from cholinergic neurons.

In addition, tacrine may moderate cholinergic activity by acting as a partial agonist through direct binding to nicotinic receptors and, with greater affinity, to muscarine receptors.

Additionally, tacrine inhibits monoamine oxidase (MAO)—MAO-A to a greater extent than MAO-B. Tacrine may also inhibit the reuptake of norepinephrine, serotonin, and dopamine.

Because of its mechanism of action, tacrine has the potential to interfere with the activity of anticholinergic medications. A synergistic effect is expected when tacrine is given concurrently with succinylcholine, cholinesterase inhibitors, or cholinergic agonists, such as bethanecol. Coadministration of tacrine with theophylline increases theophylline elimination half-life and average plasma concentrations.

Overdosage with cholinesterase inhibitors can cause a cholinergic crisis characterized by severe nausea, vomiting, salivation, sweating, bradycardia, hypotension, and seizures. Increasing muscle weakness may occur and can result in death if respiratory muscles are involved. Tertiary anticholinergics, such as atropine, may be used as an antidote for tacrine overdosage.

Four inhibitors of acetylcholinesterase (AChE) currently are approved by the FDA for treatment of Alzheimer's disease: **tacrine** (1,2,3,4-tetrahydro-9-ammoacridine; Cognex), **donepezil** (Aricept), **rivastigmine** (Exelon), and **galantamine** (Razadyne). Tacrine is a potent centrally acting inhibitor of AChE. Studies of oral tacrine in combination with lecithin have confirmed that there is, indeed, an effect of **tacrine** on some measures of memory performance, but the magnitude of improvement observed with the combination of lecithin and tacrine is modest, at best. The side effects of tacrine often are significant and dose-limiting; abdominal cramping, anorexia, nausea, vomiting, and diarrhea are observed in up to one-third of patients receiving therapeutic doses, and elevations of serum transaminases are observed in up to 50% of those treated. Because of significant side effects, tacrine is not used widely clinically. Donepezil is a selective inhibitor of AChE in the CNS with little effect on AChE in peripheral tissues. It produces modest improvements in cognitive scores in Alzheimer's disease patients and has a long half-life, allowing once-daily dosing. Rivastigmine and galantamine are dosed twice daily and produce a similar degree of cognitive improvement. Adverse effects associated with donepezil, rivastigmine, and galantamine are similar in character but generally less frequent and less severe than those observed with tacrine; they include nausea, diarrhea, vomiting, and insomnia. Donepezil, rivastigmine, and galantamine are not associated with the hepatotoxicity that limits the use of tacrine.

TACROLIMUS
(Prograf capsules 0.5 mg, capsules 1 mg, capsules 5 mg, injection 5 mg/mL, Protopic ointment 0.3%, ointment 0.1%)

Tacrolimus is an immunosuppressive/immunomodulator. It suppresses cell-mediated immune reactions and some humoral immunity.

Tacrolimus, a novel macrocyclic lactone with potent immunosuppressive properties, is currently available as an intravenous formulation and as a capsule for oral use.

Tacrolimus (0.05 to 0.1 mg/kg/day) is used in organ liver rejection prophylaxis. Perhaps the most effective immunosuppressive drugs in routine use are the **calcineurin inhibitors**, **cyclosporine** and **tacrolimus**, which target intracellular signaling pathways induced as a consequence of T-cell-receptor activation. Although they are structurally unrelated and bind to distinct, albeit related molecular targets, they inhibit normal T-cell signal transduction essentially by the same mechanism. Cyclosporine and tacrolimus do not act *per se* as immunosuppressive agents. Instead, these drugs bind to an immunophilin (cyclophilin for cyclosporine or FKBP-12 for tacrolimus), resulting in subsequent interaction with calcineurin to block its phosphatase activity. Calcineurin-catalyzed dephosphorylation is required for movement of a component of the nuclear factor of activated T-lymphocytes (NFAT) into the nucleus NFAT, in turn, is required to induce a number of cytokine genes, including that for interleukin-2 (IL-2), a prototypic T-cell growth and differentiation factor.

Tacrolimus (Prograf, FK506) is a macrolide antibiotic produced by *Streptomyces tsukubaensis*.

Like cyclosporine, **tacrolimus** inhibits T-cell activation by inhibiting calcineurin. Tacrolimus binds to an intracellular protein, FK506-binding protein—12 (FKBP-12), an immunophilin structurally related to **cyclophilin**. A complex of tacrolimus-FKBP-12, Ca^{2+} calmodulin, and calcineurin then forms, and calcineurin phosphatase activity is inhibited. The inhibition of phosphatase activity prevents dephosphorylation and nuclear translocation of NFAT and inhibits T-cell activation. Thus, although the intracellular receptors differ, cyclosporine and **tacrolimus** target the same pathway for immunosuppression.

Tacrolimus is available for oral administration as capsules (0.5, 1, and 5 mg) and as a sterile solution for injection (5 mg/mL). Immunosuppressive activity resides primarily in the parent drug. Because of intersubject variability in pharmacokinetics, individualized dosing is required for optimal therapy. Whole blood, rather than plasma, is the most appropriate sampling compartment to describe tacrolimus pharmacokinetics. For tacrolimus, the C_0 level seems to correlate better with clinical events than it does for cyclosporine. Target concentrations in many centers are 200 to 400 ng/mL in the early preoperative period and 100 to 200 ng/mL 3 months after transplantation. Unlike cyclosporine, more frequent tacrolimus dosing has not been formally evaluated. Gastrointestinal absorption is incomplete and variable. Food decreases the rate and extent of absorption. Plasma-protein binding of tacrolimus is 75 to 99%, involving primarily albumin and α_1-acid glycoprotein. Its half-life is about 12 hours. Tacrolimus is extensively metabolized in the liver by CYP3A, with a half-life of 12 hours; at least some of the metabolites are active. The bulk of excretion of the parent drug and metabolites is in the feces. Less than 1% of administered tacrolimus is excreted unchanged in the urine.

Tacrolimus is indicated for the prophylaxis of solid-organ allograft rejection in a manner similar to cyclosporine and as rescue therapy in patients with rejection episodes despite "therapeutic" levels of cyclosporine. The recommended starting dose for tacrolimus injection is 0.03 to 0.05 mg/kg/day as a continuous infusion. Recommended initial oral doses are 0.15 to 0.2 mg/kg/day for adult kidney transplant patients, 0.1 to 0.15 mg/kg/day for adult liver transplant patients, and 0.15 to 0.2 mg/kg/day for pediatric liver transplant patients in two divided doses 12 hours apart. These dosages are intended to achieve typical blood trough levels in the 5- to 15-ng/mL range. Pediatric patients generally require higher doses than do adults.

Nephrotoxicity, neurotoxicity (tremor, headache, motor disturbances, seizures), GI complaints, hypertension, hyperkalemia, hyperglycemia, and diabetes are all associated with tacrolimus use. As with cyclosporine, nephrotoxicity is limiting. **Tacrolimus** has a negative effect on pancreatic islet beta cells, and glucose intolerance and diabetes mellitus are well-recognized complications of tacrolimus-based immunosuppression. As with other immunosuppressive agents, there is an increased risk of secondary tumors and opportunistic infections. Notably, tacrolimus does not adversely affect uric acid or LDL cholesterol.

Because of its potential for nephrotoxicity, tacrolimus blood levels and renal function should be monitored closely, especially when tacrolimus is used with other potentially nephrotoxic drugs. Coadministration with **cyclosporine** results in additive or synergistic nephrotoxicity; therefore, a delay of at least 24 hours is required when switching a patient from cyclosporine to tacrolimus. As **tacrolimus** is metabolized mainly by CYP3A, the potential interactions described above for **cyclosporine** also apply for tacrolimus.

TADALAFIL
(Cialis tablets 5 mg)

Tadalafil is a phosphodiesterase type 5 inhibitor that enhances the effect of nitric oxide at the nerve ending and endothelial cells in the corpus cavernosum by inhibiting phosphodiesterase type 5 in the corpus cavernosum of the penis. This results in vasodilation, increased inflow of blood into the corporus cavernosum, and ensuing penile erection upon sexual stimulation. It is used for the treatment of erectile dysfunction.

Erectile dysfunction is a frequently encountered problem whose risk factors parallel those of coronary artery disease. Thus, many men desiring therapy for erectile dysfunction already may be receiving (or may require, especially if they increase physical activity) antianginal therapy. The combination of sildenafil and other phosphodiesterase 5 (PDE5) inhibitors with organic nitrate vasodilators can cause extreme hypotension.

Cells in the corpus cavernosum produce NO during sexual arousal in response to nonadrenergic, noncholinergic neurotransmission. NO stimulates the formation of cyclic GMP, which leads to relaxation of smooth muscle of the corpus cavernosum and penile arteries, engorgement of the corpus cavernosum, and erection. The accumulation of cyclic GMP can be enhanced by inhibition of the cyclic GMP-specific PDE5 family. **Sildenafil** (**Viagra**) and congeners inhibit PDE5 and have been demonstrated to improve erectile function in patients with erectile dysfunction. Not surprisingly, PDE5 inhibitors have assumed the status of widely used recreational drugs. Since the introduction of sildenafil, two additional PDE5 inhibitors have been developed for use in therapy of erectile dysfunction. **Tadalafil** (**Cialis**) and **vardenafil** (**Levitra**) share similar therapeutic efficacy and side-effect profiles with sildenafil; tadalafil has a longer time to onset of action and a longer therapeutic half-life than the other PDE5 inhibitors. Sildenafil has been the most thoroughly characterized of these compounds, but all three PDE5 inhibitors are contraindicated for patients taking organic nitrate vasodilators or adrenergic-receptor antagonists.

The side effects of sildenafil and other PDE5 inhibitors are largely predictable on the basis of their effects on PDE5. Headache, flushing, and rhinitis may be observed, as may dyspepsia owing to relaxation of the lower esophageal sphincter. Sildenafil and vardenafil also weakly inhibit PDE6, the enzyme involved in photoreceptor signal transduction, and can produce visual disturbances, most notably changes in the perception of color hue or brightness. **Tadalafil** inhibits PDE11, a widely distributed phosphodiesterase isoform, but the clinical importance of this effect is not clear. The most important toxicity of all these PDE5 inhibitors is hemodynamic. When given alone to men with severe coronary artery disease, these drugs have modest effects on blood pressure, producing less than a 10% fall in systolic, diastolic, and mean systemic pressures and in pulmonary artery systolic and mean pressures. However, sildenafil, tadalafil, and vardenafil all have a significant and potentially dangerous interaction with organic nitrates, the therapeutic actions of which are mediated *via* their conversion to NO with resulting increases in cyclic GMP. In the presence of a PDE5 inhibitor, nitrates cause profound increases in cyclic GMP and can produce dramatic reductions in blood pressure. Compared with controls, healthy male subjects pretreated with sildenafil or the other PDE5 inhibitors exhibit a much greater decrease in systolic blood pressure when treated with sublingual glyceryl trinitrate, and in many subjects a fall of more than 25 mm Hg was detected. This drug class toxicity is the basis for the warning that PDE5 inhibitors should not be prescribed to patients receiving any form of nitrate and dictates that patients should be questioned about the use of PDE5 inhibitors within 24 hours before nitrates are administered. A period of longer than 24 hours may be needed following administration of a PDE5 inhibitor for safe use of nitrates, especially with **tadalafil** because of its prolonged half-life. In the event that patients develop significant hypotension following combined administration of sildenafil and a nitrate, fluids and adrenergic receptor agonists, if needed, should be used for support.

Sildenafil, **tadalafil**, and **vardenafil** are metabolized via cytochrome P450 (CYP3A4), and their toxicity may be enhanced in patients who receive other substrates of this enzyme, including macrolide and imidazole antibiotics, some statins, and antiretroviral agents. PDE5 inhibitors also may prolong cardiac repolarization by blocking the I_{Kr}. Although these interactions and effects are important clinically, the overall incidence and profile of adverse events observed with PDE5 inhibitors, when used without nitrates, are consistent with the expected background frequency of the same events in the treated population. In patients with coronary artery disease whose exercise capacity indicates that sexual activity is unlikely to precipitate angina and who are not currently taking nitrates, the use of PDE5 inhibitors can be considered. Such therapy needs to be individualized, and appropriate warnings must be given about the risk of toxicity if nitrates are taken subsequently for angina; this drug interaction may persist for approximately 24 hours for sildenafil and vardenafil and for considerably longer with tadalafil. Alternative nonnitrate antianginal therapy, such as β-adrenergic receptor antagonists, should be used during these time periods.

TALC, STERILE POWDER
(Sclerosol aerosol 4 g talc, Sterile talc powder 5 g talc)

Talc, sterile powder, is an antineoplastic agent, that induces an inflammatory reaction, which promotes adherence of the visceral and parietal pleura, obliterating the pleural space and preventing reaccumulation of pleural fluid. It decreases or prevents recurrence of malignant pleural effusions.

TAMOXIFEN CITRATE
(Nolvadex tablets 10 mg)

Tamoxifen citrate is an antiestrogen. A nonsteroidal agent with antiestrogenic properties, tamoxifen (10 to 20 mg morning and evening) is indicated for treatment of axillary node-negative breast cancer in women following total mastectomy or segmental mastectomy, axillary dissection, and breast irradiation; for treatment of node-positive breast cancer in postmenopausal women following total mastectomy or segmental mastectomy, axillary dissection, and breast irradiation; and for the treatment of metastatic breast cancer in men and women.

In addition, tamoxifen has been used in the treatment of mastalgia (10 mg/day for 4 months) and for decreasing the size and pain of gynecomastia.

Tamoxifen is a competitive inhibitor of estradiol binding to the estrogen receptors. When bound to estrogen receptor, tamoxifen induces a change in the three-dimensional shape of the receptor, inhibiting its binding to the estrogen-responsive element on DNA. Under normal physiological conditions, estrogen stimulation increases tumor cell production of transforming growth factor beta (TGF-beta), an autocrine inhibitor of tumor cell growth. By blocking these pathways, the net effect of tamoxifen treatment is to decrease the autocrine stimulation of breast cancer growth, capturing the cell in G_1. In addition, tamoxifen decreases the local production of insulin-like growth factor 1(IGF-1) by surrounding tissues; IGF-1 is a paracrine growth factor for the breast cancer cell (see also Figure 36).

Tamoxifen is metabolized mostly to *N*-desmethyl tamoxifen, which is an active metabolite, and to a small extent to 4-hydroxytamoxifen. The hypoprothrombinemic effects of anticoagulants may be increased by concomitant administration of tamoxifen.

Bromocriptine may elevate serum tamoxifen and *N*-desmethyl tamoxifen.

Adverse reactions to tamoxifen are relatively mild and rarely require discontinuation of therapy. If adverse reactions are severe, it is sometimes possible to control severe adverse reactions by dosage reduction without losing control of the disease.

The most frequently occurring side effects of tamoxifen are hot flashes, nausea, and vomiting (up to 25%, rarely severe). The less often occurring side effects of tamoxifen are vaginal bleeding, vaginal discharge, menstrual irregularities, and skin rash.

Hypercalcemia, peripheral edema, food distaste, pruritus vulvae, depression, dizziness, lightheadedness, headache, retinopathy, thrombocytopenia, leukopenia, and hair thinning have been reported on rare occasions.

TAMSULOSIN HYDROCHLORIDE (Flomax capsules 0.4 mg)

Tamsulosin is an alpha$_1$-adrenergic blocker that selectively blocks alpha$_1$-adrenergic receptors, causing relaxation of prostate smooth muscle resulting in an increase in urinary flow rate and a reduction in symptoms of BPH. It is used in the treatment of signs and symptoms of benign prostatic hyperplasia (BPH).

Alpha receptor antagonists have a wide spectrum of pharmacological specificities and are chemically heterogeneous. Some of these drugs have markedly different affinities for α_1 and α_2 receptors. For example, **prazosin** is much more potent in blocking α_1 than α_2 receptors (i.e., α_1 selective), whereas **yohimbine** is α_2 selective; **phentolamine** has similar affinities for both of these receptor subtypes. More recently, agents that discriminate among the various subtypes of a particular receptor have become available; for example, **tamsulosin** has higher potency at α_{1A} than at α_{1B} receptors.

Tamsulosin (Flomax), a benzenesulfonamide, is an α receptor antagonist with some selectivity for α_{1A} (and α_{1D}) subtypes compared to α_{1B} subtype. This selectivity may favor blockade of α_{1A} receptors in prostate. **Tamsulosin** is efficacious in the treatment of BPH with little effect on blood pressure. Tamsulosin is well absorbed and has a half-life of 5 to 10 hours. It is extensively metabolized by CYPs. Tamsulosin may be administered at a 0.4-mg starting dose; a dose of 0.8 mg ultimately will be more efficacious in some patients. Abnormal ejaculation is an adverse effect of **tamsulosin**.

Tamsulosin has efficacy in BPH owing to relaxation of smooth muscle in the bladder neck, prostate capsule, and prostatic urethra. These drugs rapidly improve urinary flow, whereas the actions of finasteride are typically delayed for months. Recent studies show that combination therapy with doxazosin and finasteride reduces the risk of overall clinical progression of BPH significantly more than treatment with either drug alone. **Prazosin**, **terazosin**, **doxazosin**, **tamsulosin**, and **alfuzosin** have been studied extensively and used widely in patients with benign prostatic hyperplasia. With the exception of tamsulosin, the comparative efficacies of each of these drugs, especially in comparison with relative adverse effects such as postural hypotension, appear similar, although direct comparisons are limited. **Tamsulosin** at the recommended dose of 0.4 mg daily is less likely to cause orthostatic hypotension than are the other drugs. There is growing evidence that the predominant α_1-receptor subtype expressed in the human prostate is the α_{1A} receptor. Developments in this area will provide the basis for the selection of receptor antagonists with specificity for the relevant subtype of α_1 receptor. However, the possibility remains that some of the symptoms of BPH are due to α_1 receptors in other sites, such as bladder, spinal cord, or brain.

Although anecdotal evidence suggested that prazosin might be useful in the treatment of patients with variant angina (Prinzmetal's angina) due to coronary vasospasm, several small controlled trials have failed to demonstrate a clear benefit. Some studies have indicated that prazosin can decrease the incidence of digital vasospasm in patients with Raynaud's disease; however, its relative efficacy as compared with other vasodilators (e.g., Ca^{2+}-channel blockers) is not known. Prazosin may have some benefit in patients with other vasospastic disorders. Prazosin decreases ventricular arrhythmias induced by coronary artery ligation or reperfusion in laboratory animals; the therapeutic potential for this use in humans is not known. Prazosin also may be useful for the treatment of patients with mitral or aortic valvular insufficiency, presumably because of reduction of afterload.

TAZAROTENE (Avage cream 0.1%, Tazorac cream 0.05%, cream 0.1%, gel 0.05%, gel 0.1%)

Tazarotene is a retinoid that inhibits cornified envelope formation, which is an element of psoriatic scales. It is indicated in the treatment of **acne** (Tazorac cream and gel), psoriasis (Tazorac gel); as an adjunctive agent in mitigation of **facial fine wrinkling**, **facial mottled hyper- and hypopigmentation**, and benign facial lentigines in patients who use comprehensive skin care and sunlight avoidance programs (Avage).

Retinoids include natural compounds and synthetic derivatives of retinol that exhibit vitamin A activity. Retinoids have many important functions throughout the body, including roles in vision, regulation of cell proliferation and differentiation and bone growth, immune defense, and tumor suppression. Because vitamin A affects normal epithelial differentiation, it was investigated as a treatment for cutaneous disorders but was abandoned initially because of unfavorable side effects. Molecular modifications yielded compounds with vastly improved margins of safety. First-generation retinoids include **retinol**, **tretinoin** (all-*trans*-retinoic acid), **isotretinoin** (13-*cis*-retinoic acid), and alitretinoin (9-*cis*-retinoic acid). Second-generation retinoids, also known as **aromatic retinoids**, were created by alteration of the cyclic end group and include acitretin. Third-generation retinoids contain further modifications and are called **arotinoids**. Members of this generation include **tazarotene** and **bexarotene**. **Adapalene**, a derivative of naphthoic acid with retinoid-like properties, does not fit precisely into any of the three generations.

Tazarotene (Tazorac) is a third-generation retinoid approved for the treatment of **psoriasis** and **acne vulgaris**. This retinoid binds to all three RARs. In mice, tazarotene blocks ornithine decarboxylase activity, which is associated with cell proliferation and hyperplasia. In cell culture, it suppresses markers of epidermal inflammation and inhibits cornification of the keratinocyte.

Tazarotene gel, applied once daily to dry skin, may be used as monotherapy or in combination with other medications, such as topical corticosteroids, for the treatment of localized plaque psoriasis. This is the first topical retinoid approved by the Food and Drug Administration (FDA) for the treatment of psoriasis. Side effects of burning, itching, and skin irritation are relatively common, and patients should avoid sun exposure.

TEGASEROD MALEATE
(Zelnorm tablets 2 mg, tablets 6 mg)

Tegaserod maleate is a GI agent that binds with high affinity to human 5-HT_4 receptors, acting as an agonist at neuronal 5-HT_4 receptors to trigger the release of neurotransmitters. Activation of 5-HT_4 receptors in the GI tract stimulates peristaltic reflex and intestinal secretion, and inhibits visceral sensitivity. It is used for short-term treatment of women with irritable bowel syndrome (IBS) whose primary symptom is constipation; and in treatment of patients younger than 65 years of age with chronic idiopathic constipation.

Tegaserod (Zelnorm), an aminoguanidine indole, is structurally related to serotonin and is a partial 5-HT_4 agonist with negligible affinity for other receptor subtypes. Tegaserod has multiple effects on the GI tract. It stimulates motility and accelerates transit in the esophagus, stomach, small bowel, and ascending colon. It also stimulates chloride secretion. Thus far, the clinical efficacy of tegaserod has been proven only in female patients with constipation-predominant IBS; however, the drug is being tested in a variety of other conditions, including **gastroparesis**. In patients with constipation, tegaserod results in a statistically significant but mild to modest improvement in stool frequency, with less consistent effects on other parameters such as stool form, bloating, and pain. The absolute improvement is modest at best, with a difference of only about one to two bowel movements per week between the drug and placebo groups. It is not clear that the drug has any greater efficacy in this regard than other agents used for constipation. Males with constipation also may respond to tegaserod, but existing studies did not include enough men to demonstrate a statistically significant effect.

In clinical trials, tegaserod also reduced bloating (a prominent symptom in patients with irritable bowel syndrome) and pain, but it is not clear whether this represents an independent effect on sensory nerves or simply a consequence of decreased fecal or air distention of the colon. As yet, there is no evidence for significant modulation of nociceptive signaling by 5-HT_4 receptors.

Tegaserod is available for oral administration in 2-mg and 6-mg tablets and approved for use in women with constipation-dominant irritable bowel syndrome at a dose of 6 mg twice daily. **Tegaserod** also has been approved for the treatment of chronic constipation. Higher doses have been suggested for other prokinetic effects (e.g., stimulation of gastric emptying) but such uses have not been validated clinically.

After oral administration, **tegaserod** is partially absorbed from the gut, reaching peak-plasma levels after 1 to 1.3 hours. Absorption is slowed by the presence of food in the stomach, so tegaserod is best taken on an empty stomach. Once in circulation, tegaserod is approximately 98% bound to plasma proteins. Tegaserod is degraded by acid hydrolysis before absorption from the stomach, and by oxidation and glucuronidation in the liver to three inactive N-glucuronide metabolites. Approximately two-thirds of the orally administered dose of tegaserod is excreted unchanged in feces, with the remainder excreted in urine; the drug has an estimated half-life of about 11 hours.

Diarrhea and headache are the most common side effects of tegaserod, occurring in about 10% of patients. Tegaserod does not appear to have any significant cardiac toxicity, and no clinically relevant drug–drug interactions have been identified. No dosage adjustment is required in elderly patients or those with mild to moderate hepatic or renal impairment; however, tegaserod should not be used in patients with severe hepatic or renal impairment.

TELENZEPINE

Vagal impulses elicit the release of acetylcholine in the parietal cells and in the gastric mucosal cells containing gastrin, a peptide hormone. Both the directly released acetylcholine and the indirectly released gastrin then stimulate the parietal cells to secrete hydrogen ions into the gastric lumen.

The most useful anticholinergic drugs are propantheline (Pro-Banthine), pirenzepine, and telenzepine, which antagonize muscarinic cholinergic receptors (M_1 receptors). All three agents depress gastric motility and secretion. The production of pepsin is also reduced. Propantheline may be used as adjunctive therapy with antacids but not as a sole agent. The side effects and contraindications of propantheline use are identical to those of atropine (prostatic hypertrophy, urinary retention, glaucoma, and cardiac arrhythmias). The timing of medication is critical in ulcer therapy. Anticholinergic drugs should be given about 30 minutes before meals, and antacids about 1 hour after meals. A double dose of an antacid is often taken just before bedtime (see Figure 12).

TELITHROMYCIN
(Ketek tablets 400 mg)

Telithromycin is a ketolide, which interferes with microbial protein synthesis. It is indicated in the treatment of acute bacterial exacerbation of chronic bronchitis, acute bacterial sinusitis, and community-acquired pneumonia caused by strains of susceptible organisms.

Ketolides, of which **telithromycin** (**Ketek**) is the only one currently approved, are semisynthetic derivatives of erythromycin. Telithromycin differs from erythromycin in that a 3-keto group replaces the α-L-cladinose of the 14-member macrolide ring, and there is a substituted carbamate at C11-C12. These modifications render ketolides less susceptible to methylase-mediated (erm) and efflux-mediated (mef or msr) mechanisms of resistance. Ketolides therefore are active against many macrolide-resistant Gram-positive strains.

Ketolides and **macrolides** have very similar antibacterial properties. **Telithromycin** is active against staphylococci, streptococci, *S. pneumoniae*, *Haemophilus* spp., *Moraxella catarrhalis*, *Mycoplasma*, *Chlamydia*, and *Legionella*. It is slightly more active by weight than erythromycin. MIC breakpoints for telithromycin are ≤0.25 μg/ml for *S. aureus*, ≤1 μg/ml for *S. pneumoniae*, and ≤4 μg/ml for *H. influenzae*.

Ketolides and **macrolides** have the same ribosomal target site. The principal difference between the two is that structural modifications within ketolides neutralize the common resistance mechanisms that make macrolides ineffective. Introduction of the 3-keto function converts a methylase-inducing macrolide into a noninducing ketolide. This moiety also prevents drug efflux, probably because it generates a less-desirable substrate. The carbamate substitution at C11-C12 enhances binding to the ribosomal target site, even when the site is methylated, by introducing an extra interaction of the ketolide with the ribosome. Inducible and constitutive methylase-producing strains of *S. pneumoniae* are, therefore, telithromycinsusceptible. However, constitutive methylase-producing strains of *S. aureus* and *S. pyogenes* are telithromycin-resistant because the strength of the ketolide interaction with the fully methylated ribosomal binding site is insufficient to overcome resistance. Constitutive methylase producers can be selected from strains with the inducible erm phenotype.

Telithromycin is formulated as a 40-mg tablet for oral administration. There is no parenteral form. It is well absorbed with approximately 60% bioavailability. Peak serum concentrations, averaging 2μg/mL following a single, 800-mg oral dose, are achieved within 30 minutes to 4 hours. With a half-life of 9.8 hours, the drug can be given once daily. It is 60 to 70% bound by serum protein, principally albumin. It penetrates well into most tissues, exceeding plasma concentrations by approximately two- to tenfold or more. **Telithromycin** is concentrated into macrophages and white blood cells, where concentrations of 40 μg/mL (500 times the simultaneous plasma concentration) are maintained 24 hours after dosing. The drug is cleared primarily by hepatic metabolism, 50% by CYP3A4 and 50% by CYP-independent metabolism. No adjustment of the dose is required for hepatic failure or mild to moderate renal failure. No dose has been established for patients in whom creatinine clearance is less than 30 mL/minute, although a reduction in dosage probably is advisable.

Given its spectrum of activity and based on its noninferiority against a number of comparators, **telithromycin** is approved for treatment of respiratory tract infections, including acute exacerbation of **chronic bronchitis** (5-day regimen), acute **bacterial sinusitis** (5-day regimen), and **community-acquired pneumonia** (7- to 10-day regimen). Although telithromycin is not indicated for treatment of severe pneumonia or bacteremia, almost 90% of patients who proved to have pneumococcal bacteremia were clinically cured after taking it. In premarketing trials of telithromycin on patients with community-acquired pneumonia caused by multiple-drug-resistant strains of *S. pneumoniae* (resistant to **penicillins**, **cephalosporins**, **macrolides**, **tetracyclines**, or **trimethoprim-sulfamethoxazole**) over 90% of patients were cured.

Telithromycin generally is well tolerated. Nausea, vomiting, and diarrhea are the most common side effects, occurring in 3 to 10% of treatment courses. Visual disturbances due to slowed accommodation occur in about 1% of treatment courses, and include blurred vision, difficulty focusing, and diplopia. Reversible hepatic dysfunction with elevated transaminases or hepatitis has been reported. Pseudomembranous colitis has been reported. **Telithromycin** is not recommended for routine use in patients with myasthenia gravis due to reports of disease exacerbation in telithromycin-treated patients.

Telithromycin may cause clinically significant QTc prolongation and increased risk of ventricular arrhythmia in predisposed patients. It should not be used in patients with prolonged QT syndrome, uncorrected hypokalemia or hypomagnesemia, profound bradycardia, or in patients receiving certain antiarrhythmics (e.g., quinidine, procainamide, amiodarone) or other agents that prolong QTc (e.g., **cisapride**, **pimozide**).

Telithromycin has several clinically significant drug interactions similar to those for erythromycin. It is both a substrate and a strong inhibitor of CYP3A4. Coadministration of rifampin, a potent inducer of CYP, decreases the serum concentrations of telithromycin by 80%. CYP3A4 inhibitors (e.g., itraconazole) increase peak serum concentrations of telithromycin. Serum concentrations of CYP3A4 substrates (e.g., pimozide, cisapride, midazolam, statins, cyclosporine, phenytoin) are increased by telithromycin. **Telithromycin** also increases peak serum concentrations of metoprolol and digoxin.

TELMISARTAN
(Micardis tablets 20 mg)

Telmisartan is an angiotensin-II-receptor antagonist. It antagonizes the effect of angiotensin II (vasoconstriction and aldosterone secretion) by blocking the angiotensin II (AT_1 receptor) in vascular smooth muscle and the adrenal gland, producing decreased BP. It is indicated in the treatment of hypertension.

There are two distinct **subtypes of angiotensin II receptors**, designated as type 1 (AT_1) and type 2 (AT_2). The AT_1-angiotensin-II-receptor subtype is located predominantly in vascular and myocardial tissue and also in brain, kidney, and adrenal glomerulosa cells, which secrete aldosterone.

The AT_2 subtype of angiotensin-II receptor is found in the adrenal medulla, kidney, and in the CNS, and may play a role in vascular development. Because the AT_1 receptor mediates feedback inhibition of renin release, renin and angiotensin II concentrations are increased during AT_1-receptor antagonism. The clinical consequences of increased angiotensin II effects on an uninhibited AT_2 receptor are unknown; however, emerging data suggest that the AT_2 receptor may elicit antigrowth and antiproliferative responses.

The importance of angiotensin II in regulating cardiovascular function has led to the development of nonpeptide antagonists of the AT_1-angiotensin-II receptor for clinical use. **Losartan** (Cozaar), **candesartan** (Atacand), **irbesartan** (Avapro), **valsartan** (Diovan), **telmisartan** (Micardis), and **eprosartan** (Teveten) have been approved for the treatment of hypertension. By antagonizing the effects of angiotensin II, these agents relax smooth muscle and thereby promote vasodilation, increase renal salt and water excretion, reduce plasma volume, and decrease cellular hypertrophy. Angiotensin-II-receptor antagonists also theoretically overcome some of the disadvantages of ACE inhibitors, which not only prevent conversion of angiotensin I to angiotensin II but also prevent ACE-mediated degradation of **bradykinin** and **substance P**.

The angiotensin-II-receptor blockers (ARBs) available for clinical use bind to the AT_1 receptor with high affinity and generally are more than 10,000-fold selective for the AT_1 receptor versus the AT_2 receptor. The rank-order affinity of the AT_1 receptor for ARBs is **candesartan** = **omesartan** > **irbesartan** = **eprosartan** > **telmisartan** = **valsartan** = EXP 3174 (the active metabolite of losartan) > losartan. Although binding of ARBs to the AT_1 receptor is competitive, the inhibition by ARBs of biological responses to angiotensin II often is insurmountable; i.e., the maximal response to angiotensin II cannot be restored in the presence of the ARB regardless of the concentration of angiotensin II added to the experimental preparation. Of the currently available ARBs, candesartan suppresses the maximal response to angiotensin II the most, whereas insurmountable blockade by irbesartan, eprosartan, **telmisartan**, and valsartan is less. Although losartan antagonism is surmountable, its active metabolite, EXP 3174, causes some degree of insurmountable blockade. The mechanism of insurmountable antagonism by ARBs may be due to slow dissociation kinetics of the compounds from the AT_1 recent however, a number of other factors may contribute, such as ARB-induced receptor internalization and alternative binding sites for ARBs on the AT_1 receptor. Regardless of the mechanism insurmountable antagonism has the theoretical advantage of sustained receptor blockade even with increased levels of endogenous ligand and with missed doses of drug. Whether this theoretical advantage translates into an enhanced clinical performance remains to be determined.

ARBs potently and selectively inhibit, both *in vitro* and *in vivo*, most of the biological effects of angiotensin II, including angiotensin-II-induced (1) contraction of vascular smooth muscle, (2) rapid pressor responses, (3) slow pressor responses, (4) thirst, (5) vasopressin release, (6) aldosterone secretion, (7) release of adrenal catecholamines, (8) enhancement of noradrenergic neurotransmission, (9) increases in sympathetic tone, (10) changes in renal function, and (11) cellular hypertrophy and hyperplasia. ARBs reduce arterial blood pressure in animals with renovascular and genetic hypertension, as well as in transgenic animals overexpressing the renin gene. ARBs, however, have little effect on arterial blood pressure in animals with low-renin hypertension (e.g., rats with hypertension induced by NaCl and deoxycorticosterone).

A critical issue is whether or not ARBs are equivalent to ACE inhibitors with regard to therapeutic efficacy. Although both classes of drugs block the renin-angiotensin system, ARBs differ from ACE inhibitors in several important aspects: (1) ARBs reduce activation of AT_1 receptors more effectively than do ACE inhibitors. ACE inhibitors reduce the biosynthesis of angiotensin II produced by the action of ACE on angiotensin I but do not inhibit alternative non-ACE angiotensin-II-generating pathways. Because ARBs block the AT_1 receptor, the actions of angiotensin II *via* the AT_1 receptor are inhibited regardless of the biochemical pathway leading to angiotensin II formation. (2) In contrast to ACE inhibitors, ARBs permit activation of AT_2 receptors.

Telmisartan (Micardis): Peak plasma levels are obtained approximately 0.5 to 1 hour after oral administration and the plasma half-life is about 24 hours. **Telmisartan** is cleared from the circulation mainly by biliary secretion of intact drug. The plasma clearance of telmisartan is affected by hepatic but not renal insufficiency. The recommended oral dosage of telmisartan is 40 to 80 mg once daily.

TELMISARTAN/HYDROCHLOROTHIAZIDE (Micardis HCT tablets 40 mg telmisartan and 12.5 mg hydrochorothiazide, tablets 80 mg telmisartan and 12.5 mg hydrochlorothiazide)

Telmisartan/hydrochlorothiazide is an antihypertensive combination. **Telmisartan** antagonizes the effect of angiotensin II (vasoconstriction and aldosterone secretion) by blocking the angiotensin II (AT_1 receptor) in vascular smooth muscle and the adrenal gland, producing decreased BP. **Hydrochlorothiazide** (HCTZ) increases chloride, sodium, and water excretion by interfering with transport of sodium ions across renal tubular epithelium. It is indicated in the treatment of hypertension.

TEMAZEPAM (Restoril capsules 7.5 mg, capsules 15 mg, capsules 22.5 mg, capsules 30 mg)

Temazepam is a benzodiazepine, which potentiates action of GABA (gamma-aminobutyric acid), an inhibitory neurotransmitter, resulting in increased neuronal inhibition and CNS depression, especially in the limbic system and reticular formation.

Temazepam (15 to 30 mg p.o. 30 minutes before bedtime) is indicated in the treatment of insomnia.

Temazepam depresses the CNS at the limbic and subcortical levels of the brain. It produces a sedative-hypnotic effect by potentiating the effect of the neurotransmitter gamma-aminobutyric acid (GABA) on its receptor in the ascending reticular activating system, which increases inhibition and blocks both cortical and limbic arousal (see Table 9 and Figure 50).

Temazepam is metabolized principally by conjugation, though a minor metabolic pathway involves its *N*-demethylation to oxazepam. The absorption of temazepam is complete but may depend greatly on the pharmaceutical preparation used. Protein binding with temazepam is 96 to 98%, and the elimination half-life varies between 8 and 13 hours.

Temazepam potentiates the CNS depressant effects of phenothiazines, narcotics, antihistamines, monoamine oxidase inhibitors, barbiturates, alcohol, general anesthetics, and antidepressants.

Heavy smoking accelerates temazepam metabolism, thus lowering clinical effectiveness. Benzodiazepines block the therapeutic effects of levodopa. Temazepam may decrease plasma levels of haloperidol.

Clinical manifestations of overdose include somnolence, confusion, hypoactivity or absent reflexes, dyspnea, labored breathing, hypotension, bradycardia, slurred speech, unsteady gait or impaired coordination, and ultimately, coma.

Flumazenil, a specific benzodiazepine antagonist, may be useful.

TEMOZOLOMIDE
(Temodar capsules 5 mg, capsules 20 mg, capsules 100 mg, capsules 250 mg)

Temozolomide is an imidazotetrazine derivative. Temozolomide is a prodrug that undergoes rapid nonenzymatic conversion to the reactive compound MTIC. Cytotoxicity and antiproliferative activity against tumor cells are thought to be primarily caused by alkylation (methylation) of specific guanine-rich areas of DNA that initiates transcription. It is indicated for refractory anaplastic astrocytoma; and treatment of newly diagnosed glioblastoma multiforme concomitantly with radiotherapy and then as maintenance treatment.

Temozolomide (Temodar) is a recently introduced triazene that has significant activity in patients with malignant gliomas, where it is the standard agent in combination with radiation therapy. **Temozolomide**, like **dacarbazine**, forms the methylating metabolite MTIC and kills cells in all phases of the cell cycle.

Temozolomide is administered orally and its bioavailability approaches 100%. Maximum drug concentration reaches 5 μg/mL, or about 10 μM in plasma, approximately 1 hour after administration of a dose of 200 mg, and declines with an elimination half-life of 1.2 hours. The primary active metabolite MTIC reaches a maximum plasma concentration of 150 ng/mL 90 minutes after a dose, and declines with a half-life of 2 hours. Little intact drug is recovered in the urine, the primary urinary metabolite being the inactive imidazole carboxamide. The pharmacokinetics of temozolomide are linear over the dose range of 100 to 260 mg/m^2.

Clinical toxicity: The toxicities of **temozolomide** mirror those of dacarbazine (DTIC). The toxicity of DTIC includes nausea and vomiting in more than 90% of patients; vomiting usually develops 1 to 3 hours after treatment and may last up to 12 hours. Myelosuppression, with both leukopenia and thrombocytopenia, usually is mild to moderate. A flu-like syndrome consisting of chills, fever, malaise, and myalgias, may occur during treatment with DTIC. Hepatotoxicity, alopecia, facial flushing, neurotoxicity, and dermatologic reactions also have been reported.

TENIPOSIDE
(Vumon injection concentrate 50 mg/5 mL)

Teniposide is a podophyllotoxin derivative. Teniposide is a phase-specific cytotoxic drug, acting in the late S or early G_2 phase of the cell cycle, thus preventing cells from entering mitosis. Teniposide causes single- and double-stranded breaks in DNA and DNA:protein cross-links. The mechanism of action appears to be related to the inhibition of type II topoisomerase activity. The terminal half-life is 5 hours. The volume of distribution is 3 to 11 L in children and 8 to 44 L in adults. Renal elimination is 44%, fecal elimination is up to 10%, and 4 to 12% is excreted unchanged in the urine. **Adult**: used in refractory childhood acute lymphoblastic leukemia. **Pediatric**: used in refractory acute lymphoblastic leukemia (ALL).

Teniposide (Vumon) is administered intravenously. It has a multiphasic pattern of clearance from plasma. After distribution, half-lives of 4 hours and 10 to 40 hours are observed. Approximately 45% of the drug is excreted in the urine, but in contrast to etoposide, as much as 80% is recovered as metabolites. Anticonvulsants such as **phenytoin** increase the hepatic metabolism of teniposide and reduce systemic exposure. Dosage does not need to be reduced for patients with impaired renal function.

Teniposide is available for treatment of refractory ALL in children and appears to be synergistic with cytarabine. It is administered by intravenous infusion in doses that range from 50 mg/m^2 per day for 5 days to 165 mg/m^2 per day twice weekly. The clinical spectrum of activity includes acute leukemia in children, particularly monocytic leukemia in infants, as well as glioblastoma, neuroblastoma, and brain metastases from small cell carcinomas of the lung. Myelosuppression, nausea, and vomiting are its primary toxic effects.

Teniposide, a podophyllotoxin with antineoplastic properties, is indicated in acute lymphocytic leukemia in childhood.

TENOFOVIR DISOPROXIL FUMARATE
(Viread tablets 300 mg (equivalent to tenofovir disoproxil 245 mg))

Tenofovir disoproxil fumarate is a nucleotide analog reverse transcriptase inhibitor. Tenofovir disoproxil fumarate is a prodrug of tenofovir, which inhibits the activity of HIV-1 reverse transcriptase by competing with deoxyadenosine 5′-triphosphate and by DNA chain termination after incorporation into DNA. It is indicated in the treatment of HIV-1 infection in combination with other antiretroviral agents.

The HIV-encoded, RNA-dependent DNA polymerase, also called **reverse transcriptase**, converts viral RNA into proviral DNA that is then incorporated into a host cell chromosome. Available inhibitors of this enzyme are either nucleoside/nucleotide analogs or nonnucleoside inhibitors.

Like all available antiretroviral drugs, nucleoside and nucleotide reverse transcriptase inhibitors prevent infection of susceptible cells but have no impact on cells that already harbor HIV. Nucleoside and nucleotide analogs must enter cells and undergo phosphorylation to generate synthetic substrates for the enzyme. The fully phosphorylated analogs block replication of the viral genome both by competitively inhibiting incorporation of native nucleotides and by terminating elongation of nascent proviral DNA because they lack a 3-hydroxyl group.

All but one of the drugs in this class are nucleosides that must be triphosphorylated at the 5′-hydroxyl to exert activity. The sole exception, **tenofovir**, is a nucleotide monophosphate analog that requires two additional phosphates to acquire full activity. These compounds inhibit both HIV-1 and HIV-2, and several have broad-spectrum activity against other human and animal retroviruses; **emtricitabine**, **lamivudine**, **zalcitabine**, and **tenofovir** are active against hepatitis B virus (HBV) *in vitro*, and tenofovir also has activity against herpes viruses.

The selective toxicity of these drugs depends on their ability to inhibit the HIV reverse transcriptase without inhibiting host cell DNA polymerases. Although the intracellular triphosphates for all these drugs have low affinity for human DNA polymerase-α and -β, some are capable of inhibiting human DNA polymerase-γ which is the mitochondrial enzyme. As a result, the important toxicities common to this class of drugs result in part from the inhibition of mitochondrial DNA synthesis. These toxicities include anemia, granulocytopenia, myopathy, peripheral neuropathy, and pancreatitis. Lactic acidosis with or without hepatomegaly and hepatic steatosis is a rare but potentially fatal complication seen with stavudine, zidovudine, didanosine, and zalcitabine; it is probably not associated independently with the other drugs. Phosphorylated emtricitabin, lamivudine, and tenofovir have low affinity for DNA polymerase-γ and are largely devoid of mitochondrial toxicity.

Tenofovir is a derivative of adenosine 5′-monophosphate lacking a complete ribose ring and is the only nucleotide analog currently marketed for the treatment of HIV infection. Because the parent compound had very poor oral bioavailability, tenofovir is available only as the disoproxil fumarate prodrug, which has improved oral absorption and cellular penetration substantially. Like lamivudine and emtricitabine, tenofovir is active against HIV-1, HIV-2, and HBV. The IC_{50} of tenofovir disoproxil fumarate against laboratory strains of HIV-1 ranges from 2 to 7 nM, making the prodrug about 100-fold more active *in vitro* than the parent compound.

Tenofovir disoproxil fumarate is hydrolyzed rapidly to tenofovir and then is phosphorylated by cellular kinases to its active metabolite, tenofovir diphosphate; the active moiety is, in fact, a triphosphate compound because the parent drug starts out as the monophosphate. The intracellular diphosphate is a competitive inhibitor of viral reverse transcriptases and is incorporated into HIV DNA to cause chain termination because it has an incomplete ribose ring. Although **tenofovir** diphosphate has broad-spectrum activity against viral DNA polymerases, it has low affinity for human DNA polymerases-α, -β, and -γ, which is the basis for its selective toxicity.

Tenofovir disoproxil fumarate has an oral bioavailability of 25%. A high-fat meal increases the oral bioavailability to 39%, but the drug can be taken without regard to food. Tenofovir is not bound significantly to plasma proteins. The plasma elimination half-life ranges from 14 to 17 hours. The reported half-life of intracellular tenofovir diphosphate is 11 hours in activated peripheral blood mononuclear cells and 49 hours or longer in resting cells. The drug, therefore, can be dosed once daily. Tenofovir undergoes both glomerular filtration and active tubular secretion. Between 70% and 80% of an intravenous dose of tenofovir is recovered unchanged in the urine. Doses should be decreased in those with renal insufficiency.

Tenofovir generally is well tolerated, with few significant adverse effects reported except for flatulence. In placebo-controlled, double-blinded trials, the drug had no other adverse effects reported more frequently than with placebo after treatment for up to 24 weeks; tenofovir was significantly less toxic than stavudine. Unlike the antiviral nucleotides adefovir and cidofovir, **tenofovir** is not toxic to human renal tubular cells *in vitro*. However, rare episodes of acute renal failure and **Fanconi's syndrome** have been reported with tenofovir, and this drug should be used with caution in patients with preexisting renal disease. Because tenofovir also has activity against HBV and may lower plasma HBV DNA concentrations, caution is warranted in using this drug in patients coinfected with HBV: discontinuation of tenofovir may be associated with a rebound of HBV replication and exacerbation of hepatitis.

Tenofovir is not metabolized to a significant extent by CYPs and is not known to inhibit or induce these enzymes. However, tenofovir has been associated with a few potentially important pharmacokinetic drug interactions. A 300-mg dose of tenofovir increased the didanosine AUC by 44 to 60% probably as a consequence of inhibition of the enzyme purine nucleoside phosphorylase by both tenofovir and tenofovir monophosphate. These two drugs probably should not be used together, or if this is essential, the dose of didanosine should be reduced from 400 to 250 mg/day.

Although tenofovir is not known to induce CYPs, it has been reported to reduce the atazanavir AUC by approximately 26%. In addition, low-dose ritonavir (100 mg twice daily) increases the tenofovir AUC by 34%, and atazanavir increases the tenofovir AUC by 25%. The mechanism of these interactions is unknown.

Tenofovir is FDA approved for treating HIV infection in adults in combination with other antiretroviral agents. The use of tenofovir in antiretroviral-experienced patients resulted in a further sustained decrease in HIV plasma RNA concentrations of 4.5 to 7.4 times relative to placebo after 48 weeks of treatment. Several large trials have confirmed the antiretroviral activity of tenofovir in three-drug regimens with other agents, including other nucleoside analogs, protease inhibitors, and/or NNRTIs. In a randomized, double-blind comparison trial in which treatment-naive patients also received lamivudine and efavirenz, tenofovir 300 mg once daily was as effective and less toxic than stavudine 40 mg twice daily.

TERAZOSIN HYDROCHLORIDE (Hytrin)

Terazosin (initially 1 mg at bedtime) alone or in combination with other antihypertensive agents such as diuretics or beta-adrenergic-receptor-blocking agents is indicated in the management of hypertension.

In addition, terazosin is used in the symptomatic treatment of benign prostatic hyperplasia. It improves urinary flow.

Terazosin has a peripheral postsynaptic $alpha_1$-adrenergic-blocking action, which is thought to account primarily for its effects (see Figure 37).

Terazosin produces vasodilation and reduces peripheral resistance but generally has little effect on cardiac output. Antihypertensive effect with chronic dosing is usually not accompanied by reflex tachycardia. There is little or no effect on renal blood flow or glomerular filtration rate.

Relaxation of smooth muscle in the bladder neck, prostate, and prostate capsule produced by $alpha_1$-adrenergic blockade results in a reduction in urethral resistance and pressure, bladder outlet resistance, and urinary symptoms.

Terazosin may affect serum lipids. The most consistent changes observed are a decrease in levels of serum total cholesterol and low density lipoprotein (LDL) cholesterol plus very-low-density lipoprotein (VLDL) cholesterol fraction.

A "first-dose orthostatic hypotensive reaction" sometimes occurs, most frequently 30 minutes to 2 hours after the initial dose of terazosin, and may be severe. Syncope or other postural symptoms, such as dizziness, may occur. Subsequent occurrence with dosage increases is also possible. Incidence appears to be dose-related; thus, it is important that therapy be initiated with a 1 mg dose given at bedtime. Patients who are volume-depleted or sodium-restricted may be more sensitive to the orthostatic hypotensive effects of terazosin, and the effect may be exaggerated after exercise.

TERBINAFINE (Lamisil tablets 250 mg, Lamisil AT cream 1%)

Terbinafine is an infective/antifungal agent that inhibits squalene epoxidase, resulting in ergosterol deficiency and a corresponding accumulation of squalene within the fungal cell leading to fungal cell death. It is indicated in the treatment of onychomycosis of the toenail or fingernail caused by dermatophytes. **Topical**: used in interdigital tinea pedis, tinea cruris, or tinea corporis caused by *E. floccosum*, *T. mentagrophytes*, or *T. rubrum*.

Terbinafine is a synthetic allylamine, structurally similar to the topical agent naftifine.

Terbinafine is well absorbed, but bioavailability is decreased to about 40% because of first-pass metabolism in the liver. Proteins bind more than 99% of the drug in plasma. Drug accumulates in skin, nails, and fat. The initial half-life is about 12 hours but extends to 200 to 400 hours at steady state. Drug can be found in plasma for 4 to 8 weeks after prolonged therapy. Terbinafine is not recommended in patients with marked azotemia or hepatic failure, because in the latter condition, **terbinafine** plasma levels are increased by unpredictable amounts. **Rifampin** decreases and **cimetidine** increases plasma **terbinafine** concentrations. The drug is well tolerated, with a low incidence of gastrointestinal distress, headache, or rash. Rarely, hepatotoxicity, severe neutropenia, **Stevens–Johnson syndrome**, or toxic epidermal necrolysis may occur. The drug is contraindicated in pregnancy. It is recommended that systemic terbinafine therapy for onychomycosis be postponed until after pregnancy is complete. Its mechanism of action is probably inhibition of fungal squalene epoxidase, blocking ergosterol biosynthesis.

Terbinafine (Lamisil), given as one 250-mg tablet daily, is at least as effective for nail onychomycosis as 200 mg daily of itraconazole, and slightly more effective than pulse itraconazole therapy (see above). Duration of treatment varies, with the site being treated but typically is 3 months. Although not approved for this use, terbinafine (250 mg daily) also is effective in ringworm elsewhere on the body. No pediatric formulation is available, so there is little experience with the drug in tinea capitis, usually a disease of children.

Terbinafine 1% cream or spray is applied twice daily and is effective in tinea corporis, tinea cruris, and tinea pedis. Terbinafine is less active against *Candida* species and *Malassezia furfur*, but the cream also can be used in cutaneous candidiasis and tinea versicolor. In European studies, oral terbinafine has appeared to be effective in treatment of ringworm, and in some cases of onychomycosis. The systemic use of terbinafine is discussed above.

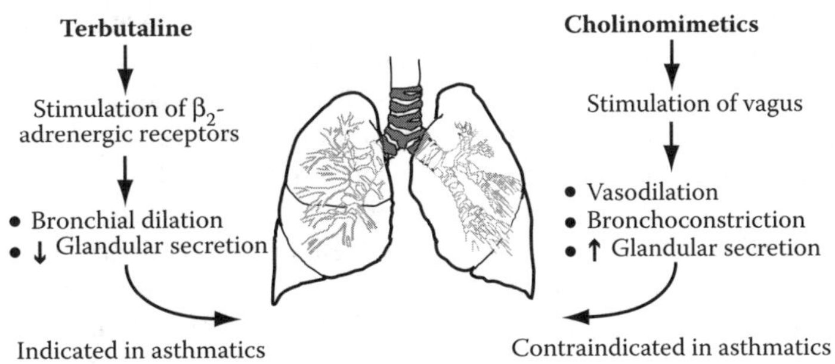

FIGURE 94 The selective beta$_2$-adrenergic stimulants cause bronchodilation without cardiac acceleration. **Metaproterenol** and **terbutaline** are available in tablet form, and terbutaline is also available for subcutaneous injection. Metaproterenol and albuterol are available in metered-dose inhalers.

TERBUTALINE SULFATE
(Brethine)

Terbutaline, a bronchodilator (5 mg given p.o. at 6 hour intervals 3 times during waking hours), is indicated for relief of bronchospasm in patients with reversible obstructive airway disease (see Figure 94); and terbutaline, a tocolytic agent (10 mcg/minutes IV), is also used in managing premature labor.

Terbutaline acts directly on beta$_2$-adrenergic receptors to relax bronchial smooth muscle, relieving bronchospasm and reducing airway resistance. Cardiac and CNS stimulation may occur with high doses.

When used in premature labor, it relaxes uterine smooth muscle, which in turn inhibits uterine contractions.

Terbutaline is contraindicated in patients with diabetes, hypertension, hyperthyroidism, or cardiac disease (especially when associated with arrhythmias).

When used concomitantly with other sympathomimetics, terbutaline may potentiate the adverse cardiovascular effects of the other drugs; however, as an aerosol bronchodilator (adrenergic-stimulator type), concomitant use may relieve acute bronchospasm in patients on long-term oral terbutaline therapy.

Beta-blockers may antagonize the bronchodilating effects of terbutaline. Use of monoamine oxidase inhibitors within 14 days of terbutaline or the concomitant use of tricyclic antidepressants may potentiate terbutaline's effects on the vascular system.

TERCONAZOLE
(Femstat, Terazol 3, Terazol 7, Terazol 3, vaginal cream 0.8%, vaginal suppositories 80 mg, Terazole 7 vaginal cream 0.4%)

Terconazole is a vaginal antifungal agent. It alters permeability of fungus cell membrane, allowing leakage of essential intracellular components. Terconazole and butoconazole nitrate (Femstat) are available as a 2% vaginal cream for local treatment of vulvovaginal candidiasis (moniliasis). These drugs are used at bedtime for 3 days in nonpregnant females. There is a slower response during pregnancy, which requires a 6-day course of treatment.

Terconazole (Terazol, others) is a ketal triazole with structural similarities to ketoconazole. The mechanism of action of terconazole is similar to that of the imidazoles. The 80-mg vaginal suppository is inserted at bedtime for 3 days, whereas the 0.4% vaginal cream is used for 7 days and the 0.8% cream for 3 days. Clinical efficacy and patient acceptance of both preparations are at least as good as for clotrimazole in patients with vaginal candidiasis.

TERFENADINE
(Seldane)

Terfenadine, an H_1-histamine receptor antagonist (60 mg p.o. q. 8 to 12 hours), is indicated for the treatment of rhinitis and symptoms associated with allergy.

Terfenadine, astemizole, loratadine, and cetirizine are second-generation antihistaminic agents that are relatively nonsedating. Other H_1-receptor antagonists currently undergoing clinical trials are azelastine, ebastine, and levocabastine.

Terfenadine, like other antihistamines, compete with histamine for histamine H_1-receptor sites on the smooth muscle of the bronchi, GI tract, uterus, and large blood vessels. By binding to cellular receptors, they prevent access of histamine and suppress histamine-induced allergic symptoms, even though they do not prevent its release.

Inhaled selective beta$_2$-adrenergic-receptor agonists (albuterol, terbutaline, fenoterol, and bitolterol) have a rapid onset of action and are effective for 3 to 6 hours. Formoterol and salmeterol are longer-acting agents (12 hours) and may prove useful in treating nocturnal symptoms.

Terfenadine is absorbed well from the GI tract, distributed mainly into the lungs, liver, GI tract, spleen, and bile; lower concentrations have been detected in the blood, kidneys, and heart. Terfenadine does not cross the blood–brain barrier and hence causes no sedation. It becomes bound to plasma proteins to the extent of 97%, is metabolized in the liver, and the metabolites are excreted in the feces (60%) and urine (40%).

Terfenadine is contraindicated in patients with impaired hepatic function (for example, alcoholic cirrhosis, hepatitis) or in those who take drugs such as ketoconazole, itraconazole, clarithromycin, erythromycin, troleandomycin, or other potent inhibitors of the hepatic cytochrome P450 isoenzyme. Terfenadine should not be given to patients with electrolyte abnormalities such as hypokalemia or hypomagnesemia, who take diuretics with potential for inducing electrolyte abnormalities, or who have congenital QT syndrome.

It should be used with caution in patients with asthma or other lower respiratory diseases, because its mild anticholinergic effects might aggravate these conditions. It should also be used with caution in patients with underlying cardiac disease because of the potential development of ventricular tachyarrhythmia while taking terfenadine.

Unlike other antihistamines, terfenadine has minimal anticholinergic activity and does not potentiate the CNS effects of alcohol, antianxiety agents, or other CNS depressants.

TERIPARATIDE
(Forteo injection 250 mcg/mL)

Teriparatide is a parathyroid hormone, which regulates bone metabolism, renal tubular reabsorption of calcium and phosphate, and intestinal calcium reabsorption. It is indicated in the treatment of postmenopausal women with **osteoporosis** who are at high risk for fracture (e.g., history of osteoporotic fracture); and to increase bone mass in men with primary or hypogonadal osteoporosis who are at high risk of fracture (e.g., history of osteoporotic fracture).

Continuous administration of PTH or high circulating PTH levels achieved in primary hyperparathyroidism causes bone demineralization and osteopenia. However, intermittent PTH administration promotes bone growth. Beginning in the 1970s, studies focused on the anabolic action of PTH, culminating with FDA approval of synthetic human 34-amino-acid amino-terminal PTH fragment [hPTH(l-34), **teriparatide**] for use in treating severe osteoporosis. Full-length PTH(1-84) is likely to be approved in the near future; its benefits over PTH(1-34) are unclear.

Pharmacokinetics and systemic actions of teriparatide on mineral metabolism are the same as for PTH. **Teriparatide** is administered by once-daily subcutaneous injection of 20 μg into the thigh or abdomen. With this regimen, serum PTH concentrations peak at 30 minutes after the injection and decline to undetectable concentrations within 3 hours, whereas the serum calcium concentration peaks at 4 to 6 hours after administration. Based on aggregate data from different dosing regimens, **teriparatide** bioavailability averages 95%. Teriparatide clearance averages 62 L/hour in women and 94 L/hour in men, which exceeds normal liver plasma flow, consistent with both hepatic and extrahepatic PTH removal. The serum half-life of teriparatide is approximately 1 hour when administered subcutaneously versus 5 minutes when administered intravenously. The longer half-life following subcutaneous administration reflects the time required for absorption from the injection site. The elimination of PTH(1-34) and full-length PTH proceeds by nonspecific enzymatic mechanisms in the liver, followed by renal excretion.

In postmenopausal women with osteoporosis, teriparatide increases BMD and reduces the risk of vertebral and nonvertebral fractures. Several laboratories have examined the effects of intermittent PTH on BMD in patients with osteoporosis. In these studies, **teriparatide** increased axial bone mineral, although initial reports of effects on cortical bone were disappointing. Coadministration of hPTH(l-34) with estrogen or synthetic androgen led to impressive gains in vertebral bone mass or trabecular bone. However, in some early studies there was only maintenance or even loss of cortical bone. Vitamin D insufficiency in patients at baseline or pharmacokinetic differences involving bioavailability or circulating half-life may have contributed to observed differences on cortical bone. The most comprehensive studies to date established the value of daily hPTH(l-34) administration on total BMD, with significant elevations of BMD in lumbar spine and femoral neck and with significant reductions of vertebral and nonvertebral fracture risk in osteoporotic women and men.

Candidates for **teriparatide** treatment include women who have a history of osteoporotic fracture, who have multiple risk factors for fracture, or who failed or are intolerant of previous osteoporosis therapy. Teriparatide should not be used in patients who are at increased baseline risk for **osteosarcoma** (including those with **Paget's disease of bone**, unexplained elevations of alkaline phosphatase, open epiphyses, or prior radiation therapy involving the skeleton). Full-length PTH(1-84), which is in clinical trials, has not been associated with osteosarcomas. Other adverse effects have included exacerbation of **nephrolithiasis** and elevation of serum uric acid levels.

TERPIN HYDRATE

Terpin hydrate, an aliphatic alcohol with expectorant properties (5 to 10 ml of elixir p.o. q. 4 to 6 hours), is used in excessive bronchial secretions.

TESTOLACTONE
(Teslac)

Testolactone, an androgen with antineoplastic effectiveness (250 mg p.o. q.i.d.), is used in advanced postmenopausal breast cancer.

TESTOSTERONE
(Aandro 100, Andronaq-50, Histerone, Testaqua, Testoject-50)

TESTOSTERONE CYPIONATE
(Andro-Cyp 100, Andro-Cyp 200, Andronate, dep Andro 100, dep Andro 200, Depo-Testosterone, Duratest 100, Testa-C, Testoject-LA)

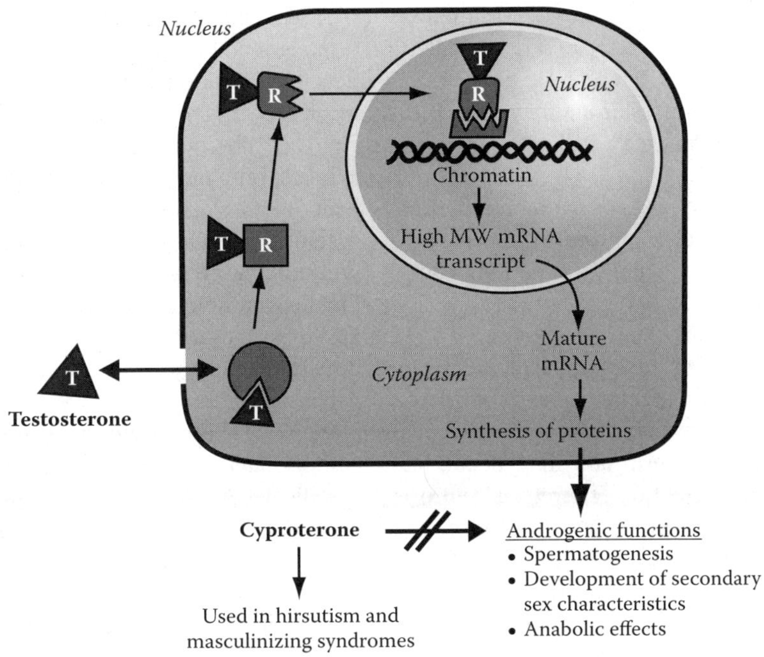

FIGURE 95 Testosterone is used in primary or hypogonadotrophic hypogonadism in men age 18 and older.

TESTOSTERONE ENANTHATE (Andro L.A. 200, Andryl, Delatestryl, Everone, Testone L.A., Testrin-P.A.)

TESTOSTERONE PROPIONATE (Testex)

Testosterone, an androgen, is used in male hypogonadism, delayed puberty in males, postpartum breast pain and engorgement, and in inoperable breast cancer (see also Table 8 and Figure 95).

TESTOSTERONE TRANSDERMAL SYSTEM (Testoderm)

Testosterone transdermal system (4 mg/day) is used in primary or hypogonadotropic hypogonadism in men age 18 and older.

Testosterone (25 to 100 mg/mL) is available in suspension, and testosterone cypionate, testosterone enanthate, and testosterone propionate are supplied in oil.

Testosterone is indicated in male hypogonadism, in delayed puberty in males, in postpartum breast pain and engorgement, and in inoperable breast cancer.

At many sites of action, testosterone is not the active form of the hormone. It is converted by steroid 5a-reductases in target tissues to the more active dihydrotestosterone. Steroid 5a-reductase 1 is located largely in nongenital skin and liver, and steroid 5a-reductase 2 is present principally in the urogenital tract of the male and in the genital skin of both sexes.

Testosterone or dihydrotestosterone binds to an intracellular protein receptor, and the hormone-receptor complex is attached in the nucleus to specific hormone regulatory elements on the chromosomes and acts to increase the synthesis of specific RNAs and proteins. The human androgen receptor is a typical member of the superfamily of steroid and thyroid hormone receptors. It is encoded by a gene on the X chromosome and contains androgen-binding, DNA-binding, and functional domains (see Figure 95).

Testosterone, the male sex hormone, is responsible for the development and maintenance of the male sex organs (the penis, prostate gland, seminal vesicle, and vas deferens) and secondary sex characteristics. In addition, testosterone has anabolic effects. Similar to progesterone, testosterone is metabolized very rapidly by the liver by the first-pass mechanism, and hence requires structural modifications in order to be effective. For example, the 17–OH group of testosterone may be modified by the addition of propionic acid, which yields testosterone propionate, cyclopentylpropionic acid, which yields testosterone cypionate, or enanthate, which yields testosterone enanthate. In addition, the 17 position may be methylated to yield methyltestosterone, or a fluorine and a methyl group may be inserted to yield fluoxymesterone. In general, these agents are more effective when given orally and have a longer duration of action than testosterone itself (see also Table 8).

Testosterone and its derivatives are used in the treatment of hypogonadism (eunuchoidism), hypopituitarism, accelerated growth, aging in men, osteoporosis, anemia, endometriosis, promotion of anabolism, suppression of lactation, and breast carcinoma.

Hormonal therapy with testosterone should be reserved primarily for patients with hypogonadal disorders. There are two important warnings about the indiscriminate use of intramuscular testosterone in patients with serum testosterone levels in the normal range. First, many impotent patients are older and may have adenocarcinoma of the prostate, thus exogenous testosterone may accelerate the growth of the neoplasm. Second, although testosterone may induce a marked increase in libido, patients may still be unable to achieve adequate erection.

Although hypogonadism and sexual dysfunction are common in alcoholic cirrhotic males, currently there are no effective medications to treat the sexual dysfunction. Vitamin A therapy has not proved effective.

One of the side effects of testosterone compounds is masculinization in women (such as hirsutism, acne, depression of menses, and clitoral enlargement) and of their female offspring. Therefore, androgens are contraindicated in pregnant women. Prostatic hypertrophy may occur in males, which leads to urinary retention. Therefore, androgens are contraindicated in men with prostatic carcinoma.

Cyproterone inhibits the action of androgens (see Figure 95), and gossypol prevents spermatogenesis without altering the other endocrine functions of the testis.

TETANUS AND DIPHTHERIA TOXOIDS (ADULT STRENGTH, TD)

Tetanus and diphtheria toxoids induce antibodies against toxins made by *Corynebacterium diphtherias* and *Clostridium tetani*. It is indicated for achievement of active immunity against diphtheria and tetanus. Tetanus and diphtheria toxoids (Td) for adult use are the preferred agents for immunizing most adults and children after 7 years.

Immunization may be active or passive. **Active immunization** involves stimulation with an antigen to develop immunologic defenses against a future exposure. **Passive immunization** involves administration of preformed antibodies to an individual who is already exposed or is about to be exposed to an antigen.

Active immunization, vaccination, involves administration of an antigen as a whole, killed organism, attenuated (live) organism, or a specific protein or peptide constituent of an organism. Booster doses often are required, especially when killed (inactivated) organisms are used as the immunogen. In the United States, vaccination has sharply curtailed or practically eliminated a variety of major infections, including diphtheria, measles, mumps, pertussis, rubella, **tetanus**, *Haemophilus influenzae* type b, and pneumococcus.

Although most vaccines have targeted infectious disease, a new generation of vaccines may provide complete or limited protection from specific cancers or autoimmune diseases. Because T-cells optimally are activated by peptides and costimulatory ligands, both of which are present on antigen-presenting cells (APCs), one approach for vaccination has consisted of immunizing patients with APCs expressing a tumor antigen. The first generation of anticancer vaccines used whole cancer cells or tumor-cell lysates as a source of antigen in combination with various adjuvants, relying on host APCs to process and present **tumor-specific antigens**.

These anticancer vaccines resulted in occasional clinical responses and are being tested in prospective clinical trials. Second generation anticancer vaccines utilized specific APCs incubated *ex vivo* with antigen or transduced to express antigen and subsequently reinfused into patients. In laboratory animals, immunization with dendritic cells previously pulsed with MHC class I-restricted peptides derived from tumor-specific antigens led to pronounced antitumor cytotoxic T-lymphocyte responses and protective tumor immunity. Finally, multiple studies have demonstrated the efficacy of DNA vaccines in small-arid large-animal models of infectious diseases and cancer. The advantage of **DNA vaccination** over peptide immunization is that it permits generation of entire proteins, enabling determinant selection to occur in the host without having to restrict immunization to patients bearing specific HLA alleles. However, a safety concern about this technique is the potential for integration of the plasmid DNA into the host genome, possibly disrupting important genes and thereby leading to phenotypic mutations or carcinogenicity. A final approach to generate or enhance immune responses against specific antigens consists of infecting cells with recombinant viruses that encode the protein antigen of interest. Different types of viral vectors that can infect mammalian cells, such as vaccinia, avipox, lentivirus, adenovirus or adenovirus-associated virus, have been used.

Passive immunization is indicated when an individual is deficient in antibodies because of a congenital or acquired immunodeficiency, when an individual with a high degree of risk is exposed to an agent and there is inadequate time for active immunization (e.g., measles, rabies, hepatitis B), or when a disease is already present but can be ameliorated by passive antibodies (e.g., botulism, diphtheria, tetanus). Passive immunization may be provided by several different products. Nonspecific immunoglobulins or highly specific immunoglobulins may be provided based upon the indication. The protection provided usually lasts from 1 to 3 months. Immune globulin is derived from pooled plasma of adults by an alcohol-fractionation procedure. It contains largely IgG (95%) and is indicated for antibody-deficiency disorders, exposure to infections such as hepatitis A and measles, and specific immunologic diseases such as **immune thrombocytopenic purpura** and **Guillain-Barre syndrome**. In contrast, specific immune globulins ("hyperimmune") differ from other immune globulin preparations in that donors are selected for high titers of the desired antibodies.

TETANUS IMMUNE GLOBULIN, (TIG) (Hyper-Tet, Baytet solution 250 units/syringe)

Tetanus immune globulin is an immune globulin, which directly neutralizes toxin excreted by *Clostridium tetani*. It is indicated as a passive, transient protection against tetanus in any person that may be contaminated with tetanus spores when: (1) a patient's personal history of immunization with tetanus toxoid is unknown or uncertain, (2) a person received less than 2 a prior doses of tetanus toxoid, or (3) a person received 2 prior doses of tetanus toxoid, but a delay of more than 24 hours occurred between the time of injury and initiation of tetanus prophylaxis. This tetanus prophylaxis agent is used in primary immunization (absorbed formulation), primary immunization (fluid formulation), and tetanus prophylaxis in wound management.

Tetanus immune globulin, an immune serum with tetanus prophylaxis effectiveness, is used in tetanus exposure and tetanus treatment.

TETRACYCLINES

Tetracyclines, which are bacteriostatic, have the broadest spectrum of activity and are effective against infections with Gram-positive and Gram-negative bacteria: *Rickettsia*, *Mycoplasma*, amoeba, and *Chlamydia*. These agents consist of:

Tetracycline (Achromycin and Panmycin)
Chlortetracycline (Aureomycin)
Oxytetracycline (Terramycin)
Demeclocycline (Declomycin)
Doxycycline (Vibramycin)
Minocycline (Minocin and Vectrin)
Methacycline (Rondomycin) (see Figure 96)

Tetracyclines enter bacterial cells by both passive diffusion and active transport, and then accumulate intracellularly. This does not occur in mammalian cells. The tetracyclines bind to the 30S subunit of the bacterial ribosome in such a way that the binding of the aminoacyl-transfer RNA to the acceptor site on the messenger RNA ribosome complex is blocked.

The resistant mutant bacteria do not transport or accumulate tetracycline. This plasmid-controlled resistance is transmitted by transduction or by conjugation.

Structural formulas of the tetracyclines

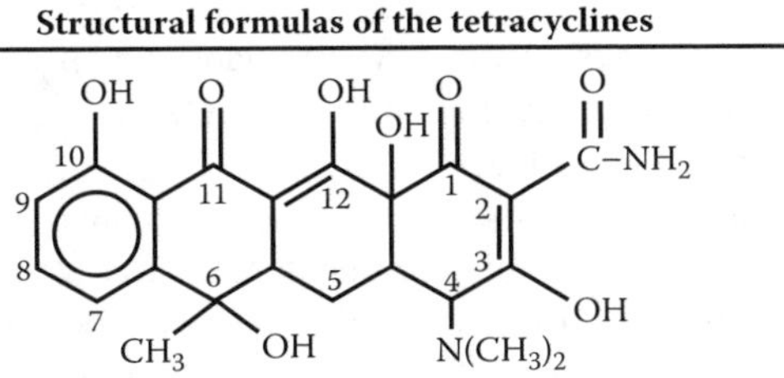

Tetracycline

Congeners	Substituent(S)	Position(S)
Chlortetracycline	–CI	(7)
Oxytetracycline	–OH, –H	(5)
Demeclocycline	–OH, –H; –C	(6; 7)
Methacycline	–OH, –H; = CH_2	(5; 6)
Doxycycline	–OH, –H; –CH_3, –H	(5; 6)
Minocycline	–H, –H; –$N(CH_3)_2$	(5; 7)

FIGURE 96 Tetracyclines, which are bacteriostatic, have the broadest spectrum of activity and are effective against infections with Gram-positive and Gram-negative bacteria, *Rickettsia*, *Mycoplasma*, amoeba, and *Chlamydia*.

The absorption of tetracyclines from the gastrointestinal tract is nonuniform. Up to 30% of chlortetracycline is absorbed. The absorption for tetracycline, oxytetracycline, and demeclocycline ranges between 60 and 80%, whereas as much as 90 to 100% of doxycycline and minocycline is absorbed. The unabsorbed tetracycline may modify the intestinal flora. The absorption of tetracyclines is impaired by divalent cations (calcium, magnesium, and ferrous iron), by aluminum, and by extremely alkaline pHs. Tetracyclines are distributed widely throughout the body fluid, cross the placental barrier, and can accumulate in growing bones. The concentrations of chlortetracycline in spinal fluid are only one-fourth of those in plasma. Minocycline, a more lipid-soluble tetracycline, reaches a high concentration in tears and saliva and can eradicate the meningococcal carrier state. The tetracyclines are metabolized in the liver and excreted mainly by the bile and urine. The concentrations of tetracyclines in the bile are ten times higher than those in serum.

Tetracyclines are effective in the treatment of Rocky Mountain spotted fever, murine typhus, recrudescent epidemic typhus, scrub typhus, Q fever, lymphogranuloma venereum, psittacosis, tularemia, brucellosis, gonorrhea, certain urinary tract infections, granuloma inguinale, chancroid, syphilis, and disease due to *Bacteroides* and *Clostridium*.

Tetracyclines in general cause toxic and hypersensitivity reactions. These consist commonly of gastrointestinal irritations that are disabling and may necessitate discontinuation of the medications. With continuous usage, tetracyclines may alter the normal flora, allowing the growth of *Pseudomonas*, *Proteus*, staphylococci-resistant coliforms, *Clostridium*, and *Candida* organisms. These superinfections should be recognized and treated appropriately with vancomycin (see Figure 96) and other drugs.

Tetracyclines have been known to cause hepatic necrosis, especially when given in large intravenous doses or when taken by pregnant women or patients with preexisting liver impairment.

Tetracycline preparations whose potency has expired can cause renal tubular acidosis. With the exception of doxycycline, tetracyclines accumulate in patients with renal impairment. Tetracyclines also produce nitrogen retention, especially when given with diuretics.

The systemic administration of demeclocycline elicits photosensitization to ultraviolet light or sunlight. Minocycline causes vertigo and dizziness. The intravenous administration of tetracyclines has been observed to cause venous thrombosis.

Tetracyclines bind to calcium and then become deposited in bone, causing damage to developing bone and teeth.

TETRACYCLINES

Chlortetracycline	Minocycline
Demeclocycline	Oxytetracycline
Doxycycline	Tetracycline
Methacycline	

TETRAHYDROZOLINE HYDROCHLORIDE (Collyrium Fresh, Murine Plus, Ocu-Drop, Soothe, Tyzine Pediatric, Visine)

Tetrahydrozoline, a sympathomimetic agent with vasoconstrictor properties, is used in nasal congestion and conjunctival congestion.

TETRANDRINE

Tetrandrine, a traditional medicinal alkaloid, has been used in China for the treatment of hypertension, cardiac arrhythmia, and angina pectoris. Recently, it has been shown that tetrandrine blocks voltage activated L-type Ca^{++} channels in a variety of excitable cells including cardiac tissue. The binding site of tetrandrine is located at the benzothiazepine receptor on the a_1-subunit of the channel. It is clear that tetrandrine's actions in the treatment of cardiovascular diseases, including hypertension and supraventricular arrhythmia, are due primarily to its blocking of voltage activated L-type and T-type Ca^{++} channels.

THALIDOMIDE (Thalomid capsules 50 mg)

Thalidomide is an immunomodulator that is indicated for acute treatment of cutaneous manifestations of moderate to severe **erythema nodosum leprosum** (ENL); and maintenance therapy for prevention and suppression of cutaneous manifestations of ENL recurrence.

Thalidomide originally was developed in the 1950s for the treatment of pregnancy-associated morning sickness, but withdrawn from the market due to the tragic consequences of teratogenicity and dysmyelia (**stunted limb growth**). However, it has since been reintroduced to clinical practice, initially because of its clinical efficacy as an oral agent for the management of **erythema nodosum leprosum**, which the FDA approved in 1998. Meanwhile, the realization of thalidomide's antiangiogenic and immunomodulatory effects, including the inhibition of TNF-α signaling, triggered an expansion of thalidomide uses in other disease settings, most notably **multiple myeloma** (MM). Indeed, significant clinical experience has been acquired on the activity of thalidomide in both newly diagnosed and heavily pretreated relapsed/refractory MM patients. In addition, **thalidomide** has shown clinical activity in patients with **myelodysplastic syndromes** and ongoing clinical studies are addressing the potential role of thalidomide in the therapeutic management of other neoplasias. Although the precise mechanism(s) of antitumor activity of thalidomide remain(s) to be fully elucidated, substantial insight has been generated by extensive preclinical studies in MM. New analogs derived from thalidomide now are in clinical trials for MM and myelodysplasia.

Thalidomide exists at physiologic pH as a nonpolar racemic mixture of cell-permeable and rapidly interconverting S(-) and R(+) isomers, the former being associated with the teratogenic, and the latter with the sedative properties of **thalidomide**. **Thalidomide** absorption from the GI tract is slow and highly variable (4 hours mean time to reach peak concentration [t_{max}], with a range of 1 to 7 hours). Thalidomide is widely distributed throughout most tissues and organs, without significant binding to plasma proteins, and with a large apparent volume of distribution (V_d). Importantly, thalidomide is detected in the semen of patients after a period of 4 weeks of therapy, with levels that correlate with serum levels. **Thalidomide** metabolism via the hepatic CYP system is limited, and no induction of its own metabolism is noted with prolonged use. However, thalidomide undergoes rapid and spontaneous nonenzymatic hydrolytic cleavage at physiologic pH, generating >50 metabolites, most of which are unstable *in vitro* or *in vivo*. Importantly, there are substantial species-specific differences in the patterns and profiles of thalidomide metabolites in mice compared with humans, which likely explains why teratogenicity of thalidomide was not detected in preclinical murine models.

Elimination of **thalidomide** is mainly by spontaneous hydrolysis, which occurs in all body fluids, with an apparent mean clearance of 10 L/hour for the (R)-enantiomer and 21 L/hour for the (S)-enantiomer in adult subjects. This leads to higher blood concentrations of the (R)-enantiomer compared to those of the (S)-enantiomer. Thalidomide and its metabolites appear to be rapidly excreted in the urine, whereas the nonabsorbed portion of the drug is excreted unchanged in feces, but clearance is primarily nonrenal. Studies of both single and multiple dosing of thalidomide in elderly prostate cancer patients showed significantly longer half-life at higher doses (1200 mg daily) versus lower doses (200 mg daily). Conversely, no effect of increased age on elimination half-life was identified in the age range of 55 to 80 years. The impact of renal or hepatic dysfunction on thalidomide clearance remains to be fully elucidated.

Thalidomide's interactions with other drugs have not been systematically addressed, except for lack of significant interaction with oral contraceptives and **thalidomide's** effect in enhancing the sedative effects of barbiturates and alcohol and the catatonic effects of chlorpromazine and reserpine. Conversely, CNS stimulants (such as methamphetamine and methylphenidate) counteract the depressant effects of thalidomide.

Lenalidomide constitutes a lead compound in the new class of immunomodulatory thalidomide derivatives (IMIDs) and exhibits a constellation of pharmacological properties, including stimulation of T-cells and NK-cells, inhibition of angiogenesis and tumor cell proliferation, and modulation of hematopoietic stem-cell differentiation. This orally administered agent has been tested in MM, myelodysplastic syndrome, and an expanding array of other clinical settings, because of preclinical data suggesting more potent activity than its parent compound, as well as less toxicity and a lack of teratogenic effects as compared to thalidomide. Lenalidomide is rapidly absorbed following oral administration, with peak-plasma levels occurring between 0.6 and 1.5 hours postdose. The C_{max} and AUC values increased proportionately with an increasing dose, both over a single-dose range of 5 to

400 mg and after multiple dosing with 100 mg daily. The half-life increases with dose, from approximately 3 hours at the 5-mg dose, to approximately 9 hours at the 400-mg dose (the higher dose is believed to provide a better estimate of the half-life due to the prolonged elimination phase). Approximately 70% of the orally administered dose of lenalidomide is excreted by the kidney. Ongoing studies are characterizing the adverse-effect profile of lenalidomide use and are addressing the potential for drug interactions with other agents. More extensive clinical experience is required to determine whether lenalidomide is completely devoid of some of thalidomide's side effects.

The precise mechanisms responsible for thalidomide's clinical activity remain to be completely elucidated. Its enantiomeric interconversion and spontaneous cleavage to multiple short-lived and poorly characterized metabolites, as well as its species-specific *in vivo* metabolic activation, confound the interpretation of preclinical *in vitro* and *in vivo* mechanistic studies. At least four distinct, but potentially complementary, mechanisms have been proposed to explain the antitumor activity of thalidomide and its derivatives: (1) direct antiproliferative/proapoptotic antitumor effects, probably mediated by one or more metabolites of thalidomide, that include inhibition of the transcriptional activity of NF-κB and its antiapoptotic target genes, including the caspase inhibitors FLIP, cIAP-2 (cellular inhibitor of apoptosis-2), or the antiapoptotic Bcl-2 family member Al/Bfl-1; (2) indirect targeting of tumor cells by abrogation of the protection conferred to tumor cells by their cell-adhesion-molecule or cytokine (e.g., IL-6)-mediated interactions with bone marrow stromal cells; (3) inhibition of cytokine production, release, and signaling, leading to antiangiogenic effects; and (4) immunomodulatory effects, including enhanced natural killer (NK) cell-mediated cytotoxicity against tumor cells, contributing to potentiated antitumor immune response. It is conceivable that because NF-κB protects MM cells from the proapoptotic effects of steroids or cytotoxic chemotherapeutics, the inhibitory effect of thalidomide and its derivatives on NF-κB activity could account for the ability of its combination with dexamethasone or cytotoxic chemotherapeutics to achieve synergistic antitumor responses.

Generally, **thalidomide** is well tolerated at doses below 200 mg daily. The most common adverse effects reported in cancer patients are sedation and constipation, while the most serious one is treatment-emergent peripheral sensory neuropathy, which occurs in 10 to 30% of patients with MM or other malignancies in a dose- and time-dependent manner. **Thalidomide-related neuropathy** is an asymmetric, painful, peripheral paresthesia with sensory loss, commonly presenting with numbness of toes and feet, muscle cramps, weakness, signs of pyramidal tract involvement, and carpal tunnel syndrome. The incidence of peripheral neuropathy increases with higher cumulative doses of thalidomide, especially in elderly patients. Although clinical improvement typically occurs upon prompt drug discontinuation, long-standing residual sensory loss can occur. Particular caution should be applied in cancer patients with preexisting neuropathy (e.g., related to diabetes) or prior exposure to drugs that can cause peripheral neuropathy (e.g., vinca alkaloids or bortezomib), especially since there has been little progress in defining effective strategies to alleviate neuropathic symptoms. An increasing incidence of thromboembolic events in thalidomide-treated patients has been reported, but mostly in the context of thalidomide combinations with other drugs, including steroids and particularly anthracycline-based chemotherapy, and with very low incidence with single-agent thalidomide treatment.

THEOPHYLLINE
(Aerolate, Bronkodyl, Constant-T, Elixophylin, Slo-bid, Slo-Phyllin, Somophyllin-T, Sustaire, Theobid, Theoclear, Theo-Dur, Theolair, Theophyl, Theospan-SR, Theo-24, Theovent, Uniphyl)

THEOPHYLLINE SODIUM GLYCINATE
(Synophylate)

Theophylline, a bronchodilator, is indicated for the symptomatic relief of bronchospasm in patients not currently receiving theophylline who require rapid relief of acute symptoms and for prophylaxis of bronchial asthma, bronchospasm of chronic bronchitis, and emphysema (see also Figure 94).

The methylxanthines consist of aminophylline, dyphylline, enprofylline, and pentoxifylline. Aminophylline (theophylline ethylenediamine) is the most widely used of the soluble theophyllines. Its main therapeutic effect is bronchodilation. In addition, it causes central nervous system stimulation, cardiac acceleration, diuresis, and gastric secretion. Aminophylline is available in an oral, rectal (pediatric), or intravenous solution, which is used in the treatment of status asthmaticus. Although aminophylline is a less effective bronchodilator than beta-adrenergic agonists, it is particularly useful in preventing nocturnal asthma.

Mechanisms of xanthine-induced physiologic and pharmacological effects have included (1) inhibition of phosphodiesterases, thereby increasing intracellular cyclic AMP, (2) direct effects on intracellular calcium concentration, (3) indirect effects on intracellular calcium concentrations via cell membrane hyperpolarization, (4) uncoupling of intracellular calcium increased with muscle contractile elements, and (5) antagonism of adenosine receptors. A large body of evidence suggests that adenosine receptor antagonism is the most important factor responsible for the most pharmacological effects of methylxanthines in doses that are administered therapeutically or consumed in xanthine-containing beverages.

Xanthines are biotransformed in the liver (85 to 90%) to 1,3-dimethyluric acid, 3-methylxanthine, and 1-methyluric acid; 3-methylxanthine accumulates in concentrations approximately 25% of those of theophylline.

Dyphylline, a chemical derivative of theophylline, is not a theophylline salt as are the other agents. It is about one tenth as potent as theophylline. Following oral administration, dyphylline is 68 to 82% bioavailable.

Aminoglutethimide, rifampin, barbiturates, charcoal, ketoconazole, smoking (cigarettes and marijuana), sulfinpyrazone, and sympathomimetics (beta-agonists)—all decrease the plasma levels of theophylline, whereas allopurinol, beta-blockers (nonselective), calcium-channel blockers, cimetidine, contraceptives, corticosteroids, disulfiram, ephedrine, interferon, macrolides, mexiletine, quinolones, and thiabendazole all increase the plasma levels of theophylline.

When used concomitantly, theophylline increases the excretion of lithium. Also, cimetidine, allopurinol (high dose), propranolol, erythromycin, and troleandomycin may cause an increase in serum concentrations of theophylline by decreasing the hepatic clearance. Barbiturates and phenytoin enhance hepatic clearance and hepatic metabolism of theophylline, decreasing plasma levels. Beta-adrenergic blockers exert an antagonistic pharmacologic effect.

THIABENDAZOLE
(Mintezol)

Thiabendazole, an anthelmintic (22 mg/kg t.i.d. after meals), is indicated for the treatment of strongyloidiasis (threadworm infection), cutaneous larva migrans (creeping eruption), and visceral larva migrans.

Thiabendazole is vermicidal or vermifugal against *Enterobius vermicularis* (pinworm), *Ascaris lumbricoides* (roundworm), *Strongyloides stercoralis* (threadworm), *Necator americanus* and *Ancylostoma duodenale* (hookworm), *Trichuris trichiura* (whipworm), *Ancylostoma braziliense* (dog and cat hookworm), and *Toxocara canis* and *Toxocara cati* (ascarids).

Thiabendazole's effect on larvae of *Trichinella spiralis* that have migrated to muscle is questionable. It suppresses egg and larval production and may inhibit the subsequent development of those eggs or larvae that are passed in the feces. Although the exact mechanism is unknown, the drug inhibits the helminth-specific enzyme fumarate reductase. The anthelmintic activity against *Trichuris trichiura* (whipworm) is least predictable.

Thiabendazole is absorbed rapidly from the gastrointestinal tract. It is metabolized by hydroxylation and conjugation with glucuronic acid. The commonly occurring side effects are anorexia, nausea, and dizziness. It should be used with caution in patients with decreased hepatic function.

THIAMINE HYDROCHLORIDE
(Vitamin B_1) (Biamine)

Thiamine, a water-soluble vitamin, is indicated in beriberi, anemia secondary to thiamine deficiency, polyneuritis secondary to alcoholism, pregnancy or pellagra, Wernicke's encephalopathy, and "wet beri-beri" with myocardial failure.

THIAZIDE DIURETICS

The thiazide diuretics, also called sulfonamide or benzothiadiazide diuretics, vary in their actions. For instance, the potency of hydrochlorothiazide (Hydro Diuril and Esidrix) is ten times greater than that of chlorothiazide (Diuril), but the drugs have equal efficacy. The duration of action of hydrochlorothiazide, which is 6 to 12 hours, equals that of chlorothiazide. On the other hand, chlorthalidone (Hygroton) has a duration of action lasting 48 hours. Some thiazide derivatives inhibit carbonic anhydrase, which is unrelated to their diuretic activity. Those that are active in this respect may, at sufficient doses, have the same effect on bicarbonate excretion as does acetazolamide. They cause a moderate loss of sodium (5 to 10% of the filtered load), chloride, and water, and the clearance of free water is impaired. They may cause metabolic alkalosis (resorption of bicarbonate and loss of hydrogen ions), hyperuricemia (enhanced resorption of uric acid), or hyperglycemia (due to directly inhibited insulin release and to hypokalemia).

Thiazide diuretics are used in the treatment of edema of cardiac and gastrointestinal origin and bring about a state of intravascular volume depletion. Because this depleted intravascular volume is replenished from the interstitial (edematous) sites, the thiazide diuretics should not be administered too frequently. For example, hydrochlorothiazide is given every other day and chlorthalidone is given once every 2 to 3 days (Table 25).

TABLE 25
Sites of Action of Diuretics

Drugs	Sites of Action
Sulfonamide diuretics	
Hydrochlorothiazide	Thick ascending limb (cortical) of the loop of Henle or distal tubule
Chlorthalidone	
Loop diuretics	
Furosemide	Thick ascending limb (medullary) of the loop of Henle
Ethacrynic acid	
Potassium-sparing diuretics	
Spironolactone (Aldactone)	Distal tubules
Triamterene	
Amiloride	
Uricosuric diuretics	
Tienilic acid	Thick ascending limb (cortical) of the loop of Henle
Osmotic diuretics	Proximal tubules, descending limb of the loop of Henle, and collecting tubule
Urea	
Mannitol	
Carbonic anhydrase inhibitors	Proximal tubules
Acetazolamide	
Ethoxzolamide	(See Figure 4)
Dichlorphenamide	

In small doses, thiazide diuretics are extremely effective in controlling essential hypertension. They exert their effects initially by bringing about volume depletion, then they reduce the peripheral resistance and sensitivity of vascular receptor sites to catecholamine. Thiazide diuretics are also used in conjunction with antihypertensive medications.

The thiazides decrease the urinary calcium concentration by diminishing glomerular filtration and also enhance the urinary magnesium level.

The thiazide diuretics can reduce free water formation in patients with diabetes insipidus, in whom large amounts of free water are eliminated.

The loss of potassium can produce hypokalemia, which is particularly dangerous in patients receiving digitalis because it increases the risk of arrhythmias. Hypokalemia can be offset either by giving a potassium supplement (potassium chloride), or by the concurrent use of a potassium-sparing diuretic. However, both measures should not be adopted because hyperkalemia will result. Hyperglycemia is a potential hazard for patients with diabetes mellitus. Hyperuricemia can precipitate an acute attack of gout, but usually only in those patients who either have already had gout or have the propensity for it. As thiazides can cause a decrease in the GFR, they should not be used in patients whose renal function is less than one third of normal. The risk of thiazide-induced hypercalcemia should be kept in mind in patients with conditions such as malignancies or hyperparathyroidism that are associated with hypercalcemia (see Table 25).

THIAZOLIDINEDIONE DERIVATIVES

Thiazolidinedione derivatives, namely ciglitazone, englitazone, pioglitazone, and troglitazone, which lower blood glucose by improving peripheral insulin resistance, are a newly developed group of oral antihyperglycemic agents that are completely different from sulfonylurea compounds. This class of drugs shows promise for use in clinical practice for treatment of patients, especially older patients, with non-insulin-dependent diabetes mellitus (see also Tables 1 and 19).

THIETHYLPERAZINE
(Vesprin)

Thiethylperazine (10 to 30 mg daily in divided doses) is indicated for relief of nausea and vomiting, especially emesis associated with surgery, cancer chemotherapy, radiation therapy, and toxins.

The physiologic purpose of nausea is to discourage food intake, and vomiting is meant to expel food or other toxic substances present in the upper part of the gastrointestinal tract. Protracted vomiting may not only cause electrolyte imbalance, dehydration, or a malnutrition syndrome, but may also lead to mucosal laceration and upper gastrointestinal hemorrhage (Mallory–Weiss syndrome).

Nausea and vomiting may occur when the stomach is overly irritated, stimulated, or distended (from overeating). In addition, nausea and vomiting may occur when the chemoreceptor trigger zone for emesis or the vomiting center, or both, are directly stimulated (see Figure 73).

Pharmacologic agents such as aspirin and levodopa may cause vomiting by directly irritating the stomach. Agents such as aminophylline, isoniazid, reserpine, antiinflammatory steroids, and caffeine may also elicit vomiting in susceptible individuals by causing the release of hydrochloric acid. This drug-induced emesis may be avoided by having patients take the drugs with meals. Antiemetics are not effective in rectifying these conditions, and their use is not justified.

In addition to agents that stimulate or irritate the stomach, many other factors may be responsible for inducing emesis centrally. The central control of vomiting is vested in two areas:

1. The vomiting center, which is located in the lateral reticular formation in the midst of a group of cells governing such activities as salivation and respiration.
2. The chemoreceptor trigger zone, which is a narrow strip along the floor of the fourth ventricle located close to the vomiting center.

The functions of these two areas are distinct but interdependent.

The vomiting center is activated by impulses that originate from the gastrointestinal tract and other peripheral structures. In addition, there are unidentified tracts that extend from the cerebral cortex to the vomiting center, such that emotional trauma and unpleasant olfactory and visual stimuli may cause nausea and vomiting.

Stimulation of the vestibular apparatus that responds to movements of the head, neck, and eye muscles may also cause nausea and vomiting by stimulating the vomiting center. On the other hand, circulating chemicals, toxins, virus, and ions may provoke nausea and vomiting by first stimulating the chemoreceptor zone for emesis, which in turn stimulates the vomiting center.

The nausea and vomiting associated with circulating physical agents (radiation therapy and virus particles) and chemical agents (toxins and cancer chemotherapeutic agents) are treated with phenothiazine derivatives such as chlorpromazine, perphenazine, prochlorperazine, promethazine, triethylperazine, and triflupromazine. These agents block the dopamine receptors in the area postrema (see Figure 73).

THIOGUANINE
(6-Thioguanine, 6-TG, Thioguanine tabloid)

Thioguanine, a purine antimetabolite (2 mg/kg daily p.o.), is indicated in the treatment of acute lymphoblastic and myelogenous leukemia, and chronic granulocytic leukemia.

Thioguanine is not effective in chronic lymphocytic leukemia, Hodgkin's lymphoma, multiple myeloma, or solid tumors. Although thioguanine is one of several agents with activity in the treatment of the chronic phase of chronic myelogenous leukemia, more objective responses are observed with busulfan; therefore, busulfan is usually regarded as the preferred drug.

6-Mercaptopurine (6MP) and 6-thioguanine are analogs of the purines, hypoxanthine and guanine, which must be activated by nucleotide formation according to the following scheme:

6-MP + phosphoribosylpyrophosphate (PRPP)

$$\xrightarrow{\textit{Hypoxathine–guanine phosphoribosyl transferase}} \text{6 ThiolMP}$$

$$\text{6TG + PRPP} \longrightarrow \text{6 ThioGMP}$$

Thioguanine competes with hypoxanthine and guanine for the enzyme hypoxanthine-guanine phosphoribosyltransferase (HGPTRase) and is converted to 6-thioguanylic acid (TGMP). TGMP interferes at several points with the synthesis of guanine nucleotides; it inhibits *de novo* purine biosynthesis by inhibiting glutamine-6-phosphoribosylpyrophosphate aminotransferase. Thioguanine nucleotides are incorporated into both RNA and DNA by phosphodiester linkages, and incorporation of such fraudulent bases may contribute to the cytotoxicity of thioguanine.

Thioguanine has multiple metabolic effects. Its tumor inhibitory properties may be due to one or more of its effects on feedback inhibition of *de novo* purine synthesis: inhibition of purine nucleotide interconversions; or incorporation into DNA and RNA. The net consequence of its actions is a sequential blockade of the synthesis and utilization of the purine nucleotides.

Resistance may result from the loss of HGPRTase activity (inability to convert thioguanine to TGMP) or increased catabolism of TGMP by a nonspecific phosphatase. Although it is variable, cross-resistance with mercaptopurine usually occurs.

The adverse reactions of thioguanine are nausea, vomiting, anorexia, and stomatitis. The rapid cell lysis causes hyperuricemia which should be minimized by taking allopurinol, a xanthine oxidase inhibitor which prevents the formation of uric acid.

Myelosuppression is the most frequent adverse reaction to thioguanine.

THIOPENTAL SODIUM
(Pentothal)

Thiopental, an ultra-short-acting barbiturate, is indicated for induction of anesthesia in short surgical procedures, for supplementing the actions of other anesthetic agents, and for creating a hypnotic state. Thiopental may be used to control convulsive states and in neurosurgical patients with increased intracranial pressure. In addition, it has been used rectally as a suspension to cause narcosis to take care of minor procedures where muscular relaxation and analgesia are not required. The onset of action is 10 minutes.

The ultra-short-acting barbiturates, thiopental, thiamylal, and methohexital, quickly cross the blood–brain barrier but are rapidly redistributed from the brain to other body tissues, first to highly perfused visceral organs (liver, kidneys, heart) and muscle, and later to fatty tissues.

These agents produce anesthesia within one minute. Recovery after a small dose is rapid, with somnolence and retrograde amnesia. Muscle relaxation occurs at the onset of anesthesia. The duration of anesthetic activity following a single IV dose is 20 to 30 minutes for thiopental and thiamylal, and somewhat shorter for methohexital.

THIORIDAZINE
(Mellaril)

Thioridazine (50 to 100 mg p.o. t.i.d.) is indicated in psychosis. Thioridazine has potent anticholinergic properties and causes heavy sedation. However, it produces a very low incidence of extrapyramidal reactions such as akathisia, dystonia, parkinsonism, tardive dyskinesia, and neuroleptic malignant syndrome. Thioridazine is metabolized to mesoridazine, which is an active antipsychotic (see Table 19).

Because of its potent anticholinergic properties, thioridazine should be used cautiously in patients with cardiac diseases such as congestive heart failure, arrhythmias, angina pectoris, or heart block; in encephalitis, Reye's syndrome, head injury, respiratory disease, epilepsy and other seizure disorders, glaucoma, prostatic hypertrophy, urinary retention, Parkinson's disease, and pheochromocytoma because the drug may exacerbate these conditions; and in hypocalcemia because it increases the risk of extrapyramidal reactions.

Concomitant use of thioridazine with sympathomimetics, including epinephrine, phenylephrine, phenylpropranolamine, and ephedrine (often found in nasal sprays), and with appetite suppressants may decrease their stimulatory and pressor effects. Thioridazine, having alpha-adrenergic-receptor-blocking effects, may cause epinephrine reversal, where the administration of epinephrine would cause only hypotension.

Thioridazine may inhibit blood pressure response to centrally acting antihypertensive drugs, such as guanethidine, guanabenz, guanadrel, clonidine, methyldopa, and reserpine. Additive effects are likely after concomitant use of thioridazine with CNS depressants, including alcohol, analgesics, barbiturates, narcotics, tranquilizers, anesthetics (general, spinal, or epidural), and parenteral magnesium sulfate (oversedation, respiratory depression, and hypotension), antiarrhythmic agents, including quinidine, disopyramide, and procainamide (increased incidence of cardiac arrhythmias and conduction defects); atropine and other anticholinergic drugs, including antidepressants, MAO inhibitors, antihistamines, meperidine, and antiparkinsonian agents (oversedation, paralytic ileus, visual changes, and severe constipation); nitrates (hypotension) and metrizamide (increased risk of seizures).

Beta-blocking agents may inhibit thioridazine metabolism, increasing plasma levels and toxicity.

Concomitant use with propylthiouracil increases risk of agranulocytosis; concomitant use with lithium may result in severe neurologic toxicity with an encephalitis-like syndrome and in decreased therapeutic response to thioridazine.

Thioridazine may antagonize the therapeutic effect of bromocriptine on prolactin secretion; it also may decrease the vasoconstricting effects of high-dose dopamine and may decrease effectiveness and increase toxicity of levodopa (by dopamine blockade). Thioridazine may inhibit metabolism and increase toxicity of phenytoin.

Overdose of thioridazine causes CNS depression characterized by deep, unarousable sleep and possible coma, hypotension or hypertension, extrapyramidal symptoms, abnormal involuntary muscle movements, agitation, seizures; arrhythmias, ECG changes, hypothermia or hyperthermia, and autonomic nervous system dysfunction.

THIOTEPA
(Thioplex powder for injection 15 mg)

Thiotepa is an alkylating agent, which is a cell-cycle nonspecific alkylating agent related to nitrogen mustard. Its radiomimetic action is believed to occur through the release of ethylenimine radicals, which disrupt the bonds of DNA. TEPA possesses cytotoxic activity.

Thiotepa, an alkylating agent with antineoplastic properties, is indicated in breast, lung, and ovarian cancer, Hodgkin's disease, lymphomas, and in bladder tumor and neoplastic effusions.

In addition to effects on the hematopoietic system, alkylating agents are highly toxic to dividing mucosal cells, leading to oral mucosal ulceration and intestinal denudation. The mucosal effects are particularly significant in high-dose chemotherapy protocols associated with bone marrow reconstitution, as they predispose to bacterial sepsis arising from the gastrointestinal tract. In these protocols, **cyclophosphamide**, **melphalan**, and **thiotepa** have the advantage of causing less mucosal damage than the other agents. In high-dose protocols, however, a number of additional toxicities become limiting.

Thiotepa (Thioplex) is composed of three ethyleneimine groups stabilized by attachment to the nucleophilic thiophosphoryl base. Its current use is primarily for high-dose chemotherapy regimens.

Both thiotepa and its desulfurated primary metabolite, **triethylenephosphoramide** (TEPA), to which it is rapidly converted by hepatic CYPs, form DNA cross-links. The aziridine rings open after protonation of the ring-nitrogen, leading to a reactive molecule.

TEPA becomes the predominant form of the drug present in plasma within hours of thiotepa administration. The parent compound has a plasma half-life of 1.2 to 2 hours, as compared to a longer half-life of 3 to 24 hours for TEPA. Thiotepa pharmacokinetics are essentially the same in children as in adults at conventional doses (up to 80 mg/m^2), and drug and metabolite half-lives are unchanged in children receiving high-dose therapy of 300 mg/m^2 per day for 3 days. Less than 10% of the administered drug appears in urine as the parent drug or the primary metabolite. Multiple secondary metabolites and chemical degradation products account for the remainder of the parent.

The toxicities of **thiotepa** are essentially the same as those of the other alkylating agents, namely myelosuppression and to a lesser extent mucositis. Myelosuppression tends to develop somewhat later than with **cyclophosphamide**, with leukopenic nadirs at 2 weeks and platelet nadirs at 3 weeks. In high-dose regimens thiotepa produces neurotoxic symptoms, including coma and seizures.

THIOTHIXENE HYDROCHLORIDE
(Intensol)

Thiothixene (2 mg t.i.d. in mild cases) is indicated in the management of psychotic disorders. Thiothixene and chlorprothixene are thioxanthene antipsychotics. Their select pharmacological properties are compared with chlorpromazine and haloperidol and are shown in Table 2.

THROMBIN
(Thrombinar, Thrombogen, Thrombostat)

Thrombin, a topical hemostatic, is indicated in bleeding from parenchymatous tissue, cancellous bone, dental sockets, during nasal and laryngeal surgery, and in plastic surgery and skin-grafting procedures.

THYROGLOBULIN
(Proloid)

In the treatment of hypothyroidism, levothyroxine (Levothroid and Synthroid Sodium; 2 to 25 µg/kg) is given for replacement therapy in patients with hypothyroidism. Following are other thyroid preparations:

- Thyroglobulin (Proloid) is purified from hog thyroid gland and standardized to yield a T_4 to T_3 ratio of 2.5 to 1.
- Liothyronine (Cytomel and Cytomine) has a short half-life and hence is used diagnostically in the T_3 suppression test.
- Liotrix (Euthyroid, Thyrolar) is a combination of T_4 and T_3, and is standardized to yield a T_4 to T_3 ratio of 4 to 1.

THYROID USP (DESICCATED)
(Armour Thyroid, Dathroid, Delcoid, S-P-T, Thermoloid, Thyrar, Thyrocrine, Thyroid Strong, Thyro-teric)

Thyroid hormone is used in adult hypothyroidism, in adult myxedema, and in cretinism and juvenile hypothyroidism.

Thyroid USP affects protein and carbohydrate metabolism, promotes gluconeogenesis, increases the utilization and mobilization of glycogen stores, stimulates protein synthesis, and regulates cell growth and differentiation. The major effect of thyroid is to increase the metabolic rate of tissue.

THROMBOLYTIC AGENTS: A Need for Improvement

Cardiovascular diseases, comprising acute myocardial infarction, stroke, and venous thromboembolism, have, as their immediate underlying cause, thrombosis of critically situated blood vessels with loss of blood flow to vital organs. One approach to the treatment of thrombosis consists of pharmacologic dissolution of the blood clot via the intravenous infusion of plasminogen activators that activate the blood fibrinolytic system.

Despite their widespread use in patients with acute myocardial infarction, all currently available thrombolytic agents suffer from a number of significant limitations, including resistance to reperfusion, the occurrence of acute coronary reocclusion, and bleeding complications. Therefore, the quest continues for thrombolytic agents with a higher thrombolytic potency, specific thrombolytic activity, and/or a better fibrin selectivity.

The fibrinolytic system comprises an inactive proenzyme, plasminogen, which is converted by plasminogen activators to the active enzyme, plasmin, which degrades fibrin. Two immunologically distinct plasminogen activators have been identified: tissue-type plasminogen activator (t-PA) and urokinase-type plasminogen activator (u-PA). Plasminogen activation is regulated by specific molecular interactions between its main components, as well as by controlled synthesis and release of plasminogen activator inhibitors, primarily from endothelial cells. The observed association between abnormal fibrinolysis and a tendency toward bleeding or thrombosis demonstrates the (patho)physiological importance of the fibrinolytic system. Transgenic animals are a suitable experimental model in which to examine the *in vivo* impact of fibrinolytic components in thrombosis and thrombolysis. Inactivation, by homologous recombination, of the tissue-type plasminogen activator genes in mice impairs thrombolysis in a significant manner, whereas inactivation of the plasminogen activator-1 gene enhances the rate of spontaneous lysis.

Several lines of research toward improvement of thrombolytic agents are being explored, including the construction of mutants and variants of plasminogen activators, chimeric plasminogen activators, conjugates of plasminogen activators with monoclonal antibodies, or plasminogen activators from animal or bacterial origin.

Thyroid USP is contraindicated in patients with thyrotoxicosis, acute myocardial infarction, or uncorrected adrenal insufficiency.

Thyroid USP should be used cautiously in patients with angina or other cardiovascular disease because of the risk of increased metabolic demands.

Concomitant use of thyroid USP with adrenocorticoids or corticotropin causes changes in thyroid status, and changes in thyroid dosages may require adrenocorticoid or corticotropin dosage changes as well. Concomitant use with anticoagulants may alter anticoagulant effect; an increased thyroid USP dosage may necessitate a lower anticoagulant dose.

Use with tricyclic antidepressants or sympathomimetics may increase the effects of these medications or of thyroid USP, possibly leading to coronary insufficiency or cardiac arrhythmias. Use with oral antidiabetic agents or insulin may affect dosage requirements of these agents. Estrogens, which increase serum thyroxine-binding globulin levels, raise thyroid USP requirements.

Hepatic enzyme inducers (for example, phenytoin) may increase hepatic degradation of levothyroxine, causing increased dosage requirements of levothyroxine. Concomitant use with somatrem may accelerate epiphyseal maturation. Intravenous phenytoin may release free thyroid from thyroglobulin. Cholestyramine and colestipol may decrease absorption.

Overdosage with thyroid USP causes exaggerated signs and symptoms of hyperthyroidism, including weight loss, increased appetite, palpitations, nervousness, diarrhea, abdominal cramps, sweating, tachycardia, increased pulse and blood pressure, angina, cardiac arrhythmias, tremor, headache, insomnia, heat intolerance, fever, and menstrual irregularities.

THYROID PREPARATIONS

Thyroid, USP	Desiccated hog, beef, or sheep thyroid gland
Armour Thyroid, 1/4, 1/2, 11/2, 2, 3, 4, and 5 grain tablets	
Thyroglobulin	Partially purified hog thyroglobulin
32 mg (1/2 grain), 65 mg (1 grain), 100 mg (11/2 grain), 130 mg (2 grain), and 200 mg (3 grain)	
L-Thyroxine	Synthetic T_4
Synthroid, Levothroid, 25, 50, 75, 100, 125, 150, 175, 200, and 300 μg tablets; 100 μg/mL, 5 mL	
Liothyronine	Synthetic T_3
Cytomel, 5, 25, and 50 μg tablets	
Liotrix	Synthetic T_4:T_3 in 4:1 ratio
Euthyroid, Thyrolar, 1/4-, 1/2-, 1-, 2-, and 3-strength tablets	

THYROTROPIN

(Thyroid-stimulating hormone, or TSH) (Thytropar)

Thyrotropin is indicated in diagnosis of thyroid cancer remnant with ^{131}I after surgery (see Table 20); in the differential diagnosis of primary and secondary hypothyroidism; in protein-bound iodine or ^{131}I uptake determinations for differential diagnosis of subclinical hypothyroidism or low thyroid reserve; as therapy for thyroid carcinoma (local or

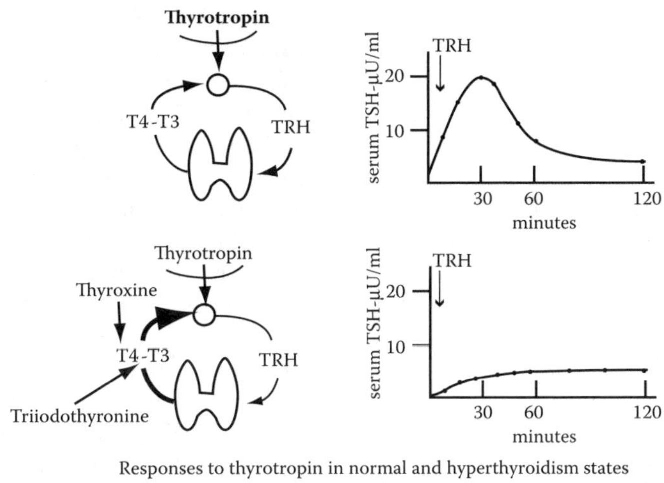

FIGURE 97 The production of thyroid hormones is regulated in two ways: (1) by **thyrotropin**, and (2) by a variety of nutritional, hormonal, and illness-related factors.

metastatic) with ^{131}I; and to determine the thyroid status of patients receiving thyroid therapy (see Figures 97 and 98).

THYROTROPIN-RELEASING HORMONE (TRH)

The production of thyroid hormones is regulated in two ways: (1) by thyrotropin and (2) by a variety of nutritional, hormonal, and illness-related factors. The secretion of thyrotropin is regulated by the circulating levels of T_4 and by thyrotropin-releasing hormone (TRH), as shown in Figure 98.

Thyrotropin is synthesized by thyrotrophs located in the anterior pituitary gland and consists of two peptide subunits, the alpha subunit (see also Luteinizing Hormone, Follicle-Stimulating Hormone, and Chorionic Gonadotropin), and the beta subunit, which determines the biologic activities of thyrotrophs. T_3 and T_4 inhibit both the synthesis and release of thyrotropin.

The concentration of TSH increases rapidly following the administration of TRH. In hyperthyroidism, the high levels of T_3 and T_4 inhibit the action of TSH and cause a lack of response to TRH.

THYROXINE (T_4)

The ingested iodide (100 to 150 μg/day) is actively transported to (iodide trapping) and then accumulates in the thyroid gland. Following this, the trapped iodide is oxidized by a peroxidase system to active iodine, which iodinates the tyrosine residue of glycoprotein to yield monoiodotyrosine (MIT) and diiodotyrosine (DIT). This process is called iodide organification. The MIT and DIT combine to form T_3, whereas two molecules of DIT combine to form T_4. T_3 and T_4 are released from thyroglobulin through the actions of pinocytosis and the proteolysis of thyroglobulin by lysosomal enzymes. In the circulation, 75% of T_4 is

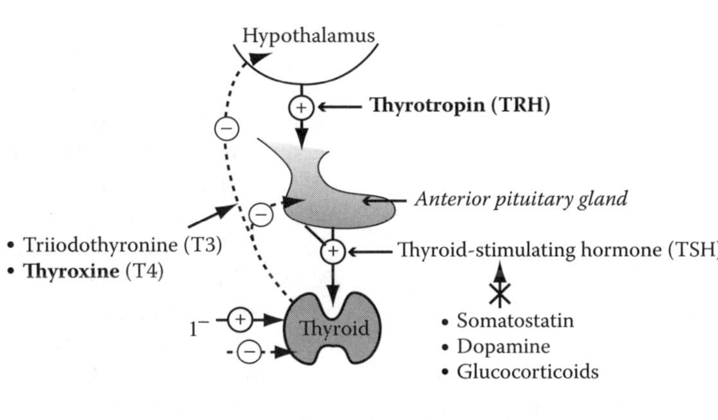

FIGURE 98 The secretion of thyrotropin is regulated by the circulating levels of T_4 and by thyrotropin-releasing hormone (TRH).

bound to thyroxine-binding globulin (TBG), and the remainder is bound mostly to thyroxine-binding prealbumin (TBPA). Approximately 0.05% of T_4 remains free. T_3 is similarly bound to TBG, allowing only 0.5% of it to remain in the free form.

T_4 may undergo deamination, decarboxylation, and glucuronic acid conjugation. However, it is mostly deiodinated in one of two ways: it may either be deiodinated to 3,5,3′-triiodothyronine, which is more efficacious than T_4, or it may be deiodinated to the pharmacologically inactive 3,3′,5′-triiodothyronine (reverse T_3).

TIAGABINE HYDROCHLORIDE
(Gabitril Filmtabs tablets 4 mg)

Tiagabine hydrochloride is an anticonvulsant, which blocks GABA uptake into presynaptic neurons, allowing more GABA to be available for binding with the GABA receptor of postsynaptic cells. It is effective as an adjunctive treatment for partial seizures.

Tiagabine (Gabitril) is a derivative of nipecotic acid and was approved by the FDA in 1998 for treating partial seizures in adults when used in addition to other drugs.

Tiagabine inhibits the GABA transporter, GAT-1, and thereby reduces GABA uptake into neurons and glia. In CA1 neurons of the hippocampus, tiagabine increases the duration of inhibitory synaptic currents, findings consistent with prolonging the effect of GABA at inhibitor synapses through reducing its reuptake by GAT-1. Tiagabine inhibits maximum electroshock seizures and both limbic and secondarily generalized tonic-clonic seizures in the kindling model, results suggestive of clinical efficacy against partial and tonic-clonic seizures.

Tiagabine is rapidly absorbed after oral administration, extensively bound to serum or plasma proteins, and metabolized mainly in the liver, predominantly by CYP3A. Its half-life of about 8 hours is shortened by 2 to 3 hours when coadministered with hepatic enzyme-inducing drugs such as phenobarbital, phenytoin, or carbamazepine.

Double-blind, placebo-controlled trials have established tiagabine's efficacy as add-on therapy of refractory partial seizures with or without secondary generalization. Its efficacy for monotherapy for newly diagnosed or refractory partial and generalized epilepsy has not been established.

The principal adverse effects include dizziness, somnolence, and tremor; they appear to be mild to moderate in severity and appear shortly after initiation of therapy. The fact that tiagabine and other drugs thought to enhance effects of synaptically released GABA can facilitate spike-and-wave discharges in animal models of absence seizures raises the possibility that tiagabine may be contraindicated in patients with generalized absence epilepsy. Patients with a history of spike-and-wave discharges have been reported to have exacerbations of their EEG abnormalities.

TICARCILLIN/CLAVULANATE POTASSIUM
(Timentin powder for injection 3 g ticarcillin (as disodium) and 0.1 g clavulanic acid (as potassium) (contains 4.75 mEq sodium and 0.15 mEq potassium/g), injection solution 3 g ticarcillin (as disodium) and 0.1 g clavulanic acid (as potassium) per 100 mL (contains 18.7 mEq sodium and 0.5 mEq potassium per 100 mL))

Ticarcillin/clavulanate potassium is an extended-spectrum penicillin. **Ticarcillin** inhibits bacterial cell wall mucopeptide synthesis. **Clavulanate** lactamase enzymes are commonly found in microorganisms resistant to ticarcillin. They are indicated in the treatment of bacterial septicemia, skin and skin structure infections, lower respiratory tract infections, bone and joint infections, GU and gynecologic infections, and intra-abdominal infections caused by susceptible strains of bacteria.

TICARCILLIN DISODIUM
(Ticar)

Ticarcillin, extended-spectrum penicillin, alpha-carboxypenicillin, is indicated for the treatment of bacterial septicemia, skin and soft-tissue infections, acute and chronic respiratory tract infections caused by susceptible strains of *Pseudomonas aeruginosa*, *Proteus* species (both indole-positive and indole-negative), and *Escherichia coli*; and for genitourinary tract infections (complicated and uncomplicated) due to susceptible strains of *P. aeruginosa*, *Proteus* species (both indole-positive and indole-negative), *E. coli*, *Enterobacter*, and *Streptococcus faecalis* (enterococcus).

Ticarcillin disodium/clavulanate potassium (Timentin) is an extended-spectrum penicillin and inhibits beta-lactamase.

Ampicillin, amoxicillin, carbenicillin, ticarcillin, piperacillin, mezlocillin, and azlocillin differ from penicillin G in having greater activity against Gram-negative bacteria, but they are inactivated by beta-lactamases.

Carbenicillin resembles ampicillin but has more activity against *Pseudomonas* and *Proteus* organisms, though *Klebsiella* species are usually resistant. In susceptible populations of *Pseudomonas*, resistance to carbenicillin may emerge rapidly. Therefore, in *Pseudomonas* sepsis (e.g., burns, immunosuppressed patients), carbenicillin, 12 to 30 g/d intravenously (300 to 500 mg/kg/d), is usually combined with an aminoglycoside, e.g., gentamicin, 5 to 7 mg/kg/d intramuscularly, to delay emergence of resistance and perhaps to obtain synergistic effects. Carbenicillin contains Na^+, 4.7 mEq/g. Carbenicillin indanyl sodium is acid-stable and can be given orally in urinary tract infections. Ticarcillin resembles carbenicillin in single and combined activity, but the dose may be lower, e.g., 200 to 300 mg/kg/d intravenously. Piperacillin, mezlocillin, azlocillin, and others resemble ticarcillin and claim special effectiveness against Gram-negative aerobic rods, including *Pseudomonas*. However, in serious *Pseudomonas* infections, they should be used in combination with an aminoglycoside.

Ampicillin, amoxicillin, ticarcillin, and others in this group can be protected from destruction by beta-lactamases if they are administered together with beta-lactamase inhibitors such as clavulanic acid, sulbactam, or tazobactam. Such mixtures have been employed against lactamase-producing *H. influenzae* or coliform organisms.

Ticarcillin is excreted primarily (80 to 93%) in urine by renal tubular secretion and glomerular filtration; it is also excreted in bile and in breast milk. Therefore, it should be used cautiously in patients with renal impairment because it is excreted in urine.

Aminoglycoside and ticarcillin are physically and chemically incompatible and are inactivated when mixed or given together.

The clinical signs of overdosage with ticarcillin include neuromuscular hypersensitivity or seizures resulting from CNS irritation by high drug concentrations.

TICARCILLIN DISODIUM/CLAVULANATE POTASSIUM

(Timentin)

Ticarcillin, an extended-spectrum penicillin that inhibits beta lactamase, is indicated in infections of the lower respiratory tract, urinary tract, bones and joints, skin and skin structures, and septicemia when caused by susceptible organisms.

TICLOPIDINE HYDROCHLORIDE

(Ticlid tablets 250 mg)

Ticlopidine is an antiplatelet, which produces time- and dose-dependent inhibition of both platelet aggregation and release of platelet granule constituents as well as prolongation of bleeding time; interferes with platelet membrane function by inhibiting platelet-fibrinogen binding and subsequent platelet–platelet interactions. It is indicated for reduction of risk of thrombotic stroke in patients who have experienced stroke precursors and in patients who have had completed thrombotic stroke. It is reserved for patients intolerant to aspirin because of greater risk of adverse reactions.

Mortality in patients with peripheral vascular disease is most commonly due to cardiovascular disease, and treatment of coronary disease remains the central focus of therapy. Many patients with advanced peripheral arterial disease are more limited by the consequences of peripheral ischemia than by myocardial ischemia. In the cerebral circulation, arterial disease may be manifest as stroke or transient ischemic attacks. The painful symptoms of peripheral arterial disease in the lower extremities (**claudication**) typically are provoked by exertion, with increases in skeletal muscle O_2 demand exceeding blood flow impaired by proximal stenoses. When flow to the extremities becomes critically limiting, peripheral ulcers and rest pain from tissue ischemia can become debilitating.

Most of the therapies shown to be efficacious for treatment of coronary artery disease also have a salutary effect on progression of peripheral artery disease. Reductions in cardiovascular morbidity and mortality in patients with peripheral arterial disease have been documented with antiplatelet therapy using aspirin or with ADP antagonists such as **clopidogrel** or **ticlopidine**, administration of ACE inhibitors, and treatment of hyperlipidemia. Interestingly, neither intensive treatment of diabetes mellitus nor antihypertensive therapy appears to alter the progression of symptoms of claudication. Other risk factor and lifestyle modifications remain cornerstones of therapy for patients with claudication: physical exercise, rehabilitation, and smoking cessation have proven efficacy. Drugs used specifically in the treatment of lower extremity claudication include **pentoxyfylline** and **cilastozol**. Pentoxifylline is a methylxanthine derivative that has been termed a **rheologic modifier** for its effects on increasing the deformability of red blood cells. However, the effects of pentoxifylline on lower extremity claudication appear to be modest. Cilastozol is an inhibitor of PDE3 and promotes accumulation of intracellular cyclic AMP in many cells, including blood platelets. Cilastozol-mediated increases in cAMP inhibit platelet aggregation and promote vasodilation. The drug is metabolized by CYP3A4 and has important drug interactions with other drugs metabolized via this pathway. Cilastozol treatment improves symptoms of claudication but has no effect on cardiovascular mortality. As a PDE3 inhibitor, **cilastozol** is placed in the same drug class as **milrinone**, which had been used as an inotropic agent for patients with heart failure. Milrinone therapy was associated with an increase in sudden cardiac death, and the drug was withdrawn from the market. Cilastozol, therefore, is contraindicated in patients with heart failure, conditions that lead to myocardial infarction, stroke, and peripheral vascular thromboses. Potent inhibitors of platelet function have been developed in recent years. These drugs act by discrete mechanisms, and thus in combination their effects are additive or even synergistic. Their availability has led to a revolution in cardiovascular medicine, whereby angioplasty and vascular stenting of lesions now is feasible with low rates of restenosis and thrombosis when effective platelet inhibition is employed.

Purinergic receptors respond to extracellular nucleotides as agonists. Platelets contain two purinergic receptors, $P2Y_1$ and $P2Y_{12}$; both are GPCRs for ADP. The ADP-activated platelet $P2Y_1$ receptor couples to the G_q-PLC-IP-Ca^{2+} pathway and induces a shape change and aggregation. The $P2Y_{12}$ receptor couples to G_i and, when activated by ADP, inhibits adenylyl cyclase, resulting in lower levels of cyclic AMP and thereby less cyclic AMP-dependent inhibition of platelet activation. Based on pharmacological studies, it appears that both receptors must be stimulated to result in platelet activation, and inhibition of either receptor is sufficient to block platelet activation. Ticlopidine (Ticlid) is a thienopyridine that inhibits the $P2Y_{12}$ receptor. **Ticlopidine** is a prodrug that requires conversion to the active thiol metabolite by a hepatic cytochrome P450 enzyme. It is rapidly absorbed and highly bioavailable.

It permanently inhibits the $P2Y_{12}$ receptor by forming a disulfide bridge between the thiol on the drug and a free cysteine residue in the extracellular region of the receptor and thus has a prolonged effect. Like aspirin it has a short half-life with a long duration of action, which has been termed "hit-and-run pharmacology." Maximal inhibition of platelet aggregation is not seen until 8 to 11 days after starting therapy. Thus, "loading doses" of 500 mg sometimes are given to achieve a more rapid onset of action. The usual dose is 250 mg twice per day. Inhibition of platelet aggregation persists for a few days after the drug is stopped.

The most common side effects are nausea, vomiting, and diarrhea. The most serious is severe neutropenia (absolute neutrophil count [ANC] <1500/μL), which occurred in 2.4% of stroke patients given the drug during premarketing clinical trials. Fatal agranulocytosis with thrombopenia has occurred within the first 3 months of therapy; therefore, frequent blood counts should be obtained during the first few months of therapy, with immediate discontinuation of therapy should cell counts decline. Platelet counts also should be monitored, as thrombocytopenia has been reported. Rare cases of **thrombotic thrombocytopenic purpura-hemolytic uremic syndrome** (TTP-HUS) have been associated with ticlopidine with a reported incidence of 1 in 1600 to 4800 patients when the drug is used after cardiac stenting; the mortality associated with these cases is reported to be as high as 18 to 57%. Remission of TTP has been reported when the drug is stopped.

Ticlopidine has been shown to prevent cerebrovascular events in secondary prevention of stroke and is at least as good as aspirin in this regard. It also reduces cardiac events in patients with unstable angina; however, its only FDA-approved indication is to reduce the risk of thrombotic stroke in patients who have experienced stroke precursors, and in patients who have had a completed thrombotic stroke. Since ticlopidine has a mechanism of action distinct from that of aspirin, combining the drugs might be expected to provide additive or even synergistic effects. This appears to be the case, and the combination has been used in patients undergoing angioplasty and stenting for coronary artery disease, with a very low frequency of stent thrombosis occurring over a short, 30-day follow-up (<1%). As ticlopidine is associated with life-threatening blood dyscrasias and a relatively high rate of TTP, it is generally reserved for patients who are intolerant or allergic to aspirin or who have failed aspirin therapy.

Ticlopidine, a platelet aggregation inhibitor possessing antithrombotic effects (250 mg p.o. b.i.d.), is used to reduce the risk of thrombotic stroke in patients with a history of stroke or who have experienced stroke precursors (see also Figures 13 and 93). Ticlopidine, a thienopyridine derivative, and a new antiplatelet agent for secondary prevention of stroke, causes potent inhibition of adenosine diphosphate (ADP)-induced platelet aggregation and moderate inhibition of aggregation induced by collagen, epinephrine, thrombin, and platelet-activating factor.

TICNILIC ACID
(Ticrynafen)

Ticnilic acid, which is a uricosuric diuretic, is chemically related to ethacrynic acid, but pharmacologically it resembles the thiazide diuretics. Ticnilic acid is as efficacious as hydrochlorothiazide, but it is superior in enhancing uric acid excretion, which is a problem with most effective diuretics. The usefulness of this agent in medicine awaits confirmation.

TIGECYCLINE
(Tygacil powder for injection 50 mg)

Tigecycline is an antiinfective/glycylcycline, which inhibits protein transportation in bacteria by binding to the 30S ribosomal subunit and blocking entry of amino-acyl tKNA molecules into the A site of the ribosome. This prevents incorporation of amino-acid residues into elongating peptide chains. Glycylcycline class antibiotics are structurally similar to tetracycline class antibiotics and may have similar adverse reactions.

It is indicated in the treatment of complicated skin and skin structure infections and complicated intra-abdominal infections caused by susceptible strains of specific microorganisms.

The glycylcyclines are synthetic analogs of the tetracyclines, with the most promising compound being the 9-tert-butyl-glyclyamido derivative of minocycline, tigecycline. The glycylcyclines exhibit antibacterial activities typical of earlier tetracyclines, and also display activity against tetracycline-resistant organisms containing genes responsible for efflux mechanisms or ribosomal protection. The glycylcyclines also appear to be active against other resistant pathogens including methicillin-resistant *S. aureus* and *S. epidermidis*, penicillin-resistant *S. pneumoniae*, and vancomycin-resistant enterococci.

TILUDRONATE DISODIUM
(Skelid tablets 240 mg (eq. to 200 mg tiludronic acid))

Tiludronate disodium is a bisphosphonate that inhibits normal and abnormal bone resorption. It is indicated in the treatment of **Paget's disease of bone**.

Several bisphosphonates are available in the United States. Etidronate sodium (Didronel) is used for treatment of Paget's disease and may be used parenterally to treat hypercalcemia. As etidronate is the only bisphosphonate that inhibits mineralization, it has been supplanted largely by pamidronate and zoledronate for treating hypercalcemia. Pamidronate (Aredia) is approved for management of hypercalcemia but also is effective in other skeletal disorders. Pamidronate is available in the United States only for parenteral administration. For treatment of hypercalcemia, pamidronate may be given as an intravenous infusion of 60 to 90 mg over 4 to 24 hours.

Several newer bisphosphonates have been approved for treatment of Paget's disease. These include **tiludronate** (Skelid), **alendronate** (Fosamax), and **risedronate** (Actonel). Although the drug is approved only for treating hypercalcemia of malignancy, a single injection of **zoledronate** (Zometa) decreased bone turnover markers for 90 days in patients with Paget's disease. **Tiludronate** and the potent bisphosphonate **ibandronate** currently are under development for treatment of women with osteoporosis, with encouraging preliminary results

TIMOLOL MALEATE
(Timoptic-XE) Timolol Maleate (Biocarden)

Timolol (10 mg t.i.d.) alone or in combination with other antihypertensive agents, such as thiazide diuretics, is used in the management of hypertension. Timolol is indicated for the treatment of myocardial infarction and prophylaxis of migraine headaches. Timolol (1 drop of 0.25% solution twice daily) is effective in lowering intraocular pressure in patients with chronic open-angle glaucoma.

Timolol's beta-blocking action decreases the production of aqueous humor, thereby decreasing intraocular pressure.

Timolol is a nonselective beta-adrenergic-blocking agent; the affinity to $beta_1$- and $beta_2$-receptors is almost equal. In currently recommended dosages, it has no membrane-stabilizing and only negligible partial agonist activity. In humans, it is 8 to 10 times more potent than propranolol in reducing resting heart rate and 14 times more potent in suppressing tachycardia induced by isoproterenol infusion.

When timolol tablets are administered orally, 90 to 100% of the drug is rapidly absorbed, uninfluenced by food ingestion. Between 5 and 10% is excreted unchanged in the urine; the rest is broken down into several inactive metabolites that are subsequently excreted through the kidneys. Plasma half-life is not influenced by a moderate degree of renal failure.

Timolol is an effective antihypertensive agent. It improves exercise tolerance in patients with angina pectoris. It substantially reduces the long-term risk of sudden death and reinfarction in patients surviving acute myocardial infarction. It has been shown to reduce the size of an acute myocardial infarction when given intravenously within 4 hours after the onset of symptoms. Timolol is effective in the treatment of supraventricular arrhythmias and in certain cases of recurrent ventricular tachycardia.

Similar to other beta-adrenergic-blocking agents, timolol reduces systemic blood pressure mainly through a decrease in cardiac output. In hypertensive patients with normal cardiac function, the stroke index remains largely unaffected. Maximum blood pressure reductions usually occur after several days of therapy, when the initial rise in total peripheral resistance begins to fall toward pretreatment levels.

Similar to other nonselective beta-adrenergic-blocking agents, timolol causes a decrease in plasma renin activity.

In hypertension, timolol may be used either alone or in combination with most other antihypertensive agents. The combination with angiotensin-converting enzyme inhibitors is probably less useful because both agents exert part of their effect by diminishing the activity of the renin-angiotensin system. Combination with verapamil should be avoided because of the effect on AV nodal conduction.

In angina pectoris, doses of 5 mg b.i.d. may prove sufficient for optimal increase of exercise tolerance, especially in elderly patients.

Timolol seems particularly indicated in patients with hypertension, angina, or both after acute myocardial infarction because of the drug's combined effect on those conditions. It also has a well-documented protective effect in diabetic patients who have had myocardial infarction.

Timolol is contraindicated in patients with unstabilized cardiac failure or bronchial obstruction, AV conduction disturbances of the second and third grade, unstable insulin-dependent diabetes, and severe peripheral arterial obstruction. The most common side effects are muscular fatigue, cold hands and feet, symptomatic hypotension, and bradycardia.

TINIDAZOLE
(Tindamax tablets 250 mg, tablets 500 mg)

Tinidazole is an antiprotozoal. It is indicated in the treatment of **trichomoniasis** caused by *T. vaginalis*, giardiasis caused by *G. duodenalis*, and amebiasis caused by *E. histolytica*.

The cornerstone of therapy for amebiasis is the nitroimidazole compound **metronidazole** or its analogs **tinidazole** and **ornidazole**. Metronidazole and tinidazole are the only nitroimidazoles available in the United States and are the drugs of choice for the treatment of amebic colitis, amebic liver abscess, and any other extraintestinal form of amebiasis. Other agents, such as **dehydroemetine** and chloroquine, are now used rarely in the treatment of amebic colitis or amebic liver abscess and are reserved for only very unusual cases where metronidazole is contraindicated. Because metronidazole is so well absorbed in the gut, levels may not be therapeutic in the colonic lumen, and it is less effective against cysts. Hence, patients with amebiasis (amebic colitis or amebic liver abscess) also should receive a luminal agent to eradicate any *E. histolytica* trophozoites residing within the gut lumen. Luminal agents are also used to treat asymptomatic individuals found to be infected with *E. histolytica*. The nonabsorbed aminoglycoside paromomycin and the 8-hydroxy-quinoline compound iodoquinol are two effective luminal agents. Diloxanide furoate, previously considered the luminal agent of choice for amebiasis, is no longer available in the United States. Nitazoxanide (Alinia), a drug approved in the United States for the treatment of cryptosporidiosis and giardiasis, is also active against *E. histolytica*.

TINZAPARIN SODIUM
(Innohep injection 20,000 IU/mL)

Tinzaparin sodium is a low-molecular-weight heparin that inhibits reactions leading to the clotting of blood, including the formation of fibrin clots. It is indicated in the treatment of acute symptomatic **deep vein thrombosis** with or without pulmonary embolism when administered with **warfarin**.

Enoxaparin (Lovenox), **dalteparin** (Fragmin), **tinzaparin** (Innohep, others), **ardeparin** (Normiflo), **nadroparin** (fraxiparine, others), and **reviparin** (Clivarine) differ considerably in composition, and it cannot be assumed that two preparations that have similar antifactor Xa activity will produce equivalent antithrombotic effects. The more predictable pharmacokinetic properties of low-molecular-weight heparins, however, permit administration in a fixed or weight-adjusted dosage regimen once or twice daily by subcutaneous injection. Since they have a minimal effect on tests of clotting *in vitro*, monitoring is not done routinely. Patients with end-stage renal failure may require monitoring with an antifactor Xa assay because this condition may prolong the half-life of low-molecular-weight heparin. Specific dosage recommendations for various low-molecular-weight heparins may be obtained from the manufacturer's literature.

TIOCONAZOLE
(Vagistat-1)

Tioconazole, an imidazole derivative with antifungal activity (vaginal ointment 6.5%), is used in the treatment of vulvovaginal candidiasis.

TIOPRONIN
(Thiola)

Tiopronin, a thiol compound that stabilizes the cystine moiety, is used in prevention of urinary cystine stone formation in patients with severe homozygous cystinuria (urinary cystine excretion exceeding 500 mg daily) unresponsive to other therapies.

TIOTROPIUM BROMIDE
(Spiriva powder for inhalation 18mcg (as base))

Tiotropium bromide is an anticholinergic that inhibits smooth muscle receptors, leading to bronchodilation. It is indicated for long-term, maintenance treatment of bronchospasm associated with COPD, including chronic bronchitis and emphysema.

The class of drugs referred to as **muscarinic receptor antagonists** includes (1) the naturally occurring alkaloids, **atropine** and **scopolamine**; (2) semisynthetic derivatives of these alkaloids, which primarily differ from the parent compounds in their disposition in the body or their duration of action; and (3) synthetic congeners, some of which show selectivity for particular subtypes of muscarinic receptors. Noteworthy agents among the synthetic derivatives are **homatropine** and **tropicamide**, which have a shorter duration of action than atropine, and **methylatropine**, **ipratropium**, and **tiotropium**, which are quaternized and do not cross the blood–brain barrier or readily cross membranes. The latter two agents are given by inhalation in the treatment of **chronic obstructive pulmonary disease** and are pending approval for use in bronchial asthma. Ipratropium also has an FDA-approved indication for perennial- and common-cold-associated rhinorrhea. The synthetic derivatives possessing partial receptor selectivity include **pirenzepine**, used in the treatment of **acid-peptic disease** in some countries, and **tolterodine**, **oxybutynin**, and several others, used in the treatment of urinary incontinence.

TIPRANAVIR
(Aptivus capsules 250 mg)

Tipranavir is a protease inhibitor. Tipranavir is a nonpeptide protease inhibitor that prevents formation of mature virions by inhibiting virus-specific processing of the viral Gag and Gag-Pol polyproteins in HIV-1 infected cells. It is indicated in combination with **ritonavir** 200 mg for the treatment of HIV-1 infected adult patients with evidence of viral replication, who are highly treatment-experienced or have HIV-1 strains resistant to multiple protease inhibitor.

TIZANIDINE

Tizanidine is a clonidine derivative that has been introduced recently for treatment of spasticity. It is more effective than buclofen. It is a centrally acting myorelaxant with predominantly $alpha_2$-adrenergic properties. Tizanidine is an imidazole derivative that exhibits central muscle relaxant activity principally affecting spinal polysynaptic reflexes. This action arises from agonistic activity of the compound at noradrenergic $alpha_2$ receptors resulting in both direct impairment of excitatory amino-acid release from spinal interneurons and a concomitant inhibition of facilitatory coeruleospinal pathways. Tizanidine has received widespread acceptance in the treatment of spasticity and rheumatological conditions associated with painful muscle spasm (see also Figure 31).

TOBRAMYCIN SULFATE
(Nebcin)

Tobramycin is available in ophthalmic ointments and solutions. Tobramycin (1 mg/kg initially, to be adjusted thereafter) is indicated in the treatment of:

- Serious infections caused by susceptible strains of *Pseudomonas aeruginosa*, *Escherichia coli*, *Proteus* sp. (indole-positive and indole-negative) including *P. mirabilis*, *Morganella morganii* and *P. vulgaris*, *Providencia* sp. including *P. rettgeri*, the *Klebsiella-Enterobacter-Serratia* group, *Citrobacter* sp. and staphylococci, including *S. aureus* (coagulase-positive and coagulase-negative)
- Septicemia (neonates, children, and adults) caused by *P. aeruginosa*, *E. coli*, and *Klebsiella* sp.

- Lower respiratory tract infections caused by *P. aeruginosa*, *Klebsiella* sp., *Enterobacter* sp., *Serratia* sp., *E. coli*, and *S. aureus* (penicillinase- and nonpenicillinase-producing strains)
- Serious CNS infections (meningitis) caused by susceptible organisms
- Intra-abdominal infections, including peritonitis, caused by *E. coli*, *Klebsiella* sp., and *Enterobacter* sp.
- Skin, bone, and skin structure infections caused by *P. aeruginosa*, *Proteus* sp., *E. coli*, *Klebsiella* sp., *Enterobacter* sp., and *S. aureus*
- Complicated and recurrent urinary tract infections (UTIs) caused by *P. aeruginosa*, *Proteus* sp. (indole-positive and indole-negative), *E. coli*, *Klebsiella* sp., *Enterobacter* sp., *Serratia* sp., *S. aureus*, *Providencia* sp., and *Citrobacter* sp., the drug is not indicated in uncomplicated initial episodes of UTIs unless the organisms are not susceptible to less toxic antibiotics

The antimicrobial activity and pharmacokinetic properties of tobramycin are very similar to those of gentamicin. Tobramycin may be given either intramuscularly or intravenously. Dosages are identical to those for gentamicin. When doses of 1.5 mg/kg are given intravenously every 8 hours, peak concentrations in plasma are typically 5 to 8 μg/ml, and minimal concentrations are 1 to 2 μg/ml. Toxicity is most common at minimal (trough) concentrations that exceed 2 μg/ml for a prolonged period. The latter observation usually requires reduction of dosage.

Tobramycin, like other aminoglycosides, causes both nephrotoxicity and ototoxicity. However, tobramycin may be less toxic to hair cells in the cochlear and vestibular end organs and cause less renal tubular damage than does gentamicin.

TOCAINIDE HYDROCHLORIDE
(Tonocard)

Tocainide, an antiarrhythmic (initially 400 mg t.i.d.), is indicated in the treatment of life-threatening ventricular arrhythmias.

Tocainide may be beneficial in the treatment of myotonic dystrophy (800 to 1200 mg/day) and trigeminal neuralgia (20 mg/kg/day in three divided doses). Tocainide is a class 1B antiarrhythmic with electrophysiologic properties similar to those of lidocaine (see Figure 84). In patients with cardiac disease, tocainide produces no clinically significant changes in sinus nodal function, effective refractory periods, or intracardiac conduction times. Tocainide does not prolong QRS duration or QT intervals. Theoretically, it may be useful for ventricular arrhythmias associated with a prolonged QT interval.

Tocainide produces a small degree of depression on left ventricular function and left ventricular end diastolic pressure.

Tocainide does not change heart rate or blood pressure. Tocainide is contraindicated in patients with second- or third-degree AV block in the absence of an artificial ventricular pacemaker.

Cimetidine (but not ranitidine) or rifampin reduces the plasmic level of tocainide, whereas metoprolol has added effects with tocainide on wedge pressure and cardiac index.

The most frequent adverse reactions following tocainide are dizziness, vertigo, nausea, paresthesia, and tremor. However, fatal agranulocytosis, bone marrow depression, leukopenia, neutropenia, aplastic/hypoplastic anemia, thrombocytopenia, interstitial pneumonitis, fibrosing alveolitis, pulmonary edema, and pneumonia have occurred in patients receiving tocainide.

TOLAZAMIDE
(Tolinase)

Tolazamide, a sulfonylurea oral hypoglycemic agent (100 mg p.o. daily with breakfast), is indicated as an adjunct to diet to lower blood glucose levels in patients with non-insulin-dependent diabetes mellitus (type II), and it is indicated as a medication for switching patients from insulin to oral therapy (see Table 1).

Oral hypoglycemic agents have advantages over insulin because, by releasing insulin and decreasing the release of glucagon, they mimic physiologic processes and cause fewer allergic reactions. Furthermore, they are effective in an oral form, thus eliminating the need for daily injections.

The mechanisms that underlie the hypoglycemic actions of sulfonylureas are:

Pancreatic
- Improved insulin secretion
- Reduced glucagon secretion

Extrapancreatic
- Improved tissue sensitivity to insulin
- Direct
  - Increased receptor binding
  - Improved postbinding action
- Indirect
  - Reduced hyperglycemia
  - Decreased plasma free fatty-acid concentrations
  - Reduced hepatic insulin extraction

Tolazamide is five times more potent than tolbutamide but is considerably weaker than glipizide and glyburide.

Tolazamide is metabolized by the liver and is excreted by the kidneys. It has diuretic effects but possesses no disulfiram-like properties.

Tolazamide should not be used in patients with burns, acidosis, diabetic coma, severe infection, ketosis, or severe trauma, or in those who are undergoing major surgery, because such conditions of severe physiologic stress require insulin for adequate blood glucose control.

Concomitant use with anticoagulants may increase plasma levels of both drugs and, after continued therapy, may reduce the plasma levels of anticoagulant effects. Use with chloramphenicol, guanethidine, insulin, monoamine oxidase inhibitors, probenecid, salicylates, or sulfonamides may enhance the hypoglycemic effect by displacing tolazamide from its protein-binding sites.

Concomitant use with beta-adrenergic-blocking agents may increase the risk of hypoglycemia, mask its symptoms (rising pulse rate and blood pressure), and prolong it by blocking gluconeogenesis. Use with drugs that may increase blood glucose levels (adrenocorticoids, glucocorticoids, amphetamines, baclofen, corticotropin, epinephrine, ethacrynic acid, furosemide, phenytoin, thiazide diuretics, triamterene, and thyroid hormones) may require dosage adjustments.

Because smoking increases corticosteroid release, smokers may require higher doses of tolazamide.

Clinical manifestation of overdosage with tolazamide includes low blood glucose levels, tingling of lips and tongue, hunger, nausea, decreased cerebral function (lethargy, yawning, confusion, agitation, nervousness), increased sympathetic activity (tachycardia, sweating, tremor), and ultimately, seizures, stupor, and coma.

TOLAZOLINE HYDROCHLORIDE
(Priscoline)

Tolazoline, an alpha-adrenergic-receptor-blocking agent with vasodilating properties (1 to 2 mg/kg IV via a scalp vein over 10 minutes), is indicated in persistent pulmonary vasoconstriction and hypertension of the newborn (persistent fetal circulation).

TOLBUTAMIDE
(Oramide, Orinase, SK-Tolbutamide)

Tolbutamide, a sulfonylurea antidiabetic agent (1 to 2 g p.o. daily), is indicated in stable, maturity-onset nonketotic diabetes mellitus uncontrolled by diet alone and previously untreated.

TOLCAPONE
(Tasmar tablets 100 mg, tablets 200 mg)

Tolcapone is an antiparkinson agent that inhibits **catechol-O-methyl transferase** (COMT), thus blocking the degradation of catechols including dopamine and levodopa. This may lead to more sustained levels of dopamine and consequently a more prolonged antiparkinson's effect. It is indicated as an adjunct to levodopa/carbidopa for the management of signs and symptoms of Parkinson's disease.

Two COMT inhibitors presently are available for this use in the United States, **tolcapone** (Tasmar) and **entacapone** (Comtan). Both these agents have been shown in double-blind trials to reduce the clinical symptoms of "**wearing off**" in patients treated with levodopa/carbidopa. Although the magnitude of their clinical effects and mechanisms of action are similar, they differ with respect to pharmacokinetic properties and adverse effects. Tolcapone has a relatively long duration of action, allowing for administration two to three times a day, and appears to act by both central and peripheral inhibition of COMT. The duration of action of entacapone is short, around 2 hours, so it usually is administered simultaneously with each dose of levodopa/carbidopa. The action of entacapone is attributable principally to peripheral inhibition of COMT. The common adverse effects of these agents are similar to those observed in patients treated with levodopa/carbidopa alone and include nausea, orthostatic hypotension, vivid dreams, confusion, and hallucination. An important adverse effect associated with tolcapone is hepatotoxicity. In clinical trials, up to 2% of the patients treated had increases in serum alanine aminotransferase and aspartate transaminase; after marketing, three fatal cases of fulminant hepatic failure in patients taking tolcapone were observed, leading to addition of a warning to the label. At present, tolcapone should be used only in patients who have not responded to other therapies and with appropriate monitoring for hepatic injury. Entacapone has not been associated with hepatotoxicity and requires no special monitoring. Entacapone also is available in fixed-dose combinations with levodopa/carbidopa (Stalevo).

TOLFENAMIC ACID

Tolfenamic acid is an effective nonsteroidal antiinflammatory drug which belongs to the fenamate group. Tolfenamic acid possesses analgesic, antipyretic, and antiinflammatory properties (see Table 3), and tolfenamic acid inhibits cyclic AMP and cyclic GMP phosphodiesterase. It inhibits cyclooxygenase, reducing the formation of prostaglandin; and inhibits lipoxygenase, leading to formation of leukotriene (see also Figure 13).

TOLMETIN SODIUM
(Tolectin 200 tablets 200 mg (as sodium), Tolectin 600 tablets 600 mg (as sodium))

Tolmetin sodium is a NSAID, which decreases inflammation, pain, and fever, probably through inhibition of cyclooxygenase activity and prostaglandin synthesis. It is indicated in the treatment of chronic and acute rheumatoid arthritis and **osteoarthritis** and **juvenile rheumatoid arthritis. Tolmetin** and **ketorolac** are structurally related heteroaryl acetic acid derivatives with different pharmacological features. Diclofenac is a phenylacetic acid derivative that was developed specifically as an antiinflammatory agent.

Tolmetin is an antiinflammatory, analgesic, and antipyretic agent introduced into clinical practice in the United States in 1976. Tolmetin, in recommended doses (200 to 600 mg three times a day), appears to be approximately equivalent in efficacy to moderate doses of aspirin. **Tolmetin** possesses typical tNSAID properties and side effects

Tolmetin demonstrates rapid and complete absorption, extensive plasma-protein binding, and a short half-life. It undergoes extensive hepatic metabolism, mostly by oxidation of the para-methyl group to a carboxylic acid.

Metabolites are excreted in the urine. Accumulation of the drug in synovial fluid begins within 2 hours and persists for up to 8 hours after a single oral dose.

Tolmetin (tolmetin sodium; Tolectin) is approved in the United States for the treatment of osteoarthritis, rheumatoid arthritis; and juvenile rheumatoid arthritis; it also has been used in the treatment of **ankylosing spondylitis**. In general, tolmetin is thought to have similar therapeutic efficacy to aspirin. The maximum recommended dose is 2 g per day, typically given in divided doses with meals, milk, or antacids to lessen abdominal discomfort. However, peak plasma concentrations and bioavailability are reduced when the drug is taken with food.

Side effects occur in 25 to 40% of patients who take **tolmetin**, and 5 to 10% discontinue use of the drug. Gastrointestinal side effects are the most common (15%) and gastric ulceration has been observed. CNS side effects similar to those seen with indomethacin and aspirin occur, but they are less common and less severe.

Tolmetin (400 mg t.i.d.) is indicated in the treatment of acute flares and long-term management of rheumatoid arthritis and osteoarthritis. In addition, it is effective in the treatment of juvenile rheumatic arthritis (see also Table 3).

Tolmetin has analgesic, antipyretic, and antiinflammatory properties.

Tolmetin is rapidly and completely absorbed after oral administration. Peak concentrations are achieved 20 to 60 minutes after oral administration, and the half-life in plasma is about 5 hours. Accumulation of the drug in synovial fluid begins within 2 hours and persists for up to 8 hours after a single oral dose.

After absorption, tolmetin is extensively (99%) bound to plasma proteins. Virtually all of the drug can be recovered in the urine after 24 hours; some is unchanged, but most is conjugated or otherwise metabolized. The major metabolic transformation involves oxidation of the para-methyl group to a carboxylic acid.

The most common side effects of tolmetin are gastrointestinal side effects consisting of epigastric pain, dyspepsia, nausea, and vomiting. Tolmetin is able to cause gastric erosion and to prolong bleeding time.

Tolmetin is contraindicated in patients in whom aspirin or other nonsteroidal antiinflammatory drugs (NSAIDs) induce symptoms of asthma, urticaria, or rhinitis.

Serious GI toxicity, especially ulceration or hemorrhage, can occur at any time in patients on chronic NSAID therapy. Tolmetin should be used cautiously in patients with a history of GI bleeding or GI ulcer because the drug may irritate the GI tract; in patients with renal disease because the drug may be nephrotoxic; or in patients with cardiac disease because it may cause peripheral edema, sodium retention, and hypertension.

Patients with known "triad" symptoms (aspirin hypersensitivity, rhinitis/nasal polyps, and asthma) are at high risk of cross-sensitivity to tolmetin with precipitation of bronchospasm.

The signs and symptoms of acute infection (fever, myalgias, erythema) may be masked by the use of tolmetin.

The actions of anticoagulants and thrombolytic drugs may be potentiated by the platelet-inhibiting effect of tolmetin. Concomitant use of tolmetin with highly protein-bound drugs (for example, phenytoin, sulfonylureas, warfarin) may cause displacement of either drug and adverse effects. Concomitant use with other GI-irritating drugs (such as steroids, antibiotics, NSAIDs) may potentiate the adverse GI effects of tolmetin.

Antacids and food can delay and decrease the absorption of tolmetin. NSAIDS are known to decrease renal clearance of lithium carbonate, thus increasing lithium serum levels and risks of adverse effects. Concomitant use of tolmetin and aspirin may decrease plasma levels of tolmetin.

TOLNAFTATE

(Absorbine Athlete's Foot cream 1%, Absorbine footcare spray liquid 1%, Aftate for Athlete's Foot gel 1%, spray powder 1%, spray liquid 1%, Aftate for Jock Itch gel 1%, spray powder 1%, Blis-To-Sol liquid 1%, Genaspor cream 1%, NP-27 liquid 1%, Quinsana Plus foot powder 1%, Tinactin cream 1%, solution 1%, powder 1%, spray powder 1%, spray liquid 1%, Tinactin for Jock Itch cream 1%, spray powder 1%, Ting cream 1%)

Tolnaftate is an antifungal agent that distorts hyphae and inhibits mycelial growth in susceptible fungi. It is indicated in the treatment and prophylaxis of tinea pedia (**athlete's foot**); treatment of tinea cruris (**jock itch**) or tinea corporis (**ringworm**) caused by specific fungi; treatment of onchomycosis, chronic scalp infections, palm and sole infections with kerion formation; and treatment of tinea versicolor.

Tolnaftate is a thiocarbamate. **Tolnaftate** is effective in the treatment of most cutaneous mycoses caused by *T. rubrum*, *T. mentagrophytes*, *T. tonsurans*, *E. floccosum*, *M. canis*, *M. audouinii*, *Microsporum gypseum*, and *M. furfur*, but it is ineffective against *Candida*. In tinea pedis, the cure rate is around 80%, compared with about 95% for miconazole. Toxic or allergic reactions to tolnaftate have not been reported.

Tolnaftate (Aftate, Tinactin, others) is available in a 1% concentration as a cream, gel, powder, aerosol powder, and topical solution, or as a topical aerosol liquid. The preparations are applied locally twice a day. Pruritus is usually relieved in 24 to 72 hours. Involution of interdigital lesions caused by susceptible fungi is very often complete in 7 to 21 days.

Tolnaftate (1% cream, solution and gel) is indicated for treatment of tinea pedis (athlete's foot), t. cruris (jock itch), or t. corporis (ringworm) due to infection with *Trichophyton rubrum*, *T. mentagrophytes*, *T. tonsurans*, *Microsporum canis*, *M. audouini*, and *Epidermophyton floccosum*, and as treatment for tinea versicolor due to *Malassezia furfur*.

In onychomycosis, in chronic scalp infections in which fungi are numerous and widely distributed in skin and hair follicles, where kerion has formed, and in fungus infections of palms and soles, tolnaftate may be used concurrently for adjunctive local benefit in these lesions.

TOLTERODINE TARTRATE

(Detrol tablets 1 mg, tablets 2 mg, Detrol LA capsule, extended-release 2 mg, capsule, extended-release 4 mg)

Tolterodine tartrate is an anticholinergic agent that antagonizes the muscarinic receptor, which mediates urinary bladder contraction and salivation. It is in indicated in the treatment of overactive bladder with symptoms of urinary frequency, urgency, or urge incontinence.

TOPIRAMATE

(Topamax tablets 25 mg, tablets 50 mg, tablets 100 mg, tablets 200 mg, capsules, sprinkle 15 mg, capsules, sprinkle 25 mg)

Topiramate is an anticonvulsant that blocks repetitively elicited action potentials, affects the ability of chloride ion to move into neurons, and antagonizes an excitatory amino acid receptor. It is indicated as an adjunctive therapy for partial onset seizures; primary generalized tonic–clonic seizures; seizures associated with Lennox-Gastaut syndrome; and prophylaxis of migraine headache.

Topiramate (Topamax) is a sulfamate-substituted monosaccharide.

Topiramate reduces voltage-gated Na^+ currents in cerebellar granule cells and may act on the inactivated state of the channel in a manner similar to that of **phenytoin**. In addition, **topiramate** activates a hyperpolarizing K^+ current, enhances postsynaptic $GABA_A$-receptor currents, and also limits activation of the AMPA-kainate-subtype(s) of glutamate receptor. **Topiramate** also is a weak carbonic anhydrase inhibitor. Topiramate inhibits maximal electroshock and **pentylenetetrazol-induced seizures** as well as partial and secondarily generalized tonic–clonic seizures in the kindling model, findings predictive of a broad spectrum of antiseizure actions clinically.

Topiramate is rapidly absorbed after oral administration, exhibits little (10 to 20%) binding to plasma proteins, and is mainly excreted unchanged in the urine. The remainder undergoes metabolism by hydroxylation, hydrolysis, and glucuronidation with no single metabolite accounting for more than 5% of an oral dose. Its half-life is about 1 day. Reduced estradiol plasma concentrations occur with concurrent topiramate, suggesting the need for higher doses of oral contraceptives when coadministered with topiramate.

A double-blind study revealed topiramate to be equivalent to valproate and carbamazepine in children and adults with newly diagnosed partial and primary generalized epilepsy. Additional studies disclosed topiramate to be effective as monotherapy for refractory partial epilepsy and refractory generalized tonic–clonic seizures. Topiramate also was found to be significantly more effective than placebo against both drop attacks and tonic–clonic seizures in patients with Lennox-Gastaut syndrome.

Topiramate is well tolerated. The most common adverse effects are somnolence, fatigue, weight loss, and nervousness. It can precipitate renal calculi, which is most likely duc to inhibition of carbonic anhydrase. **Topiramate** has been associated with cognitive impairment and patients may complain about a change in the taste of carbonated beverages.

TOPOTECAN HYDROCHLORIDE

(Hycamtin powder for injection 4 mg)

Topotecan hydrochloride is a DNA topoisomerase inhibitor. Topotecan hydrochloride is an antitumor drug with topoisomerase I-inhibitory activity. It is indicated in metastatic carcinoma of the ovary after failure of initial or subsequent chemotherapy; small-cell-lung-cancer-sensitive disease after failure of first-line chemotherapy.

The **camptothecins** are potent, cytotoxic antineoplastic agents that target the nuclear enzyme **topoisomerase I**. The lead compound in this class, camptothecin, was isolated from the Chinese tree ***Camptotheca acuminata*** in 1966. Initial efforts to develop the compound as a sodium salt were compromised, despite evidence of promising preclinical and clinical antitumor activity, by severe and unpredictable toxicity, principally myelosuppression and hemorrhagic cystitis. Elucidation of the mechanism of action and a better understanding of its physicochemical properties during the 1980s led to the development of more soluble and less toxic analogs. **Irinotecan** and **topotecan**, currently the only camptothecin analogs approved for clinical use, have established activity in colorectal, ovarian, and **small-cell lung cancer**.

Topotecan (Hycamtin) is indicated for previously treated patients with ovarian and small-cell lung cancer. Its significant hematological toxicity, though, has limited its use in combination with other active agents in these diseases (e.g., cisplatin). Promising antitumor activity also has been observed in hematological malignancies, particularly in CML and in myelodysplastic syndromes.

The recommended dosing regimen of topotecan is a 30-minute infusion of 1.5 mg/m^2 per day for 5 consecutive days every 3 weeks. As a significant fraction of the topotecan administered is excreted in the urine, severe toxicities have been observed in patients with decreased creatinine clearance. Therefore, the dose of topotecan should be reduced to 0.75 mg/m^2 per day in patients with moderate renal dysfunction (creatinine clearance 20 to 40 mL/minute), and **topotecan** should not be administered to patients with severe renal impairment (creatinine clearance <20 mL/minute). Topotecan clearance and toxicity are not significantly altered in patients with hepatic dysfunction, and therefore no dose reduction is necessary in these patients.

Approved dosage schedules of irinotecan (Camptosar) in the United States include: 125 mg/m^2 as a 90-minute infusion administered weekly for 4 out of 6 weeks; 350 mg/m^2 given every 3 weeks; 100 mg/m^2 every week; or 150 ing/m^2 every other week. Irinotecan has significant clinical activity in patients with advanced colorectal cancer. It now is the treatment of choice in combination with **fluoropyrimidines** for **advanced colorectal cancer** in patients who have not received chemotherapy previously or as a single agent following failure on a 5-FU regimen. Encouraging results from different phase II studies suggest that irinotecan may have an increasing role in the treatment of other solid tumors, including small-cell and non-small-cell lung cancer, cervical cancer, ovarian cancer, gastric cancer, and brain tumors.

Topotecan: The dose-limiting toxicity with all schedules is neutropenia, with or without thrombocytopenia. The incidence of severe neutropenia at the recommended phase II dose of 1.5 mg/m^2 daily for 5 days every 3 weeks may be as high as 81%, with a 26% incidence of febrile neutropenia. In patients with hematological malignancies, gastrointestinal side effects such as mucositis and diarrhea become dose limiting. Other less common and generally mild topotecan-related toxicities include nausea and vomiting, elevated liver transaminases, fever, fatigue, and rash.

The dose-limiting toxicity with all schedules is delayed diarrhea, with or without **neutropenia**. In the initial studies up to 35% of patients experienced severe diarrhea. Adoption of an intensive loperamide regimen (4 mg of **loperamide** starting at the onset of any loose stool beginning more than a few hours after receiving therapy, followed by 2 mg every 2 hours) has effectively reduced this incidence by more than half. However, once severe diarrhea does occur, standard doses of antidiarrheal agents tend to be ineffective, although the diarrhea episode generally resolves within a week and, unless associated with fever and neutropenia, is rarely fatal.

The second most common irinotecan-associated toxicity is **myelosuppression**. Severe neutropenia occurs in 14 to 47% of the patients treated with the every-3-week schedule, and is less frequently encountered among patients treated with the weekly schedule. Febrile neutropenia is observed in 3% of patients, and may be fatal, particularly when associated with concomitant diarrhea. A cholinergic syndrome resulting from the inhibition of acetylcholinesterase activity by irinotecan may occur within the first 24 hours after irinotecan administration. Symptoms include acute diarrhea, diaphoresis, hypersalivation, abdominal cramps, visual accommodation disturbances, lacrimation, rhinorrhea, and less often, asymptomatic bradycardia. These effects are short lasting and respond within minutes to atropine. Atropine may be prophylactically administered to patients who have previously experienced a cholinergic reaction, prior to the administration of additional cycles of irinotecan. Other common and generally manageable toxicities include nausea and vomiting, fatigue, vasodilation or skin flushing, mucositis, elevation in liver transaminases, and alopecia. Finally, there have been case reports of dyspnea and interstitial pneumonitis associated with irinotecan therapy in Japanese patients with lung cancer.

TOREMIFENE CITRATE
(Fareston oral tablets 60 mg)

Toremifene citrate is an antiestrogen, which is a nonsteroidal antiestrogen that blocks the growth-stimulating effects of estrogen in the tumor. It is indicated in **metastatic breast cancer in postmenopausal women**.

Toremifene (Fareston) is a triphenylethylene derivative of tamoxifen and has a similar pharmacological profile. Toremifene is indicated for the treatment of breast cancer in women with tumors that are ER-positive or of unknown receptor status.

In preclinical models, **toremifene** has activity against breast cancer cells *in vitro* and *in vivo* similar to that of tamoxifen. Unlike tamoxifen, however, toremifene is not hepatocarcinogenic in experimental animals. Two adjuvant studies were initiated to compare efficacy of these two agents, and in particular, long-term tolerability and safety in early-stage breast cancer. In the largest of these studies, 1480 postmenopausal patients with lymph node-positive disease were randomized to receive adjuvant tamoxifen (20 mg daily) or toremifene (40 mg daily) for 5 years. Although longer follow-up is needed, there were no significant differences in efficacy or tolerability after a median follow-up of 4.4 years, and the number of subsequent second cancers was similar. Other head-to-head comparisons of toremifene and tamoxifen in prospective, randomized clinical trials have shown that toremifene has generally similar efficacy and adverse events to tamoxifen. However, *in vitro* in a low-estrogen environment, toremifene has an approximately 40 times lower estrogen agonist effect than tamoxifen. This may make toremifene more effective in combination with an aromatase inhibitor than tamoxifen, and this is the subject of ongoing clinical trials.

Tamoxifen, **raloxifene**, and **toremifene** are selective estrogen receptor modulators, or SERMs are compounds with tissue-selective actions. The pharmacological goal of these drugs is to produce beneficial estrogenic actions in certain tissues (e.g., bone, brain, and liver) during postmenopausal hormone therapy, but antagonist activity in tissues such as breast and endometrium, where estrogenic actions (e.g., carcinogenesis) might be deleterious. Currently approved drugs in the United States in this class are **tamoxifen citrate** (Nolvadex, others), **raloxifene hydrochloride** (Evista), and **toremifene** (Fareston), which is chemically related and has similar actions to tamoxifen. Tamoxifen and toremifene are used for treatment of breast cancer, and raloxifene is used primarily for prevention and treatment of osteoporosis.

TORSEMIDE
(Demadex tablets 5 mg, tablets 10 mg, tablets 20 mg, tablets 100 mg, injection 10 mg/mL)

Torsemide is a loop diuretic that inhibits the sodium/ potassium/chloride carrier system in the ascending loop of Henle, resulting in increased urinary excretion of sodium, chloride, and water. It does not significantly alter glomerular filtration rate, renal plasma flow, or acid-base balance. It is indicated in the management of edema associated with CHF, hepatic cirrhosis, and renal disease; and treatment of hypertension.

Of the loop diuretics currently available, furosemide (Lasix), **bumetanide** (Bumex), and **torsemide** (Demadex) are widely used in the treatment of heart failure. Due to the increased risk of ototoxicity, **ethacrynic acid** (Edecrin) should be reserved for patients who are allergic to sulfonamides or who have developed interstitial nephritis on alternative drugs.

TOSITUMOMAB AND IODINE ^{131}I-TOSITUMOMAB (Bexxar injection kits)

Tositumomab and iodine ^{131}I-tositumomab is a monoclonal antibody that blocks (complement-dependent cytotoxicity) CD20 antigen, which is found on the surface of normal and malignant B lymphocytes. Cell death is associated with ionizing radiation from the radioisotope. It is indicated in the treatment of patients with CD20-positive, follicular, **non-Hodgkinr's lymphoma**, with and without transformation, whose disease is refractory to rituximab and has relapsed following chemotherapy.

TRACE MINERALS ESSENTIAL FOR HEALTH

Elements	Sign of Deficiency
Zinc	Dermatitis, hypogeusia, alopecia, diarrhea, apathy, depression
Copper	Neutropenia, hypochromic anemia, osteoporosis, decreased hair and skin pigmentation, dermatitis, anorexia, diarrhea
Chromium	Glucose intolerance, peripheral neuropathy, increased free fatty acid levels, low respiratory quotient
Manganese	Nausea, vomiting, dermatitis, color changes in hair, hypocholesterolemia, growth retardation
Selenium	Muscle weakness and pain, cardiomyopathy
Molybdenum	Tachycardia, tachypnea, altered mental status, visual changes, headache, nausea, vomiting
Iodine	Hyperthyroid goiter, hypothyroidism

TRAMADOL HYDROCHLORIDE (Ultram tablets 50 mg)

Tramadol hydrochloride is an opioid analgesic that binds to certain opioid receptors and inhibits reuptake of norepinephrine and serotonin; its exact mechanism of action is unknown. It is indicated for relief of moderate to moderately severe pain.

TRAMADOL HYDROCHLORIDE/ACETAMINOPHEN (Ultracet tablets 325 mg acetaminophen/37.5 mg tramadol hydrochloride)

Tramadol hydrochloride/acetaminophen is a nonnarcotic analgesic combination. **Tramadol**: the exact mechanism is unknown; however, it binds to certain opioid receptors and inhibits reuptake of norepinephrine and serotonin. **Acetaminophen**: inhibits prostaglandin in CNS and reduces fever through direct action on the hypothalamic heat-regulating center.

Tramadol (Ultram) is a synthetic codeine analog that is a weak μ-opioid receptor agonist. Part of its analgesic effect is produced by inhibition of uptake of norepinephrine and serotonin. In the treatment of mild to moderate pain, tramadol is as effective as morphine or meperidine. However, for the treatment of severe or chronic pain, **tramadol** is less effective. Tramadol is as effective as meperidine in the treatment of labor pain and may cause less neonatal respiratory depression.

Tramadol is 68% bioavailable after a single oral dose and 100% available when administered intramuscularly. Its affinity for the μ-opioid receptor is only 1/6000 that of morphine. However, the primary *O*-demethylated metabolite of tramadol is two to four times as potent as the parent drug and may account for part of the analgesic effect. **Tramadol** is supplied as a racemic mixture that is more effective than either enantiomer alone. The (+)-enantiomer binds to the μ receptor and inhibits serotonin uptake. The (−)-enantiomer inhibits norepinephrine uptake and stimulates α_2-adrenergic receptors. The compound undergoes hepatic metabolism and renal excretion, with an elimination half-life of 6 hours for tramadol and 7.5 hours for its active metabolite. Analgesia begins within an hour of oral dosing and peaks within 2 to 3 hours. The duration of analgesia is about 6 hours. The maximum recommended daily dose is 400 mg.

Common side effects of **tramadol** include nausea, vomiting, dizziness, dry mouth, sedation, and headache. Respiratory depression appears to be less than with equianalgesic doses of morphine, and the degree of constipation is less than that seen after equivalent doses of codeine. Tramadol can cause seizures and possibly exacerbate seizures in patients with predisposing factors. Although tramadol-induced analgesia is not entirely reversible by naloxone, tramadol-induced respiratory depression can be reversed by naloxone. However, the use of naloxone increases the risk of seizure. Physical dependence on and abuse of tramadol have been reported. Although its abuse potential is unclear, tramadol probably should be avoided in patients with a history of addiction. Because of its inhibitory effect on serotonin uptake, tramadol should not be used in patients taking monoamine oxidase (MAO) inhibitors.

TRANDOLAPRIL (Mavik tablets 1 mg, tablets 2 mg tablets 4 mg)

Trandolapril is an angiotensin-converting enzyme (ACE) inhibitor that reduces the formation of the vasopressor hormone angiotensin II by inhibiting ACE. It Results in decreased BP and reduced sodium reabsorption and potassium retention. **Heart failure post-MI/left-ventricular dysfunction post-MI**: used for stable patients who have evidence of left-ventricular systolic dysfunction (identified by wall motion abnormalities) or who are symptomatic from CHF within the first few days after sustaining acute MI. **Hypertension**: used in treatment of hypertension either alone or in combination with other antihypertensive drugs.

TRANDOLAPRIL/VERAPAMIL HYDROCHLORIDE

(Tarka tablets 1 mg trandolapril and 240 mg verapamil, tablets 2 mg trandolapril and 180 mg verapamil, tablets 2 mg trandolapril and 240 mg verapamil, tablets 4 mg trandolapril and 240 mg verapamil)

Trandolapril/verapamil hydrochloride is an antihypertensive combination, which **Trandolapril** reduces formation of the vasopressor hormone angiotensin II by inhibiting angiotensin-converting enzyme (ACE), resulting in decreased BP and reduced sodium reabsorption and potassium retention. **Verapamil** inhibits movement of calcium ions across cell membrane, resulting in depression of mechanical contraction of myocardial and vascular smooth muscle and depression of both impulse formation (automaticity) and conduction velocity. They are indicated in the treatment of hypertension.

Angiotensin II is an important regulator of cardiovascular function. The ability to reduce levels of angiotensin II with orally effective inhibitors of **angiotensin-converting enzyme** (ACE) represents an important advance in the treatment of hypertension. **Captopril** (Capoten) was the first such agent to be developed for the treatment of hypertension. Since then, **enalapril** (Vasotec), **lisinopril** (Prinivil), **quinapril** (Accupril), **ramipril** (Altace), **benazepril** (Lotensin), **moexipril** (Univasc), **fosinopril** (Monopril), **trandolapril** (Mavik) and **perindopril** (Aceon) also have become available These drugs have proven to be very useful for the treatment of hypertension because of their efficacy and their very favorable profile of adverse effects, which enhances patient adherence.

The ACE inhibitors appear to confer a special advantage in the treatment of patients with diabetes, slowing the development and progression of **diabetic glomerulopathy**. They also are effective in slowing the progression of other forms of chronic renal disease, such as **glomerulosclerosis**, and many of these patients also have hypertension. An ACE inhibitor is the preferred initial agent in these patients. Patients with hypertension and ischemic heart disease are candidates for treatment with ACE inhibitors; administration of ACE inhibitors in the immediate postmyocardial infarction period has been shown to improve ventricular function and reduce morbidity and mortality.

TRANYLCYPROMINE SULFATE

(Parnate)

Tranylcypromine, a monoamine oxidase alpha inhibitor (30 mg/day in divided doses), is indicated for the treatment of depression (see Figure 37).

Monoamine oxidase can metabolize monoamines by oxidative deamination and convert them to inactive acidic derivatives. Monoamine oxidase inhibitors seem to compete with physiologically active monoamine for the active site of the enzyme. In general, not only do these agents inhibit the oxidase that metabolizes amines, but they also inhibit the oxidase that metabolizes drugs and essential nutrients. Hence, the incidence of drug–drug and drug–food interactions is extremely high with these agents. Monoamine oxidases have various applications. They may be used as a local anesthetic (cocaine), an antihistaminic (diphenylhydramine), or an antidepressant (tranylcypromine). Monoamine oxidase inhibitors have been used in the treatment of hypertension (direct blockade of sympathetic ganglion), angina pectoris (coronary dilation), narcolepsy (stimulating the reticular-activating system), and depression (increasing the brain's norepinephrine pool). Needless to say, these agents should be used with extreme caution in conjunction with sympathomimetic amines, ganglionic blocking agents, procaine, and anesthetic agents. They are contraindicated in patients with hyperthyroidism and in combination with tricyclic antidepressants. In the event of poisoning, adrenergic-blocking agents such as phentolamine may be effective for combating the hypertensive crisis.

The high incidence of drug–food and drug–drug interactions rules out monoamine oxidase inhibitors as antidepressants of first choice. However, there are circumstances in which these agents may be used effectively and successfully. These are:

- When a patient has not responded to a tricyclic antidepressant for an adequate trial period and with an appropriate dosage
- When a patient has developed allergic reactions to tricyclics
- When a patient has had previous depressive episodes that responded well to monoamine oxidase inhibitors

TRASTUZUMAB

(Herceptin powder for injection, lyophilized 440 mg)

Trastazumab is a monoclonal antibody. It is a recombinant DNA-derived humanized monoclonal antibody that selectively binds with high affinity to the extracellular domain of the HER2. It inhibits the proliferation of human tumor cells that over express HER2 and mediates antibody-dependent cellular cytotoxicity (ADCC). It is indicated in breast cancer.

Trastuzumab (Herceptin) is a humanized monoclonal antibody against the HER2/neu (ErbB-2) member of the epidermal growth factor family of cellular receptors. The internal domain of the HER2/neu glycoprotein encodes a tyrosine kinase that activates downstream signals and enhances metastatic potential and inhibits apoptosis. HER2/neu is overexpressed in up to 30% of breast cancers and is associated with clinical resistance to cytotoxic and hormone therapy. A number of mechanisms of action have been proposed, which may lead to both cytostatic and cytotoxic effects. Downregulation of HER2/ neu expression may inhibit cell proliferation, potentially through induction of p27 and reduction of cyclin Dl, and is associated with antiangiogenetic effects. **Trastuzumab** also can initiate FC-receptor-mediated antibody-dependent cellular cytotoxicity and directly induce apoptosis.

Trastuzumab is the first monoclonal antibody to be approved for the treatment of a solid tumor. Currently, trastuzumab is approved for HER2/neu overexpressing metastatic breast cancer in combination with **paclitaxel** as initial treatment or as monotherapy following chemotherapy relapse. **Trastuzumab** also is synergistic with other cytotoxic agents, but expectedly, this is only observed in HER2/neu-overexpressing cancers. Phase III studies are randomizing patients between chemotherapy with or without trastuzumab to assess the optimum regimen. HER2/neu expression also is found in other solid tumors and responses have been reported in colorectal and non-small cell lung cancer. Clinical trials of trastuzumab in other tumors that express HER2/neu at relatively high frequency, such as pancreas and stomach, are likely.

Trastuzumab has dose-dependent pharmacokinetics with a mean half-life of 5.8 days at the 2 mg/kg maintenance dose. Steady-state levels were achieved between the 16th and the 32nd weeks with mean trough and peak concentrations of approximately 79 and 123 μg/ml, respectively. The infusional effects of trastuzumab are typical of other monoclonal antibodies and include fever, chills, nausea, dyspnea, and rashes. Allergic reactions also may be observed. Cardiac dysfunction is an unexpected and potentially serious side effect that was observed in the pivotal trial of **trastuzumab** and chemotherapy. Left ventricular dysfunction was seen most commonly in those patients who received doxorubicin and cyclophosphamide. In a murine model, mice with a ventricular-restricted deletion of the HER2/neu gene developed cardiomyopathy, indicating that HER2/neu signaling is important for cardiac muscle.

TRAVOPROST
(Travatan solution 0.004%)

Travoprost is a prostaglandin agonist that may reduce intraocular pressure (IOP) by increasing uveoscleral outflow. It is indicated for reduction of IOP in patients with open-angle glaucoma or ocular hypertension who are intolerant of other IOP-lowering agents or insufficiently responsive to other IOP-lowering medications.

The goal is to prevent **progressive glaucomatous optic-nerve damage** with minimum risk and side effects from either topical or systemic therapy. With these general principles in mind, a stepped medical approach may begin with a topical prostaglandin analog. Due to their once-daily dosing, low incidence of systemic side effects, and potent intraocular pressure lowering effect, prostaglandin analogs have largely replaced β-adrenergic-receptor antagonists as first-line medical therapy for glaucoma. The prostaglandin analogs consist of **latanoprost** (Xalatan), **travoprost** (Travatan), **bimatoprost** (Lumigan), and **unoprostone** (Rescula).

TRAZODONE HYDROCHLORIDE
(Desyrel)

Trazodone (150 mg/day) is indicated in the treatment of depression. Trazodone selectively inhibits serotonin reuptake in the brain, causes beta-receptor subsensitivity, and induces significant changes in serotonin-receptor binding with only a slight effect on alpha-adrenergic receptors. Also, trazodone potentiates the action of 5-hydroxytryptophan, the precursor of serotonin (see also Tables 5 through 7).

Trazodone is perhaps the most sedative antidepressant available, being more sedative than amitriptyline, trimipramine, doxepan, or imipramine. Therefore, death has occurred in patients taking trazodone with alcohol, chloral hydrate, diazepam, chlordiazepoxide, meprobamate, or amobarbital.

The most severe reactions reported with overdose of trazodone alone have been priapism, respiratory arrest, seizures, and ECG changes.

TREFOIL PEPTIDES

Trefoil peptides constitute a rapidly growing family of peptides containing one or more characteristic trefoil domains. A trefoil domain is defined as a sequence of 38 or 39 amino acid residues in which 6 cysteine residues are disulfide-linked in the configuration 1–5, 2–4, and 3–6 when the cysteines are numbered from the N-terminal end of the peptide. The amino acid sequence together with the disulfide bonds thus forms a distinctive three-leafed structure giving the peptide family its name.

Although trefoil peptides have been cloned or isolated from a series of different organs and tissues from several species, recent evidence indicates that trefoil peptides may have their main function in association with the mucous layer of the gastrointestinal tract. Trefoil peptides have thus been suggested as possible naturally occurring healing factors for peptic ulcers, inflammatory bowel disease, and other diseases in the gastrointestinal tract involving mucosal injury.

TRETINOIN (VITAMIN A ACID)
(Avita cream 0.025%, gel 0.025%, Renova cream 0.02%, cream 0.05%, Retin-A cream 0.025%, cream 0.05%, cream 0.1%, gel 0.025%, gel 0.01%, Retin-A Micro gel 0.04%, gel 0.1%, Vesanoid capsules 10 mg)

Tretinoin is a retinoid, which decreases cohesiveness and stimulates mitotic activity and turnover of follicular epithelial cells, resulting in decreased formation and increased extrusion of comedones. **PO** induces maturation of acute promyelocytic leukemia cells followed by a repopulation of the bone marrow and peripheral blood by normal, polyclonal hematopoietic cells in patients achieving complete

TRAVELER'S DIARRHEA: Prevention of

Diarrhea is by far the most common medical problem among people traveling to the tropical and semitropical areas of Latin America, parts of the Caribbean, such as Haiti and the Dominican Republic, southern Asia, and North, East, and West Africa.

Bacterial enteropathogens cause as least 80% of traveler's diarrhea, which explains the prophylactic and therapeutic effects of antibacterial drugs. Although different organisms predominate in different regions, the principal agents in most of the high-risk areas are, in decreasing order of importance, enterotoxigenic *Escherichia coli*, *Shigella* species, *Campylobacter jejuni*, *Aeromonas* species, *Plesiomonas shigelloides*, salmonella species, and noncholera *Vibrios*. Doxycycline and trimethoprim-sulfamethoxazole may be used for prophylaxis.

Other approaches to the prevention of traveler's diarrhea are the use of lactobacillus preparations or bismuth subsalicylate. Lactobacilli are bacteria that metabolize dietary carbohydrate to lactic acid and other organic acids, reducing the intraluminal pH and inhibiting the growth of enteropathogens.

Bismuth subsalicylate has short-term intraluminal antimicrobial action, but it must be given four times daily, with meals and at bedtime.

Drugs	Dose
Bismuth subsalicylate	Tablets chewed four times a day
Fluoroquinolone antibiotics	
Norfloxacin	400 mg daily
Ciprofloxacin	500 mg daily
Ofloxacin	300 mg daily
Fleroxacin	400 mg daily
Trimethoprim-sulfamethoxazole	160 mg of trimethoprim and 800 mg of sulfamethoxazole once daily
Doxycycline	100 mg daily

remission. It is indicated in the topical treatment of acne vulgaris; as an adjunctive agent for use in the mitigation of fine wrinkles, mottled hyperpigmentation, and tactile roughness of facial skin; and PO treatment for **acute promyelocytic leukemia** (APL).

The most important of these for cancer treatment is **tretinoin** (all-*trans* retinoic acid; ATRA), which induces a high rate of complete remission in APL as a single agent, and in combination with anthracyclines, has become part of a curative regimen for this disease.

Retinoids include natural compounds and synthetic derivatives of retinol that exhibit vitamin A activity. Retinoids have many important functions throughout the body, including roles in vision, regulation of cell proliferation and differentiation and bone growth, immune defense, and tumor suppression. Because vitamin A affects normal epithelial differentiation, it was investigated as a treatment for cutaneous disorders but was abandoned initially because of unfavorable side effects. Molecular modifications yielded compounds with vastly improved margins of safety. First-generation retinoids include retinol, **tretinoin** (all-*trans*-retinoic acid), isotretinoin (13-*cis*-retinoic acid), and alitretinoin (9-*cis*-retinoic acid). Second-generation retinoids, also known as aromatic retinoids, were created by alteration of the cyclic end group and include acitretin. Third-generation retinoids contain further modifications and are called arotinoids. Members of this generation include tazarotene and bexarotene. Adapalene, a derivative of naphthoic acid with retinoid-like properties, does not fit precisely into any of the three generations.

Retinoic acid (RA) exerts its effects on gene expression by activating two families of receptors—retinoic acid receptors (RARs) and the retinoid X receptors (RXRs)—that are members of the thyroid/steroid hormone receptor superfamily. Retinoids (ligands) bind transcription factors (nuclear receptors), and the ligand-receptor complex then binds to the promoter regions of target genes to regulate their expression. The gene products formed contribute to the desirable pharmacological effects of these drugs and their unwanted side effects. Additional complexity arises because each receptor has three iso-forms (α, β and γ) that form homo- and heterodimers. Retinoid-responsive tissues express one or more RAR and RXR subtypes in various combinations that determine activity locally. Human skin contains mainly RARα and RARβ.

First- and second-generation retinoids can bind to several retinoid receptors because of the flexibility imparted by their alternating single and double bonds. This relative lack of receptor specificity may lead to greater side effects. The structures of third-generation retinoids are much less flexible than those of earlier-generation retinoids and therefore interact with fewer retinoid receptors.

Acute retinoid toxicity is similar to vitamin A intoxication. Side effects of retinoids include dry skin, nosebleeds from dry mucous membranes, conjunctivitis, and hair loss. Less frequently, musculoskeletal pain, pseudotumor cerebri, and mood alterations occur. Oral retinoids are potent teratogens and cause severe fetal malformations. Because of this, systemic retinoids should be used with great caution in females of childbearing potential.

Retinoids are used in the treatment of diverse diseases and are effective in the treatment of inflammatory skin disorders, skin malignancies, hyperproliferative disorders, photoaging, and many other disorders. Topical retinoids can normalize disordered keratinization in sebaceous follicles and reduce inflammation, and they may enhance the penetration of other topical medications. Specific retinoids and their uses in the treatment of dermatologic disorders are discussed below.

Tretinoin (Retin-A, others) has been used in the treatment of acne vulgaris for almost four decades. A primary use for tretinoin is to reduce the hyperkeratinization that leads to microcomedone formation, the initial lesion in acne. Follicular comeocytes become less cohesive as a result of shedding of desmosomes, decreasing tonofilaments and increasing keratinocyte autolysis and intracellular deposition of glycogen.

In addition to treating acne, tretinoin improves photodamaged human skin. Epidermal effects include increased epidermal and granular layer thickness, decreased melanocytic activity, and increased secretion of a glycosaminoglycan-like substance into the intercellular space. In the dermis, blood vessel vasodilation and angiogenesis and increased papillary dermal collagen synthesis have been documented. Clinically, this translates to modest attenuation of fine and coarse wrinkling, smoother texture, increased pinkness, and diminished hyperpigmentation. In clinical trials, wrinkling, mottled hyperpigmentation, and roughness improved in most patients treated with retinoids, a response rate roughly twice that of control subjects who used sunscreens and emollients. Ultraviolet radiation also activates growth factor and cytokine receptors on epidermal keratinocytes and dermal cells. These receptors stimulate mitogen-activated protein kinases (MAP kinases), which, in turn, induce c-Jun expression. This transcription factor heterodimerizes with c-Fos to form activated AP-1 complexes that induce the transcription of metalloproteinases that degrade dermal collagens and other proteins.

Tretinoin is approved for the treatment of acne vulgaris and as an adjunctive agent for treating photoaging. Topical preparations contain from 0.01% to 0.1% tretinoin in cream, gel, and solution formulations. Initiation of therapy with lower-strength preparations and progression to higher strengths may be useful because individual sensitivity is unpredictable. **Tretinoin** formulations with cream base are indicated for dry skin, whereas gel-based formulations are indicated for oily skin. The medication is applied once daily before bedtime to minimize photodegradation. Maximum clinical response in acne may require several months, and maintenance therapy is necessary. A formulation of tretinoin with active drug incorporated into microsponges (Retin-A Micro) has been developed. The microsponges not only decrease irritation by slowing the release of the medication but also may enhance efficacy by targeting delivery to the sebaceous follicle.

A 0.5% emollient cream formulation of tretinoin (Renova) is one formulation approved for treatment of photoaged skin. Nightly application produces maximum response within 1 year, and application one to three times weekly is said to maintain improvement. Treatment must be combined with a rigorous program of photoprotection, including sunscreens, sun avoidance, and photoprotective clothing.

TRIAMCINOLONE (SYSTEMIC)
(Aristocort, Kenacort)

TRIAMCINOLONE ACETONIDE
(Kenalog, Kenalone, Triam-A)

TRIAMCINOLONE ACETONIDE (ORAL INHALANT)
(Azmacort)

Triamcinolone (2 inhalations t.i.d.) is indicated in the treatment of steroid-dependent asthma.

TRIAMCINOLONE ACETONIDE (TOPICAL)
(Aristocort, Flutex, Kenalog, Kenalog in Orabase, Triacet)

Topical triamcinolone (cream, lotion, aerosol, and paste 0.025 to 0.5%) is indicated in the treatment of inflammation of corticosteroid-responsive dermatoses.

TRIAMCINOLONE DIACETATE
(Amcort, Aristocort, Aristocort Forte, Aristocort Intralesional, Articulose LA, Cenocort Forte, Cinalone, Kenacort, Triam-Forte, Triamolone, Tristoject)

TRIAMCINOLONE HEXACETONIDE
(Aristospan intra-Articular, Aristospan intralesional)

Triamcinolone, a glucocorticoid (4 to 12 mg p.o. daily), is indicated in adrenal insufficiency; and triamcinolone (4 to 60 mg p.o. daily) is indicated for severe inflammation and immunosuppression.

The glucocorticoids possess a plethora of physiologic actions, including a role in differentiation and development. They are vital in the treatment of adrenal insufficiency and are used extensively in large pharmacologic doses as antiinflammatory and immunosuppressive agents. Some of the nonendocrine conditions for which they may be used include arthritis, tenosynovitis, systemic lupus erythematosus, acute rheumatic carditis, bronchial asthma, organ transplantation, ulcerative colitis, cerebral edema, and myasthenia gravis.

The relative antiinflammatory potency and sodium-retaining properties of several steroids are listed in Table 14.

Glucocorticoids have an anti-insulin effect and aggravate the pathologic consequences of diabetes mellitus. They increase gluconeogenesis, inhibit the peripheral utilization of glucose, and cause hyperglycemia and glucosuria. Cortisol's effect, for example, is opposite to that of insulin's.

Glucocorticoids promote the breakdown of proteins and inhibit protein synthesis. This leads to muscle wasting in the quadriceps-femoris groups, and muscular activities may become difficult as a result.

The effects of glucocorticoids on glycogen accumulation appear to be predominantly, although not exclusively, insulin-dependent, as glycogen accumulation is markedly reduced in pancreatectomized animals. Glucocorticoid-stimulated increases in insulin secretion promote further glycogen accumulation.

Glucocorticoids cause the abnormal deposition of a fat pad called "buffalo hump." Glucocorticoids cause hypernatremia, hypokalemia, and hypercalciurea. Glucocorticoids cause hyperuricemia by suppressing the renal tubular resorption of uric acid. Glucocorticoids promote the production of gastric hydrochloric acid, and, like epinephrine, they augment the coagulability of blood.

Glucocorticoids exert their antiinflammatory effects in part by blocking the release and action of histamine. In addition, they decrease the migration of polymorphonuclear leukocytes.

Glucocorticoids produce eosinophilia and cause the involution of lymphoid tissues. They bring about lymphocytopenia, monocytopenia, and eosinopenia. In addition, glucocorticoids block a number of lymphocytic functions.

Although considered to be immunosuppressive, therapeutic doses of glucocorticoids do not significantly decrease the concentration of antibodies in the circulation. Furthermore, during glucocorticoid therapy, patients exhibit a nearly normal antibody response to antigenic challenge.

Glucocorticoids, which do penetrate the blood-brain barrier, affect behavior, mood, and neural activity, and are able to regulate the permeability of the blood–brain barrier to other substances. Hence they are used to treat brain edema. Both glucocorticoid deficiency and excess may cause mood swings and rarely psychosis. Patients receiving glucocorticoids have a feeling of well-being. On the other hand, patients with spontaneously evolving Cushing's syndrome, which involves the overproduction of glucocorticoids, are commonly depressed. Patients with Addison's disease, which is caused by a deficiency of cortisol and aldosterone, tend to be depressed, negativistic, irritable, seclusive, and apathetic. Patients with Addison's disease also suffer from anorexia, whereas a glucocorticoid excess stimulates the appetite. In addition, high doses of glucocorticoids can affect sleep, with a trend toward increased wakefulness, a reduction in rapid-eye-movement (REM) sleep, increase in stage II sleep, and an increase in the time to the first REM sleep.

Glucocorticoids affect bone metabolism in a variety of ways. Mild hyperkalemia can occur in Addison's disease. Conversely, glucocorticoids are used to treat certain hypercalcemias—largely granulomatous conditions such as sarcoidosis, in which the steroid blocks the formation of 1-alpha,25-dihydroxycholecalciferol [1-alpha,25-$(OH)_2D_3$] by the granulomatous tissues. However, most hypercalcemias are not glucocorticoid responsive and, in general, glucocorticoid excess does not result in lower serum calcium levels. Serum phosphate levels are lowered and urinary calcium and phosphorous concentrations are elevated in glucocorticoid excess states. Glucocorticoid excess ultimately leads to osteoporosis, the major limitation to their long-term use.

Besides the adverse effects just described, glucocorticoid therapy is contraindicated under the following circumstances: diabetes mellitus, digitalis therapy, glaucoma, hypertension, infection, osteoporosis, peptic ulcer, tuberculosis, and viral infection.

TRIAZOLAM
(Halcion)

Triazolam, a benzodiazepine derivative (0.125 to 0.25 mg p.o.), is indicated in insomnia. Triazolam, a short-acting hypnotic sedative, depresses the CNS at the limbic and subcortical levels of the brain. It produces a sedative-hypnotic effect by potentiating the effect of the neurotransmitter gamma-aminobutyric acid (GABA) on its receptor in the ascending reticular-activating system, which increases inhibition and blocks both cortical and limbic arousal (Table 9).

Triazolam is absorbed well orally, exerts its sedative effects in 15 minutes, is distributed widely in the body, is bound to plasma proteins to the extent of 90%, is metabolized to 6-hydroxytriazolam, which is subsequently conjugated with glucuronic acid and is excreted in the urine.

Triazolam is contraindicated in patients in coma, because the drug's hypnotic or hypotensive effect may be prolonged or intensified; in pregnant patients, because it may be fetotoxic; and in patients with acute alcohol intoxication who have depressed vital signs, because the drug will worsen CNS depression.

Triazolam should be used cautiously in patients with impaired hepatic function, which prolongs elimination of the drug; in elderly or debilitated patients, who are usually more sensitive to the drug's CNS effects; and in individuals prone to addiction or drug abuse.

Triazolam potentiates the CNS depressant effects of phenothiazines, narcotics, antihistamines, MAO inhibitors, barbiturates, alcohol, general anesthetics, and antidepressants. Enhanced amnestic effects have been reported when combined with alcohol (even in small amounts).

Concomitant use with cimetidine and possibly disulfiram causes diminished hepatic metabolism of triazolam, which increases its plasma concentration.

Heavy smoking accelerates triazolam metabolism, thus lowering clinical effectiveness. Benzodiazepines may decrease the therapeutic effects of levodopa. Triazolam may decrease serum levels of haloperidol. Erythromycin decreases clearance of triazolam.

The clinical manifestations of overdosage with triazolam are somnolence, confusion, hypoactive reflexes, dyspnea, labored breathing, hypotension, bradycardia, slurred speech, unsteady gait, or impaired coordination, and, ultimately, coma.

Flumazenil, a specific benzodiazepine-receptor antagonist will antidote and reverse the deleterious effects of triazolam (see Figure 50).

TRICHLORMETHIAZIDE
(Diurese, Metahydrin, Naqua, Trichlorex)

Trichlormethiazide, a thiazide diuretic (1 to 4 mg p.o. daily), is used in treating hypertension.

TRIENTINE HYDROCHLORIDE
(Syprine capsules 250 mg, Cuprid)

Trientine hydrochloride is a chelating agent, which forms chelate with copper, facilitating removal from the body. It is indicated in the treatment of **Wilson's disease** in patients intolerant of **penicillamine**.

Penicillamine is the drug of choice for treatment for Wilson's disease. However, the drug produces undesirable effects, and some patients become intolerant. For these individuals, **trientine** (triethylenetetramine dehydrochloride, Cuprid) is an acceptable alternative. Trientine is an effective **cupriuretic agent** in patients with Wilson's disease, although it may be less potent than penicillamine. The drug is effective orally. Maximal daily doses of 2 g for adults or 1.5 g for children are taken in two to four divided portions on an empty stomach. **Trientine** may cause iron deficiency; this can be overcome with short courses of iron therapy, but iron and trientine should not be ingested within 2 hours of each other.

Trientine, a heavy-metal-chelating agent (750 to 1250 mg in divided doses), is used in Wilson's disease in patients who are intolerant of penicillamine.

TRIETHANOLAMINE POLYPEPTIDE OLEATE-CONDENSATE
(Cerumenex)

Triethanolamine, an oleic acid derivative with cerumenolytic properties, is used in impacted cerumen.

TRIFLUOPERAZINE HYDROCHLORIDE
(Stelazine)

Trifluoperazine, a phenothiazine antipsychotic with antiemetic properties (2 to 5 mg p.o. t.i.d.), is indicated in the management of manifestations of psychotic disorders (see Table 2).

Trifluoperazine exerts its antipsychotic effects by postsynaptic blockade of CNS dopamine receptors, thereby inhibiting the action of dopamine.

Trifluoperazine's antiemetic effects are attributed to dopamine-receptor blockade in the medullary chemoreceptor trigger zone (see also Figure 73).

Trifluoperazine exhibits low incidences of sedative and anticholinergic properties, but causes a high incidence of extrapyramidal movement disorders including akathisia, dystonia, parkinsonism, tardive dyskinesia, and neuroleptic malignant syndrome.

Concomitant use of trifluoperazine with sympathomimetics, including epinephrine, phenylephrine, phenylpropanolamine, and ephedrine (often found in nasal sprays), and appetite suppressants may decrease their stimulatory and pressor effects. Using epinephrine as a pressor agent in patients taking trifluoperazine may result in epinephrine reversal or further lowering of blood pressure.

Trifluoperazine may inhibit blood pressure response to centrally acting antihypertensive drugs, such as guanethidine, guanabenz, guanadrel, clonidine, methyldopa, and reserpine. Additive effects are likely after concomitant use of trifluoperazine with CNS depressants, including alcohol, analgesics, barbiturates, narcotics, tranquilizers, anesthetics (general, spinal, epidural), and parenteral magnesium sulfate (oversedation, respiratory depression, and hypotension); antiarrhythmic agents, quinidine, disopyramide, and procainamide (increased incidence of cardiac arrhythmias and conduction defects); atropine and other anticholinergic drugs, including antidepressants, monoamine oxidase inhibitors, phenothiazines, antihistamines, meperidine, and antiparkinsonian agents (oversedation, paralytic ileus, visual changes, and severe constipation); nitrates (hypotension); and metrizamide (increased risk of seizures).

The clinical manifestations of overdosage of trifluoperazine include CNS depression characterized by deep, unarousable sleep and possible coma, hypotension or hypertension, extrapyramidal symptoms, dystonia, abnormal involuntary muscle movements, agitation, seizures, arrhythmias, ECG changes, hypothermia or hyperthermia, and autonomic nervous system dysfunction.

TRIFLUPROMAZINE HYDROCHLORIDE
(Vesprin)

Triflupromazine (60 mg IM, up to 150 mg/day) is indicated in the management of manifestations of psychotic disorders; and triflupromazine (5 to 15 mg q. 4 hours) is used to control severe nausea and vomiting.

Triflupromazine causes heavy sedation and has potent anticholinergic properties. It causes a moderate degree of extrapyramidal movement disorders such as akathisia, dystonia, Parkinson's disease, tardive dyskinesia, and neuroleptic malignant syndrome.

Triflupromazine, possessing strong anticholinergic properties, is contraindicated in patients with cardiac diseases such as congestive heart failure, arrhythmias, angina pectoris, and heart block; in encephalitis; Reye's syndrome; head injury; respiratory disease; epilepsy and other seizure disorders; glaucoma; prostatic hypertrophy; urinary retention; Parkinson's disease and pheochromocytoma, because it may exacerbate these conditions; in patients with hypocalcemia, because the drug increases the risk of extrapyramidal reactions; and in patients with hepatic or renal dysfunction (diminished metabolism and excretion cause the drug to accumulate).

Triflupromazine, possessing potent sedative properties, is contraindicated in patients with disorders accompanied by coma, brain damage, CNS depression, circulatory collapse, or cerebrovascular disease (additive CNS depression and adverse blood pressure effects); and in patients taking adrenergic-blocking agents or spinal or epidural anesthetics (excessive respiratory, cardiac, and CNS depression).

As is the case with trifluoperazine, concomitant use of triflupromazine with sympathomimetics, including epinephrine, phenylephrine, phenylpropanolamine, ephedrine (often found in nasal sprays), and appetite suppressants may decrease their stimulatory and pressor effects. Using epinephrine as a pressor agent in patients taking triflupromazine may result in epinephrine reversal or further lowering of blood pressure.

Triflupromazine may inhibit blood pressure response to centrally acting antihypertensive drugs, such as guanethidine, guanabenz, guanadrel, clonidine, methyldopa, and reserpine. Additive effects are likely after concomitant use of triflupromazine with CNS depressants, including alcohol, analgesics, barbiturates, narcotics, tranquilizers, anesthetics (general, spinal, epidural), and parenteral magnesium sulfate (oversedation, respiratory depression, and hypotension); antiarrhythmic agents, quinidine, disopyramide, and procainamide (increased incidence of cardiac arrhythmias and conduction defects); atropine and other anticholinergic drugs, including antidepressants, monoamine oxidase inhibitors, phenothiazines, antihistamines, meperidine, and antiparkinsonian agents (oversedation, paralytic ileus, visual changes, and severe constipation); nitrates (hypotension); and metrizamide (increased risk of seizures).

The clinical manifestations of overdosage with triflupromazine are characterized by deep, unarousable sleep and possible coma, hypotension and hypertension, extrapyramidal symptoms, dystonia, abnormal involuntary muscle movements, agitation, seizures, arrhythmias, ECG changes, hypothermia or hyperthermia, and autonomic nervous system dysfunction.

TRIFLURIDINE (Viroptic)

Trifluridine, an antiviral agent (1 drop of 1% solution onto the cornea), is used every 2 hours while awake until the corneal ulcer has reepithelialized completely. Trifluridine is indicated for primary keratoconjunctivitis and recurrent epithelial keratitis due to herpes simplex virus types 1 and 2. In addition, it is used for epithelial keratitis that has not responded clinically to topical idoxuridine, or when ocular toxicity or hypersensitivity to idoxuridine has occurred.

The antiviral mechanism of action of trifluridine involves inhibition of viral DNA synthesis. Trifluridine monophosphate irreversibly inhibits thymidylate synthetase, and trifluridine triphosphate is a competitive inhibitor of thymidine triphosphate incorporation into DNA by DNA polymerases. Trifluridine is incorporated into viral and cellular DNA. Trifluridine-resistant HSV with altered thymidine kinase substrate specificity can be selected *in vitro*, and resistance in clinical isolates has been described.

The most frequent adverse reactions reported are mild, transient burning or stinging upon instillation and palpebral edema.

TRIHEXYPHENIDYL HYDROCHLORIDE (Artane)

Trihexyphenidyl, an anticholinergic agent (1 mg p.o. daily), is indicated as an adjunct with other medications in the treatment of Parkinson's disease, and especially in drug-induced parkinsonism.

Belladonna alkaloids, antagonists of muscarinic cholinergic receptors, were initially used in the treatment of Parkinson's disease before the discovery of levodopa. It seems likely that trihexyphenidyl acts within the neostriatum, through the receptors that normally mediate the response to the intrinsic cholinergic innervation of this structure, which arises primarily from cholinergic striatal interneurons. Several muscarinic cholinergic receptors have been cloned, and like the dopamine receptors, these are proteins with seven transmembrane domains that are linked to second-messenger systems by G proteins. Five subtypes of muscarinic receptor have been identified; at least four, and probably all five, subtypes are present in the striatum, although each has a distinct distribution.

Neurochemically, Parkinson's syndrome is considered a striatal dopamine-deficiency syndrome, and the main extrapyramidal symptoms—tremor, akinesia, and rigidity—correlate positively with the degree of this deficiency. Although eight separate neurotransmitters interact in the nigro-striato-nigral loop, the basic therapeutic problem in parkinsonism has been to find suitable compounds that (1) increase the concentration of dopamine, (2) stimulate the dopamine receptor sites directly, or (3) suppress the activity at cholinergic receptor sites.

Trihexyphenidyl blocks central cholinergic receptors, helping to balance cholinergic activity in the basal ganglia. It may also prolong dopamine's effects by blocking dopamine reuptake and storage at central receptor sites.

Trihexyphenidyl is contraindicated in patients with narrow-angle glaucoma because drug-induced cycloplegia and mydriasis may increase intraocular pressure; in patients with cardiac disorders, arteriosclerosis, renal disorders, hepatic disorders, hypertension, obstructive GI or genitourinary tract disease, or suspected prostatic hypertrophy because the drug may exacerbate these conditions.

Concomitant use with amantadine may amplify trihexyphenidyl's anticholinergic adverse effects, causing confusion and hallucinations. Concomitant use with haloperidol or phenothiazines may decrease the antipsychotic effectiveness of these drugs, possibly from direct CNS antagonism; concomitant phenothiazine use also increases the risk of anticholinergic adverse effects.

Concomitant use with CNS depressants, such as tranquilizers, sedative-hypnotics, and alcohol, increases trihexyphenidyl's sedative effects. When used with levodopa, dosage of both drugs may need adjustment because of synergistic anticholinergic effects and possible enhanced gastrointestinal metabolism of levodopa from reduced gastric motility and delayed gastric emptying. Antacids and antidiarrheals may decrease trihexyphenidyl's absorption.

Overdosage with trihexyphenidyl causes clinical symptoms consisting of central stimulation followed by depression, with such psychotic symptoms as disorientation, confusion, hallucinations, delusions, anxiety, agitation, and restlessness. Peripheral effects may include dilated, nonreactive pupils, blurred vision, flushed, dry, hot skin, dry mucous membranes, dysphagia, decreased or absent bowel sounds, urinary retention, hyperthermia, headache, tachycardia, hypertension, and increased respiration.

TRIIODOTHYRONINE

The steps involved in the synthesis of thyroid hormones are depicted in Figure 56. First the ingested iodide (100 to 150 μg/day) is actively transported (iodide trapping) and then accumulates in the thyroid gland. Following this, the trapped iodide is oxidized by a peroxidase system to active iodine, which iodinates the thyrosine residue of glycoprotein to yield monoiodotyrosine (MIT) and diiodo-tyrosine (DIT). This process is called iodide organification. The MIT and DIT combine to form triiodothyronine T_3, whereas two molecules of DIT combine to form thyroxine T_4. T_3 and T_4 are released from thyroglobulin through the actions of pinocytosis and the proteolysis of thyroglobulin by lysosomal enzymes. In the circulation, 75% of T_4 is bound to thyroxine-binding globulin (TBG), and the remainder is bound mostly to thyroxine-binding prealbumin (TBPA). Approximately 0.05% of T_4 remains free. T_3 is similarly bound to TBG, allowing only 0.5% of it to remain in the free form.

T_4 may undergo deamination, decarboxylation, and glucuronic acid conjugation. However, it is mostly deiodinated in one of two ways: it may either be deiodinated to 3,5,3′-triiodothyronine, which is more efficacious than T_4, or it may be deiodinated to the pharmacologically inactive 3,3′,5′-triiodothyronine (reverse T_3) (see Figure 66).

TRILOSTANE
(Modrastane)

Trilostane, a glucocorticoid suppressant (30 mg p.o. q.i.d.), is used in the treatment of adrenocortical hyperfunction in Cushing's syndrome.

TRIMAZOSIN

The newer selective $alpha_1$-adrenoreceptor-blocking agents, such as trimazosin, doxasozin, and terazosin, display a pharmacologic profile virtually identical to that of prazosin, but pharmacokinetic differences between the various $alpha_1$-blockers exist.

The bioavailability, plasma half-life (3 hours), and extensive metabolism of trimazosin are similar to those of prazosin. 1-Hydroxytrimazosin, a major metabolite in human beings, may have antihypertensive efficacy, and the delayed onset of the peak hypotensive effect of trimazosin may reflect the rate of formation of this metabolite. Although therapeutic doses of trimazosin are ten- to fifty-fold higher than those of prazosin, the drug is highly selective for $alpha_1$-adrenergic receptors. However, high doses of trimazosin may produce vasodilation directly (see also Figure 37).

TRIMEPRAZINE TARTRATE
(Temaril)

Trimeprazine, a phenothiazine antihistaminic possessing antipruritic activity (25 mg p.o. q.i.d.), is used in pruritis.

TRIMETHADIONE
(Tridione)

Trimethadione (300 mg p.o. t.i.d.) is indicated in the treatment of refractory absence seizures. The oxazolidine derivatives consist of trimethadione and paramethadione (Paradione).

Trimethadione is rapidly absorbed when given orally, and its binding to plasma proteins is negligible. Trimethadione is demethylated to dimethadione, which is an active anticonvulsant. The rate of conversion of trimethadione to dimethadione is rapid, but its rate of elimination is slow. As a result, the plasma ratio of dimethadione to trimethadione is 20 to 1.

Like ethosuximide, dimethadione inhibits T-type Ca^{2+} currents in dissociated thalamic neurons in therapeutically relevant concentrations. This provides a plausible explanation of the anti-absence seizure effects of trimethadione.

The consequences of trimethadione toxicity consist of hematologic side effects (neutropenia, pancytopenia), hemeralopia (day blindness), photophobia, diplopia, dermatologic side effects (rash and erythema multiform), CNS side effects (drowsiness and tolerance), nephrotoxic syndrome (albuminuria), and teratogenic effects such as fetal trimethadione syndrome. From this it is apparent that trimethadione is only indicated for the control of absence seizures that are not responsive or have become refractory to treatment with less toxic substances such as ethosuximide or valproic acid.

TRIMETHAPHAN CAMSYLATE
(Arfonad)

Trimethaphan (500 mg/10 ml by IV infusion) is indicated for the production of controlled hypotension during surgery, for the short-term acute control of blood pressure in hypertensive emergencies, and in the emergency treatment of pulmonary edema in patients with pulmonary hypertension associated with systemic hypertension. In addition, trimethaphan has been used in patients with dissecting aortic aneurysm or in ischemic heart disease when other agents could not be used.

Trimethaphan camsylate is a ganglionic-blocking drug that inhibits both sympathetic and parasympathetic autonomic activities. It has a rapid onset and brief duration of action and must be administered by continuous intravenous infusion with constant monitoring of blood pressure. Trimethaphan camsylate is particularly useful in aortic dissection because it can be titrated carefully to permit smooth control of blood pressure and because it decreases cardiac output and left ventricular ejection rate. Tachyphylaxis develops rapidly, making early transition to oral antihypertensive agents mandatory.

Adverse effects including blurred vision, exacerbation of glaucoma due to mydriasis and cycloplegia, dry mouth, respiratory depression, nausea, constipation, fetal meconium ileus, paralytic ileus, impairment of renal blood flow with azotemia, and urinary retention frequently complicate therapy with trimethaphan camsylate. Because of the frequency and severity of the side effects associated with this drug and the availability of more effective agents, it is now rarely used.

TRIMETHOBENZAMIDE HYDROCHLORIDE

(Pediatric Tiban pediatric suppositories 100 mg, T-Gen, pediatric suppositories 100 mg, adult suppositories 200 mg, Tebamide pediatric suppositories 100 mg, adult suppositories 200 mg, Ticon injection 100 mg/mL, Tigan capsules 100 mg, capsules 250 mg, pediatric suppositories 100 mg, adult suppositories 200 mg, injection 100 mg/mL, Triban adult suppositories 200 mg, Trimazide pediatric suppositories 100 mg, adult suppositories 200 mg)

Trimethobenzamide hydrochloride is an anticholinergic that is believed to directly affect the medullary chemoreceptor trigger zone to inhibit nausea. It is indicated in the prevention and treatment of nausea and vomiting.

Trimethobenzamide (250 mg t.i.d.) is indicated for controlling nausea and vomiting. The modest antiemetic effects of trimethobenzamide appear to result from blockade of dopamine receptors mediated through the chemoreceptor trigger zone for emesis. The direct impulse to the vomiting center is not inhibited.

Trimethobenzamide is contraindicated in patients with hypersensitivity to benzocaine, or other local anesthetics. The injectable form is contraindicated in neonates and premature infants.

Encephalitis, gastroenteritis, dehydration, electrolyte imbalance and CNS reactions have occurred when used, especially in children and debilitated elderly patients.

The drug's antiemetic effect may mask signs of overdose of toxic agents, intestinal obstruction, brain tumor, or other conditions. Antiemetics should not be the sole therapy of severe emesis. Restoration of fluid and electrolyte balance and relief of the underlying disease process are critical.

Alcohol and other CNS depressants, including tricyclic antidepressants, antihypertensives, phenothiazines, and belladonna alkaloids may increase trimethobenzamide toxicity.

Overdosage with trimethobenzamide may produce clinical symptoms consisting of severe neurologic reactions such as opisthotonos, seizures, coma, and extrapyramidal reactions.

TRIMETHOPRIM

(Proloprim, Trimpex)

Trimethoprim, a synthetic folate antagonist (100 mg p.o. q. 12 hours), is used in the treatment of uncomplicated urinary tract infections and in prophylaxis of chronic and recurrent urinary tract infections.

TRIMETHOPRIM SULFATE/POLYMYXIN B SULFATE

(Polytrim ophthalmic solution 1 mg/mL trimethoprim sulfate and 10,000 units/g polymyxin B sulfate)

Trimethoprim sulfate/polymyxin B sulfate is an antibiotic combination. **Trimethoprim** blocks production of tetrahydrofolic acid by inhibiting the enzyme dihydrofolate reductase. **Polymyxin B** interacts with phospholipid components of bacterial cell membranes, increasing cell-wall permeability. They are indicated in the treatment of surface ocular bacterial infections, including acute bacterial conjunctivitis and blepharoconjunctivitis caused by susceptible organisms.

TRIMETHOPRIM/SULFAMETHOXAZOLE (TMP-SMZ)

(Bactrim tablets 80 mg trimethoprim and 400 mg sulfamethoxazole, Bactrim D.S. tablets, double-strength 160 mg trimethoprim and 800 mg sulfamethoxazole, Bactrim IV injection 80 mg trimethoprim and 400 mg sulfamethoxazole/5 mL, Bactrim pediatric oral suspension 40 mg trimethoprim and 200 mg sulfamethoxazole/5 mL, Cotrim tablets 80 mg trimethoprim and 400 mg sulfamethoxazole, Cotrim D.S. tablets, double-strength 160 mg trimethoprim and 800 mg sulfamethoxazole, Cotrim pediatric oral suspension 40 mg trimethoprim and 200 mg sulfamethoxazole/5 mL, Septra tablets 80 mg trimethoprim and 400 mg sulfamethoxazole, oral suspension 40 mg trimethoprim and 200 mg sulfamethoxazole/5 mL, Septra DS tablets, double-strength 160 mg trimethoprim and 800 mg sulfamethoxazole, Septra IV injection 80 mg trimethoprim and 400 mg sulfamethoxazole/5 mL, Sulfatrim oral suspension 40 mg trimethoprim and 200 mg sulfamethoxazole/5 mL, Uroplus DS tablets 160 mg trimethoprim and 800 mg sulfamethoxazol, Uroplus SS tablets 80 mg trimethoprim and 400 mg sulfamethoxazole)

Trimethoprim/sulfamethoxazole is an antibiotic combination. **Sulfamethoxazole** (SMZ) inhibits bacterial synthesis of dihydrofolic acid by competing with PABA. **Trimethoprim** (TMP) blocks production of tetrahydrofolic acid by inhibiting the enzyme dihydrofolate reductase. This combination blocks two consecutive steps in bacterial biosynthesis of essential nucleic acids and proteins and is usually bactericidal.

PO/parenteral: used in treatment of UTIs caused by susceptible strains of bacteria, shigellosis enteritis, and Pneumocystis carinii pneumonitis. **PO**: used in treatment of acute otitis media and acute exacerbations of chronic bronchitis; and treatment of traveler's diarrhea.

The combination of trimethoprim and sulfamethoxazole (usually five parts sulfamethoxazole to one part trimethoprim) interferes with the synthesis of active folic acid by means of two separate reactions. In the first, sulfonamides compete with p-aminobenzoic acid and prevent its conversion to dihydrofolic acid. In the second, trimethoprim, by inhibiting the activity of dihydrofolic acid reductase, prevents the conversion of dihydrofolic acid into tetrahydrofolic acid, which is necessary for the synthesis of DNA.

These drug combinations have the following therapeutic advantages:

They cause synergistic antibacterial effects.
They have bactericidal activity.
The emergence of bacterial resistance is decreased.
The spectrum of antibacterial activity is enhanced.
Toxicity is reduced.

Folic acid deficiency may occur either following prolonged usage of methotrexate or in patients with preexisting folic acid deficiency. Folinic acid may be administered to overcome the folic-acid deficiency-related megaloblastic anemia.

Orally administered trimethoprim is used in the treatment of chronic recurring urinary tract infection. Oral forms of trimethoprim-sulfamethoxazole are used in *Shigella* and some *Salmonella* infections, particularly when they are resistant to ampicillin and chloramphenicol. High doses of oral trimethoprim-sulfamethoxazole are used in *Pneumocystis* pneumonia. This combination, along with polymyxin, has been shown to be effective in treating sepsis caused by *Serratia* or *Pseudomonas* organisms.

Intravenously administered trimethoprim-sulfamethoxazole is indicated in severe cases of *Pneumocystis carinii* pneumonia, Gram-negative bacterial sepsis, and shigellosis.

Oral trimethoprim in combination with sulfonamide has been used in the treatment of leishmaniasis, toxoplasmosis, and falciparum malaria.

TRIMETREXATE GLUCURONATE
(Neutrexin powder for injection, lyophilized 25 mg)

Trimetrexate glucuronate is a folate antagonist that inhibits dihydrofolate reductase necessary for DNA, RNA, and protein synthesis, leading to cell death. Following a single-dose of 10 to 130 mg/m^2 the alpha phase $t_{1/2}$ was about 57 minutes followed by a terminal phase with a $t_{1/2}$ of approximately 16 hours. Clearance has been reported as about 53 mL/min and about 32 mL/min following single-dose administration. It is indicated as an alternative therapy, with concurrent leucovorin administration, for treatment of moderate to severe *Pneumocystis carinii* pneumonia in immunocompromised patients in whom trimethoprim-sulfamethoxazole cannot be used.

Trimetrexate, an inhibitor of dihydrofolate reductase, is available for hospital use in treatment of patients with *Pneumocystis carinii* pneumonia and who have exhibited serious (severe or life-threatening) intolerance to both co-trimazole and pentamidine.

TRIMIPRAMINE MALEATE
(Surmontil)

Trimipramine, a tricyclic antidepressant (75 mg/day in divided doses), is indicated in the management of depression and enuresis. Trimipramine exerts its antidepressant effects by equally inhibiting reuptake of norepinephrine and serotonin in CNS nerve terminals, which results in increased concentration and enhanced activity of these neurotransmitters in the synaptic cleft. Trimipramine also has anxiolytic effects and inhibits gastric acid secretion (see Tables 5 through 7).

Trimipramine exhibits moderate affinity for alpha$_1$-adrenergic receptors and muscarinic-cholinergic receptors, and a very strong affinity for H_1-histamine receptors. Trimipramine causes heavy sedation, has strong anticholinergic properties, and exhibits a moderate degree of orthostatic hypotension.

Trimipramine is contraindicated in patients with known hypersensitivity to tricyclic antidepressants, trazodone, and related compounds; in the acute recovery phase of myocardial infarction (MI), because the drug depresses cardiac function and causes dysrhythmia in patients in coma or severe respiratory depression (additive CNS and respiratory depression); and during or within 14 days of therapy with monoamine oxidase inhibitors.

Trimipramine should be used cautiously in patients with other cardiac disease (arrhythmias, CHF, angina pectoris, valvular disease, or heart block), respiratory disorders, seizure disorders, scheduled electroconvulsive therapy, bipolar disease, glaucoma, hyperthyroidism, and parkinsonism; in patients taking thyroid replacement; in patients with diabetes types I and II; in patients with prostatic hypertrophy, paralytic ileus, or urinary retention because the drug may worsen these conditions; in patients with hepatic or renal dysfunction because diminished metabolism and excretion causes the drug to accumulate; and in patients undergoing surgery using general anesthesia because the drug may increase cardiac sensitivity to the effects of general anesthetics or pressor agents.

Concomitant use of trimipramine with sympathomimetics, including epinephrine, phenylephrine, phenylpropanolamine, and ephedrine (often found in nasal sprays) may increase blood pressure. Use with warfarin may increase prothrombin time and cause bleeding.

Concomitant use with thyroid medication, pimozole, and antiarrhythmic agents (quinidine, disopyramide, procainamide) may increase incidence of cardiac arrhythmias and conduction defects.

Trimipramine may decrease hypotensive effects of centrally acting antihypertensive drugs, such as guanethidine, guanabenz, quanadrel, clonidine, methyldopa, and reserpine.

Concomitant use with disulfiram or ethchlorvynol may cause delirium and tachycardia.

Additive effects are likely after concomitant use of trimipramine with CNS depressants, including alcohol, analgesics, barbiturates, narcotics, tranquilizers, and anesthetics (oversedation), atropine and other anticholinergic drugs, including phenothiazines, antihistamines, meperidine, and antiparkinsonian agents (oversedation, paralytic ileus, visual changes, and severe constipation), and metrizamide (increased risk of seizures).

Barbiturates and heavy smoking induce trimipramine metabolism and decrease therapeutic efficacy; phenothiazines and haloperidol decrease its metabolism, thus decreasing therapeutic efficacy; methylphenidate, cimetidine, oral contraceptives, propoxyphene, and beta-blockers may inhibit trimipramine metabolism, increasing plasma levels and toxicity.

Overdosage with trimipramine causes CNS stimulation followed by CNS depression. The first 12 hours after acute ingestion are a stimulatory phase characterized by excessive anticholinergic activity (agitation, irritation, confusion, hallucinations, parkinsonian symptoms, seizure, urinary retention, dry mucous membranes, pupillary dilatation, constipation, and ileus). This is followed by CNS depressant effects, including hypothermia, decreased or absent reflexes, sedation, hypotension, cyanosis, and cardiac irregularities (including tachycardia, conduction disturbances, and quinidine-like effects on the ECG).

TRIPELENNAMINE CITRATE
(PBZ)

TRIPELENNAMINE HYDROCHLORIDE
(PBZ, PBZ-SR, Pelamine)

Tripelennamine, an ethylene-diamine-derivative antihistamine (25 to 50 mg p.o. q. 4 to 6 hours), is indicated in rhinitis, allergy symptoms, allergic reactions to blood or plasma, and as an adjunct to epinephrine in anaphylaxis.

In addition, it is used in pruritis, minor burns, insect bites, sunburn, and skin irritations. Tripelennamine competes with histamine for the H_1 receptor, thereby ameliorating histamine effects in target tissues, but does not prevent the release of histamine.

Tripelennamine is contraindicated in patients with known hypersensitivity to similar chemical structures, such as pyrilamine; in neonates, other infants, and breastfeeding women because young children may be more susceptible to the toxic effects of antihistamines; during asthma attacks because it thickens bronchial secretions; and in patients who have taken MAO inhibitors within the preceding two weeks.

Because of the significant anticholinergic effects, tripelennamine should be used with caution in patients with narrow-angle glaucoma; in those with pyloroduodenal obstruction or urinary bladder obstruction from prostatic hypertrophy or narrowing of the bladder neck; and in patients with cardiovascular disease or hypertension because the drug may cause palpitations.

MAO inhibitors interfere with the detoxification of antihistamines and phenothiazines and thus prolong and intensify their central depressant and anticholinergic effects; additive CNS depression and sedation may occur when tripelennamine is administered with other CNS depressants, such as alcohol, barbiturates, tranquilizers, sleeping aids, or antianxiety agents.

Overdosage with tripelennamine may include manifestations such as either CNS depression (sedation, reduced mental alertness, apnea, and cardiovascular collapse) or CNS stimulation (insomnia, hallucinations, tremors, or seizures). Anticholinergic symptoms, such as dry mouth, flushed skin, fixed and dilated pupils, and GI symptoms, are common especially in children. Children may also experience fever, excitement, ataxia, and athetosis.

TRIPROLIDINE HYDROCHLORIDE
(Actidil, Myidyl, Zymine liquid 1.25 mg per 5 mL)

Triprolidine hydrochloride is an alkylamine (nonselective) that competitively blocks histamine at H_1-receptor sites. It is indicated in symptomatic relief of perennial and seasonal allergic rhinitis; vasomotor rhinitis; allergic conjunctivitis caused by inhalant allergens and foods; and mild uncomplicated allergic skin manifestations of urticaria and angioedema.

TRIPTORELIN PAMOATE
(Trelstar Depot microgranules for injection, lyophilized equivalent to 3.75 mg triptorelin peptide base, Trelstar LA microgranules for injection, lyophilized equivalent to 11.25 mg triptorelin peptide base)

Triptorelin pamoate, a synthetic analog of GnRH, acts as a potent inhibitor of gonadotropin secretion. It is indicated as a palliative treatment of advanced prostate cancer and as an alternative treatment for prostate cancer when orchiectomy or estrogen administration are not indicated or are unacceptable to the patient.

TROLEANDOMYCIN
(TAO)

Troleandomycin, a macrolide antibiotic (250 to 500 mg p.o. q. 6 hours), is used in pneumonia or respiratory tract infection caused by sensitive pneumococci or group A betahemolytic streptococci.

TROMETHAMINE
(THAM)

Tromethamine is indicated for prevention and correction of system acidosis such as metabolic acidosis associated with cardiac bypass surgery; the correction of acidity of acid citrate dextrose (ACD) blood in cardiac bypass surgery or cardiac arrest.

Tromethamine, a highly alkaline, sodium-free organic amine, acts as a proton acceptor to prevent or correct acidosis. When administered IV as an 0.3 M solution, it combines with hydrogen ions from carbonic acid to form bicarbonate and a cationic buffer. It also acts as an osmotic diuretic, increasing urine flow, urinary pH, and excretion of fixed acids, carbon dioxide, and electrolytes.

Tromethamine is contraindicated in anuria or uremia.

TROPICAMIDE
(Mydriacyl)

Tropicamide, an anticholinergic agent causing mydriasis and cycloplegia, is used for cycloplegic refractions and fundus examinations.

TROSPIUM CHLORIDE
(Sanctura tablets 20 mg)

Trospium chloride is an anticholinergic that antagonizes effects of acetylcholine on muscarinic receptors in cholinergically innervated organs. Its parasympatholytic action reduces tonus of smooth muscle in the bladder. It is indicated in the treatment of overactive bladder with symptoms of urinary incontinence, urgency, and urinary frequency.

Overactive urinary bladder disease can be successfully treated with muscarinic receptor antagonists. These agents can include synthetic substitutes of atropine, such as tolterodine and **trospium chloride**, which lower intravesicular pressure, increase capacity, and reduce the frequency of contractions by antagonizing parasympathetic control of the bladder. There is renewed interest in muscarinic antagonists as a modality for treating this increasingly common disorder, as well as for treating enuresis in children, particularly when a progressive increase in bladder capacity is the objective. These agents also are used to reduce **urinary frequency in spastic paraplegia** and to increase the capacity of the bladder.

Trospium is a quaternary amine long used in Europe and approved recently for use in the United States for treatment of overactive bladder. It has been shown to be as effective as **oxybutynin** with better tolerability. **Solifenacin** is newly approved for overactive bladder with a favorable efficacy: side effect ratio. Stress urinary incontinence has been treated with some success with **duloxetine** (Yentreve), which acts centrally to influence serotonin and norepinephrine levels.

Tripitramine and darifenacin are selective antagonists for M_2 and M_3 muscarinic receptors, respectively. They are of potential utility in blocking cholinergic bradycardia (M_2) and smooth muscle activity or epithelial secretions (M_3).

TRYPSIN/BALSAM PERU/CASTOR OIL
(Granulex aerosol 0.12 mg trypsin/87 mg balsam peru/788 mg castor oil per g)

Trypsin/balsam peru/castor oil is a topical enzyme combination that physiologically debrides tissue and improves epithelization by reducing premature epithelial desiccation and cornification. It is used in acute and chronic conditions such as varicose ulcers, decubital ulcers, eschar, dehiscent wounds and sunburn; relieves pain and promotes healing; debrides eschar and necrotic tissue; stimulates vascular bed; improves epithelization; and reduces odor from necrotic wounds.

TUBERCULIN, PURIFIED PROTEIN DERIVATIVE (PPD)
(Tuberculin purified protein derivative Aplisol injection 5 TU/0.1 mL, Tubersol injection 1 TU/0.1 mL, injection 5 TU/0.1 mL, injection 250 TU/0.1 mL, Tuberculin PPD multiple puncture device Aplitest injection 5 TU activity/test, Tine test PPD injection 5 TU activity/test)

Tuberculin, a purified protein derivative, is an *in vivo* diagnostic biological agent that contains soluble products from *Mycobacterium*, which react with lyphocytes to release mediators of cellular hypersensitivity. Some of these mediators induce inflammatory response. A positive reaction is consistent with previous or current tuberculosis infection or previous BCG vaccination.

This *Mycobacterium tuberculosis* and *Mycobacterium bovis* antigen is used for diagnosis of tuberculosis and evaluation of immunocompetence in patients with cancer or malnutrition. It is indicated for detection of delayed hypersensitivity to *Mycobacterium tuberculosis*; as an aid in diagnosis of infection with *M. tuberculosis*; in routine testing for tuberculosis; in testing individuals suspected of having contact with active tuberculosis; and for follow-up verification testing in individuals who have had reactions to tuberculin multipuncture devices used as screening test.

TUBERCULOSIS: Treatment of

Drugs	Main Adverse Effects
Isoniazid (INH)	Hepatic toxicity, peripheral neuropathy
Rifampin	Hepatic toxicity, flu-like syndrome
Pyrazinamide	Arthralgias, hepatic toxicity, hyperuricemia
Ethambutol	Optic neuritis
Streptomycin	Vestibular toxicity, renal damage
Combinations	
Rifamate (isoniazid 150 mg, rifampin 300 mg)	
Rifater (isoniazid 50 mg, rifampin 120 mg, pyrazinamide 300 mg)	
Second-Line Drugs	
Capreomycin	Auditory and vestibular toxicity, renal damage
Kanamycin	Auditory toxicity, renal damage
Amikacin	Auditory toxicity, renal damage
Cycloserine	Psychiatric symptoms, seizures
Ethionamide	Gastrointestinal and hepatic toxicity, hypothyroidism
Ciprofloxacin	Nausea, abdominal pain, restlessness, confusion
Ofloxacin	Nausea, abdominal pain, restlessness, confusion
Aminosalicylic acid (PAS)	Gastrointestinal disturbance

Tuberculosis continues to be a major problem, particularly in areas of the world where drug resistance is common. Treatment should be continued 12 to 24 months after the culture becomes negative.

TUBERCULOSIS SKIN TEST ANTIGENS

TUBERCULIN PURIFIED PROTEIN DERIVATIVE (PPD)
(Aplisol, Tubersol)

D-TUBOCURARINE CHLORIDE
(Tubarine)

Tubocurarine (6 to 9 mg IV) is indicated as an adjunct to general anesthesia to induce skeletal muscle relaxation, facilitate intubation, and reduce fractures and dislocations.

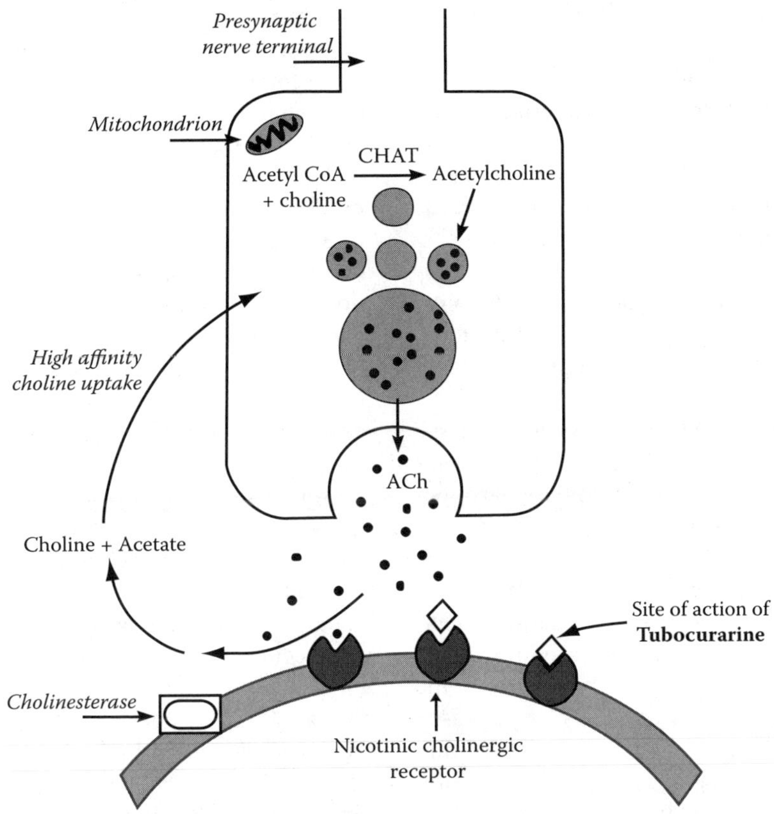

FIGURE 99 Agents such as **tubocurarine** and **pancuronium** compete with acetylcholine for the cholinergic receptors at the end plate. They combine with the receptors but do not activate them. Competitive or nondepolarizing agents are antagonized by neostigmine.

Agents such as tubocurarine and pancuronium compete with acetylcholine for the cholinergic receptors at the end plate. They combine with the receptors but do not activate them. Competitive or nondepolarizing agents are antagonized by neostigmine (see Figure 99).

Neuromuscular blockade takes place in the following sequence: rapidly contracting muscles (eyes, fingers, and toes) followed by slowly contracting muscles (diaphragm, limbs, and trunk). The onset and duration of action of succinylcholine are 1 and 5 minutes, respectively. The onset and duration of action of tubocurarine are 5 and 20 minutes, respectively.

The skeletal muscle relaxants have quaternary ammonium groups, are ionized at the physiologic pH, and are highly water soluble. They have a limited volume of distribution and do not readily cross the placenta or blood–brain barrier. After intravenous administration, their concentration rises and then falls rapidly.

Antiarrhythmic agents such as quinidine, procainamide, and propranolol have been shown to augment *d*-tubocurarine-induced blockade. Quinidine has also been reported to unmask or worsen the symptoms of myasthenia gravis and to cause postoperative respiratory depression after the use of muscle relaxants.

Diuretics such as thiazides, ethacrynic acid, and furosemide intensify the effects of nonpolarizing muscle relaxants, possibly because of a diuresis-induced reduction in the volume of distribution and an associated electrolyte imbalance, such as hypokalemia.

The local anesthetics procaine and lidocaine enhance the neuromuscular block produced by nonpolarizing and depolarizing muscle relaxants.

Phenytoin has been shown to interfere with neuromuscular transmission, and the drug has been reported to exacerbate myasthenia gravis. Lithium augments the effects of both depolarizing and nondepolarizing muscle relaxants and also reportedly unmasks myasthenia gravis.

Chlorpromazine has been shown to potentiate nondepolarizing relaxants The administration of steroids may lead to a transient worsening of symptoms in patients with myasthenia gravis, but the mechanism by which they interfere with neuromuscular transmission is unknown. The antagonism of pancuronium-induced blockade by hydrocortisone has also been reported. d-Penicillamine, which is used in the treatment of Wilson's disease, may cause a myasthenia gravis-like syndrome. These patients have elevated serum levels of antibody to acetylcholine receptors, suggesting that an immunologic mechanism is involved in this drug-induced syndrome. Azathioprine antagonizes nondepolarizing neuromuscular blockade, possibly by inhibiting phosphodiesterase.

Calcium ions play an important role in the presynaptic release of acetylcholine, and prolonged neuromuscular blockade has been reported after calcium antagonist administration during anesthesia that includes concurrent nondepolarizing neuromuscular blockade. Ketamine potentiates neuromuscular blockade produced by tubocurarine but not that produced by succinylcholine.

All of the inhalational agents augment both the degree and duration of the neuromuscular blockade induced by the nondepolarizing muscle relaxants. Possible mechanisms by which they exert their effect include depression of the central nervous system, presynaptic inhibition of acetylcholine mobilization and release, postsynaptic receptor desensitization, or an action imposed on the muscle at some point distal to the cholinergic receptor.

The generation of action potentials by muscle and nerve results from changes in the conductance of their membranes to sodium and potassium, and normal neuromuscular function depends on the maintenance of the correct ratio between intracellular and extracellular ionic concentrations.

An acute decrease in the extracellular potassium concentration tends to elevate the end-plate transmembrane potential, causing hyperpolarization and an increased resistance to depolarization, together with a greater sensitivity to the nondepolarizing muscle relaxants. Conversely, an increased extracellular potassium concentration lowers the resting end-plate transmembrane potential and thereby partially depolarizes the membrane, which should augment the effects of the depolarizing agents and oppose the action of the nondepolarizing drugs. Diuretic-induced chronic hypokalemia reduces the pancuronium requirements for neuromuscular blockade, and thus more neostigmine is required to achieve antagonism.

The release of acetylcholine from the motor nerve terminal is also affected by calcium and magnesium ion concentrations, which have opposing effects. Calcium increases the quantal release of acetylcholine from the nerve terminal, decreases the sensitivity of the postjunctional membrane to transmitter, and enhances the excitation-contraction coupling mechanisms of muscle. In contrast, magnesium decreases acetylcholine release and reduces the sensitivity of the postjunctional membrane to acetylcholine. Consequently, the action of the nondepolarizing muscle relaxants can be accentuated by low calcium and high magnesium levels. In addition, magnesium augments the block produced by depolarizing relaxants. Therefore, the dose of a muscle relaxant should be reduced in patients who have toxemia associated with pregnancy and are undergoing magnesium replacement therapy.

Respiratory acidosis enhances *d*-tubocurarine- and pancuronium-induced neuromuscular block and opposes reversal by neostigmine.

Hypothermia prolongs the neuromuscular blockade produced by *d*-tubocurarine and pancuronium.

The plasma concentrations of *d*-tubocurarine and pancuronium are increased in patients with impaired liver function because liver disease interferes with the metabolism of pancuronium.

Neonates are more sensitive to nondepolarizing muscle relaxants, and the response of the small infant to some extent resembles that of an adult patient with myasthenia gravis.

Although the main site of action of the neuromuscular blocking agents is the nicotinic receptor of striated muscle, they may act at other cholinergic receptor sites throughout the body, such as the nicotinic receptors in the autonomic ganglia and the muscarinic receptors in the heart.

Succinylcholine may cause tachycardia, cardiac arrhythmias, and hypertension, which is brought about by stimulation of the sympathetic ganglia. It may also provoke bradycardia, caused by stimulation of muscarinic receptor sites in the sinus node of the heart. This effect is more pronounced following a second dose of succinylcholine. The bradycardia may be blocked by thiopental, atropine, and ganglionic-blocking agents.

Succinylcholine increases intraocular pressure transiently. It can also cause muscle pain, which may be due to fasciculation and uncoordinated muscle contraction. The prior administration of a competitive blocking agent may prevent both fasciculation and pain.

Patients with myotonia congenita and myotonia dystrophica respond differently to succinylcholine, in that their muscles are contracted rather than relaxed.

Tubocurarine, metocurine, and succinylcholine have all been shown to elicit histamine release in humans. However, histamine release is less common with pancuronium and alcuronium. Vecuronium does not cause histamine release.

TYPHOID VACCINE

This bacterial vaccine is used for primary immunization (exposure to typhoid carrier or plans to travel to an area endemic for typhoid fever).

U

UNDECYLENIC ACID

(Desenex)

Undecylenic acid is available as a foam, ointment, cream, powder, soap, and liquid, all administered topically. It is indicated as an antifungal and antibacterial agent for tinea pedis (athlete's foot), exclusive of the nails and hairy areas. It is also recommended for relief and prevention of diaper rash, itching, burning and chafing, prickly heat, tinea cruris (jock itch), excessive perspiration, and irritation in the groin area and bromhidrosis.

Zinc undecylenate is marketed in combination with other ingredients. The zinc provides an astringent action that aids in the suppression of inflammation. Compound undecylenic acid ointment contains both undecylenic acid (about 5%) and zinc undecylenate (about 20%). Calcium undecylenate (Caldesene, Cruex) is available as a powder. At best, the clinical "cure" rate is about 50% and is thus much lower than that obtained with the imidazoles, haloprogin, or tolnaftate.

URACIL MUSTARD

Uracil mustard, an alkylating agent with antineoplastic activity (1 to 2 mg p.o. daily for three months), is indicated in treatment of chronic lymphocytic and myelocytic leukemia; Hodgkin's disease, non-Hodgkin's lymphomas of the histiocytic and lymphocytic types; reticulum cell sarcoma; lymphomas; mycosis fungoides; polycythemia vera; and ovarian, cervical, and lung cancer.

URAPIDIL

Urapidil is an alpha$_1$-adrenoreceptor antagonist that also has a central antihypertensive effect. Its plasma half-life is about 5 hours. Urapidil reduces peripheral resistance and has no significant effect on cardiac output; there is no reflex tachycardia. Comparative clinical studies have shown that urapidil (30 to 90 mg/day) and acebutalol (200 to 400 mg/day) were effective in lowering blood pressure by about the same level, but acebutalol significantly reduced heart rate, whereas urapidil did not. Urapidil causes arteriolar vasodilation and may have some venous dilator effects. The hypotensive action of urapidil results from blockade of vascular postsynaptic alpha$_1$-adrenoreceptors, and a central hypotensive effect occurs by a mechanism not yet completely elucidated but which appears to be unrelated to alpha-adrenoreceptors. The central mechanism is not the same as that of clonidine and other alpha$_2$-adrenoreceptor antagonists, and appears to be unrelated to activity at central alpha$_2$- or alpha$_1$-adrenoreceptors or at histamine (H_1 and H_2), dopamine (DA_2), muscarine (M_1), serotonin (5-HT_2), or opioid receptors. It is possible that some central 5-HT_{1A}-antagonist activity occurs, but the pharmacologic implications of this are not clear.

UREA

(Carbamide, Ureaphil)

Urea, an osmotic diuretic (1 to 1.5 g/kg as a 30% solution given by slow IV infusion over two hours) is indicated for reducing intracranial or intraocular pressure. The osmotic diuretics and related agents consist of mannitol (Osmitrol), glycerin (Glycerol, Osmoglyn), and isosorbide (Hydronol). Mannitol and urea are nonelectrolytes that are freely filterable and undergo very little or no metabolism or renal tubular resorption. When given in sufficient quantities, these drugs increase the osmolarity of plasma and the amount of both the glomerular filtrate and the renal tubular fluid. The presence of such a drug in the lumen prevents the resorption of much of the water; hence the urine volume is increased. They do not prevent the active resorption of sodium from the tubular fluid, but some additional sodium is excreted as a normal constituent of the increased volume of urine.

UPPER RESPIRATORY TRACT INFECTION: Treatment of

Antibiotic*	*Streptococcus pneumoniae*	*Haemophilus influenzae* β-Lactamase Negative	*Haemophilus influenzae* β-Lactamase Positive	*Moraxella catarrhalis* β-Lactamase Negative	*Moraxella catarrhalis* β-Lactamase Positive	Group A β-hemolytic streptococci
Ampicillin	+	+	—	+	—	+
Amoxicillin	+	+	—	+	—	+
Erythromycin-sulfisoxazole	+	+	+	+	+	+
Trimethoprim-sulfamethoxazole	+	+	+	+	—	—
Amoxicillin/clavulanate	+	+	+	+	+	+
Cefaclor	+	+	+	+	±	+
Cefixime	+	+	+	+	+	+
Cefuroxime axetil	+	+	+	+	+	+

* Spectrum of activity

Osmotic diuretics are not effective in removing the edematous fluid caused by sodium retention but can maintain the flow of urine even when the GFR is decreased. Osmotic diuretics are given by intravenous infusion in a hypertonic solution, and they are excreted by glomerular filtration.

The osmotic diuretics may be used for any of the following conditions:

- In congestive glaucoma, to reduce intraocular pressure
- In neurosurgery, to reduce the pressure and volume of cerebrospinal fluid and hence decrease the intracranial pressure
- In acute renal failure, to maintain urine flow
- In drug poisoning, to prevent nephrotoxicity

These agents should not be used in edematous states associated with diminished cardiac reserve because any increase in the extracellular fluid volume constitutes a hazard.

URINARY TRACT INFECTIONS: Treatment of

ORAL THERAPY	
Sulfonamides	
Trimethoprim-sulfamethoxazole	
Penicillins	
Ampicillin	Amoxicillin-clavulanic acid
Amoxicillin	Carbenicillin indanyl
Cephalosporins	
Cephalexin	Cefadroxil
Cephradine	Cefuroxime
Cefaclor	Cefixime
Tetracyclines	
Tetracycline	Oxytetracycline
Doxycycline	Minocycline
Quinolones	
Nalidixic acid	Ciprofloxacin
Oxolinic acid	Norfloxacin
Cinoxacin	Ofloxacin
Nitrofurantoin	
Methenamine hippurate	
Methenamine mandelate	
PARENTERAL THERAPY	
Aminoglycosides	
Gentamicin	Amikacin
Tobramycin	Netilmicin
Penicillins	
Ampicillin	Mezlocillin
Carbenicillin	Piperacillin
Ticarcillin	
Cephalosporins	**Imipenem/cilastatin**
First, second, and third generation	Aztreonam

UROFOLLITROPIN

(Bravelle powder for injection, lyophilized 75 units follicle-stimulating hormone (FSH) activity)

Urofollitropin is a gonadotropin that stimulates ovarian follicular growth in women who do not have primary ovarian failure. It is to be administered in conjunction with **human chorionic gonadotropin** (hCG) for ovulation induction and multiple follicular development (controlled ovarian stimulation) during assisted reproductive technology (ART) cycles in patients who have previously received pituitary suppression.

Gonadotropins are purified from human urine or prepared using recombinant DNA technology. Several preparations of urinary gonadotropins have been developed. Chorionic gonadotropin (Pregnyl, Novarel, Profasi, others), which mimics the action of luteinizing hormone (LH), is obtained from the urine of pregnant women. Urine from postmenopausal women is the source of menotropins (Pergonal, Repronex), which contain roughly equal amounts of FSH and LH, as well as a number of other urinary proteins. Because of their relatively low purity, menotropins are administered intramuscularly to decrease the incidence of hypersensitivity reactions. **Urofollitropin** (uFSH; Bravelle) is a highly purified FSH prepared by immunoconcentration with monoclonal antibodies and pure enough to be administered subcutaneously.

Recombinant preparations of gonadotropins are assuming an increasing role in clinical practice. Recombinant FSH (rFSH) is prepared by expressing cDNAs encoding the α and β subunits of FSH in a mammalian cell line, yielding products whose glycosylation pattern mimics that of FSH produced by gonadotropes. The two rFSH preparations that are available (follitropin α [GONAL-F] and follitropin β [Puregon, Follistim]) differ slightly in their carbohydrate structures; both exhibit less inter-batch variability than do preparations purified from urine and can be administered subcutaneously, because they are considerably purer. The recombinant preparations are more expensive than the naturally derived hormones, and their relative advantages (i.e., efficacy, lower frequency of side effects such as ovarian hyperstimulation) have not been definitively established despite much debate in the published literature.

Recombinant forms of hCG (choriogonadotropin alfa, Ovidrel) and LH (Luveris, Lhadi) also have been developed and are being investigated for the treatment of infertility. Provided their cost-benefit ratios are favorable, it is likely that these recombinant gonadotropin preparations will have an increasing role in the future, possibly replacing the urinary preparations entirely. In addition, recombinant technology is likely to lead to improved forms of gonadotropins with increased half-lives or higher clinical efficacy.

UROKINASE

(Abbokinase)

Urokinase, a thrombolytic enzyme (4400 IU/kg over 10 minutes followed by 4400 IU/kg hourly), is indicated for lysis of acute massive pulmonary emboli and of pulmonary emboli accompanied by unstable hemodynamics. In addition, urokinase (6000 IU/minute of urokinase intra-arterial via a coronary artery catheter) is indicated for the treatment of coronary artery thrombosis. Urokinase is a two-chain serine protease containing 411 amino acid residues. It is isolated from cultured human kidney cells. It has a half-life of 15 to 20 minutes and is metabolized by the liver. Like streptokinase, it lacks fibrin specificity and therefore readily induces a systemic lytic state. Saruplase (prourokinase, single-chain urokinase) does display selectivity for clots by binding to fibrin before activation.

Urokinase is contraindicated in patients with ulcerative wounds, active internal bleeding, and recent trauma with possible internal injuries, pregnancy and the first 10 days postpartum, ulcerative colitis, diverticulitis, severe hypertension, acute or chronic hepatic or renal insufficiency, uncontrolled hypocoagulation, chronic pulmonary disease with cavitation, subacute bacterial endocarditis or rheumatic valvular disease and recent cerebral embolism, thrombosis, or hemorrhage, or diabetic hemorrhagic retinopathy, because of the potential for excessive bleeding.

Concomitant use with anticoagulants may cause hemorrhage; heparin must be stopped and its effects allowed to diminish. It may also be necessary to reverse effects of oral anticoagulants before beginning therapy. Concomitant use with aspirin, indomethacin, phenylbutazone, or other drugs affecting platelet activity increases the risk of bleeding.

Aminocaproic acid inhibits urokinase-induced activation of plasminogen (see Figure 45).

URSODIOL

(Actigall capsules 300 mg, URSO 250 tablets 250 mg, URSO Forte tablets 500 mg)

Ursodiol is a gallstone solubilizing agent, which suppresses hepatic synthesis and cholesterol secretion and inhibits intestinal absorption of cholesterol.

Ursodiol (ursodeoxycholic acid—UDCA), a bile acid with gallstone-stabilizing properties (8 to 10 mg/kg/day), is used for dissolution of radiolucent gallbladder stones and to increase the flow of bile in patients with bile duct prosthesis or stents.

It is used in dissolution of gallstones in patients with radiolucent, noncalcified, gallbladder stones less than 20 mm at their greatest diameter, in whom elective cholecystectomy would be undertaken except for the presence of increased surgical risk due to systemic disease, advanced age, idiosyncratic reaction to general anesthesia, or for patients refusing surgery (capsules only); prevention of gallstone formation in obese patients experiencing rapid weight loss (capsules only); treatment of patients experiencing rapid weight loss (capsules only); and treatment of patients with primary biliary cirrhosis (tablets only).

Bile acids and their conjugates are essential components of bile that are synthesized from cholesterol in the liver. Bile acids induce bile flow, feedback-inhibit cholesterol synthesis, promote intestinal excretion of cholesterol, and facilitate the dispersion and absorption of lipids and fat-soluble vitamins. After secretion into the biliary tract, bile acids are largely (95%) reabsorbed in the intestine (mainly in the terminal ileum), returned to the liver, and then again secreted in bile (enterohepatic circulation). **Cholic acid**, **chenodeoxycholic acid**, and **deoxycholic acid** constitute 95% of bile acids, whereas lithocholic acid and ursodeoxycholic acid are minor constituents. The bile acids exist largely as glycine and taurine conjugates, the salts of which are called bile salts. Colonic bacteria convert primary bile acids (cholic and chenodeoxycholic acid) to secondary acids (mainly deoxycholic and lithocholic acid) by sequential deconjugation and dehydroxylation. These secondary bile acids also are absorbed in the colon and join the primary acids in the enterohepatic pool.

Dried bile from the **Himalayan bear** (Yutan) has been used for centuries in China to treat liver disease. UDCA (ursodiol, Actigall) is a hydrophilic, dehydroxylated bile acid that is formed by epimerization of the bile acid, chenodeoxycholic acid (CDCA; Chenodiol), in the gut by intestinal bacteria. It comprises approximately 1 to 3% of the total bile acid pool in human beings but is present at much higher concentrations in bears. When administered orally, litholytic bile acids, such as chenodiol and ursodiol, can alter relative concentrations of bile acids, decrease biliary lipid secretion, and reduce the cholesterol content of the bile so that it is less lithogenic. Ursodiol also may have cytoprotective effects on hepatocytes and effects on the immune system that account for some of its beneficial effects in cholestatic liver diseases.

Bile acids were first used therapeutically for gallstone dissolution. For this indication, a functional gallbladder is required because the modified bile must enter the gallbladder to interact with gallstones. To be amenable to dissolution, the gallstones must be composed of cholesterol monohydrate crystals and generally must be smaller than 15 mm in diameter to provide a favorable ratio of surface to size. For these reasons, the overall efficacy of litholytic bile acids in the treatment of gallstones has been disappointing (partial dissolution occurs in 40 to 60% of patients completing therapy and is complete in only 33 to 50% of these). Although a combination of chenodiol and ursodiol probably is better than either agent alone, ursodiol is preferred as a single agent because of its greater efficacy and less-frequent side effects (e.g., hepatotoxicity).

Primary biliary cirrhosis is a chronic, progressive, cholestatic liver disease of unknown etiology that typically affects middle-aged to elderly women. Ursodiol (administered at 13 to 15 mg/kg per day in two divided doses) reduces the concentration of primary bile acids and improves biochemical and histological features of primary biliary cirrhosis. Ursodiol also has been used in a variety of other cholestatic liver diseases, including primary sclerosing cholangitis, and in cystic fibrosis. In general, it is less effective in these conditions than in primary biliary cirrhosis.

UVEITIS: Management of

Inflammation of the uveal tract has many causes and may involve one or all three portions simultaneously, as in sarcoidosis. The most frequent form of uveitis is acute anterior uveitis (iritis), usually unilateral and characterized by a history of pain, photophobia, and blurring of vision; a red eye (circumcorneal flush) without purulent discharge; and a small or irregular pupil.

The treatment of uveitis includes reduction of inflammation, relief of symptoms, and an attempt to restore or preserve vision. Idiopathic uveitis (autoimmune) requires the systemic administration of corticosteroids, cyclosporin, and cytotoxic agents.

The arsenal of immunosuppressive agents available for the treatment of uveitis has expanded recently to include: tacrolimus, sirolimus (rapamycin), and mycophenolate mofetil.

V

VACCINIA IMMUNE GLOBULIN IV (HUMAN)

(Vaccinia immune globulin intravenous (Human) solution for injection 50 mg/mL (immunoglobulin 2500 mg/vial))

Vaccinia immune globulin IV is a vaccinia-specific immunoglobulin G (IgG), which directly neutralizes vaccinia virus. It is indicated in treatment and/or modification of aberrant infections induced by vaccinia virus (including accidental implantation in eyes, mouth, or other areas where vaccinia infection would constitute a special hazard), eczema vaccinatum, progressive vaccinia, severe generalized vaccinia, and vaccinia infections in individuals who have skin conditions such as burns, impetigo, varicella-zoster, or poison ivy, or in individuals with eczematous skin lesions. Treat complications that include vaccinia keratitis with caution.

VAGINAL CANDIDIASIS: Treatment of

Drugs	Formulations
Butoconazole	2% cream
	Clotrimazole
Gyne-Lotrimin (OTC)	100 mg vaginal tablet
	1% cream
Mycelex-G	100 mg vaginal tablet
	500 mg vaginal tablet
	1% cream
	Miconazole
Monistat-7	2% cream
	100 mg vaginal suppository
Monistat-3	200 mg vaginal suppository
Nystatin	
Mycostatin	100,000 U vaginal tablet
Nilstat	100,000 U vaginal tablet
	Terconazole
Terazol-7	0.4% cream
Terazol-3	80 mg vaginal suppository or 0.8% cream
Tioconazole	
Vagistat	6.5% ointment

All regimens of topical antifungal drugs are safe and effective for most patients with vulvovaginal candidiasis. Burning and itching can occur with all of the topical antifungal drugs used for vaginal candidiasis. Other adverse effects include contact dermatitis, irritation, vulval edema, dysuria, and dyspareunia.

VALACICLOVIR

Acyclovir was the first antiherpetic agent to selectively inhibit herpes virus replication while maintaining an excellent safety profile, and currently constitutes the standard therapy for the management of herpes virus infections. Research to improve the oral bioavailability of acyclovir has resulted in the development of its L-valyl ester, valaciclovir. Oral valaciclovir is rapidly and extensively converted to acyclovir, substantially increasing acyclovir bioavailability, and thus it has the potential for improved efficacy and more convenient dosing than oral acyclovir (see also Figure 16).

Ganciclovir (9-[1,3-dihydroxy-2-propoxymethyl] guanine) is an acyclic guanine nucleoside analog that is similar in structure to acyclovir except in having an additional hydroxymethyl group on the acyclic side chain. **Valganciclovir** is the L-valyl ester prodrug of ganciclovir.

This agent has inhibitory activity against all herpesviruses but is especially active against CMV. Inhibitory concentrations are similar to those of acyclovir for HSV and VZV but 10 to 100 times lower for human CMV strains (0.2 to 2.8 μg/mL).

Inhibitory concentrations for human bone marrow progenitor cells are similar to those inhibitory for CMV replication, a finding predictive of ganciclovir's myelotoxicity during clinical use. Inhibition of human lymphocyte blastogenic responses also occurs at clinically achievable concentrations of 1 to 10 μg/mL.

Ganciclovir inhibits viral DNA synthesis. It is monophosphorylated intracellularly by viral thymidine kinase during HSV infection and by a viral phosphotransferase encoded by the UL97 gene during CMV infection. Ganciclovir diphosphate and ganciclovir triphosphate are formed by cellular enzymes. At least tenfold higher concentrations of ganciclovir triphosphate are present in CMV-infected than in uninfected cells. The triphosphate is a competitive inhibitor of deoxyguanosine triphosphate incorporation into DNA and preferentially inhibits viral rather than host cellular DNA polymerases. Ganciclovir is incorporated into both viral and cellular DNA. Incorporation into viral DNA causes eventual cessation of DNA chain elongation.

Intracellular ganciclovir triphosphate concentrations are tenfold higher than those of acyclovir triphosphate and decline much more slowly, with an intracellular half-life of elimination exceeding 24 hours. These differences may account in part for ganciclovir's greater anti-CMV activity and provide the rationale for single daily doses in suppressing human CMV infections.

CMV can become resistant to ganciclovir by one of two mechanisms: reduced intracellular ganciclovir phosphorylation owing to mutations in the viral phosphotransferase encoded by the UL97 gene and mutations in viral DNA polymerase. Resistant CMV clinical isolates have 4 to more than 20 times the increases in inhibitory concentrations. Resistance has been associated primarily with impaired phosphorylation but sometimes only with DNA polymerase mutations. Highly resistant variants with dual UL97 and polymerase mutations are cross-resistant to cidofovir and variably to foscarnet. Ganciclovir also is much less active against acyclovir-resistant thymidine kinase-deficient HSV strains.

The oral bioavailability of ganciclovir averages 6 to 9% following ingestion with food. Peak and trough plasma levels are about 0.5 to 1.2 and 0.2 to 0.5 μg/mL, respectively, after 1000-mg doses every 8 hours. Oral valganciclovir is well absorbed and hydrolyzed rapidly to ganciclovir. The bioavailability of ganciclovir averages 61% following valganciclovir. Food increases the bioavailability of **valganciclovir** by about 25%, and peak ganciclovir concentrations average 6.1 μg/mL after 875-mg doses. High oral **valganciclovir** doses in the fed state provide ganciclovir exposures comparable to intravenous dosing. Following intravenous administration of 5 mg/kg doses of ganciclovir, peak and trough plasma concentrations average 8 to 11 and 0.6 to 1.2 μg/mL, respectively. Following intravenous dosing, vitreous fluid levels are similar to or higher than those in plasma and average about 1 μg/mL. Vitreous levels decline with a half-life of 23 to 26 hours. Intraocular sustained-release ganciclovir implants provide vitreous levels of about 4.1 μg/mL.

The plasma half-life is about 2 to 4 hours in patients with normal renal function. Over 90% of ganciclovir is eliminated unchanged by renal excretion through glomerular filtration and tubular secretion. Consequently, the plasma half-life increases almost linearly as creatinine clearance declines and may reach 28 to 40 hours in those with severe renal insufficiency.

Myelosuppression is the principal dose-limiting toxicity of ganciclovir. Neutropenia occurs in about 15 to 40% of patients and thrombocytopenia in 5 to 20%. Neutropenia is observed most commonly during the second week of treatment and usually is reversible within 1 week of drug cessation. Persistent, fatal neutropenia has occurred. Oral valganciclovir is associated with headache and gastrointestinal (GI) disturbance (i.e., nausea, pain, and diarrhea) in addition to the toxicities associated with intravenous ganciclovir, including neutropenia. Recombinant granulocyte colony-stimulating factor (G-CSF, filgrastim, lenograstim) may be useful in treating ganciclovir-induced neutropenia.

CNS side effects occur in 5 to 15% of patients and range in severity from headache to behavioral changes to convulsions and coma. About one-third of patients have had to interrupt or prematurely stop intravenous ganciclovir therapy because of bone marrow or CNS toxicity. Infusion-related phlebitis, azotemia, anemia, rash, fever, liver function test abnormalities, nausea or vomiting, and eosinophilia also have been described.

Teratogenicity, embryotoxicity, irreversible reproductive toxicity, and myelotoxicity have been observed in animals at ganciclovir dosages comparable to those used in human beings. Ganciclovir is classified in pregnancy as category C.

Zidovudine, and probably other cytotoxic agents, increase the risk of myelosuppression, as do nephrotoxic agents that impair ganciclovir excretion. Probenecid and possibly acyclovir reduce renal clearance of ganciclovir. Zalcitabine increases oral ganciclovir exposure by an average of 22%. Oral ganciclovir increases the absorption and peak-plasma concentrations of didanosine approximately twofold and that of zidovudine by about 20%.

Ganciclovir is effective in treatment and chronic suppression of CMV retinitis in immunocompromised patients and for prevention of CMV disease in transplant patients. In CMV retinitis, initial induction treatment (5 mg/kg intravenously every 12 hours for 10 to 21 days) is associated with improvement or stabilization in about 85% of patients. Reduced viral excretion is usually evident by 1 week, and funduscopic improvement is seen by 2 weeks. Because of the high risk of relapse, AIDS patients with retinitis require suppressive therapy with high doses of ganciclovir (30 to 35 mg/kg week). Oral ganciclovir (1000 mg three times daily) is effective for suppression of retinitis after initial intravenous treatment. Oral **valganciclovir** (900 mg twice daily for 21 days initial treatment) is comparable with intravenous dosing for initial control and sustained suppression (900 mg daily) of CMV retinitis.

Intravitreal ganciclovir injections have been used in some patients, and an intraocular sustained-release ganciclovir implant (Vitrasert) is more effective than systemic dosing in suppressing retinitis progression.

Ganciclovir therapy (5 mg/kg every 12 hours for 14 to 21 days) may benefit other CMV syndromes in AIDS patients or solid-organ transplant recipients. Response rates of 67% or higher have been found in combination with a decrease in immunosuppressive therapy. The duration of therapy depends on demonstrating clearance of viremia; an early switch from intravenous ganciclovir to oral valganciclovir is feasible. Recurrent CMV disease occurs commonly after initial treatment. In bone marrow transplant recipients with CMV pneumonia, ganciclovir alone appears ineffective. However, ganciclovir combined with intravenous immunoglobulin or CMV immunoglobulin reduces the mortality of CMV pneumonia by about one-half. Ganciclovir treatment may benefit infants with congential CMV disease, and further studies are in progress.

Ganciclovir has been used for both prophylaxis and preemptive therapy of CMV infections in transplant recipients. In bone marrow transplant recipients, preemptive ganciclovir treatment (5 mg/kg every 12 hours for 7 to 14 days followed by 5 mg/kg every day up to days 100 to 120 after transplant), starting when CMV is isolated from bronchoalveolar lavage or from other sites, is highly effective in preventing CMV pneumonia and appears to reduce mortality in these patients. Initiation of ganciclovir at the time of engraftment also reduces CMV disease rates but does not improve survival, in part because of infections due to ganciclovir-related neutropenia.

Intravenous ganciclovir, oral ganciclovir, and oral valganciclovir reduce the risk of CMV disease in solid-organ transplant recipients. Oral ganciclovir (1000 mg three times daily for 3 months) reduces CMV disease risk in liver transplant recipients, including high-risk patients with primary infection or those receiving antilymphocyte antibodies. Oral valganciclovir prophylaxis generally is more effective than high-dose oral acyclovir. Oral valganciclovir (900 mg once daily) provides somewhat greater antiviral effects and similar reductions in CMV disease as oral ganciclovir in mismatched solid-organ transplant recipients.

In advanced HIV disease, oral ganciclovir (1000 mg three times daily) may reduce the risk of CMV disease, and possibly mortality, in those not receiving didanosine. The addition of oral high-dose ganciclovir (1500 mg three times daily) to the intraocular ganciclovir implant further delays the time to retinitis progression and reduces the risk of new CMV disease and, possibly, the risk of Kaposi's sarcoma.

VALDECOXIB

(Bextra tablets 10 mg, tablets 20 mg)

Valdecoxib is a nonsteroidal antiinflammatory drug (NSAID) that inhibits inflammation, pain, and fever, probably by inhibition of cyclooxygenase-2 (COX-2). It is indicated in the relief of signs and symptoms of osteoarthritis and adult rheumatoid arthritis; and treatment of primary dysmenorrhea.

VALPROIC ACID

(Depakote)

Valproic acid, a broad-spectrum anticonvulsant (initially 15 mg/kg/day p.o.), is indicated as a sole and adjunctive therapy in simple (petit mal) and complex absence seizures. Also, it is used adjunctively in patients with multiple seizure types, including absence seizures.

In addition, valproic acid has shown effectiveness against myoclonic and grand mal seizures, and possibly against atonic, complex partial, and infantile spasm seizures. Moreover, it has been used effectively in preventing recurrent febrile seizures in children and in treating rapidly cycling bipolar affective disorders. The mechanism of action of valproic acid has been postulated to be its enhancement of gamma aminobutyric acid (GABA) ergic transmission. Valproic acid is rapidly absorbed orally, rapidly distributed, and highly bound (90%) to plasma proteins, primarily albumin. Increases in dose may decrease protein binding. Significantly reduced plasma-protein binding has occurred in renal insufficiency, cirrhosis, and acute viral hepatitis. The drug is primarily metabolized in the liver and is excreted as the glucuronide. Elimination of valproic acid and its metabolites occurs principally in the urine. Very little unmetabolized drug is excreted in the urine and feces.

Chlorpromazine, cimetidine, and salicylates decrease the clearance of valproic acid and increase its half-life. Addition of valproic acid to phenobarbital may result in an increased phenobarbital level and an increase in CNS effects.

The side effects of valproic acid are gastrointestinal in nature, consisting of transient and inconsequential nausea and vomiting. In addition, sedation occurs (50%), especially when the drug is taken in combination with phenobarbital. Additional rare side effects include hepatic toxicity, pancreatitis, alopecia, and hematologic problems.

Hepatic failure resulting in fatalities has occurred in patients receiving valproic acid and its derivatives. Children less than 2 years of age are at considerable increased risk of developing fatal hepatotoxicity, especially those on multiple anticonvulsants, those with congenital metabolic disorders, those with severe seizure disorders accompanied by mental retardation, and those with organic brain disease.

VALSARTAN

(Diovan capsules 80 mg, capsules 160 mg)

Valsartan is an angiotensin-II-receptor antagonist that antagonizes the effect of angiotensin II (vasoconstriction and aldosterone secretion) by blocking the angiotensin-II receptor (AT_1 receptor) in vascular smooth muscle and the adrenal gland, producing decreased BP. It is indicated in the treatment of hypertension, either alone or in combination with other antihypertensive drugs; and heart failure.

VALSARTAN/HYDROCHLOROTHIAZIDE

(Diovan HCT tablets 12.5 mg hydrochlorothiazide and 80 mg valsartan, tablets 12.5 mg hydrochlorothiazide and 160 mg valsartan, tablets 25 mg hydrochlorothiazide and 160 mg valsartan)

Valsartan is an antihypertensive combination. **Valsartan** antagonizes the effect of angiotensin II (vasoconstriction and aldosterone secretion) by blocking the angiotensin-II receptor (AT_1 receptor) in vascular smooth muscle and the adrenal gland, producing decreased BP. **Hydrochlorothiazide** (HCTZ) increases chloride, sodium, and water excretion by interfering with transport of sodium ions across renal tubular epithelium. They are used in hypertension.

VANADIUM

Vanadium is a transitional metal found in relative abundance in nature. It can readily change its oxidation state and take an anionic or a cationic form. Vanadium has insulin-like effects in that it induces a sustained fall in blood glucose level in insulin-dependent animals. Recent short-term trials with vanadium salts seem promising in type II (non-insulin-dependent) diabetic patients in whom liver and peripheral insulin resistance was attenuated, indicating the therapeutic potential of vanadium salts.

VANCOMYCIN

(Vancocin)

Vancomycin (500 mg IV q. 6 hours) is indicated for the treatment of severe staphylococcal infections, when other antibiotics are ineffective or contraindicated. Vancomycin (125 to 500 mg p.o. q. 6 hours for 7 to 10 days) is indicated for the treatment of antibiotic-associated pseudomembranous and staphylococcal enterocolitis; and vancomycin (1 g IV given slowly over 1 hour, starting 1 hour before a procedure) is indicated for endocarditis prophylaxis for dental, GI, biliary, and genitourinary instrumentation procedures; and

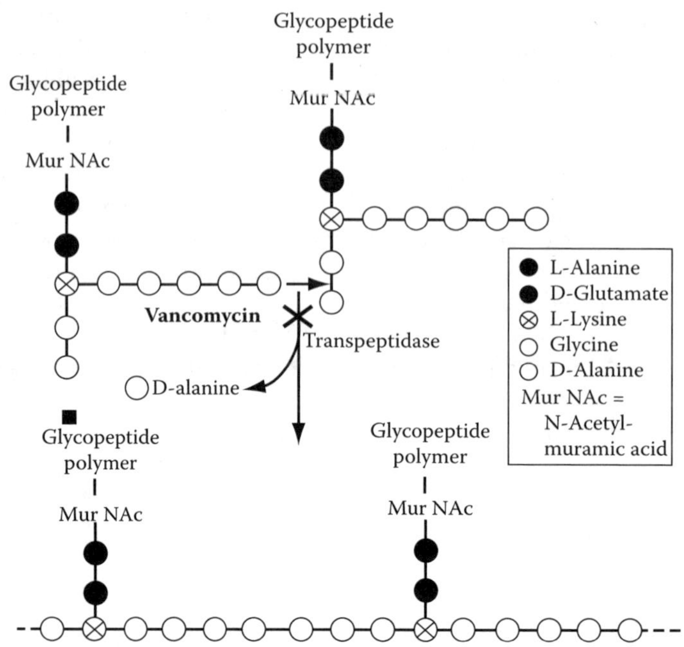

FIGURE 100 Vancomycin, a bactericidal antibiotic, inhibits cell-wall synthesis in Gram-positive bacteria. It is effective against methicillin-resistant organisms and as an alternate to semisynthetic penicillins or cephalosporins in patients with severe staphylococcal infections.

as surgical prophylaxis in patients allergic to penicillin. It is indicated in the treatment of serious or severe infections not treatable with other antimicrobials, including the penicillins and cephalosporins (see Figure 100).

Vancomycin is an antibiotic produced by *Streptococcus orientalis*, an actinomycete isolated from soil samples. Other glycopeptide antimicrobial agents, daptomycin and teicoplanin, are available. Vancomycin is primarily active against Gram-positive bacteria. *Staphylococcus aureus* and *Staphylococcus epidermidis*, including strains resistant to methicillin, are usually inhibited by concentrations of 1.0 to 5.0 µg/mL. Synergism between vancomycin and gentamicin or tobramycin occurs against *S. aureus*, including methicillin-resistant strains *Streptococcus pyogenes*, *Streptococcus pneumoniae*, and viridans streptococci are highly susceptible, as are most strains of *Enterococcus* spp. Vancomycin is not generally bactericidal for *Enterococcus* spp., and the addition of a synergistic aminoglycoside is necessary to produce a bactericidal effect. *Corynebacterium* spp. (diphtheroids) are inhibited by less than 0.04 to 3.1 µg/mL of vancomycin; most species of *Actinomyces* by 5 to 10 µg/mL; and *Clostridium* spp. by 0.39 to 6 µg/mL. Vancomycin inhibits the synthesis of the cell wall in sensitive bacteria by binding with high affinity to the *d*-alanyl-*d*-alanine terminus of cell-wall precursor units (Figure 100). The drug is rapidly bactericidal for dividing microorganisms.

Vancomycin has caused reversible neutropenia, nephrotoxicity, hypotension (rapid bolus injection), and pseudomembranous colitis (rare). The concomitant use of vancomycin with aminoglycosides increases the risk of nephrotoxicity. Vancomycin potentiates the neuromuscular blocking effects of nondepolarizing skeletal muscle relaxants such as *d*-tubocurarine.

VARDENAFIL HYDROCHLORIDE

(Levitra tablets 2.5 mg, tablets 5 mg, tablets 10 mg, tablets 20 mg)

Vardenafil hydrochloride is a phosphodiesterase type 5 inhibitor. It enhances the effect of nitric oxide at the nerve ending and endothelial cells in the corpus cavernosum by inhibiting phosphodiesterase type 5 in the corpus cavernosum of the penis. This results in vasodilation, increased inflow of blood into the corpora cavernosa, and ensuing penile erection upon sexual stimulation. It is used to treat erectile dysfunction.

VARICELLA-ZOSTER IMMUNE GLOBULIN (VZIG)

This immune substance is used for passive immunization of susceptible patients, primarily patients who are immunocompromised owing to exposure to varicella (chicken pox or herpes zoster).

VASODILATORS

The vasodilators may be classified as ventodilators, arterial dilators, or balanced-type vasodilators (Table 26).

The rationale for vasodilation in the management of congestive heart failure is based on the increased arteriolar vasotone that occurs. This initiates a vicious circle in which cardiac function is further depressed by an increase in afterload and in resistance to ejection.

TABLE 26
Classification of Vasodilators by Peripheral Site of Action

Sites of Action	Agents
Venodilators	Nitrates/nitroglycerin (low dose)
	Molsidomine
Arterial dilators	Hydralazine, dihydralazine, endralazine
	Minoxidil
	Calcium antagonists
	Phentolamine
	Fenoldopam
Balanced-type vasodilators	Prazosin, trimazosin
	Nitrates/nitroglycerin (high dose)
	Angiotensin-converting enzyme inhibitors
	Phosphodiesterase inhibitors
	Nitroprusside
	Flosequinan

Vascular tone is regulated by the cytosolic calcium level, the interaction of calcium and calmodulin with myosin light-chain kinase, and the subsequent myosin light-chain phosphorylation, which promotes the interaction of myosin with actin and finally leads to contraction.

Receptor-dependent vasodilation may also take place in a more indirect way through the presynaptic modulation of the release of neurotransmitters such as norepinephrine and acetylcholine. In addition to its effects on postsynaptic receptors, norepinephrine stimulates the presynaptic alpha$_2$-receptor, thereby inhibiting further transmitter release. Moreover, the activation of other presynaptic receptors such as the muscarinic cholinergic, dopaminergic, purinergic, serotoninergic, and histaminergic receptors leads to diminished norepinephrine release and subsequent vasodilation.

A number of vasodilators, such as acetylcholine, bradykinin, adenine nucleosides, thrombin, histamine, or serotonin, need an intact vascular endothelium in order to exert their effects. For example, stimulation of endothelial cholinergic receptors causes the release of endothelium-derived relaxing factors (EDRFs), which may involve arachidonic acid formation and compartmentalization via the lipoxygenase pathway. EDRF, which is identical to nitric oxide, activates guanylate cyclase and enhances the formation of cyclic guanosine monophosphate (cyclic GMP) in smooth muscle. Tetranoic acid (a vasoconstrictor), thromboxane A$_2$ (a vasoconstrictor), and prostacycline (a vasodilator) are formed through the lipoxygenase pathway.

The vasodilating properties of captopril or hydralazine (antihypertensive agents) are mediated by the formation of EDRF, or prostaglandin, or both. On the other hand, the vasodilating properties of nitroprusside (an antihypertensive agent) result directly from the formation of cyclic GMP (see also Figure 24).

Vasodilators: Effects on Cardiac Output (CO)

Drugs	CO
Venous vasodilators	
Isosorbide dinitrate	0/+
Arterial vasodilators	
Hydralazine	+
Minoxidil	+
Nifedipine	+
Diltiazem	+
Mixed arterial–venous vasodilators	
Prazosin	+
Captopril	+
Enalapril	+
Lisinopril	+

Abbreviations: + = increase; 0 = no change.

VASOPRESSIN
(Pitressin)

The second hormone that originates from the posterior pituitary gland is antidiuretic hormone, or vasopressin. It has the following amino-acid sequence:

```
Gln–Asn–Cys–Pro–Arg–Gly
|       |
Phe - - - -Tyr
```

With the exception of two amino acids, vasopressin resembles oxytocin in structure. Oxytocin contains leucine and isoleucine, and vasopressin contains phenylalanine and arginine. The sites of synthesis, storage, and release of vasopressin are identical to those described for oxytocin. Many agents alter the secretion or action of vasopressin, and these are listed in Figures 101 and 102.

The loss of the neurosecretory neurons that make up the neurohypophysis eliminates the secretion of vasopressin, and this produces diabetes insipidus. Some of the various causes of neurogenic diabetes insipidus are the following:

Acquired
- Idiopathic
- Trauma (accidental or surgical)
- Tumor (craniopharyngioma, metastasis, or lymphoma)
- Granuloma (sarcoid or histiocytosis)
- Infectious (meningitis or encephalitis)
- Vascular (Sheehan's syndrome, aneurysm, or aortocoronary bypass)

Familial (autosomal dominant)

Another form of diabetes insipidus is a vasopressin-insensitive or nephrogenic diabetes insipidus, and it stems from the following causes:

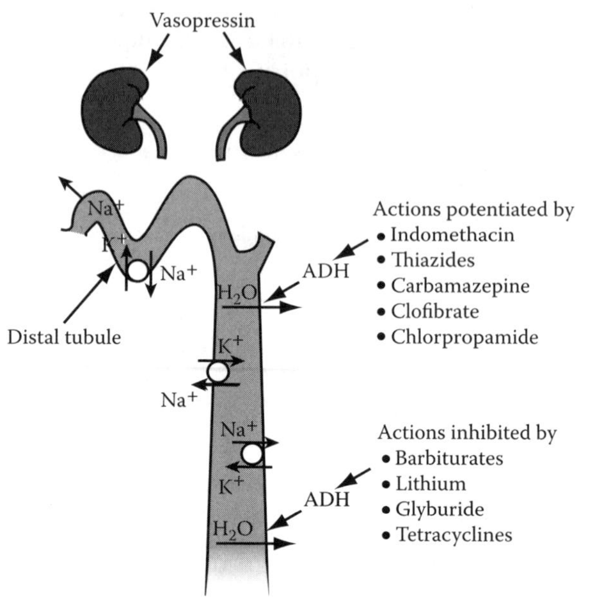

FIGURE 101 Many agents alter the secretion or actions of antidiuretic hormone (ADH).

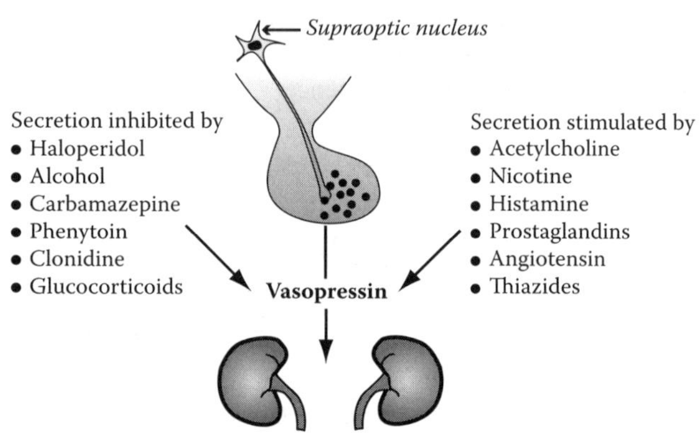

FIGURE 102 Many agents alter the secretion or actions of vasopressin.

Acquired

- Infectious (pyelonephritis)
- Postobstructive (prostatic or ureteral)
- Vascular (sickle cell disease or trait)
- Infiltrative (amyloid)
- Cystic (polycystic disease)
- Metabolic (hypokalemia or hypercalcemia)
- Granuloma (sarcoid)
- Toxic (lithium, demeclocycline, or methoxyflurane)
- Solute overload (glucosuria or postobstructive)

Familial (X-linked recessive)

Agents that cause the syndrome of inappropriate antidiuretic secretion consist of the following:

- Carbamazepine
- Chlorpropamide
- Clofibrate
- Cyclophosphamide
- Haloperidol
- Monoamine oxidase inhibitors
- Nicotine
- Oxytocin
- Phenothiazine derivatives
- Thiazide diuretics
- Tricyclic antidepressants
- Vincristine

Vasopressin may be administered either subcutaneously or intramuscularly. It has a duration of action of 2 to 8 hours. Vasopressin tannate (Pitressin tannate) is a suspension and should be injected intramuscularly only. It has a duration of action of 2 to 3 days. Desmopressin acetate (DDAVP) is used topically. Lypressin (Diapid) is administered as an intranasal spray. All these agents may be used in the treatment of central diabetes insipidus (vasopressin-sensitive).

VENLAFAXINE

(Effexor tablets 25 mg, tablets 37.5 mg, tablets 50 mg, tablets 75 mg, tablets 100 mg, Effexor XR capsules, extended-release 37.5 mg, capsules, extended-release 75 mg, capsules, extended-release 150 mg)

Venlafaxine is a serotonin and norepinephrine reuptake inhibitor that potentiates norepinephrine, serotonin, and dopamine neurotransmitter activity in the CNS by inhibiting their neuronal reuptake. **Effexor, Effexor XR**: are used in treatment of major depressive disorder. **Effexor XR**: is used in treatment of generalized anxiety disorder; and treatment of social anxiety disorder.

VENLAFAXINE HYDROCHLORIDE

(Effexor)

Venlafaxine, an antidepressant blocking the uptake of serotonin, dopamine, and norepinephrine (75 mg p.o. daily), is used in the treatment of depression. Venlafaxine has no significant affinity for muscarinic cholinergic, histaminergic, or alpha$_1$-adrenergic receptors. Venlafaxine is as efficacious as tricyclic antidepressants and trazodone; however, because it has fewer side effects, it is better tolerated (see Tables 5 through 7).

VERAPAMIL HYDROCHLORIDE

(Calan, Calan SR, Isoptin, Isoptin SR, Verelan)

Verapamil (80 mg p.o. q. 6 to 8 hours) is indicated in the management of Prinzmetal's or variant angina or unstable or chronic, stable angina pectoris; verapamil (0.075 to 0.15 mg/kg IV push over a 2-minute period) is indicated in the treatment of supraventricular tachyarrhythmias; verapamil (240 to 480 mg p.o. daily) is indicated in the prevention of recurrent paroxysmal supraventricular tachycardia; verapamil (240 to 320 mg p.o. daily) is indicated in the control of the ventricular rate in digitalized patients with chronic atrial flutter and/or fibrillation; and verapamil (80 mg p.o. t.i.d.) is indicated in the management of hypertension.

Verapamil blocks both activated and inactivated calcium channels. Thus, its effect is more marked in tissues that fire

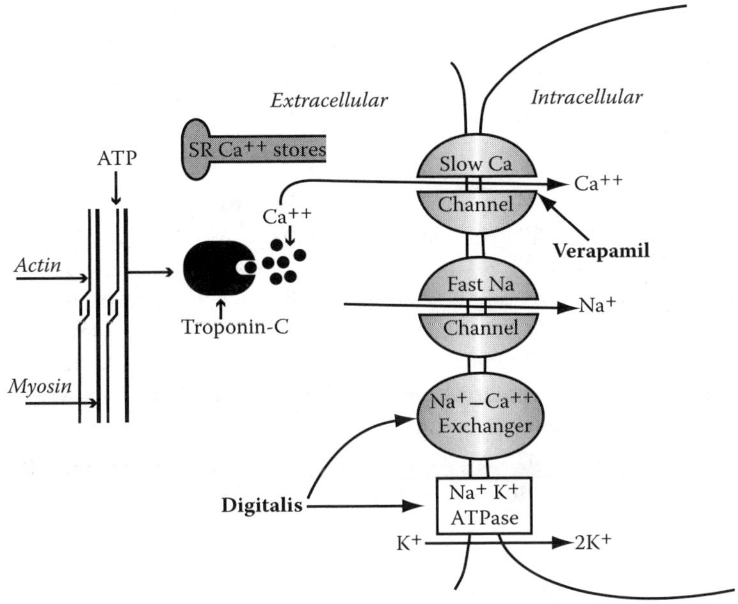

FIGURE 103 Verapamil is used in the management of Prinzmetal's or variant angina. ATP = adenosine triphosphate; SR = sarcoplasmic reticulum.

frequently, those that are less completely polarized at rest, and those in which activation depends exclusively on the calcium current, such as the sinoatrial and atrioventricular nodes. It is therefore not surprising that verapamil has marked effects on these tissues. Atrioventricular (AV) nodal conduction and effective refractory period are invariably prolonged by therapeutic concentrations. Verapamil usually slows the sinoatrial node by its direct action, but its hypotensive action may occasionally result in a small reflex increase of sinoatrial nodal rate (Figure 103).

Verapamil can suppress both early and delayed depolarizations and may antagonize slow responses arising in severely depolarized tissue.

Verapamil causes peripheral vasodilation, which may be beneficial in hypertension and peripheral vasospastic disorders. Its effects upon smooth muscle produce a number of extracardiac effects (see Figure 103 and Table 21).

Verapamil's cardiotoxic effects are dose related and usually avoidable. A common error has been to administer intravenous verapamil to a patient with ventricular tachycardia misdiagnosed as supraventricular tachycardia. In this setting, hypotension and ventricular fibrillation can occur.

Verapamil's negative inotropic effects may limit its clinical usefulness in damaged hearts. Verapamil can lead to atrioventricular block when used in large doses or in patients with partial atrioventricular block. This block can be treated with atropine, beta-receptor stimulants, or calcium. In patients with sinus node disease, verapamil can precipitate sinus arrest.

Verapamil is absorbed rapidly and completely from the GI tract after oral administration; however, only about 20 to 35% of the drug reaches systemic circulation because of the first-pass effect. Verapamil is *N*-methylated to norverapamil, which is an active metabolite. The half-lives of calcium-blocking agents increase in hepatic cirrhosis and in older patients.

Verapamil is contraindicated in patients with severe hypotension (systolic blood pressure below 90 mmHg) of cardiogenic shock, because of the drug's hypotensive effect; in patients with second- or third-degree AV block or sick-sinus syndrome (unless a functioning artificial ventricular pacemaker is in place), because of the drug's effects on the cardiac conduction system; in patients with severe left-ventricular dysfunction (indicated by pulmonary wedge pressure above 20 mmHg and left-ventricular ejection fraction below 20%), unless heart failure results from supraventricular tachycardia, because the drug may worsen the condition in patients with ventricular dysfunction or AV abnormalities who are receiving beta-adrenergic blocks, as a result of the drug's negative inotropic effect and inhibition of the cardiac conduction system.

Concomitant use of verapamil with adrenergic-receptor beta blockers may cause additive effects leading to congestive heart failure, conduction disturbances, arrhythmias, and hypotension.

Concomitant use of oral verapamil with digoxin may increase serum digoxin concentration by 50 to 75% during the first week of therapy. Concomitant use with antihypertensives may lead to combined antihypertensive effects, resulting in clinically significant hypotension. Concomitant use with drugs that attenuate alpha-adrenergic response (such as prazosin and methyldopa) may cause excessive blood pressure (BP) reduction. Concomitant use with disopyramide may cause combined negative inotropic effects. Use with quinidine to treat hypertrophic cardiomyopathy may cause excessive hypotension; use with carbamazepine, may cause increased serum carbamazepine levels and subsequent toxicity; with rifampin, it may substantially reduce verapamil's oral bioavailability. Verapamil therapy may inhibit the clearance and increase the plasma levels of theophylline. Overdosage of verapamil causes heart block asystole and hypotension.

VERCURONIUM BROMIDE

(Norcuron)

Vercuronium, a nondepolarizing neuromuscular-blocking agent (0.08 to 0.10 mg/kg IV), is indicated as an adjunct to anesthesia to facilitate intubation and to provide skeletal muscle relaxation during surgery or mechanical ventilation. Vercuronium prevents acetylcholine from binding to receptors on the motor end plate, thus blocking depolarization. Vercuronium exhibits minimal cardiovascular effects and does not appear to alter heart rate or rhythm, systolic or diastolic blood pressure, cardiac output, systemic vascular resistance, or mean arterial pressure. It has little or no histamine-releasing properties (see also Figure 99).

Vercuronium is an intermediate-acting nondepolarizing muscle relaxant. It has a wide margin of safety and does not produce undesirable hemodynamic effects. Its onset of action is similar to atracurium's, but not as short as succinylcholine's.

VIDARABINE

(Adenine Arabinoside; ARA-A)

Vidarabine, an antiviral agent (10 to 15 mg/kg/day for 5 to 10 days), is indicated in the treatment of herpes simplex virus encephalitis, neonatal herpes simplex virus infections, and herpes zoster in immunosuppressed patients. In addition, vidarabine (ophthalmic ointment: 3% vidarabine monohydrate [equivalent to 2.8% vidarabine]) is indicated in the treatment of acute keratoconjunctivitis and recurrent epithelial keratitis due to herpes simplex virus types 1 and 2, or superficial keratitis caused by herpes simplex virus that has not responded to topical idoxuridine or when toxic or hypersensitivity reactions to idoxuridine have occurred.

Vidarabine is an inhibitor of viral DNA synthesis. Cellular enzymes phosphorylate vidarabine to the triphosphate, which inhibits viral DNA polymerase activity in a manner that is competitive with deoxyadenosine triphosphate. Vidarabine triphosphate is incorporated into both cellular and viral DNA, where it may act as a chain terminator. Vidarabine triphosphate also inhibits ribonucleoside reductase, RNA polyadenylation, and *S*-adenosylhomocysteine hydrolase, an enzyme involved in transmethylation reactions. Resistant variants due to mutations in viral DNA polymerase can be selected *in vitro*.

The main metabolite, arabinosyl hypoxanthine (Ara-Hx) has approximately 1/20 the activity of vidarabine. In renal impairment, the excretion of Ara-Hx is decreased, requiring dose adjustment. Allopurinol, a xanthine oxidase inhibitor, may interfere with the metabolism of vidarabine (see also Figure 18).

Vidarabine has caused nausea, vomiting, anorexia, diarrhea; decreased reticulocytes, hemoglobin, hematocrit, WBC, and platelets; and tremor, dizziness, headache, hallucinations, confusion, psychosis, and ataxia. These side effects are more pronounced in patients with impaired hepatic or renal functions.

VIGABATRIN

(VGB, Sabril)

Vigabatrin is a new antiepileptic drug used for treatment of partial and secondarily generalized tonic–clonic seizures. Vigabatrin acts as an irreversible substrate for GABA transaminase that leads to elevated brain GABA levels. Adverse effects on the nervous system include drowsiness and fatigue, primarily during the first weeks of treatment (Figure 104).

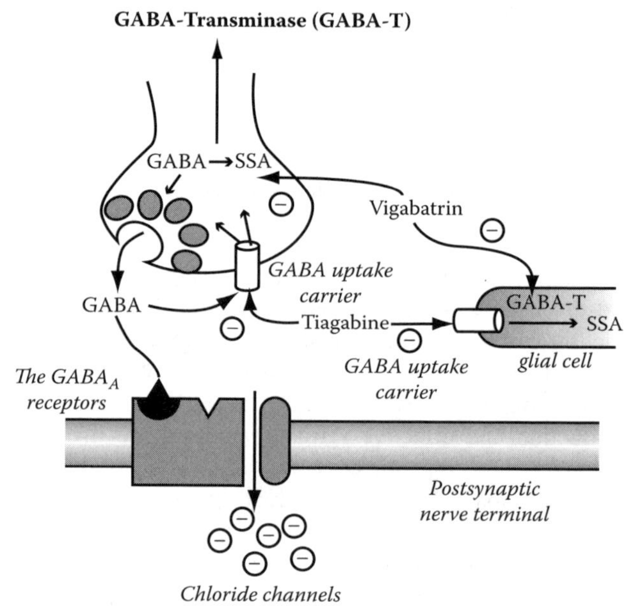

FIGURE 104 Vigabatrin inhibits GABA transaminases and has anticonvulsant properties.

VINBLASTINE

(VLB)

Vinblastine (initially 3.7 mg/m^2) is indicated in the treatment of frequently responsive malignancies such as generalized Hodgkin's disease (stages III and IV, Ann Arbor modification of the Rye staging system) and lymphocytic lymphoma (nodular and diffuse, poorly differentiated); histiocytic lymphoma; mycosis fungoides (advanced stages); advanced testicular carcinoma; Kaposi's sarcoma, and Letterer–Siwe disease (histiocytosis X). Less frequently, the drug is used in responsive malignancies such as choriocarcinoma resistant to other chemotherapy and breast cancer unresponsive to surgery and hormonal therapy.

Vinblastine is an alkaloid derived from *Vinca rosea*, the periwinkle plant. Its mechanism of action involves depolymerization of microtubules, which are an important part of the cytoskeleton and the mitotic spindle. The drug binds specifically to the microtubular protein tubulin in dimeric form; the drug–tubulin complex joins to the forming end of the microtubules to terminate assembly, and depolymerization of the microtubules then occurs. This results in mitotic arrest at metaphase, dissolution of the mitotic spindle, and interference with chromosome segregation.

The combination of vinblastine and mitomycin C has caused shortness of breath and bronchospasm. Vinblastine reduces the level and, hence, the effectiveness of phenytoin, requiring increased dosage. Vinblastine produces nausea and vomiting and marrow depression as well as alopecia (see Figure 15).

VINCA ALKALOIDS

The vinca alkaloids (vinblastine, vincristine, and vindesine), which bind to tubulin, block mitosis with metaphase arrest. Vinca alkaloids are used for the following types of cancer:

Acute lymphoid leukemia: In the induction phase, vincristine is used with prednisone.
Acute myelomonocytic or monocytic leukemia: Cytarabine, vincristine, and prednisone.
Hodgkin's disease: Mechlorethamine, Oncovin (vincristine), procarbazine, and prednisone (MOPP).
Nodular lymphoma: Cyclophosphamide, Oncovin (vincristine), and prednisone (CVP).
Diffuse histiocytic lymphoma: Cyclophosphamide, adriamycin (doxorubicin), vincristine, and prednisone (CHOP); bleomycin, adriamycin (doxorubicin), cyclophosphamide, Oncovin (vincristine), and prednisone (BACOP); or cyclophosphamide, Oncovin (vincristine), methotrexate, and cytarabine (COMA).
Wilm's tumor: Dactinomycin and vincristine.
Ewings' sarcoma: Cyclophosphamide, dactinomycin, or vincristine.
Embryonal rhabdomyosarcoma: Cyclophosphamide, dactinomycin, or vincristine.
Bronchogenic carcinoma: Doxorubicin, cyclophosphamide, and vincristine.

The chief toxicity associated with vinblastine use is bone marrow depression. The toxicity of vincristine consists of paresthesia, neuritic pain, muscle weakness, and visual disturbances. In addition, both vinblastine and vincristine may cause alopecia (see Figure 15).

VINCRISTINE SULFATE

(VCR:LCR)

Vincristine (1.4 to 2.0 mg/m^2) is indicated in the treatment of acute leukemia and in combination therapy for Hodgkin's disease, non-Hodgkin's malignant lymphomas (lymphocytic, mixed-cell, histiocytic, undifferentiated, nodular, and diffuse types), rhabdomyosarcoma, neuroblastoma, and Wilm's tumor. In addition, vincristine has been used in the treatment of idiopathic thrombocytopenic purpura, Kaposi's sarcoma, breast cancer, and bladder cancer. The intrathecal administration of vincristine is fatal.

Vincristine is an alkaloid derived from *Vinca rosea*, the periwinkle plant. Its mechanism of action involves depolymerization of microtubules, which are an important part of the cytoskeleton and the mitotic spindle. The drug binds specifically to the microtubular protein tubulin in dimeric form; the drug–tubulin complex adds to the forming end of the microtubules to terminate assembly, and depolymerization of the microtubules then occurs. This results in mitotic arrest at metaphase, dissolution of the mitotic spindle, and interference with chromosome segregation.

Within 15 to 30 minutes following IV administration, more than 90% of the drug is distributed from blood into tissue, where it remains tightly, but not irreversibly, bound. Penetration across the blood–brain barrier is poor. The liver is the major excretory organ; about 80% of an injected dose appears in the feces, and 10 to 20% in the urine. Hepatic dysfunction may alter the elimination kinetics and augment toxicity, which limits its use to short courses. It occasionally produces bone marrow depression (see Figure 15).

VINORELBINE TARTRATE

(Navelbine solution for injection 10 mg/mL)

Vinorelbine is a vinca alkaloid. Vinorelbine interferes with microtubule assembly primarily by inhibiting mitosis at metaphase through its interaction with tubulin. It is indicated in unresectable, advanced non-small-cell lung cancer.

Vinorelbine (Navelbine, others) is administered in normal saline as an intravenous (IV) infusion of 30 mg/m^2 given over 6 to 10 minutes. A lower dose (20 to 25 mg/m^2) may be required for patients who have received prior chemotherapy. When used alone, it is initially given every week until progression of disease or dose-limiting toxicity. When used with cisplatin for the treatment of non-small-cell lung carcinoma, it is given every 3 weeks. As with the other vincas, it is eliminated by hepatic metabolism, and has an elimination half-life of 24 hours. Its primary toxicity is granulocytopenia, with only modest thrombocytopenia and less neurotoxicity than other vinca alkaloids. It may cause allergic reactions and mild, reversible changes in liver enzymes. In experimental studies, it has been given in an oral capsule, but bioavailability is only 30 to 40%. As with the other vincas, doses should be reduced in patients with elevated bilirubin or with over 75% liver replacement by metastatic disease.

VITAMIN A

(Retinol) (Aquasol A)

Vitamin A, a fat-soluble vitamin, is indicated for severe vitamin A deficiency with xerophthalmia.

VITAMIN E

(Alpha Tocopherol) (Aquasole E, CEN-E, Eprolin Gelseas, Episilan-M, E-Vital, Pheryl-E 400, Tocopher-Caps, Vita-Plus E, Vitera E)

Vitamin E, a fat-soluble vitamin, is used in vitamin E deficiency in premature infants and in patients with impaired fat absorption (including patients with cystic fibrosis) and in biliary atresia.

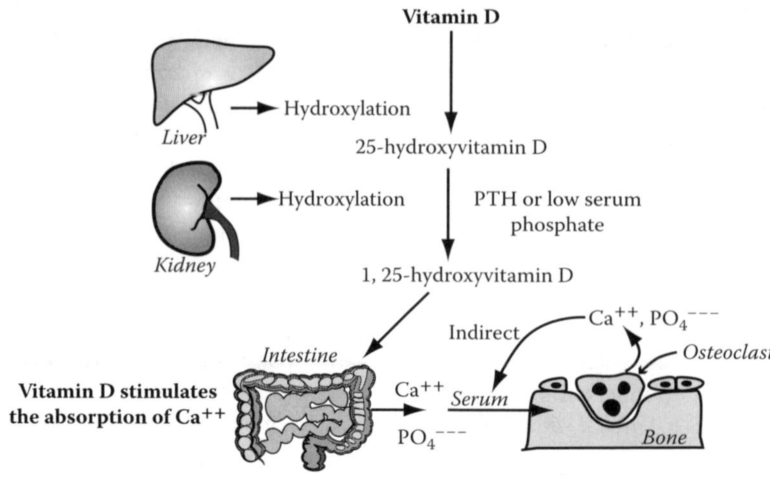

FIGURE 105 Vitamins D_3 and D_2 are produced by ultraviolet irradiation of animal skin and plants, respectively. The precursor of vitamin D_3 in skin is 7-dehydrocholesterol, or **provitamin D**. In humans, the storage, transport, metabolism, and potency of vitamins D_2 and D_3 are identical, and the net biologic activity of vitamin D *in vivo* results from the combined effects of the hydroxylated derivatives of vitamins D_2 and D_3.

VITAMIN K DERIVATIVES

MENADIOL SODIUM DIPHOSPHATE (Synkayvite)

PHYTONADIONE

(Aquamephyton, Konakion, Mephyton)

Vitamin K derivatives are used in treating hypoprothrombinemia secondary to vitamin K malabsorption or drug therapy, or when oral administration is desired and bile secretion is inadequate; in hypoprothrombinemia secondary to vitamin K malabsorption, drug therapy, or excess vitamin A; hypoprothrombinemia secondary to the effect of oral anticoagulants; prevention of hemorrhagic disease in neonates; differentiation between hepatocellular disease or biliary obstruction as a source of hypoprothrombinemia; prevention of hypoprothrombinemia related to vitamin K deficiency in long-term parenteral nutrition; and prevention of hypoprothrombinemia in infants receiving less than 0.1 mg/L vitamin K in breast milk or milk substitutes (see also Tables 17 and 18).

VITAMINS

Vitamins are organic dietary substances necessary for the maintenance of normal metabolic function. Only small amounts of the vitamins are required for normal health. In the body, they act as components of the important enzyme systems that catalyze the reactions by which protein, fat, and carbohydrate are metabolized. Some of the vitamins (e.g., vitamin K) may be formed by bacteria in the gut, whereas vitamin D is synthesized by exposure of the skin to sunlight. With these exceptions, the vitamins must be ingested in the food, and restricted diets or disorders of the gastrointestinal tract, interfering with absorption, lead to vitamin deficiency. When pronounced, such deficiencies give rise to easily recognizable clinical syndromes (beriberi, pellagra, rickets, scurvy) that have long been recognized. Milder forms of avitaminosis are much more common and also cause disability and ill health.

The fat-soluble vitamins are A, D, E, and K. The water-soluble vitamins are thiamine (vitamin B_1), riboflavin, nicotinic acid (niacin) and nicotinamide, pyridoxine (vitamin B_6), pantothenic acid, biotin, paraaminobenzoic acid, choline, inositol and other lipotropic agents, ascorbic acid (vitamin C), the riboflavonoids, folate, and vitamin B_{12} (see Figures 105 and 106).

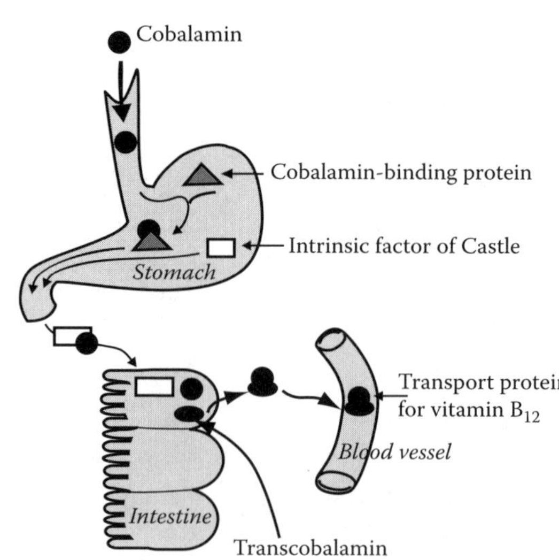

FIGURE 106 Both **vitamin B_{12}** and **folic acid** are essential for the synthesis of DNA, and this process is impaired in patients with megaloblastic anemia.

VITAMINS: Their Coenzymatic Functions

	Fat-Soluble Vitamins
A, retinol	Rhodopsin, visual cycle, night vision
K, menadiol	Blood-clotting factors II, VII, IX, and X
D, calciferol	Calcium and phosphorous homeostasis
E, tocopherol	Antioxidant, glutathione oxidase
	Water-Soluble Vitamins
C, ascorbate	Antioxidant, regulation of intracellular oxidation-reduction potentials, hydroxylation reactions that require copper or iron
B_1, thiamin	Oxidative decarboxylation of amino acids, transketolase
B_2, riboflavin	Flavin mononucleotide and flavin adenine dinucleotide, essential for oxidative systems and oxygen transport
B_3, pantothenic acid	As CoA precursor, necessary for acyl transfers
B_5, niacin	Endogenous source for tryptophan; component of NAD and its phosphorylate, NADP; assists in hydrogen transfer of glycolysis, fatty acid synthesis, and tissue respiration
B_6, pyridoxine	Nitrogen metabolism: transamination, racemization, decarboxylation, cleavage, synthesis, dehydration, and desulfhydration
B_{12}, cyanocobalamin	Methylation of homocysteine to methionine, conversion of methyl malonyl CoA to succinyl CoA
Biotin	Cofactor for some carboxylases; acetyl CoA carboxylase, pyruvate carboxylase, b-methylcrotonyl carboxylase, and methylmalonyl carboxylase
Folic acid	Transport of single carbon fragments, especially nucleic acid synthesis and metabolism of some amino acids

VOMITING CAUSED BY ANTINEOPLASTIC AGENTS

Severe Vomiting	Moderate Vomiting	Mild Vomiting
Cisplatin	Carboplatin	Bleomycin
Cyclophosphamide	Carmustine	Chlorambucil
Cytarabine	Cyclophosphamide	Cytarabine
Dacarbazine	Dactinomycin	Etoposide
Mechlorethamine	Daunorubicin	Fluorouracil
Streptozocin	Doxorubicin	Hydroxyurea
	Idarubicin	Melphalan
	Ifosfamide	Methotrexate
	Lomustine	Paclitaxel
	Mitomycin	Plicamycin
	Mitoxantrone	Thioguanine
	Pentostatin	Vinblastine
	Procarbazine	Vincristine

The incidence and severity of vomiting depends on the dosage and route of administration of antineoplastic agents. Intravenous ondansetron (Zofran) plus dexamethasone and lorazepam is the most effective treatment available for prevention of severe vomiting due to antineoplastic agents (see also Figure 73).

VORICONAZOLE

(Vfend tablets 50 mg, tablets 200 mg, powder for injection, lyophilized 200 mg, powder for oral suspension 45 g (40 mg/mL after reconstitution))

Voriconazole is a triazole antifungal. It causes inhibition of fungal cytochrome P450-mediated 14-alpha-lanosterol demethylation, an essential step in fungal ergosterol biosynthesis. It is indicated in the treatment of invasive aspergillosis; treatment of *Scedosporium apiospermum* and *Fusarium* spp., including *Fusarium solani*, in patients intolerant of or refractory to other therapy; treatment of esophageal candidiasis.

Voriconazole (Vfend; UK-109,495) is a triazole with a structure similar to fluconazole but has increased activity *in vitro*, an expanded spectrum, and poor aqueous solubility (pregnancy risk category C).

Oral bioavailability is 96% and protein binding 56%. Gastric acid is not necessary for absorption. Volume of distribution is high (4.6 L/kg), with extensive drug distribution in tissues. Metabolism occurs through the hepatic CYPs, particularly CYP2C19 and to a lesser extent CYP2C9. CYP3A4 plays a limited role. Less than 2% of native drug is recovered from urine, though 80% of the inactive metabolites are secreted in the urine. The oral dose does not have to be adjusted for azotemia or hemodialysis. Peak-plasma concentrations after oral doses of 200 mg orally twice daily are about 3 μg/mL. CSF concentrations of 1 to 3 μg/mL have been reported in a patient with fungal meningitis.

The plasma elimination half-life is 6 hours. **Voriconazole** exhibits nonlinear metabolism so that higher doses cause greater-than-linear increases in drug exposure. Genetic polymorphisms in CYP2C19 can cause up to fourfold differences in drug exposure; 15 to 20% of Asians are homozygous poor metabolizers, compared to 2% of Caucasians and African-Americans. Patients older than 65 years had 86% higher plasma AUC than patients aged 18 to 45. Patients with mild or moderate hepatic insufficiency had an average AUC that was 223% of age- and weight-matched controls. Patients with cirrhosis should receive the same loading dose of voriconazole but half the maintenance dose. There are no data to guide dosing in patients with severe hepatic insufficiency.

The intravenous formulation of voriconazole contains sulfobutyl ether β-cyclodextrin (SBECD). When voriconazole is given intravenously, SBECD is excreted completely by the kidney. Significant accumulation of SBECD occurs with a creatinine clearance below 50 mL/minute. Because toxicity of SBECD at high plasma concentrations is unclear, oral voriconazole is preferred in azotemic patients.

Voriconazole is metabolized by, and inhibits, CYP2C19, CYP2C9, and CYP3A4. The affinity of voriconazole is highest for CYP2C19, followed in rank order by CYP2C9 and CYP3A4. The major metabolite of voriconazole, the voriconazole *N*-oxide, also inhibits the metabolic activity of CYP2C9, CYP3A4, and to a lesser extent, CYP2C19. Inhibitors or inducers of these three enzymes may increase or decrease voriconazole plasma concentrations, respectively. In addition, there is potential for voriconazole and its major metabolite to increase the plasma concentrations of other drugs metabolized by these enzymes.

Coadministration with rifampin, rifabutin, or ritonavir is contraindicated because of accelerated **voriconazole** metabolism. **Efavirenz,** and perhaps other nonnucleoside reverse transcriptase inhibitors (NNRTIs), significantly increase voriconazole metabolism and slow the metabolism of the NNRTI. When given with phenytoin, the voriconazole dose should be doubled. Drugs that significantly accumulate in patients receiving voriconazole include cyclosporine, tacrolimus phenytoin, rifabutin, warfarin, and sirolimus. Because the sirolimus AUC increases 11-fold when voriconazole is given, coadministration is contraindicated. An omeprazole dose should be reduced by half if 40 mg or more per day is given. Until more experience with voriconazole is gained, it is prudent to be observant for the drug interactions known to occur with other azoles.

In an open, randomized trial, **voriconazole** provided superior efficiency to C-AMB in the primary therapy of invasive aspergillosis. In a secondary analysis, survival also was superior in the voriconazole arm. Voriconazole was compared to Ambisome in an open randomized trial in the empirical therapy of neutropenic patients whose fever did not respond to more than 96 hours of antibacterial therapy. Because the 95% confidence interval in this noninferiority trial permitted the possibility that voriconazole might be more than 10% worse than Ambisome, the FDA did not approve voriconazole for this use. However, in a secondary analysis, there were fewer breakthrough infections with voriconazole (1.9%) than with Ambisome (5%). Voriconazole is approved for use in esophageal candidiasis on the basis of a double-blind, randomized comparison with fluconazole. Voriconazole is also approved for use as salvage therapy in patients with *Pseudallescheria boydii* (*Scedosporium apiospermum*) and *Fusarium* infections.

Voriconazole is teratogenic in animals and contraindicated in pregnancy. Although voriconazole is generally well tolerated, occasional cases of hepatotoxicity have been reported and liver function should be monitored. Voriconazole, similar to some other azoles, causes a prolongation of the QTc interval, which can become significant in patients with other risk factors for torsade de pointes. Patients must be warned about possible visual effects. Approximately 30% of patients note transient visual changes beginning about half an hour after administration and lasting for another half hour. Blurred vision, altered color perception, and photophobia have been reported. Activities that require keen vision should be avoided when vision is altered. No sequelae occur. Uncommonly, confusion or transient visual hallucinations occur. Patients receiving their first intravenous infusion have had anaphylactoid reactions, with faintness, nausea, flushing, feverishness, and rash. In such patients, the infusion should be stopped. Rash has been reported in 5.8% of patients.

W

WARFARIN SODIUM

(Coumadin Panwarfin, Sofarin)

Warfarin (initially 10 to 15 mg p.o. for three days) is indicated as an anticoagulant in pulmonary emboli, deep-vein thrombosis (DVT), myocardial infarction (MI), rheumatic heart disease with heart valve damage, and atrial arrhythmias.

In the presence of cardiac arrhythmias, when the heart is beating rapidly but inefficiently, the formation of clots in atrial appendages is common. When converting to a normal sinus rhythm, the clots may be freed and become lodged in vital organs. To avoid this, patients with arrhythmias may be treated with anticoagulants before and after conversion of the arrhythmia to a sinus rhythm.

The oral anticoagulants are antagonists of vitamin K. Coagulation factors II, VII, IX, and X and the anticoagulant proteins C and S are synthesized mainly in the liver and are biologically inactive unless 9 to 12 of the amino-terminal glutamic acid residues are carboxylated. The gamma-carboxyglutamate residues confer Ca^{2+}-binding properties on these proteins that are essential for their assembly into an efficient catalytic complex. This reaction requires carbon dioxide, molecular oxygen, reduced vitamin K, and a precursor form of the target protein containing a propeptide recognition site. It is catalyzed in the rough endoplasmic reticulum by a 758-residue protein that has been purified, cloned, and characterized. Carboxylation is directly coupled to the oxidation of vitamin K to the epoxide.

Reduced vitamin K must be regenerated from the epoxide for sustained carboxylation and synthesis of biologically competent proteins. Warfarin is rapidly and completely absorbed from the gastrointestinal (GI) tract. It is highly bound to plasma protein, especially albumin; the drug crosses the placenta but does not appear to accumulate in breast milk. Warfarin is hydroxylated by the liver into inactive metabolites. Metabolites are reabsorbed from bile and excreted in urine. Duration of action is 2 to 5 days—more closely reflecting the drug's half-life.

The use of anticoagulants is contraindicated in the presence of active hemorrhage, potential hemorrhage (acid-pepsin disease), and hemorrhagic disorders (hemophilia).

Anticoagulants should be used with extreme caution in patients with traumatic injuries to the central nervous system or the eyes because it is very difficult to control hemorrhage in these areas.

Anticoagulant therapy during pregnancy is indicated for the treatment and prophylaxis of venous thromboembolic disease and systemic embolism associated with valvular heart disease or prosthetic heart valves. However, there are special problems that need to be considered when deciding on optimal anticoagulant therapy in pregnant women. Heparin does not cross the placenta and is probably safe for the fetus. However, long-term heparin therapy is occasionally associated with maternal hemorrhage and rarely with symptomatic osteoporosis. Coumarin derivatives cross the placenta and are potentially teratogenic, particularly in the first trimester. Neonatal hemorrhage is a risk if warfarin is administered to the pregnant mother near term.

The possible existence of an aneurysm must be considered in an untreated hypertensive patient.

Anticoagulant therapy should be monitored carefully in patients with severe hepatic or renal failure, vitamin K deficiency, or alcoholism, and those with arthritis who are taking acetylsalicylic acid in large quantities. Furthermore, anticoagulants are extensively metabolized and their metabolites excreted, which can have an important bearing in patients suffering from renal disorders.

The incidence of interactions between the oral anticoagulants and other drugs, especially barbiturates, salicylates, and phenylbutazone, are numerous and at times may be life threatening. All aspects of the pharmacokinetics may be involved.

Various drugs can augment the properties of oral anticoagulants in a variety of ways:

- By displacing extensively bound anticoagulants from the plasma albumin (e.g., chloral hydrate, clofibrate, and phenylbutazone)
- By inhibiting hepatic microsomal enzymes (e.g., chloramphenicol and clofibrate)
- By reducing the availability of vitamin K (e.g., anabolic steroids and broad-spectrum antibiotics)
- By inhibiting clotting factor synthesis (e.g., anabolic steroids and salicylates)

There are also a number of agents that can diminish the response to oral anticoagulants, and they accomplish this by the following means:

- By inhibiting absorption of anticoagulants (e.g., griseofulvin and clofibrate)
- By inducing hepatic microsomal enzymes (e.g., barbiturates, ethchlorvynol, and glutethimide)
- By stimulating clotting factor synthesis (e.g., vitamin K)

These interactions have not been reported to occur with regard to heparin, however.

WILSON'S DISEASE: Treatment of

Wilson's disease is an autosomal recessive disorder of copper metabolism that produces neurological and hepatic dysfunction. The gene defect has been localized to the long arm of chromosome 13. Although the precise nature of the biochemical abnormality in Wilson's disease is unknown, its pathogenesis appears to involve decreased binding of copper to the transport protein ceruloplasmin. As a result, large amounts of unbound copper enter the circulation and are subsequently deposited in tissues, including the brain, liver, kidney, and cornea. There are four drugs used in the treatment of Wilson's disease. These are zinc, which blocks intestinal absorption of copper, penicillamine and trientine, both of which are chelators that increase urinary excretion of copper, and tetrathiomolybdate, which forms a tripartite complex with copper and protein and can block copper absorption from the intestine or render blood copper nontoxic.

WOUND INFECTION AND SEPSIS IN SURGICAL PATIENTS: Treatment of

Nature of Operation	Pathogens	Recommended Drugs
	Clean	
	Cardiac	
Prosthetic valve, coronary artery bypass, other open-heart surgery, pacemaker implant	*Staphylococcus epidermidis*, *S. aureus*, *Corynebacterium*, enteric Gram-negative bacilli	Cefazolin or cefuroxime or vancomycin
Noncardiac thoracic	*S. aureus*, *S. epidermidis*, streptococci, enteric Gram-negative bacilli	Cefazolin or cefuroxime or vancomycin
	Vascular	
Arterial surgery involving the abdominal aorta, a prosthesis, or a groin incision	*S. aureus*, *S. epidermidis*, enteric Gram-negative bacilli	Cefazolin or vancomycin
Lower-extremity amputation for ischemia	*S. aureus*, *S. epidermidis*, enteric Gram-negative bacilli, clostridia	Cefazolin or vancomycin
	Neurosurgery	
Craniotomy	*S. aureus*, *S. epidermidis*	Cefazolin or vancomycin
	Orthopedic	
Total joint replacement, internal fixation of fractures	*S. aureus*, *S. epidermidis*	Cefazolin or vancomycin
	Ophthalmic	
	S. aureus, *S. epidermidis*, streptococci, enteric Gram-negative bacilli, *Pseudomonas*	Gentamicin or tobramycin or neomycin-gramicidin/polymyxin B, cefazolin
	Clean–Contaminated	
	Head and neck	
Entering oral cavity or pharynx	*S. aureus*, streptococci, oral anaerobes	Cefazolin or clindamycin ± gentamicin
	Abdominal	
Gastroduodenal	Enteric Gram-negative bacilli, Gram-positive cocci	High risk only: cefazolin
Biliary tract	Enteric Gram-negative bacilli, enterococci, clostridia	High risk only: cefazolin
Colorectal	Enteric Gram-negative bacilli, anaerobes	Oral: neomycin + erythromycin base Parenteral: cefoxitin or cefotetan
Appendectomy	Enteric Gram-negative bacilli, anaerobes	Cefoxitin or cefotetan
	Gynecologic and Obstetric	
Vaginal or abdominal hysterectomy	Enteric Gram-negative, anaerobes, Gram-positive *B strep*, enterococci	Cefazolin or cefotetan or cefoxitin
Cesarean section	Same as for hysterectomy	High risk only: cefazolin

WOUND INFECTION AND SEPSIS IN SURGICAL PATIENTS: Treatment of (Continued)

Nature of Operation	Pathogens	Recommended Drugs
Abortion	Same as for hysterectomy	First trimester, high risk only: aqueous penicillin G or doxycycline Second trimester: cefazolin
	Dirty Surgery	
Ruptured viscus	Enteric Gram-negative bacilli, anaerobes, enterococci	Cefoxitin or cefotetan ± gentamicin or clindamycin + gentamicin
Traumatic wound	*S. aureus*, *Gram-positive A strep*, clostridia	Cefazolin

X

XAMOTEROL

(Carwin)

Xamoterol (200 mg t.i.d.) has been shown to improve left ventricular systolic and diastolic function in most patients with mild to moderate heart failure. Xamoterol (±)-*N*-[2-[[2-hydroxy-3-(*p*-hydro-xyphenoxy)proprylamino] ethyl]-4-morpholine carboxamide is a beta$_1$-adrenoreceptor partial agonist with a pK_a of 8.2.

In the normal heart during exertion, xamoterol increases the force of myocardial contraction and the rate of myocardial relaxation and lowers left-ventricular filling pressure, whereas the drug has little effect on the heart rate at rest. At high levels of sympathetic stimulation (e.g., with strenuous exercise) xamoterol reduces heart rate. Improved myocardial performance is maintained during submaximal exercise. There is no evidence of downregulation of the beta$_1$-adrenoreceptors during prolonged administration of the drug.

Approximately 9% of an oral dose of xamoterol is absorbed from the gastrointestinal tract. The low absorption rate of the drug results from its hydrophilic nature, which limits penetration of the gastrointestinal wall to the bloodstream, but not absorption from extensive hepatic phase I metabolism. The only metabolism appears to be sulfate conjugation of the 4-hydro group, occurring primarily in the gut wall after oral administration and in the liver after intravenous administration. Xamoterol is cleared from the blood by renal excretion, and some tubular excretion may be involved. After oral administration, 56% of the conjugate, which is pharmacologically inactive, is excreted in urine. There is no evidence of enterohepatic circulation.

XANTHINE OXIDASE INHIBITORS

Gout is a hyperuricemic state (>6 mg/dL) that is effectively diagnosed through the detection of monosodium urate crystals in the synovial fluid of the involved joint. Conditions causing hyperuricemia include the excessive synthesis of uric acid, the excessive synthesis of purine precursor to uric acid, a high dietary intake of purine (shellfish, organ meat, anchovies, and wild game), diminished renal excretion of uric acid, and tissue destruction following injury or therapeutic irradiation.

Numerous agents, when used in therapeutic doses, can also cause hyperuricemia. This includes an analgesic dose of aspirin, thiazide diuretics, nicotinic acid, chronic consumption of alcohol, and antineoplastic agents.

If left untreated, the hyperuricemic state may precipitate an acute attack of gout, which first appears in metatarsal phalangeal joints. Ultimately, tophaceous deposits form in the joints and soft tissues such as the kidneys. The hyperuricemic state may be corrected either by inhibiting the synthesis of uric acid by allopurinol or by enhancing the elimination of uric acid by uricosuric agents.

Allopurinol (Zyloprim) reduces the synthesis of uric acid by inhibiting the activity of xanthine oxidase, according to the scheme shown in Figure 18.

The reduction in the uric acid pool occurs slowly. Because xanthine and hypoxanthine are more soluble than uric acid, they are easily excreted.

Allopurinol not only is used in treating the hyperuricemia associated with gout, but also in the secondary hyperuricemia associated with the use of antineoplastic agents. However, allopurinol may interfere with the metabolism of antineoplastic agents such as azathioprine and 6-mercaptopurine.

XANTHINES

(Caffeine, theobromine, and theophylline)

In a number of plants used in different parts of the world to make beverages and condiments, there are found the xanthine compounds, caffeine, theobromine, and theophylline (Theocin), which are also employed in therapeutics, and have, therefore, acquired a double importance as drugs and as articles of diet.

Caffeine, theobromine, and theophylline are purine derivatives closely related to the xanthine bodies found in the urine and tissues of animals. Xanthine is 2:6 dioxypurine; caffeine is 1:3:7 trimethylxanthine; theobromine is 3:7 dimethylxanthine; and theophylline is 1:3 dimethylxanthine.

These all resemble each other in most points of their pharmacological action, but they differ markedly in the relative intensity of their action on various functions. Thus, caffeine is the most potent central nervous system (CNS) stimulant of the group; theobromine exerts the greatest action on the muscles; and theophylline is the most effective diuretic and coronary dilator. Theobromine has comparatively little effect on the CNS, whereas theophylline has no action on the muscles.

Coffee is not used in medicine but is of great dietetic importance. The coffee bean contains about 1 to 2% caffeine, and a cup of coffee is equivalent to 0.1 to 0.2 g of caffeine along with some volatile substances, such as furfuralcohol, produced by the roasting; these have been called Coffeon and resemble the volatile oils in their action.

Tea leaves contain more caffeine than the coffee bean, but because a relatively smaller quantity of leaves is used in preparing tea, this beverage contains slightly less caffeine than does coffee. In green tea there is a considerable quantity of a volatile oil that also passes into the infusion, and the flavor of black tea also arises from volatile substances (theon). Both black and green tea contain about 7% tannic acid, but this is extracted only slowly. The bitter taste in tea that has been prepared too long is due to the tannic acid.

The wakefulness and the relief from fatigue produced by tea and coffee are undoubtedly due to the caffeine contained in them. On the other hand, the feeling of well-being and comfort produced by coffee after a full meal is similar to the carminative effects of the volatile oils and appears to be due to the local action in the stomach of the volatile constituents of coffee. There is a widespread belief that excessive tea drinking disturbs gastric digestion, and this has generally been attributed to the tannic acid contained in it. It is not unlikely that the caffeine and theophylline may also play a part in this gastric action by causing irritation of the mucous membrane. Excessive consumption of tea or coffee may produce, in addition to digestive disturbances, increased nervousness, excitability, tremor, palpitation, and insomnia—effects directly due to the caffeine content of these beverages.

Chocolate contains theobromine (0.5 to 1%) instead of caffeine, and a large amount of fat (cacao-butter, 15 to 50%), starch, and albumins as well. The theobromine does not possess the stimulant action of caffeine on the nervous system, and chocolate may therefore be taken without producing wakefulness. The starch and fat are assimilated by the tissues, so that chocolate is a true food.

XYLOMETAZOLINE HYDROCHLORIDE

(Chlorohist-LA-neo-spray long acting, Neo-Synephrine II, Otrivin)

Xylometazoline (spray 1% solution to nasal mucosa every 8 to 10 hours) is used as a nasal decongestant. Xylometazoline acts on alpha-adrenergic receptors in nasal mucosa to produce constriction, thereby decreasing blood flow and nasal congestion.

Xylometazoline is contraindicated in patients with narrow-angle glaucoma, because the drug may increase intraocular pressure, and in patients receiving tricyclic antidepressants, because of the potential for adverse cardiovascular effects.

Xylometazoline should be used with caution in patients with hyperthyroidism, cardiac disease, hypertension, diabetes mellitus, or advanced arteriosclerosis.

Y

YELLOW FEVER VACCINE

(YF-Vax)

This viral vaccine is used for primary vaccination.

YOHIMBINE HYDROCHLORIDE

(Yohimex)

Yohimbine, an alpha$_2$-adrenergic-receptor-blocking agent has no medical indications. Urologists have used yohimbine in determining the nature of male erectile impotence; and internists have used it successfully (18 mg/day) to treat impotence associated with vascular or diabetic origins.

Yohimbine, an indolalkylamine alkaloid, is chemically similar to reserpine. It is the principal alkaloid of the bark of the West African *Corynanthe yohimbe* tree and is also found in *Rauwolfia serpentina*. It is believed to have properties similar to rauwolfia alkaloids.

Yohimbine is primarily an alpha$_2$-adrenergic blocker. It blocks presynaptic alpha$_2$-adrenoreceptors causing release of norepinephrine, and hence has been used in the treatment of postural hypotension.

Symptoms of dizziness and syncope due to postural hypotension may result from dehydration, blood loss, and myocardial disease. However, the most important cause of chronic recurrent symptomatic postural hypotension is failure of the autonomic nervous system. The drug treatment for postural hypotension is difficult because the response varies and tolerance to drugs develops. Patients with autonomic abnormalities may suffer symptoms after eating, and this further hampers treatment.

Z

ZACOPRIDE

In addition to agents that stimulate or irritate the stomach, many other factors may be responsible for inducing emesis centrally. The central control of vomiting is vested in two areas:

- The vomiting center, which is located in the lateral reticular formation in the midst of a group of cells governing such activities as salivation and respiration.
- The chemoreceptor trigger zone, which is a narrow strip along the floor of the fourth ventricle located close to the vomiting center (see also Figure 73).

The functions of these two areas are distinct but interdependent.

The vomiting center is activated by impulses that originate from the gastrointestinal (GI) tract and other peripheral structures. In addition, there are unidentified tracts that extend from the cerebral cortex to the vomiting center, such that emotional trauma and unpleasant olfactory and visual stimuli may cause nausea and vomiting.

Stimulation of the vestibular apparatus, which responds to movements of the head, neck, and eye muscles, may also cause nausea and vomiting by stimulating the vomiting center. On the other hand, circulating chemicals, toxins, virus, and ions may provoke nausea and vomiting by first stimulating the chemoreceptor zone for emesis, which in turn stimulates the vomiting center.

The nausea and vomiting associated with circulating physical agents (radiation therapy and virus particles) and chemical agents (toxins and cancer chemotherapeutic agents) are treated with phenothiazine derivatives such as chlorpromazine, perphenazine, prochlorperazine, promethazine, triethylperazine, and triflupromazine. These agents block the dopamine receptors in the area postrema.

A new class of antiemetic agents, the serotonin antagonists, has been identified. These agents could be clinically useful in a wide range of areas. Selective antagonists of the serotonin (5-hydroxytryptamine) type 3 (5-HT_3) receptor, such as batanopride, granisetron, ondansetron, or zacopride, have proved in early clinical trials to be potent antiemetic agents in patients undergoing cytotoxic chemotherapy. Their efficacy has been shown to be comparable or superior to that of conventional phenothiazine antiemetics. The toxic effects observed so far with these agents have been modest (see also Figure 73).

ZAFIRLUKAST

(Accolate tablets 10 mg, tablets 20 mg)

Zafirlukast is a leukotriene receptor antagonist that inhibits three leukotriene receptor types. Leukotrienes have been associated with the longer, inflammatory component of asthma. It is indicated as a prophylaxis and chronic treatment of asthma in adults and children 5 years of age and older. **Zafirlukast** (Accolate) and **montelukast** (Singulair) are leukotriene-receptor antagonists. Zileuton (Zyflo) is an inhibitor of 5-lipoxygenase, which catalyzes the formation of leukotrienes from arachidonic acid.

The leukotriene-modifying drugs are administered orally. **Zafirlukast** is absorbed rapidly, with greater than 90% bioavailability. At therapeutic plasma concentrations, it is over 99% protein-bound. **Zafirlukast** is metabolized extensively by hepatic CYP2C9. The parent drug is responsible for its therapeutic activity, with metabolites being less than 10% as effective. The half-life of zafirlukast is approximately 10 hours.

Montelukast is absorbed rapidly, with about 60 to 70% bioavailability. At therapeutic concentrations, it is highly protein-bound (99%). It is metabolized extensively by CYP3A4 and CYP2C9. The half-life of montelukast is between 3 and 6 hours.

Zileuton is absorbed rapidly on oral administration and is metabolized extensively by CYPs and by UDP-glucuronosyltransferases. The parent molecule is responsible for its therapeutic action. Zileuton is a short-acting drug with a half-life of approximately 2.5 hours and also is highly protein-bound (93%).

Leukotriene-modifying drugs act either as competitive antagonists of leukotriene receptors or by inhibiting the synthesis of leukotrienes.

Leukotriene-receptor antagonists: Cysteinyl leukotrienes (cys-LTs) include leukotriene C4 (LTC4), leukotriene D4 (LTD4), and leukotriene E4 (LTE4). All the cys-LTs are potent constrictors of bronchial smooth muscle. On a molar basis, LTD4 is approximately 1000 times more potent than is histamine as a bronchoconstrictor. The receptor responsible for the bronchoconstricter effect of leukotrienes is the cys-LTl receptor. Although each of the cys-LTs is an agonist at the cys-LTl receptor, LTE4 is less potent than either LTC4 or LTD4. Zafirlukast and montelukast are selective high-affinity competitive antagonists for the cys-LTl receptor. Pranlukast is another cys-LTl-receptor antagonist used in some countries in the treatment of asthma, but it is not approved for use in the United States. Inhibition of cys-LT-induced bronchial smooth-muscle contraction likely is involved in the therapeutic effects of these agents in relieving the symptoms of asthma.

Leukotriene-synthesis inhibitors: The formation of leukotrienes depends on lipoxygenation of arachidonic acid by 5-lipoxygenase. Zileuton is a potent and selective inhibitor of 5-lipoxygenase activity and thus inhibits the formation of all 5-lipoxygenase products. Thus, in addition to inhibiting the formation of the cys-LTs, zileuton also inhibits the formation of leukotriene B4 (LTB4), a potent chemotactic autacoid, and other eicosanoids that depend on leukotriene A4 (LTA4) synthesis. In theory the therapeutic effects of a 5-lipoxygenase inhibition would include all those observed with the cys-LTl-receptor antagonists, as well as other effects that may result from inhibiting the formation of LTB4 and other 5-lipoxygenase products.

There are few adverse effects directly associated with inhibition of leukotriene synthesis or function. This likely is due to the fact that leukotriene production is limited predominantly to sites of inflammation.

Although leukotriene inhibitors are effective prophylactic treatment for mild asthma, their role in asthma therapy is not clearly defined. Most clinical trials with these drugs have studied patients with mild asthma who were not taking glucocorticoids. In general the studies show a modest but significant improvement in pulmonary function and a decrease in symptoms and asthma exacerbations. In a meta-analysis of clinical trials with **zafirlukast**, all studies showed some decrease in the rate of asthma exacerbations, with an average reduction of 50%. When zafirlukast was compared with low-dose inhaled glucocorticoid therapy, the improvement in lung function and decreased dependence on short-acting β_2-adrenergic-receptor-agonist therapy was found to be greater in the glucocorticoid-treated subjects. There was little difference, however, between the steroid- and montelukast-treated subjects in the reduction in rate of asthma exacerbations. Clinical trials with antileukotriene drugs have revealed considerable heterogeneity in response to therapy, with patients falling into "responder" and "non-responder" groups. For those who respond to antileukotriene therapy, the National Heart, Lung, and Blood Institute recognizes these drugs as alternatives to low-dose inhaled steroids for control of mild chronic asthma.

ZALCITABINE

(Dideoxycytidine, ddC, Hivid tablets 0.375 mg, tablets 0.75 mg)

Zalcitabine is a nucleoside reverse transcriptase inhibitor that inhibits replication of DNA in HIV. It is indicated in combination therapy for the treatment of selected patients with advanced HIV infection.

Zalcitabine (2′,3′ dideoxycytidine; ddC) is a synthetic cytosine analog reverse-transcriptase inhibitor. It is active against HIV-1, HIV-2, and hepatitis B virus (HBV). The *in vitro* IC_{50} of zalcitabine against HIV-1 ranges from 2 nM in monocytes–macrophage cell lines to 0.5 μM in human peripheral blood mononuclear cells. Zalcitabine has considerably more antiretroviral activity in monocytes–macrophage cell lines than other nucleoside analogs, but the potential clinical utility of this observation is uncertain.

Zalcitabine enters cells by both carrier-mediated transport and passive diffusion. It is converted to the monophosphate by deoxycytidine kinase and undergoes further phosphorylation by deoxycytidine monophosphate kinase and nucleoside diphosphate kinase to yield dideoxycytidine 5′-triphosphate, which is the active anabolite. Zalcitabine is more efficiently phosphorylated in resting cells and therefore is more potent in resting cells than other nucleoside analogs, although the clinical relevance of this is unknown. As with other dideoxynucleoside analogs, dideoxycytidine 5′-triphosphate terminates the elongation of proviral DNA because it is incorporated by reverse transcriptase into nascent HIV DNA but lacks a 3′-hydroxyl group. Zalcitabine inhibits human DNA polymerases-β and γ and also decreases intracellular deoxycytidine triphosphate pools, factors that may contribute to its cellular and host toxicity.

High-level resistance has not been reported in patients receiving **zalcitabine** as a sole nucleoside analog or in combination with zidovudine. However, low to moderate *in vitro* resistance is seen with four mutations associated with zalcitabine use that occur at reverse transcriptase codons 65, 69, 74, and 184. The K65R substitution is associated with cross-resistance to didanosine, abacavir, and tenofovir, as well as the cytosine analogs lamivudine and emtricitabine. The M184V substitution is also associated with the use of lamivudine or emtricitabine and enhances HIV-1 sensitivity to zidovudine *in vitro*; the presence of this mutation is associated with improved long-term suppression of viremia when zidovudine is combined with lamivudine or emtricitabine, although a similar effect has not been demonstrated for the combination of zalcitabine and zidovudine. The T69D substitution is unique to zalcitabine but overlaps a recently described mutation at codon 69 (typically T69S) followed by a 2-amino-acid insertion that produces cross-resistance to all current nucleoside and nucleotide analogs.

The oral bioavailability of zalcitabine is greater than 80%, and 60 to 80% of the parent compound is recovered unchanged in the urine. Food has a negligible effect on oral bioavailability. Clearance is greatly diminished in patients with compromised renal function, and daily doses should be reduced in this population. The half-life of intracellular dideoxycytidine 5′-triphosphate is estimated to be 2 to 3 hours. It is therefore recommended that zalcitabine be administered every 8 hours in patients with normal renal function. The CSF-plasma concentration ratio ranges from 0.09 to 0.37, although the clinical significance of CSF penetration is not known.

Zalcitabine toxicities are similar to those of the other dideoxynucleoside analogs didanosine and stavudine. Severe peripheral neuropathy has been reported in up to 15% of patients. Peripheral neuropathy is dose related and more common with preexisting HIV-associated neuropathy and advanced HIV disease. This is a symmetrical distal sensory neuropathy that begins in the feet but may progress to a stocking/glove distribution. Other specific risk factors for neuropathy include alcohol consumption, diabetes, and low vitamin B_{12} concentrations. If the drug is stopped as soon as symptoms appear, the neuropathy usually stabilizes and should improve or resolve. Pancreatitis occurs rarely with zalcitabine therapy and appears to be less frequent than with didanosine.

One toxicity unique to zalcitabine is oral ulceration and stomatitis, suggesting that this drug may have toxicity in rapidly dividing mucosal cells. Ulcerations of the buccal mucosa, soft palate, tongue, or pharynx occur in up to 4% of patients but may resolve with continued therapy. An erythematous maculopapular rash is reported commonly during the first 14 days of therapy but generally is self-limited and mild. Other reported toxicities include cardiomyopathy, arthralgias, myalgias, and elevated hepatic transaminases.

Lamivudine inhibits the intracellular phosphorylation of zalcitabine and antagonizes zalcitabine's antiretroviral activity *in vitro*, although the clinical significance of this interaction is unknown. Probenecid increases the zalcitabine AUC by about 50%, probably through inhibition of tubular secretion; cimetidine increases the AUC by 36% via an unknown mechanism. Zalcitabine should be avoided in patients with a history of pancreatitis or neuropathy because the risk and severity of both complications increase. Coadministration of other drugs that cause pancreatitis or neuropathy also will increase the risk and severity of these symptoms. Ethambutol, isoniazid, vincristine, cisplatin, and pentamidine, as well as the antiretroviral drugs didanosine and stavudine, therefore, should be avoided.

Zalcitabine has long-term efficacy in three-drug combination regimens. For example, the combination of zalcitabine, zidovudine, and saquinavir was superior to two-drug regimens in a prospective, randomized clinical trial. Zalcitabine is used infrequently in the United States because it is the only nucleoside analog that still must be administered every 8 hours, carries significant toxicity risks, and has inferior antiviral activity compared with more convenient agents.

Zalcitabine, a potent nucleoside analog inhibitor of reverse transcriptase with antiviral properties, is used in patients with advanced human immunodeficiency virus (HIV) infection (CD4 count below 300 cells/mm^3) who have demonstrated significant clinical or immunologic deterioration. It is approximately tenfold more potent than zidovudine (AZT) and causes reversible peripheral nephropathy (see Figure 107).

ZALEPLON

(Sonata capsules 5 mg, capsules 10 mg)

Zaleplon is a sedative and hypnotic that interacts with the gamma-aminobutyric acid-receptor complex. It is indicated in the short-term treatment of insomnia.

ZANAMIVIR

(Relenza Blisters of powder for oral inhalation 5 mg)

Zanamivir is an antiviral agent that inhibits influenza virus neuraminidase, with the possibility of alteration of virus particle aggregation and release. It is indicated in uncomplicated acute illness caused by influenza A and B virus in adults and pediatric patients of at least 7 years of age who have been symptomatic for no longer than 2 days.

Hypnotics in this class include **zolpicone** (not available in the United States), **zolpidem** (Ambien), **zaleplon** (Sonata), and **indiplon**. Although the chemical structures of these compounds do not resemble those of benzodiazepines, it is assumed that their therapeutic efficacies are due to agonist effects on the benzodiazepine site of the $GABA_A$ receptor.

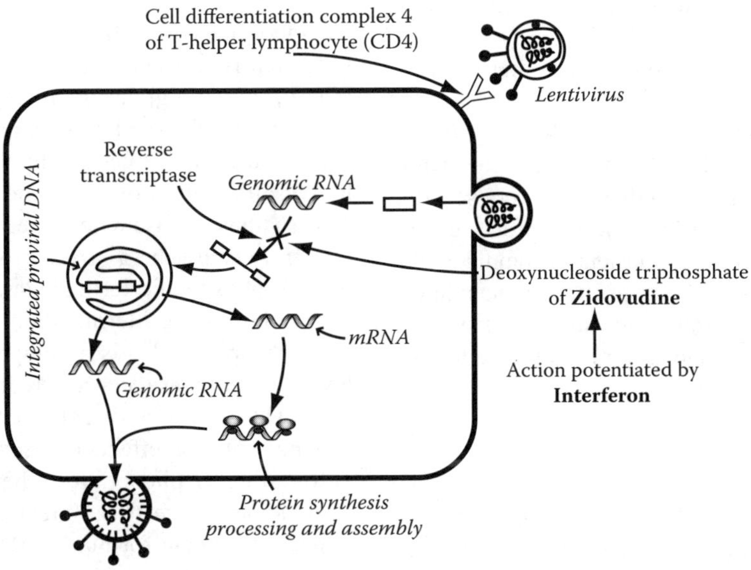

FIGURE 107 Patients with a clinical diagnosis of AIDS should undergo long-term therapy with zidovudine (AZT, 1200 mg q. 4 hrs). **Acyclovir** may potentiate the beneficial effects of AZT. In addition, patients should be treated prophylactically for *Pneumocystis carinii* pneumonia; such regimens include **sulfadoxine** and **pyrimethamine** (Fansidar), **dapsone**, or aerosolized **pentamidine**. **Dextran sulfate** is also useful because it blocks the binding of HIV to target cells.

Zaleplon and **zolpidem** are effective in relieving sleep-onset insomnia. Both drugs have been approved by the FDA for use for up to 7 to 10 days at a time. Zaleplon and zolpidem have sustained hypnotic efficacy without occurrence of rebound insomnia on abrupt discontinuation. Both have similar degrees of efficacy. Zolpidem has a half-life of about 2 hours, which is sufficient to cover most of a typical 8-hour sleep period, and is presently approved for bedtime use only. **Zaleplon** has a shorter half-life, about 1 hour, which offers the possibility for safe dosing later in the night, within 4 hours of the anticipated rising time. As a result, it is approved for use immediately at bedtime or when the patient has difficulty falling asleep after bedtime. Because of its short half-life, zaleplon has not been shown to be different from placebo in measures of duration of sleep and number of awakenings. Zaleplon and zolpidem may differ in residual side effects; late-night administration of zolpidem has been associated with morning sedation, delayed reaction time, and anterograde amnesia, whereas zaleplon has no more side effects than placebo.

Zaleplon (Sonata) is a nonbenzodiazepine and is a member of the pyrazolopyrimidine class of compounds.

Zaleplon preferentially binds to the benzodiazepine-binding site on gamma-aminobutyric acid ($GABA_A$) receptors containing the α_1-receptor submit. It is absorbed rapidly and reaches peak-plasma concentrations in about an hour. Its half-life is approximately 1 hour. Its bioavailability is approximately 30% because of presystemic metabolism. **Zaleplon** has a volume of distribution of approximately 1.4 L/kg and plasma-protein binding of approximately 60%. It is metabolized largely by aldehyde oxidase and to a lesser extent by CYP3A4. Its oxidative metabolites are converted to glucuronides and eliminated unchanged in urine. Less than 1% of zaleplon is excreted unchanged in urine. None of zaleplon's metabolites is pharmacologically active.

Zaleplon (usually administered in 5-, 10-, or 20-mg doses) has been studied in clinical trials of patients with chronic or transient insomnia. Studies have focused on its effects in decreasing sleep latency. Zaleplon-treated subjects with either chronic or transient insomnia have experienced shorter periods of sleep latency than have placebo-treated subjects. Tolerance to zaleplon does not appear to occur, nor do rebound insomnia or withdrawal symptoms after stopping treatment.

ZICONOTIDE

(Prialt solution 25 mcg/mL, solution 100 mcg/mL)

Ziconotide is an analgesic. Animal data indicate that ziconotide blocks N-type calcium channels by binding to them, which leads to blockade of excitatory neurotransmitter release in primary afferent nerve terminals and antinociception. It is indicated in the management of severe chronic pain in patients for whom intrathecal therapy is warranted, and who are intolerant of or refractory to other treatment.

ZIDOVUDINE (COMPOUND S)

(Retrovir tablets 300 mg, capsules 100 mg, syrup 50 mg/5 mL, injection 10 mg/mL)

Zidovudine is a nucleoside reverse transcriptase inhibitor that inhibits replication of retroviruses, including HIV. It is indicated in combination with other antiretroviral agents for the treatment of HIV infections; and prevention of maternal–fetal HIV transmission.

ZIDOVUDINE

(Zaidothymidine, AZT, Retrovir)

Zidovudine (200 mg every 4 hours) is indicated in the management of patients with HIV infection who show evidence of impaired immunity. Trimethoprim-sulfamethoxazole, pyrimethamine, and acyclovir may be necessary for the management or prevention of opportunistic infections. Zidovudine (3′-azido-3′-deoxythymidine, commonly referred to as AZT) is a thymidine analog with antiviral activity against HIV-1, HIV-2, human T-lymphotropic (or leukemia) virus (HTLV)-I, and other retroviruses. Low concentrations (<0.001 to 0.04 μg/ml) inhibit acute HIV-1 infection in human T-cell lines and peripheral blood lymphocytes. Zidovudine is less active in human monocyte–macrophages or quiescent cells but inhibits HIV replication in human brain macrophages. Zidovudine is also inhibitory for HBV and EBV.

Low concentrations of zidovudine inhibit human myeloid and erythroid progenitor cell growth (0.3 to 0.6 μg/ml) and blastogenesis in peripheral blood mononuclear cells.

Following diffusion into host cells, the drug is initially phosphorylated by cellular thymidine kinase. The rate-limiting step is conversion to the diphosphate by thymidylate kinase, so that high levels of the monophosphate but much lower levels of di- and triphosphates are present in the cells. Zidovudine triphosphate, which has an intracellular half-life of elimination of 3 to 4 hours, competitively inhibits reverse transcriptase with respect to thymidine triphosphate (TTP). Because the 3′-azido group prevents the formation of 5′-3′-phosphodiester linkages, zidovudine incorporation causes DNA-chain termination (Figure 107). Zidovudine monophosphate also is a competitive inhibitor of cellular thymidylate kinase, causing reduced intracellular levels of TTP. This effect may contribute to its cytotoxicity and enhance antiviral effects by decreasing the competition for zidovudine triphosphate. The antiviral selectivity of zidovudine is due to its greater affinity for HIV reverse transcriptase than for human DNA polymerases, although low concentrations inhibit DNA polymerase gamma (see Figure 107).

Resistant mutants with 10- to over 100-fold decreases in susceptibility have been recovered from treated patients and can be produced by site-directed mutagenesis of the reverse transcriptase. Resistance is associated with point mutations leading to amino-acid substitutions at multiple sites in reverse transcriptase, particularly codons 41, 67, 70, 215, and 219. Resistance mutations appear sequentially, and multiple ones are required to confer high-level resistance.

Zidovudine is rapidly absorbed from the GI tract with peak serum concentrations occurring within 30 to 90 minutes. It binds to plasma proteins to the extent of 35 to 40%. Zidovudine is rapidly metabolized in the liver to the inactive 3′-azido-3′-deoxy-5′-0-beta-D-glucopyranuronosylthymidine (GAZT), which has an apparent elimination half-life of 1 hour. Zidovudine undergoes glomerular filtration and active tubular secretion. Coadministration of zidovudine with agents such as dapsone, pentamidine, amphotericin B, flucytosine, vincristine, vinblastine, adriamycin, and interferon with potential to cause nephrotoxicity or cytotoxicity to hematopoietic elements, enhance its risk of adverse effects. Probenecid will inhibit the renal excretion of zidovudine.

Fluconazole, acetaminophen, aspirin, or indomethacin competitively inhibit the glucuronidation of zidovudine, increasing the risk of causing agranulocytosis. The major toxicities of zidovudine are granulocytopenia and anemia. The risk of hematologic toxicity increases with lower CD4 counts, more advanced disease, higher zidovudine doses, and prolonged therapy. Severe headache, nausea, emesis, insomnia, and myalgia occur commonly during initiation of zidovudine therapy.

ZILEUTON

(Zyflo tablets 600 mg)

Zileuton is a leukotriene formation inhibitor, which attenuates bronchoconstriction by inhibiting leukotriene-dependent smooth muscle contractions. It is indicated in prophylaxis and chronic treatment of asthma.

ZINC

(Medizinc, Orazinc, Scrip Zinc, Verazine, Zinc 15, Zinc 220, Zincate, Zinkaps-220)

ZINC SULFATE (OPHTHALMIC)

(Eye-Sedophthalmic, Op-Thal-Zin)

Zinc (200 to 220 mg p.o. t.i.d.) is used in zinc-deficiency states and as an adjunct in ulcers, acne, ear granulomata, rheumatoid arthritis, hypogeusia, anosmia, vitamin A therapy, and acrodermatitis enteropathica. In addition, zinc has antiinfective properties and hence is used twice a day as an ophthalmic solution (1 to 2 drops). Zinc sulfate ophthalmic solution exhibits astringent and weak antiseptic activity, which may result from precipitation of protein by the zinc ion and by clearing mucus from the outer surface of the eye. This drug has no decongestant action and produces mild vasodilation.

Zinc, which serves as a cofactor for numerous enzymes, facilitates wound healing, normal growth rates, and normal skin hydration, and helps maintain the senses of taste and smell.

Adequate zinc provides normal growth and tissue repair. In patients receiving total parenteral nutrition with low plasma levels of zinc, dermatitis has been followed by alopecia. Zinc is an integral part of many enzymes important to carbohydrate and protein mobilization of retinal-binding protein.

Zinc sulfate is absorbed poorly from the GI tract; only 20 to 30% of dietary zinc is absorbed. After administration, zinc resides in muscle, bone, skin, kidney, liver, pancreas, retina, prostate, and, particularly, red and white blood cells. Zinc binds to plasma albumin, alpha-2 macroglobulin, and some plasma amino acids including histidine, cysteine, threonine, glycine, and asparagine.

Major zinc stores are in the skeletal muscles, skin, bone, and pancreas. After parenteral administration, 90% of zinc is excreted in the stool, urine, and sweat. After oral use, the major route of excretion is secretion into the duodenum and jejunum. Small amounts are also excreted in the urine (0.3 to 0.5 mg/day) and in sweat (1.5 mg/day).

Concomitant use of oral zinc with tetracycline will impair antibiotic absorption. When zinc sulfate ophthalmic solution is used with sodium borate, precipitation of zinc borate may occur; glycerin may prevent this interaction. Zinc sulfate ophthalmic solution has a dehydrating effect on methylcellulose suspensions, causing precipitation of methylcellulose. Zinc sulfate ophthalmic solution may also precipitate acacia and certain proteins.

Parenteral use of zinc sulfate is contraindicated in patients with renal failure or biliary obstruction.

ZIPRASIDONE

(Geodon capsules 20 mg (as hydrochloride), capsules 40 mg (as hydrochloride), capsules 60 mg (as hydrochloride), capsules 80 mg (as hydrochloride), powder for injection 20 mg/mL (as Mesylate) (after reconstitution)

Ziprasidone is a benzisoxazole derivative with antipsychotic activity, apparently because of dopamine and serotonin-receptor antagonism. It is indicated in the treatment of schizophrenia; treatment of acute manic or mixed episodes associated with bipolar disorder; and treatment of acute agitation in schizophrenic patients (injection only).

ZOLEDRONIC ACID

(Zometa powder for injection 4.264 mg)

Zoledronic acid is a bisphosphonate that causes inhibition of bone resorption. It is indicated in the treatment of hypercalcemia of malignancy; treatment of patients with multiple myeloma and bone metastases from solid tumors in conjunction with standard antineoplastic therapy.

ZOLMITRIPTAN

(Zomig tablets 2.5 mg, tablets 5 mg, Zomig spray, nasal 5 mg, Zomig ZMT tablets, orally disintegrating 2.5 mg)

Zolmitriptan is a serotonin 5-HT$_1$-receptor antagonist that is a selective agonist for the vascular serotonin (5-HT)-receptor subtype, causing vasoconstriction of cranial arteries and inhibition of proinflammatory neuropeptide release. It is indicated in the short-term treatment of migraine attacks with/without aura.

ZOLPIDEM TARTRATE

(Ambien tablets 5 mg, tablets 10 mg)

Zolpidem is an imidazopyridine whose mechanism of action may involve subunit modulation of the aminobutyrate activase (GABA) receptor chloride channel macromolecular complex. It is indicated for short-term treatment of insomnia.

ZOLPIDEM TARTRATE

(Ambien)

Zolpidem, an imidazopyridine (10 mg p.o. at bedtime), is used in short-term management of insomnia (see also Table 9).

ZONISAMIDE

(Zonegran capsules 25 mg, capsules 50 mg, capsules 100 mg)

Zonisamide is an anticonvulsant/sulfonamide that may exert its anticonvulsant effects through action at sodium and calcium channels. It is indicated as an adjunctive therapy in the treatment of partial seizures in adult epileptic patients.

ZOPICLONE

Zopiclone, the first compound of the cyclopyrrolone class to be marketed, possesses anticonvulsant, anxiolytic, muscle relaxant, and sedative properties. It causes no dependence and no rebound insomnia. Zopiclone interacts with GABA receptors (see Figure 50). It is rapidly absorbed from the GI tract, and with an oral dose of 7.5 mg, it produces a peak-plasma concentration of 50 to 80 μg/L. Zopiclone becomes metabolized to *N*-demethylzopiclone (inactive) and zopiclone-*N*-oxide (active). Zopiclone exhibits a high affinity for benzodiazepine-binding sites in the cerebral cortex, hippocampus, and cerebellum, but does not interact with the peripheral benzodiazepine-binding sites.

INDEX

A

B

C

D

E

F

G

H

I

J

K

L

M

N

O

P

Q

R

S

T

U

V

W

X

Y

Z